S0-BXN-334

Tumours of Infancy and Childhood

To the children of
today and tomorrow,
with help from
the children of
yesterday

Tumours of Infancy and Childhood

BY THE STAFF OF THE
ROYAL CHILDREN'S HOSPITAL
MELBOURNE

EDITED BY

PETER G. JONES

MS(Melb), FRCS(Eng), FRACS, FACS
Senior Surgeon, Royal Children's Hospital, Melbourne

AND

PETER E. CAMPBELL

MBBS(Melb), FRCPA
Director of Anatomical Pathology, Royal Children's Hospital, Melbourne
Member of the Committee on Cancer in Children, of the Commission on Epidemiology, UICC

FOREWORD BY

HARVEY E. BEARDMORE

BSc, MD, CM, FRCS(C), FACS, FAAP
Associate Surgeon
The Montreal Children's Hospital
Associate Professor of Surgery
Faculty of Medicine
McGill University, Montreal

BLACKWELL SCIENTIFIC PUBLICATIONS
OXFORD LONDON EDINBURGH MELBOURNE

Osney Mead, Oxford
8 John Street, London WC1
9 Forrest Road, Edinburgh
P.O. Box 9, North Balwyn, Victoria, Australia

ISBN 0 63209 380 3

First published 1976

Distributed in the United States of America by
J. B. Lippincott Company, Philadelphia
and in Canada by
J. B. Lippincott Company of Canada Ltd., Toron o.

Printed in Great Britain by
Adlard & Son, Ltd.
Dorking, Surrey
and bound by
Mansell (Bookbinders) Ltd.
Witham, Essex

Contents

APPENDIXES

Contributors

Members of the staff of the Royal Children's Hospital, Melbourne

ALEX W. AULDIST MBBS(Melb), FRACS
Surgeon
Paediatric Surgeon, Austin Hospital, Melbourne
Chapters (16) (20)

F. A. BILLSON FRCS(Edin), FRCS(Eng), FRACS, DLO
Ophthalmologist
Chapter 15

PETER E. CAMPBELL MBBS, FRCPA
Director of Anatomical Pathology*
Chapters 2, 5, (10), (11), (13), (14), (15), (16), (17), (18), (19), (20), (21), (22), (23), (24), (25)
Appendix I

A. MURRAY CLARKE FRCS, FRACS, DCH
Consultant (formerly Senior) Surgeon*
Chapter 19

J. H. COLEBATCH MD(Melb), FRCP(Lond), FRACP, DCH
Kilpatrick Cancer Research Fellow, Anti-Cancer Council of Victoria
Head, Haematology Research Unit, Royal Children's Hospital Research Foundation
Consultant (formerly Director), Haematology Clinic*
Chapters 9, 10, (13), (14), (16), (17), (18), (19), (20), (21), (23), (24), (25)
Appendix III

W. G. DOIG FRCS(Eng), FRACS
Senior Assistant Orthopaedic Surgeon
Chapter (22)

H. EKERT MBBS, FRACP
Director, Clinical Haematology*
Chapters 6, 11, (22)

R. S. FERGUSON MB, ChB(Otago), FRACS
Formerly Senior Surgical Registrar
Chapter (14B)

J. H. FLOYD FRACS, DLO
Formerly Senior Assistant Ear, Nose and Throat Surgeon
Chapter (14D, E, F)

( ) indicates contributor to chapter.
* indicates Past Chairman of the Combined Therapy Clinic.

NIGEL GRAY MBBS(Melb), FRACP, FACMA
Director, Anti-Cancer Council of Victoria
Formerly Deputy Medical Director
Chapter 1A

G. S. GUNTER MS(Melb), FRCS, FRACS
Plastic Surgeon
Chapter (24)

ROGER K. HALL MDSc(Melb), FRACDS
Chief Dental Officer
Honorary Senior Clinical Assistant, Royal Dental Hospital, Melbourne
Chapter (14C)

H. G. HILLER MD, BS, FRACP, FRACR
Formerly Director of Radiology*
Chapter 4A (14), (16), (17), (18), (19), (21), (22), (23)

REGINALD HOOPER MS, FRCS, FRACS
Formerly Senior Neurosurgeon
Chapter 13

PETER G. JONES MS, FRACS, FRACS, FACS
Senior Surgeon*
Chapters 1B; 4B; 8; 12; 14A, B, C, E, F, G; 16B, C, D, E; 18; (20); 22; 23; 24; 25
Appendixes IV and V

DAVID G. JOSE MBBS(Adel), MRACP
C. J. Martin Research Fellow, NH & MRC (Australia)
Royal Children's Hospital Research Foundation, Melbourne
Chapter 3; (9), (10)

JUSTIN H. KELLY FRACS, Surgeon
Chapter (10)

MAX KENT MBBS(Melb), FRACS
Surgeon*
Chapter 16A

C. C. J. MINTY MBBS, DTR, FFR, FRACR
Radiotherapist*
Chapters 7, (10), (14), (15), (16), (17), (18), (19), (20), (22), (23)

N. A. MYERS FRCS, FRACS
Hunterian Professor, 1973
Chairman, Department of Surgery*
Professorial Associate, University of Melbourne
Chapter 17

J. N. SANTAMARIA MBBS, FRACP
Assistant Haematologist
Chapter (23)

( ) indicates contributor to chapter.
* indicates Past Chairman of the Combined Therapy Clinic.

E. DURHAM SMITH MD, MS(Melb), FRACS, FACS
Surgeon*
Chapter 21

JOHN R. SOLOMON FRCS(Eng), FRACS
Surgeon
Chapter (19), 20, (21)

GEOFFREY P. TAURO MBBS(Syd), FRCPA
Director, Haematology Laboratory
Appendix II

( ) indicates contributor to chapter.
* indicates Past Chairman of the Combined Therapy Clinic.

Foreword

Nowhere in the field of paediatric surgery has individually guided treatment been dispersed more widely than in the care of the paediatric patient with a malignant tumour. In the most advanced paediatric centres this dispersal has been greatest. This collective form of treatment control has been named, in some parts of the world, the 'Combined Therapy Clinic' in other parts of the world, the 'Tumour Board'.

A 'Combined Therapy Clinic' may be comprised of fourteen or more members, each individual having expertise in some area of patient care. When this body of specialists functions well, it represents the most advanced form of care for the cancer patient. A 'Tumour Board' can create or adhere to a treatment protocol, and it can collect, store and report the hard data that are so necessary to further progress in this field.

In many areas on this earth, indeed in many universities and children's hospitals, paediatric physicians and surgeons, medical students and ancillary personnel do not have access to a 'Tumour Board' at all, or at best only occasionally, and it appears to me that this is the void which this new book fills so adequately, and for so many people.

Peter Jones and Peter Campbell, in editing not only their own major contributions to the text, but also the thoughts and writings of the many members of the staff of The Royal Children's Hospital, Melbourne, have succeeded, unquestionably, in producing a lucid, well-stylized adequately illustrated edition.

The title has been well chosen, for the book contains not only information about the benign tumour masses so characteristically encountered in the paediatric patient but includes statistically-based data relating to the original working title of the book, 'Malignant Disease in Childhood'.

It is a no-nonsense book, clearly delineating the differential diagnoses and hopefully raising the index of suspicion for the early diagnosis of malignant tumours in infants and children.

This much needed, clinically-oriented text places its reader on a plateau from which he will be better able to grasp and understand the innovations in cancer therapy which must inevitably appear in the not too distant future.

Harvey E. Beardmore MD, CM

Preface

In the last two decades the medical profession has gradually realized the implications of the changing order of causes of death in children; in many parts of the world malignant disease is now the second commonest cause of death (after accidents) in children more than one year old.

Even when taken as a whole, the three major categories, brain tumours, leukaemias and 'solid tumours', are still uncommon enough to engender a low index of suspicion in clinical practice. Delays in investigation and diagnosis make the outlook worse, and survival rates in some malignancies could be significantly improved by earlier diagnosis and prompt action.

No other kind of illness requires the participation of so many in such a variety of fields, or makes greater demands on their humanity or their time. The family doctor is often the first (and not infrequently the last) to be involved; the paediatrician or paediatric surgeon, the radiologist, clinical biochemist, histopathologist, immunologist, radiotherapist, chemotherapist, nurses, medical social workers and, depending on the type of disease, the haematologist, neurosurgeon, orthopaedic surgeon or other specialist: each has a contribution to make.

Regular and frequent meetings of a multidisciplinary consultative clinic make it possible for the patient to derive maximum benefit from their expertise in planning and carrying out a carefully integrated regime of treatment. Such a team functions most effectively when each member plays his part at the appropriate time, while one doctor retains complete responsibility for the overall care of the child, and for close and continuing contact with the parents.

The publisher's invitation to compile this book was the stimulus to review the experience of the Combined Therapy Clinic established at the Royal Children's Hospital in 1964. Data from earlier cases have also been reviewed, and histological material from more than 1600 children has been re-examined, and reclassified where necessary, in the light of current diagnostic criteria.

We have attempted to bring together and summarize information scattered in journals and textbooks, and continually augmented by developments in many diverse fields. As a compilation, no claim is made that it is encyclopaedic, nor a comprehensive review of the literature in all the related fields, nor simply a report of some 1600 cases. Where our experience is limited or nonexistent, the lacuna has been partially filled by data from recent articles; where our experience differs significantly from the usual, this is noted and individual patients whose history illustrates particular points are briefly described.

The original working title, 'Malignant Disease in Childhood', remains the central theme, but it became apparent that if differential diagnosis was to be covered adequately and in proper perspective, a host of much more common non-malignant or non-neoplastic swellings should be included, and the original title could be thought to be misleading.

The fields represented by brain tumours and leukaemias are disciplines in their own right, and these have been broadly surveyed by senior clinicians of great experience.

The 'solid' tumours of infancy and childhood, although collectively the largest category comprising 45% of the total, have, perhaps, been covered less than adequately in some books on cancer in childhood. The greater part of this book is devoted to tumours which may arise anywhere in the broad field of general paediatric surgery, or in what might be considered 'special' areas such as the thorax, the eye, or the nose and throat.

At the risk of displeasing some who might prefer more orthodox taxonomy, solid tumours have been grouped on a clinical regional basis and, where possible, according to modes of presentation rather than a strictly anatomical or pathological plan.

This book has been written for paediatricians and paediatric surgeons, but realizing that specialized paediatric facilities for children with a tumour are not everywhere available, material has been included which may be useful to clinicians, radiologists, pathologists, chemotherapists and radiotherapists, whose practice is chiefly concerned with adults, and who may welcome information concerning the markedly different tumours and needs of children.

P.G.J.
P.E.C.

December, 1975

Acknowledgements

We are grateful to the staff of the Royal Children's Hospital, and some further afield; in addition to the contributors, they gave, unstintingly, permission to draw upon their experience, case notes and records, which were retrieved by Miss J. Brady, Medical Records Librarian, Miss L. Robertson, Radiology Librarian, and Mrs. Noelle Ely, Secretary to the Combined Therapy Clinic. Colleagues who helped are too numerous to list in full, but particular thanks are due to the following: Dr. Kester Brown, Director of Anaesthesia, for assistance with Chapter 18, Dr. John Court (Chapter 20), Dr. John Connelly (Chapter 18), Dr. Geoffrey Tauro (illustrations, Chapter 9; Appendix II), Dr. John Andrews, Director of the Department of Nuclear Medicine, Royal Melbourne Hospital, and his staff, for arranging scans for our patients, for information incorporated in Chapter 4, and for Fig. 14.17. Dr. James Arey of St. Christopher's Hospital, Philadelphia, suggested the 'check lists' of benign and malignant swellings in each area, and supplied preliminary material subsequently altered so that any inappropriate inclusions or omissions are ours.

Dr. R. W. Miller of the National Cancer Institute, Bethesda, Maryland, kindly supplied data for the graphs of the age incidence of individual tumours in Chapters 2, 10, 13, 15, 17, 18, 19, 20, 22 and 23.

We are indebted to Urban and Schwartzenberg, Berlin, for permission on reproduce illustrations from *Recent Advances in Paediatric Surgery*, Vol. 7, 1974, and acknowledged in Chapter 19; and to the Editor of *Pathology* for the source of Fig. 21.14.

The Department of Radiology under successive Directors Dr. H. G. Hiller and Dr. Fred Jensen provided the films for many of the illustrations; Mr. Bert Winther supplied negatives from his meticulously kept files in the Department of Pathology. The artwork, line drawings, charts and diagrams were drawn by the medical artist, Mrs. Vivienne James, with her customary skill and clarity. These and other sources were processed by Mrs. Edna Cottrell, Head of the Department of Photography, and by Mr. Joe Szcsepanski.

The drafts of the manuscript were typed (and retyped) accurately and speedily by Mrs. Margaret Harrison, and additional material by our secretaries, Mrs. Ruki Guneratne, Mrs. Gloria Nassau and Mrs. Paola Murdoch.

Mrs. Peg Stormont did the Index.

We would also like to thank Mr. Per Saugman, Managing Director of Blackwell Scientific Publications Limited, for commissioning the book;

Mr. John Robson, Production Manager, for agreeing to suggestions concerning typography and accepting additional material at the galley proof stage so that the text might be as up to date as possible, and Mrs. Lucinda Gerson, supervising editor, and the publishers and printers for their usual excellent standards of production.

Chapter 1. Malignant disease in childhood

A. CAUSES, STATISTICS AND SURVIVAL

Although cancer is a rarity in childhood, it kills more children than any other disease, and is second only to accidents (of all kinds) as the commonest cause of death between one and fourteen years of age. Its lethal nature, insidious onset, emotional impact, and the increasing prospects of cure make it one of the most challenging aspects of paediatric practice.

The chief characteristic of a malignant tumour is the ability of its cells to grow and multiply in excess of the normal rate, free of controls normally concerned with maintaining tissue repair and limiting the rate and extent of tissue growth. Although these control mechanisms are not fully understood, their existence is obvious when one considers the body's ability to grow and to stop growing, to heal and to stop healing, and to replace cells dying of old age with new cells in such numbers as to maintain the *status quo*. Uncontrolled multiplication theoretically progresses more and more rapidly as each generation of cells continues to divide, leading to a 'cell doubling time' which would more or less halve with each generation. However, the growth of a tumour is an extremely complex biological phenomenon; increase in size depends on many factors, including the specific type of tumour, its rate of growth and the body's defence mechanisms.

The rate of growth depends upon the size of the fraction of cells (the growth fraction) in the process of active proliferation. The size of this fraction represents the number of cells vulnerable at any point in time, to cytotoxic agents, which exert their maximum anti-tumour effect on cells in the 'cell cycle', and specifically in different phases of the cycle (Fig. 6.1, p. 101). The rate of growth is also influenced by any factor which causes cell death, such as infarction following vascular accidents, and by the phenomenon of apoptosis whereby cells die and are removed.

An enlarging primary growth encroaches upon its environment and eventually produces, in most cases, a clinical picture determined largely by its site, or its size, or in some cases by substances it secretes. Sooner or later, clumps of cells leave the parent body and metastasize, by direct spread or via blood vessels or lymphatic channels, to establish secondary deposits elsewhere.

Metastasis may occur early in the life of a tumour, or late. The time relationship between the development of the primary and the occurrence of metastasis is a critical factor affecting the results of treatment, and in many tumours tends to be one of its more constant features. In such cases both treatment and prognosis are less haphazard than they might otherwise be.

The histological and behavioural characteristics of individual tumours also tend to be reasonably consistent. Thus a therapeutic attack on a secondary deposit from a slowly growing tumour may be worthwhile, whereas it may not be warranted when the metastasis comes from a rapidly growing primary. Despite a general tendency to be consistent, there are examples of a very broad spectrum of behaviour within one type of tumour. Histologically, cells vary from the grossly anaplastic to the barely abnormal; cellular and biochemical function may be virtually normal or bizarre. The clinical features may also vary from the predictable to the extraordinary; the management is consequently difficult and the prognosis impossible to predict in cases which deviate markedly from the usual pattern.

ETIOLOGY

The etiology of cancer is complicated, usually multifactorial, and may never be fully understood. However, it is possible that some etiological factors are common to all forms of cancer; it is not unreasonable to expect that research may reveal that a particular biological process occurs as an indispensable part of the chain of causation in all forms of cancer, and that this process may be blocked, diverted or otherwise hindered by some means. We would then have a method of control which might effectively rid mankind of the disease. As an example, one possibility concerns the acquisition of a blood supply. Until a tumour reaches a diameter of 1 to 2 mm (varying with the cell type), it exists in an 'avascular' phase, the cells being nourished from tissue fluids. Beyond this critical size, a 'vascular phase' is essential for continuing growth, and solid tumours have been demonstrated to secrete an 'angiogenesis' factor (Folkman, 1975); without it, failure to convey nutrients and remove wastes limits growth to a few millimetres in diameter, a point of control which might be achieved by inhibiting angiogenesis.

Research into changes in the structure and constitution of nucleic acid in cancer cells may uncover a single cause operating at a molecular level which might then be attacked on a relatively narrow front. A new theory of oncogenesis, recently proposed by Comings (1973), links genetic and viral factors, and attributes neoplasia to inactivation of regulatory genes which normally prevent the action of growth-stimulating genes.

The activities of the molecular biologists and anti-smoking propagandists represent the outer edges of a broad approach to the control of cancer, which is based on knowledge of at least some of the facts related to etiology. Information already available indicates that environmental factors are varied and widespread, but potentially identifiable, and in many cases removable. Research workers took a long time to realize that cancer of the lung was largely dependent on something which was inhaled (Doll, Muir & Waterhouse, 1970), and even longer to start looking for causes of intestinal cancer in things we eat. A great deal of current cancer research has its origins in simple epidemiological observations which showed that certain groups of people with a high incidence of certain types of cancer had specific habits or habitats. A high rate of lung cancer has been correlated with the habit of smoking (*U.S. Public Health*, No. 1696); a high rate of cancer of the stomach with residence in Japan (Haenszel & Kurihara, 1968); and cancer of the large bowel with residence in developed countries with a 'western' type of diet. Not many of the environmental causes of cancer so far identified (cigarettes excepted) are of a kind which public health measures could reduce appreciably. Nevertheless, some of the facts collected provide glimpses of the biological aspects of carcinogenesis.

Ionizing radiation

Information linking radiation to cancer has been available for centuries. The mining communities of Schneeburg (Germany) and Joachimstal (Czechoslovakia) were known to suffer from 'mountain sickness' since the sixteenth century, diagnosed as lung cancer at the end of the nineteenth century. In due course the disease was shown to be caused by radioactive materials present in the mines. Later it was noted that the pioneer radiologists were unduly prone to skin cancer and leukaemia, and later again that their patients were also at risk when large doses of x-rays were used therapeutically (*International Atomic Energy Agency*, 1969; Clemmesen, 1965).

The tragic experience of Hiroshima confirmed these effects, and established that whole body irradiation produced cancers in various tissues, such as thyroid (p. 370), bone and stomach. Observations of the effects of irradiation *in utero* suggest that the risk of cancer is directly proportional to the radiation dose, and there is probably no safe threshold (Stewart & Barber, 1971). The long term effects of nuclear fallout on the survivors of Hiroshima (Bizzozero, Johnson *et al.*, 1966), have clearly demonstrated a specific leukaemogenic effect, as well as a general carcinogenetic effect. The National Research Council Report reveals a 1·48 fold excess over the expected rate of deaths due to cancers, other than leukaemia, in survivors who received 200 rads or more of ionizing radiation. In more recent years the excess has been even greater (× 1·84), suggesting an increasing rate of carcinogenetic effects. An important finding is that there is a dose-response relationship which leads to the logical conclusion that even minimal doses of radiation may be harmful (Stewart & Barber, 1971). The possibility that nucleic acid repair mechanisms may counteract the effect of low doses should not allow the unnecessary use of any dose of radiation with confidence.

Diagnostic radiation during fetal life has recently been implicated as a hazard causing an increased incidence of leukaemia and some other cancers in childhood.

Bross & Natarajan (1972) have reported variable susceptibility of children to intrauterine irradiation, with a higher incidence of leukaemia in those children who had asthma or hives. Eczema was not mentioned as a possible predisposing cause, but the association with hives and asthma is taken by the authors to reflect altered immunological surveillance which could render the subject more susceptible to mutations resulting in the emergence of cancer cells. However, as pointed out by Miller (1973) the leukaemic child might be predisposed to allergies rather than the allergic state predisposing to leukaemia, and more data are required.

Therapeutic irradiation in relatively large doses has long been used in the treatment of ankylosing spondylitis (Clemmesen, 1965), and this had led to a substantial increase in the risk of aplastic anaemia and myeloid leukaemia among patients so treated. In childhood, radiotherapy for 'thymic hyperplasia' has been responsible for a number of carcinomas of the thyroid gland (p. 370).

Nuclear 'accidents' have occurred and even well-designed colour television sets can deliver undesirably high doses. The use of radio-nucleides in the investigation of patients (p. 75), and in research, is increasing and requires careful control. It should also be remembered that careless use of x-rays is a major risk to the staff involved and is relatively common.

Sunlight

It has long been known that skin cancer occurs most frequently on the exposed parts of the body. Modern social custom has, to a degree, changed the patterns of body exposure and in the future we may see a wider distribution of skin cancers, but the face, arms and hands will presumably continue to be the major sites, as they are in xeroderma pigmentosum in children.

The incidence of all forms of skin cancer, including malignant melanoma, particularly in fair-skinned Europeans, in the clear, hot, dry air on the inland slopes of the Dividing Range in Queensland, is the highest anywhere in the world (Gordon, Silverstone & Smithurst, 1972), and increases progressively with cumulative exposure, and hence with age.

Ultraviolet radiations of wavelength 2900–3300 Å are carcinogenic in experimental animals, and probably in humans as well, for example in xeroderma pigmentosum (p. 839). Various sun-screening agents now freely available minimize the penetration of these rays and may be capable of reducing the incidence of skin cancer.

Environmental Hazards

The number of environmental factors known to be involved in the development of cancer is steadily increasing.

An association recently suggested links exposure to the solvent vinyl chloride, used extensively in the plastic industry in the manufacture of polyvinyl chloride (PVC), with angiosarcoma of the liver (Lee & Harry, 1974; *Lancet Annotation*, 1974b).

Unfortunately, environmental carcinogens are difficult to identify because of the complexity of the human condition, diet, social habits and occupations, and particularly because of the long latent period between exposure to a carcinogen and the development of a tumour. Some substances are of such a low carcinogenic potential that they require remarkably high dosages or prolonged exposure; for example, acquisition of a high risk of lung cancer may require the consumption of thirty or more cigarettes daily for thirty years or more, a total of more than 300,000 cigarettes. Yet such a dose, while conferring a high risk of lung cancer, produces only a small though real risk of bladder cancer. Although other factors such as genetic influences may also be important, the beneficial effects of giving up smoking suggest that cancer may be controlled successfully (in co-operative patients) by quite simple means, once the carcinogen has been identified.

Transplacental carcinogens are even more difficult to identify and to convict as causes of neoplasms in childhood (Fraumeni, 1974) or late adolescence.

A recently recognized example of chemical carcinogenesis in the fetus is the development of clear-cell adenocarcinoma of the vagina (less commonly of the cervix) eighteen to twenty-two years after the mother was treated for threatened miscarriage with diethyl stilboestrol in high dosage early in the pregnancy (Herbst *et al.*, 1972; *Lancet Annotation*, 1974a; Herbst *et al.*, 1975).

The presenting symptom in the first cases detected was vaginal bleeding, but on careful examination of others at risk, some were found to have hyperplasia of mucosal cells ('microadenosis') which appears to be pre-cancerous. The incidence of this carcinoma in those at risk has yet to be determined and is currently the subject of several national studies (in Australia conducted by the Royal College of Obstetricians and Gynaecologists). Screening of girls at risk should probably commence at the menarche, firstly by means of vaginal and cervical smears for exfoliated cells, endoscopy when smears are positive, and biopsy of any 'velvety' areas of hyperplastic mucosa. There is some evidence that areas of adenosis may be inhibited or dispelled by progesterone (Herbst, Poskanzer, Robboy *et al.*, 1975).

Such observations offer scope for identifying etiological possibilities, and similar data can be expected to accumulate as the search for potential transuterine carcinogens intensifies. Information of this kind has been collected in *Evaluation of Carcinogenic Risk of Chemicals to Man*, Vol. 1., published by the I.A.R.C.

Genetic Factors

Cancer rarely runs in families, although, as a relatively common disease, it is likely to occur in more than one member of a family. Peculiar associations not explicable by chance are being uncovered, mainly by epidemiologists investigating familial incidence of cancer; for example, seven of the women in one family developed a carcinoma of the ovary (Li, Rapaport *et al.*, 1970). In other families several members have developed the same kind of rare neoplasm, adrenocortical carcinoma in one kindred, rhabdomyosarcoma in another, and these associations have been detected by studying death certificates of children dying of cancer (Miller, 1971). The meaning of these observations is not yet clear, but the information is already of practical significance in counselling, and in detecting other associations in the siblings at risk.

In childhood, the tumours and premalignant conditions in which there is a genetic influence strong enough to require counselling parents concerning further children are retinoblastoma (p. 727), xeroderma pigmentosum (p. 839), glioma of the optic nerve (p. 262), familial polyposis of the colon (p. 650), intestinal polyposis (syn. Gardner's syndrome, p. 656), familial medullary carcinoma of the thyroid and phaeochromocytoma (Sipple's syndrome, p. 562), and in some families, von Recklinghausen's disease (p. 830).

Much remains to be learnt of the neurocutaneous syndromes generally, and in particular their association with neoplasia. Vinken and Bruyn (1972) have recently reviewed the present knowledge concerning the phakomatoses.

Certain populations have quite specific cancer risks which persist regardless of emigration and changes in social customs; nasopharyngeal cancer among Chinese is a clear example (*W.H.O.*, 1972). In Singapore the incidence of this tumour in Chinese is ten to fifty times higher than in Indians. However, considering only Chinese, there is a very high incidence in those originating in South China, and in certain areas such as Kwantung Province there is a maximum rate well above those in other parts of China. There is little doubt that genetic factors are important in the development of this cancer, even though the Epstein-Barr virus has been implicated as a co-factor.

A similar high incidence of nasopharyngeal carcinoma has recently been described in Tunisians (Cammoun *et al.*, 1974), but the etiological factors have yet to be determined.

Viruses

No evidence is yet available as proof that viruses are a cause of human cancer, in spite of numerous studies showing frequent associations between cancer and viruses, such as nasopharyngeal cancer and other tumours with the Epstein-Barr virus (*W.H.O.*, 1972); despite the discovery of the same virus in association with Burkitt's lymphoma (p. 328) which has an epidemiological pattern suggestive of an insect-borne infection; despite the discovery of virus-like particles in the milk from patients with breast cancer (Editorial, *Lancet*, 1972); and despite the demonstration in humans of an enzyme mechanism potentially capable of allowing the incorporation of viral nucleic acid components in the nucleic acid of the human cell (Temin & Mizutani, 1970).

Hodgkin's disease has long been thought of as a possible result of a virus infection, and recent data from Albany, N.Y., has suggested that it may be transmitted by healthy carriers (Vianna, Greenwald & Davies, 1971), but the theory remains speculative.

Fedrick & Alberman (1972) have described six unrelated children with leukaemia, whose mothers had influenza during pregnancy; the expected incidence in the exposed group was only 0·7. The numbers are small, but potentially very significant, and similar relationships will no doubt be further explored. The probability exists that viruses play a part in human cancer, but no more can be said at present.

CONGENITAL MALFORMATIONS ASSOCIATED WITH CANCER

Some tumours in childhood are closely associated with developmental anomalies, particularly those related to excessive growth; both Wilms' tumour and hepatoblastoma may occur in association with hemihypertrophy, and also with Beckwith's syndrome (exomphalos, macroglossia and visceral cytomegaly). Less striking but significant associations are adrenal cortical carcinoma and syndromes of excess growth, and more will be uncovered by closely questioning parents of children with tumours concerning causes of illness and death in other members of the family.

A common etiological factor may be at work producing a tumour, and also causing disordered development, in the one patient, or in the same sibship or kindred.

CANCER STATISTICS

Registration

Epidemiological observations, frequently quite simple ones, have been responsible for the direction of much current cancer research. Percival Pott's original discovery of an increased incidence of scrotal cancer in chimney-sweeps was such an observation, and led to the identification of soot as the first environmental carcinogen. Various types of cancer registry have been established around the world to measure the incidence, survival patterns and mortality rates in selected groups, or in the population at large. Mortality rates are relatively easy to obtain, and data of considerable accuracy are available from government agencies in many countries. Cancer incidence, on the other hand, is both difficult and expensive to assess. Survival rates may also be difficult to determine because they depend on careful follow-up over long periods.

Incidence registries

Some countries, for example Norway, have a highly developed national system of registration; each citizen has an identifying number and consequently cancer incidence can be estimated with sufficient accuracy to detect quite small changes in incidence rates. Larger populations pose more problems because many cases escape registration, and some educated guesswork may be required to estimate the percentage of patients who have been missed. If only a small percentage of affected patients are first identified from a study of death certificates, then registration will have been fairly complete. Incidence registries tend to concentrate on circumscribed populations within larger countries, e.g. Manchester, Connecticut, Birmingham, South London.

Follow-up registries

Sampling a population is often adequate for assessing survival rates. Such samples usually include some bias, but this poses no serious problem as long as it is known. Meticulous follow-up of cancer patients to death, while a vital aspect of caring for the patient, is also essential in evaluating regimes of treatment. Care and experience in abstracting information from patient records is important, and the presentation of survival rates should usually include 90–95% of all patients in the initial sample.

Survival and mortality rates

Both survival and mortality rates are required to obtain a complete picture of a tumour. Mortality rates tell us the number of people who die each year from the various forms of cancer, but they do not tell us how long the patients lived after diagnosis. Survival rates tell us this, and hence they reflect certain characteristics of the particular tumour and the response to treatment.

Survival for five years is frequently taken as an index of the effectiveness of treatment, even though survival for this period does not always imply a cure. Absolute survival rates (i.e. crude survival rates) refer to patients known to have cancer and who died of cancer *or* of other causes, and these are satisfactory for normal purposes. Since the death rates from causes other than cancer are quite well known, it is possible to allow for them and to modify 'crude survival' rates to produce 'relative' rates of survival. It is sometimes desirable to further modify relative rates by 'age adjustment', bringing the age spectrum of the patients involved into relation with the number of people in the various age groups in a 'standard' community, thus allowing international comparisons.

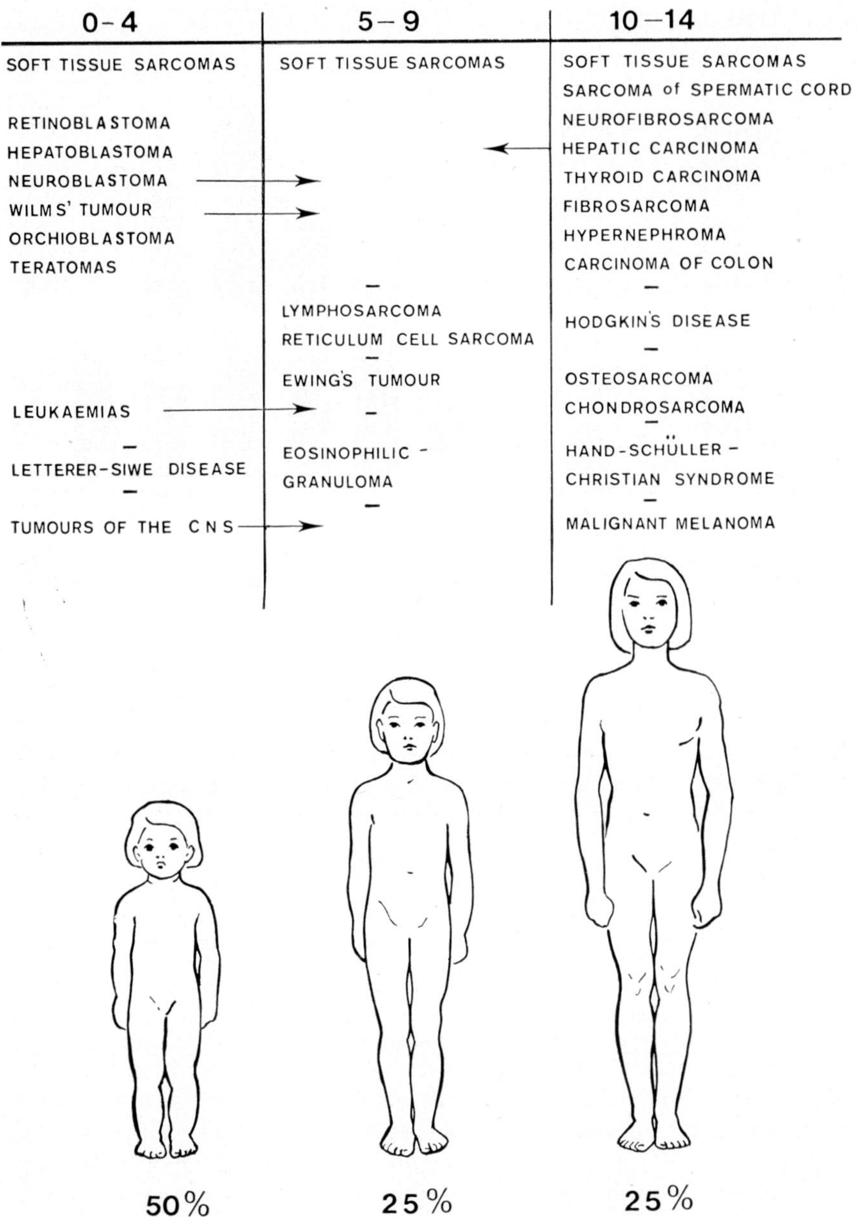

Figure 1.1. THE THREE QUINQUENNIA OF CHILDHOOD, showing the proportion of malignant tumours occurring in each five-year period, and some of the malignant conditions typically associated with a particular quinquennium are listed.

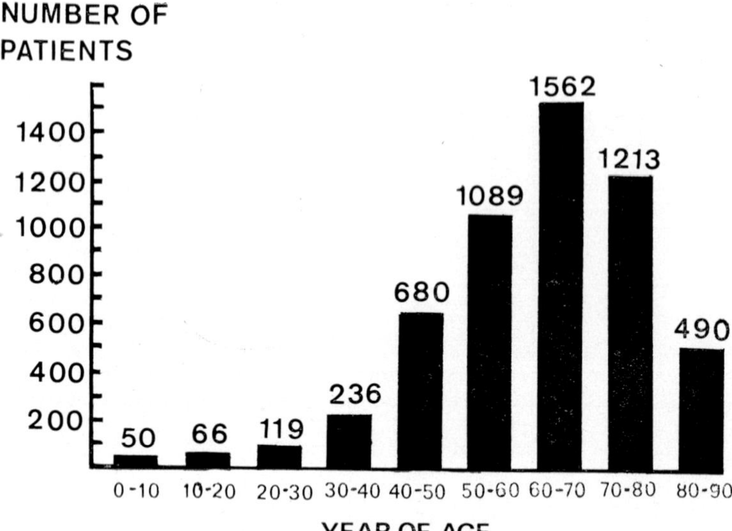

Figure 1.2. INCIDENCE RELATED TO AGE, showing a progressive increase in the incidence of malignant disease in relation to age (Victorian Cancer Registry).

The influence of age and sex

The risk of most types of cancer increase progressively with age, except of course, the cancers of childhood, in which there are nevertheless correlations with a particular quinquennium (Fig. 1.1). Figure 1.2 shows increasing incidence with age in over 5,000 residents of Victoria who developed cancer in 1969.

Differences between the sexes are significant (Fig. 1.3), even in some cancers which affect organs other than the genitalia. Sex differences in the incidence of lung cancer can be attributed to smoking habits.

CANCER CONTROL

Cancer is responsible for approximately one-sixth of all deaths in Australia, America and Britain. In spite of many improvements in surgical technique, more effective radiotherapy and the introduction of chemotherapy and immunotherapy, survival rates in adults have improved, overall, only slightly. Future improvement will depend not only on research aimed at finding more causes, but also on improved methods of early detection and prevention.

In childhood, however, the last decade has seen significant improvements in the survival rates in several tumours, e.g. Wilms' tumour, leukaemia and rhabdomyosarcoma (p. 792) and in the latter, advances in chemotherapy,

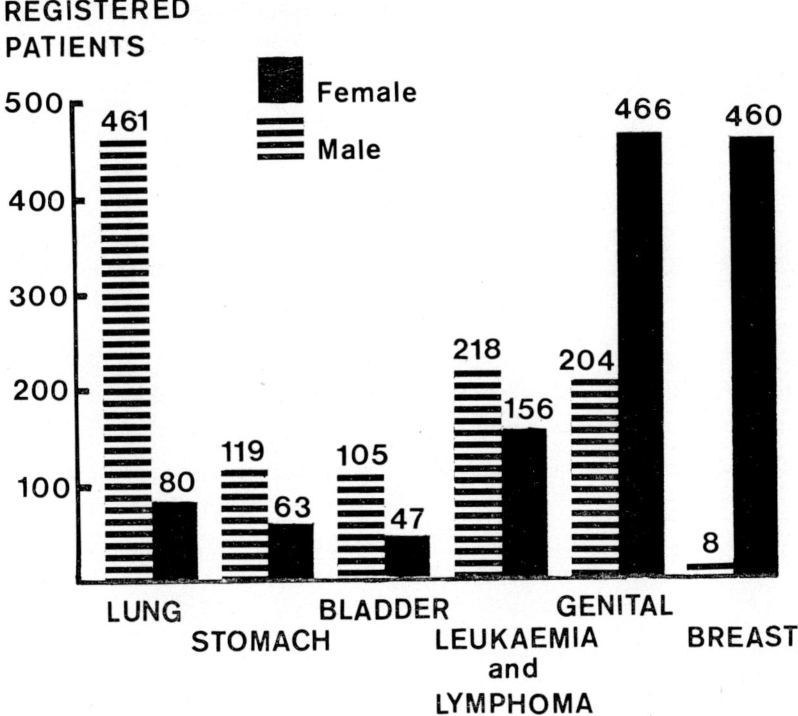

Figure 1.3. INCIDENCE RELATED TO SEX; differences in the incidence of various cancers in males and females (Victorian Cancer Registry).

particularly combination chemotherapy and recurrent courses for up to two years, have probably been largely responsible for improved results.

In some countries, some cancers follow a pattern which is conducive to better control. A decision to embark on a campaign to control cancer involves careful assessment of incidence rates, of the efficiency of screening techniques, of survival rates and of morbidity. However, the public, the politicians, and their purse, are the final arbiters. In Japan (Gutmann, 1971), the incidence of carcinoma of the stomach is so high that radiological and endoscopic screening programmes are acceptable, and have been shown to provide detection and more effective treatment. The incidence in Japan is 164 per 100,000 males between 35 and 64 years, whereas in New Zealand it is 22 per 100,000 males, and it is highly unlikely that the same programme would be acceptable, or as successful, in a country with a low incidence. Similar considerations apply to screening for cancers of the lung, breast, cervix and large bowel.

Difficulties in screening are represented, in miniature, by three situations in childhood: (i) in the early detection of a retinal tumour in the siblings of a child with a retinoblastoma (p. 424); (ii) the surveillance of an infant found to have aniridia and who may develop a Wilms' tumour at any time in the following ten years (p. 506); and (iii) the early detection of leukaemia in the second of identical twins after the first has developed leukaemia. In these circumstances, the need for frequent re-examinations is obvious and warranted by the predicted incidence, but in general, the incidence of malignant disease in children is so small that screening them for tumours is not practical. Nevertheless, frequent re-examinations as part of 'well baby care' provide an opportunity to detect an abdominal mass, and hence earlier diagnosis, of the two commonest solid tumours in childhood, Wilms' tumour and neuroblastoma.

The development of a reliable test for increased excretion of catecholamines in the urine (p. 551) also offers an opportunity to 'screen' children presenting

Table 1.1 Variations in Incidence and Types of Malignant Tumours. Geographic (and/or racial) differences in the incidence of paediatric tumours in various populations

	Australia*		United Kingdom†		Africa‡		Papua New Guinea§	
Type of tumour	No.	%	No.	%	No.	%	No.	%
Leukaemia	615	36·0	293	29·5	54	7·0	37	10·0
Lymphomas	178	11·0	86	9·0	377	50·0	151	42·0
Tumours of C.N.S.	345	20·0	169	17·0	10	1·5	10	3·0
Retinoblastoma	9	0·5	31	3·0	57	7·5	34	9·5
Bone and soft tissue sarcomas	142	8·5	141	14·0	116	15·0	52	14·0
Neuroblastoma and other neural crest tumours	144	8·5	75	7·5	17	2·0	24	7·0
Wilms' tumour	112	6·5	54	5·5	56	7·5	13	3·5
Teratoma	79	5·0	41	4·0	10‖	1·0	11	3·0
Ovary	4	0·5	7	0·5	14	2·0	7	2·0
Testis	7	0·5	9	1·0	6	1·0	3	1·0
Liver	20	1·0	3	0·5	12	1·5	12	3·0
Miscellaneous	34	2·0	85	8·5	32	4·0	6	2·0
	n=1689 1952–72		n=994 1953–63		n=761 1964–68		n=360 1960–70	

* Australia : Index Series, Royal Children's Hospital.

† United Kingdom : figures from *Tumours in Children*, H.B. Marsden & J.K. Steward. Springer-Verlag Stuttgart & New York, 1969.

‡ Africa : figures from Tumors in a Tropical Country. In *Childhood tumours*, by Davies, J.N.P., Chapter 19. Springer-Verlag, Stuttgart & New York, 1973.

§ Papua-New Guinea : Tumour Registry, Port Moresby.

‖ Figure for extragonadal teratomas only.

with symptoms of 'malignant malaise' (p. 549), a small proportion of whom may have a latent neuroblastoma.

GEOGRAPHIC AND RACIAL VARIATIONS

There are considerable variations in both incidence and death rates in national populations, differences which emphasize the complex etiology of malignant disease and make comparisons of results somewhat difficult. An appreciation of these differences is important in considering screening programmes and regimes of management. Table 1.1 shows the marked variations in the incidence of some selected tumours.

CANCER IN CHILDREN

The characteristics of malignant tumours in childhood differ greatly from those in adults (see p. 35). No doubt this is partly due to the well-known capacity of the child's body to repair itself and to resist to a remarkable degree the assaults of the environment. It may also be due to the fact that such carcinogens as act in childhood are focused on tissues which are growing and developing at a very rapid rate. The age incidence, with a considerable number of embryonal cancers occurring near birth, indicates that fetal life is a period of relatively high risk (Miller & Dalager, 1974).

Incidence in Children

Since cancer in this age group is rare, it is difficult to estimate incidence rates accurately. Table 1.2 shows the percentage ('relative') incidence rates of the seven major categories of tumour in childhood in a sample of 1023 children registered with the Victorian Cancer Registry between 1960 and 1969.

The relatively constant proportion of various groups of tumours is also illustrated by the figures in Figure 1.4 which show that 20–25% of malignant tumours arise in the central nervous system and the eye, 35% are leukaemias, and 40–45% are solid tumours (individually uncommon except for Wilms' tumour and neuroblastoma) which when taken together nevertheless comprise the largest group of malignant conditions in childhood. The figures are in accord with the relative incidence in the Index Series (Appendix I, p. 911), and Table 1.2 contains data which substantiate the following conclusions.

1. The four commonest classes of malignant tumours of infancy and childhood, in rank order are leukaemia, tumours of the CNS, neuroblastoma and Wilms' tumour.
2. All four have their maximal incidence in the first quinquennium; 84% of neuroblastomas and 80% of Wilms' tumours develop in this age group.

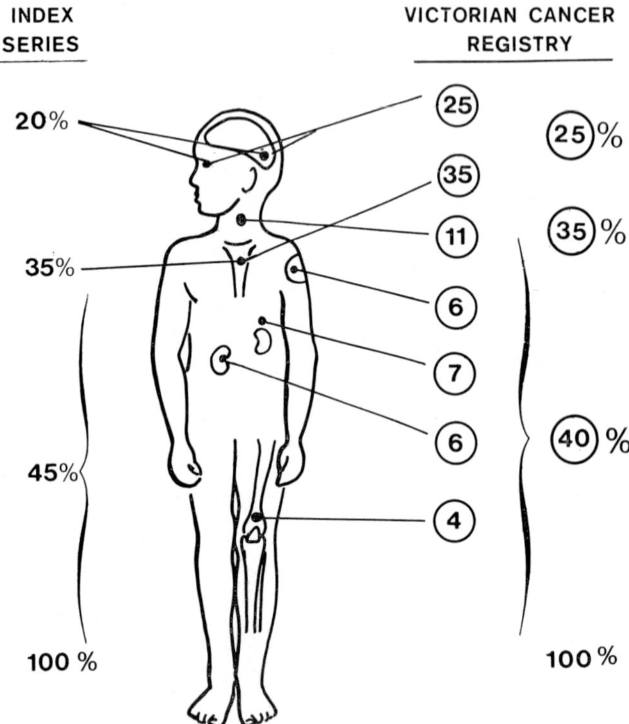

Figure 1.4. RELATIVE INCIDENCE OF DIFFERENT CATEGORIES OF TUMOURS IN CHILDHOOD; left: in the 1689 cases in the Index Series (1950–1972), and right: in 1023 tumours in the Victorian Tumour Registry (1960–1969).

3. The first quinquennium contains 45·9% of all malignant disease of childhood.

Differences in the incidence of the various categories in each quinquennium are even more marked when the grouping of tumours is refined, for example:
(a) if Hodgkin's disease alone were considered in the category 'lymphoma', the percentage in the third quinquennium would be very much greater than 42%;
(b) if Ewing's tumour were excluded from 'bone sarcoma', the proportion of the latter in the third quinquennium would be much greater than 67%.

The great preponderance of malignant tumours arising in the first quinquennium has been attributed to immaturity, or at least partial incompetence, of the immune surveillance mechanisms, which may be responsible for the successful establishment of clones of malignant cells

Table 1.2. Incidence of Tumours according to Age. The relative incidence of malignant tumours in 1023 children (Victorian Cancer Registry, Melbourne, 1960–1969) analysed according to age (the three quinquennia of childhood) and to type of tumour (major categories)

AGE	EYE and CNS	SOFT TISSUE SARCOMA	LYMPHOMA	NEURO BLASTOMA	WILMS' TUMOUR	LEUKAEMIA	BONES	OTHERS	
0–4	25% 117 (44)%	5% 23 (40)%	5% 22 20%	13% 63 (84)%	11% 50 (81)%	37% 173 (49)%	– 2 5%	4% 18 31%	100% 468 = 46%
5–9	27% 81 30%	7% 20 34%	14% 42 38%	3% 8 11%	4% 11 18%	36% 107 30%	3% 10 27%	6% 19 32%	100% 298 = 29%
10–14	27% 69 26%	6% 15 26%	18% 47 (42)%	1% 4 5%	– 1 1%	29% 74 21%	10% 25 (68)%	9% 2 37%	100% 257 = 25%
TOTALS	267 100% [25%]	58 100% [6%]	111 100% [11%]	75 100% [7%]	62 100% [6%]	354 100% [35%]	37 100% [4%]	59 100% [6%]	1023 OF ALL TUMOURS

(%) PERCENTAGE OF EACH TUMOUR OCCURRING IN EACH AGE GROUP

[%] PERCENTAGE OF ALL TUMOURS IN PAEDIATRIC AGE GROUP

(p. 57). Further, it raises the probability that paediatric carcinogens, whatever they are, exert their influence during intrauterine life or early infancy.

In contrast, sarcomas of bone and the lymphomas are more common in the second and third quinquennia, while soft tissue sarcomas are evenly distributed throughout all three quinquennia.

The information in this table has obvious diagnostic importance.

Prenatal carcinogenesis

The development of a cancer cell presumably depends upon 'mutation' occurring in normal tissues, either 'accidentally' or in response to a stimulus. Such a mutant cell must survive and replicate in order to become a tumour. The prenatal human lacks, at least initially, the normal immune surveillance system (p. 57) which appears to be at least partly capable of dealing with such mutations in the adult. Thus the chance of a cancer cell surviving is probably greater during fetal life. Developing tissue is, of course, undergoing a process of controlled but rapid and progressive differentiation, a milieu which may favour the creation and survival of malignant cells. Some mutations may be lethal and never appear postnatally, and such are certainly recorded post mortem from time to time; or the process may be successful but not lethal, and thereby result in the birth of a child with an established tumour which may or may not be detectable at birth, or even in the first quinquennium.

Much of the carcinogenesis in adults depends on environmental factors; we know little about those operative in the intrauterine environment, but some things are clear. Whole body irradiation *in utero* can cause cancer which substantially develops within the first seven to eight years of life. Genetic predisposition to cancer, and dominant or recessive inheritance of certain tumours, are also well known. One type of retinoblastoma occurs in significant associations with mental retardation, other malformations, and an excess tendency to develop a second primary cancer without requiring the stimulus of postnatal irradiation, and in even greater excess when therapeutic radiation has been used.

It is quite possible that environmental carcinogens other than x-rays are important in the prenatal period, although proof is lacking. Some viruses and other micro-organisms are known to cross the placental barrier and cause maldevelopment of the fetus, for example, the rubella virus. There is no reason why other viruses or chemical substances or maternal metabolites, could not contribute to the development of a cancer. Very large epidemiological surveys would be necessary to detect such effects.

Postnatal carcinogenesis

While the presence of tumours at birth indicates the existence of a prenatal influence, the development of other types of tumours in older children in the second and third quinquennia, suggests that postnatal carcinogens may also exert their effects during childhood.

Association between tumours and disturbances in development are well known (Table 1.3), and more are identified as time goes by. It is conceivable that noxious influences *in utero* may have a short term, almost immediate, effect on embryonic development causing congenital abnormalities, and long-term carcinogenic effects as well.

Table 1.3 Developmental Anomalies and Malignant Tumours; some associations observed in childhood

Wilms' tumour	Congenital hemihypertrophy
	Hamartoma
	Adrenocortical neoplasia
	Aniridia
	Microcephaly
	Mental retardation
	Facial dysostosis
Leukaemia	Mongolism
	Immune deficiency syndromes
	Blooms' syndrome
	Fanconi's aplastic anaemia
Adrenocortical carcinoma	Hemihypertrophy
	Astrocytoma
Neuroblastoma	None known
Glioma of the optic nerve	Congenital defects of spine
	Tuberous sclerosis
	Multiple neurofibromatosis
Medulloblastoma	Basal cell naevus syndrome
Lymphoma	Immune deficiency syndromes
Gonadoblastoma	Gonadal dysgenesis

Ionizing radiation

Ionizing radiation is the only known carcinogen to contribute to the development of cancer in childhood.

The most recent evidence of the role of ionizing radiation in causing tumours in childhood is the report of Modan, Baidatz *et al.* (1974) from Israel, following the treatment of 16,473 immigrant children with approximately 140 rads to the scalp as part of treatment for ringworm. Among the 10,902 reviewed, there was a significant increase in the incidence of both benign and malignant tumours of the head and neck, notably meningioma, carcinoma of the thyroid (1·1 per thousand treated) and tumours of the parotid gland.

The effects of postnatal irradiation are seen in similar 'mutations', but the latent period is longer (cancers continue to develop for more than 25 years after nuclear irradiation) and the types of cancer are more likely to be those which usually arise in adults, e.g. of the stomach and breast. As children exposed to nuclear fallout are followed for another three decades, the long-term effects will become more clear.

Latency

Some cancers have a long latent period, in others the period is relatively short. The differences are probably related to the nature of the carcinogenic stimulus, to the tissue affected, and to other factors as yet unknown. Some asbestos workers develop cancer ten years after three months exposure, while workers exposed to wood dust seem to require exposure for much longer periods, and the latent period is longer.

The existence of long latent periods and the difficulty of establishing significant correlations after the passage of many years, poses an epidemiological problem, but clinicians should be aware of the associations, and avoid unnecessary radiation or new drugs, for this and many other good reasons.

IMMUNOLOGICAL SURVEILLANCE

The excess incidence of cancer in patients with syndromes due to deficiencies in their immune mechanisms (Gatti & Good, 1971) is clear evidence that the immune system is important in the prevention of cancer (see Chapter 3). Approximately 10 % of patients with congenital agammaglobulinaemia develop a lymphoma or leukaemia; about the same percentage of patients with ataxia telangiectasia develop a lymphoma, leukaemia or other cancers; a similar proportion of patients with the Wiskott-Aldrich syndrome develop a lymphoreticular malignancy, and about one-tenth of patients with acquired agammaglobulinemia develop cancers of diverse types.

Although immune defence mechanisms are immature in the fetus, they may still be sufficiently competent to overcome some tumours. The occurrence of neuroblastoma *in-situ* at autopsy in neonates (p. 538), in far greater numbers than neuroblastoma tumours, may be an example of effective immunosurveillance and the eradication of tumours while they are still literally microscopic (p. 58).

SURVIVAL IN CHILDREN WITH CANCER

In many tumours the pattern of survival is peculiar to childhood and, in general, a two-year survival can be equated with a five-year survival in an adult. However, the most useful survival figure in childhood varies from one tumour to another and has a bearing on the optimum duration of chemotherapy. For example, late recurrence or the first appearance of metastases in Stage I Wilms' tumour is most unusual after an interval of one year from the time of definitive treatment; this is the basis for continuing recurrent courses of chemotherapy for fifteen months. In other types of tumour, such as rhabdomyosarcoma, local recurrences or metastases are known to occur as late as three years after commencing treatment, and the plan of treatment calls for prolonged maintenance chemotherapy (p. 112).

The patient's age at the time of diagnosis is another factor which has a significant effect on the prognosis in some tumours. In children with neuroblastoma, there appear to be fairly precise limits to the period with the most favourable prognosis, and in the Index Series these limits were after the age of three months and before the age of fifteen months; the underlying reason(s) are the subject of debate, and may be related to the variations in the level of immune defences.

Neuroblastoma is one of the very few tumours which undoubtedly undergo complete maturation and remission (p. 539), although this occurs in less than 3% of cases, and is most likely to occur in patients less than two years of age.

In general, very young children enjoy a clear survival advantage. Babies who develop a retinoblastoma have a two-year survival rate of over 80%. The results of treatment in children with a Wilms' tumour are improving progressively; they have already reached a two-year survival rate of 80%, and are approaching 95% in Stage I. With modern methods of intensive and aggressive treatment, even those with pulmonary metastasis may have a 50% two-year survival rate (p. 528). Survival rates for leukaemia have also improved over the past decade (p. 165).

The results in tumours of central nervous system remain disappointing, primarily because of their site rather than their degree of malignancy; early diagnosis is difficult because of the low index of suspicion of the medical profession at large, and the extraordinary adaptability of young children who ignore and compensate remarkably for progressive loss of sight.

CANCER AS A CAUSE OF DEATH

The real incidence of cancer in children has probably not altered greatly over the past four or five decades. However, it now represents a much more important percentage of the spectrum of deaths because of the relative decrease in other causes, for example, infectious diseases. The fact that the percentage of deaths due to cancer has increased slightly is probably due to better diagnosis, as well as better treatment of the bacterial infections which may have previously masked an underlying tumour. Children with malignant disease are a very obvious part of the hospital population today, for a number of reasons: the relatively short time required to control infective, infectious and other diseases; the intensive supervision necessary with modern methods of treatment sometimes undesirably prolongs the stay in hospital, and

Table 1.4. Causes of Death in Childhood. The relative frequency of various causes of death in children between one and fourteen years of age in Australia. The figures are the number of deaths per 100,000 of the relevant (childhood) population, in three census years (1933, 1954, 1971) arranged in rank order for 1971

Statistical categories	1933		1954		1971		Rank Order
Accidents:							
Motor vehicle accidents	7·05	31·00	9·41	26·73	10·69	21·29	1
Other accidents	23·95		17·32		10·60		
Malignant disease		4·35		8·57		7·31	2
Congenital malformations		4·64		6·89		4·85	3
Infectious and parasitic diseases		42·39		8·96		3·94	4
Pneumonia and influenza		32·51		6·83		2·88	5
Heart disease		5·11		1·15		0·59	6
Tuberculosis		7·82		0·77		0·06	7

because treatment often includes a research component requiring careful monitoring of the effects of cytotoxic agents, and other parameters.

The changing patterns of deaths in childhood in Australia are in accord with those in other 'western' populations in 'developed' countries. The major groups are compared in Table 1.4, taking 1933, 1954 and 1971 as examples because they were census years for which information is most comprehensive. Over a period of nearly forty years there has been a clear and dramatic reduction in deaths from infectious disease; motor vehicle accidents show a surprisingly small increase in incidence while other accidents are now only half as common. Taking children of all ages malignant disease is the sixth most common cause of death; when only those more than one year of age are considered (thereby excluding most deaths from developmental abnormalities, pneumonia, prematurity etc.), malignant disease is the second commonest cause of death in childhood (Table 1.4), after 'accidents' (of all types).

B. THE TACTICS OF CANCER THERAPY

As a basis for analysing the rationale of the treatment of cancer, the stages in the evolution of a hypothetical tumour are depicted diagrammatically in Fig. 1.5. Among the several unknowns, are the length of the intervals A, B and C, i.e. the time between the instant of malignant transformation, the point at which the tumour becomes detectable clinically, and when the first cells break away from the primary to establish metastases.

Several factors bear on the length of these intervals.

1. The rate of replication and the cell death rate

It has been estimated that a tumour generally contains 1×10^{12} cells when it is first detected, whereas a tumour of 1×10^{9} cells is usually too small to be recognized. The rates of replication and cell death are relatively constant characteristics of each particular tumour; the intervals A, B and C are probably shortest in rapidly growing embryonal tumours, and possibly longest in papillary carcinomas of the thyroid gland (p. 381), although a palpable metastasis may nevertheless be more common as the mode of presentation than a palpable primary tumour (p. 373).

2. The accessibility of the tumour

This is obviously an important factor; there is a very wide range of possibilities and the extremes are represented by a tumour in the skin of the face, and one in the retroperitoneal tissues of the posterior abdominal wall where a tumour may grow to a huge size before it emerges from beneath the costal margins to become palpable.

3. The effects of the tumour

The tumour itself may produce effects which favour early detection and hence a more favourable prognosis.

(*a*) *Secretory function*

In particular, the elaboration of highly potent metabolites or hormones producing clinical effects, can call attention to a small and deeply situated tumour, e.g. an adenocarcinoma 2–2.5 cm in diameter in the adrenal cortex has been diagnosed by its endocrine effects, and successfully removed.

(*b*) *Pressure on sensitive structures*

Pressure close to the site of a tumour, e.g. on a nerve root causing severe pain, or on the spinal cord causing paraplegia, demands attention at an early stage. Among the group of tumours with the most favourable outlook are those which cause paraplegia (p. 561) while the tumour is only a few cubic centimetres in size.

4. The clinician's index of suspicion

This is one of the most important factors; if it is low, it will almost certainly add to any preceding delays—e.g. delay in recognizing the presence of a painless swelling, or progressive loss of sight in an uncomplaining toddler, or the parents' procrastination in seeking medical advice.

NOMENCLATURE AND STAGING

Recently a more complex and more precise system of staging, the 'TNM' nomenclature, has been proposed, and it can be adapted to fit almost every tumour (Veronesi *et al.*, 1973). It is essentially a classification expressed in 'shorthand' of the presenting clinical findings, supplemented by radiographic and endoscopic evidence. One of its disadvantages is that

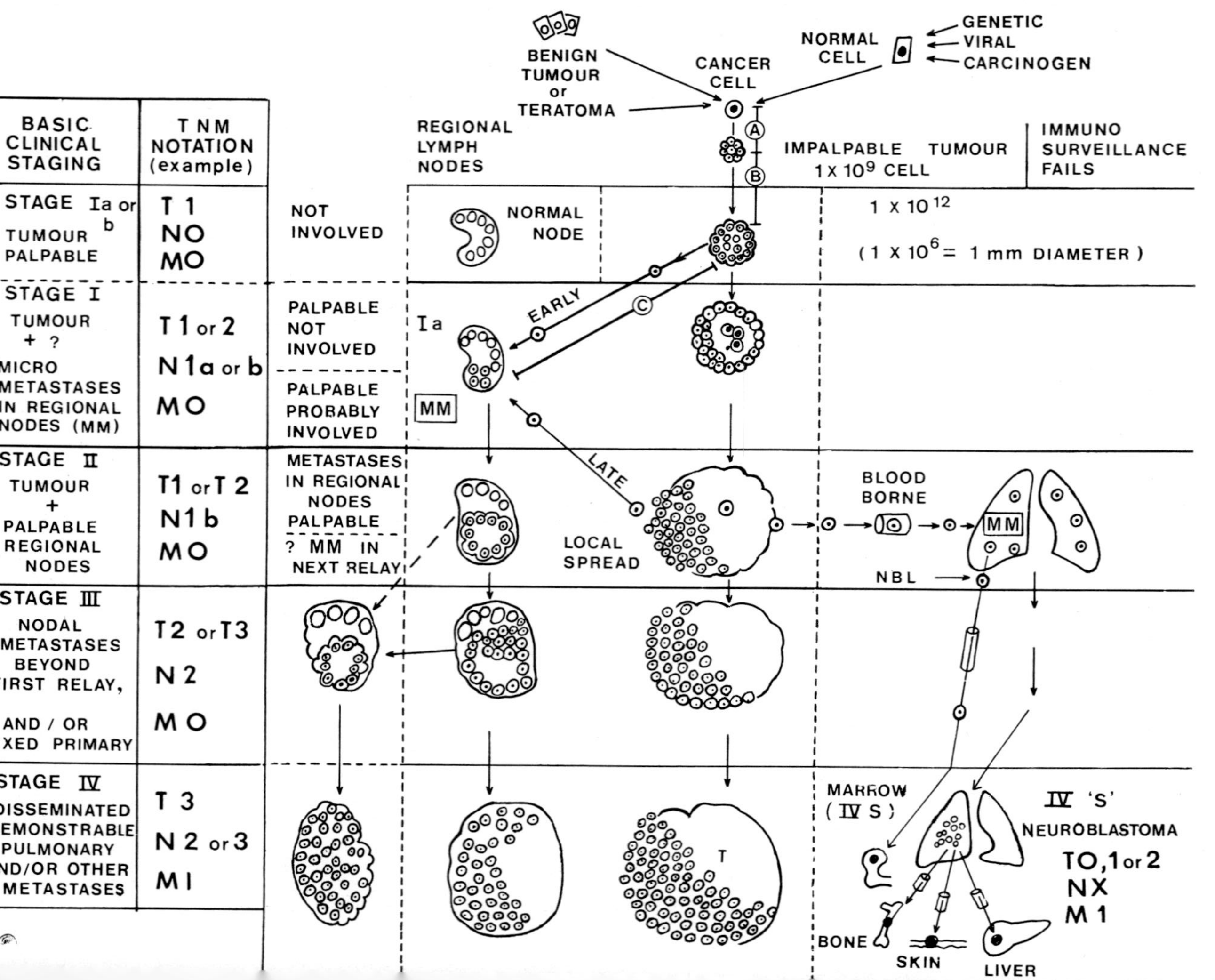
BASIC CLINICAL STAGING
TNM NOTATION (example)
STAGE Ia or b
TUMOUR PALPABLE
T 1 NO MO
NOT INVOLVED
STAGE I
TUMOUR + ?
MICRO METASTASES IN REGIONAL NODES (MM)
T 1 or 2
N 1a or b
MO
PALPABLE NOT INVOLVED
PALPABLE PROBABLY INVOLVED
STAGE II
TUMOUR + PALPABLE REGIONAL NODES
T1 or T 2
N1 b
MO
METASTASES IN REGIONAL NODES PALPABLE
? MM IN NEXT RELAY
STAGE III
NODAL METASTASES BEYOND FIRST RELAY,
AND / OR FIXED PRIMARY
T2 or T3
N 2
M O
STAGE IV
DISSEMINATED DEMONSTRABLE PULMONARY AND/OR OTHER METASTASES
T 3
N 2 or 3
M I
BENIGN TUMOUR or TERATOMA
CANCER CELL
NORMAL CELL
GENETIC
VIRAL
CARCINOGEN
REGIONAL LYMPH NODES
NORMAL NODE
A
B
C
IMPALPABLE TUMOUR 1 X 10^9 CELL
IMMUNO SURVEILLANCE FAILS
1 X 10^12
(1 X 10^6 = 1 mm DIAMETER)
Ia
MM
EARLY
LATE
LOCAL SPREAD
BLOOD BORNE
MM
NBL
T
MARROW (IV S)
IV 'S' NEUROBLASTOMA
TO,1 or 2
NX
M 1
BONE
SKIN
LIVER

retrospective information derived from operative findings is deliberately excluded in establishing the various categories (Appendix V, p. 953).

The TNM notation is included in the stages of a hypothetical tumour depicted in Fig. 1.5, and in this instance, is as follows:

T Represents the findings in the tumour.
TO No tumour palable.
T1 Tumour less than 2 cm in maximum dimension.
T2 Tumour more than 2 cm but less than 5 cm in diameter.
T3 Tumour more than 5 cm in maximum diameter, or fixed to adjacent structures.

N Expresses the clinical findings in the regional lymph nodes.
N0 No regional nodes palpable (when accessible).
NX Regional nodes not capable of clinical assessment (e.g. when intra-abdominal or intrathoracic).
N1 Mobile homolateral lymph nodes palpable enlarged.
N1a ; palpable but not considered to contain metastases.
N1b ; palpable and enlargement considered to be due to metastases.
N2 Mobile contralateral (or second relay) nodes palpable and involved.
N3 Non-mobile (fixed) unilateral (homolateral) nodes.
N4 Non-mobile contralateral or bilateral nodes palpable and involved.

M Represents evidence or absence of distant metastases.
M0 No evidence of distant metastases (e.g. in lungs).
M1 Demonstrable distant metastases (in lungs and/or elsewhere).

STAGE I

According to the general schema, Stage I (in TNM notation : T1 N0 M0) represents the point at which the primary tumour is the only abnormality on clinical examination, and this raises the following questions:

1. Is the swelling a neoplasm?
2. If so, what type is it, and hence what is its expected behaviour?
3. If it is malignant, how far has it spread?

1. Management

Management depends firstly on a proven diagnosis, for it is a basic rule that no treatment should be given until the risks can be justified by proof (usually by histological examination) that the patient has a malignant tumour. With a few notable exceptions (see p. 554), biopsy of the primary tumour is the first step; whenever possible, depending on its site and size, *excision-biopsy* (p. 950), removing the lesion *in toto* together with a safe margin of

---

Figure 1.5. A MALIGNANT TUMOUR : diagram of its evolution, including clinical stages and examples of the TNM notation (see Appendix IV, p. 945).

macroscopically uninvolved tissue, is always preferable to *incision-biopsy* (p. 140), i.e. excision of part of the tumour (see Colour plates following p. 140).

The prognosis of any tumour is unquestionably best when the primary is the only abnormality present. In reviewing the histories of children who presented with a tumour in a later stage, it is often apparent that a swelling had been present for weeks, months or even years before medical advice was sought, or before appropriate action was taken. In the hope that the latter delay can be eliminated or materially reduced by a higher index of suspicion, the dictum reiterated by the late Sidney Farber (1969) is reproduced here:

> 'Every solid, or semisolid, semicystic mass in an infant or child should be regarded as a malignant tumour until its exact nature is determined by histological examination of the removed tumour.
>
> 'This generalization is still useful. The words not only indicate the most reliable means of early recognition of a malignant tumor but also imply the ideal treatment. When a solid mass is found in a patient, the surgeon, the radiotherapist, the chemotherapist, the pathologist, the hematologist, and any other experts whose opinions might be of value in determining the nature of the tumor and the ideal form of treatment, should conduct a rapid study. The ideal treatment for any patient with cancer, and particularly the child with a malignant tumor, should be selected after discussion by a group of experts in a number of different disciplines. It follows from this that the best treatment for a given patient will be mapped out from the moment of recognition of the tumor and subsequent therapeutic procedures will depend on the response to treatment. Optional methods should be recorded far in advance of need. This approach, which is embodied in the 'total care' of the patient with cancer, makes use of all available knowledge from the very beginning and brings together in a logical and co-ordinated program the talents and knowledge of representatives of many different disciplines. Such an approach replaces the traditional one which is unfortunately still in wide use, i.e. sequential, unco-ordinated treatment first by the surgeon; later, possibly, by the radiotherapist; and finally, after metastases have occurred, by the chemotherapist'.
>
> Sidney Farber (1969).

BIOPSY

Surgical manipulation of a malignant tumour raises the possibility of disseminating viable tumour cells by lymphatic or vascular channels, although experimental evidence has shown that liberation of tumour cells into the blood stream occurs only in the more advanced stages and is virtually never seen in Stages I and II; even in Stage III it can be demonstrated in only 3–8% of cases, and at least some of the circulating cells are non-viable or incapable of establishing metastases, a consequence which depends partly on the extent of the patient's immune response to the tumour.

Chemotherapy 'cover'

There are theoretical advantages in having cytotoxic agents present in the bloodstream ready to act upon any viable cells liberated by a surgical procedure, and thus prevent the establishment of metastases; this is the basis for the still debatable use of chemotherapy to 'cover' surgical biopsy or definitive excision. Cytotoxic agent administered for this purpose will act upon the primary tumour as well as on any cells circulating in the blood.

Studies of the number of circulating malignant cells in adults with cancer suggest that the maximum chemotherapeutic 'cover' can be obtained by giving the cytotoxic agent one or two days before the operative procedure, as is our routine for Wilms' tumour. However, if an agent which acts by arresting mitoses in the metaphase (p. 102) is given as early as 48 hours before biopsy, there is a temporary accumulation of cells in mitosis in the primary tumour, and the consequent increase in the mitotic index can make the histologist's task of interpreting the biopsy more difficult. Vincristine (p. 106) is a potential hazard in this respect if it is given more than twelve hours before a biopsy, for its maximum effect on dividing cells is reached in six to twelve hours. This disadvantage of pre-biopsy chemotherapy can be reduced by giving vincristine only a few hours before biopsy. It can also be overcome by choosing an alternative agent; actinomycin D, daunorubicin and cyclophosphamide are three of the drugs which can be used instead of vincristine, because they have little or no action on mitosis. However, the policy of chemotherapy to 'cover' a biopsy is still controversial, especially as the lesion may prove to be benign.

Other arguments against preoperative chemotherapy are that there is, as yet, a lack of objective evidence that metastasis is thereby diminished (a large controlled trial would be necessary to obtain such evidence). There is also a risk of undesirable effects, such as damage to the marrow and immuno-suppression which might, theoretically, enhance seeding of tumour cells during operation. In practice, there is almost no risk of these complications following a single pre-biopsy dose of a cytotoxic agent in a child with a benign lesion and whose bone marrow and immune functions are normal, although there may be some (justifiable) risk in a child whose bone marrow is already involved by metastases. Finally, there is experimental evidence in mice that cyclophosphamide may predispose to anaesthetic complications and even death (Bruce, 1973).

A compromise which may sometimes be justifiable is to defer the chemotherapy 'cover' until the index of suspicion of cancer has been heightened by the macroscopic appearances of the lesion as seen at biopsy or exploration.

2. The histological diagnosis

The probable behavioural characteristics of the tumour, as indicated in the histological diagnosis, may be a relatively easy matter to determine or one of great difficulty requiring a variety of specialized techniques to derive as much information as possible from the material available (Chapter 5).

3. Investigations designed to determine the extent of dissemination

These are a vital step in the assessment of the patient, in planning treatment and in estimating the prognosis. All available information is assembled, from x-rays of the chest, angiography, including lymphangiography where practical, scanning with radionucleides (Chapter 4) and marrow biopsy. Biochemical investigations of the products of tumour metabolism, e.g. catecholamines, or tumour-related antibodies may be particularly important in diagnosis, in monitoring the response to treatment and in detecting evidence of recurrence.

Lymph node metastasis

For the purposes of discussion, Stage I can be sub-divided on hypothetical pathological grounds into two stages Ia and Ib which, however, cannot be distinguished with certainty on clinical evidence alone; Stage 1b (T1 N1a M0) represents micrometastases in regional lymph nodes not sufficiently enlarged to be regarded as clinical Stage II (T1 N1b M0).

Lymphatic metastasis occurring before blood-borne metastases to the lungs is a characteristic of carcinomas rather than sarcomas, but in spite of the preponderance of sarcomas among malignant tumours of childhood (p. 35), metastasis to the regional lymph nodes is not uncommon in children, not only in the two commonest embryonal tumours, Wilms' tumour and neuroblastoma, but also in otherwise characteristic sarcomas, e.g. rhabdomyosarcoma (p. 787), synovial sarcoma (p. 804), and also in malignant lymphomas (p. 173).

In common tumours in adults, sufficient data has been collected from operative specimens to allow accurate predictions of the incidence of lymph node metastases according to the specific sites involved. In an adult with a primary tumour in the head and neck and no palpable lymph node metastases, micrometastases will be found in 15–23% of the apparently normal relevant nodes (Novak, 1967). Further, correlations have also been made between the incidence of palpable and impalpable metastases; when only one clinically positive node is present, in almost 50% of cases there will also be micrometastases in several other nodes in the same group; if more than one node is palpably involved, in 75% of cases there will be impalpable micrometastases in several additional nodes (Gowen and Desuto-Nagy, 1963). These figures vary according to the type of tumour, the site of the primary and the age of the patient, and they should not be looked upon as generally applicable.

Nevertheless, the surgical implication is that as it is probable (and in some tumours very likely) that there are micrometastases in clinically normal regional nodes (Stage Ia). Consideration should be given to removing the first relay of regional nodes in continuity with the primary tumour when this is feasible; this has long been a general principle of radical surgery for cancer in adults, as exemplified in the classical Halsted radical mastectomy, now less commonly employed.

The desirability of preserving and acting in concert with the body's natural defences raises the possibility that unnecessary excision of regional nodes (i.e. those subsequently be shown to be uninvolved) may remove a significant mechanical and biological filter (Song *et al.*, 1971; Fisher & Fisher, 1972) in the path of disseminating cells, as this could conceivably impair the patient's ability to cope with metastases both locally and generally (Hammond & Rolley, 1970). Some of the experimental evidence (McCredie, Inch & Cowie, 1973) indicates that excision of regional nodes does not weaken the general immunodefence mechanisms (Fisher, Saffer & Fisher, 1974); on the other hand there is little or no evidence that 'prophylactic' removal of regional lymph nodes in Stage Ia increases survival rates, except in malignant melanoma (p. 861).

Experiments in animals (Crile, 1968; Crile & Deodhar, 1971) have shown that metastasis may be actually enhanced if the filtering regional nodes are excised or irradiated, but only when these measures are applied four to ten days after the establishment of a primary tumour by transplantation.

Lymphangiography

This is one means of assessing whether there are metastases in regional lymph nodes (or in inaccessible abdominal nodes, p. 190), but has not yet been refined to the point where it is a reliable means of distinguishing between Stages Ia and Ib.

Sampling the relevant nodes

The separate procedure of sampling the relevant nodes by selective biopsy, is another possibility, and theoretically preferable to routine 'prophylactic' clearance of regional nodes *en bloc*, but the feasibility of sampling depends on whether the related nodes are anatomically accessible, whether they lend themselves to a relatively minor additional procedure, and whether the findings in the sample can be taken as reliably representative. Sampling forms part of the plan in the Cardiff Breast Trial (p. 905), in which a particular subgroup of the axillary nodes is sampled at the conclusion of simple mastectomy (Roberts *et al.*, 1973); when the nodes are found to contain tumour cells, this determines the plan of subsequent treatment.

Regional nodes other than those in the axilla, the neck or the groin, are not accessible (NX), but the selection of the optimum plan of treatment may be so dependent on determining the exact extent of nodal and other metastases that a major procedure (such as laparotomy and biopsies of the liver, spleen and lymph nodes in Hodgkin's disease, p. 191) may be justifiable, or even essential for proper treatment.

In many instances sampling cannot be conveniently performed at the same time as, or as a prelude to, excision of the primary tumour, and there are then three options open:

(i) The nodes are left undisturbed, for they may not be involved (Stage Ia), or if they are (Stage Ib), the micrometastases may be left to be dealt with by the patient's immunodefence mechanisms, which are known to be facilitated by removal of most or all of the primary tumour. Alternatively, immunotherapy (p. 65) may be employed to stimulate the body's defences to overcome the metastases.

(ii) The decision may be made to rely on chemotherapy and/or radiotherapy to control presumptive micrometastasis, but these forms of treatment are rarely employed without definite indications (e.g. the type of tumour, or confirmation of regional micrometastases) because there are risks in either method which require some supporting evidence or high probability of metastases to become acceptable, and also because most cytotoxic agents cause some temporary immunosuppression (p. 59) even when administered intermittently. In addition, there are vulnerable epiphyses (p. 124) closely related to the axilla and the groin, and in a child, epiphyseal damage may follow their irradiation.

(iii) Often the decision is made to restrict the operation to removal of the primary tumour, and to rely on surveillance, by careful and regular re-examination of the regional nodes, to detect the first signs of metastases.

STAGE II (T1 or 2 N1b M0)

The requirements of treatment are immediately altered when the regional nodes are significantly enlarged. The first step is to determine whether the enlargement is, in fact, the result of metastasis or due to other causes.

(i) Even the minor trauma and healing inherent in simple excision-biopsy of the primary tumour, or mild inflammation in the biopsy wound may cause non-malignant enlargement of the regional nodes.

(ii) In sites where the primary is in contact with bacterial flora, such as the mouth or pharynx, enlargement of the related regional nodes may be entirely inflammatory rather than metastatic, even when biopsy has not been performed.

(iii) A third possibility is 'reactive hyperplasia' or sinus histiocytosis, a phenomenon presumed to be stimulated by the primary tumour as a function of the immunodefence mechanisms and, by definition, not due to micrometastases. Although it may be a favourable prognostic index of the patient's resistance, it can lead to uncertainty as to whether the nodes should be classified as N1a or N1b. This distinction can only be made with certainty on histological grounds, and in a patient with a proven malignant tumour, 'significant' clinical enlargement of the regional nodes should be taken as presumptive evidence of metastasis when planning treatment. This frequently includes block dissection of the nodes, ideally at the same time as and in continuity with the primary tumour or, alternatively, as a separate operation, e.g. a formal block dissection of the cervical nodes.

Another aspect of Stage II is the possibility that there are already micrometastases in the lungs. The same arguments against active treatment of regional nodes in Stage I can be raised against 'prophylactic' radiotherapy of the lungs, unless there are demonstrable pulmonary metastases. However, if histological study of the operative specimens shows that the regional nodes *were* involved, and depending on the known behaviour of the particular tumour, consideration should be given to a course of cytotoxic agents to control micrometastases in the lungs (and elsewhere). A full primary course of chemotherapy is indicated in this situation, and repeated courses or 'pulses' of chemotherapy for the following one to two years, have been shown to significantly improve survival rates (Donaldson *et al.*, 1973).

Finally, in some tumours, notably neuroblastoma (p. 554), distant metastases, e.g. in the marrow (Fig. 1.5) are frequently present, without demonstrable pulmonary metastases; the marrow and/or bone metastases are assumed to come from micrometastases in the lungs (i.e. T1 NX M1, or T0 NX M1 if the primary is latent).

STAGE III

When the tumour has reached this stage (i.e. with demonstrable distant metastases) at the time of diagnosis, the prognosis is poor but not invariably hopeless. The surgical implication of Stage III is that the tumour and its extensions are obviously beyond the scope of excisional surgery. It is a general rule, and a sound one, that no radical surgical treatment of the primary tumour is warranted unless there are grounds for believing that distant metastases can be controlled.

This rule is often waived in the case of neuroblastoma, and some other tumours, because of special considerations. One is the role of the host's immunodefence mechanisms; there is experimental and clinical evidence that metastases can undergo significant and prolonged regression (as supported by a decrease in humoral blocking-antibody in the patient's serum) following excision, or even subtotal but substantial removal of most of the primary tumour, thus diminishing the total number of tumour cells to a point where the body's defences (or cytotoxic agents) may be able to cope with those remaining.

A variation of Stage III exists when pulmonary metastases first appear after the primary tumour has been completely removed; in many instances the pulmonary secondaries are the only evidence of metastasis. The prospects of treatment depend very largely on the behavioural pattern of the particular tumour. For example, in Wilms' tumour, the appearance of pulmonary metastases within one year of removal of the tumour is a recognized possibility and forms the basis of recurrent courses of chemotherapy, usually continued for fifteen months after nephrectomy (*Childrens' Cancer Study Group A*, 1968). Radiographs of the lungs are therefore taken at monthly intervals to detect the appearance of metastases as early as possible. When they appear, intensive treatment of pulmonary metastases by radiotherapy (p. 520) are warranted by the results obtained in Wilms' tumour (Vietti *et al.*, 1970; O'Gorman Hughes *et al.*, 1973), but not necessarily in other tumours, for example osteosarcoma.

When curative treatment is decided upon in Stage III, the methods available are deployed according to their particular usefulness; operative removal of the primary tumour (and also, possibly, of lymph node metastases), chemotherapy and immunotherapy, which have the advantage of reaching all secondary deposits throughout the entire body, and radiotherapy, when indicated, for suitable localized areas of metastasis.

STAGE IV

In Stage IV, the basis for selecting methods of treatment is much the same as in Stage III. A variation of Stage IV occurs in the majority of children with a neuroblastoma, in which there is often distant dissemination (in the marrow in 50%; Rice, 1966) without demonstrable pulmonary metastases (Fig. 1.5). Another mode of presentation is multiple metastatic nodules of neuroblastoma in the skin and subcutaneous soft tissues (Stage IV S, p. 558).

In the management of a patient in Stage IV, the major decision may be whether curative treatment should be attempted at all because of the poor prognosis and the price to the patient in pain or discomfort inherent in heroic measures. Nevertheless, the extraordinary and successful response to treatment which sometimes occurs unexpectedly, is always a possibility to be considered. A wholehearted attempt at curative treatment is usually justified in almost every case, subject to continuous assessment of the effects on the patient and the response of the tumour.

In children with a disseminated tumour, the principles of curative (as opposed to palliative) treatment are:

1. Identification of the primary tumour, as to site, cytology and extent.
2. Treatment of the primary, often combining all three modes of treatment including:
   (*a*) chemotherapy, which will also reach all sites of metastasis,
   (*b*) radiation of selected sites,

(*c*) surgical excision of the primary if and when this becomes feasible, and
(*d*) repeated courses of chemotherapy to maintain control of cells in various stages of the cell cycle (p. 102).

3. Simultaneous or sequential treatment of metastases by:
(*a*) chemotherapy,
(*b*) radiotherapy, for selected sites, and
(*c*) surgical excision when justified.

SUBTOTAL EXCISION

It is always a source of disappointment to a surgeon when he is unable to remove a tumour *in toto*, but it is some consolation that the removal of the greater part of a malignant tumour may yet benefit the patient and lead to a cure. In experimental models in both animals and in man, residual tumour can be eradicated by the immunological responses of the host. In general, this process is an 'all or none' phenomenon, but only effective against a certain maximum number of tumour cells. In contrast, the 'cell-kill', of chemotherapeutic agents and radiotherapy is always a 'fractional-kill', affecting only that fraction of the tumour cells which are in a vulnerable phase at the time they are administered. The immune system acts best and most effectively as a surveillance mechanism, eliminating neoplastic cells soon after their transformation and before they have had an opportunity to multiply to the point where the mechanisms are no longer capable of effectively overwhelming them.

It follows that if total surgical removal is impossible, the removal of as many tumour cells as possible is the secondary objective. Subtotal removal is then followed by radiotherapy in increments spread over several weeks, not only to dilute the effects of radiation on normal tissues, but also to catch as many cells as possible in successive vulnerable phases as their component cohorts proceed through the process of DNA synthesis and cell division (Fig. 6.1, p. 101). With the same objective, cytotoxic agents are given in divided doses and in recurring cycles, with suitable pauses to allow recovery of the marrow and, equally important, recovery of immunological responses.

REFERENCES

A. Causes: statistics and survival

Bizzozero, O.J., Johnson, K.G. *et al.* (1966). Radiation-related leukaemia in Hiroshima and Nagasaki, 1946–1964, I. Distribution incidence and appearance times. *New Engl. J. Med.*, **274** : 1095.

Bross, I.D.J. & Natarajan, N. (1972). Leukaemia from low level radiation : identification of susceptible children. *New Engl. J. Med.*, **287** : 107.

CAMMOUN, M., HOERNER, G.V. & MOURALI, M. (1974). Tumors of the nasopharynx in Tunisia; an anatomic and clinical study based on 143 cases. *Cancer*, **33** : 184.

CLEMMESEN, J. (1965). *Statistical studies in malignant neoplasms*, Vol. 1, Munksgaard, Kovenhavn.

COMINGS, D.E. (1973). A general theory of carcinogenesis. *Proc. Natl. Acad. Sci.*, **70** : 3324.

DOLL, R., MUIR, C.S. & WATERHOUSE, J.A.H. (1970). *Cancer incidence in five continents*, Vol. 2. U.I.C.C., Geneva.

DAVIES, J.N.P. (1973). Childhood tumours. In *Tumours in a Tropical Country* (Ed. Templeton, A.C.). *Recent Results in Cancer Research*. Ch. 19, p. 306. Heinemann Medical Books, London; Springer Verlag, Berlin, Heidelberg, New York.

EDITORIAL (1972). *The Lancet*, **1** : 359.

FEDRICK, J. & ALBERMAN, E.D. (1972). Reported influenza in pregnancy and subsequent cancer in the child. *Brit. Med. J.*, **2** : 485.

FOLKMAN, J. (1975). Tumor angiogenesis : a possible control point in tumour growth. *Ann. Int. Med.*, **82** ; 96.

FRAUMENI, J.F. (1974). Chemicals in human teratogenesis and transplacental carcinogenesis. *Pediatrics* (*Supplement*), **53** : 807.

GATTI, R.A. & GOOD, R.A. (1971). Occurrence of malignancy in immunodeficiency diseases : a literature review. *Cancer*, **28** : 89.

GORDON, D., SILVERSTONE, H. & SMITHIRST, B.A. (1971). The epidemiology of skin cancer in Australia. *Proceedings of the International Cancer Conference, Sydney*. N.S.W. Government Printer.

GUTMANN, RENE A. (1971). Early diagnosis of gastric cancer. *Am. J. Gastroenterol.*, **56** ; 248.

HAENSZEL, W. & KURIHARA, M. (1968). Studies of Japanese migrants. I. Mortality from cancer and other diseases among Japanese in United States. *J. Nat. Cancer Inst.*, **40** : 43.

HERBST, A.L., POSKANZER, D.C., ROBBOY, S.J. *et al.* (1975). Prenatal exposure to stilbestrol : a prospective study. *New Eng. J. Med.*, **292** : 334.

HERBST, A.L., KURMAN, R.J., SCULLY, R.E. & POSKANZER, D.C. (1972). Clear-cell adenocarcinoma of the genital tract in young females ; Registry report. *New Eng. J. Med.*, **287** ; 1259.

I.A.R.C. MONOGRAPH, Vol. 1. (1972). Evaluation of carcinogenic risks of chemicals to man. International Agency for Research on Cancer, Lyon.

INTERNATIONAL ATOMIC ENERGY AGENCY, Vienna (1969). Radiation induced cancer. *Proceedings of a Symposium*, Athens.

LANCET, ANNOTATION (1974a). Vaginal adenocarcinomas and maternal oestrogen ingestion. **1** : 250.

LANCET, ANNOTATION (1974b) *Lancet*, **1** : 1323.

LEE, F. I. & HARRY, D. S. (1974). Angiosarcoma of the liver in a vinyl-chloride worker. *Lancet*, **1** : 1316.

LI, F.P., RAPAPORT, A.H., FRAUMENI, J.F.Jr. & JENSEN, R.D. (1970). Familial ovarian carcinoma. *J. Amer. Med. Assoc.*, **214** : 1559.

MILLER, R. W. (1971). Deaths from childhood leukaemia and solid tumours among twins and other sibs in the United States, 1960–1967. *J. Nat. Cancer Inst.*, **46** : 203.

MILLER, R.W. (1974). How environmental effects on child health are recognized. *Pediatrics* (*Supplement*), **53** : 792.

MILLER, R.W. (1973). Proceedings. New hypothesis on the etiology of cancer. *Proc. Natl. Cancer Conf., Epidemiology* **7** : 653.

MILLER, R.W. & DALAGER, N.A. (1974). U.S. Childhood cancer deaths by cell type, 1960–1968. *J. Pediat.*, **85** : 664.

MODAN, B., BAIDATZ, D. *et al.* (1974). Radiation induced head and neck tumours. 1974. *Lancet*, 1 : 277.

STEWART, ALICE & BARBER, RENATE. (1971). Epidemiological importance of childhood cancer. *British Medical Bulletin*, **27** : 64.

TEMIN, H.M. & MIZUTANI, S. (1970). RNA dependent DNA polymerase in virions of Rous sarcoma virus. *Nature* (London), **226** : 1211.

U.S. PUBLIC HEALTH SERVICE PUBLICATION NO. 1696. *The Health Consequences of Smoking*, Ch. 3.

VIANNA, N.J., GREENWALD, P. & DAVIES, J.N.P. (1971) Extended epidemic of Hodgkin's disease in high school students. *Lancet*, **1** : 1209.

VINKEN, P.J. & BRUYN, G.W. (eds). (1972). The Phakomatoses. In *Handbooks of Clinical Neurology*, Vol. 14. American Elsevier, New York.

WORLD HEALTH ORGANIZATION (1972). *Health Hazards of the Human Environment*, p. 219. Geneva.

WORLD HEALTH ORGANIZATION (1972–1973). International Agency for Cancer Research, *Annual Report*, p. 56, Geneva.

B. The Tactics of Cancer Therapy

BRUCE, D.L. (1973). Anaesthetic-induced increase in mortality from cyclophosphamide. *Cancer*, **31** : 361.

CHILDRENS' STUDY GROUP A (1968). Single versus multiple dose Dactinomycin therapy in Wilms' tumour. *New Engl. J. Med.*, **279** : 290.

CRILE, G. (1968). The effect on metastases of removing or irradiating region nodes in mice. *Surg. Gynec. Obstet.*, **126** : 1270.

CRILE, G. & DEODHAR, S.D. (1971). Role of preoperative irradiation in prolonging con-commitant immunity and preventing metastasis in mice. *Cancer*, **27** : 629.

DONALDSON, S.S., CASTRO, J.R., WILBUR, J.R. & JESSE, R.H. (1973). Rhabdomyosarcoma of head and neck in children. *Cancer*, **31** : 26.

FARBER, S. (1969). The Heath Memorial Lecture. In *Neoplasia in childhood.* Year Book Medical Publishers Inc., Chicago.

FISHER, B. & FISHER, E.R. (1972). Studies concerning the regional lymph nodes in cancer. II. Maintenance of immunity. *Cancer*, **29** : 1496.

FISHER, B., SAFFER, E. & FISHER, E.R. (1974). Studies concerning the regional lymph nodes in cancer. IV. Tumor inhibition by regional lymph node cells. *Cancer*, **33** : 631.

GOWEN, G.F. & DE SUTO-NAGY, G. (1963). The incidence and sites of metastasis in head and neck carcinoma. *Surg. Gynec. Obstet.*, **116** : 603.

HAMMOND, W.G. & ROLLEY, R.T. (1970). Retained regional lymph nodes : effect on metastases and recurrence after tumour removal. *Cancer*, **25** : 368.

MCCREDIE, J.A., INCH, W.R. & COWIE, H.C. (1973). Effect of excision on local radio-therapy to a tumour and its regional nodes on metastases. *Cancer*, **31** : 983.

NOVAK, A.J. (1967). Incidence and significance of metastases to the lymph nodes in unilateral neck dissections. In *Cancer of the head and neck*. Butterworth, Washington, D.C.

O'GORMAN HUGHES, D.W., BOWRING, A.C. *et al.* (1973). Wilms' tumour : increasing hopes for survival. *Med. J. Aust.*, **2** : 917.

RICE, M.S. (1966). Neuroblastoma in childhood : a review of 69 cases. *Aust. paediat. J.*, **2** : 1.

ROBERTS, M.M., FORREST, A.P.M. *et al.* (1973). Simple versus radical mastectomy : Preliminary report of the Cardiff Breast Trial. *Lancet*, **1** : 1073.

SONG, J., FROM, P., MORRISSEY, W.J. & SAMS, J. (1971). Circulating cancer cells : pre and post chemotherapy observations. *Cancer*, **28** : 553.

VERONESI, U. (Chairman) *et al.* (1973). *Clinical Oncology*. UICC, Springer-Verlag. Berlin, New York.

VIETTI, T., SULLIVAN, M. *et al.* (1970). Vincristine sulphate and radiotherapy in metastatic Wilms' tumour. *Cancer*, **25** : 12.

Chapter 2. Paediatric neoplasia

A. TUMOURS

Most tumours in children are sarcomas; if leukaemias are excluded, more than 90% of tumours in childhood are derived from mesenchymal cells. Tumours of epithelium, whether of surface cells or glandular acini, are relatively rare in children, and in this respect the distribution of neoplasia in childhood is in very striking contrast to the pattern seen in adults.

ETIOLOGY

As most paediatric tumours are sarcomatous and embryonal in type and arise in internal organs, it is unlikely that the etiological mechanisms in children are the same as in adults. In the latter most tumours are epithelial in origin, on the surface or in glands, and extrinsic carcinogens have been clearly implicated in many of them. In childhood it is probable that neoplasms arise from internal stimuli related to growth and differentiation of immature tissues in the fetus and young child. These stimuli may well be carcinogens too, possibly acting on the fetus via the maternal circulation, or by ingestion during childhood. There is little concrete evidence for this, but in experimental models in animals a variety of tumours resembling those seen in children can be produced by manipulating the intrauterine environment, e.g. by feeding the pregnant mother certain toxic chemical substances.

Infection by viruses, either overt and latent, has been suggested as the cause of some childhood neoplasms, e.g. lymphoma and leukaemia. The evidence is scanty, but the hypothesis is based on well documented parallel situations in animals. However, epidemiological evidence which is accumulating would support the possibility of an infective agent in the etiology of human leukaemia, in which seasonal or regional clustering of cases is difficult to explain on the basis of chance. Similarly, the increased incidence of Hodgkin's disease in children who have had their tonsils removed may indicate an infective agent which might gain access through a pharynx deprived of the defences offered by lymphoid tissue in an intact Waldeyer's ring.

BIOLOGICAL BEHAVIOUR

Recent studies on cell doubling times have shed some light on the rate of growth of tumours in general, and can be applied to those arising in children. While some appear to grow very rapidly, others enlarge only slowly; the growth rate varies from a linear relationship to time, to those which seem to be exponential. In general, embryonal tumours appear to grow most rapidly, and this is certainly consistent with their immature histological appearance and vigorous mitotic activity. The most rapidly growing embryonal tumours are rhabdomyosarcoma, Wilms' tumour and neuroblastoma. Some malignant bone tumours, e.g. Ewing's and osteosarcoma, grow extremely quickly, both the primary and at metastatic sites. There are exceptions which are difficult to explain solely on the basis of histological appearance.

Cytotoxic agents currently used in cancer chemotherapy can have dramatic effects on growth; they seem to be capable of holding a tumour in a state of suspended growth for months, following which the tumour may be completely destroyed, or it may recommence growth at the initial rate, or at a faster or slower rate.

A different and almost unique property of growth and differentiation is illustrated by neuroblastoma which in rare instances (estimated at between 2% and 5%) is capable of undergoing spontaneous arrest of growth, with or without maturation into ganglioneuroma (p. 539). This phenomenon is of great biological interest and has still not been satisfactorily explained. The nerve growth factor, described by Burdman & Goldstein (1964) as the agent causing maturation, has recently been shown to have no biological effect *in vivo* (Kumar *et al.*, 1972).

CLASSIFICATION

Many attempts have been made to classify tumours encountered mainly in childhood, but as yet no universally acceptable basis has been adopted (Marsden & Steward, 1968; Willis, 1962). Some have been based on the type of cell produced, or on the histogenesis of the tumour cells, or according to the site of origin. The purpose of a classification is to group together similar neoplasms so that a study of their clinical and pathological features can provide a clearer understanding of their nature, their natural history or their response to treatment. Ideally, a classification should arrange tumours in order of frequency in groups according to their histogenetic origin, and in such a way that very similar tumours can be considered together. In practice this does not seem to be possible; the histogenesis of many tumours is still unknown; common tumours often share close similarities with those which are very rare, and they should be considered together. The simplest classification tends to become burdened with single examples of rare tumours which are included for the sake of completeness.

There are at least three possible bases for classification:

1. From the point of view of the pathologist, the safest method is a classification based on *histological appearances*, but difficulties arise when the cells of a tumour are so undifferentiated that they cannot be recognized.

2. A second method is based on *histogenesis*, but this requires assumptions as to the origin of the tumour cell, and difficulties arise when the origin is in dispute. In practice, tumours can be classified by either of these methods, although a histogenetic emphasis predominates in the classification of paediatric neoplasms.

3. A third method of grouping tumours is based on *the organ or tissue of origin*, but several different kinds of tumour can arise in one organ or tissue.

The classification used in the chapters which follow is a combination of all three methods, i.e. according to site of origin, to the histological appearances, or to the histogenesis where this is known. Such a classification involves some repetition, because the same type of tumour can arise in one of several tissues or organs. In childhood, however, there is a remarkable constancy of association between each organ and the tumour which commonly arises in it, e.g. Wilms' tumour and the kidney, neuroblastoma and sympathetic nervous tissue, hepatoblastoma and the liver and so on. A practical classification is thus possible, the only problem being those tumours which can arise in several different tissues, e.g. the malignant lymphomas and histiocytoses, and this difficulty can be met by treating them as distinct entities. A chapter has been devoted to each of them, the lymphomas in Chapter 10, and the histiocytoses in Chapter 11.

Malignant tumours in children can be divided into two major classes:

(*a*) embryonal (embryonic) tumours, and
(*b*) tumours composed of cells resembling mature tissue.

(*a*) In the embryonal group are:

Medulloblastoma
Medullo-epithelioma
Retinoblastoma
Neuroblastoma
Germinoma
Malignant teratoma
Yolk sac tumours (embryonal carcinomas, including orchioblastomas)
Nephroblastoma (Wilms' tumour)
Hepatoblastoma
Rhabdomyosarcoma
Mesenchymoma

(*b*) Tumours composed of cells resembling mature tissues are:

Astrocytoma
Ependymoma
Oligodendroglioma
Carcinomas of the
- Renal pelvis
- Bowel
- Skin
- Endocrine glands
- Bile ducts and liver cells
- Salivary glands

Meningioma
Neurofibroma and Neurilemmoma

Sarcomas:
- Fibrosarcoma
- Leiomyosarcoma
- Haemangiosarcoma
- Liposarcoma
- Osteosarcoma

There are, in addition, tumours which are not obviously embryonal yet have no recognizable counterpart in mature tissue and cannot logically be fitted into either of the above groups. Examples of this group are:

Ewing's tumour of bone.
Melanotic progonoma (syn. neuroectodermal tumour of infancy)
Lymphomas
Histiocytoses

Embryonal Tumours

Willis (1962) has given a clear account of embryonal tumours. Most of them are easily recognized by a preponderance of immature components resembling fetal tissues or organs as seen at an early stage of differentiation and growth. Although unquestionably malignant, these neoplasms closely resemble rapidly growing fetal tissues, and the concept that they represent errors in differentiation (or in the control of differentiation) during critical phases of organ growth, is simple and acceptable, even if the mechanism whereby control of the growing organism is relinquished is completely unknown.

Embryonal tumours can also be recognized by their site and appearance. The differential diagnosis of some of them can be extremely difficult, especially when there is little or no pattern of differentiation, because the component cells all look very similar, i.e. large cells with active, hyperchromatic nuclei and relatively scanty cytoplasm. Electron microscopy may reveal evidence of cellular differentiation, and so may the presence of certain enzymes, but in practice the cornerstone of diagnosis is still the paraffin section. However, in a difficult case, considerable help may be obtained by electron microscopy, enzyme histochemistry, cell cultures (p. 86), and by other techniques in the course of development.

While the tumours in childhood which differ markedly from those of adults are embryonal in type, most of the tumours of childhood derived from mature tissues are very similar to their adult counterparts, and these present few difficulties in diagnosis. However, there are two further aspects of paediatric pathology which can cause difficulties, first, the relatively high incidence of hamartomas (or choristomas), and second, the occurrence of a group/borderline tumours with an appearance of hypercellularity, and behaviour which combines both benign and malignant characteristics.

Hamartomas

Hamartomas are defined as tumour-like malformations composed of excess amounts of tissue normally present in the affected part. In childhood they are extremely common; the majority of naevi, lymphangiomas and haemangiomas are, in all probability, not true neoplasms at all but focal abnormalities of growth which, by their localized nature and their ability to grow as the child grows, give the impression of being tumours. Most cause no problems in either clinical or pathological diagnosis, but others (e.g. some haemangiomas of infancy) infiltrate widely, are very cellular, with anaplasia and considerable mitotic activity. Some naevi, too, in particular the juvenile melanoma (spindle-cell/epitheloid naevus), may be quite alarming clinically and cytologically. Some hamartomas by virtue of their site, e.g. in the liver or the central nervous system, can simulate a malignant tumour.

Choristomas

These are tumour-like malformations composed of tissue *not* normally present in the affected part, and they are therefore potentially misleading. Some entities, e.g. aberrant islands of cartilage or brain tissue in the tongue, or the nose (the so-called nasal 'glioma', p. 348), cause diagnostic problems by virtue of their bizarre site or inappropriate tissue components. When a hamartoma or a choristoma in a young child is also highly cellular, it may be particularly difficult to identify correctly.

Hypercellularity

Hypercellularity is a feature of benign neoplasms in children; they also have more nuclear hyperchromatism, considerably more mitotic activity, and even pleomorphism, than would be acceptable in benign tumours in adults. These features can probably be explained by the general immaturity and more rapid growth rate of children's tissues. Examples are adrenal cortical adenomas and phaeochromocytomas, many of which show considerable nuclear pleomorphism and yet, in spite of this, appear in most instances to be benign; other examples are mesenchymal hamartomas of the kidney (see p. 510), tumours and tumour-like accumulations of adipose tissues (p. 811) (Chung & Enzinger, 1973), fibrous tissue (p. 798), and some brain tumours (p. 242).

HISTOLOGICAL DIAGNOSIS OF MALIGNANCY

The decision as to whether a tumour is innocent or malignant depends upon two important aspects:

(*a*) The tissue pattern, and

(*b*) The structure (including ultrastructure) of individual tumour cells, and in some cases their extracellular products.

(a) Tissue pattern

The general criteria which are helpful in determining whether a tumour is benign or malignant are listed in Table 2.1. When applied to neoplasms in childhood however, these general criteria are not, individually, always valid.

The histopathologist recognizes a tumour by its tissue pattern, but tends to rely more on cytological features when deciding whether the tumour is

Table 2.1. Histological features typical of benign and malignant neoplasms, and the basis of their differentiation

	Benign	Malignant
Structure	Orderly, resembles tissue of origin	Irregular, disorderly, atypical of parent tissue. Tumour formations show loss of normal polarity; secretion may accumulate.
Type of growth	Slow, usually expansive, compresses adjacent structures	Usually rapid and infiltrating rather than compressing.
Metastasis	Absent	Usually occurs at some stage of the growth of the tumour.
Necrosis	Unusual	Common.
Vascularity	Slight, vessels normal	Increased, vessels often tortuous and fragile.
Inflammatory reaction and fibrosis	Unusual	Common

Cytological findings suggestive of malignancy:

Pleomorphism of cells.	Nuclear hyperchromasia, irregularity and clumping of chromatin.
Anaplasia of cells.	Increased nucleus/cytoplasm ratio.
Loss of polarity of cells.	Abnormal mitotic figures, e.g. tripolar, bizarre, fragmented.
Increased nucleolus/nucleus ratio.	Abnormalities of cell function (e.g. histochemical evidence).
Increased numbers of mitoses.	

benign or malignant, and also when assessing the degree of malignancy. However, the tissue pattern can sometimes be of help in making this distinction, for example, in distinguishing a fibrosarcoma from a fibromatosis, or an adrenal carcinoma from an adenoma. In fibrosarcomas, even when well differentiated, the component cells are arranged in a pattern of interlacing bundles similar to the structure of herring-bone tweed, or the branches of a fir tree. By contrast, no such regular pattern is seen in the fibromatoses of childhood, even though in young children these lesions may be extremely cellular (indeed more cellular than many fibrosarcomas). The cells of a fibromatosis tend to be plump and active (see p. 800).

In adrenal cortical tumours the pattern, i.e. the arrangement of cells in cords mimicking the normal adrenal cortex, is of paramount importance in deciding whether a given tumour is an adenoma or a carcinoma, in which loss of columnation of the cells is a significant feature. This is particularly important because bizarre cells commonly occur in adenomas, and their irregular, giant, hyperchromatic nuclei can easily be mistaken for malignant cells. This cytological peculiarity is seen also in other endocrine tumours e.g. a parathyroid, pituitary and pancreas (islet cell tumours).

Embryonal tumours are usually identified by their tissue pattern, for example, in recognizing a fetal hamartoma of the kidney in an infant. This lesion presents as a discrete renal mass and therefore raises the problem of distinguishing it from a Wilms' tumour. Much has been written on these lesions (see p. 515), but the correct diagnosis is usually made from a study of the tissue pattern, which closely mimics that of a malformed kidney. If this is ignored and attention is concentrated on the individual cells, an erroneous diagnosis of Wilms' tumour may be made, because hamartomas occur in young children, at a time when there is active synthesis of DNA, and sometimes considerable mitotic activity (which is however, always regular and normal).

Where a tumour has no recognizable tissue pattern, a precise diagnosis on this basis may be impossible, and evidence of differentiation of individual tumour cells should then be sought, e.g. myofilaments in a rhabdomyosarcoma, or melanosomes in a malignant melanoma. Here tissue differentiation is supplanted by cell differentiation in making a diagnosis, and ultrastructure is of great assistance in such cases.

On occasions the tissue pattern may be misleading by assuming a differentiated pattern indicative of benignancy, e.g. in sacrococcygeal teratomas; their teratomatous nature (p. 45) is usually obvious, but in spite of being composed of differentiated tissues, they should not be assumed to be 'benign'. Both local recurrence and distant metastases can occur, sometimes many years after apparently total excision.

Type of growth

Some malignant tumours in childhood have an expansive rather than an infiltrative pattern of growth and, on the other hand, several non-malignant conditions have extremely ill-defined and apparently infiltrating margins. Thus there are exceptions to the usual benign/encapsulation, malignant/infiltration patterns. Examples of the 'expansile' pseudo-encapsulated malignant tumours are Wilms' tumour and some hepatoblastomas, while examples of benign conditions with infiltrative margins are the fibromatoses, eosinophilic granuloma of bone, capillary haemangiomas (particularly in infants), ganglioneuromas, and some hamartomas and choristomas.

Infiltration of the capsule or invasion of veins or lymphatics is sometimes the only indication of malignancy in a structurally well-differentiated tumour, e.g. a carcinoma of the thyroid gland or the adrenal cortex.

The rate of growth is usually a reliable index of malignancy, but chemotherapy can inhibit the growth of a malignant tumour to a remarkable degree.

Local infiltration is a very common feature in lymphosarcoma, embryonal rhabdomyosarcoma of the genito-urinary tract, and in most tumours of the central nervous system.

Local spread is also quite common in malignant teratomas, osteosarcoma, and some soft tissue sarcomas, e.g. fibrosarcoma; in rhabdomyosarcoma a local recurrence is occasionally an unwelcome consequence of inadequate excision of the primary tumour.

Metastasis

The spread in tumours in children follows the classical pathways, but there are some notable exceptions and variations.

Lymph node metastasis is very common in embryonal tumours, especially neuroblastoma and Wilms' tumour, and in fact, the four commonest abdominal tumours of childhood (Wilms' tumour, neuroblastoma, lymphosarcoma and rhabdomyosarcoma) all show a strong predilection to spread to regional nodes. Hepatoblastomas rarely involve lymph nodes but spread directly to the lungs; hepatocarcinomas, on the other hand, frequently produce metastases in lymph nodes, even when the primary is occult.

Between a third and a half of the soft tissue sarcomas encountered in childhood also spread to regional lymph nodes, sometimes relatively early, and this occurs with sufficient frequency to justify treatment of the regional lymph nodes (by dissection or radiotherapy) as part of the management of these neoplasms.

Haematogenous spread is the commonest and most significant route of metastasis in tumours of childhood, and is virtually always to the lungs. Some neoplasms, notably Wilms' tumour, invade and proliferate within large veins, producing macroscopic masses of tumour and thrombus which can break off and form emboli. In most tumours however, invasion of vessels is on a microscopic scale. In neuroblastoma it usually occurs early, and produces widespread metastasis while the primary tumour is still quite small. Selective sparing of the lungs by neuroblastoma metastases is a unique and unexplained phenomenon; pulmonary metastases are so rare that the presence of parenchymal pulmonary metastases virtually rules out the possibility that the tumour is a neuroblastoma. However, invasion and metastasis to the visceral and parietal pleura does occur in neuroblastoma, and the reason for this localization is also obscure.

In general, venous invasion leads first to pulmonary metastasis and thence to dissemination in bone and other tissues by tertiary spread. However, except in the terminal stages, bone metastasis in children with a malignant tumour is uncommon, the notable exception being the neuroblastoma, which presents, in a significant percentage of cases (p. 554), with evidence of deposits in the bone or in the marrow. A rhabdomyosarcoma occasionally produces bone metastasis in the absence of other obvious secondary deposits, but in general, and with the exception of neuroblastoma, biopsy of the bone marrow is of limited value as an aid to the diagnosis of a solid tumour in childhood.

Ewing's tumour of bone is another tumour with an unusual pattern of metastasis; not infrequently it produces isolated metastases in other bones, without evidence of disease elsewhere, such as in the lungs. A similar phenomenon occasionally occurs in osteosarcoma, and may be an expression of multifocal origin.

Tumours of the central nervous system rarely extend outside the cranial cavity; this is occasionally reported in medulloblastoma, but usually in artificial circumstances, e.g. in the presence of a ventriculo-atrial shunt which could carry tumour cells into the systemic circulation. Likewise, a retinoblastoma is occasionally disseminated widely through the body, but usually only after it has invaded extra-ocular tissues and thus the systemic venous system. Rarely, a malignant astrocytoma metastasizes outside the skull; the route is thought to be via the meningeal veins and only occurs when the tumour has spread to involve the meninges (p. 242). The most commonly encountered form of local spread is to the spinal meninges, and this occurs with medulloblastoma, ependymoma and some malignant astrocytomas.

Necrosis is usually a reliable indication of a rapidly-growing and therefore malignant tumour, but there are exceptions in both directions, e.g. a proportion of Wilms' tumours attain a considerable size before developing areas of necrosis and haemorrhage, so that they have a uniform and homogenous appearance on cut surface.

On the other hand, some benign tumours in children have a great propensity to undergo necrosis, notably eosinophilic granuloma of bone. Necrosis and degeneration are also common in cerebellar astrocytomas, and this does not indicate a malignant potential.

Necrosis in a tumour occurs as the result of rupture or occlusion of vessels, and in general, malignant tumours have thin-walled, often tortuous, aneurysmal vessels prone to damage. In some tumours, in particular cerebral tumours, necrosis may follow endothelial hyperplasia of the arteries in the tumour. Necrosis may be followed by calcification, as in neuroblastoma, occasionally in Wilms' tumour and in some astrocytomas, and radiographic signs of calcification is indirect evidence of necrosis and the likelihood of malignancy.

Inflammatory response of the host to the tumour is seen as lymphocytic infiltration at the growing margin of the tumour. It is a particular feature of tumours of the skin, but rarely prominent in other solid tumours in children, so that it is of little practical importance. It has been suggested that the extent of lymphocytic accumulations in neuroblastomas may be of prognostic significance, but it is our belief that this phenomenon is very common and not usually helpful. Neuroblastomas tend to metastasize to lymph nodes, and quite often the lymphoid tissue in these tumours represents residual lymphoid tissue following replacement of a lymph node. Quite obviously the body's immune mechanisms are extremely important in the resistance of the host to tumour growth, but morphological evidence of this process, particularly in well-established tumours, is absent.

(b) Cytological indicators of malignancy

The appearance of both the nucleus and cytoplasm are vitally important in assessing the degree of malignancy of a particular tumour. All the classical features listed in Table 2.1 can be helpful in deciding whether a tumour is benign or malignant, but they lie in the province of general pathology rather than in this chapter. In general, much the same weight can be given to these criteria in assessing a paediatric tumour as in an adult neoplasm. However, each of the features listed has its exceptions.

A high mitotic ratio is often seen in children's tumours, particularly in infants, and should not be allowed to sway the diagnosis towards malignancy, e.g. in juvenile fibromatosis, infiltrating capillary haemangiomas or in the mesonephric hamartomas of infancy. On the other hand, in older children (over the age of two years) the number of mitoses is helpful in assessment, particularly in cerebral tumours.

The artificial and potentially misleading accumulation of mitoses following the administration of vincristine is well known, and should be ruled out as a possible cause before accepting the number of mitotic figures as an index of malignancy in a given tumour (p. 25).

Pleomorphism of nuclei is occasionally seen in some benign tumours, and notorious examples are adenoma of the adrenal cortex, parathyroid glands and pancreatic islets. In these tumours the cause of pleomorphism is not clear although it has been attributed to degeneration. The large, hyperchromatic, irregular nuclei found in benign tumours can sometimes be very striking and easily mistaken for malignant cells.

Prominent nucleoli are seen in the cells of several childhood tumours, and in general are an indication of malignancy, e.g. the dark-staining and prominent nucleoli in reticulum cell sarcoma, synovial sarcoma, some rhabdomyosarcomas and melanomas. Large, bizarre eosinophilic nucleoli, resembling viral inclusions, are a prominent feature of the reticulum cells in Hodgkin's disease.

The naevus cells of spindle/epithelioid cell naevi (juvenile 'melanoma') may have a very prominent nucleolus, also seen in cellular blue naevi, and such lesions may mistakenly be labelled as malignant (p. 846).

B. TERATOMAS

Teratomas form another group of neoplasms which have a prominent place among the tumours of childhood, although they are, of course, not confined to children. The teratomas on file in the pathology department of the Royal Children's Hospital (1949 to 1973 inclusive) are listed in Table 2.2. The time span is greater than in the Index Series, and hence the figures differ slightly from those given for teratomas in Appendix I. They are described in this chapter because a teratoma is a form of embryonal tumour. They occur in various sites and the more common are mentioned briefly below; they are also described in the appropriate chapters according to their site or organ of origin.

Table 2.2. Teratomas in childhood. The sites and the nature of a consecutive series of 94 cases (Royal children's Hospital, Melbourne, 1949–1973)

Site	Benign	Malignant	Male	Female	Totals	Comments
Ovary	32	5	–	37	37	Approx. 13% malignant
Sacro-coccygeal	26	9	4	31	35	9 malignant (8 female; 1 male) approx. 25%
Mediastinum	8	2	4	6	10	2 malignant (1 male; 1 female)
Brain	4	—	2	2	4	None histologically malignant
Testis	1	—	1	—	1	—
Other sites	6	1	2	5	7	3 retroperitoneal 2 spinal 1 spermatic cord 1 'epignathus'
Totals	77 (84%)	17 (15%)				

It can be seen that teratomas of the ovary and sacrococcygeal region are by far the most common and together they account for 77% of all the teratomas seen. Those behaving in a benign fashion accounted for 84% of the total, but a significant 16% were judged to be malignant, either from the outset or from their subsequent behaviour. It is our practice to avoid the adjective 'benign' in reporting teratomas, even the common cystic ovarian teratoma. We prefer to refer to them as 'differentiated' because of the possibility of subsequent malignant behaviour in a histologically 'benign' tumour, of which there are several examples in the Index Series.

A female infant presented with a sacral mass at birth. The mass was excised on day seven, apparently completely. Histologically it was well differentiated with areas of nervous tissue, fat, smooth muscle, bronchial epithelium and glands, cartilage, skin and skin

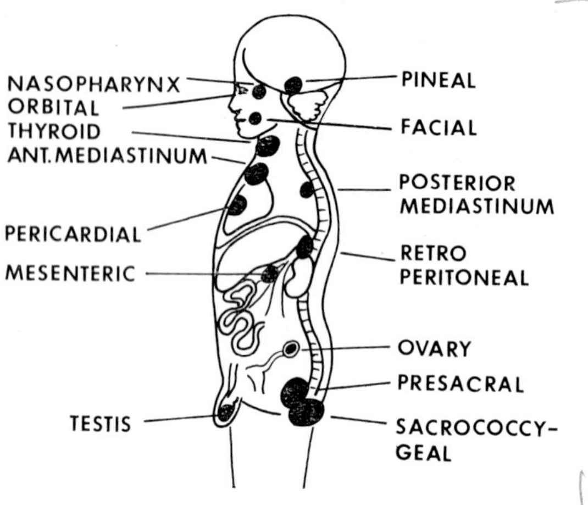

TERATOMAS — R.C.H. SERIES

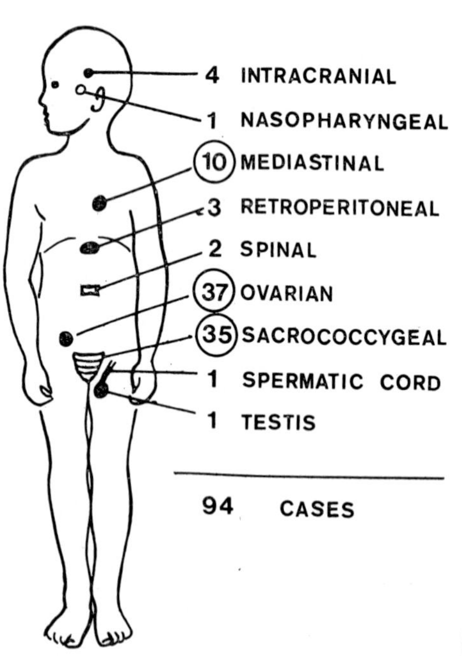

Figure 2.1. TERATOMAS, (*a*) sites reported in the literature; (*b*) the relative incidence as shown in 94 consecutive cases on file in the Department of Pathology, Royal Children's Hospital 1949–1973.

appendages. The stroma in some places appeared embryonic, but there were no mitoses. Six years later the child developed metastases in lymph nodes and the liver, and rapidly deteriorated. Biopsy of the metastatic deposits in the liver showed the microscopic structure of an embryonal papillary carcinoma.

The nature and origin of teratomas is still disputed. The word means 'monstrous tumour', and some contain tissues so well organized macroscopically that they bear a fanciful resemblance to a deformed fetus. The majority, however, show only microscopic features of differentiation. Teratomas are true tumours, that is their growth is progressive and unrestrained, although often slow and indolent, and they are composed of a variety of tissues foreign to the part in which they arise. Neuroectodermal derivatives are almost invariably present, as well as a variable amount of mesodermal tissues such as bone, cartilage, fat, muscle, and epithelia of endodermal origin (Mahour *et al.*, 1974).

The ability of the cells of a teratoma to differentiate in the direction of all three germ layers is unique, and the chief feature which sets them apart from other 'mixed' tumours, for example mesodermal mixed tumours of the uterus, and mesenchymomas (p. 812).

Ashley (1973) has recently suggested that there are two groups of teratomas: (*a*) a group comprising those which develop in the gonads (and possibly in the posterior abdominal wall) which he suggests arise by a process of parthenogenesis from germ cells; and (*b*) those in the sacrococcygeal region, the cranium and the thorax, which he believes may arise from a group of cells separated from the blastula before differentiation into the three germ layers has occurred; the sequestered cells thus escape the controlling and differentiating influences leading to growth and development of the remainder of the (normal) embryo. In other words the second group represents a form of incomplete conjoined twins. By whatever process they arise, their component cells retain an ability to grow and differentiate across the boundary lines separating 'ectoderm', 'mesoderm' and 'endoderm'.

By definition, teratomas are congenital tumours and present at birth, although not always manifest at that time. Some appear much later, sometimes not until adult life, and this is one aspect which is difficult to explain. Their occasionally unpredictable malignant behaviour is also puzzling.

While some are obviously malignant when first seen, others, notably those presenting as a sacrococcygeal mass, may recur locally or present as metastasis many years after removal. When this occurs the malignant tissue is usually a papillary embryonal adenocarcinoma with a very immature appearance resembling choroid plexus, but we have seen a malignant sacrococcygeal teratoma with pulmonary metastases which contained a variety of partially differentiated 'embryonal' tissues including neuroectoderm, chondroid tissue, and poorly formed glandular elements resembling endodermal derivatives, a pattern which was also present in the original primary tumour.

When all age groups are included the peak incidence of malignant teratoma is in the third decade, chiefly due to teratomas of the testis. There is also a distinct if lesser peak in the first quinquennium (Fig. 2.2), mostly attributable to malignant sacrococcygeal and pre-sacral teratomas (p. 715).

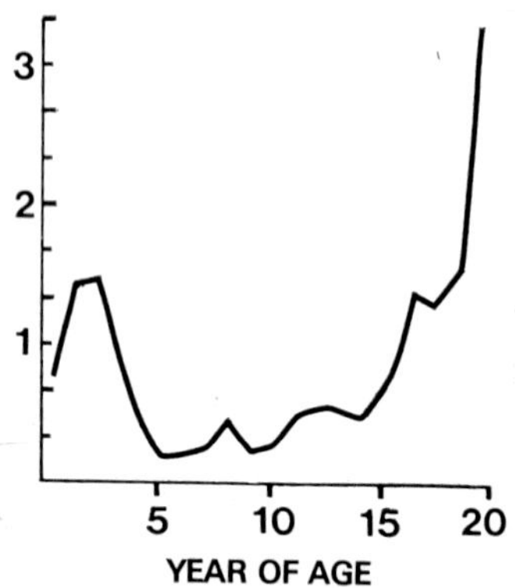

Figure 2.2. MALIGNANT TERATOMAS; the incidence according to age. The data for this and graphs of the age incidence of tumours described in other chapters, have been abstracted from illustrations based on mortality rates per million per annum for 1960–1968, in white children in the U.S.A., after Miller & Dalager (1974)*. The data are used with permission of the authors.

Sacrococcygeal Teratomas (Donnellan & Swenson, 1968; Dillard *et al.*, 1970)
These teratomas appear to present as one of three clinical groups:

Group I

This group contains those with a mass growing backwards from the sacrum and obvious at birth. These lesions may be very soft, ulcerated, and macroscopically and even microscopically malignant, especially when they contain much neuroglial tissue. This tissue is often soft, grey and jelly-like, and microscopically can be extremely cellular and undifferentiated. However, experience has shown that tissue with these features does not behave in accord with its malignant appearance. Similar tissue is sometimes found in ovarian teratomas, and here again the prognosis seems to be better than the structure and extreme cellularity would indicate.

The majority of Group I sacrococcygeal teratomas are cystic and solid, and well differentiated. However, as noted by Berry *et al.* (1969) and Donnellan & Swenson (1968), they have a malignant potential, and should be excised as soon as possible after birth.

*Miller, R. W. & Dalager, N. C. (1974).

Group II

Group II contains those few lumbosacral teratomas associated with spina bifida. Occasionally they grow inwards, into the pelvis or retroperitoneum. It is important that they should not be confused with lipomyelomeningoceles or with myelomeningoceles which contain neuroectodermal tissue, fat, and sometimes vascular and smooth muscle tissue; both are quite common but are not true teratomas, and entirely benign.

Group III

The third group comprises sacrococcygeal teratomas which present in the latter part of the first quinquennium (or later) as a mass in the pelvis or the buttock. They are more common in girls, and almost all of this group are malignant; they account for more than half of all the malignant teratomas in our series (Table 2.2). Histologically they are papillary embryonal carcinomas with a very characteristic appearance. Their teratomatous origin is not always evident, i.e. it is not often that other tissues can be identified, the malignant component being all that can be found.

Ovarian Teratomas (p. 688)

These teratomas usually present later in childhood (see p. 690) and the great majority (87% in our series) were differentiated and clinically benign. In many of them, squamous epithelium and its derivatives dominate the histological structure, giving rise to the inaccurate term 'dermoid cyst'. Malignant ovarian teratomas are usually solid, but may be both solid and cystic (Wisniewski & Deppisch, 1973). Differentiated tissues may be present, but the malignant component, either papillary embryonal carcinoma or a mixture of immature embryonal tissues, overruns the differentiated component. An unusual variant consists largely of neuroglial tissues, and although it has a sinister histological appearance, it behaves in a relatively benign fashion (Favara & Franciosi, 1973).

Mediastinal Teratomas (p. 456)

Mediastinal teratomas often appear to arise from the base of the heart, the root of the great vessels or the pericardium; a few are intrapericardial (p. 483). Sometimes the lesion has a long pedicle and comes to occupy one or other pleural cavity (usually the left). Most are differentiated and benign, but malignant variants occur and in the present series there were two, both of which had a papillary embryonal carcinoma pattern.

Teratoma of the Testis (p. 882)

The rarity of the testis as a site for a teratoma in children is well known, as is the comparatively greater frequency of teratomas in the testis of young adults (Beard & Cooner, 1966). While those in adults are usually malignant, testicular teratomas in childhood are almost invariably 'benign', i.e. histologically differentiated. These contradictory patterns of incidence and behaviour must be telling us something about the etiology of teratoma in general, but the significance has so far eluded discovery. It has been suggested (Berry *et al.*, 1969) that malignant change develops later in gonadal teratomas.

Teratomas of the Brain

Intracranial teratomas may present at any time in childhood, but there are two peaks : in infancy and in the third quinquennium. As might be expected, those in infants are composed of immature, poorly differentiated tissues; their site and their large size usually result in a fatal outcome, even though the tumours are probably not truly malignant. In older children the tumour is commonly well differentiated, cystic and solid, and encapsulated.

The relationship between these easily recognizable teratomas and the very malignant intracranial germinoma (atypical teratoma of Russell) is not clear. Russell & Rubinstein (1971) believed that the latter were examples of one-sided development of a teratoma. But the type of cell of which they are composed, a cell with histochemical and ultrastructural properties almost identical with seminoma, together with the great rarity of seminomatous tissue in most malignant teratomas, argues against this. If Ashley's theory is true, however, it is possible that malignant germinomas arise from extremely primitive cells which have lost the ability to respond to organizers, and thus to differentiate. Further support for the teratomatous origin of 'germinomas' comes from the similar nuclear morphology of the cells comprising the embryonal carcinoma component of malignant teratomas, tissue which seems almost certainly teratomatous in origin. Because of their disputed histogenesis, we have not included germinomas with the teratomas described in this chapter, but they are described in Chapter 13 (p. 273).

Teratomas in Other Sites

Teratomas are occasionally found in the neck (Stone *et al.*, 1967), usually in the midline anteriorly and related to the thyroid isthmus (p. 388), in the nasopharynx (teratomatous epignathus p. 323) on the face (p. 316), in the retroperitoneal tissues (Engel *et al.*, 1968) of the posterior abdominal wall (p. 584), in the spinal region remote from the sacrococcygeal area, in the orbit (p. 406), and very rarely in the stomach (Atwell *et al.*, 1967; Matias & Huang, 1973).

In all of these sites their development could be explained by their presumed origin during the blastula stage of development. Most of the tumours in these uncommon sites have been found to be well differentiated and clinically benign, for example, all thirty of the teratomas of the stomach.

Teratomas and Congenital Anomalies

The high frequency of developmental abnormalities of the lower part of the body associated with teratomas, both benign and malignant, has been noted by Fraumeni, Li & Dalager (1973). These included anomalies of the vertebrae, the genito-urinary system, and the ano-rectum, and the association was interpreted by the authors to suggest that a teratoma may result from the same stimulus as produces the associated anomaly. However, as they point out, this possibility does not resolve the question of which type of cells the teratomas are derived from: undifferentiated cells which escape the control of organizers or from germ cells displaced during migration into the primitive gonads.

THE INDEX SERIES

The opinions expressed in this chapter, and throughout this book, are based on experience with 1689 children with a malignant tumour treated at the Royal Children's Hospital in the last 23 years (p. 911). Their ages ranged from birth to fourteen years of age, and it is appreciated that fourteen years is a rather artificial and arbitrary cut off point. It appears that tumours are not particularly common in adolescents between fourteen and sixteen years of age, and although some reviews have included patients up to sixteen years of age, the increase in numbers and alterations in proportional incidence resulting from the inclusion of these two years is negligible, and for practical purposes such series can be considered as comparable with our own.

The numbers of tumours in the Index Series represent, fairly accurately, their actual relative frequencies, i.e. the total experience of the community (Victoria), although the figures for brain tumours may be a little high, and ocular tumours a little low because of the existence of other facilities for children with tumours of these types.

All the tumours of the central nervous system in the Index Series (see Chapter 13) have been reviewed and reclassified. In keeping with usual practice, we have included cases in which a biopsy was not performed but in which the clinical, investigational and follow-up evidence strongly suggested a tumour; the largest group in this category are those with a glioma of the brain stem (p. 254). In almost all other instances, histological evidence was required for inclusion in the series. Unsatisfactory or equivocal histological material was, in some cases, all that could be obtained, and these have been listed as histologically unclassified.

INCIDENCE OF PAEDIATRIC TUMOURS

The true incidence of tumours in a community is extremely difficult to establish, chiefly because of defects in documentation and the incomplete nature of surveys. Expression of the incidence in relation to the live birth rate, or in terms of the number of tumours per year per 100,000 total population of children at risk, is complicated by the fact that children with cancer are not all treated in one centre; furthermore there are always some who are referred for treatment from outside the defined community. Figures obtained from death certificates (and autopsy reports) can be used to obtain the number of deaths per million for each year of age. One of the chief reasons for calculating incidence figures is to obtain data which can be compared with figures from other parts of the world. This raises other difficulties such as the need for uniform criteria for establishing the diagnosis, and also an acceptable classification of all the tumours encountered.

Inevitably there are inconsistencies in a classification based on cell type, but such a classification does not necessarily infer origin from the tissue which the tumour cells resemble, and there is the added advantages that this requires a minimum of changes as knowledge of the exact origins of specific tumours is established.

TERMINOLOGY

A comprehensive list of benign swellings and malignant tumour has been placed at the head of each chapter or subsection, and we are grateful to Dr James Arey of St Christopher's Hospital, Philadelphia, for the idea. The terminology has been taken from the series of classifications published by the W.H.O. (see pp. 53–4). In addition to these, the fascicles produced by the Armed Forces Institute of Pathology, Washington D.C., are an indispensable reference library for the diagnostic histopathologist, although the lack of a fascicle devoted to paediatric tumours is a notable deficiency. The relevant fascicles are listed on pp. 54–6.

Although this book is primarily concerned with malignant tumours, consideration of their clinical and histological features without reference to the more common and therefore equally important non-malignant conditions would be incomplete from the point of view of a clinician presented with a diagnostic problem; the clinical aspects and histological patterns of benign neoplasms and non-neoplastic conditions are described wherever relevant.

REFERENCES

General

BURDMAN, J.A. & GOLDSTEIN, M.N. (1964). Longterm tissue culture of neuroblastomas. 3. In vitro studies of nerve growth—stimulating factor in sera of children with neuroblastoma. *J. Nat. Cancer Inst.*, **33** : 123.

CHUNG, E.B. & ENZINGER, F.M. (1973). Benign lipoblastomatosis : an analysis of 35 cases. *Cancer*, **32** : 482.

KUMAR, S., STEWARD, J.K. & WAGHE, M. (1972). Nerve-growth factor in human teratomas. *Lancet*, **2** : 234.

MARSDEN, H.B. & STEWARD, J.K. (1968). *Tumours in Children. Recent Advances in Cancer Research, No.* **13**. Springer-Verlag. Berlin, Heidelberg, New York.

MILLER, R.W. (1973). Proceedings. New hypothesis on the etiology of cancer. *Proc. Natl. Cancer Conf. Epidemiology*. **7** ; 653.

MILLER, R.W. & DALAGER, N.A. (1974). U.S. childhood cancer deaths by cell type, 1960–1968. *Pediat*, **85**: 664.

WILLIS, R.A. (1962). *Tumors of Childhood.* Charles C. Thomas, Springfield.

Teratomas

ASHLEY, D.J.B. (1973). Origin of Teratomas. *Cancer*, **32** : 390.

ATWELL, J.D., CLAIRAUX, A.E. & NIXON, H.H. (1967). Teratoma of the stomach in the newborn. *J. Pediat. Surg.*, **2** : 197.

BEARD, J.H. & COONER, W.H. (1966). Teratoma of the testis in an infant. *Southern. Med. J.*, **59** ; 627.

BERRY, C.L., KEELING, J. & HILTON, C. (1969). Teratomas in infancy and childhood : a review of 91 cases. *J. Path.*, **98** : 241.

DILLARD, B.M., MAYER, J.H., MCALISTER, W.H., MCGAVRIN, M. & STROMINGER, D.B. (1970). Sacrococcygeal teratoma in children. *J. Ped. Surg.*, **5** : 53.

DONNELLAN, W.A. & SWENSON, O. (1968). Benign and malignant sacrococcygeal teratomas. *Surgery*, **64** : 834.

ENGEL, R.M., ELKINS, R.C. & FLETCHER, B.D. (1968). Retroperitoneal teratoma. *Cancer*, **22** : 1068.

FAVARA, B.E. & FRANCIOSI, R.A. (1973). Ovarian teratoma and neuroglial implants on the peritoneum. *Cancer*, **31** : 678.

FRAUMENI, J.F. Jr., LI, F.P. & DALAGER, N. (1973). Teratomas in childhood : epidemiological features. *J. Natl. Cancer Inst.*, **51** : 1425.

MAHOUR, G.H., WOOLEY, M.M., TRIVEDI, S.N. & LANDING, B.H. (1974). Teratomas in infancy and childhood : experience with 81 cases. *Surgery*, **76** : 309.

MATIAS, I.C. & HUANG, Y.C. (1973). Gastric teratoma in infancy ; report of a case and review of the world literature. *Ann. Surg.*, **178** : 631.

RUSSELL, D.S. & RUBINSTEIN, L.J. (1971). *Tumours of the Central Nervous System*, 3rd ed. Edward Arnold, London.

STONE, H.H., HENDERSON, W.D. & GUIDIO, F.A. (1967). Teratomas of the neck. *Amer. J. Dis. Child.*, **113** : 222.

WISNIEWSKI, M. & DEPPISCH, L.M. (1973). Solid teratomas of the ovary. *Cancer*, **32** : **440**.

Cytological typing and Classification

Throughout this book the pathological classifications have followed as closely as possible the W.H.O. publications listed below.

W.H.O. PUBLICATIONS

Chapters 9: 10: 11

MATHÉ, G. & RAPPAPORT, H. with O'CONOR, G.T., TORLONI, H. (1973). *Histological and Cytological Typing of Neoplastic Diseases of Haematopoietic and Lymphoid Tissues*. W.H.O., Geneva.

Chapter 14

B.

THACKRAY, A.C. & SOBIN, L.H. (1972). *Histological Typing of Salivary Gland Tumours.* W.H.O., Geneva.

C.

WAHI, P.N. with COHEN, B., LUTHRA, U.K., TORLONI, H. (1971). *Histological Typing of Oral and Oropharyngeal Tumours*. W.H.O., Geneva.

PINDBORG, J.J. & KRAMER, I.R.H. with TORLONI, H. (1971). *Histological Typing of Odontogenic Tumours, Jaw Cysts, and Allied Lesions*. W.H.O., Geneva.

E.

HEDINGER, CHR. & SOBIN, L.H. (1974). *Thyroid Tumours*. W.H.O., Geneva.

Chapter 16

KREYBERG, L. with LIEBOW, A.A., UEHLINGER, E.A. (1967). *Histological Typing of Lung Tumours*. W.H.O., Geneva.

Chapter 21

RIOTTON, G. & CHRISTOPHERSON, W.M. with LUNT, R. (1973). *Cytology of the Female Genital Tract*. W.H.O., Geneva.

SEROV, S.F. & SCULLY, R.E., SOBIN, L.H. (1973). *Histological Typing of Ovarian Tumours*. W.H.O., Geneva.

MOSTOFI, F.K. with SOBIN, L.H., TORLONI, H. (1973). *Histological Typing of Urinary Bladder Tumours*. W.H.O., Geneva.

Chapter 22

SCHAJOWICZ, F., ACKERMAN, L.V. & SISSONS, H.A. with SOBIN, L.H., TORLONI, H. (1972). *Histological Typing of Bone Tumours*. W.H.O., Geneva.

Chapter 23

ENZINGER, F.M. with LATTES, R. & TORLONI, H. (1969). *Histological Typing of Soft Tissue Tumours*. W.H.O., Geneva.

Chapter 24

TEN SELDAM, R.E.J. & HELWIG, E.B., SOBIN, L.H., TORLONI, H. (1974). *Skin Tumours*. W.H.O., Geneva.

Chapter 25

SCARFF, R.W. & TORLONI, H. (1968). *Histological Typing of Breast Tumours*. W.H.O. Geneva.

ARMED FORCES INSTITUTE OF PATHOLOGY PUBLICATIONS

The Leukaemias
The Malignant Lymphomas
The Histiocytoses

RAPPAPORT, H. (1966). *Atlas of Tumor Pathology: Tumors of the Hemopoietic System, Parts* 1 *and* 2. Armed Forces Institute of Pathology, Washington D.C.

TUMOURS OF THE HEAD AND NECK

B. Tumours of the Face

FOOTE, F.W. Jr., & FRAZELL, E.L., (1954). *Atlas of Tumor Pathology: Tumors of the Major Salivary Glands*. Armed Forces Institute of Pathology, Washington D.C.

C. Tumours of the Mouth and Oro Pharynx

BERNIER, J.L. (1960). *Atlas of Tumor Pathology: Tumors of the Odontogenic Apparatus and Jaws*. Armed Forces Institute of Pathology, Washington D.C.

DOCKERTY, M.B. *et al.* (1968). *Atlas of Tumor Pathology: Tumors of the Oral Cavity and Pharynx*. Armed Forces Institute of Pathology, Washington D.C.

D. Tumours of the Nasopharynx and Ear

ASH, J.E., BECK, M.R., WILKES, J.D. (1964). *Atlas of Tumor Pathology: Tumors of the Upper Respiratory Tract and Ear.* Armed Forces Institute of Pathology, Washington D.C.

E. Cervical Tumours

CASTLEMAN, B. (1952). *Atlas of Tumor Pathology: Tumors of the Parathyroid Glands.* Armed Forces Institute of Pathology, Washington D.C.

LE COMPLE, P.M. (1951). *Atlas of Tumor Pathology: Tumors of the Carotid Body and Related Structures.* Armed Forces Institute of Pathology, Washington D.C.

WARREN, S. & MEISSNER, W.A. (1953). *Atlas of Tumor Pathology: Tumors of the Thyroid Gland.* Armed Forces Institute of Pathology, Washington D.C.

WILLIS, R.A. (1951). *Atlas of Tumor Pathology: Teratomas.* Armed Forces Institute of Pathology, Washington D.C., 1951.

Ocular and Orbital Tumours

REESE, A.B. (1956). *Atlas of Tumor Pathology: Tumors of the Eye and Adnexa.* Armed Forces Institute of Pathology, Washington D.C.

Intrathoracic Tumours

CASTLEMAN, B. (1955). *Atlas of Tumor Pathology: Tumors of the Thymus Gland.* Armed Forces Institute of Pathology, Washington D.C.

LANDING, B.H. & FARBER, S. (1956). *Atlas of Tumor Pathology: Tumors of the Cardio-vascular System.* Armed Forces Institute of Pathology, Washington D.C.

LIEBOW, A.A. (1952). *Atlas of Tumor Pathology: Tumors of the Lower Respiratory Tract.* Armed Forces Institute of Pathology, Washington D.C.

SCHLUMBERGER. (1951). *Atlas of Tumor Pathology: Tumors of the Mediastinum.* Armed Forces Institute of Pathology, Washington D.C.

Tumours of the Kidney

LUCKE, B. & SCHLUMBERGER, H.G. (1957). *Atlas of Tumor Pathology: Tumors of the kidney renal pelvis and ureter.* Armed Forces Institute of Pathology, Washington D.C.

Tumours of the Adrenal Gland and Retroperitoneum

ACKERMAN, L.V. (1954). *Tumors of the Retroperitoneum, Mesentery and Peritoneum.* Armed Forces Institute of Pathology, Washington D.C.

KARSNER, H.T. (1950). *Atlas of Tumor Pathology: Tumors of the Adrenal.* Armed Forces Institute of Pathology, Washington D.C.

Tumours of the Liver and Bile Ducts

EDMONDSON, H.A. (1958). *Atlas of Tumor Pathology: Tumors of the Liver and Intrahepatic Bile Ducts.* Armed Forces Institute of Pathology, Washington D.C.

EDMONDSON, H.A. (1967). *Atlas of Tumor Pathology: Tumors of the Gall Bladder and Extrahepatic Bile Ducts.* Armed Forces Institute of Pathology, Washington D.C.

Tumours of the Alimentary Canal and Pancreas

FRANTZ, V.K. (1959). *Atlas of Tumor Pathology: Tumors of the Pancreas.* Armed Forces Institute of Pathology, Washington, D.C.

STOUT, A.P. (1953). *Atlas of Tumor Pathology: Tumors of the Stomach.* Armed Forces Institute of Pathology, Washington D.C.

WOODS, D.A. (1967). *Atlas of Tumor Pathology: Tumors of the Intestines.* Armed Forces Institute of Pathology, Washington D.C.

Pelvic Tumours and Sacral Masses

DIXON, F.J. & MOORE, R.A. (1952). *Atlas of Tumor Pathology: Tumors of the male sex organs*. Armed Forces Institute of Pathology, Washington D.C.

FRIEDMAN, N.B. & ASH, J.E. (1959). *Atlas of Tumor Pathology: Tumors of the Urinary Bladder*. Armed Forces Institute of Pathology, Washington D.C.

Part I. HERTIG A.T. & MANSELL, H. (1956) Hydatidiform Mole and Choriocarcinoma.

Part II. HERTIG, A.T. & GORE, H. (1960) (with supplement) Vulva, Vagina and Uterus.

Part III. HERTIG, A.T. & GORE, H. (1961) Ovary and Fallopian Tube. *Atlas of Tumor Pathology: Tumors of the Female Sex Organs*. Armed Forces Institute of Pathology, Washington D.C.

SPJUT, H.J., DORFMAN, H.D., FECHNER, R.E. & ACKERMAN, L.V. (1971). *Atlas of Tumor Pathology: Tumors of Bone and Cartilage*. Armed Forces Institute of Pathology, Washington D.C.

WILLIS, R.A. (1951). *Atlas of Tumor Pathology: Teratomas*. Armed Forces Institute of Pathology, Washington D.C.

Bone Tumours

SPJUT, H.J., DORFMAN, H.D., FECHNER, R.E. & ACKERMAN, L.V. (1971). *Atlas of Tumor Pathology: Tumors of Bone and Cartilage*. Armed Forces Institute of Pathology, Washington D.C.

Sarcomas of Soft Tissues

HARKIN, J.C. & REED, R.J. (1969). *Atlas of Tumor Pathology: Tumors of the Peripheral Nervous System*. Armed Forces Institute of Pathology, Washington D.C.

STOUT, A.P. & LATTES, R. (1967). *Atlas of Tumor Pathology: Tumors of the Soft Tissues*. Armed Forces Institute of Pathology, Washington D.C.

Tumours of the Skin

LUND. H.Z. (1957). *Atlas of Tumor Pathology: Tumors of the Skin*. Armed Forces Institute of Pathology, Washington D.C.

LUND, J.Z. & KRAUS, J.M. (1962). *Atlas of Tumor Pathology: Melanotic Tumors of the Skin*. Armed Forces Institute of Pathology, Washington D.C.

Tumour of the Testis and Breast

DIXON, B.J. & MOORE, R.A. (1952). *Atlas of Tumor Pathology: Tumors of the Male Sex Organs*. Armed Forces Institute of Pathology, Washington D.C.

MCDIVITT, R.W., STEWART, F.W. & BERG, J.W. (1966). *Atlas of Tumor Pathology: Tumors of the Breast*. Armed Forces Institute of Pathology, Washington D.C.

Chapter 3. Immunobiology and malignant disease

The immune system has long been recognized as playing a cardinal role in the defences of the host by detecting and eliminating invading organisms or foreign substances. Lower animals such as the invertebrates eliminate infecting organisms by coating them with host protein (e.g. by 'opsonization'—opsonein, Greek: 'to prepare victuals for'), followed by phagocytosis, intracellular killing and biochemical degradation. Less palatable substances are eliminated by localizing them, walling them off, and subsequently extruding them to exterior. In man, these two primitive reactions still constitute a fundamental defence mechanism against foreign invasion and in vertebrates, the evolution of 'immunological memory' and specificity has greatly increased the efficiency of this defence (Good *et al.*, 1970).

IMMUNE SURVEILLANCE

The detection and elimination of mutated, malignant or abnormal cells, or clones of cells arising from the host's own tissues, has been suggested as a second major function of the immune system (Burnet, 1970a). The chief agents of immune surveillance are lymphocytes (Fig. 3.1) derived from the thymus

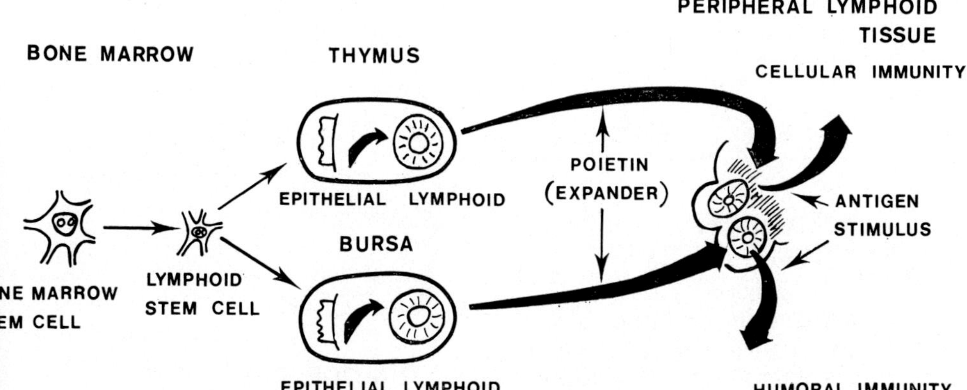

Figure 3.1. DEVELOPMENT OF THE LYMPHOID SYSTEM. The lymphoid stem cell gives rise to two types of epithelial lymphoid cells which populate the thymus and the 'bursa', and from these the thymus-derived (T) and bursal (B) lymphocytes are formed. In response to stimulation by antigen they produce 'cellular' and 'humoral' immunity respectively.

(T-lymphocytes) which occupy the deep cortical areas of lymph nodes, the parafollicular areas of the spleen, and Peyer's patches. These cells comprise 30 to 70% of circulating lymphocytes, and they form a flying squad of immunocompetent cells continually circulating through the blood, the tissues and lymphatic channels until they are activated by cells or organisms which they recognize as foreign (Fig. 3.2). Their activation starts a sequence of events which includes cell replication and the emergence of 'killer' lymphocytes (Fig. 3.2c) which specifically attack the abnormal cell, the production of long-lived 'memory cells', and the generation of chemical mediators (lymphokines), from activated T-cells. The lymphokines initiate inflammation, attract, localize and activate powerful phagocytic macrophages, and stimulate other systems, such as fibroblasts, and the production of interferon. Other aspects of these cellular reactions include delayed skin hypersensitivity, graft rejection, elimination of virus-infected cells, and the initiation of graft-versus-

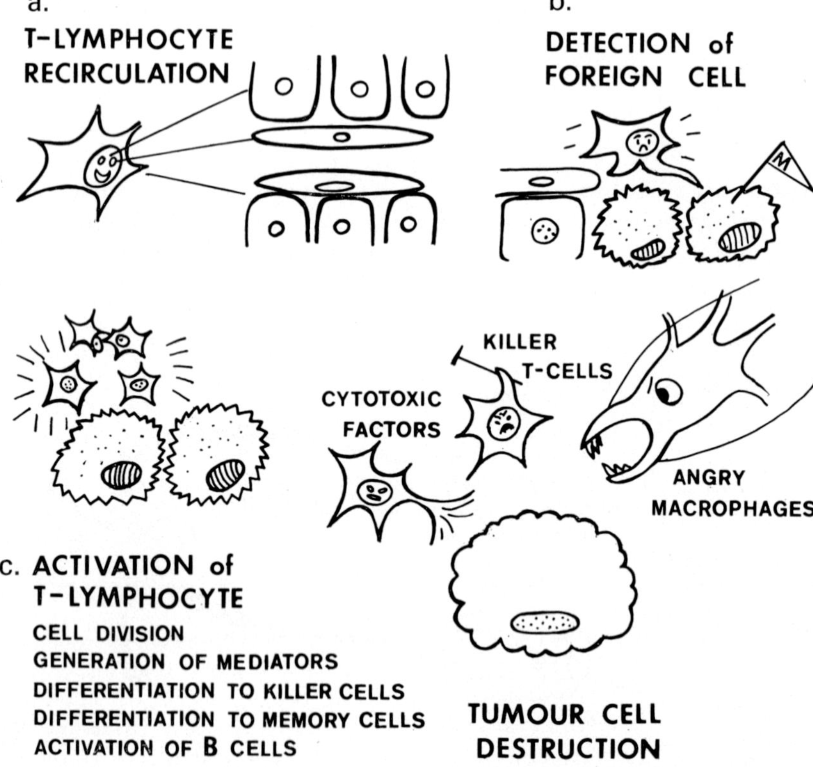

Figure 3.2. IMMUNE SURVEILLANCE; (*a*) Circulating T-lymphocyte; (*b*) T-lymphocyte recognizing malignant transformation (M); (*c*) Immune mechanisms called into action include opsonins, 'killer' B-lymphocytes, and macrophages to remove debris by phagocytosis.

host disease. This extraordinarily efficient system may also detect and eliminate a great number of newly-emerged malignant clones during a normal person's lifetime.

THE THYMUS

The role of the thymus and the intimate association it has with the peripheral lymphoid system and the development of malignancy, can be illustrated by several experimental and clinical situations. In primitive vertebrates, both the capacity for true malignant change and the appearance of a thymus occurred at about the same stage of evolution. In rodents, the removal of the thymus at birth prevents the differentiation and population of the thymus-dependent peripheral lymphoid system, and these thymectomized animals consequently have a greatly increased incidence of malignancy.

In man, the highest incidence of malignant disease occurs at the extremes of life, in the very young and the old, when immune responses are either immature or declining in vigour. In children born without a thymus-derived lymphoid system, the incidence of malignancy is approximately 10,000 times greater than in normal children at the same age (Gatti & Good, 1971). Almost every one of the recognized congenital immunologic abnormalities is now associated with a distinctive constellation of malignant conditions (Waldmann *et al.*, 1973).

The prolonged administration of immunosuppressive drugs to renal transplant patients is accompanied by a 100-fold increase in the frequency of primary malignancies. At least eight cancers have been inadvertently transplanted from the donor of the kidney to the recipient, and in four of these cases the disseminated tumours regressed (along with rejection of the kidney) when immunosuppressive drugs were discontinued (Smith & Landy, 1970).

Another provocative association is the finding that carcinogens, whether chemical, viral or related to irradiation, are also immunosuppressive, and further, minor changes in the molecular structure of chemical carcinogens which ablate their immunosuppressive function, also destroy their carcinogenic propensities.

THE MALIGNANT CHANGE

A decade ago many investigators regarded the primary event in the malignant transformation of a cell as an irreversible genetic mutation. Recent observations suggest that in at least some animal and human tumours, the genetic material responsible for malignancy may be separable from host DNA, and appear in the form of a DNA or RNA oncogenic 'virus'. In the mouse, virus-like agents have been causally associated with leukaemia, sarcomas, lymphomas and other malignant tumours. Many tumours caused by a particular virus have several shared antigens on their cell membranes, whereas tumours induced by chemical carcinogens frequently have antigens which are unique to that tumour. Transmission of these viruses appears to be longitudinal, from one generation to the next, from mother to the fetus *in utero*, or to the newborn.

The mouse mammary tumour is one illuminating example. This adenocarcinoma of the breast develops in over 90% of the females of the C_3H inbred strain when they are between nine and eighteen months of age (middle to old age for the mouse). A B-type RNA virus, the mammary tumour virus or 'Bittner' milk agent, is found in the breast milk of the nursing mouse mothers and also in the malignant cells of the tumours they induce. If the litter of an infected mother is delivered by caesarian section and foster-nursed by mice of a virus-free strain, no tumours develop. Particles morphologically and antigenically similar to the mouse mammary tumour virus have been found in the breast milk of human mothers from families with a high incidence of breast cancer (Moore *et al.*, 1971). Although no proof of a causative association exists in the human, might it not be reasonable to discourage breast feeding of female babies by mothers from families with a high incidence of breast cancer? Other strains of mice also carry the mammary tumour virus, and transmission from one generation to the next occurs by way of the germ cells or the placenta, as well as via breast milk.

Some human malignant tumours have been associated with the presence of virus-like particles (Table 3.1) and in addition, several human malignant

Table 3.1. Viruses and Malignant Disease. Some associations reported in humans

Morphology	Human cells
DNA viruses	
Herpes	Burkitt's lymphoma
(Epstein-Barr virus)	Infectious mononucleosis
	Nasopharyngeal carcinoma
Herpes type 2	Carcinoma of cervix
Herpes-like agent	Hodgkin's disease
RNA particulates	
RNA viruses	
B type	Human milk
	Breast cancer
C type	Osteosarcoma
	Lymphoma
	Liposarcoma
A type varied	Chondrosarcoma
	Fibrosarcoma
	Leukaemia

tumours carry common antigens on the surface of their cells, a feature of virus-induced tumours in animals. These human tumours include neuroblastoma, malignant melanoma, osteosarcoma, acute leukaemia and Wilms' tumour. Parents and immediate relatives of children with neuroblastoma or with various types of sarcoma have been proved to have antibodies or cellular immunity to tumour-associated antigens.

The demonstration that the enzyme 'RNA-dependent DNA polymerase' (reverse transcriptase) is associated with known oncogenic RNA viruses has proved to be a vital missing link in showing how an RNA virus can insert virus information into the DNA of the host cell. The virus-coded DNA in the host cell may lie dormant for years, possibly for generations, until, in response to an appropriate stimulus, these genes 'turn on' and instruct the cell to become malignant, or to produce infectious virus, or both. Using suitable nucleotide probes, together with virus-specific reverse transcriptase, viral genetic information can now be detected in mammalian cells. Under suitable conditions, malignant cells may be instructed to produce infectious oncogenic virus. Antibody to reverse transcriptase administered to pregnant mice of a strain highly prone to cancer, results in a marked reduction in the incidence of cancer in the offspring.

TUMOUR-ASSOCIATED ANTIGENS

One of the cellular changes which follow malignant transformation is the appearance of new molecular structures (antigens) which are then perceived by the host as being foreign. These tumour-associated antigens have been demonstrated in cells from most types of tumours. They occur within the cell nucleus, in the cytoplasm, and the cell membrane, or as extracellular products.

Studies of the antigenic substances on the surface of living tumour cells reveal a system of great complexity. While many tumour-associated antigens elicit from the host both cellular and humoral responses, some of these antigens are detectable only by antibody, some only by cellular immunity. Some of these antigens resemble those normally only present in foetal tissues, while others only appear at certain stages of the cell cycle, e.g. during replication (p. 101). Antigens may be highly specific for a particular tumour, for most tumours histologically similar, for a group of tumours, or for a great range of malignant cells. Tumour-associated antigens which cross-react with components of normal tissue may generate, in the host, immune responses which cause many puzzling clinical phenomena in cancer patients, for example, encephalopathy, neuropathy, myositis or pneumonitis.

Circulating antigen-antibody complexes have been shown to play a role in causing the cachexia seen in patients with advanced malignancy.

THE CHILD WITH A MALIGNANT TUMOUR

A child with a malignant tumour has a neoplasm which has already escaped the immune surveillance mechanism. However, control by immune mechanisms still plays a very significant role in restricting the rate of local and metastatic spread of the tumour. Marked changes in the rate of growth, or the disappearance of metastatic deposits following removal of the primary tumour, or related to a severe infection, have been attributed to changes in the immunity of the host. Over 130 well documented cases of regression of a human malignant tumour have been described in the literature (Burnet, 1970b). Measures which depress the immunity of the host without affecting the cells of the tumour have resulted in the rapid and widespread dissemination of metastases.

Patients with progressively growing malignant tumours have in their bloodstream circulating lymphoid cells (T-lymphocytes) which can completely destroy cells from their tumour, when tested *in vitro*. The addition of the patient's serum to this *in vitro* test completely or partially inhibits the killing capacity of the patient's lymphocytes. This 'blocking antibody' in the serum has been shown to be specific for the particular tumour (Hellstrom *et al.*, 1969). As the tumour progresses, the number of killer cells in the blood declines and the degree of specific blocking increases, until the terminal phase in which a decrease in blocking may occur, and other factors which cause a general depression of all immune responses may appear in blood. No free tumour-specific antibody can be detected in patients with progressively growing tumours.

If the major part of a malignant tumour is excised surgically, or severely damaged by irradiation or chemotherapy, free antibody to the tumour's antigens appears in the blood, the number of specifically sensitized killer cells increases, and the blocking activity of the serum disappears. This may explain regression of metastases following subtotal removal of a primary neuroblastoma.

Blocking antibody has recently been defined as circulating, soluble immune complexes of tumour-membrane-antigen and host tumour-specific antibody of IgG gamma 1 or gamma 3 class. By using highly sensitive techniques, free tumour antigen and antigen-antibody complexes can be identified in blocking serum from patients with a growing tumour. The specificity of these immune complexes forms the basis of an immunodiagnostic test for cancer. After removal of the tumour, antigen is no longer found in the blood, and previously bound antibody becomes free antibody (Jose & Seshadri, 1974).

CARCINOGENESIS

One of the major questions in cancer immunology is how the malignant clone escapes destruction by the immune surveillance mechanism. Most patients who develop cancer have no detectable deficiencies in their immune mechanisms when tested early in the course of their disease. Exceptions have been found mainly in lymphatic leukaemia and in other lymphoreticular malignancies. A genetically determined inability to react to the antigens of a particular tumour has been suggested as one possibility (Laroye, 1974). Perhaps a more attractive alternative is that specific blocking antibody plays a critical role by inhibiting the major immune mechanisms forming the host's defences during the early stages of the clonal development of a tumour. Inhibition of blocking antibody by nutritional deprivation, or by anti-plasma cell serum, is associated with a very great reduction in the incidence of spontaneous and carcinogen-induced malignant tumours in animals (Jose & Good, 1973). The injection into rats with growing Rous sarcoma of large doses of serum from rats with excised sarcomas, abolishes specific blocking by the recipients' serum, and is followed by a high rate of tumour regression (Sjögren & Bansal, 1971). Further evaluation of the immunologic mechanisms of patients with malignant tumours may lead to more effective means of intervening in the course of human malignancy.

THE IMMUNOLOGIST IN THE CANCER CLINIC

While rapid advances in experimental cancer research continue, the clinical immunologist can already provide direct assistance in the management of a patient with a malignant tumour. The immunodiagnosis of malignant tumours is based on the following observations.

1. Extracellular substances

Such substances secreted by cells of particular types of tumour are frequently best detected by immunological methods. Examples of these include the monoclonal spikes of gamma globulin secreted by some lymphoid or plasma cell tumours, and the α-feto-protein secreted by the cells of a malignant hepatoma.

2. Carcino-embryonic antigen

CEA in the blood is associated with a group of malignant tumours which occur in adults, such as carcinoma of the colon, lung and breast. CEA can be detected by a highly sensitive method of radioimmuno-assay.

3. Membrane antigens

Many malignant tumours have membrane antigens which are similar to but distinct from a protein antigen found in myelin. Patients with these tumours have cellular sensitivity, but no demonstrable antibody to this antigen. The full range of tumours with this property has yet to be determined, but it seems probable that a general screening test for the presence of a wide variety of malignant conditions can be developed. The assay involves a rather complex technique which measures changes in the electrophoretic mobility of macrophages in the presence of factors in the supernatant fluid from cultures of the patient's lymphocytes, and an 'encephalitogenic factor'.

4. The specific diagnosis

The specific diagnosis of a malignant tumour is becoming practical by determining the antigenic specificity of immune complexes circulating in the blood of most patients with an actively growing tumour. By means of a highly sensitive method of radio-immune-electrophoresis, these complexes can be split into their respective components, i.e. tumour antigen and antibody, and their specificity determined by a radio-precipitation reaction. This rapid assay, which can be performed on a very small sample of serum, may make it possible to determine whether a tumour has been completely ablated, and may also be helpful in detecting the presence of recurrences.

5. Other tests

Several tests can be used in selected cases including (*a*) measurement of free antibody by complement fixation, immunofluorescence or other conventional methods; (*b*) the assessment of the cytotoxic activity of killer cells by using one of several microcytotoxicity tests or by measuring the production of factors which inhibit cellular migration; and (*c*) by measuring tumour specific and non-specific inhibitors of cellular immunity in the serum of the patient.

ASSESSMENT OF GENERAL IMMUNORESISTANCE

Patients with many types of cancer show clinical evidence of decreased resistance to infection. The most florid examples of this phenomenon occur in malignant reticuloendothelial or lymphoid tumours such as myeloma, in which the high incidence of pyogenic bacterial infections suggests that there is a deficiency in antibody (B*-cell) function, and in Hodgkin's disease, in which there is depression of cell-mediated (T-cell) function associated with viral, protozoal, fungal or intracellular bacterial infections.

In addition to depression of the immune mechanisms caused by the disease itself, many therapeutic agents are also profoundly immunosuppressive; chemotherapy and irradiation may produce visible regression of the tumour mass, but the accompanying profound depression of immunoresistance may not be appreciated until secondary infection or widespread recurrence of the tumour occurs. Supportive therapy such as active immunization, or passive immunization with hyperimmune serum, gammaglobulin, or specific lymphocyte transfer factor, may correct the defect in the resistance to infection.

*Bursal equivalent', i.e. lymphocytes of the B type; in man these are formed in the marrow; in lower animals in the bursa of Fabricius.

Table 3.2. Assessment of General Immune Functions

B-cell function

1 Quantitation of serum immunoglobulins.
2 Serum antibody response to suitable vaccine, e.g. tetanus, polio, typhoid, influenza, flagellin.
3 Numbers of B-lymphocytes in blood (by membrane fluorescence or indirect rosette techniques).
4 Opsonic studies with specific organisms.

T-cell function

1 Skin delayed sensitivity to ubiquitous organisms, candida, streptokinase-streptodornase, mumps, trichophyton.
2 Contact sensitization and challenge with 2, 4-dinitrochlorobenzene.
3 Proportion of T-lymphocytes in blood (direct sheep cell rosettes).
4 Response of blood lymphoid cells to phytohaemagglutinin or allogeneic cells.

General cellular function

Bone marrow function.
Phagocytosis, metabolic and killing activity of neutrophils.

Regular monitoring of immune function during treatment can improve clinical judgement, allow a rational plan of chemotherapy and irradiation, and provide a basis for supportive or tumour immunotherapy. A selection of tests of immunofunction is shown in Table 3.2.

IMMUNOTHERAPY

The possibility of stimulating the host's immune system to react more vigorously against a tumour (Sokal *et al.*, 1974) is based on experiments which show that a growing tumour does not evoke a maximal immune response. Many methods of immunotherapy have been reported in animals and in man, and those most successful in man are listed in Table 3.3.

The general principles of immunotherapy, common to all methods, are as follows:

1. *Reduction of the tumour to the minimal number of cells*, by conventional means of treatment. The elimination of tumour masses containing more than 1×10^6 cells by immunotherapy alone is uncommon.

2. *Ensuring that the host's responses are not depressed* by continuous chemotherapy. Intermittent chemotherapy and immunotherapy may depress the growth of tumour cells and at the same time utilize to maximum effect, the phenomenon of rebound of immune responsiveness.

3. *Avoiding methods of treatment known to increase the level of blocking antibodies* which lead to enhancement of tumour growth.

Table 3.3. Immunotherapy; some selected techniques reported to have produced objective responses in man

		No. of patients	No. with objective responses
I Immunization with tumour or tumour products			
Living autologous tumour DNA extract, adjuvant		232	22
Allogeneic leukaemia blasts, BCG		75	42
Irradiated autologous tumour cells, with BCG		18	3
Irradiated cell membrane or homogenate of autologous sarcoma		15	6
II Cross transplant and cross transfusion with lymphocytes specifically sensitized in vivo			
Antigen	Lymphocyte source	No. of patients	No. with objective responses
1–2 ml of similar tumour	Matched partner	118	23
0·5 ml of similar tumour	Matched partner	35	3
$1–5 \times 10^6$ tumour cells from culture			
1 ml tumour homogenate	Matched partner	113	27
III Transfusion of non-specifically stimulated lymphocytes			
PHA	Autologous cells in culture	10	3
None	Autologous and allogeneic cells	31	2
None	Allogeneic spleen cells	8	?3
IV Non-specific stimulation of immune mechanisms			
BCG		25	20
BCG		9	7
Vaccinia		19	5
BCG		8	5

Several regimens of immunotherapy have already been shown to be safe, and occasionally bring about objective clinical responses in human cancer. Many of these studies were performed without monitoring the immune responses of the host.

THE FUTURE

Immunotherapy of cancer in man ranks fourth after surgery, radiotherapy and chemotherapy in some centres. Further improvement in the efficacy of therapeutic tumour antigens and adjuvants, and the design of protocols of immunotherapy adequately documented by both clinical and immunological data, may lead to wider clinical application. Identification and isolation of human tumour viruses might lead to the production of a vaccine which would prevent many types of human cancer. Thus the application of established immunological principles and techniques to the problem of cancer holds promise of precise diagnosis, long remissions induced by immunotherapy (Krementz *et al.*, 1974) and, ultimately, prevention by specific vaccination.

REFERENCES AND SUGGESTED READING

BURNET, F.M. (1970a). *Immunologic Surveillance*, Pergamon Press, Oxford and Sydney.

BURNET, F.M. (1970b). *Cellular Immunology*, Melbourne University Press, Melbourne.

GATTI, R.A. & GOOD, R.A. (1971). Occurrence of malignancy in immunodeficiency diseases : a literature review. *Cancer*, **28** : 89.

GOOD, R.A., FINSTAD, J. & GATTI, R.A. (1970). Bulwarks of the host defence. In *Infectious Agents and Host Reactions* (ed. Mudd, S.). Saunders. p. 76.

HELLSTROM, K.E. & HELLSTROM, I. (1969). Cellular immunity against human tumor antigens. *Advances in Cancer Research*, **12** : 167.

JOSE, D.G. & GOOD, R.A. (1963). Quantitative effects of nutritional protein and calorie deficiency upon immune responses to tumours. *Cancer Research*, **33** : 874.

JOSE, D.G. (1974). Mechanisms of immune defence. *Aust. paediat. J.*, **10** : 1.

JOSE, D.G. & SESHADRI, R. (1974). Circulating immune complexes in human neuroblastoma: direct assay and role in blocking specific cellular immunity. *Int. J. Cancer*, **13** ; 824.

LAROYE, G.J. (1973). Cancer caused by an inherited selective defect in immunological surveillance. *Lancet*, **1** : 641.

LAROYE, G.J. (1974). How efficient is immunological surveillance against cancer and why does it fail? *Lancet*, **1** : 1097.

KREMENTZ, E.T., MANSELL, P.W.A. & HORNUNG, M.O. *et al.* (1974). Immunotherapy of malignant disease : the use of viable sensitized lymphocytes or transfer factor prepared from sensitized lymphocytes. *Cancer*, **33** : 394.

MOORE, D.H., CHARNEY, J. & KRAMARSKY, B. (1971). Search for a human breast cancer virus. *Nature* (*Lond.*), **229** : 611.

SJÖGREN, H.O. & BANSAL, S.C. (1971). Antigens in virally induced tumors. *Progress in Immunology*, **1** : 921.

SMITH, R.T. & LANDY, M. (Eds.) (1970). *Immune Surveillance*. Academic Press, New York.

SOKAL, J.E., AUNGST, C.W. & SNYDERMAN, M. (1974). Delay in progression of malignant lymphoma after B.C.G. vaccination. *New Eng. J. Med.*, **291** ; 1226.

WALDMANN, T.A., STROBER, W. & BLAESE, R.M. (1973). Immunodeficiency disease and malignancy. *Ann. Internal Med.*, **77** : 605.

Chapter 4. Radiological techniques

A. ANGIOGRAPHY AND OTHER TECHNIQUES

Following the development of cardiac catheterization and angiocardiography, the basic techniques involved have been adapted to other areas where the demonstration of blood vessels by contrast media has proved to be helpful in diagnosis and management. The Seldinger technique (Seldinger, 1953), slightly modified for use in childhood, is now well established and its use in percutaneous angiography has become one of the most valuable means of investigating patients with solid malignant tumours (Tank *et al.*, 1973).

Other standard radiological procedures are also helpful in specific situations, and in this chapter both the older methods and more recently developed angiographic techniques in the investigation of infants and children with a tumour in the abdomen, or in other sites, are briefly described.

ANGIOGRAPHY

Selective arteriography, aortography, venography and lymphangiography all have their particular applications (Wallace, 1969; Gyepes, 1974).

ARTERIOGRAPHY

This is probably the most generally useful and the following information can be obtained.

1. *A diagnosis* of a malignant tumour can, in many cases, be made by demonstrating distinctive wandering vessels with an irregular lumen (Fig. 22.11), capillary and venous pooling, or arteriovenous shunting, in an area which displaces or distorts the normal vascular pattern of the organ or the tissue concerned (Hiller & MacDonald, 1968).
2. *Identification of the vessel or vessels supplying the tumour* shows clearly the organ in which it has arisen (Hiller & Kennedy *et al.*, 1970).
3. *The type of tumour* can often be determined by its distinctive site and typical radiographic features, because in childhood there is an overwhelming preponderance of one particular tumour in each viscus. The precise diagnosis can be made with a high degree of accuracy on the clinical and radiographic findings, e.g. 97% accuracy in Wilms' tumour (p. 507).

4. *The size and extent of the tumour* are depicted, and this is helpful in planning treatment, especially surgical procedures, when displacement of the major vessels is clearly demonstrated (Fig. 17.5, p. 508).
5. *In planning radiotherapy*, the exact area to be irradiated can be gauged and this is important in the treatment of sarcomas of bone or soft tissues (Fig. 23.1, p. 780).
6. *The response to irradiation or chemotherapy* can be assessed by comparing the initial films with subsequent angiograms. This has been of considerable value in hepatoblastomas, some of which were initially considered inoperable but have been successfully removed after a second angiogram showed that resection was now feasible.

Technique

A modification of the Seldinger catheter technique can be used to enter the femoral artery and the aorta, to reach and inject a radio-opaque medium into virtually any artery in the body. The hepatic, splenic, renal, the superior, and often the inferior mesenteric arteries, can all be cannulated by this route.

Similarly, the carotid, subclavian and left vertebral artery can be reached from the arch of the aorta. Alternatively, the catheter can also be passed across the aortic bifurcation into the opposite common iliac artery and thence into the internal iliac artery in the investigation of pelvic tumours. The bronchial and coronary arteries can be opacified by this technique.

The age of the patient does not limit the usefulness of the method, and with experience the femoral artery in a newborn infant can be readily cannulated with a No. 90 Seldinger needle. This size is used in children up to one year of age, and in older children the artery can accommodate a No. 160 needle.

Disposable Teflon-sheathed needles are now available and their greater sharpness make for even easier insertion. Size 20 for infants, and size 18 for older children, require a slightly thinner guide wire than the corresponding Seldinger needles, but the catheters passed over the guide wire have the same dimensions as the Seldinger series. The most suitable and adaptable catheter is black radio-opaque Teflon tubing which can be purchased in bulk, cut to the desired length, and the tip pre-formed as desired. This tubing is so resistant to heat that a soldering iron is required to make the flange to fit the Luer-lok® connection. It is not easy to puncture the smaller sizes of tube to make a side hole, but this can be readily made in the larger sizes, a side hole being useful for midstream aortic injections.

Pre-formed curves are made by autoclaving the tubing with a curved metal guide inserted in the end of the catheter.

Anaesthesia is not as a rule required in very young infants; they are held firmly by padded bandages to a plywood frame and given a dummy covered with a mixture of brandy and sugar. The skin over the site of the puncture is infiltrated with a local anaesthetic and the procedure as described below is completed without disturbing the infant. Older infants and children require sedation with omnopon and scopalamine in a dose calculated from the patient's weight. More recently, Ketamine® anaesthesia has proved to be particularly suitable for very apprehensive children. Cerebral and peripheral arteriography require general anaesthesia because of the unpleasant sensation of heat, and sometimes pain, produced by the injection of the opaque medium.

Percutaneous needling

With full aseptic ritual the needle is introduced by puncturing the skin 1–2 cm below the point of entry into the artery; the needle is then angulated, and pushed upward to enter the lumen; this method has been virtually 100% successful in the paediatric age group. The guide wire is then introduced through and beyond the needle, and the needle is withdrawn. The catheter is then passed over the guide wire into the artery, and the guide is withdrawn. The catheter is then advanced to the required site under fluoroscopic control with an image-intensifier, and displayed on closed loop television.

In abdominal tumours, the first step is a midstream aortic injection to demonstrate the exact anatomy of the major arteries so that they can be entered more easily. In infants, a size 90 Teflon end-opening catheter is used and the injection is performed by hand, but in older children size 160 tubing with a side hole is preferred and a pressure injector produces better results. Preliminary midstream aortography is not required for cerebral or peripheral arteriography, and the catheter is advanced straight to the vessel selected.

After carefully inspecting the midstream aortic films, the definitive arteriogram is performed, substituting a catheter with a preformed curve if necessary, or inserting a curved guide wire to a point just short of the catheter tip, in order to reach and enter the particular artery chosen.

A test hand injection of 1 ml or so of the contrast medium is then made and observed on the screen to ensure that the catheter is patent, properly placed, and does not block the lumen of the vessel. This step is of the utmost importance, and will also give some idea of the amount of dye required to outline the area selected. The optimum volume of medium to be injected depends on the size of the patient, the viscus and the tumour, and no precise figures can be stated. In general, a midstream aortogram requires 4–5 ml in a newborn, rising to 25 ml for an adolescent. Selective arteriography requires from 1 ml for the renal artery in a newborn to 20 ml for the hepatic artery in an older child with a large tumour. Angiografin® is the dye recommended, mainly because it is a methyl glucosamine compound which appears to be less toxic than the sodium or mixed compounds.

The selective arteriogram is performed by hand injection to avoid damage to the tissues, and biplanar films are exposed with the film changer set at four to six films per second. A period of one to one and a half seconds is required to catch both the arterial and the capillary phases, and when the venous phase is desired, a further period of two seconds may be required, during which the rate can be reduced to two films per second.

Biplanar films are preferred to cine-angiography because they permit better interpretation and more precise localization of the tumour and the vessels supplying it.

Blood vessels developing in a malignant tumour are described as larger than capillaries, without differentiating into 'arterioles' or 'venules' and lacking a muscular coat. Recent reports of 'pharmaco-angiography' suggest that absence of muscle in the wall of these vessels and consequent lack of response to either vasoconstrictors or dilators can be employed to obtain better opacification of tumour vessels. The injection of angiotensin (Ekelund & Lunderquist, 1974), or priscoline (Hawkins & Hudson, 1974) into the artery supplying the tumour, immediately before contrast arteriography, is reported to produce better filling and greater detail in the vasculature of the tumour.

Percutaneous catheterization of major arteries requires skill, and experience, catheters of appropriate size and structure, careful technique and attention to the site of puncture when the procedure has been completed. As with any special investigations the value of the information obtained has to be weighed against the incidence of complications such as diminished flow in or occlusion of the artery employed (Jacobsson *et al.*, 1973). The area should be observed carefully and when indicated early surgical thrombectomy should be performed.

VENOGRAPHY

This has a special application in the investigation of abdominal tumours by delineating the inferior vena cava (IVC) in a vena cavogram. By itself, the information it yields is limited, but in conjunction with arteriography it provides useful additional information. It is most important in cases of Wilms' tumour, in which the presence or absence of an extension of the tumour along a renal vein and into the IVC can be demonstrated as a filling defect (Fig. 17.5b, p. 508).

Deviation, compression or obstruction of the IVC can be demonstrated, obstruction being almost confined to hepatic tumours.

Inferior cavography is performed by needling the femoral vein in the same way as the arterial cannulation described above, except that it is carried out while there is an opaque catheter in the femoral artery and displayed on the television screen, the intra-arterial catheter being used as a guide during insertion of the needle into the vein lying parallel and medial to it. This method is a distinct improvement on needling or cutting down on a superficial vein at the ankle, a method which also required a tourniquet on the opposite leg during the injection.

Only a short length of straight Teflon catheter is required and the tip is positioned in the common iliac vein or in the lower end of the IVC. One, or at the most two, biplanar films are then taken.

A common error is to accept as genuine an appearance of caval obstruction when there is a large abdominal tumour. Whenever caval obstruction is apparent in the supine position, the procedure should be repeated with the patient lying prone or on one side. This will often show that the apparent obstruction is due to the weight of the tumour pressing the IVC against the front of the vertebrae. In the prone or lateral position, apparent obstruction disappears, while real obstruction can still be demonstrated.

LYMPHANGIOGRAPHY

This plays a rather limited role in the paediatric age group partly because of the technical difficulties in inserting the cannula, and is largely restricted to Hodgkin's disease, and to sarcomas arising in the lower part of the body.

The technique is the same as used for adults, although the very much smaller lymphatics in children can be extremely difficult to locate and enter; keen eyesight and a very steady hand are essential.

In young children even these may not suffice, and direct injection into palpable nodes in the groin can be used as an alternative.

PYELOGRAPHY AND CYSTOGRAPHY

In the investigation of abdominal tumours, an excretory pyelogram is now rarely performed as a separate procedure because an adequate pyelogram is obtained at the conclusion of any form of abdominal arteriography. As a separate procedure, no special preparation of the patient is necessary except restriction of fluid intake for the previous four to six hours. Instead of enemas or laxatives, the patient is given Coca Cola®, or some other effervescent drink, to produce gaseous dilatation of the stomach which displaces the intestinal shadows from in front of the kidneys and gives an unobstructed view of the pelvicalyceal systems.

CYSTOGRAPHY

The outlining of pelvic tumours by arteriography has already been mentioned, but cystography as a separate procedure can provide additional information by demonstrating fixation, compression or displacement of the bladder or the bladder neck. This is particularly informative in children with pelvic tumours such as rhabdomyosarcomas, sacrococcygeal teratomas and prostatic tumours (see Chapter 21).

The bladder is catheterized aseptically with a soft rubber catheter or a sterile disposable feeding tube. It is then filled to its maximum capacity with a sterile 20% solution of methyl glucosamine containing an added antibiotic. Antero-posterior, lateral and oblique views are then taken, and further films are exposed during micturition, for these are particularly useful in delineating prostatic tumours.

BARIUM STUDIES OF THE ALIMENTARY CANAL

BARIUM MEAL

Because of the extreme rarity of carcinoma of the stomach and alimentary canal in the paediatric age group, this investigation has a rather restricted use. However, a barium swallow may outline deviation or compression of the oesophagus by a mediastinal tumour, and the follow-through has on some occasions helped to demonstrate a tumour of the small bowel (e.g. a lymphosarcoma) or to differentiate a choledochal cyst from an abdominal tumour.

BARIUM ENEMA

Again, owing to the rarity of carcinoma of the colon or rectum in children, a barium enema is used chiefly in the investigation of pelvic tumours, in which it complements cystography in demonstrating any displacement and/or compression of the rectum or sigmoid colon (p. 710).

It is also an essential step in demonstrating polyps or polyposis in the colon or rectum (see p. 646) by means of 'double contrast' enemas (i.e. using barium and air) after careful cleansing of the distal bowel.

MYELOGRAPHY

Primary tumours of the spinal cord and its coverings are rare (p. 287) and the chief value of myelography is in the investigation of a possible extension of a thoracic or retroperitoneal neuroblastoma into the spinal theca. Depending on whether there is evidence of a complete spinal block, the contrast medium is introduced via the lumbar or the cisternal route. Myodil® is injected with the patient lying on a tilting table. Fluoroscopic control with an image intensifier and television display make it possible to demonstrate any encroachment on the spinal theca, and the level of any obstruction can be seen and recorded precisely (Fig. 16.10a).

SIALOGRAPHY

A sialogram is occasionally useful in the diagnosis of tumours in the region of the parotid gland. The duct opening is quite easily cannulated with an olive-tipped cannula (23 gauge); a very small amount (0·1–0·3 ml) of Lipiodol (Ultra fluid)® is then injected, and anteroposterior and oblique views are obtained.

B. SCANNING

The methods available for investigating patients with a suspected tumour include scintillography, the detection of gamma rays emitted by various kinds of radionucleides. Areas with different rates of emission are surveyed by a rectilinear scanner or a gamma camera, and the results can be depicted graphically on sensitized film, or as a dot print out in which each dot represents a certain number of scintillations received over a particular area. The rectilinear scanner is a motorized sensor which surveys an area of the body by passing systematically to and fro, and moving forwards in regular steps. It is more accurate but also more time consuming (average 30 min) than a gamma camera (average 10 min), and with latter, dynamic studies, such as tracking the movement of tagged substances within the body, can be performed (Loken, 1969; Samuels, 1971; James *et al.*, 1974).

The information obtained by scanning depends upon the creation of a rate of emission by a tumour which differs from that of the tissue in which it lies, and the method of establishing this differential varies with the area being investigated, with the technique chosen, and hence the most appropriate radionucleide (Riccioni *et al.*, 1968; Andrews *et al.*, 1973).

In general, the ideal nucleide has a short half-life, is readily eliminated from the body, and the quantity required for the scan should deliver a minimal or at least a tolerable dose of radiation, in most cases less than the amount received in many standard radiological procedures. The degree of resolution currently obtainable by scintillography makes it possible to detect lesions approximately 2 cm in diameter in favourable circumstances.

Since 1972, the diagnosis of brain tumours in infants and young children has been greatly facilitated by access to the 'EMI brain scanner' (computerized transverse axial tomography).

The techniques used in specific areas are as follows.

BRAIN TUMOURS

The differential emission required for a brain scan is obtained by selecting a nucleide which does not pass the blood-brain barrier, is therefore not taken up by normal brain tissue and does not appear in the CSF, but which diffuses readily into tumour tissue where it is detected as a 'hot' area.

The nucleide most commonly used is the soluble salt sodium pertechnitate containing ($^{99m}TcO_4$)$^-$. The notation 'm' indicates that this isotope of technetium is a metastable substance which decays to ^{99}Tc, giving off a gamma ray, but without any particulate emission which would add to the radiation dosage. ^{99m}Tc is the daughter product of de-excitation of Molybdenum (^{99m}Mo).

^{99m}Tc has a half-life of six hours and is taken up selectively by much the same tissues as take up iodine (the thyroid, parotid, stomach and choroid plexus), and as a preliminary step, uptake by these tissues is decreased by giving a dose of 200 mgm of potassium chloride orally, at least one hour before injecting ^{99m}Tc intravenously. A blocking effect can also be achieved by atropine, and when the brain stem is to be scanned, both KCl and atropine are given.

The amount of the nucleide administered is calculated according to the body weight, and also on the basis of experience, so that an optimal differential in emission by the lesion and the background is obtained. The child is sedated, and because of the time required for scanning and the need for immobility, an anaesthetist stands by to give a short acting anaesthetic if required.

Scanning the posterior fossa in a child is easier and more accurate than in an adult; the critical diameter of a detectable lesion is 2–3 cm and the accuracy of a positive result in childhood is greater than 90%. A brain scan for a posterior fossa tumour is at least as accurate as any single radiological contrast study, and has the added advantage of causing less disturbance to the patient, with none of the unpleasant effects of, for example, a ventriculogram, or the dangers in a patient with raised intracranial pressure.

Scanning the brain stem is more difficult and the accuracy is approximately 60% in this area, which is notoriously difficult for any type of radiological investigation aiming to demonstrate a small area of diffuse infiltration, in a short segment of cylindrical structure.

Brain scans have proved to be most useful as a preliminary step in investigation, and they are helpful in planning the next steps by indicating whether cerebral angiography or a ventriculogram should be performed next.

ABDOMINAL TUMOURS

Several techniques are available, for example a 'tumour scan' using gallium citrate (^{67}Ga) which is selectively taken up by a variety of tumours, e.g. Hodgkin's tissue, Wilms' tumour and tumours of the testis (p. 881). However, angiography is so accurate (approximately 70%) in Wilms' tumour (p. 507) that scanning can provide little additional information. It may nevertheless prove to be valuable in demonstrating the presence of local recurrences after nephrectomy.

Malignant lymphomas also have a special affinity for gallium, and this has recently been found to be helpful in assessing the extent of Hodgkin's disease in the upper part of the abdomen (in the liver and spleen); thus it complements and may replace lymphangiography, which is most informative concerning the lower half of the abdomen. A gallium scan may eventually eliminate the need for laparotomy in Hodgkin's disease.

A gallium scan may also prove to be the most reliable method of depicting a lymphosarcoma of the bowel at an early stage, a notoriously difficult task using standard radiological procedures such as a barium meal and 'follow through'.

A liver scan, more accurately a 'Kupfer cell' scan, can be performed using a sulphurated compound of ^{99m}Tc joined to a colloid of critical and predetermined molecular size. This is taken up by reticulo-endothelial cells, in the liver and the spleen (and also in the marrow), so that the size and shape of these viscera can be delineated (Rosenthal, 1974). Where reticulo-endothelial cells are missing, i.e. being pushed aside by a cyst or tumour, a 'cold' spot is registered. The presence of primary (or secondary) malignant tumour deep in the substance of the liver can thus be demonstrated, and the clarity or irregularity of the margin can, in some cases, indicate whether a cold spot is a sharply defined benign lesion or an irregular infiltrating malignant tumour. Rarely, a false positive result is obtained when non-malignant disease of the liver is focal or nodular (p. 525).

A 'blood pool' scan of the liver or spleen can provide additional information, in this case by using a nucleide such as Indium (^{113m}In) which remains for a time entirely in the bloodstream. It is thus a measure of vascularity and can be used to distinguish the 'cold' spot of a large and relatively avascular lesion (e.g. a cystic hamartoma or hydatid cyst) from a highly vascular lesion such as a hepatic tumour, which registers as a 'hot' spot (Suzuki *et al.*, 1972).

A 'biliary scan' can be performed by using another method and a further refinement which makes dynamic studies possible. The substance Rose Bengal is selectively taken up in the liver and excreted in the bile and, when tagged with ^{125}I or ^{131}I, and scanned at suitable intervals, its passage as an identifiable 'bolus' into the gall-bladder, then into the common bile duct, and finally into the duodenum, can be followed as a series of 'hot' spots. Obstructive lesions, such as a choledochal cyst or a tumour, the size and shape of the gallbladder, and the patency of the ampulla of Vater can all be demonstrated by this means.

BONE LESIONS

Scanning of bones or marrow can add to the information obtained from plain films or angiograms. ^{99m}Tc-polyphosphate and ^{18}Fe, and can be used to show increased vascularity and metabolic activity, and hence the site and the extent of primary bone tumours, metastases from neuroblastomas, or leukaemic infiltrations, in many cases before plain radiographs of the affected area show any abnormality. Bone scans are most useful where plain radiographs are most difficult to interpret, i.e. in the vertebral column, but they can also be used with advantage in lesions of the limb girdles or long bones, in which it is desirable to determine accurately the nature of the progress of a particular lesion.

THE THYROID GLAND

Scanning the thyroid, using ^{99m}Tc or ^{131}I, has long been established as the valuable method of investigating thyroid nodules or thyroid ectopia. When a nodule corresponds with a 'hot spot' as demonstrated by the uptake of technetium or iodine, the nodule is interpreted as a functioning adenoma and a malignancy can generally be excluded; in a 'cold' nodule the probability of malignancy is correspondingly greater (although it may be a cyst) and in adults, about 20% of cold nodules are malignant (p. 374). ^{131}I or ^{125}I can also be given in therapeutic doses when a primary thyroid carcinoma or its metastases have been shown to take up iodine.

A technique using perchlorate washout after iodine uptake has also been developed for the investigation of patients with Hashimoto's disease (p. 375).

In general, caution is dictated by the carcinogenetic long term effects of iodine nucleides, particularly in the thyroid and especially in children, in whom exploration is usually preferable.

The scope of nuclear medicine is expanding rapidly and nucleides play an increasingly important role in the investigation, treatment, and subsequent monitoring of patients with malignant disease.

REFERENCES AND RECOMMENDED READING

A. Radiology

EKELUND, L. & LUNDERQUIST, A. (1974). Pharmaco-angiography with angiotensin. *Radiol.*, **110** : 533.

GYEPES, M.T. (1974). *Angiography in Infants and Children.* Grune and Stratton, Inc., New York.

HAWKINS, I.F. & HUDSON, T. (1974). Priscoline in bone and soft-tissue angiography. *Radiol.*, **110** : 541.

HILLER, H.G., KENNEDY, J.C. & MCDONALD, P. (1970). The role of angiography in suspected abdominal tumours in childhood. *GANN Monograph*, No. 9, 91.

HILLER, H.G. & MACDONALD, P. (1968). Angiography in abdominal tumours in children with particular reference to neuroblastoma and Wilms' tumour. *Clin. Radiol.*, **19** : 1.

JACOBSSON, B., CARLGREN, G., *et al.* (1973). A review of children after arterial catheterization. *Pediat. Radiol.*, **1** : 96.

SELDINGER, S.I. (1953). Catheter replacement of needle in percutaneous arteriography. A new technique. *Acta Radiol.*, **39** : 368.

TANK, E.S., POZNANSKI, A.K. & HOLT, J.E. (1973). The radiologic discrimination of abdominal masses in infants. *J. Urol.*, **109** : 128.

WALLACE, S. (1969). Angiography in childhood neoplasia. In *Neoplasia in Childhood.* Year Book Medical Publishers, Inc., Chicago.

B. Scintillography

ANDREWS, J.T., STEVEN, L.W., ARKLES, L.B., SEPHTON, R.G. & MARTIN, J.J. (1973). Reticulo-endothelial and blood pool scanning in the diagnosis and differentiation of space occupying lesions of the liver. *Aust. N.Z. J. Surg.*, **43** : 14.

JAMES, A.E., WAGNER, H.M. & COOKE, R.E. (1974). *Pediatric Nuclear Medicine.* W.B. Saunders, Philadelphia.

LOKEN, M.L. (1969). Evaluation of neoplasia in childhood with techniques in nuclear medicine. In *Neoplasia in Childhood.* Year Book Medical Publishers, Inc., Chicago.

RICCIONI, N., BECCHINI, M.F., NAVALESI, R. *et al.* (1968). The use of radiofibrin in the evaluation of the cold areas of the hepatic scans. *J. Nucl. Med.*, **12** : 101.

ROSENTHAL, L. (1974). Imaging the liver. In *Pediatric Nuclear Medicine*. W.B. Saunders, Philadelphia.

SAMUELS, L.D. (1971). Organ scan diagnosis of abdominal masses in children. *J. Pediat. Surg.*, **6** : 124.

SUZUKI, T., SARUMARU, S., KAWABE, E. & HONJO, I. (1972). Study of vascularity of tumors of the liver. *Surg. Gynec. Obstet.*, **134** : 27.

Chapter 5. Biopsies and histological techniques

A. BIOPSY

This is often the last and the definitive step in the diagnosis of a tumour. It should be preceded by thorough clinical, radiological, and when indicated, biochemical and other specific investigations, so that all the relevant data are available before proceeding to biopsy. This ensures that the equipment required for various histological techniques is available, and the biopsy can then be made to yield as much information as possible.

Whenever feasible, the pathologist should be present when the biopsy is taken. His knowledge of macroscopic pathology is usually greater, and his experience of tumours wider, than the individual surgeon's; the need for frozen sections should be discussed beforehand, and the amount and extent of tissue to be removed should be decided when the lesion has been displayed.

General anaesthesia

With the possible exception of drill biopsy in older children, tissue from a suspected tumour should always be removed under general anaesthesia; the patient is motionless, the necessity for haste is removed, and this favours the least distortion of the sample of tissue obtained. Infiltration of tissues with local anaesthetic can produce considerable deformation and introduce artefacts which may make diagnosis difficult.

The principles of surgical biopsy

(*a*) The tissue removed should be adequate in amount, representative, viable, and unmarred by rough handling.

(*b*) The histological techniques to be employed and the processing of the material obtained should be decided before biopsy; there is no point in placing the material obtained in formalin if it is proposed to culture the cells or to study their enzyme content. Not all enzymes are destroyed by formalin, but most are completely inactivated very rapidly.

Electron microscopy requires the appropriate fixing fluid, as well as other equipment such as sharp razor blades, fine forceps and a dissecting microscope, all of which should be available for immediate use on the freshly removed tissue.

Imprints require clean glass slides, ready and labelled, to minimize delay in imprinting the cut surface of the tumour.

Biochemical studies. Arrangements should be made beforehand with the laboratories in which the studies are to be carried out on part of the tissue excised. The biochemist is not concerned with morphology, and is usually content with tissue which may have been damaged during removal; even when material is unsuitable for histology, it may still be perfectly adequate for assays, which usually involve homogenization of the specimen.

In obtaining a biopsy there are two over-riding considerations; one concerns the surgeon, the other the pathologist.

(*a*) *The surgeon* should handle the tissue with the greatest care and gentleness to avoid disruption and distortion of soft, friable, poorly cohesive tumour cells, which occur very easily. The various types of surgical biopsy are described in Appendix IV, p. 945.

(*b*) *The pathologist* is chiefly concerned with adequate fixation, and the fixative must be able to gain access to the tissue as quickly as possible. A large amount of tissue placed in a small volume of fixing fluid is inimical to adequate histological examination. All too often a diagnosis is attempted on poorly fixed and poorly prepared material, and this may make the histological diagnosis, at best, an inspired guess. With co-operation between the surgeon and the pathologist, this should not occur; there should be the closest liaison and sharing of all the information obtained up to the time of biopsy.

Once the specimen has been removed, there are sometimes conflicting requirements; photographs of the biopsy, or an operative specimen, are desirable for record purposes and for teaching; time spent in photography may conflict with the need for fresh tissue for electron microscopy or enzyme histochemistry. If the pathologist has his own photographic equipment delay is minimal. It is usually possible to excise a piece of the tumour without diminishing the value of the specimen as photographic material, and it is best if the pathologist himself selects the portion of the specimen to be excised.

B. HISTOLOGICAL TECHNIQUES

These are described in the usual order in which material is studied and are as follows.

1. IMPRINT CYTOLOGY

The basis of histological diagnosis is undoubtedly the architectural pattern of the tumour, particularly in childhood neoplasms in which there are close similarities between the cells of different types of embryonal tumours. However, the morphology of individual cells can also be extremely important in reaching a diagnosis in some tumours (p. 47).

To obtain good cell preparations for histological study, imprints should be made with minimal delay. A suitable piece of the tumour is selected; a clean cut is made with a sharp scalpel or a razor blade, and clean glass slides are touched *gently* on the raw surface. It is simpler to hold the tissue in forceps and bring the slide down on to the tissue than to bring tissue to the slide. Any lateral movement at the moment of contact may produce numerous artefactual 'string cells' which can be confused with neurofibrillary processes in neuroblastoma, or strap cells in rhabdomyosarcoma.

The imprints are then air-dried and stained with a Romanowsky stain, or fixed in formalin vapour, ethyl alcohol, or other suitable fixative, and stained with a variety of agents, e.g. haematoxylin and eosin, PAS for glycogen and mucus, and Sudan stain for fat. Alternatively, the slides can be freeze-dried and used for immunofluorescence studies when a suitable antibody is available.

Imprint cytology has proved to be of the greatest value in lymphomas (particularly lymphosarcoma), in Hodgkin's disease and reticulum cell sarcoma, in eosinophilic granuloma of bone, and also in Ewing's tumour in which tissue sections are often difficult to interpret. It is our experience that in Ewing's tumour a good imprint is of more diagnostic value than histological sections. The presence of glycogen in the cytoplasm of delicate cells with small amounts of lacy cytoplasm, and oval nuclei with a fine chromatin pattern showing delicate condensations are practically diagnostic of Ewing's tumour of bone (Table 5.1).

2. PARAFFIN SECTIONS

The principles of preparing paraffin sections are well known, but it is worth noting that adequate fixation requires twenty times as much formalin (by

Table 5.1. Imprint Cytology. Differentiation of Ewing's tumour, neuroblastoma, lymphosarcoma and rhabdomyosarcoma

Type of tumour	Leishman's stain			Oil red 0	P.A.S.
	Nucleus	Chromatin	Cytoplasm	Fat	Glycogen
Lymphosarcoma	Round	Coarse, uniform	Moderate blue to grey	0 to ++++ (Burkitt's tumour)	+ (fine droplets)
Ewing's tumour	Round or ovoid	Fine, dusty	Very pale lilac	0	++++
Neuroblastoma	Irregularly oval	Coarse, irregular	Pale blue	0	0
Rhabdomyosarcoma	Irregular	Coarse, irregular	Pink	0	+++

volume) as the amount of tissue to be fixed. The tumour is best cut into slices no more than 4 mm thick to ensure adequate penetration by the formalin. Buffered formalin produces the best results by avoiding the formation of formalin pigment; this complicates the histological picture in tissues fixed in unbuffered formalin in which the pH is often quite acid. However, this technique may result in some loss of clarity in the nuclei.

Mercurial fixatives improve the sharpness and density of membranes generally and are used routinely in some laboratories. Disadvantages are the problem of disposing of spent solutions, the extra steps required to remove mercury pigments, and the risk of toxicity when handling mercury salts.

Stains

The range of stains available is almost limitless, and the most useful are as follows:

(*a*) Haematoxylin and eosin (or its equivalent).

(*b*) A stain for collagen, e.g. Masson or van Gieson.

(*c*) A stain for fibrin and myofibrils, e.g. phosphotungstic acid haematoxylin (PTAH).

(*d*) Silver impregnation, to demonstrate reticulin, is occasionally required, and our preference is a modification of Foot's method.

Sections stained with haematoxylin and eosin (or its equivalent) are the cornerstone of diagnosis. The importance of obtaining thin sections of good quality, cut with care and precision, cannot be over-emphasized. Special stains, such as those mentioned above, are used to confirm the presence of specific intra- or extracellular components, or substances which may be indistinguishable in sections treated with routine stains. (Another advantage of special stains is that the pathologist is thereby compelled to examine more sections of the specimen.) In most cases the diagnosis can be readily made with haematoxylin and eosin stains, but occasionally special stains are required. It is desirable to confine these to a few (such as those listed above), and it is important that the pathologist should be familiar with the special stains and their vagaries.

The diagnosis of a tumour is based on the recognition of tissue patterns, and cytological features such as nuclear and cytoplasmic morphology. These are discussed in detail on p. 39.

3. ENZYME HISTOCHEMISTRY

Enzymes are occasionally helpful in confirming the diagnosis, as shown in a list of histochemical findings in 120 tumours studied in the past ten years (Table 5.2). However, the patterns of the enzymes present show considerable variation, and diagnosis rarely rests on this evidence alone.

Studies of glycolytic enzyme activity by microchemical methods on cerebral tumours reveal different enzyme patterns in different tumours. In general, the more malignant the tumour, the greater the glycolytic activity. Similar techniques have been applied to oxidative enzymes, but they are of little help in differential diagnosis.

Table 5.2. Histochemical reactions of some common paediatric tumours. Positive reactions (first numbers) and group totals (second numbers) are set out for various substances and enzymes studied on frozen (cryostat) sections of fresh tumour tissues.

The most useful was the simple P.A.S. stain, with and without digestion of diastase, to demonstrate the presence of glycogen. In malignant ependymomas, a positive reaction with acid phosphatase was helpful in confirming the diagnosis. Succinic dehydrogenase and esterase appear to be relatively non-specific.

	Fat	Glyc.[1]	Acid[2] P'ase	Alk[3] P'ase	SD'ase[4]	Esterase[5]
Neuroblastoma	3/24	4/24	16/23	7/24	18/23	17/18
Wilms' tumour	12/21	6/21	19/21	10/21	20/21	11/17
Astrocytoma	10/14	5/10	11/15	10/15	7/11	12/13
Medulloblastoma	1/9	2/9	2/9	3/9	6/8	5/7
Ependymoma	1/7	6/8	8/8	1/8	6/9	4/5
Rhabdomyosarc.	4/9	12/12	9/12	6/11	6/10	7/9

1. Glycogen demonstrated by positive P.A.S. stain and diastase lability.
2. Acid phosphatase (method of Gomori described by Pearse)
3. Alkaline phosphatase (method of Gomori described by Pearse)
4. Succinic dehydrogenase (method of Pearse)
5. Esterase; substrate α-naphthyl acetate (Thompson)

4. ELECTRON MICROSCOPY

Ultra-structure is increasingly used in studying childhood neoplasms, especially in making the final differentiation between two very similar types of cell, e.g. fibrocytes and leiomyocytes, and in tumours such as rhabdomyosarcoma, melanoma, fibrosarcoma, leiomyosarcoma and chondromyxoid fibroma. No doubt with increasing experience this list will rapidly lengthen, but in most laboratories the time required to process tissue for electron microscopy removes it from routine diagnostic use.

In the last few years there have been a great number of reports in the literature describing the ultrastructure of a variety of tumours in childhood. A selected list of references in the recent literature concerned mainly with the tumours of childhood is included for those seeking accounts and illustration of their ultrastructure (see references p. 90).

5. TISSUE CULTURE

This can be useful in confirming the diagnosis, e.g. in neuroblastoma in which characteristic neurofibrils elaborated by the tumour cells form in the culture medium. This technique may also be useful in the diagnosis of some cerebral tumours, and in clarifying the types of histiocytic tumours which occur in childhood (see histiocytoses, p. 205).

As with electron microscopy, tissue culture techniques are time consuming, unsuitable for routine use, and rarely helpful in diagnosis.

6. IMMUNOFLUORESCENCE

Although of limited value in routine diagnosis, this technique is useful in research because of the specificity of the reactions. It may eventually prove to have particular diagnostic applications in paediatric neoplasia (Johnson *et al.*, 1965; Nairn, 1969).

7. FROZEN SECTIONS

There is rarely a need for immediate histological diagnosis in paediatric practice. The only situation when a frozen section is required is when the result will materially and directly influence immediate treatment. The chief contra-indication to frozen sections is the possibility that the pathologist may misinterpret the findings because the preparation is of poor quality, the biopsy is not representative, or the pathologist lacks experience in interpreting frozen sections. In cryostat sections a tumour may appear less cellular than in conventional paraffin sections, partly because cryostat sections tend to be fairly thin, and there is virtually no artefactual shrinkage; indeed there may be swelling so that the cells appear further apart.

In neurosurgery frozen sections are used most often to distinguish the more malignant medulloblastomas and ependymomas from the more benign astrocytomas. When the diagnosis is an astrocytoma, an attempt is usually made to remove the tumour completely, whereas with a medulloblastoma while total removal may still be attempted (though less likely to be complete) it is not mandatory because radiotherapy and intrathecal chemotherapy can control the tumour adequately.

Frozen sections are also used extensively in some centres in the treatment of *bone tumours*. According to the plan proposed by Dahlin (1967) at the Mayo Clinic, a biopsy of a suspected bone tumour is taken distal to an occluding tourniquet. On the basis of the diagnosis made on frozen section, amputation is performed when the tumour is malignant.

An immediate diagnosis may occasionally be required to determine the diagnosis of a *very large tumour* which is not easily resectable, e.g. a tumour of the liver, in which lobectomy may be indicated. However, most paediatric tumours are amenable to 'excision biopsy' (p. 950), and this is the procedure of choice in most cases when a tumour is suspected.

Frozen sections are also important in *distinguishing inflammatory conditions* from tumours. In all but very experienced hands, however, it is probably wiser and safer to await the result of properly prepared, carefully stained and thoroughly studied paraffin sections before embarking on what may be an extensive and radical operation, or on intensive radiotherapy.

The two main techniques are (i) the long-established method of rapid formalin (heated) fixation, and cutting sections on a 'freezing' microtome, and (ii) the more recently adopted technique of cutting unfixed tissue on a cryostat, followed by fixation (usually in formalin) for two to three minutes before staining. Sections cut on a freezing microtome tend to be thick; there is much shrinkage, and some nuclear and cytoplasmic artefacts caused by rapid fixation; small specimens (e.g. needle biopsies) and soft or friable tissues are not easy to handle in this way.

Sections cut in a cabinet freezing microtome, using fresh or unfixed tissue, have largely supplanted the older methods. Very small pieces of tissue can be used, supporting them if necessary in a block of agar or other inert material such as egg albumen.

Cryostat sections are comparable in thickness with paraffin sections and resemble them more closely than pre-fixed freezing microtome sections; tumours cut by the former method may appear less cellular than they actually are, and may thus mislead the inexperienced. Cryostat sections are also used for enzyme histochemistry and for fluorescent antibody techniques.

8. SMEAR TECHNIQUES AND SQUASH PREPARATIONS

Some soft textured tumours are suitable for making squash or smear preparations (Russell, 1951). A minute piece of the fresh tumour is squeezed firmly between two glass slides which are then pulled apart with a sliding motion; the slides are then dried, fixed and stained. The advantages of this technique are its speed, and the partial preservation of tissue architecture. In addition, individual cells can be studied in the thin parts of the preparation. The technique is of particular usefulness in brain tumours, but can also be applied to other soft tumours, e.g. eosinophilic granuloma, Wilms' tumour and neuroblastoma. However, experience with the technique is essential for accurate interpretation, and practice with preparations from known tumours should be studied to become competent with this method.

9. EXFOLIATIVE CYTOLOGY

The two fluids most often examined for tumour cells in paediatric pathology are cerebrospinal fluid (including ventricular fluid) and pleural fluid.

Method of preparation

The fluid must be fresh, and the method originally described by Sayk (1960) is recommended, using a heavy glass plastic cylinder, containing 0·5 ml of the fluid, held down by a weighted lever on a ring of blotting paper. The cells settle on to the surface of a glass microscope slide underneath the cylinder, through a hole in the blotting paper. The paper absorbs the fluid and the resultant preparation produces excellent cell detail with minimal distortion. Recently the cytocentrifuge has replaced this manual method, and has the added advantage that multiple preparations can be made.

CSF

Tumours which spread in the CSF are medulloblastoma, ependymoma, some malignant astrocytomas and retinoblastoma (p. 429). Papillomas of the choroid plexus readily shed cells, and these often look quite alarming. The technique is most useful for detecting recurrences of tumours already identified and treated, and is also useful in monitoring the effectiveness of postoperative treatment with intrathecal mothotrexatt (p. 283).

Pleural fluid

Malignant cells from a lymphosarcoma of the thymus or mediastinum can be readily detected by cytological examination of pleural fluid. When obtaining pleural fluid, it is essential that it is collected into a heparinized tube, for clotting due to a high protein content renders the material useless for cytology.

Aqueous humour

When a retinoblastoma is suspected, it is possible to confirm the diagnosis in some cases by examining fluid aspirated from the anterior chamber of the eye and prepared by Sayk's method.

Peritoneal fluid, urine and other exudates and effusions, such as joint fluid, can also be examined for malignant cells. Examination of ascitic fluid aspirated from patients in whom a lymphosarcoma of the bowel is suspected, has been useful in demonstrating malignant lymphoma cells, but laparotomy is nevertheless required to determine the resectability of the tumour (p. 637).

Vaginal, gastric and sputum cytology have little application in childhood because of the rarity of carcinomas.

10. DRILL BIOPSY

This method can be very useful in diagnosis. The advantages are:
(i) Minimal handling and disturbance of the tumour, and hence less risk of dissemination.
(ii) Deep seated tumours (e.g. in the cerebral hemispheres) can be reached without an extensive surgical procedure.

The disadvantages are:
(i) The drill may miss the tumour, producing negative findings.
(ii) The sample is small, and inadequate for a full range of studies.

The technique involves puncture of the skin and passage of the needle and obturator down to the tumour. The De Soutter air driven drill and a smooth cutting-edge hollow biopsy needle are used; the diameter of the needle chosen is determined by the site of the tumour and the risk of haemorrhage. A syringe is used to apply suction to the needle while it is being withdrawn. The method is most applicable in deep seated cerebral and cerebellar tumours, suspected tumours of the prostate (p. 708), hepatic tumours, bone tumours and swellings of the parotid gland.

11. RAPID TECHNIQUES

Brain tumours

The soft texture of most cerebellar and cerebral tumours makes them suitable for 'smear' or 'squash' preparations. These are not advocated as substitutes for frozen sections, but the delicacy of the nuclei, the relationship of cells to their vascular supply, and the intrinsic fibril content of the tumour can be appreciated more easily in smears than in cryostat sections.

Bone tumours

The rapid diagnosis of bone tumours remains a difficult problem for the pathologist occasionally called upon for the diagnosis. Our experience is limited by the rarity of bone tumours (an average of two per year in the Index Series), and paraffin sections are relied on. Good quality paraffin sections can be prepared within 24 hours without decalcifying the biopsy, because most biopsies of bone tumours contain soft portions which can be selected under a dissecting microscope, and processed overnight. Imprints can also be made from this softer material. The remainder, composed of spicules of bone etc., can be fixed, decalcified, and processed without haste to confirm the diagnosis made on the softer material.

Haematoxylin and eosin stain is almost always adequate for a diagnosis, but if a Ewing's tumour or a metastasis from a neuroblastoma is suspected, the sections should be stained for glycogen (see colour plates following p. 170).

REFERENCES

GENERAL

American Registry of Pathology (1968). *Manual of Histologic Staining Methods of the Armed Forces Institute of Pathology*, 3rd ed. McGraw Hill.

Bancroft, J.D. (1967). *Introduction to Histochemical Technique*. Appleton, New York.

Baker, J.R. (1966). *Cytological Technique*. Methuen & Co., Ltd., London.

Carleton, H.M. (1967). *Carleton's Histological Technique*, 4th ed. Oxford University Press.

Cohen, H.J. (1965). *Biological Stains*. Williams & Wilkins, Baltimore.

Culling, C.F. (1963). *Handbook of Histopathological Technique*, 2nd ed. Appleton, New York.

Dahlin, D.C. (1967). *Bone Tumors* 2nd ed. Charles C. Thomas, Springfield.

Johnson, W., Jurand, J. & Hiramoto, R. (1956). Immunohistologic studies of tumors containing myosin. *Am. J. Path.*, **47** ; 1139.

Kolar, O. & Zerman, W. (1968). Spinal fluid cytomorphology. *Arch. Neurol.*, **18** : 44.

Lillie, R.D. (1965). *Histopathologic Technique and Practical Histochemistry*, 3rd ed. McGraw Hill.

Nairn, R. C. (1969). *Fluorescent Protein Tracing*. 3rd ed. Livingstone, Edinburgh & London.

Neustein, H.B. (1973). Electron microscopy in diagnostic pathology. In *Perspectives in Pediatric Pathology*, **1** : Vol. 1, p. 369. Year Book Medical Publishers, Chicago.

Pearse, A.G. (1969). Histochemistry; Theoretical & Applied. 2 vols. (3rd ed.). Williams & Wilkins, Baltimore.

Russell, D. S. (1951). The wet-film technique in neurosurgery. In *Recent Advances in Clinical Pathology* 2nd ed. Dyke, S.C.—Ed. J. & A. Churchill Ltd. London. pp. 455–462.

Sayk, J. (1960). *Cytologie der Cerebro-spinalflüssigkeit*. Fischer-Verlag, Jena.

Spurr, A.R. (1969). A low viscosity epoxy resin embedding medium for electron microscopy. *J. Ultrastruct. Res.*, **26** ; 31.

Thompson, S.W. (1966). *Selected Histochemical and Histopathological Methods*. Charles C. Thomas, Springfield.

ULTRASTRUCTURE

Leukaemia

Dmochowski, L. (1965). Electron microscopic observations of leukemia in animals and in man. *Cancer Res.*, **25** : 1654.

Dmochowski, L., Yumoto, T., Grey, C.E., Hales, R.L., Langford, P.L., Taylor, H.G., Freireich, E.J., Shullenberger, C.C., Shively, J.A. & Howe, C.D. (1967). Electron microscopic studies of human leukemia and lymphoma. *Cancer*, **20** : 760.

Freeman, A.I. & Journey, L.J. (1971). Ultrastructural studies on monocytic leukaemia. *Brit. J. Haematol.*, **20** : 225.

Foa, R., Perrimond, H., Orsini, A. & Muratore, R. (1970). Cytochemical and ultrastructural study of a case of acute monocytic leukosis. *C.R. Soc. Biol.* (*Paris*), **164** : 593.

Johnson, D.E., Griep, J.A. & Baehner, R.L. (1973). Histiocytic leukemia following lifelong infection and thrombocytopenia : histologic, metabolic and bactericidal studies. *J. Pediat.* **82** : 664.

NARANG, H.K. (1973). Surface particles on leukemic lymphocytes. *Brit. Med. J.*, **2** : 422.

ROSS, A. & HARNDEN, D. (1969). Ultrastructural studies on normal and leukaemic and human haematopoietic cells. *Europ. J. Cancer* **5** : 349.

SCHUMACHER, H.R., SZEKELY, I.E. & PARK, S.A. (1972). Ultrastructural studies on the acute leukemic myeloblast. *Blut.*, **25** : 169.

TANAKA, Y., BELL, W.R. & BRINDLEY, D. (1967). Pseudoviral inclusion bodies in acute leukemia. A report of two cases. *J. Nat. Cancer Inst.* **38** : 629.

VAN HOOSIER, G.L. Jr., STENBACK, W.A., MUMFORD, D.M., HILL, W.A., DUNN, S.C., MACDONALD, E.J., MACDONALD, M.C., TAYLOR, H.G. & TRENTIN, J.J. (1968). Epidemiological findings and electron microscopic observations in human leukemia and canine contacts. *Int. J. Cancer*, **3** : 7.

WITZLEBEN, C.L., DRAKE, W.L., Jr., SAMMON, J. & MOHABBAT, O.M. (1970). Gaucher's cells in acute leukemia of childhood. *J. Pediat.*, **76** : 129.

YUMOTO, T. (1969). Electron microscopic study of virus-like particles in human leukemia and allied disease. *Acta Haemat. Jap.*, **32** : 578.

Lymphomas and Histiocytoses

BASSET, F. & NEZELOF, C. (1969). Histiocytosis X., electron microscopy 'In vitro' culture and histoenzymology. Apropos of 21 cases. *Rev. Franç. Étud. Clin. Biol.*, **14** : 31.

CHAVES, E. (1970). Burkitt's tumour. A cytologic and histological study of three cases. *Arch. Ital. Patol. Clin. Tumori*, **13** : 65.

CHAVES, E. (1973). Hodgkin's disease in the first decade. *Cancer*, **31** : 925.

COHNEN, G., DOUGLAS, S.D., KONIG E. & BRITTINGER, G. (1973). In vitro lymphocyte response to phytohemagglutinin and pokeweed mitogen in Hodgkin's disease. An electron microscopic and functional study. *Cancer*, **31** : 1346.

DE MAN, J.C. (1968). Rod-like tubular structures in the cytoplasm of histiocytes in 'histiocytosis X'. *J. Path. Bact.*, **95** : 123.

DORFMAN, R.F. (1967). The fine structure of a malignant lymphoma in a child from St. Louis, Missouri. *J. Nat. Cancer Inst.*, **38** : 491.

DORFMAN, R.F. (1968). Diagnosis of Burkitt's tumour in the United States. *Cancer*, **21** : 563.

FARRIAUX, J.P., BOURY, G., FOVET-POINGT, D., FONTAINE, G., CLAY, A., DUPONT, A. & GOSSELIN, B. (1970). Disseminated forms of histiocytosis X: 10 cases. *Pédiatrie*, **25** : 359.

FISHER, E.R., SIERACKI, J.C. & GOLDENBERG, D.M. (1970). Identity and nature of isolated lymphoid tumors (so-called nodal hyperplasia, hamartoma, and angiomatous hamartoma) as revealed by histologic, electron microscopic and heterotransplantation studies. *Cancer*, **25** : 1286.

GIANOTTI, F. (1972). Histiocytosis with cells containing vermiform intracytoplasmic particles, 2nd case in an infant. *Bull. Soc. Franç. Dermatol. Syphiligr.*, **79** : 244.

GILLOT, F., TUSQUES, J., COLLET, M., PRADAL, G. & BODIN, G. (1968). Recent case of histiocytosis X with electron microscopy study. *Arch. Franç. Pédiat.*, **25** : 1073.

GRISLAIN, J.R., TUSQUES, J., BERRANGER, P. & DE PRUDAL, G. (1969). A recent case of reticulosis X studies by optic and electron microscopy. *Pédiatrie*, **24** : 87.

IMAMURA, M., SAKAMOTO, S. & HANAZONO, H. (1971). Malignant histiocytosis : a case of generalized histiocytosis with infiltration of Langerhans' granule-containing histiocytes. *Cancer*, **28** : 467.

LEVINE, G.D. & DORFMAN, R.F. (1975). Nodular lymphoma ; an ultrastructural study of its relationship to geminal centres and a correlation of light and electron microscopic findings. *Cancer*, **35** ; 148.

POPE, J.H., ACHONG, B.G. & EPSTEIN, M.A. (1968). Cultivation and fine structure of virus-bearing lymphoblasts from a second New Guinea Burkitt lymphoma : establishment of sublines with unusual cultural properties. *Int. J. Cancer*, **3** : 171.

Pope, J.H., Achong, B.G., Epstein, M.A. & Biddulph, J. (1967). Burkitt lymphoma in New Guinea : establishment of a line of lymphoblasts in vitro and description of their fine structure. *J. Nat. Cancer Inst.*, **39** : 933.

Schnitzer, B., Nishiyama, R.H., Heidelberger, K.P. & Weaver, D.K. (1974). Hodgkin's disease in children. *Cancer*, **31** : 560.

Steel, C.M. & Edmond, E. (1971). Human lymphoblastoid cell lines. I. Culture methods and examination for Epstein-Barr virus. *J. Natl., Cancer Inst.*, **47** : 1193.

Toshima, S., Takagi, N., Minowada, J., Moore, G.E. & Sandberg, A.A. (1967). Electron microscopic and cytogenetic studies of cells derived from Burkitt's lymphoma. *Cancer Res.*, **27** : 753.

Yumoto, T. & Dmochowski, L. (1968). Hodgkin's disease and viruses : an electron microscopic study. *Acta Path. Jap.*, **18** : 394.

Central Nervous System and Eye

Carter, L.P., Beggs, J. & Waggener, J.D. (1972). Ultrastructure of three choroid plexus papillomas. *Cancer*, **30** : 1130.

Castaigne, P., David, M., Pertuiset, B., Ecourolle, R. & Poirier, J. (1968). L'ultrastructure des hémangioblastomes du système nerveux central. *Rev. neurol.*, **118** : 5.

Font, R.L. & Zimmerman, L.E. (1972). Electron microscopic verification of primary rhabdomyosarcoma of the iris. *Am. J. Ophthalmol.*, **74** : 110.

Fu, Y.S., Chen, A.T.L., Kay, S. & Young, H.F. (1974). Is subependymoma (subependymal glomerate astrocytoma) an astrocytoma or ependymoma? A comparative ultrastructural and tissue culture study. *Cancer*, **34** : 1992.

Goebel, H.H. & Cravioto, H. (1972). Ultrastructure of human and experimental ependymomas. *J. Neuropath. Exp. Neurol.*, **31** : 54.

Gonatas, N.K., Martin, J. & Evangelista, I. (1967). The osmiophilic particles of astrocytes. Viruses, lipid droplets or products of secretion? *J. Neuropath. Exp. Neurol.*, **26** : 369.

Gullotta, F. & Kersting, G. (1972). The ultrastructure of medulloblastoma in tissue culture. *Virchow's Arch.* (*Pathol. Anat.*), **356** : 111.

Hadfield, M.G. & Silverberg, S.G. (1972). Light and electron microscopy of giant-cell glioblastoma. *Cancer*, **30** : 989.

Hassoun, J., Tripier, M.F., Pellissier, J.F., Berard, M., Choux, R. & Toga, M. (1973). Ultrastructural study of a pseudosarcomatous glioma of the cerebellum. *Arch. Anat. Pathol.* (*Paris*), **21** : 73.

Hirano, A., Ghatak, N.R. & Zimmerman, H.M. (1973). The fine structure of ependymoblastoma. *J. Neuropath. Exp. Neurol.*, **32** : 144.

Hogan, M.J. & Wood, I. (1972). Orbital rhabdomyosarcoma : An electron microscopic study. *Trans. Am. Ophthalmol.* Soc., **70** : 131.

Iwamoto, T., Witmer, R. & Landolt, E. (1967). Diktyoma : A clinical histological and electronmicroscopical observation. *von Graefe Arch. Klin. Exp. Ophthal.*, **172** : 293.

Kadin, M.E., Rubinstein, L. J. & Nelson, J.S.(1970). Neonatal cerebellar medulloblastoma originating from the fetal external granular layer. *J. Neuropathol. Exp. Neurol.*, **29** : 583.

Lee, J.C. & Glasauer, F.E. (1968). Ganglioglioma : Light and electron microscopic study. *Neurochirurgia* (*Stuttgart*), **11** : 160.

Luse, S.A. (1960). Electron microscopic studies of brain tumours. *Neurology*, **10** : 881.

Maunoury, R., Vedrenne, C., Arnoult, J., Constans, J.P. & Febvre, H. (1972). Culture in vitro de tissue glial normal et néoplasique. *Neuro-chirurgie*, **18** : 101.

Misugi, K. & Liss, L. (1970). Medulloblastoma with cross-striated muscle. A fine structural study. *Cancer*, **25** : 1279.

NAPOLITANO, L., KYLE, R. & FISHER, E.R. (1964). Ultrastructure of meningiomas and the derivation and nature of their cellular components. *Cancer*, **17** : 233.

NEUSTEIN, H.B. (1967). Fine structure of a melanotic progonoma or retinal anlage tumor of the anterior fontanel. *Exp. Molec. Path.*, **6** : 131.

POIRIER, J., ESCOUROLLE, R. & CASTAIGNE, P. (1968). Les neurofibromes de la maladie de Recklinghausen. *Acta neuropath.*, **10** : 279.

RAIMONDI, A.J. (1966). Ultrastructure and the biology of human brain tumors. *Progress in neurological surgery*, Vol. 1. Year Book Medical Publishers. Inc., Chicago.

RAMSEY, H.J. (1965). Ultrastructure of a pineal tumor. *Cancer*, **18** : 1014.

SATO, K., FUJIKURA, T., KAWAI, S. & NUKUI, H. (1969). Retinoblastoma with intracranial extension—an autopsy case with light and electron microscope. *Acta Path. Jap.*, **19** : 103.

SPENCE, A.M. & RUBINSTEIN, L.J. (1975). Cerebellar capillary haemangioblastoma ; its histogenesis studied by organ culture and electron microscopy. *Cancer*, **35** ; 362.

SUMI, S.M. & REIFEL, E. (1971). Unusual nuclear inclusions in astrocytoma. *Arch. Pathol.*, **92** : 14.

TANI, E. & AMETANI, T. (1970). Polygonal crystalline structures in human ependymoma cells. *Acta Neuropath. (Berlin)*, **15** : 359.

VOIGT, W.H. (1968). Elektronenmikroskopische Beobachtungen an menschlichen Medulloblastomen. *Deutsch. Z. Nervenheilk.*, **192** : 290.

ZIMMERMAN, L.E., FONT, R.L. & ANDERSEN, S.R. (1972). Rhabdomyosarcomatous differentiation in malignant intraocular medulloepitheliomas. *Cancer*, **30** : 817.

Jaws and Related Tissues

HANSEN, J. & KOBAYASI, T. (1970). Ultrastructural studies of odontogenic cysts. I. Non-keratinizing cysts. *Acta Morphol. Neerl., Scand.*, **8** : 29.

HANSEN, J. & KOBAYASI, T. (1970). Ultrastructural studies of odontogenic cysts. II. Keratinizing cysts. *Acta Morphol. Neerl., Scand.*, **8** : 43.

TAKAGI, M. (1967). Adenomatoid ameloblastoma. An analysis of nine cases by histopathological and electron microscopic study. *Bull. Tokyo Med. Dent. Univ.*, **14** : 487.

Salivary Glands

ERLANDSON, R.A. & TANDLER, B. (1972). Ultrastructure of acinic cell carcinoma of the parotid gland. *Arch. Pathol.*, **93** : 130.

FUKUSHIMA, M. (1968). An electron microscopic study of human salivary gland tumors. Pleomorphic adenoma and adenoid cystic carcinoma. *Bull. Tokyo Med. Dent. Univ.*, **15** : 387.

Thyroid Gland

GOULD, V.S., GOULD, N.S. & BENDITT, E.P. (1972. Ultrastructural aspects of papillary and sclerosing carcinomas of the thyroid. *Cancer*, **29** : 1613.

Kidney

FAVARA, B.E., JOHNSON, W. & ITO, J. (1968). Renal tumors in the neonatal period. *Cancer*, **22** : 845.

FU, Y. & KAY, S. (1973). Congenital mesoblastic nephroma and its recurrence. *Arch. Pathol.*, **96** : 66.

GARCIA-BUNUEL, R. & BRANDES, D. (1970). Fetal hamartoma of the kidney : case report, with ultrastructural cytochemical observations. *Johns Hopkins Med. J.*, **127** : 213.

PRATT-THOMAS, H.R., SPICER, S.S., UPSHUR, J.K. & GREENE, W.B. (1973). Carcinoma of the kidney in a 15 year old boy. Unusual histologic features with formation of microvilli. *Cancer*, **31** : 719.

TREMBLAY, M. (1971). Ultrastructure of a Wilms' tumour and myogenesis. *J. Pathol.*, **105** : 269.

Neuroblastoma and Ganglioneuroma

GOLDSTEIN, M.N. (1971). Annulate lamellae in cultured human neuroblastoma cells. *Cancer Res.*, **31** : 209.

GULLOTTA, F., FLIEDNER, E., WUELLENWEBER, R. & ORF, G. (1973). Tissue culture, electron microscopic and enzyme histochemical investigations on a sympathetic ganglioneuroblastoma. *Acta Neuropathol.* (*Berl*)., **24** : 107.

KAHN, L.B. (1974). Esthesioneuroblastoma ; a light and electron microscopic study. *Human Path.* **5** ; 364.

MISUGI, K., MISUGI, N. & NEWTON, W.A. Jr. (1968). Fine structural study of neuroblastoma, ganglioneuroblastoma and pheochromocytoma. *Arch. Path.* (*Chicago*), **86** : 160.

ROSENTHAL, I.M., GREENBERG, R., KATHAN, R., FALK, C.S. & WONG, R. (1969). Catecholamine metabolism of a ganglioneuroma : correlation with electronmicrographs. *Pediat. Res.*, **3** : 413.

STALEY, N.A., POLEKSY, H.F. & BENSCH, K.G. (1967). Fine structural and biochemical studies on the malignant ganglioneuroma. *J. Neuropath. Exp. Neurol.*, **26** : 634.

TAZAWA, K., SOGA, J. & ITO, H. (1971). Fine structure of neuroblastoma—a case report. *Acta Pathol. Jap.*, **21** : 257.

YOKOYAMA, M., OKADA, K., TOKUE, A., TAKAYASU, H. & YAMADA, R. (1971). Ultrastructural and biochemical study of neuroblastoma and ganglioneuroblastoma. *Invest. Urol.*, **9** : 156.

Adrenal Gland

BLASCHKO, H., JERROME, D.W., ROBB-SMITH, A.H., SMITH, A.D. & WINKLER, H. (1968). Biochemical and morphological studies on catecholamine storage in human phaeochromocytoma. *Clin. Sci.*, **34** : 453.

BROWN, W.J., BARAJAS, L., WAISMAN, J. & DE QUATTRO, V. (1972). Ultrastructural and biochemical correlates of adrenal and extra-adrenal pheochromocytoma. *Cancer*, **29** : 744.

HOSHINO, M. (1969). 'Polysome-lamellae complex' in the adenoma cells of the human adrenal cortex. *J. Ultrastruct. Res.*, **27** : 205.

ROSENTHAL, I.M., GREENBERG, R., GOLDSTEIN, R., KATHAN, R. & CADKIN, L. (1966). Catecholamine metabolism in a pheochromocytoma. Correlation with electron micrographs. *Amer. J. Dis. Child.*, **112** : 389.

Alimentary including Pancreas

BALSAM, M.J., BAKER, L., BISHOP, H.C., HUMMELER, K., YAKOVAC, W.C. & KAYE, R. (1972). Beta cell adenoma in a child with hypoglycemia controlled with diazoxide. *J. Pediatr.*, **80** : 788.

FRABLE, W.J., STILL, W.J. & KAY, S. (1971). Carcinoma of the pancreas, infantile type. A light and electron microscopic study. *Cancer*, **27** : 667.

GROSFELD, J.L., CLATWORTHY, H.W. Jr. & HAMOUDI, A.B. (1970). Pancreatic malignancy in children. *Arch. Surg.* (*Chicago*), **101** : 370.

HAMOUDI, A.B., MISUGI, K., GROSFELD, J.L. & REINER, C.B. (1970). Papillary epithelial neoplasm of pancreas in a child. Report of a case, with electron microscopy. *Cancer*, **26** : 1126.

UEI, Y., KIM, U. & ITATSU, Y. (1968). An autopsy case of islet-cell carcinoma with Cushing's syndrome. *Acta. Path. Jap.*, **18** : 333.

WELLER, R.O. & MCCOLL, I. (1966). Electron microscope appearances of juvenile and Peutz-Jeghers polyps. *Gut.*, **7** : 265.

Liver

GEISER, C.F., BAEZ, A., SCHINDLER, A.M. & SHIH, V.E. (1970). Epithelial hepatoblastoma associated with congenital hemihypertrophy and cystathioninuria : presentation of a case. *Pediatrics*, **46** : 66.

GONZALEZ-CRUSSI, F. & MANZ, H.J. (1972). Structure of a hepatoblastoma of pure epithelial type. *Cancer*, **29** : 1272.

ITO, J. & JOHNSON, W.W. (1969). Hepatoblastoma and hepatoma in infancy and childhood. Light and electron microscopic studies. *Arch. Path.* (*Chicago*), **87** : 259.

MISUGI, K., OKAJIMA, H., MISUGI, N. & NEWTON, W.A. Jr. (1967). Classification of primary malignant tumors of liver in infancy and childhood. *Cancer*, **20** : 1760.

RUEBNER, B.H., GONZALEZ-LICEA, A. & SLUSSER, R.J. (1967). Electron microscopy of some human hepatomas. *Gastroenterology*, **53** : 18.

Ovary and Female Genitalia

LUSE, S.A. & VIETTI, T. (1968). Ovarian teratoma. Ultrastructure and neural component. *Cancer*, **21** : 38.

MURAD, T.M., MANCINI, R. & GEORGE, J. (1973). Ultrastructure of a virilizing ovarian Sertoli-Leydig cell tumour with familial incidence. *Cancer*, **31** ; 1440.

SILVERBERG, S.G. & DEGIORGI, L.S. (1972). Clear cell carcinoma of the vagina : a clinical, pathologic and electron microscopic study. *Cancer*, **29** : 1680.

WOYKE, S., DOMAGALA, W. & OLSZEWSKI, W. (1972). Mesonephroma of the uterine cervix. Submicroscopical study and comparison with fine structure of endocervical adenocarcinoma. *Virchow's Arch.* (*Pathol. Anat.*), **355** : 29.

Soft Tissue Tumours

BATTIFORA, H. & HINES, J.R. (1971). Recurrent digital fibromas of childhood. An electron microscope study. *Cancer*, **27** : 1530.

BURRY, A.F., KERR, J.F. & POPE, J.H. (1970). Recurring digital fibrous tumour of childhood : an electron microscopic and virological study. *Pathology*, **2** : 287.

CLARK, M.A. & O'CONNELL, K.J. (1973). An ultrastructural study of embryonal rhabdomyosarcoma (sarcoma botryoides) of the bladder. *J. Urol.*, **109** : 897.

DEHNER, L.P., ENZINGER, F.M. & FONT, R.L. (1972). Fetal rhabdomyoma. An analysis of nine cases. *Cancer*, **30** : 160.

FISHER, E.R. & VUZEVSKI, V.D. (1968). Cytogenesis of Schwannoma (neurilemoma), neurofibroma, dermatofibroma and dermatofibrosarcoma as revealed by electron microscopy. *Amer. J. Clin. Path.*, **49** : 141.

FISHER, E.R. & REIDBORD, H. (1971). Electron microscopic evidence suggesting the myogenous derivation of the so-called alveolar soft part sarcoma. *Cancer*, **27** : 150.

FREEMAN, A.I. & JOHNSON, W.W. (1968). A comparative study of childhood rhabsomyosarcoma and virus-induced rhabdomyosarcoma in mice. *Cancer Res.*, **28** : 1490.

GONZALEZ-CRUSSI, F. (1970). Ultrastructure of congenital fibrosarcoma. *Cancer*, **26** : 1289.

GRUNNET, N., GENNER, J., MOGENSEN, B. & MYRE-JENSEN, O. (1973). Recurring digital fibrous tumour of childhood. Case report and survey. *Acta Pathol. Microbiol. Scand.* (*A*), **81** : 167.

HASHIMOTO, K. & PRITZKER, M.S. (1973). Electron microscopic study of reticulohistiocytoma. An unusual case of congenital, self-healing reticulohistiocytosis. *Arch. Dermatol.*, **107** : 263.

HOGAN, M.J. & WOOD, I. (1972). Orbital Rhabdomyosarcoma : an electron microscopic study. *Trans. Am. Ophthalmol. Soc.*, **70** : 131.

HOSODA, S., SUZUKI, H., KAWABE, Y., WATANABE, Y. & ISOJIMA, G. (1971). Embryonal rhabdomyosarcoma of the middle ear. *Cancer*, **27** : 943.

KAY, S., ELZAY, R.P. & WILLSON, M.A. (1971). Ultrastructural observations on a gingival granular cell tumor (congenital epulis). *Cancer*, **27** : 674.

KITANO, Y., HORIKI, M., AOKI, T. & SAGAMI, S. (1972). Two cases of juvenile hyalin fibromatosis. Some histological, electron microscopic, and tissue culture observations. *Arch. Dermatol.*, **106** : 877.

MEHREGAN, A.H., NABAI, H. & MATTHEWS, J.E. (1972). Recurring digital fibrous tumor of childhood. *Arch. Dermatol.*, **106** : 375.

MISUGI, K., MISUGI, N. & NEWTON, W.A. (1967). Ultrastructure of a so-called granular cell myoblastoma. *Yokohama Med. Bull.*, **18** : 225.

MORALES, A.R., FINE, G. & HORN, R.C. Jr. (1972). Rhabdomyosarcoma : an ultrastructural appraisal. *Pathol. Annual*, **7** : 81.

MORETTIN, L.B., MUELLER, E. & SCHREIBER, M. (1972). Generalized hamartomatosis, (congenital generalized fibromatosis). *Am. J. Roentgenol. Radium. Ther. Nucl. Med.*, **114** : 722.

SARKAR, K., TOLNAI, G. & MCKAY, D.E. (1973). Embryonal rhabdomyosarcoma of the prostate. An ultrastructural study. *Cancer*, **31** : 442.

SCHUSTER, S.A., FERGUSON, E.C. & MARSHALL, R.B. (1972). Alveolar rhabdomyosarcoma of the eyelid. Diagnosis by electron microscopy. *Arch. Ophthalmol.*, **87** : 646.

SOBEL, H.J., MARQUET, E., AVRIN, E. & SCHWARZ, R. (1971). Granular cell myoblastoma. An electron microscopic and cytochemical study illustrating the genesis of granules and aging of myoblastoma cells. *Am. J. Pathol.*, **65** : 59.

TOKER, C. (1968). Embryonal rhabdomyosarcoma. An ultrastructural study. *Cancer*, **21** : 1164.

WELSH, R.A., BRAY, D.M., SHIPKEY, F.H. & MEYER, A.T. (1972). Histogenesis of alveolar soft part sarcoma. *Cancer*, **29** : 191.

Vascular and Allied Tumours

HAHN, M.J., DAWSON, R., ESTERLY, J.A. & JOSEPH, D.J. (1973). Heman giopericytoma An ultrastructural study. *Cancer*, **31** : 255.

SVOBODA, D.J. & KIRCHNER, F. (1966). Ultrastructure of nasopharyngeal angiofibromas. *Cancer*, **19** : 1949.

TOKER, C. (1969). Glomangioma. An ultrastructural study. *Cancer*, **23** : 487.

VENKATACHALAM, M.A. & GREALLY, J.G. (1969). Fine structure of glomus tumor : similarity of glomus cells to smooth muscle. *Cancer*, **23** : 1176.

WALIKE, J.W. & MACKAY, B. (1970). Nasopharyngeal angiofibroma : light and electron microscopic changes after stilbesterol therapy. *Laryngoscope*, **80** : 1109.

Bone Tumours

FRIEDMAN, B. & HANAOKA, H. (1971). Round-cell sarcomas of bone. A light and electron microscopic study. *J. Bone Jt. Surg.*, **53A** : 1118.

FRIEDMAN, B. & GOLD, H. (1968). Ultrastructure of Ewing's sarcoma of bone. *Cancer*, **22** : 307.

HAYWARD, A.F., FICKLING, B.W. & LUCAS, R.B. (1969). An electron microscope study of a pigmented tumour of the jaw of infants. *Brit. J. Cancer*, **23** : 702.

HOU-JENSEN, K., PRIORI, E. & DMOCHOWSKI, L. (1972). Studies on ultrastructure of Ewing's sarcoma of bone. *Cancer*, **29** : 280.

HUVOS, A.G., MARCOVE, R.C., ERLANDSON, R.A. & MIK'E, V. (1972). Chondroblastoma of bone. A clinicopathologic and electron microscopic study. *Cancer*, **29** : 760.

KADIN, M.E. & BENSCH, K.G. (1971). On the origin of Ewing's tumor. *Cancer*, **27** : 257.

KEMPSON, R.L. (1966). Ossifying Fibroma of the long bones. A light and electron microscopic study. *Arch Path. (Chicago)*, **82** : 218.

SAPP, J.P. (1972). Ultrastructure and histogenesis of peripheral giant cell reparative granuloma of the jaws. *Cancer*, **30** : 1119.

SIRSAT, S.M., PANICKER, K.N. & POTDAR, G.G. (1971). Ultrastructure of Ewing's sarcoma of the bone. *Indian. J. Cancer*, **8** : 157.

TAKAYAMA, S. & SUGAWA, I. (1970). Electron microscopic observation of Ewing's sarcoma. A case report. *Acta Path. Jap.*, **20** : 87.

Skin Tumours

BERGER, R.S. & VOORHEES, J.J. (1971). Multiple congenital giant nevocellular nevi with halos. A clinical and electron microscopic study. *Arch. Dermatol.*, **104** : 515.

ENZINGER, F.M. (1970). Epitheloid sarcoma. A sarcoma simulating a granuloma or a carcinoma. *Cancer*, **26** : 1029.

GUERRIER, C., DEVICO, V., LUTZNER, M. & PRUNI'ERAS, M. (1972). Ultrastructural study of the skin in xeroderma pigmentosum. *Ann. Dermatol. Syphiligr. (Paris)*, **99** : 523.

SILVERBERG, G.D., KADIN, M.E., DORFMAN, R.F., HANBERY, J.W. & PROLO, D.J. (1971). Invasion of the brain by a cellular blue nevus of the scalp. A case report with light and electron microscopic studies. *Cancer*, **27** : 349.

WONG, C.K., GUERRIER, C.J., MACMILLAN, D.C. & VICKERS, H.R. (1971). An electron microscopical study of Bloch-Sulzberger syndrome (incontinentia pigmenti). *Acta Derm. Venereol. (Stockholm)*, **51** : 161.

Tumours of the Testis

LEUNG, T.K., LESBROS, F. & FEROLDI, J. (1971). Ultrastructural study of the Leydig cell. Apropos of a Leydig adenoma and a feminizing testis. *Arch. Anat. Pathol. (Paris)*, **19** : 303.

YANG, H., USHIJIMA, H. & FUKUSHIMA, T. (1969). Fine structure of embryonal carcinoma of the testis. *Kurume Med. J.*, **16** : 219.

Miscellaneous

GONZALES-CRUSSI, F. & CAMPBELL, R.J. (1970). Juvenile xanthogranuloma. Ultrastructural study. *Arch. Path.*, **89** : 65.

KAY, S. (1970). Comparative ultrastructural studies on three thymic lesions. *Arch. Pathol.*, **90** : 416.

LEVINE, G.D. (1973). Primary thymic seminoma. *Cancer*, **31** ; 729.

PRUNIERAS, M., GAZZOLO, L., DELESCLUSE, C., CHARACHON, J. & BOUCHAYER, M. (1968). Karyological and ultrastructural study of two cases of papilloma of the larynx in an infant. *Path. Biol. (Paris)*, **16** : 277.

WENTWORTH, P., LYNCH, M.J., FALLIS, J.C., TURNER, J.A., LOWDEN, J.A. & CONEN, P.E. (1968). Xanthomatous pseudotumor of lung. A case report with electron microscope and lipid studies. *Cancer*, **22** : 345.

Chapter 6. The chemotherapy of tumours

The aim of treatment with cytotoxic agents is to eradicate tumour cells as completely as possible without producing fatal toxic side effects. Although surgery and radiotherapy can in many circumstances destroy all localized tumour cells, they cannot prevent the spread of tumour cells to distant organs, or eradicate established distant metastases.

The results of experiments and clinical experience suggest that the chemotherapeutic agents presently available are most effective when the number of tumour cells in the host has been reduced to a minimum. Based on these considerations and depending on the extent of tumour spread, there are two logical approaches to the use of chemotherapy:

1. The curative approach

The aim of chemotherapy is to prevent and/or treat potential distant metastasis when the primary lesion has been eradicated by other means. In two tumours, choriocarcinoma and Burkitt's lymphoma, chemotherapy may be used as the sole curative agent. Both these tumours are associated with a recognizable and well-defined anti-tumour immunological response by the host, and are therefore rather exceptional.

2. The palliative approach

When curative treatment is not possible because of widespread local infiltration of unresectable organs or extensive distant spread, chemotherapy may be used to prolong life and relieve symptoms. Striking results of successful palliative chemotherapy have been obtained in cases of acute lymphocytic leukaemia, the malignant lymphomas, rhabdomyosarcoma and Ewing's tumour.

THE DEVELOPMENT OF CANCER CHEMOTHERAPY

Attempts to cure cancer by various forms of medication began far back in antiquity. Metals and their salts, acids, alkalis and plant extracts were all tried, mostly with little success and frequently with severe toxic effects on the patient.

Nitrogen mustard

It is a paradox of medical history that modern cancer chemotherapeutic agents originated from the development of poison gases during World War I. Sulphur 'mustard' gas, used during the 1914–1918 war, was found to have toxic effects upon the haemopoietic elements of the bone marrow. In the 1940s it was discovered that nitrogen mustards had similar suppressive effects on the marrow, and they were subsequently shown in clinical trials to have the same kind of effects on tumour cells. Research into the mode of action of these compounds has resulted in the development of new groups of agents with varying degrees of anti-tumour activity.

Folic acid

Widespread devastation and hunger during and after World War II stimulated intensive research into nutritional requirements and the causes of the various forms of nutritional anaemia. The central role of *folic acid* in the anabolism of nucleic acid was discovered, and in addition it was noted that certain non-naturally occurring pyrimidines were able to inhibit the growth of bacteria, even in the presence of folic acid. From this work came programmes for the construction of antimetabolites which blocked the synthesis of DNA by interfering with the metabolism of folic acid, or by introducing modified purines and pyrimidines into the DNA double helix. This resulted in the production of drugs such as Methotrexate ®, 6-mercaptopurine and 5-fluoro-uracil.

Subsequent developments in the group of drugs represented by the alkylating agents and antimetabolites have largely followed the incomplete and transient success of these drugs in the treatment of leukaemia and Hodgkin's disease. Despite various modifications of these drugs, based on known biochemical processes within the cell, it became apparent that these new agents did not have specific anti-tumour activity and hence were not curative.

The growing importance of cancer as one of the principal causes of death in the more technically developed nations (see p. 20) led to facilities for screening many substances for anti-tumour activity. The Cancer Chemotherapy National Service Centre in the U.S.A. has to date tested at least 250,000 compounds in model tumour systems. Using this type of approach, alkaloids of the periwinkle plant *Catharanthus roseus* (G. Donn) were found to have anti-tumour activity and this resulted in the production of vincristine and vinblastine. Similarly, the testing of filtrates of mould ferments for anti-tumour as well as anti-bacterial activity led to the discovery of actinomycin D, Mitomycin C® and Daunomycin®. Mass screening programmes also brought to light other drugs, not readily classifiable, which are useful in cancer chemotherapy, e.g. the terephthalanilides, hydroxyurea and the bisguanyl hydrazones.

The vital place of careful scientific observation in the development of chemotherapeutic agents is illustrated by Kidd's discovery (1953) of the growth dependence of certain tumours on exogenous asparagine. Unlike normal cells, certain tumour cells are unable to synthesize asparagine, or have a relatively poorly developed enzymatic mechanism for its synthesis. The growth of these cells depends upon an exogenous supply of asparagine, and l-asparaginase, by breaking down asparagine, deprives tumour cells of this amino acid. It is so far the only enzyme demonstrated to have an anti-tumour effect and the only cancer chemotherapeutic agent with an action based on a recognizable biochemical difference between normal and tumour cells.

The synthesis and testing of compounds prepared primarily for uses other than cancer chemotherapy are proceeding constantly throughout the world and the list of available drugs grows rapidly. Their multiplicity attests to our current inability to cure cancer by chemical means alone.

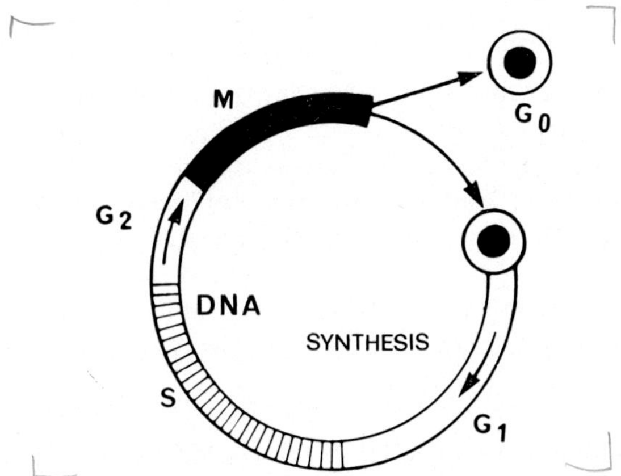

Figure 6.1. THE CELL CYCLE. The resting phase (G_1) is followed by synthesis (S) of DNA, a premitotic resting phase (G_2), mitosis (M), and division to form daughter cells which may enter a latent phase (G_0) or re-enter the cell cycle.

THE CELL CYCLE

Progress in therapy has also resulted from investigations of cellular kinetics. In most experimental tumours, and in the few human tumours that have been studied, most cells are in a latent phase (G_0), but some retain the capacity to replicate (Fig. 6.1). These cells are referred to as being in 'cell cycle', for in their case the resting phase (G_1) is followed by the synthesis of DNA (S), a premitotic resting phase (G_2), mitosis (M), and the appearance of daughter cells. The time for the cells to pass from G_1 to the appearance of daughter cells is defined as the generation time. Currently available experimental evidence indicates that in tumours of considerable size, the cycle is of long duration while in small tumours it is shorter.

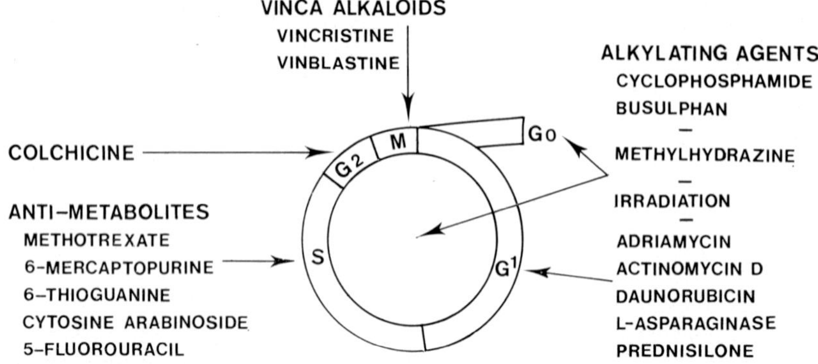

Figure 6.2. SITES OF ACTION OF CYTOTOXIC AND OTHER AGENTS, at various points in the cell cycle.

As a general rule, agents which interfere with the synthesis of DNA, its replication or the metabolic processes based on replication of RNA from DNA, are most toxic to cells which are in cell cycle. Agents which damage DNA through chemical cross-linkage are toxic to resting cells as well as those in cell cycle. Figure 6.2 illustrates the phase of the cell cycle in which the drugs exert their predominant effect in blocking the progression of tumour cells. Their cytotoxic action is mostly in 'S' and in the G_1–S interphase. It is clear that a knowledge of cellular kinetics may prove to be of considerable assistance in selecting the most effective combinations of cytotoxic drugs.

CLASSIFICATION OF CHEMOTHERAPEUTIC AGENTS

In this chapter the agents are given their commonly accepted pharmaceutical names rather than those based on their chemical structure; whenever alternative names are commonly used, these appear in brackets.

Cancer chemotherapeutic agents are usually classified on the basis of their origin or their probable mode of action. Most commonly both types of classification are combined, as in the following lists:

1. Alkylating agents, e.g. nitrogen mustard (Mustine®), cyclophosphamide (Endoxan,® Cytoxan®).
2. Anti-metabolities, e.g. methotrexate, 6-mercapto-purine.
3. Plant derivatives, e.g. vincristine, vinblastine.
4. Antibiotic derivatives, e.g. actinomycin D (Dactinomycin®), mitomycin D, daunomycin (daunorubicin, rubidomycin), adriamycin.
5. Enzymes, e.g. 1-asparaginase.
6. Miscellaneous, e.g. methyl hydrazine (procarbazine, Natulan®), hydroxyurea.

1. ALKYLATING AGENTS

This group contains some of the most active compounds in cancer chemotherapy, including substances which can be classified chemically into the following subgroups:

(*a*) Dihalogeno-alkyamines, e.g. nitrogen mustard, Nitromin®, Chlorambucil® and cyclophosphamide.

(*b*) Dimethanesulphonates, e.g. Myleran® (Busulphan®).

(*c*) Polyethylineimines, e.g. ThioTEPA, TEM.

(*d*) Di-epoxides, e.g. Ethoglucid®.

Mode of Action

Although the structure of the various alkylating agents is quite variable, they are nevertheless welded into a single group by their ability to alkylate a number of different functional groups under physiological conditions. The alkylating reaction consists of the addition of an alkyl group (e.g. CH3. CH2) either to anions or to nitrogenous bases in which an unbound pair of electrons is available to satisfy the electrophilicity of the alkylating agent.

Although alkylation of many anionic molecules, including water, may take place in the body, the anti-tumour effect results from the alkylation of nucleic acids. This consists of alkylating adjacent molecules of guanine situated at similar levels in the intertwining strand of DNA (Fig. 6.3). The ability of these drugs to damage DNA by chemical bonds permits them to

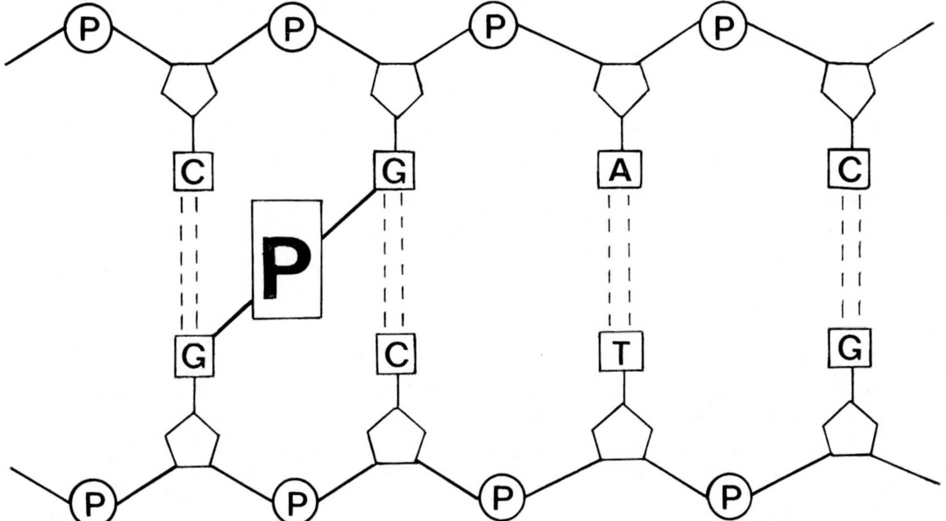

Figure 6.3. STRAND OF DNA, a diagram showing alkylation (P) of adjacent molecules of guanine (G).

act on resting cells as well as those in cell cycle. It will be apparent that the solubility of the agents, their ability to penetrate into the cell, and their retention within the cell, may all influence their potency.

Cyclophosphamide has proved to be the most effective of the family of alkylating agents. The drug was synthesized on the hypothesis that the phosphamide group would make it inactive until phosphamidases in malignant tissue liberated the active group, such as nor-HN_2, but current investigations have not confirmed that this is the mode of action, which illustrates that our knowledge of the *in vivo* metabolism and actions of the alkylating agents is far from complete.

Clinical Indications

Since they are not phase specific, they are capable of damaging the DNA in resting cells as well as in cells which are dividing. Cells in M and G_1 are most susceptible to their action. They are most likely to be effective in tumours with a high proportion of cells in prolonged G_1 or G_0, e.g. in large tumour masses which are growing slowly. In paediatric practice alkylating agents have been found to be most effective in the treatment of neuroblastoma, retinoblastoma, rhabdomyosarcoma, hepatoma, Ewing's tumour, reticulum cell sarcoma and in Hodgkin's disease Stage III and IV (see p. 198).

2. ANTI-METABOLITES

These are compounds with structural similarities to normal metabolites yet sufficiently different to interfere with cellular function when taken up into the appropriate pathway.

(*a*) **Anti-folates**

With the discovery of the essential growth-promoting activity of folic acid, it was suggested that antagonists to folic acid might retard the growth of leukaemia cells and this was proven by the successful use of the folic antagonist, aminopterin. A modification of the aminopterin molecule was later found to be clinically more useful and this is called Methotrexate® (Fig. 6.4).

Mode of Action

Folic acid is a starting point for a series of reactions, each of which results in a metabolite necessary for the synthesis of purine. In this process folic acid is enzymatically reduced to dihydrofolic acid and then to tetrahydrofolic acid which acts as a receiver and donor of extra carbon atoms. Transfer of a carbon atom from tetrahydrofolic acid is essential for the synthesis of purine, ribonucleotides, and serine, methionine and histidine, and for the methylation of uridylic acid to thymidylic acid. Methotrexate, by binding strongly to dihydrofolate reductase, prevents the formation of tetrahydrofolic

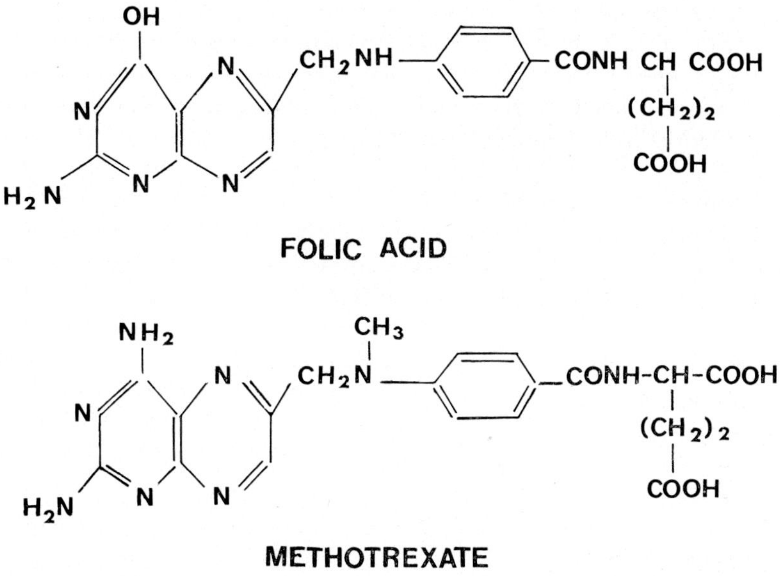

FOLIC ACID

METHOTREXATE

Figure 6.4. FOLATES AND ANTIFOLATES; (*a*) folic acid and (*b*) methotrexate, an anti-folate with a similar molecule, capable of combining with dihydrofolic reductase.

acid and thus interferes with the synthesis of nucleic acid. Citrivorum factor (5-foryml tetrahydrofolic acid) acts as an antagonist of Methotrexate by providing the N^5-N^{10}-methylene tetrahydrofolic acid, the formation of which has been blocked by Methotrexate.

Clinical Indications

Methotrexate is a 'cell-cycle' specific agent and hence most effective in tumours with a high proportion of cells going through the cell cycle and those in which the doubling time is short. In practice it has proved to be most effective in the treatment of patients with choriocarcinoma, Burkitt's tumour, malignant teratoma, lymphosarcoma, neuroblastoma and in high doses in bone tumours, particularly osteosarcoma.

(*b*) **Purine anti-metabolites**

These interfere with the synthesis of purines, being anabolized to ribonucleotide within the cell. This 'lethal synthesis' interferes with the growth of the tumour by producing defective mutant cells or by inhibiting replication. The most widely used purine antagonists are 6-mercapto-purine (6-Mp) 6-thioguanine (6-Tb) and azothioprine.

Clinical indications

Despite the major role of 6-MP and 6-Tb in the treatment of leukaemia, it has not been found useful in the chemotherapy of solid tumours or lymphomas. Azothioprine is mainly used as an immunosuppressive agent and, like 6-MP, is of little use in the treatment of tumours.

(*c*) **Pyrimidine anti-metabolites**

These interfere with the synthesis of nucleic acid, either by introducing 'lethal' metabolites or by altering the deoxyribose moiety of the pyrimidines, e.g. the same action as cytosine arabinoside.

Other *in vivo* effects have also been demonstrated, e.g. 5-fluorouracil inhibits the activity of thymidylate synthesase which is responsible for the methylation of uridylic acid to thymidylic acid. Cytosine arabinoside, in addition to inhibiting the reduction of the ribose diphosphate of cytosine to its deoxy form, also disturbs the production of DNA by inhibiting the action of DNA polymerase and this may be its most significant mode of action. The most widely used derivatives are 5-fluorouracil, 5-fluorouridine and cytosine arabinoside.

Clinical indications

5-fluorouracil and 5-fluorouridine are mainly used in the treatment of carcinoma in adults. Their results in the treatment of children with osteosarcomas have been disappointing. Cytosine arabinoside is mainly used in the treatment of leukaemia and malignant lymphoma.

3. PLANT DERIVATIVES

The vinca alkaloids extracted from the periwinkle, *Catharanthus roseus*, have proven to be particularly useful, and of the thirty alkaloids identified, vincristine and vinblastine have proved to be the most effective. Their exact mode of action is not known, but they produce arrest at the metaphase by interfering with the formation of the mitotic spindle, and with the turnover of RNA; either or both of these effects may be the basis of their anti-tumour effect, and cells in S, late G_1 and M are most susceptible to their lethal effect.

Vincristine has been of value in the treatment of Wilms' tumour, neuroblastoma, rhabdomyosarcoma, Ewing's tumour, retinoblastoma, hepatoma and malignant lymphomas. It is also used by some workers before or during diagnostic and operative procedures, with the object of preventing the dissemination and seeding of tumour cells (p. 24). Its wide range of effectiveness and relatively minor marrow toxicity make it particularly attractive.

Vinblastine, despite its minor molecular difference from vincristine, has been less useful and is primarily used in the treatment of Hodgkin's disease and histiocytosis X (see p. 220).

4. ANTIBIOTIC DERIVATIVES

The metabolism of tumour cells closely resembles that of normal cells and differs greatly from that of bacteria. It was therefore an unexpected finding that some antibiotics also have marked anti-tumour effects. The most important are those derived from the genus *Streptomyces*, namely actinomycin D and mitomycin C. Another derivative, variously known as daunomycin, rubidomycin and daunorubicin, is obtained from *Streptomyces coerulorubidus*. A modification of the daunomycin molecule by the addition of an —OH group has resulted in the development of a new agent, adriamycin which has already proved to be useful in a variety of tumours, including histiocytic lymphoma, Ewing's tumour, rhabdomyosarcoma, Wilms' tumour, carcinoma of the thyroid, and some cases of osteosarcoma.

Mode of Action

Actinomycin D seems to associate with DNA in such a manner that it inhibits the synthesis of RNA from the DNA template, and hence interferes with the synthesis of protein within dividing cells.

Mitomycin C seems to be able to crosslink strands of DNA in a similar manner to alkylating agents, and it also seems to be able to interfere with purine synthesis. It is thought that the mode of action of daunomycin is similar to that of actinomycin D. Cells in S are most susceptible to the action of adriamycin and daunomycin.

Clinical indications

Actinomycin D has been particularly useful in the treatment of Wilms' tumour (p. 527); both secondary and even large primary tumours may regress during treatment. There is also strong evidence that maintenance chemotherapy with actinomycin D during the fifteen months after removal of the tumour may prevent the occurrence of metastases. In one controlled study of patients who received maintenance therapy with actinomycin D, 86% were free of disease at two years, compared with 48% of patients who were given only a single course after operation.

Actinomycin D has also been used with variable success in the treatment of soft tissue sarcomas, particularly Ewing's tumour and rhabdomyosarcoma, and in teratomas and choriocarcinoma.

Mitomycin C is widely used in Japan where it has been reported to be useful in the treatment of hepatic tumours.

Daunomycin has been used with very limited success in the treatment of neuroblastomas and some soft tissue sarcomas, but compared with actinomycin D it has not found a secure niche in tumour therapy.

In contrast, the role of adriamycin in the treatment of tumours is being rapidly established, and it is now widely used in the treatment of the tumours mentioned above.

METHODS OF EFFECTING COMPLETE REMISSION

Complete remission has been achieved when the tumour cells have been eradicated or altered so as to return to a normal state. Theoretically this can be accomplished by the following methods:

1. *Direct and specific anti-tumour effect* by a chemotherapeutic agent, by surgery or radiotherapy.
2. *Eradication of the tumour cells* by a combined approach using surgery, radiotherapy and chemotherapy.
3. *Prolongation of the generation time* of the cells so that they become essentially dormant.
4. *Alteration of the infiltrative and metastatic properties* of neoplastic cells.
5. *Induction of host resistance* to the tumour.
6. *Correction of metabolic abnormality* which may bring the tumour cells under normal regulatory processes.
7. *Prevention of reinduction* of new malignant disease.

At present, the second is the only effective method without unacceptable impairment of the host's resistance. The other methods listed above are not yet available, although premalignant lesions can be removed surgically, and in choriocarcinoma and Burkitt's tumour, host resistance to the tumours appears to play a major role in cures obtained by chemotherapy alone.

THE SELECTION OF SPECIFIC ANTI-TUMOUR AGENTS

Although selection is still largely empirical, it should be based on some understanding of the likely cellular kinetics in the particular tumour. In general, it can be assumed that rapidly growing tumours have a large proportion of cells in cell cycle, during which they are actively synthesising DNA and may therefore be susceptible to drugs capable of acting on cells in cell cycle. The classic examples are leukaemia and malignant lymphomas.

Large tumours which present as solid masses generally have a long doubling time, and as only a small fraction of their cells are undergoing division, greater 'tumour cell kill' may be produced by agents which are not 'cell cycle specific' but are able to affect resting as well as dividing cells, e.g. the alkylating agents. In practice, most solid tumours fall into this group, even when they have become disseminated. It is possible that in solid tumours which are rapidly increasing in size, or with rapidly growing metastases, both types of cellular kinetics are present and a combination of a 'phase specific' and a 'non-phase specific' agent may be most cytotoxic. It is because our knowledge of the actual kinetics in solid tumours in man is rudimentary that the selection of chemotherapeutic agents for any particular neoplasm is still largely empirical.

The most effective agents in the treatment of particular tumours are set out in Table 6.1.

THE CONSTRUCTION OF A CHEMOTHERAPEUTIC PROGRAMME

In the treatment of children with a solid tumour it is necessary to plan a long term programme based on a knowledge of the natural behaviour of the particular tumour and on the available clinical and investigational data.

The important factors in planning such a programme are:

I The type of tumour.
II The extent of the disease.
III The availability of an effective agent for the particular tumour (as indicated in Table 6.1).
IV The known cellular kinetics of the tumour.
V Objective criteria for assessing the response to treatment.

I. THE TYPE OF TUMOUR

Without exception a histological diagnosis is a prerequisite for commencing treatment, and the usual choice of anti-tumour agent for each type of tumour is indicated in Table 6.1 and in Appendix III (p. 934).

II. THE EXTENT OF THE DISEASE

This is the most important practical point in planning a regime, and presupposes thorough investigation to demonstrate or exclude, as far as possible, the extent of local tumour spread and the presence of metastases.

(*a*) **Resectable tumour without obvious dissemination**

The primary role of chemotherapy is to prevent the growth of distant metastases, and this entails two kinds of regime:

1. *Pre-operative chemotherapy*

This provides an environment hostile to the seeding and possible multiplication of any tumour cells that may be dislodged during an operative procedure (p. 24). In the absence of a proven specific agent for this purpose, one of the currently available drugs with a wide range and little toxicity may be selected. From Table 6.1 it is apparent that vincristine and actinomycin D would appear to provide the best available cover during biopsy or definitive surgical excision. At present there is no evidence that pre-operative chemotherapy diminishes the incidence of metastases and improves the long term results of treatment. The danger of precipitating haematologic toxicity in

Table 6.1. Tumours and chemotherapy. The common tumours of childhood and anti-tumour agents usually selected for their treatment

Tumour	Chemotherapeutic agents					
	Agents most active on cells in cell cycle				Agents active on both resting cells and cells in cell cycle	
	Antifolate	Antipyrimidine	Plant derivatives	Antibiotic derivative	Alkylating Agents	Miscellaneous Agents
Wilms' tumour	—	—	Vincristine	Actinomycin D Adriamycin	?Cyclophosphamide	—
Neuroblastoma	Methotrexate	—	Vinblastine	Daunomycin Adriamycin	Cyclophosphamide	?Procarbazine
Reticulum cell sarcoma	Methotrexate	Cytosine arabinoside	Vincristine	Actinomycin D Adriamycin	Nitrogen mustard Cyclophosphamide	Procarbazine
Lymphoma	Methotrexate	Cytosine arabinoside	Vinblastine Vincristine	Adriamycin Adriamycin	Nitrogen mustard	Procarbazine
Rhabdomyosarcoma	—	—	Vincristine	Actinomycin D	Cyclophosphamide	—
Ewing's tumour	—	—	Vincristine	Actinomycin D Adriamycin	Cyclophosphamide	—
Malignant teratomas	Methotrexate	—	—	Actinomycin D Adriamycin	Chlorambucil Cyclophosphamide	—
Testicular tumours	Methotrexate	5-fluorouracil	Vincristine	Actinomycin D	Nitrogen mustard Chlorambucil Cyclophosphamide	—
Ovarian tumours	Methotrexate	—	—	Actinomycin D	Chlorambucil Cyclophosphamide	—
Retinoblastoma	—	—	Vincristine	—	TEM Cyclophosphamide	—
Hepatoma	—	—	Vincristine	Mitomycin C Actinomycin D	Cyclophosphamide	—
Osteosarcoma	Methotrexate	5-fluorouracil	Vincristine	?Adriamycin	Nitrogen mustard	—
Histiocytosis X	Methotrexate	—	Vinblastine	—	Cyclophosphamide	—
Brain tumours	Methotrexate	—	Vinblastine	—	Chlorambucil	—

the post-operative period, together with the possibility of administering marrow-suppressive drugs to a patient who may not have a neoplasm, make preoperative chemotherapy of dubious value.

2. *Definitive chemotherapy*

This appears to have been used in most successfully or relatively successfully treated neoplasms. In general 'non-cell cycle specific' agents are indicated, because solid tumours have long doubling times, i.e. a relatively small proportion of cells are 'in cycle'. Experience clearly indicates that intermittent combination chemotherapy is more effective than continuous chemotherapy.

Combination chemotherapy involves the administration of therapeutic doses of at least two agents, with different sites of action, thus producing maximum 'cell kill' without cumulative general toxic effects (Table 6.2).

Intermittent courses allow the recovery of normal cellular function, particularly in the haemopoietic and immune systems. The choice of drugs for combination therapy is based on the known effectiveness of the drug against the particular tumour, on the mode of action of the drug (Table 6.1), and its toxicity.

The simultaneous use of two drugs with similar sites of action on the cell is likely to lead to cumulative toxicity without added anti-tumour effect. Even with correctly chosen agents, combination chemotherapy is associated with a higher incidence of toxic side effects and should be undertaken in centres where there are adequate facilities for close surveillance of patients (p. 118) and for supportive measures such as transfusions of platelets and white cells. If these facilities are not available, the patient should be transferred to a centre where they are available. At present, the evidence for the

Table 6.2. Combination chemotherapy; tumours responding to combinations of two or more cytotoxic agents, indicating those commonly employed

Tumour	Agents combined
Neuroblastoma	Vincristine and cyclophosphamide
Wilms' tumour	Actinomycin D and vincristine
Reticulum cell sarcoma and lymphoblastic lymphoma	Vincristine, nitrogen mustard, procarbazine, prednisolone, cytosine arabinoside, vincristine, cyclophosphamide, prednisolone, vincristine and adriomyein
Teratomas and testicular tumours	Actinomycin D, chlorambucil and methotrexate
	Vincristine, actinomycin D, cyclophosphamide
Rhabdomyosarcoma	Actinomycin D, vincristine and cyclophosphamide
Ewing's tumour	Actinomycin D, vincristine and cyclophosphamide
	Vincristine, adriamycin, D.I.C.
Osteosarcoma	Methotrexate, vincristine and adriamycin
Histocytosis X	Vinblastine, prednisolone, methotrexate and cyclophosphamide

advantages of combination chemotherapy, compared with a single agent, is based on comparative rather than controlled studies, but is becoming more and more convincing.

The optimum duration of definitive chemotherapy is difficult to determine, but in general it should continue until the point in time when metastases from the particular tumour never, or virtually never, occur.

In Wilms' tumour this is generally at least twelve months from the time of diagnosis, or from the time of irradiation (or surgical excision) of a metastasis, and when no new lesions have appeared in the interim.

In neuroblastoma (p. 559) and the soft tissue sarcomas (p. 970), chemotherapy should be continued for at least two years because late metastases are known to occur in these tumours.

The role of chemotherapy

The primary role is to prevent the spread of the disease and to stop the growth of clinically non-apparent secondary deposits.

The secondary role is to potentiate the cytotoxic effects of radiotherapy on the cells of the primary tumour. Whenever possible chemotherapy should be given during the period of radiotherapy, for two reasons:

(i) Large infiltrative tumours usually spread to distant organs, but these metastases may not be clinically apparent when treatment is commenced. Valuable time is lost if chemotherapy is postponed until radiotherapy has been completed, for radiotherapy of the primary does not affect the growth of distant metastases.

(ii) Evidence from animal experiments suggests that destruction of tumour cells in the primary site may result in an increase in the number of cells entering the 'cell cycle' in secondary sites, and hence more rapid growth of the metastases, as well as greater sensitivity to chemotherapeutic agents.

The toxic effects of combined radiotherapy and chemotherapy can be held to a minimum by carefully monitoring the patient's blood cells (p. 117), and by reducing or omitting the next dose of the chemotherapeutic agent when indicated.

The appearance of additional metastases during maintenance chemotherapy indicates that the cells are no longer sensitive to the agents being used and alternative agents should then be substituted. The mode of action of the new agent should, of course, differ from the one to which the tumour cells have become resistant.

(*b*) **Disseminated tumours**

The place of chemotherapy in patients with disseminated tumours is controversial. An assessment of the situation in each individual, based on the clinical condition, psychological factors and family circumstances, is necessary. In some patients chemotherapy may clearly aggravate an already hopeless situation. In others, prolongation of life by the use of palliative chemotherapy is clearly desired by the patient and his family. Above all, the decision whether to use palliative chemotherapy should be made on objective grounds of maximum benefit to the patient or family, and should be free of personal bias.

Certain facts, based on the best available knowledge, may help in reaching a decision objectively. In infants less than two years of age, certain tumours (particularly neuroblastoma) may undergo spontaneous regression, even after they have given rise to widespread metastases. The advent of chemotherapy seems to have significantly improved the survival of children with these tumours. In metastatic Wilms' tumour there was a zero survival rate in 1956 when no chemotherapy was available, compared with 50% survival since 1962 when an integrated plan of treatment, including chemotherapy, came into operation.

Although chemotherapy may not cure the patient, it may significantly prolong life and maintain the patient in reasonable health during remission. This is best exemplified by steady improvement in the survival of children with acute lymphocytic leukaemia, reticulum cell sarcoma, lymphosarcoma, Stage III and IV Hodgkin's disease, rhabdomyosarcoma and Ewing's tumour. The most appropriate agent for the treatment of disseminated tumours is selected on the same basis as for operable tumours. Again, there is convincing evidence that combination chemotherapy is more effective than a single agent.

CRITERIA FOR ASSESSING RESPONSE

This is an essential aspect of chemotherapy. At present the sensitivity of a particular tumour to a particular chemotherapeutic agent cannot be predicted with certainty. Tumour cells may, by mutation or the development of new metabolic pathways, become resistant to anti-tumour agents. The effect on the tumour should be closely checked by using the best available indicators at frequent intervals. In addition to clinical examinations, serial radiological investigations of both the primary and possible metastatic sites are necessary, and estimation of the amount of identifiable tumour products (e.g. catecholamines (p. 539) in neuroblastomas, α-fetoglobulin in hepatomas and serum copper of Hodgkin's disease) may greatly aid the early recognition of recurrences.

TOXIC EFFECTS OF CANCER CHEMOTHERAPY

GENERAL TOXIC EFFECTS

Many of the side effects can be prevented by simple measures, the most important being frequent follow-up visits to the physician responsible for the chemotherapy, at intervals of not more than three to four weeks while anti-tumour agents are being administered. In addition to taking a history and performing a clinical examination, a full blood examination should be performed at each visit. Haematological side effects can be predicted and anticipated by charting the blood counts as part of monitoring the patients' response to chemotherapy (see below).

All chemotherapeutic agents suppress normal immunological responses and render the patient more liable to frequent and severe infections. Infections in children receiving chemotherapy should be treated intensively, with antibiotics when indicated, and close supervision. Infectious diseases such as chickenpox, measles, herpes zoster and herpes simplex can cause serious morbidity and even death, and their severity can be diminished by administering γ-globulin as soon as contact is confirmed. Vaccination with live organisms, particularly smallpox and measles, should be avoided during treatment.

Some side effects of anti-tumour agents may be prevented by their mode of administration; for example, the alopecia caused by vincristine can be reduced by applying a pneumatic head band, inflated to a pressure above systolic during injection and for five to ten minutes thereafter. The incidence and severity of toxic effects of cyclophosphamide on the bladder may be reduced by giving the drug early in the morning, ensuring a high fluid intake during the day, and by encouraging frequent micturition. The cardiotoxicity of daunomycin and adriamycin may be prevented by limiting the total dose of each drug to 550 mg/m^2.

SPECIFIC TOXIC EFFECTS

1. The bone marrow

All types of chemotherapeutic agents are toxic to the rapidly replicating cells of the marrow. Alkylating agents most frequently produce neutropenia, anaemia and, less frequently, thrombocytopenia.

Methotrexate and cytosine arabinoside frequently produce thrombocytopenia before neutropenia or anaemia. Vincristine causes neutropenia and anaemia, but virtually never thrombocytopenia. Vinblastine likewise seldom causes thrombocytopenia. Actinomycin D most often causes neutropenia and thrombocytopenia, and less often anaemia. Procarbazine may cause severe neutropenia and some degree of haemolytic anaemia. Overdose of any of these agents may result in temporary but severe aplasia of the bone marrow.

The appearance of haematological side effects of these drugs is an indication that the dose should be reduced or temporarily omitted. In general, the drug should be omitted if the Hb is less than 8 g/dl, the white cell count less than 1500/cmm, the neutrophil count less than 500/cmm, or the platelet count less than 50–70,000/cmm.

Reduction of the dose by 10–50% may be indicated when the Hb is 8–10 g/dl, total white cell count 1500–2500/cmm, neutrophil count 1000–1500/cmm, or the platelets 50–100,000/cmm. When combination chemotherapy is used, a falling white cell count or platelet count may be an early indication to postpone the next dose.

2. Immunological suppression

Intermittent dosage is less likely to cause profound suppression than continuous daily therapy. Both cellular and humoral immune responses are suppressed; the result is an increased tendency to infection and possibly an impaired immunological response to the tumour (see p. 64).

3. Gastrointestinal toxicity

Any chemotherapeutic agent may cause some degree of nausea and vomiting. Nitrogen mustard, cytosine arabinoside, actinomycin D and procarbazine almost always produce these side effects.

Constipation and colicky abdominal pain may follow the administration of Vincristine, particularly in doses in excess of 2·0 mg/m^2, but these may to some extent be overcome by the use of laxatives.

Methotrexate may cause mucosal ulceration, the most serious of gastrointestinal side effects. Although most obvious in the mouth, it may be widespread throughout the alimentary canal and cause severe diarrhoea. Ulceration of the mouth may be minimized by warning the patient of its occurrence, and advising that the next dose should be omitted if ulcers appear. Citrivorum factor, given intramuscularly, can be used as an antidote in the more severe cases. Methotrexate may also cause a hepatitis characterized by periportal necrosis of liver cells and elevated levels of SGOT. Mild degrees of hepatitis may be treated by reducing the dosage, but in the more severe grades the drug may have to be discontinued.

4. Renal toxicity

Cyclophosphamide seems to be the most common offender, and this usually takes the form of a haemorrhagic cystitis, possibly due to the excretion of the phosphamide radicle of the cyclophosphamide molecule. Preventive measures should be taken in all patients treated with this drug. If haematuria appears, and this is often the first sign of toxicity, the drug should be discontinued. The haemorrhagic cystitis may persist for weeks and even months after discontinuing treatment, and very rarely symptoms may be so intractable that cystectomy may be required.

5. Cutaneous toxicity

Vincristine, cyclophosphamide, and to a much lesser extent methotrexate and actinomycin D, may all produce alopecia, and this can be partially prevented by the use of a cranial tourniquet during and after administration of the drug. Alopecia is not usually an indication to reduce the dose, and the unsightly appearance can be greatly improved by wearing a wig.

Pigmentation of the skin similar to that seen in Addison's disease is an occasional side effect of myleran.

6. Cardiac toxicity

Daunomycin and adriamycin have been associated with myocardial fibrosis which may lead to irreversible cardiac failure. This side effect seldom occurs with a total dose of less than 550 mg/m^2, and it is recommended that this dose should not be exceeded. Cardiac toxicity at lower doses of adriamycin has been described in patients who have had thoracic irradiation.

7. Pulmonary toxicity

Myleran has been associated with diffuse interstitial pulmonary fibrosis and there is also evidence that methotrexate can cause an inflammatory reaction in the lungs.

8. CNS toxicity

Vincristine causes dose-related as well as non-dose-related toxicity. The former is characterized by peripheral neuritis and convulsions, and the latter by abdominal distension, inappropriate secretion of antidiuretic hormone and convulsions. These side effects usually occur 5 to 8 days after injection of vincristine, and may be fatal.

Absolute doses

In large children and adolescents, excessive doses may be administered if these are calculated on the basis of mg/m^2 rather than mg/Kg; in small infants the reverse applies. Vincristine should not be given in doses exceeding 3·6 mg, and actinomycin D in doses exceeding 600 micrograms; doses above these levels are usually associated with severe toxicity.

In the case of a large Wilms' tumour in a child less than two years of age, the weight of the excised tumour should be subtracted from the patient's preoperative weight, and the remaining doses of actinomycin recalculated, otherwise toxic effects from overdosage may occur.

MONITORING OF CYTOSTATIC DRUGS

All cytostatic drugs affect all regenerating cells, including the bone marrow. Overdoses, or too frequent administration of combination of cytostatic drugs, may have toxic effects on the haemopoietic elements of the marrow, which are reflected in peripheral blood counts.

ROYAL CHILDREN'S HOSPITAL

SOLID TUMOUR THERAPY

PAGE

RECORD TYPE 002

CLINICAL FLOW CHART

	Observation number	A	1	2	3	4	5	6	7	8
1,	Date	N								
2,	Therapy plan									
3,										
4,	Drugs 1.									
5,	2.									
6,	3.									
7,	4.									
8,	5.									
9,	6.									
10,	Temperature	N								
11,	Weight (Kg)	N								
12,	Height (Cm)	N								
13,	Primary Tumour site									
14,	Lymph nodes									
15,	Metastases									
16,	Liver									
17,	Spleen									
18,	Others									
19,	Hb. (gm%)	N								
20,	Platelets (x 10^3)	N								
21,	W.B.C. (x 10^3)	N								
22,	Granulocytes									
23,	Lymphocytes									
24,	Other (%)									
25,	B.M.A.									
26,	Lab. 1.									
27,	2.									
28,	3.									
29,	4.									
30,	5.									
31,	6.									
32,	Performance status									
33,	Toxicity 1.									
34,	2.									
35,	Response									

Acceptable character sets indicated by code in column A. N. denotes numeric values, SQ characters are 0, 1+, 2+, 3+, 4+, 5+ indicating degrees of abnormality or frequency. NP characters are NEG = negative or absent, POS = positive or present, ISQ = same, NAD = normal, QRY = query or equivocal, ABN = abnormal, IMP = improving, DET = deteriorating. Blanks acceptable in all sets.

Figure 6.5. MONITORING CHEMOTHERAPY. Form used to record effects of therapy with cytotoxic agents.

Patients receiving a single chemotherapeutic agent require a full blood examination (haemoglobin level, platelet count or an estimate of platelet number, total and differential white cell counts) at intervals of not less than three weeks. Toxic effects can be anticipated when the blood counts are charted on semi-logarithmic paper so that changes can be followed closely. It is also helpful to record the counts and the findings on examination on a specially designed therapy record, of which Fig. 6.5 is an example.

Patients receiving combination chemotherapy require a full blood count before the administration of each drug, and also on days five, eight and fourteen of each programme of combination chemotherapy. In general, the nadir of the white cell count can be expected to occur between day seven and day twelve and counts indicating recovery should become apparent by day fourteen. Again, trends in the blood counts can best be followed by charting the results. If the platelet and/or the white cell counts are falling rapidly, it can be anticipated that the next dose of cytotoxic agent will produce toxic effects, and by omitting it, serious toxicity can be prevented.

Patients who have recently received radiotherapy and are then treated with chemotherapy, require very careful monitoring, for they are particularly sensitive to chemotherapy; anticipation of trends in the blood count can usually prevent serious toxic effects.

It is important to recognize that all chemotherapeutic agents are also immunodepressants. No regular programme of immunological surveillance can be recommended at the present time, as there has been insufficient experience with the type and frequency of tests required to estimate accurately the patients' immunological status. However, if a child receiving chemotherapy is having frequent infections, fails to gain weight, or loses weight progressively without evidence of active tumour growth, investigation of both humoral and cellular immunity (p. 65) should be performed. Depression of either, or both, could be an indication for ceasing chemotherapy or a change in the drugs employed.

Bone marrow samples obtained by aspiration are not usually necessary in monitoring toxic effects of chemotherapy, but if there is any doubt whether changes in the blood picture are due to toxic effects of the drug or to infiltration of the marrow by the tumour, a specimen of marrow should be obtained, preferably by aspiration with a trephine needle, as soon as feasible.

RECOMMENDED READING

Cole, Warren H. (Ed.) (1970). *Chemotherapy of Cancer*. Lea & Febiger, Philadelphia.

Cooper, I.A., Rana, C. *et al.* (1972). Combination chemotherapy (MOPP) in the management of advanced Hodgkin's disease : a progress report on 55 patients. *Med. J. Aust.*, **1** : 41.

EVANS, AUDREY E. (1969). Chemotherapy of solid tumours. In *Pediatric Surgery*. (Eds. Mustard, W.T., Ravitch, M.M., Snyder, W.H. Jr., Welch, K.J. & Benson, C.D.). Year Book Publishing Co., Chicago.

FARBER, S. (1966). Chemotherapy in the treatment of leukaemia and Wilms' tumour. *J. Amer. Med. Assoc.*, **198** : 826.

FREI, E. (1972). III. Prospectus for chemotherapy. *Cancer*, **30** : 1656.

O'BRYAN, R.M., LUCE, J.K. *et al.* (1973). Phase II. Evaluation of adriamycin in human neoplasia. *Cancer*, **32** : 1.

SARTORELLI, A.C., & JOHNS, D.G., (1974). *Antineoplastic and Immunosuppressive Agents*. I. Springer-Verlag, Berlin, Heidelberg, New York.

SCHABEL, F.M. (1969). Cellular kinetics and its implications in cancer chemotherapy. In *Neoplasia in Childhood.* Year Book Publishers Inc., Chicago.

SUTTOW, W.W., VIETTI, T.J., & FERNBACH, D.J. (1973). *Clinical Pediatric Oncology*. C.V. Mosby Co., St. Louis.

Chapter 7. Radiotherapy

More than three millennia elapsed between the first description of cancer (in the Ebers papyrus, ca. 1500 B.C.) and the production of x-rays, but the first patient with cancer treated with x-rays was reported within three months of their discovery.

In the 1800s Conrad Roentgen was one of several scientists in different parts of the world who were investigating the electrical conductivity of gases, and Roentgen discovered a new kind of ray, produced by passing an electric current between electrodes enclosed in a glass tube containing a gas at extremely low pressures. The new rays were different from cathode rays which had been previously described, in that they caused barium platinocyanide to fluoresce brightly, even when the tube was covered with black paper. Further experiments showed that the rays were invisible, travelled in straight lines undeflected by magnetic or electrical fields, penetrated solid materials, and cast shadows on a photographic emulsion. He reported his findings to the University of Würtzburg on November 8th, 1895, and he was awarded the first Nobel Prize in Physics, in 1901.

Voigt of Hamburg is usually credited with the first therapeutic use of x-rays, on February 3rd, 1896, but on January 27th, 1896, E.H. Grubbe of Chicago sought medical advice from Dr J.F. Gilman for a rash on his hand, which had been exposed to x-rays. Dr Gilman suggested that the rays might be useful in treating cancer, and sent such a patient to Dr Grubbe on January 29th, 1896. The patient showed little improvement, and Dr Grubbe underwent several operations on his damaged hand, which was finally amputated.

The first cure of cancer by x-rays was described by Stenbeck in 1899, and the patient was still alive and well in 1925. In 1902 the first x-ray-induced cancer was recognized.

Natural radioactivity was explored by Becquerel (1896) and the Curies (1898), and the rapid progress in physics was soon reflected in the development of radiology and radiotherapy.

Artificial radioactivity was produced by Joliot and Curie in 1934, following the invention of the cyclotron (Lawrence, 1931). Later came the betatron (Kerst, 1940), megavoltage linear accelerators (Cockroft & Walton, 1947), and after 1945, atomic reactors which in turn yielded radioactive materials such as the nucleides of cobalt and strontium.

Radiations used for therapy today are electromagnetic emissions, ranging in wavelength from 40×10^{-9} metres to $0{\cdot}6 \times 10^{-9}$ metres, generated by x-ray machines or by artificial radioactive nucleides. Other radiations used in treatment include beams of electrons (β-rays), protons and neutrons.

The choice of the type and source of radiation is determined by convenience, availability, the site of the lesion to be treated, and by the need to protect normal tissues. The differences in type and source are mostly quantitative, but there are some qualitative differences which are also important. Megavoltage treatment is less absorbed in skin and bone, and so a larger dose can be given to deep-seated tumours with less damage to overlying tissues and bone. The biological effects of proton radiation are less dependant on the presence of oxygen than are x- and γ-rays.

The dose in radiotherapy means the amount of energy absorbed at a given point, and two units have been internationally accepted:

The 'Roentgen' (R) is the 'quantity of x- or γ-radiation such that the associated corpuscular emission per 0·001293 gm of air produced, in air, ions carry 1 e.s.u. (electrostatic unit) of electricity of either sign'.

The 'rad' (radiation absorbed dose), a more simply defined unit used for most clinical purposes, is defined as 'the quantity of radiation which, when absorbed, deposits 100 ergs of energy in 1 gm of tissue'.

For therapeutic purposes the quantity of radiation (i.e. the dose in rads) must be related to time, for example a single treatment of 2000 rads may produce effects similar to 6000 rads given in thirty fractions over a period of six weeks.

The biological effects of radiation are due to the ionization caused within the cell, and the results are partly due to direct interference with molecular structure, but mainly due to active radicles, e.g. hydroxyl ions and peroxides, which are formed when ionization takes place in water in the presence of oxygen. Several ionizations within a cell are required to cause its death.

The visible effects of radiation reflect the molecular damage; mitosis is suppressed and cells increase in size without division, producing giant forms. Cell populations subjected to radiation become depleted in numbers, and the surviving cells show increased sensitivity to irradiation, a prolonged intermitotic interval, and an increased incidence of chromosomal aberrations. Irradiated human tissues show a general depletion of cells, a relative increase in fibrous tissue, and infiltration by inflammatory cells. As an example, the effects on skin, depending on the dose, are:

(*a*) with low doses: epilation and dryness;
(*b*) moderate doses: delayed erythema, and
(*c*) with higher doses: vesication and loss of epithelium.

The more severe reactions are followed by the formation of a scar which is pale, atrophic, telangiectatic, and later scaly.

Sensitivity to irradiation varies from one tissue to another; bone marrow, lymph nodes and intestinal epithelium, being the most rapidly replicating, are most readily affected. The lens of the eye, the thyroid gland and the gonads are also vulnerable (i.e. highly sensitive), and also the central nervous system because there is no pool of proliferating cells to repair any injury.

All tissues and all tumours are susceptible to a variable extent, and the therapeutic effect depends upon the relatively greater susceptibility of rapidly proliferating tissues (tumour cells) and the relatively greater ability of normal tissues to repair injury. When the objective is cure, it is necessary to give the highest dose which can be tolerated by normal tissues. On the other hand, palliation and symptomatic relief can be achieved by a low or moderate dose sufficient to produce regression of the tumour by destroying a large number of malignant cells, accepting the fact that some cells will survive and later increase in number.

Control of the effects of irradiation is obtained by varying the dose and the duration of treatment. Repeated doses over a period of time are less injurious than a single large dose, and at the same time they progressively reduce the size of the surviving fraction.

The influence of oxygen tension is of considerable importance because absence of oxygen reduces the yield of active radicles produced by ionization. Anoxic tissues are therefore protected to some extent from radiation damage. Most tumours are relatively anoxic when compared with normal tissues, so that a general increase in oxygen tension will increase the damage to tumour cells. Conversely, inducing anoxia will reduce the sensitivity of normal tissues relative to tumour cells. Heat and cytotoxic agents also increase radiation damage, and metallic substances such as zinc oxide and mercurochrome on the skin will absorb radiation and emit caustic secondary rays which greatly accentuate the local reaction.

The aim of radiotherapy is simple: to irradiate a volume of tissue containing malignant cells to a dose known to produce a reasonable proportion of cures. The dose is made as uniform as possible throughout the volume treated, to avoid low-dose areas in which tumour cells might survive, and high-dose areas where normal tissues might be damaged beyond repair. A high dose in a tumour area must be achieved without damage to vulnerable tissues in the vicinity, for example the brain, spinal cord, eye, growing bone and teeth. The irradiation of large volumes of the lung, liver, kidneys, intestine and gonads, should also be avoided, and the inhibition of subsequent growth in any tissue is an extra hazard in children.

In standard techniques, treatment is given from two or more directions, thus concentrating the maximum irradiation dose and its effects where the fields intersect, directing or angling the fields so as to avoid vulnerable structures.

Filters of tin, copper or aluminium can be used to reduce high-dose areas, or to absorb rays of longer wave-length and yet allow the passage of shorter wave-lengths which are more penetrating. The objective is to localize the high dose to the tumour volume, and to ensure that the dose is distributed uniformly through the tumour.

The lethal dose for most tumours is of the order of 4000 rads in four weeks, and this dose is well tolerated by normal tissues. Some tissues are especially vulnerable. More than 2000 rads will cause serious damage if a large proportion of lung or kidney is included. Even lesser doses are injurious to particularly vulnerable tissues, e.g.

1000 rads will probably damage a growing epiphysis;
500 rads may produce opacity in the lens after some years;
500 rads will cause temporary epilation.

Damage to bone marrow depends on the amount of marrow irradiated as well as the dose; 500 rads to a large proportion of the marrow can be expected to reduce the peripheral blood count. However, vulnerable tissues can be protected by shielding with lead blocks, by the careful direction of angled fields, and when wide 'field therapy' involving the marrow is unavoidable, by monitoring the peripheral blood so that treatment can be discontinued if the neutrophils fall below 1200/cmm or the platelets below 75,000/cmm.

Shielding susceptible tissues is important. The testes can be enclosed in lead boxes during treatment, and when the pelvis is to be irradiated, one or both ovaries can be moved, at laparotomy (p. 194), out of the field to be irradiated.

Combining radiotherapy with cytotoxic agents has proved to be effective in some types of malignant tumours. The two methods are particularly appropriate and complementary when there is dissemination, by using radiotherapy for localized tumours and cytotoxic agents to reach metastases. The effects of the two methods are additive in that cytotoxic agents increase the damage to tissue caused by radiation. In some instances they are synergistic, for example the effects of 5-fluorouracil (see p. 106) combined with irradiation, produce greater effects than can be accounted for by simple addition.

The disadvantages of combining these two methods of treatment include the need to reduce the dose of irradiation to levels which are below the optimum for tumour control. Not only the local reactions are increased when both methods are used together, but general reactions such as nausea and vomiting may also be accentuated in combined therapy.

There are also theoretical disadvantages in that tumour cells are more sensitive to irradiation when in the phase of the 'cell cycle' (see p. 101), in which synthesis of protein or mitosis is occurring, and less sensitive in the intervening resting phases. Cytotoxic agents exert their effects at different points in the cycle, for example antimetabolites act during protein synthesis and alkylating agent during mitosis (see p. 102). Damaged cells may enter a resting phase and hence become temporarily insensitive to irradiation. On the other hand, the vinca alkaloids (see p. 106) cause more cells to enter the phases of nucleoprotein synthesis and mitosis together, and so may enhance sensitivity to other drugs and to irradiation.

Attempts have been made to synchronize cell division by giving colchicine to cause arrest in the metaphase and then using irradiation at a time calculated to catch more cells undergoing mitosis.

Combining cytotoxic agent with surgery and radiotherapy has achieved a remarkable increase in cures in Wilms' tumour (see p. 519), but on the other hand such combinations have actually decreased the survival rate in adult patients with ovarian or bronchial tumours.

The classification of tumours according to the degree of sensitivity to irradiation has proven useful; the degree of sensitivity for these purposes is defined as follows:

(i) High sensitivity: showing rapid regression with doses of 1500 rads,
(ii) Moderate sensitivity: regression with doses up to 4000 rads, and
(iii) Low sensitivity: showing a response to 6000 rads.

On this basis, the accompanying lists have been compiled (Table 7.1).

Table 7.1. Classification of paediatric tumours according to their sensitivity to radiation

High sensitivity	Moderate sensitivity	Low sensitivity
Wilms' tumour	Neuroblastoma	Osteosarcoma
Ewing's tumour	Retinoblastoma	Fibrosarcoma (most)
Lymphoblastic lymphosarcoma	Rhabdomyosarcoma	Chondrosarcoma
Medulloblastoma	Hepatoblastoma	Astrocytoma (grades I and II)
Acute leukaemia	Reticulum cell sarcoma	
Hodgkin's disease	Synovial sarcoma	
Follicular lymphoma	Astrocytomas (grades III and IV)	
Suprasellar germinoma	Fibrosarcoma (some)	
	Sacrococcygeal teratoma	
	Malignant melanoma	
	Ependymoma	
	Papilloma of choroid plexus	

Radiosensitivity is not synonymous with curability. The most sensitive tumours are those which proliferate most rapidly, and hence those which metastasize early arc the most malignant, and the least curable. Furthermore, different examples of the same tumour, e.g. reticulum cell sarcoma, vary greatly in their sensitivity; some are highly sensitive, while others prove to be very resistant. Co-ordination with other types of treatment, such as delayed amputation, permit the use of a high dose to a resistant tumour in a limb, e.g. an osteosarcoma, without being deterred by the delayed effects in an area which will subsequently be removed (see p. 752).

The dangerous or undesirable side-effects of radiotherapy are well recognized, and proportional to the dosage and the type of irradiation employed. Both short term serious damage to skin and soft tissues generally, and long term effects, occurred more frequently with orthovoltage radiation than with megavoltage techniques now in use. High dosage irradiation (more than 4000 rads) produces atrophy of the skin, and fibrosis of subcutaneous tissues and muscle. Heavy irradiation of bone leads to early closure of epiphyses, impaired growth, and fragility.

The effects of radiotherapy in the region of the hypothalamus and pituitary should be carefully monitored for alterations in the rate of growth and other pituitary functions.

Each tissue has its own particular expression of long term effects and radiation-induced tumours are of particular concern in children who, as survivors of a malignant disease, have before them many years of life in which a second tumour may appear. Even when the incidence of a 'spontaneous' second tumour (unrelated to treatment) is included (1 to 1·5%), the total incidence of second tumours, including those arising in irradiated areas, is less than 5%.

Skin cancer related to radiation is scarce and decreasing as radiotherapy for benign lesions is more rarely employed.

The frequent occurrence of a thyroid tumour following irradiation of the neck (p. 370) has predictably led to strict limitation of its use in this area, and to more effective shielding and lower dosages when unavoidable. However, the long term survival of many children with Hodgkin's disease in the cervical region depends upon 'upper mantle' radiotherapy (p. 198) in which the thyroid gland cannot be avoided. This also applies to irradiation of the neuraxis (p. 283) to prevent relapses affecting the central nervous system in children with leukaemia.

Sarcomas of bone may follow heavy irradiation (p. 526) and the risk is significant, particularly when the radiotherapy was given for a benign bone lesion. The onset of a radiation-induced bone tumour is typically delayed, for 7 to 10 years, and often develops in an atypical site for a bone tumour.

Soft tissue sarcomas induced by radiation, e.g. fibrosarcoma or less common types, are more rare than radiation-induced bone tumours. Leukaemia (p. 136) may follow wide field radiotherapy.

The hazards of radiation are well known, and carefully taken into consideration before deciding whether to use it all, and what form or dosage of radiotherapy should be employed for conditions which directly threaten life or carry a high probability of serious handicaps in later life. The relatively small risk is acceptable in such cases.

RECOMMENDED READING

DEELEY, T.J. (Ed.) (1974). Malignant Disease in Childhood. In *Modern Radiotherapy Series*. Butterworth, London.

EBERT, M. (1973). Molecular radiobiology. In *British Medical Bulletin*. Vol. 29. *Biological Basis of Radiotherapy* (Bleehen, N.M., Ed.) Part 1. p. 12.

LAMERTON, L.F. (1973). Tumour Cell Kinetics. In *British Medical Bulletin* Vol. 29. *Biological Basis of Radiotherapy*, **29** ; 1.

Chapter 8. Patients and parents

One of the most responsible and demanding aspects of caring for a child with a malignant disease is helping the parents to understand the nature and progress of the illness, its effects on their child, and the ways in which they can cope with the physical and emotional burdens it imposes.

Although many physicians, i.e. the family doctor, paediatrician, radiologist, surgeon, radiotherapist, and chemotherapist are necessarily involved in investigation and treatment, it is essential that only one, ideally an experienced clinician, should be in charge of the patient and bear sole responsibility for discussing with the parents the diagnosis and treatment, and for supporting and counselling them.

The possibility or likelihood of a malignancy should not be voiced too soon, so as to avoid unnecessary anguish if it is disproven, nor yet so late that the diagnosis is completely unexpected and all the more shattering. The parents' anxiety may commence as soon as symptoms or signs appear, but more commonly not until they learn that investigations should be undertaken without delay.

There is no easy way to tell parents that their child has cancer; euphemisms such as 'tumour', 'neoplasm', or 'growth' may be subconsciously adopted by the clinician to spare his own feelings, but only at the risk of causing misunderstandings. The diagnosis must, of course, be established beyond doubt before the parents are told, and when this certainty is unavoidably delayed, for example because of difficulty in interpreting histological findings, an interim explanation will be required.

THE INITIAL INTERVIEW

When the diagnosis is to be conveyed, both parents should be present and the interview should be deferred until this can be arranged. It is unreasonable to expect one to be able to give the other an accurate account of this discussion, and equally important is the strength each may draw from the other when both are present. The interview should be in complete privacy, in a room where the parents may remain as long as they wish.

At the first interview a simple statement of the diagnosis is all that is required. The possible causes, or details of treatment, should not be discussed, for experience has shown that the stunning effect on the parents usually makes it almost impossible for them to take in any complex information at this time. However, the need for prompt surgery may require immediate explanation.

The situation should not be over- or understated and a truthful straightforward statement of the diagnosis, in terms appropriate to the parents' level of understanding, is the best foundation on which to build the trust which is a vital and indispensable asset in management. Hope should not be denied, but any limitations of the treatment proposed should be pointed out.

The parents' initial reactions vary greatly. There may be disbelief and rejection of the diagnosis, anger and hostility, or feelings of guilt. The clinician must be prepared for and accept these reactions and should not allow them to disrupt his relationship with the parents. Even so, their anger or distrust sometimes leads them to transfer the care of their child to another doctor. More often their questioning of the diagnosis or the clinician's competence is short-lived and may even swing to the other extreme of adulation and unrealistic expectations.

Hostility towards the bearer of bad news is not uncommon, and yet another reason why both parents should hear it together and not one from the other, which might impair their relationship at a time when they are under considerable strain.

Feelings of guilt are almost always part of every deep emotional stress, and in the first frantic search for reasons why this has happened, many quite irrelevant but supposed short-comings may come to light.

LATER INTERVIEWS

A second interview with the parents a few days later is usually the appropriate time to go into details. The clinician should encourage the parents to ask questions, for these will reveal their particular anxieties and the kind of information they require, their needs and their individual strengths and weaknesses, as well as any baseless folklore they may have heard. As a rule, several lengthy interviews will be necessary, and parents who are confused by conflicting information, in magazines etc., or whose ways of coping include a thirst for the result of every test, will need to be given regular reports and, when justified, reassurance or at least the relief which comes from putting their fears and thoughts into words.

Specific points

Although the situation varies greatly from one patient to another, 'all cases are unique and very similar to others', and there are several matters which the parents usually raise, and if not they should be mentioned by the clinician.

A malignancy is no one's fault

With the exception of retinoblastomas (p. 423), multiple polyposis (p. 650) and xeroderma pigmentosum (p. 839), there is no certain hereditary basis for malignant disease, and feelings of guilt on this score should be dispelled by reassurance. Similarly, even if it may be debatable, it should also be firmly stated that the prognosis would not have been better if the diagnosis had been made earlier by seeking medical attention when signs or symptoms first appeared.

A thorough attempt will be made to control the disease and to cure it if possible
This attempt is warranted in practically every case, for unexpected and inexplicable regression of even advanced tumours is not unknown, particularly neuroblastomas. A reasonable level of cautious optimism is in order, and hope should not be completely denied unless or until all reasonable measures have been tried and failed.

Gaining the parents' trust is of prime importance
With it comes the receptivity which enables the clinician to give them some support, help them find the courage to carry on, or at least console them with the knowledge that everything feasible is being done. Without it, confidence and continuity may be lost, suspicions multiply, and may lead to despairing, fruitless journeys in search of unorthodox remedies.

All sources of assistance should be drawn upon
The parents may need additional support, from a medical social worker, a minister, and in a few instances from a psychiatrist. The social worker can provide therapeutic support as well as practical assistance with hospital finances, transport, accommodation, and other details so much appreciated by those under stress. Sensible friends or relatives should be asked to look after other children in the family and so enable the parents to spend as much time as reasonable with the patient.

The nursing staff can provide valuable information and assistance as well as nursing care
They should be kept fully informed of the results and implications of investigations, the prognosis, the plan of treatment, and what has been said to the parents. Only then can they discuss with the parents their child's progress, or answer questions effectively and without seeming to be evasive or contradictory.

Nurses are also in the best position to report on the patient's physical and emotional reactions to tests, treatments and parents' visits. They can also encourage (or when necessary discourage) the inevitable contacts in the ward between parents of other children, contacts which may be a source of helpful support, or needless anxiety to the patient's parents, depending on the personalities and circumstances.

Social and domestic arrangements are also important

Hospital care may not be required, for longer or shorter periods, e.g. during a remission, and it is most desirable that while the patient *is* in hospital, the medical and nursing staff should not undermine or take over the parents' role in ordering the child's life. The understandable temptation to overindulge the child should be pointed out, and the parents encouraged to continue or resume their usual roles.

The child may well be, at times, listless, apathetic or hostile as a result of investigations and treatment, and parents often need to be reassured of their competence to care for their child at home. Suggestions and guidance are welcomed and as a general rule the child's life should be as normal as possible as regards schooling, games, and all reasonable outings. The older patient may react in ways somewhat similar to the manner in which the parents cope with the illness, e.g. disbelief, hostility, anxiety, depression.

Every child should be given an adequate explanation

He should be told what is going to happen, in terms and detail determined by temperament and ability to comprehend. Precise estimates or promises concerning time, e.g. the length of stay in hospital, are best avoided; until five or six years of age 'a few days' is an elastic abstraction, and death itself is seen by many young children as being, in some strange way, impermanent. Many are too young to grasp the nature of their illness, but additional problems are presented by the discerning older child or adolescent who suspects or learns the nature of the illness. The answer to the question: 'Have I got cancer?' is primarily determined by the parents' wishes, and they should be warned that this may well be asked by a child of ten years or more.

Experience shows that evasive replies or prevarication are not good enough

One possible result is a double pretence; both parents and child feign ignorance to spare the other knowing that each is aware of the true situation; an unspoken but mutual understanding is another possibility. In some instances at least, open acknowledgement can lead to a warm and moving exchange of confidences. The parents should be encouraged, if they find it possible, to seek this frank relationship with an older child, bearing in mind that their best endeavours to keep the diagnosis from the patient may well fail because, in a hospital ward, patients learn from each other, and parents do, too.

Other children in the family should always be considered

Their reaction will depend on their age and temperament, but they are usually confused and hurt by their apparent neglect, and the loss of the time and interest their parents would normally have for them. This may cause them to resent the patient's preferential treatment and possibly to feel guilty about this resentment, an ambivalence which may be expressed in a variety of ways including hostility towards the patient or their parents. They should be allowed to participate in the family's grieving, for the realities are often less disturbing than their phantasies.

When treatment has failed, the care of the child in the final stages of the illness is at least as crucial as in any other phase

If there are no painful complications the child may be managed at home if feasible, and for as long as the parents wish. Close co-operation with the family doctor is essential, as well as clear understanding that readmission will be arranged as soon as it is requested.

Supplies of drugs or dressings should be arranged and replenished as required. Circumstances vary considerably, and death at home or in nearby hospital may, or may not, be more desirable than in a distant medical centre.

Treatment will not be pushed to the point where an uncomfortable existence is merely prolonged or made worse without prospect of improvement

The parents should be given this reassurance at some point, but not in the early interviews unless, as sometimes happens, they raise it themselves.

All pain can be relieved by one means or another and the child's death can be made free of pain

This promise can be made and must be honoured. It should probably be mentioned as soon as there is evidence that treatment will not be successful, because the prospect of an inevitably painful death is one of the chief causes of parents' distress. For children, analgesics in generous doses, hypnotics and tranquillizers, orally or in suppositories (see below) can be completely effective; it is only rarely necessary, as a last resort, to use injections.

The parents' feelings and behaviour may change in the late stages of their child's illness

Gradually, with the loss of hope of cure, their expectations usually contract from years to months, and then to weeks and days. The projection of survival becomes shorter, from the next birthday to the next party or family occasion, and the realization of this change in focus leads to grieving, or to a measure of resignation. Mourning, of a kind, begins well before death when the end can be foreseen. Sudden deep sighs, sleeplessness, irritability, or detachment and lack of interest, are recognized as normal reactions indicating a progressive and probably desirable separation in anticipation of the final loss. On the other hand, the clinician's daily visits, however brief and fruitless, may become more important to the parents.

Having previously been constant visitors, the parents may now not wish to see again a child who no longer resembles the one they would like to remember, and if this is the way they feel, it would be pointless to press them to come when the patient has ceased to benefit from their visits.

Whenever possible, the clinician they have come to know should be the one to tell the parents when death has come

It may also be desirable to tactfully ask for permission for an autopsy, even at this moment of distress, for there is usually no other opportunity. Although this may at first appear to be an extra imposition, permission is rarely withheld when a close relationship has developed and when the value of the information to future patients, and to the parents themselves, is pointed out.

The request should carry with it an offer of one or more further interviews, a month or so later. This is desirable regardless of whether permission for autopsy is granted, for it provides an opportunity to answer questions which have come from further reflection and to dispel any unfounded fears concerning other or subsequent children.

Survival not infrequently brings its own particular difficulties

As a result of improvements in treatment, many more children with a malignant disease are now surviving. Previously the quantity of life was the main concern, but problems which affect the quality of life have become apparent (Lansky, Lowman *et al.*, 1975). Some stem from strain and distress in the early stages; others result from changes in attitudes necessary when the prospect of survival becomes more certain.

The nature of the particular problems vary from one case to another: 'reattachment' to the child by parents who have withdrawn emotionally in anticipation of loss; return to normal discipline after over-indulgence; reappearance of temporarily submerged marital difficulties; 'drug dependance' in parents who have come to look upon continuation of chemotherapy as essential for their child's survival.

The patient may share embarrassment with his peers when he returns to them; other reactions include regression, school phobia, conflict with siblings, and irresponsible behaviour possibly the result of a belief in 'a short life but a gay one'.

The knowledge that difficulties of these types can arise later may help to prevent or at least minimize them by competent counselling and continuing support from the time of diagnosis.

When treatment is successful, and fortunately this is becoming more frequent, few of these grimmer aspects arise, but in other instances all of them must be faced and handled with the utmost consideration for the child and the parents. Although this involves a considerable amount of time and emotional strain, it is an integral part of the clinician's role. He will learn, and gain from the experience, and parents who have together weathered this strain may develop a closer relationship and greater mutual respect.

The following, written by a mother after the death of her four-year old daughter due to Wilms' tumour, emphasizes the importance of truth and trust.

'I cannot stress enough the extreme importance of telling the truth both to parent and patient. To the parent, the truth, no matter how bad it may be, is far easier to bear than the anguish of uncertainty. Human nature is such that the vast majority of people can face the most appalling despair and through this acceptance find the necessary fortitude to weather all that will eventually happen.

'To the child, the truth, I feel, is also of great importance. Naturally a young child will not understand the nature of the illness or the eventual outcome, but they should be told about the various types of investigations and procedures. Even a small child is much more 'adult' than we adults sometimes give credit. Because of this they are entitled to know the truth about pain; whether a procedure will hurt or not is the prime concern of a frightened child suddenly thrust away from his mother and the security of the home. To lie to a child will only lead to mistrust of hospital staff which, in turn, will lead to worry by both child and parent.'

RELIEF OF PAIN

Of the many preparations available, the following have proved to be extremely effective in relieving pain without the need of injections.

Suppository

Proladone® (Crooke's Laboratories) Suppositories contain 30 mg of oxycodeine pectinate. Half a suppository (15 mg) is suitable and effective in relieving pain in children less than five years of age; a whole suppository is required in older children.

Oral preparations

Two mixtures based on the 'Brompton Cocktail' are as follows:

<table>
<tr><th></th><th></th><th>A</th><th>B</th></tr>
<tr><td>Morphine sulph</td><td></td><td>10 mg</td><td>15 mg</td></tr>
<tr><td>Cocaine sulph.</td><td></td><td>5 mg</td><td>10 mg</td></tr>
<tr><td>Alcohol</td><td></td><td colspan="2">2 ml</td></tr>
<tr><td>Syr.</td><td></td><td colspan="2">4 ml</td></tr>
<tr><td>Aq. chlorof.</td><td>ad</td><td colspan="2">10 ml</td></tr>
<tr><td>Dose</td><td></td><td>5 or 10 ml</td><td>5 or 10 ml</td></tr>
</table>

A is suitable for children up to 35–50 Kg.
B is suitable for children over 50 Kg.

REFERENCES AND RECOMMENDED READING

Articles

BURGET, J. (1972/73). Psychological management of children with cancer, and of their families. *Paediatrician*, **1** : 311.

EASSON, W.M. (1972). The family of the dying child. *Ped. Clin. N. Amer.*, **19** : 1157.

EISEN, P. (1972). The dying child. *Australian Family Physician*, **1** : 469.
FLETCHER, A.B., MILHORAT, T.M., RANDOLPH, J.G. *et al.* (1972). The right to life and the right to die with dignity. *Clin. Proc. Child. Hosp.* (*Wash*), **28** : 233.
GREEN, M. (1967). Care of the dying child. *Pediatrics*, **40** : 492.
LANSKY, S.B., LOWMAN, J.T. *et al.* (1975). School phobia in children with malignant neoplasms. *Am. J. Dis. Child.*, **129** ; 42.
PAYNE, E.C. Jr, & KRANT, M.J. (1969). The psychosocial aspects of advanced cancer. *J. Amer. Med. Assoc.*, **210** : 1238.
RICHARDS, A.I. & SCHMALE, A.H. (1974). Psychosocial conferences in medical oncology : role in a training program. *Ann. Int. Med.*, **80** : 541.
SYMPOSIUM (1971). Dying children and adults. *Med. J. Aust.*, **1** : 1137.
SYMPOSIUM (1973). Care of the dying. *Brit. med. J.*, **1** : 29.
WAHL, C.W. (1972). The physician's treatment of the dying patient. *Ann. N.Y. Acad. Sci.*, **164** : 759.
WILLIAMS, H.E. (1963). On the teaching hospital's responsibility to counsel parents concerning their child's death. *M.J. Aust.*, **2** : 643.

Books

FEIFEL, H. (Ed.) (1969) *The Meaning of Death*. McGraw Hill, New York.
GROLMAN, E.A. (1967). *Explaining Death to Children*. Beacon Press, Boston.
HINTON, J. (1967). *Dying*. Penguin Books, Ringwood, Victoria.
KUBLER-ROSS, E. (1969). On *Death and Dying*. Macmillan, New York.
OREMLAND, E.K., & OREMLAND, J.D. (1973). The dying child. In *The Effects of Hospitalization on Children*. Charles C. Thomas, Springfield.
PROCEEDINGS of the National Conference on Cancer Nursing, U.S.A. (1974). American Cancer Society, New York.
REED, E.L. (1970). *Helping Children with the Mystery of Death*. Abingdon Press, Nashville.
ROBERTSON, J. (1970). *Young Children in Hospital*. 2nd ed. Tavistock Publications, London.
TROUP, S.B. & GREENE, W.A., (Eds). (1974). *The Patient, Death and the Family*. Scribner & Sons, New York.
WESTBERG, G.E. (1966). *Good Grief: A Constructive Attitude to the Problems of Loss*. Joint Board of Christian Education of Australia and New Zealand, Melbourne.

Chapter 9. Leukaemia

Leukaemia is by far the commonest neoplastic disease of childhood, accounting for some 35% of all paediatric malignancies, and about 40% when the closely related malignant lymphomas (see Chapter 10) are included. These two forms of reticulo-endothelial neoplasia differ so fundamentally from all other paediatric neoplasms, in their mode of presentation, in their pathology and especially in treatment, that their descriptions in this and the following chapter differ from the pattern used in those dealing with solid tumours.

DEFINITION

Leukaemia seems to be a disease which is well understood until one attempts to define it. The term 'leukaemia' (white blood), was introduced by Virchow in the 1840s following its recognition as an entity after a study of patients now regarded as examples of chronic myeloid leukaemia. Like many so-called 'blood disorders', leukaemia is not really a disease of the blood but of the blood-forming tissues. It has been defined as a 'fatal disease of unknown cause characterized by proliferation of leukocytes and their precursors', but research has been steadily changing this picture. Proliferation may be limited to primitive leucocytes in the bone marrow, and other haemopoietic tissues, not in the blood; evidence is mounting in favour of a viral aetiology, as in animal leukaemias; although death is still the expected outcome, in a small but growing proportion of leukaemic children, treatment has produced complete remissions persisting for more than ten years, and perhaps indefinitely.

So, to paraphrase the conclusions of Dameshek & Gunz (1964), leukaemia can be appropriately defined as a generalized neoplastic proliferation, slow or rapid, of one of the leukocytopoietic tissues, often associated with abnormal white blood cell counts and leading eventually to anaemia, thrombocytopenia and usually death.

ETIOLOGY

The cause of human leukaemia remains unknown, but experimental and clinical research over the past decade have provided a number of clues. Despite differences between animal and human leukaemias, there is much to suggest that the development of leukaemia in man may require three factors, as it does in mice:

1. A genetic or constitutional predisposition.
2. A viral or other infective agent.
3. One or more conditioning or trigger factors.

1. Genetic or constitutional factors

A family history of leukaemia or lymphoma occurred in 8·5% of 200 children with acute leukaemia in the Index Series, and in 8·1% of a similar series in Denmark, compared with 0·5% in controls. There are a number of reports of multiple cases in sibships though this is rare, occurring in only two of more than 700 affected families in the Index Series. When leukaemia develops in a monozygotic twin, there is one chance in five that the other twin will also develop leukaemia, usually within weeks.

In Down's syndrome the frequency of leukaemia is at least twenty times that in controls, and there is an increased risk of leukaemia in children with chromosome D group trisomy, C group abnormalities, Klinefelte's syndrome, aplastic and Fanconi's anaemia, Bloom's syndrome, hereditary ataxia-telangiectasia and other immunoglobulin disorders. A feature common to all of these is some abnormality of the chromosomes, e.g. deficiencies, trisomy and breakage.

2. Viruses

RNA viruses have been shown to be the cause of certain leukaemias in animals, particularly in fowls and mice. In human leukaemia, indications of a similar viral basis are steadily accumulating, e.g. the identification of specific leukaemia antibodies. Clustering of cases in time and place, and reports of leukaemia in cattle and cats in relation to human cases, have raised the question of infectiousness, but evidence from exhaustive epidemiological studies does not support the transmission of human leukaemia from case to case or between species.

At least one animal leukaemia is due to a virus transmitted via breast milk, but there are almost no reports of leukaemia in the offspring of pregnant women with leukaemia, and at least 10% of the Index Series of leukaemia children were never even put to the breast. Nevertheless the search for a viral cause of human leukaemia has been stimulated afresh by the finding that the Epstein-Barr virus is the cause of infectious mononucleosis, and possibly of Burkitt's lymphoma, too.

3. Conditioning factors

(*a*) *Irradiation*

Ionizing irradiation may be leukaemogenic at any age, an effect which is dose-related as shown beyond doubt by studies following the effects of the atomic bombs in Hiroshima and Nagasaki. It is also illustrated by the increased risk of leukaemia in persons who operate x-ray machines, unless appropriate protective measures are taken, and in patients irradiated for ankylosing spondylitis, though in this group constitutional predisposition may also be a factor.

There is evidence that irradiation of the thymus or the neck in early childhood, once a common practice in some centres, causes an increase in the incidence of leukaemia or cancer (p. 370); radiotherapy with nucleides such as ^{32}P and the early forms of radio-iodine has been suspected to produce the same effect, and so has high-dosage irradiation of a solid tumour (p. 126). This may have been a factor in the development in the Index Series of chronic myeloid leukaemia in a boy, five to six years after a cerebral astrocytoma was successfully irradiated with 6900 rads.

There have been extensive studies of the effect on the fetus of prenatal diagnostic radiography; if it does increase the incidence of neoplasia, this danger is probably limited to fluoroscopy in the first half of pregnancy. Of several hundred children with leukaemia treated at this hospital, less than 1% had a history even suggesting the possibility of prenatal irradiation as an etiological factor.

(*b*) *Chemical and hormonal factors*

Benzene is the only chemical agent definitely known to lead to leukaemia, in some cases after an intermediate phase of aplastic anaemia. Other chemicals which can cause aplastic anaemia have been incriminated as leukaemogenic, e.g. phenylbutazone, chloramphenicol and chlorpromazine, but the evidence against them is unconvincing. Recently the androgen oxymetholone has also been suspected, and this possibility is less easily dismissed for in experimental animals the development of leukaemia can be influenced by various steroids—corticoids, androgens and oestrogens.

The age distribution curve, with peaks in late infancy and pre-school years, around puberty and after the menopause, also suggests a hormonal influence in human leukaemia. In our epidemiological study of 200 children, there was an unexpected frequency of diabetes mellitus in the family history, and it is also possibly relevant that major emotional disturbances in the child commonly occurred four to ten months before the diagnosis of leukaemia.

INCIDENCE

Total incidence

Of 1390 children with malignant disease seen at this hospital between 1950 and 1969, 505 (36%) had leukaemia. The incidence in relation to the number of hospital admissions is also a useful index, in spite of the difficulties involved when admission policy is changed. In this hospital, approximately one of every 320 new admissions is for leukaemia; figures ranging from 1 in 250 to 1 in 800 have been reported from other paediatric hospitals. Whether the real incidence of leukaemia has increased in recent years is still not certain.

Age incidence

Leukaemia occurs at all ages, but in early childhood there is a relatively high incidence, in keeping with the general pattern of paediatric malignancies (p. 15). In fact, the incidence is higher in the first five years of life than at any stage until after the age of fifty. In this hospital 64% (201 of 316) of children with acute leukaemia were aged five years or less at the time of diagnosis, a figure almost identical with a large German series (Optiz, 1954). But only 11 of these 201 children were less than twelve months old, compared with 44 aged one year, 40 aged two years, 55 aged three years, 31 aged four years, and 20 aged five years. The obvious peak at three years of age is found in all large series reported, except (until quite recently) in American Negroes. The relatively low incidence in those less than twelve months of age reflects a decline in the incidence in young infants, a trend first noted in the 1940s. A very minor peak is also discernible in early puberty (Fig. 9.1, facing page 140). These various incidences within the paediatric age group have not yet been adequately explained.

Sex incidence

In all types of adult leukaemia, males outnumber females, but in childhood, as would be expected, the sex distribution is more nearly even. Of 316 patients with acute leukaemia in the Index Series, 165 were males and 151 females. In the earliest years there was a tendency to a female preponderance, but after the age of six years males outnumbered females by 5 : 4 (21 to 16).

CLASSIFICATION

It is clinically useful to distinguish a number of forms of leukaemia, although the terms applied to them are sometimes confusing. A practical classification (Table 9.1) is based on two main criteria:

1. the clinical picture and its natural course, and
2. the predominant type of leukaemic cell.

Both are essential for the full differentiation of the various forms.

1. The clinical picture and course

The distinction between acute and chronic leukaemia can no longer be made solely on the basis of an expected survival time. In Australia, almost all children with acute leukaemia receive sufficient treatment to give them a

Table 9.1. Leukaemia. Classification of types of leukaemia seen in childhood

A. *Acute leukaemia*
  (1) Lymphatic (lymphoblastic, lymphocytic) (Fig. 9.2)
  (2) Myeloid
    myeloblastic (granulocytic) (Fig. 9.3),
    promyelocytic (Fig. 9.4)
    myelomonocytic (Fig. 9.5)
  (3) Monocytic (monoblastic) (Fig. 9.6)
  (4) ? Stem cell (unclassified).

B. *Chronic myeloid leukaemia* (granulocytic)
  (1) Juvenile form (Fig. 9.8)
  (2) Adult form (Ph^1—positive)

C. *Miscellaneous group of uncommon forms*
  (1) Erythroleukaemia (di Guglielmo's disease) (Fig. 9.7)
  (2) Myelofibrosis with myeloid metaplasia
  (3) Eosinophilic leukaemia
  (4) Haemophagic reticulosis (Farquhar & Claireaux) (Fig. 9.9)

median survival time of the same order as for chronic leukaemia, so clinical and cytological criteria are both required.

Acute leukaemia has a short clinical history, of four weeks' median duration, with many primitive cells in the bone marrow, and a natural course (without treatment) of only a few months; chronic leukaemia has a longer history, many well differentiated leukaemic cells in the blood, and a natural course usually exceeding one year.

In childhood, no less than 19 out of every 20 cases of leukaemia are of the acute form. In our series, 96% of 259 consecutive cases were classified as acute (including a few which others might call subacute) and only 2·7% were chronic. This proportion is in marked contrast to adult leukaemia, in which 40–50% of cases are of the chronic form.

2. The predominant type of cell

Histochemical techniques, in addition to the Romanowsky stains, have made it possible to differentiate the various cell types in 99% of cases. Again, the distribution of cell types in children differs greatly from adults. Of our 247 acute cases, 201 (81%) were lymphatic, 40 (16%) myeloid, and the remainder were rare types such as monocytic and erythro-leukaemia, whereas acute cases in adults are predominantly myeloid. The few chronic cases in this hospital (2·7% of all leukaemias) were mostly chronic myeloid leukaemia. Chronic lymphatic leukaemia, so common after the age of fifty years, almost never occurs in childhood.

ACUTE LEUKAEMIA

There is relatively little clinical difference between the various cytological types of acute leukaemia. With the myeloid and monocytic forms, children are more likely to have infection in the gums, mouth, skin, anus and vulva, and much less likely to have enlarged lymph nodes, which are more common in the lymphatic form. In general, the three cytological types of acute leukaemia are clinically indistinguishable and will be discussed together.

CLINICAL FEATURES

Symptoms

The duration of symptoms attributable to leukaemia varies from only two or three days to as long as six months before the diagnosis is established. The median duration in the Index Series was four weeks, compared with six weeks in earlier reports, probably reflecting earlier diagnosis in the present leukaemia-conscious era.

Symptoms may develop abruptly, e.g. over a matter of days (15% of cases), but in the great majority the onset is insidious, and often the parents have difficulty in recalling when symptoms began.

The earliest symptoms are non-specific and usually fail to arouse suspicion. In 75% there is one or more of the following; anorexia, malaise, lassitude, fatigue, weakness and irritability (see 'malignant malaise', p. 549) mainly due to the gradual development of anaemia, with or without subclinical infection.

Fever, pain in the limbs, and pallor usually appear somewhat later. They are more likely to prompt investigations leading to the diagnosis, but these symptoms are absent in a quarter of the cases. Pain may arise in the larger joints or in bones, and in other tissues of the limbs, back, chest, neck or head, and may cause a toddler to stop walking.

Haemorrhage, usually described as a characteristic feature, develops eventually in most cases, but in our series, bleeding was absent until a late stage in 70% of cases. Ecchymoses and petechiae in skin and mucosae, epistaxis, and excessive bleeding after minor procedures or trauma are the commonest forms.

The typical symptom complex which most often leads parents to seek medical advice is a febrile illness with pain, pallor and bleeding. There may be a persistent low fever or intermittent bursts of high fever. The accompanying impairment of the immune system in children with untreated leukaemia makes them abnormally susceptible to micro-organisms, especially viruses, so that they commonly present with symptoms of infection in the upper or lower respiratory tract, or in the bowel.

Other less frequent symptoms are headache and vomiting, due to infiltration of the nervous system (5 % of all cases), puffy eyes and face (especially in infants), sore mouth and gums, infective and leukaemic skin lesions, and painless swelling of the parotid glands or the testes.

Signs

Now that the diagnosis of acute leukaemia is commonly made at an earlier stage in the course of the disease, the clinical picture regarded as characteristic at the time of diagnosis has changed. In the earliest stage, the symptoms may not suggest the diagnosis, and clinical examination may be essentially normal. The first intimation often comes from the results of blood tests or x-rays undertaken because of an infection or some other complicating disorder. Our own studies indicate that the prognosis is more favourable in cases diagnosed at such an early stage.

The commonest signs are enlargement of lymph nodes and the spleen, although the parents in four cases out of five have not been aware of such enlargement, even when it was in the cervical region.

Lymphadenomegaly

The overall incidence in childhood leukaemia (77 %) is much greater than in adults, and in the lymphatic form the incidence (85 %) is twice as high as in myeloid cases (Table 9.2).

Two special forms of lymphadenomegaly occur infrequently in childhood: (*a*) *A mediastinal tumour*, which may involve the thymus, is found on

Table 9.2. Differentiation of lymphatic from other forms of acute leukaemia

Feature	Acute lymphatic leukaemia	Acute myeloid, monocytic and erythro-leukaemia
Enlarged lymph nodes		
cervical	85%	41%
axillary	77%	35%
inguinal	75%	24%
Splenomegaly	80%	70%
Gingival and skin infection	rare	30%
W.C.C.> 50,000/cmm	14%	38%
Neutropenia	Almost always	Often
Blastaemia >3% or >100/cmm	75%	94%
Blast count in the bone marrow	93·5% (median)	51% (median)
Remission induction rate	95%	60+%
Remission maintenance	Relatively good	Usually short-lived

x-ray examination in 5% of children with acute leukaemia and more frequently in generalized lymphosarcoma. It may be associated with cough, dyspnoea and signs of mediastinal compression which may threaten life (see p. 445).
(*b*) *Mikulicz' syndrome*, i.e. bilateral enlargement of the lacrimal, parotid and submandibular salivary glands, occurs with a variable degree of related lymphadenomegaly and tenderness, mainly in lymphatic leukaemia.

Splenomegaly
The spleen is usually enlarged and soft. The lower edge is palpable in at least 80% of lymphatic cases, commonly to 2–6 cm below the costal margin, but myeloid cases tend to have less splenomegaly. It is worth noting that the spleen is usually not palpable until it is at least twice the normal size, that it lies nearer the flank in small children, and that enlargement is detectable earlier by bimanual palpation.

Hepatomegaly
In leukaemia the liver is enlarged almost as often as the spleen. Its lower edge is not usually as far below the costal margin; when the degree of hepatomegaly is disproportionately large, non-leukaemic causes such as viral infection, malnutrition and congestion should be considered.

Haemorrhage is usually in the form of large or small ecchymoses, petechiae in the skin and mucosae, and epistaxes. Less often there is bleeding from the mouth or into the retina, excessive bleeding following extraction of teeth, tonsils or adenoids and, occasionally, bleeding from the urinary, genital or gastro-intestinal tract. When the leukocyte count is above 200,000/cmm, there is a special risk of serious intracranial haemorrhage and of disseminated intravascular coagulation with hypofibrinogenaemia, particularly in acute myeloid leukaemia. Although in many cases the diagnosis of leukaemia is now made before any bleeding is apparent, in others it is the most dramatic and serious feature, and especially in young children a severe haemorrhage may cause shock, cardiac failure, coma and even convulsions.

Lesions in the mouth and skin develop in a third of the patients with myeloid and monocytic leukaemia and can be diagnostically helpful (Table 9.2). The gums may be swollen and spongy and there may be erythema with ulcerative stomatitis. Infective skin lesions occur most commonly around the mouth, vulva and anus, often becoming haemorrhagic, and occasionally reddish-purple nodular lesions of leukaemic infiltration are seen.

Bone tenderness over the sternum in children occurs less than in adults; in children, tenderness over the ends of the long bones and around the joints is often misleading, especially if the joints are also swollen, suggesting a rheumatic disorder. Radiological changes in bones (see p. 742) may be present without bone pain or tenderness, and vice versa.

Other signs infrequently found at presentation include; papilloedema, cranial nerve palsy, spinal root signs and other evidence of infiltration of the central nervous system; a 'chloromatous' tumour, most commonly involving the orbit (see p. 409); hyperuricaemia with renal failure; massive renal enlargement with little or no impairment of renal function; hypercalcaemia; and cardiac failure, but a 'haemic' systolic murmur associated with anaemia is a common and unimportant finding. As acute lymphatic leukaemia may be part of the clinical picture of a child with lymphosarcoma, signs of the latter disease will also occasionally be present, e.g., pleural effusion, enlarged thymic shadow (p. 446), abdominal mass (p. 633).

INVESTIGATIONS

1. *A full blood examination* is often diagnostic, and almost always abnormal, though not invariably so. Anaemia is found at presentation in 90% of cases, and thrombocytopenia nearly as often.
(*a*) *The anaemia* is typically normocytic and aregenerative; the reticulocyte count is usually low or at most 2–3%. The haemoglobin value may be at almost any level and is below 6 g/dl in 25% of patients.
(*b*) *The platelet count* is sometimes normal at presentation, particularly in the myeloid form, but thrombocytopenia is usually evident on the blood film, commonly less than 50,000 and sometimes as low as 1000/cmm.
(*c*) *The total white cell count* at the time of presentation varies widely. The normal range is 5000–15,000 cmm; in 100 consecutive cases the count was below normal in 28%, normal in 27% and above normal in 45%. Very high counts (above 50,000 and up to 900,000/cmm) occurred in only 14% of our lymphatic cases, but in nearly 40% of the myeloid cases (Table 9.2).
(*d*) *The differential white cell count* usually shows relative and absolute neutropenia, but this is less frequently seen in the myeloid than in the lymphatic form. Characteristic leukaemic blast cells are found in the blood in diagnostic numbers (more than 100/cmm or more than 3%) in 80% of cases; when they are not present the total white cell count is usually below normal.
2. *Aspiration of bone marrow* is essential in arriving at the diagnosis in many patients, and desirable in all. In addition to providing a definitive diagnosis, it is often essential to exclude alternative diagnoses and it provides material in which to identify the cytological type of leukaemia. The bone marrow is stuffed with leukaemic blast cells in almost all lymphatic cases (median count 93·5% of nucleated cells), but less so in myeloid cases (median count 51%). Marrow blast cell counts of at least 15% in myeloid cases and 25% in lymphatic cases are usually required to establish a diagnosis of acute leukaemia. In a few instances marrow aspiration fails to show any diagnostic features of the disease in the early stages. Histochemical as well as Romanowsky stains are used to differentiate the types of acute leukaemia (p. 145).
3. *Radiological survey of the whole skeleton* provides useful information on

the extent of bone involvement, and was positive at the time of presentation in 24% of cases in the Index Series. It is also helpful in excluding other diseases (see below).

An x-ray of the chest may reveal enlargement of the thymus or mediastinal lymph nodes, a pleural effusion or pulmonary infection.

4. *Lumbar puncture* is required if there are any indications of CNS disease, and it is part of the routine in some leukaemia clinics.

5. *Specimens for culture*, e.g. blood, urine and swabs from the nose, throat, etc. for the detection or exclusion of infection are required.

6. *Tests for disseminated intravascular thrombosis* (estimation of plasma prothrombin, partial thromboplastin time, fibrin split products in plasma, factor V assay, etc.) are indicated, particularly in myeloid leukaemia, when there is an unexpected degree of thrombocytopenia with haemorrhage.

DIAGNOSIS

In many cases the diagnosis of acute leukaemia can be made provisionally from the clinical picture alone, and sometimes from the radiological findings in the skeleton, but it cannot be established without haematological investigation. In the later stages, this usually presents no difficulty. If the blood picture is not typical or diagnostic, confirmation is obtained by bone marrow aspiration.

Urgency in making the diagnosis has been considerably heightened by therapeutic advances over the past two decades. If diagnosis is delayed until the later stages of the disease, treatment cannot be expected to do more than produce transient improvement, and it may not achieve even this.

For the best prospect of a complete remission, prolonged for several years, with the possibility of eventual cure in some cases, the diagnosis must be made early.

To quote Carl Smith (1972), 'the most important feature of the diagnosis . . . is the critical evaluation of the clinical picture so that leukemia is suspected and the peripheral blood and the bone marrow are examined'.

Any one or more of a number of clinical features should lead the clinician to think of the possibility of leukaemia, and this makes a full blood examination mandatory unless convincing evidence of an alternative diagnosis explains these features. They include persistent general ill health with 'malignant malaise' (see p. 549); pallor with suspected anaemia; bleeding from any site; bone pain or a rheumatic syndrome; persistent or recurrent infection or fever; gingivitis and/or ulcerated throat; enlargement of spleen or lymph nodes; mediastinal pressure syndrome; unusual skin infections; signs of raised intracranial pressure. In some cases characteristic lytic or periosteal lesions in a skeletal x-ray survey similarly call for a full blood examination. Leukocytosis is absent in half the cases and the blood may not show pancytopenia nor even blast cells, but it will nearly always show at least

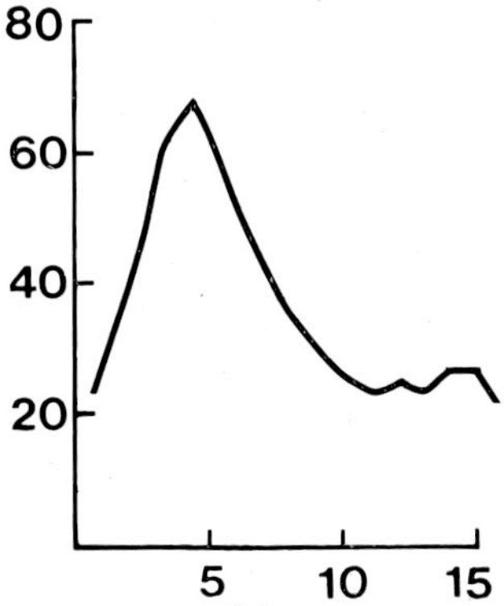

80
60
40
20
5 10 15

9.1

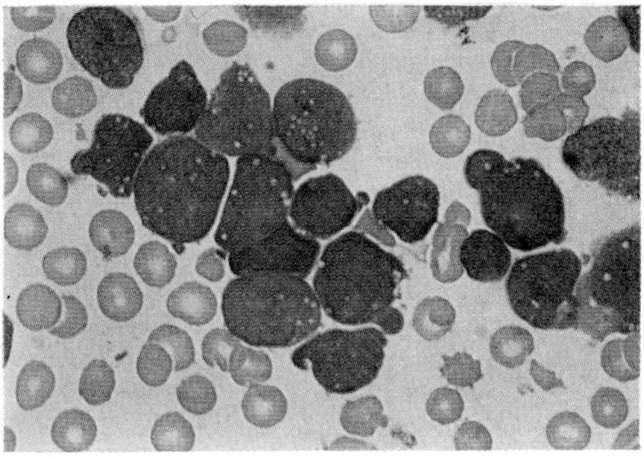

9.2(a)

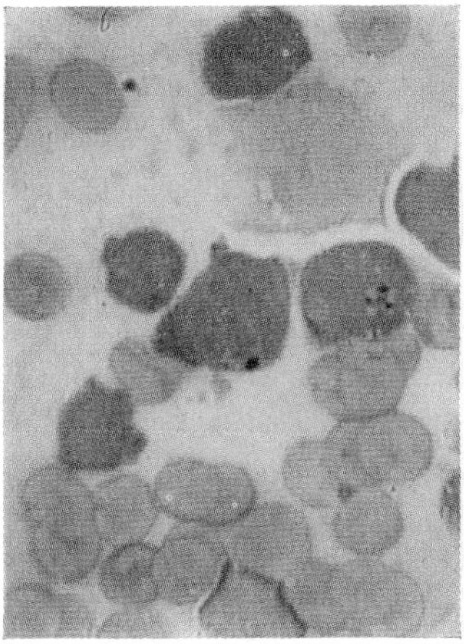

9.2(b)

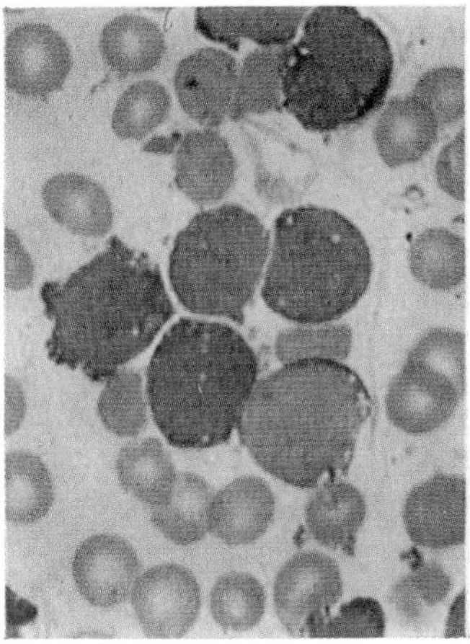

9.2(c)

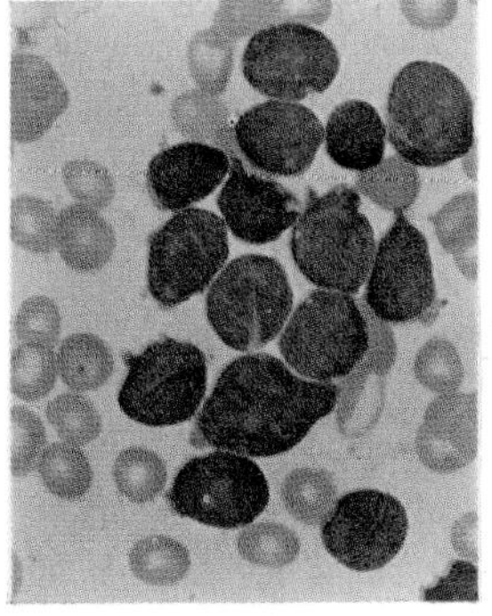

9.2(d)

Figure 9.1. LEUKAEMIA; the incidence according to age, indicating the peak in the first quinquennium (for the source of the figures see Fig. 2.2, p. 48).

Figure 9.2. ACUTE LYMPHATIC LEUKAEMIA; (*a*) the marrow, showing large cell type with a reticular nuclear chromatin pattern, up to two distinct nucleoli, many small vacuoles, and darkly staining cytoplasm; (*b*) PAS positivity; (*c*) negative Sudan black B (SBB) stain of the cells seen in (*a*); (*d*) large cell type, with 'ground glass' nuclear chromatin pattern, variably prominent nucleoli, frequent nuclear clefts and lightly staining cytoplasm.

Figure 9.2. (*e*) PAS positivity of the cells seen in (*d*); (*f*) the small cell type with dense nuclear chromatin and nucleoli seen only in the larger cells. The small blast cells resemble mature lymphocytes; (*g*) PAS positivity in cells shown in (*f*); (*h*) acute lymphatic leukaemia blast cells in the CSF.

Figure 9.3. ACUTE MYELOID LEUKAEMIA; (*a*) blast cell showing Auer rod; (*b*) blast cells in the marrow; (*c*) cells in (*b*) showing heavy overall SBB stain; (*d*) positive peroxidase stain, and (*e*) diffuse PAS staining. The SBB stain is more frequently positive than the peroxidase stain in acute myeloid leukaemia.

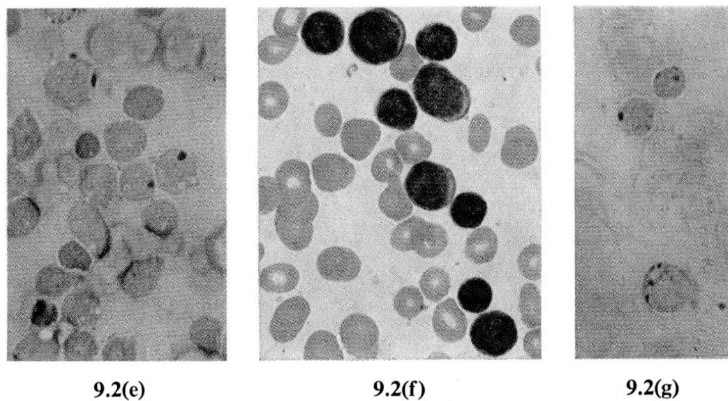

9.2(e) 9.2(f) 9.2(g)

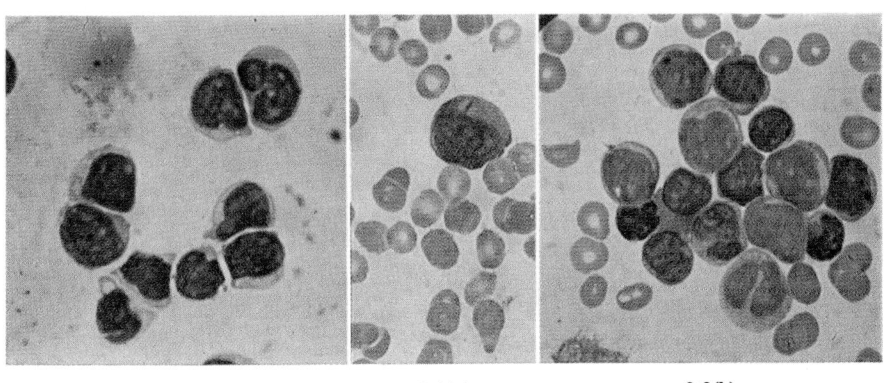

9.2(h) 9.3(a) 9.3(b)

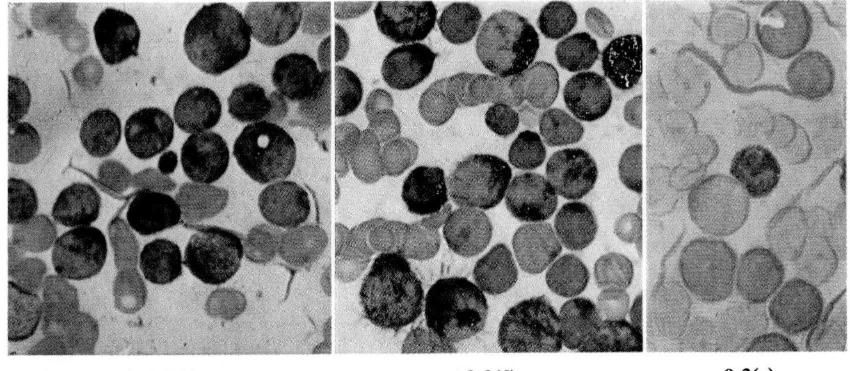

9.3(c) 9.3(d) 9.3(e)

Figure 9.4. ACUTE PROMYELOCYTE LEUKAEMIA; marrow cells showing large numbers of promyelocytes.

Figure 9.5. ACUTE MYELO-MONOCYTIC LEUKAEMIA; marrow showing a mixture of myeloblasts and monocytic blast cells.

Figure 9.6. ACUTE MONOCYTIC LEUKAEMIA; (*a*) bone marrow cells; (*b*) SBB stain of the cells seen in (*a*) showing discrete scattered granules.

Figure 9.7. ACUTE ERYTHROLEUKAEMIA; marrow showing many pro-erythroblasts.

Figure 9.8. CHRONIC MYELOID LEUKAEMIA; (*a*) peripheral blood and (*b*) marrow, showing increased granulocytes, particularly myelocytes.

Figure 9.9. HAEMOPHAGOCYTIC RETICULOSIS OF FARQUHAR AND CLAIREAUX; the marrow from two patients showing histiocytes (*a*) in a clump, and (*b*) singly, the latter showing haemophagocytosis (see also Fig. 11.6, p. 217).

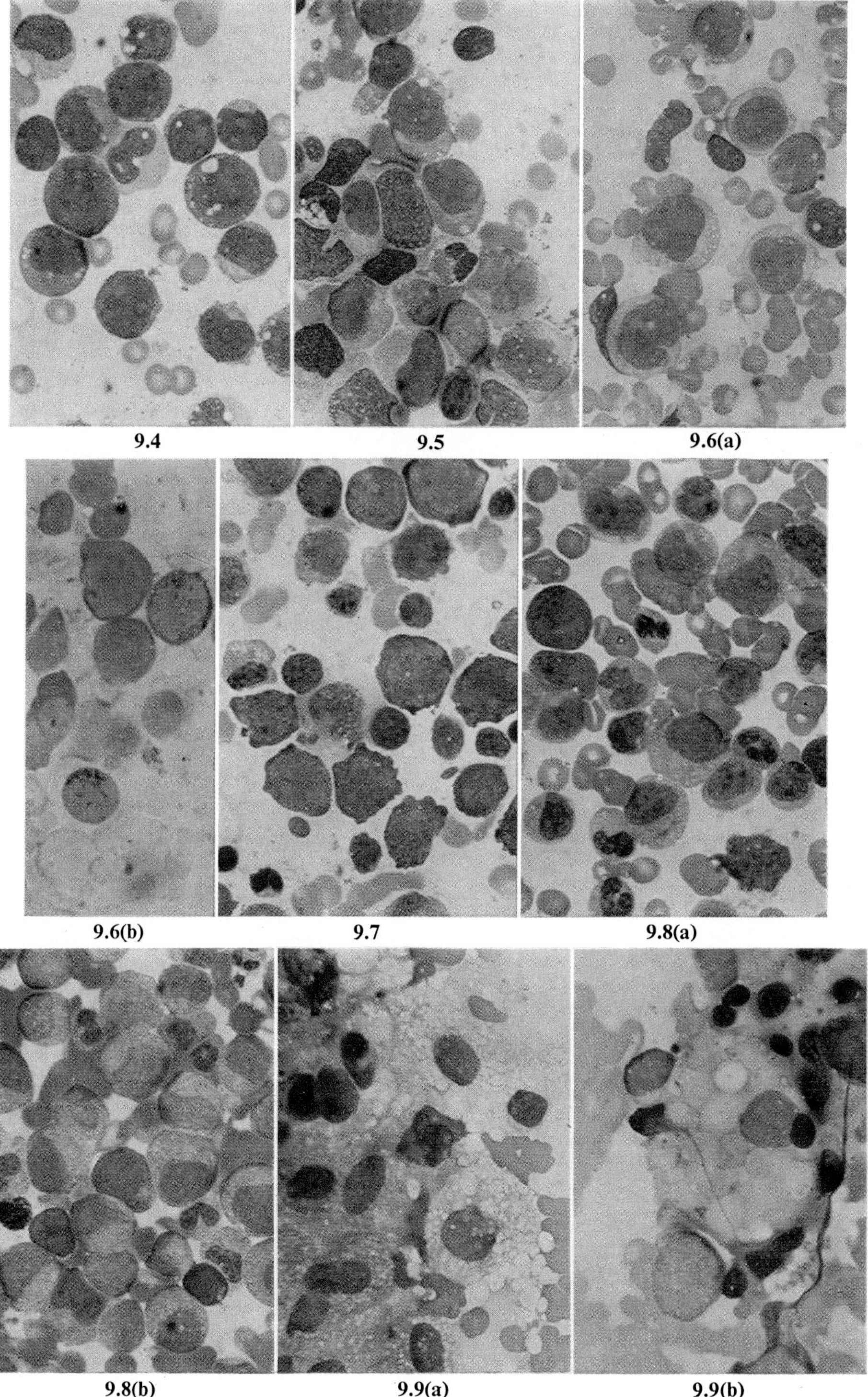

9.4 9.5 9.6(a)

9.6(b) 9.7 9.8(a)

9.8(b) 9.9(a) 9.9(b)

Figure 11.1c. EOSINOPHILIC GRANULOMA; A smear from aspirate of a lesion in the skull; large bean-shaped histocytes with delicate watery chromatin and very pale lilac cytoplasm, mingle with eosinophilic leucocytes. Free eosinophil granules are spread through the smear (H & E. × 2100).
Figure 15.15d. RETINOBLASTOMA; Cell preparation from aspirate of anterior chamber fluid; a clump of tumour cells form a closely knit mass; the nuclei are oval, with delicate chromatin (Leishman × 910).
Figure 23.3c. RHABDOMYOSARCOMA; A smear from aspirate of a metastasis in bone marrow; the abnormal cell is large, with a deeply basophilic nucleus containing even but coarse chromatin. The cytoplasm is blue and abundant, with a prominent 'tail' (Leishman × 2100).

Figure 18.7. NEUROBLASTOMA; Smear from marrow aspirate, stained with Leishman, showing a nest of metastatic neuroblasts with hyperchromatic nuclei, of various sizes. The nuclear chromatin is coarse and ropy, cytoplasm is scanty (× 1750).
Figure 18.9. NEUROBLASTOMA; An imprint stained with Leishman, for comparison with 22.11b Ewing's Tumour (below). In this preparation, also stained with Leishman, the nuclear chromatin is coarse and irregularly distributed, and cytoplasm is scanty.

Figure 14.9c. BURKITT'S LYMPHOMA; The cells have a large round nucleus, the chromatin is delicate and evenly dispersed, and the cytoplasm is deep blue with prominent vacuoles which can be shown to contain neutral fat (Leishman × 2100).

Figure 22.11. EWING'S TUMOUR. IMPRINT PREPARATIONS; (*a*) Imprint stained with Haematoxylin and Eosin. The tumour cells are oval and uniform with delicate nuclear chromatin and small inconspicuous nucleoli. Cytoplasm is moderate in amount, bubbly and pale lilac (× 847); (*b*) Imprint stained with Leishman. The round nuclei, delicate even chromatin and inconspicuous nucleoli are clearly seen. Cytoplasm is dispersed and vaculoated (× 1956); (*c*) Imprint stained with PAS. Intense red staining of the cytoplasm indicates glycogen. Prior digestion with disatase removes all positive-staining material from the cytoplasm (× 847); (*d*) Clump of neuroblasts showing rosette formation. Bone marrow aspirate. (Leishman × 847).

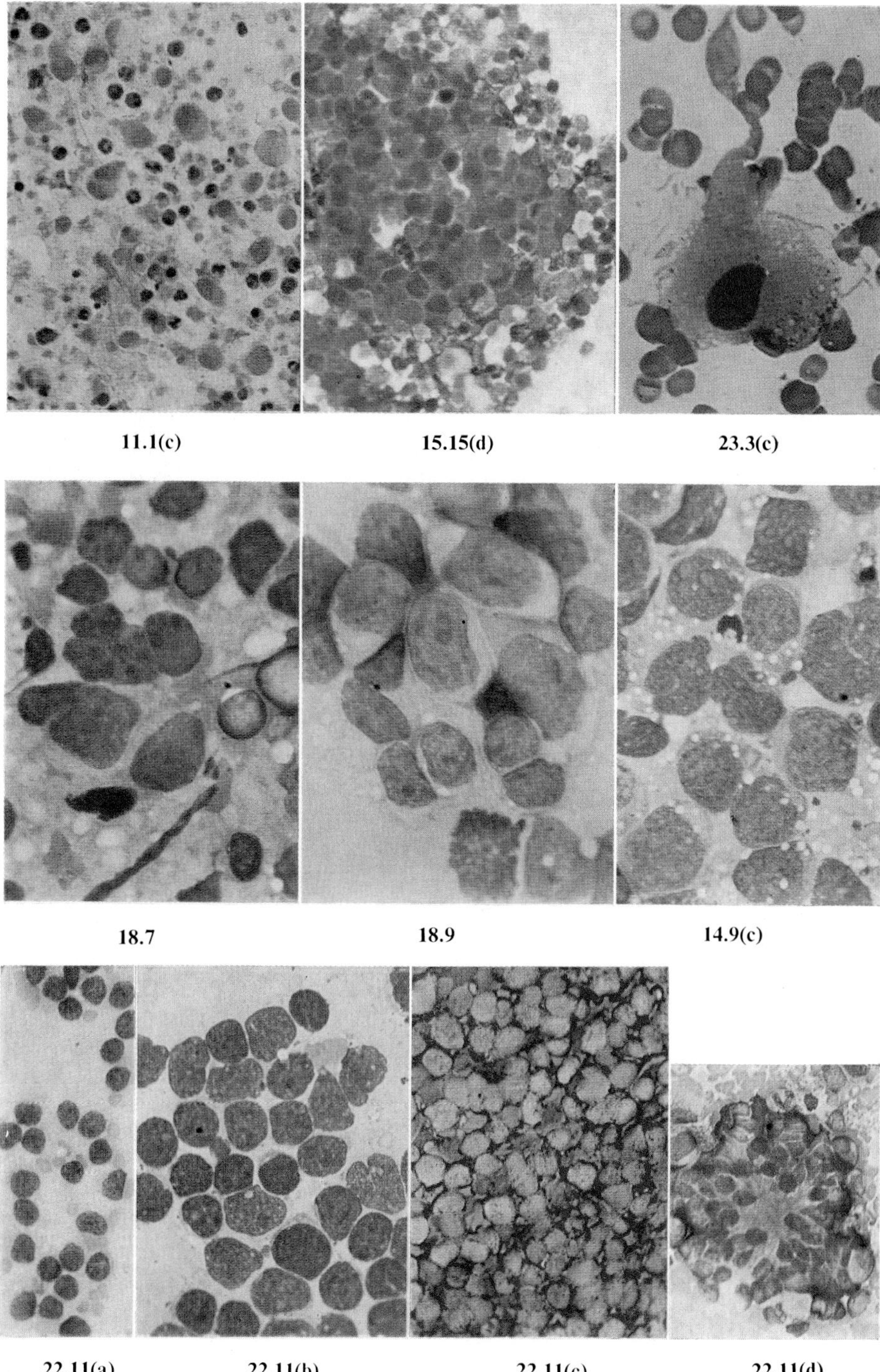

11.1(c) 15.15(d) 23.3(c)

18.7 18.9 14.9(c)

22.11(a) 22.11(b) 22.11(c) 22.11(d)

some anaemia, neutropenia or thrombocytopenia, and if any doubt remains, marrow aspiration is absolutely essential.

Whenever possible the diagnosis of acute leukaemia should include identification of the predominant cell type. This has become of practical importance because both the choice of therapy and the prognosis are influenced by the cell type. Non-lymphatic cases, for example, require radically different treatment to obtain good results. Some guides to the cell type are listed in Table 9.2. Special histochemical stains, combined with the Romanowsky stains, now make it possible for experienced laboratory workers to identify the cell type in almost every case (Figs 9.2 to 9.9).

With the Romanowsky stains, the diagnosis of the lymphatic type is favoured by a high nuclear-cytoplasmic ratio, dense nuclear chromatin pattern, less than three nucleoli per cell, and the absence of Auer bodies; the converse is usual, both in the myeloid type (with promyelocytes in the marrow) and in the monocytic type (with markedly high levels of serum muramidase or lysozyme).

Histochemical stains are required for diagnosis in 5–10%. The blast cells in acute lymphatic leukaemia are nearly always PAS-positive, Sudan black B-negative and nuclear aryl sulphatase-positive, whereas the reverse reactions are usual in the myeloid type; the pattern in monoblasts is less well defined.

DIFFERENTIAL DIAGNOSIS

No matter how strongly leukaemia is suspected on clinical and/or haematological grounds, it is important to exclude other conditions, many of which can resemble acute leukaemia clinically, while others produce a similar blood picture. The list is a long one because the leukaemias have a wide range of clinical and pathological features (Table 9.3).

Differentiation from benign conditions

Foremost among benign conditions which may closely simulate acute leukaemia, clinically and/or haematologically, are the following:

—infectious mononucleosis;

—various anaemias (aplastic, haemolytic and megaloblastic);

—thrombocytopenic purpura;

—rheumatoid disorders;

—generalized tuberculosis, and other infections.

In small children differentiation can be very difficult indeed. In the newborn, a picture closely resembling congenital leukaemia, both clinically and haematologically, can be produced by:

—erythroblastosis fetalis;

—septicaemia;

—severe infection with toxoplasmosis, cytomegalovirus, rubella or herpes simplex virus, accompanied by haemorrhage or haemolysis.

Older infants and young children, particularly those with Down's syndrome, sometimes respond to infections and other illnesses with strikingly leukaemoid blood and bone marrow pictures, including an increased number of

Table 9.3. Differential diagnosis of acute leukaemia

Common groupings of symptoms and signs	Conditions to be considered
A. *Clinically similar to acute leukaemia*	
1. *Infections*	
General ill health	Infectious mononucleosis
Fever	Viraemia (infants)
Pharyngitis	Agranulocytic angina
Ulcers in the mouth	Acute exanthemata
Rashes	Ulcerative stomatitis
Lymphadenomegaly	Septicaemia
	Respiratory, urinary and gastrointestinal infections
	Subacute bacterial endocarditis
	P.U.O.
2. *Hepatosplenomegaly*	
Splenomegaly	Infections (acute and subacute)
Hepatomegaly	Metastatic neuroblastoma
Lymphadenomegaly	Malignant lymphoma
Fever	Thalassaemia major
	Histiocytosis-X
	Portal hypertension
	Systemic lupus erythematosis
	'Hypersplenism'
3. *Haemorrhagic states*	
Purpura	Aplastic anaemia
Petechiae	Post-operative haemorrhage
Epistaxes	Purpura—thrombocytopenic, allergic or secondary
Wound bleeding	
4. '*Rheumatic*' *syndromes*	
Pains in limbs and joints, swelling, tenderness	Rheumatic fever
	Rheumatoid arthritis
Paresis	Osteomyelitis
	Poliomyelitis
	Scurvy
	Rickets
	Fractures
	Bone tumours
5. *Miscellaneous syndromes*	
Headache, vomiting, papilloedema	Cerebral tumour, meningitis, encephalitis
Mediastinal pressure	Mediastinal tumours
Abdominal pain, vomiting	Surgical abdominal emergencies

Table 9.3. continued

B. *Haematologically Similar to Acute Leukaemia* Blood picture	Disorders
1. *Leukaemoid picture*	
High W.C.C. (often <50,000/cmm)	Infectious mononucleosis
Immature leukocytes in blood smears (especially when lymph nodes and spleen are enlarged)	Viraemia (in infants)
	Pertussis
	Generalized tuberculosis
	Acute bacterial infection with bizarre response in newborns, mongols
	Septicaemia
	Erythroblastosis fetalis
	Acute haemolytic anaemia
	Metastatic tumour
2. *Pancytopenic states*	
Anaemia	Aplastic anaemia
Neutropenia and/or thrombocytopenia	Malignant lymphoma
	Metastatic tumour
	Myelosclerosis
	Megaloblastic anaemia
	Fulminating acute infections
	Generalized tuberculosis
	Idiopathic thrombocytopenic purpura
3. *Chronic leukaemic conditions*	
Immature cells in blood	Chronic myeloid leukaemia
W.C.C. often raised	Myelosclerosis
Splenomegaly	Myelofibrosis

blast cells, and these cases may be indistinguishable from acute leukaemia except by their outcome.

Some children with acute leukaemia (16% of the total) present with *a rheumatic syndrome* or pain in the limbs which simulates rheumatoid arthritis, rheumatic fever, osteomyelitis, scurvy or rickets. In these cases the presence of haemorrhages, enlarged lymph nodes and spleen, or neutropenia or thrombocytopenia, should prevent any undue delay in obtaining a diagnostic marrow aspiration.

Infectious mononucleosis may be mistaken for acute leukaemia when there are fever with a sore throat, enlarged spleen and lymph nodes, and abnormal leukocytes in the blood. The distinction is made by finding leukaemic features such as skin bleeding, neutropenia and thrombocytopenia, and by serology and cytological differentiation of leukaemic blast cells from atypical mononuclear cells.

Aplastic anaemia may be more difficult to exclude when the spleen and lymph nodes are not enlarged, but examination of aspirated marrow nearly always solves the problem; if it does not, a marrow trephine is required.

Leukaemoid reaction

This is a peripheral blood picture suggestive of leukaemia, occurring in a patient who does not have that disease. The resemblance to leukaemia is due either to a high leukocyte count, usually above 50,000/cmm, or to the presence of immature cells (myelocytes, premyelocytes, myeloblasts, lymphoblasts and often nucleated red cells) or to both. A leukaemoid reaction may simulate either acute or chronic leukaemia, and is more often myeloid than lymphatic in type.

Leukaemoid reactions are seen most frequently in younger children and infants, especially in response to acute or subacute infections, e.g. pyococcal, tuberculosis, pertussis, toxoplasmosis or viruses (see Table 9.3). Other causes include metastatic malignant disease in bone, massive haemolysis or haemorrhage, and severe allergic reactions.

The differentiation of true leukaemia from a leukaemoid reaction may be as difficult as it is important. The major differences between leukaemoid reactions and acute and chronic leukaemias are listed in Table 9.4. Although marrow smears will usually enable leukaemia to be identified or excluded, in some cases this differentiation requires serial examinations. Unrecognized leukaemoid reactions probably account for most of the cures of so-called 'leukaemia' reported before the era of modern chemotherapy.

It is important to remember that conditions which produce a leukaemoid reaction can coexist with true leukaemia.

Differentiation from other malignant conditions

These include:

—neuroblastoma (abdominal, thoracic, etc.);

—malignant lymphomas, e.g. of the mediastinum; and

—cerebral tumours.

Neuroblastoma and the other tumours which metastasize to the bone marrow, can closely resemble leukaemia both clinically and haematologically (Table 9.3), but the signs of an abdominal or thoracic mass, and investigations which demonstrate the primary tumour, e.g. angiography of the aorta and its branches (see p. 554) are often diagnostic. Marrow smears in metastatic neuroblastoma are likely to contain clusters of malignant cells with cytological features unlike those of leukaemic cells, sometimes including the presence of neurofibrillary material (see p. 545).

Lymphosarcoma of the mediastinum may be accompanied by the presence of blast cells in the blood and/or marrow, and the picture may closely resemble acute lymphatic leukaemia. The distinction can be extremely difficult, but this is seldom of practical importance because the treatment of these two closely related conditions is fundamentally the same.

A cerebral tumour may be occasionally suggested by headache, vomiting and papilloedema, or a hypothalamic syndrome when acute leukaemia

Table 9.4. Leukaemia. Differentiation between leukaemoid reactions and leukaemia

	Leukaemoid reactions	Acute leukaemia	Chronic myeloid leukaemia
Symptoms and signs	Those of the causative disorder	Enlarged spleen and nodes, fever, anaemia and haemorrhage usual	Symptoms of anaemia mainly; splenomegaly marked
Blood			
WCC	Increased or normal; usually $<100{,}000$	Variable; often $>100{,}000$	Commonly $>100{,}000$
Leukocyte morphology	Toxic changes in neutrophils if cause infective	Toxic changes rare; often 'atypical' forms as well as 'blasts'	Anisocytotic; some 'atypical' forms
Immature cells	'Blasts' not $>5\%$; myelocytes+	'Blasts' usual, often numerous	Many myelocytes. a few 'blasts'
Predominant cell type	Myeloid series most often	Lymphatic in 80%	Usually myelocytes
Leukaemic hiatus	Absent	Usually present	Usually absent
Anaemia	Little, usually; many normoblasts	Progressive, severe; normoblasts rare	Mild to moderate; normoblasts few
Thrombocytopenia	None usually	Progressive, severe	Usually none till late
Bone marrow			
Immature cells	Absent, or $<20\%$ tumour cells	'Blasts' usually $>50\%$	Myelocytes and 'blasts'
NAP* score	Normal	Normal	Low until blastic 'transformation'
Serum muramidase	Normal	High in AML, very high in monocytic	High
Course	Transient; relapse unusual	Relapsing, progressive if untreated	Very slowly progressive
Autopsy	No leukaemic infiltrations	Organs and tissues infiltrated unless death was from non-leukaemic cause	

* Neutrophil alkaline phosphatase.

presents with infiltration of the CNS, until enlarged spleen and lymph nodes, bleeding or characteristic blood changes are detected. Juvenile chronic myeloid leukaemia in the early stages may be difficult to distinguish from acute and subacute forms, in which case serial investigations are needed (see Table 9.4).

PATHOLOGY AND COMPLICATIONS

The pathology of leukaemia includes the leukaemic cell as well as the organs and tissues infiltrated or otherwise involved (Amromin, 1968). Both aspects have been greatly changed in the past two decades by the development of techniques for studying cellular pathology, and by the effects (and side-effects) of antileukaemic therapy.

The complications of leukaemia can be usefully grouped under two headings:

(*a*) *those caused by leukaemic involvement of bone marrow*, other reticulo-endothelial tissues, and of extramedullary organs and tissues, all of which are conveniently considered with the pathology; and

(*b*) *those due to the treatment* of the disease (see p. 155).

The pathology of leukaemic cells

Study of these cells was limited for a long time to sections of marrow and other reticulo-endothelial tissues, and to smears of blood and marrow stained by the Romanowsky method. In recent years the following techniques have been added:

(*i*) Histochemical methods of detecting enzyme and other chemical changes;

(*ii*) Electron microscopy;

(*iii*) Analyses of chromosomes;

(*iv*) Physical and autoradiographic methods of estimating DNA and RNA in studying cellular kinetics (see p. 101); and

(*v*) Immunological and virological techniques.

These highly specialized fields are beyond the scope of this chapter, but a few of the major discoveries of clinical importance are mentioned, together with some references for the interested reader.

Enzyme abnormalities can help to distinguish the various cell types of leukaemia, to differentiate them from leukaemoid reactions, and to detect blastic transformation in chronic myeloid leukaemia (Hayhoe *et al.*, 1964).

Cytogenetic studies more often than not reveal abnormal karyotypes in acute leukaemia and may help to define the cell type. In chronic myeloid leukaemia the 'adult' form is characterized by the presence of the Philadelphia (Ph^1) chromosome which is absent from the 'juvenile' form, and serial chromosome studies may give the first indication of blastic transformation (Whang-Peng *et al.*, 1969; Schroeder & Kurth, 1971).

Physiochemical and autoradiographic studies have shown that the accumulation of leukaemic cells is usually the result not of more rapid division but of their longer survival compared with normal cells. These studies also provide information about the cells' mitotic cycle, which has become important for the optimal timing of drug administration (Mauer, 1969).

Pathology of organs and tissues

Enlargement of the spleen, lymph nodes and liver is caused primarily by proliferation or accumulation of leukaemic cells, combined in varying degree with reticulo-endothelial hyperplasia and congestion, with haemosiderosis and with the accumulation of lipid material which is often steroid-induced. Secondary changes occur as the result of infection, haemorrhage, thrombosis and metabolic disturbances, and from the side-effects of chemotherapy.

Infarction is not uncommon in the spleen, resulting in 'perisplenitis' and adhesions, and sometimes it occurs in the brain with more serious consequences.

The central nervous system becomes involved, in one way or another, in most cases of acute leukaemia. The commonest is leukaemic infiltration, which may develop in 70–80% of children with acute leukaemia. Haemorrhage into the brain or meninges, thrombosis, infarction and necrosis also occur, especially in myeloid cases when the white cell count is more than 100,000/cmm, but with modern therapy these complications are becoming less of a problem.

CNS disease may also be iatrogenic, e.g. steroid-induced encephalopathy, myelin degeneration in craniospinal nerves from vincristine, and herpes zoster to which the child is prone because of immunosuppression by anti-leukaemic drugs.

Leukaemic infiltration of the CNS may cause clinical syndromes of the following types:

meningeal	cranial
hypothalamic	spinal
optic nerve	mixed

Over 70% of the 'clinical episodes' consist of an uncomplicated meningeal syndrome, typically with headache, vomiting, papilloedema and raised cerebrospinal fluid pressure with pleocytosis and often increased protein. Excessive appetite and weight gain associated with infiltration in the hypothalamic region occur in one sixth of the episodes. Less often cranial nerves (chiefly sixth and third) and parts of the cerebrum are infiltrated, with little or no changes in the CSF. Infiltration of the optic nerve (visible on fundoscopy) and of the spinal cord are important but uncommon syndromes. In some 20% of all clinical episodes there is a mixed syndrome, usually with meningeal involvement.

Infiltration of bone is evident radiologically in only 25% of cases at the time of diagnosis, but more commonly at autopsy. The main radiological signs are 'moth-eaten' areas of osteolysis (Fig. 22.14b, p. 744), metaphyseal bands of rarefaction and subperiosteal new bone, all of which slowly disappear in response to successful chemotherapy. A serious complication seen in recent years has been spinal osteoporosis with vertebral collapse, following excessive amounts of corticosteroids.

A chloromatous tumour, composed of myeloblasts, may develop in acute myeloid leukaemia and usually involves the cranial or facial bones (see p. 297), and an analogous lymphomatous tumour sometimes occurs in acute lymphatic leukaemia.

'*Leukaemic sanctuary*' is the term used to describe the active proliferation of leukaemic cells which sometimes occurs in one or more isolated organs or tissues, as if they were impervious to antileukaemic drugs, even during a complete haematological remission. The 'sanctuary' may be in the CNS, testes, ovaries, kidneys, and occasionally elsewhere; these lesions are sensitive to radiotherapy although often resistant to chemotherapy.

Other organs in which leukaemic infiltration can occur are the salivary glands, alimentary tract, heart, lungs, eyes and skin. In children, infiltrations in skin are almost confined to the neonatal period and to those with monocytic leukaemia.

METABOLIC AND PHYSIOLOGICAL CHANGES

The destruction of leukaemic cells and release of their nucleic acid residues presents the kidneys with an excessive load of uric acid which tends to accumulate as crystals in the pyramids and renal pelvis. The *hyperuricaemia and resultant tubular blockage* causing uraemia can be fatal if not treated promptly and adequately.

Other metabolic and physiological changes may occur, including increased metabolic rate and serum creatinine; hypercalcaemia (especially with bone lesions); hyperglycaemia; fluid and electrolyte disturbances; haemosiderosis; and impairment of growth and sexual development.

A hypercoagulation state with extensive intravascular thrombosis, resulting in depletion of coagulation factors and platelets, may be a major cause of serious haemorrhage, especially in myeloid leukaemia.

Modern therapy provides for better control of haemorrhage, but it has greatly changed the microbial pattern and the increased seriousness of infection, which is now the commonest immediate cause of death (see p. 154).

COURSE

The natural course of acute leukaemia without treatment is, in almost all cases, a relentless progress towards the overwhelming effects of leukaemic infiltration and/or its complications, ending in death within a matter of weeks. In a series of 65 leukaemic children admitted to this hospital before 1948, the median survival time was between one and two months, and more than a third died within two weeks of admission. When broad-spectrum antibiotics and transfusions of blood and then platelets become readily available, the median survival time of otherwise untreated children was increased to about four months, but only a few survived for more than a year. Spontaneous remission might occasionally occur, commonly preceded and perhaps caused by an acute infection, but such remissions were generally partial or incomplete and short-lived; for practical purposes spontaneous cure never occurred. The commonest immediate causes of death were haemorrhage, infection and anaemia, often associated with considerable pain and distress.

Therapeutic advances since the introduction of antileukaemic chemotherapy by Farber in 1948 have changed this hitherto tragic course to a remarkable degree, and the prognosis is becoming more hopeful every year. The serious complications and much of the patient's distress can be effectively treated or prevented. Recurrent relapse and reinduction of remission are the rule, but in special clinics these are so managed that children spend most of their period of survival fit for school or comparable activities. The length of survival has steadily increased, particularly with acute lymphatic leukaemia, for which the median survival time now exceeds three years and the five-year survival rate is of the order of 25%, or higher in a number of centres.

In addition, particularly in the past decade, a small but growing proportion of patients have remained so long in complete remission that the possibility of cure exists. The effects of treatment and other factors on the course and the prognosis will be discussed after the next section.

TREATMENT

No really effective treatment was discovered until ninety years after acute leukaemia was first described in 1857. While measures were virtually limited to blood transfusion and penicillin, it was common practice not to advise the use of even these because the expectation of life was in any case extremely short. This nihilistic attitude to treatment has undergone extraordinary changes during the modern era of antileukaemic chemotherapy, which began in 1948 with Farber's epoch-making report of remission in five of sixteen leukaemic children who were treated with aminopterin, a folic acid antagonist (p. 104). Since then the number of potent agents available, acting in different ways with little or no cross-reaction, has reached double figures. Along with this revolution in chemotherapy, there have developed a growing understanding of the nature and pathogenesis of leukaemia and better methods of combating its potentially fatal complications.

The prognosis is so much more hopeful now than it was even a decade ago, at least for children with acute lymphatic leukaemia (ALL), that the whole philosophy of the child's management has been transformed. The *laissez faire* attitude of the 1940s was replaced first by attempts at palliation and the induction of a clinical remission; then the aim became the production of repeated remissions; next the emphasis shifted to making remissions more complete and prolonging them with various regimens of continued chemotherapy; now the philosophy of treatment is based on total remission lasting indefinitely (tantamount to a cure), and this should be the aim, at least initially.

The objectives of treatment today are: (i) to save the child's life by arresting the natural course of the disease, (ii) to prolong life, indefinitely if possible, by eradicating the disease, and (iii) to ensure that the quality of his extended life is the best possible in the circumstances.

To achieve these objectives, the following distinct but interrelated aspects of treatment are carefully considered.

1. Control of complications.
2. Induction of remission with antileukaemic drugs.
3. Consolidation of drug-effects to maintain complete remission, indefinitely if possible.
4. General and supportive measures.

1. Treatment of complications

Complications are traditionally discussed last in standard textbooks, but in acute leukaemia the urgent need to control them justifies discussing them first. Patients who die within a few days or weeks of diagnosis usually do so as a result of complications rather than leukaemic infiltration itself. The commonest potentially fatal complications, in order of clinical significance, are infection, haemorrhage, anaemia and hyperuricaemia.

Infection is the cause of at least 75% of deaths in acute leukaemia, so great care should be taken to prevent it or to detect and treat it early. Most leukaemic children develop fever at some stage during the induction of a remission or later, especially when in a relapse, and it is now widely accepted that every febrile episode must be considered infective until proved otherwise.

Neutropenia, with counts below 500/cmm or even below 1000/cmm, predisposes the leukaemic child to bacterial infection and a count of 100/cmm or less is associated with an exceptionally high risk of septicaemia, particularly if the low count persists for more than a few days. *Staphylococcus aureus* and other Gram-positive bacteria are isolated frequently, but Gram-negative organisms occur more than twice as often and have far more serious effects, e.g. *Pseudomonas aerogenosa*, *Escherichia coli*, *Klebsiellae* and *Proteus mirabilis*.

Lymphopenia below 500/cmm likewise predisposes to infection, particularly with fungi and viruses, e.g. herpes simplex, varicella, cytomegalovirus. When active leukaemia is being treated with intensive chemotherapy, there may be such severe depression of both cellular and humoral immunity, as well as leukopenia, that the child becomes highly susceptible to all the pathogens mentioned above and to a wide range of 'opportunistic' micro-organisms, e.g. *Pneumocystis carinii*, *Toxoplasma gondii*, *Listeria monocytogenes* and *Salmonellae*. In those with serious systemic infections (excluding viruses) identified at about the time of death, 60% of 121 organisms cultivated were Gram-negative, 22% were Gram-positive and 18% fungal.

Three very important conclusions can be drawn from these observations.
1. Any serious infection may completely wreck the child's prospect of a lasting remission.
2. Because of his susceptibility and low resistance to infection, the aim must be prophylaxis, or, failing that, the earliest possible recognition and treatment of it.
3. Systemic fungal and viral infections may be as fatal as bacterial infections, and Gram-negative organisms are the greatest hazard.

As a routine on the first admission, and in any subsequent episode of fever, throat (cough) swabs, urine and blood should be cultured, and x-rays of the chest should be taken. In some cases, swabs from the nose, ear, stools or skin lesions may be indicated. Radiological shadows in films of the chest should almost never be attributed to leukaemic infiltration. Evidence of infection with viruses, fungi, and other organisms normally of low pathogenicity, should also be sought.

Positive steps to prevent infection should be taken when the neutrophils are below 500/cmm and to prevent superinfection if the child has less than 1000/cmm with clinical evidence of an infection already present. Prophylactic measures include: (1) a protected environment, provided by 'reverse' barrier nursing, and limiting visits by other than parents and essential staff; if the neutrophils fall below 200/cmm, it is mandatory to apply these measures strictly, and to nurse the child in either an isolation room, or a laminar flow over-bed unit which children usually tolerate well; (2) avoiding marrow puncture, lumbar puncture, venepuncture, and even intramuscular injections unless these are absolutely necessary; (3) Soframycin® (250–750 mg/day in divided doses by mouth), to inhibit bowel pathogens; (4) a broad-spectrum antibiotic cover when the child is ill and the neutrophils below 200/cmm (but after obtaining adequate specimens for culture); (5) if available, transfusions of leukocytes or 'buffy coat' when total agranulocytosis has persisted for more than two to three days; (6) γ-globulin if lymphopenia or a history of contact indicates a risk of a viral infection; the prophylactic dose varies from about 0·1 ml/kg for measles to 1·2 ml/kg for varicella occurring during a leukaemic relapse, preferably given intravenously if there is a risk of bleeding; (7) nystatin (0·5 gm by mouth two to four times a day) to reduce the risk of candidiasis when corticosteroids are being given.

The first suspicion of clinical infection, with or without fever, should be regarded as an emergency, the more so the lower the neutrophil count. The site of the infection must be carefully sought, fresh cultures taken and prophylactic measures instituted or intensified. It is widely accepted that appropriate antibiotics should begin as soon as material for culture has been obtained; to wait for the results of bacteriological cultures or until there are signs of shock, septicaemia or other diagnostic manifestations, is usually to wait too long.

Until the results of sensitivity tests are available, a combination of drugs should be given to cover both penicillinase-producing staphylococci and Gram-negative bacteria, especially *Pseudomonas aerogenosa*, the selection of the drugs depending on the hospital's current pattern of pathogenic flora and their sensitivities. At the present time it is our practice to commence cloxacillin and co-trimoxazole for a febrile child with neutropenia who is only mildly ill, and cephalothin and gentamycin or colistin for those who are seriously ill or have agranulocytosis. If the infection fails to respond within 36–48 hours, the chemotherapy should be reviewed, adding or substituting other antibiotics, preferably guided by information on isolates and their sensitivities. The commonest fatal infections are septicaemia, pneumonia and enterocolitis.

Infections which appear to be minor or local must nevertheless be treated seriously because they can readily and insidiously become more invasive and overwhelm a defenceless leukaemic patient in relapse. This applies to various types of infection e.g. paronychia, otorrhoea, urinary tract infection, vulvitis, oral thrush, herpetic angular stomatitis or 'cold sores'. Fatal systemic fungal infections and herpes simplex viraemia are frequently diagnosed only at autopsy.

Oral thrush should be treated vigorously with amphotericin lozenges, combined if necessary with nystatin tablets, gentian violet locally and a reduction of the dose of steroids. Courses of 5-fluorocytosine or amphotericin, IV, are necessary for systemic fungal infections. Viraemia due to herpes simplex, varicella or cytomegalovirus can be rapidly fatal during leukaemic relapse, but may respond to early treatment with cytosine arabinoside (3 mg/kg or 90 mg/m^2, IV, once or twice) and hyperimmune gammaglobulin (10 mg/kg). Infection with *Pneumocystis carinii*, which can be diagnosed with certainty only by lung biopsy, is most apt to occur as the terminal stages of leukaemia approach; early treatment with pentamidine isethionate may be effective.

Haemorrhage is far less often a serious problem or the cause of death than infection, but it occurs in some form in most cases. The major cause is thrombocytopenia, especially when the platelet count is below 20,000/cmm. Other contributory factors include vascular damage associated with infection and anaemia, disorders of platelet function, thrombosis associated with very high leukocyte counts, and disseminated intravascular coagulation. Intracranial and pulmonary haemorrhage are two very serious forms which are most often terminal. Serious gastro-intestinal haemorrhage also occurs, usually related to the administration of steroids and/or aspirin, to enterocolitis caused by fungi and Gram-negative bacteria, to thrombocytopenia of any cause, or to intestinal damage from cytotoxic drugs.

Transfusions of platelet-rich blood or platelet concentrates are so valuable that it is now unusual for a leukaemic patient under treatment to die from a major haemorrhage. Indications for platelet transfusions include (i) a platelet count below 20,000/cmm in a patient who is bleeding or needs surgery; (ii) platelet count below 10,000/cmm when a marrow or lumbar puncture are necessary; (iii) platelet count below 5000/cmm without bleeding but associated with fever, infection or when a tourniquet test or the bleeding time are abnormal. The platelets must be fresh, not frozen, and given as promptly as practicable without filtering, and a suitable dose is usually about 0·2 unit/kg body weight.

Other measures which may assist in controlling bleeding are: treatment of the leukaemia, especially the hyperleukocytosis, treatment of infection and anaemia, steroid therapy, and appropriate investigation and treatment for disseminated intravascular coagulation and for fibrinolysis. Aspirin should not be given while there is any abnormal risk of bleeding.

Hyperuricaemia

Serum uric acid levels above 8 mg/dl are often found at presentation, but at this stage it rarely causes renal complications. However, with the rapid destruction of cells by antileukaemic therapy, the serum uric acid can quickly rise to 15–60 mg/dl at which stage urate crystals may obstruct the renal tubules and cause uraemia. This risk is greatest when there is a high blast cell count, gross enlargement of lymph nodes, spleen and liver, dehydration and/or a febrile infection. The following prophylactic measures should be taken when any of these factors are present: (i) establish a good fluid intake and urinary output; (ii) do not give intensive antileukaemic therapy in full dosage until (i) has been achieved; (iii) alkalinize the urine; (iv) identify and treat infection; (v) give allopurinol (10 mg/kg/day in divided doses by mouth) for several days. Allopurinol blocks the formation of uric acid by inhibiting xanthine oxidase, an enzyme which is also involved in the breakdown of mercaptopurine, so this drug must be reduced to 25% of the usual dose when given simultaneously with allopurinol. If uric acid nephropathy with oliguria and uraemia is already present, 'prophylactic' therapy should be intensified and other measures added, such as mannitol diuresis, acetazolamide for alkalinization and dialysis to control the uraemia.

CNS leukaemia, already described in the section on pathology, is in some ways the most troublesome complication, especially to the patient. Its incidence in all forms of acute leukaemia has steadily increased as median survival times have lengthened. In 1958 it occurred in less than 15%; now 75% of children with acute lymphatic leukaemia who survive three years develop it, unless prophylactic treatment is given. It contributes to death in only 5–10% of cases, but it causes a disturbing amount of recurrent incapacity and discomfort. These can be minimized considerably by early diagnosis and treatment, and the clinician should examine the fundi at every follow-up visit;

a diagnostic lumbar puncture should be performed at the onset of any suspicious symptoms or signs, especially unexplained headache, vomiting, excess weight gain, visual disturbances, papilleodema or cranial nerve palsies. The commonest findings are raised CSF pressure and a mononuclear pleocytosis (up to 10,000/cmm); the characteristics of neoplastic or blast cells should be verified by smears, using Romanowsky-stained smears.

Treatment of a clinical episode of CNS leukaemia is usually intrathecal chemotherapy with methotrexate (10–12·5 mg/m^2, given in 10–20 ml of normal saline, and repeated every two to three days until the CSF cell count reaches a normal level of 0–4 cells/cmm). The technique calls for special care, particularly when there are cerebral signs; a fine needle, minimal trauma, withdrawal of no more than 4 ml of CSF, and the horizontal position maintained for thirty minutes afterwards. As most of the intrathecal dose reaches the bloodstream, oral or parenteral methotrexate should be reduced or omitted during intrathecal therapy. Folinic acid or citrovorum factor, a methotrexate antagonist (3–10 mg IV) can be given two hours after an intrathecal dose if there is a risk of dangerous pancytopenia. In selected cases a Rickham reservoir may be inserted to facilitate the administration of methotrexate. Cytosine arabinoside 30 mg/m^2 is a useful alternative drug for intrathecal use, and corticosteroids (particularly dexamethasone) will effectively penetrate the blood-brain barrier when given orally or parenterally.

Clinical recovery, with return of the CSF to normal occurs in most episodes after four to six doses of intrathecal therapy, but at least 10% of those with cerebral, spinal or optic nerve syndromes require irradiation (1000 rads or more), usually to the craniospinal axis (see p. 163). However, unless additional treatment is given, CNS leukaemia almost always relapses, commonly within four to eight months, or earlier if the bone marrow is also in relapse. Of over 100 children with clinical CNS leukaemia, five have had more than ten recurrences, while a few have had none for long periods. The prognostic significance of CNS leukaemia can be illustrated by evidence which suggests that in some cases recovery (or cure) of the marrow component of the disease has been followed by a relapse due apparently to dissemination from an active leukaemic focus in the 'sanctuary' of the CNS.

Prevention or complete eradication of CNS leukaemia has therefore received much attention recently. Prophylactic craniospinal or cranial irradiation (2500 rads) has been used as routine in children with acute lymphatic leukaemia at St. Jude Hospital, Memphis. Greatly improved remission and survival rates have occurred with this regimen, but it unfortunately produces total alopecia for many weeks and, usually, damage to the bone marrow, so a number of variations of this regime are currently under trial. Although eradication of established CNS disease is not yet possible, an optimal plan for its prevention should soon become clear (Haghbin *et al.*, 1975).

Other sanctuary areas where active leukaemia may progress despite remissions elsewhere include the testes, ovaries, kidneys, and occasionally the bones and the alimentary tract. The treatment of these is surgical excision where feasible, or irradiation.

2. Induction of remission (Greenwald, 1973)

This is the aim of initial treatment, by checking the growth of leukaemic cells and killing many of them, simultaneously preventing or controlling complications which may cause death or at least delay recovery. Regression allows the bone marrow to resume normal haemopoeisis, and the degree of remission is closely related to the duration of remission, and to the chances of long-term survival.

The accepted criteria of a *complete* remission are:

(i) No symptoms attributable to leukaemia.

(ii) No signs of leukaemic infiltration of organs or tissues—spleen, lymph nodes, liver, eye, skin, CNS, or elsewhere.

(iii) A peripheral blood picture within the normal range for the child's age, (i.e. granulocytes at least 1500/cmm, platelets at least 120,000/cmm, haemoglobin at least 10 gm/dl (9 gm/dl in infants, 11 gm/dl after puberty) and no leukaemic blast cells present).

(iv) Normal marrow cellularity with immature cells of all normal lines, blast cells 5% or less, and lymphocytes + blast cells 40% or less.

Lesser grades of remission (bone marrow, partial, clinical, etc.) are defined in various ways by different authors.

There are at present at least eight drugs with different actions available for treating a child with acute leukaemia. Their modes of action etc. are fully described in the chapter on Chemotherapy (p. 108) and only their essential features are mentioned here. Because most of the drugs commonly used for ALL are of only limited value in AML, the treatment of these two types of leukaemia is considered separately. The best results in any acute leukaemia are obtained by using drugs with a rapid cytocidal effect on blast cells, which are actively dividing or 'in cycle' (see p. 101) because, if unchecked, the disease may overwhelm the patient within days. It is also important to choose, whenever possible, drugs which cause least depression of the marrow, for the patient has almost no marrow reserve at the time of diagnosis or when in relapse.

The main drugs for remission induction in ALL and the complete remission rates they commonly produce, given singly and in combination, are listed in Table 9.5. No one drug is as effective as most of the combinations listed because the effects of two or more drugs with differing actions are additive. It is therefore seldom justifiable to rely on any single drug to produce a remission. Vincristine with prednisolone (or prednisone) is currently the combination of choice because both drugs act quickly and neither has much toxic effect on the bone marrow. Whether the addition of daunorubicin,

Table 9.5. Leukaemia. Cytotoxic agents. Remission induction in acute lymphatic leukaemia in children previously untreated

Single drug	Complete remission rate	Drug combination	Complete remission rate
Vincristine (VCR)	55–65%	VCR+PNL	85–92%
Prednisolone (PNL)	50–65%	DRB+PNL	75–90%
Daunorubicin (DRB)	50–65%	VCR+DRB+PNL	?95%
L-Asparaginase (APG)	45–60%	CSA+PNL	75–85%
Cytosine arabinoside (CSA)	25–35%	6MP+PNL	75–85%
Cyclophosphamide (CPA)	25–35%	6MP+MTX	40–45%
Mercaptopurine (6MP)	25–30%	MTX+PNL	75–85%
Methotrexate (MTX)	25–30%	CPA+PNL	75–85%

asparaginase, methotrexate or mercaptopurine to this combination improves the results, as some claim, has yet to be proven. The recommended dosages are as follows:

Vincristine 1·75–2·25 mg/m^2 IV once weekly.

Prednisolone 40–50 mg/m^2 PO daily for at least seven to ten days.

Daunorubicin 50 mg/m^2 IV once every seven to ten days.

L-asparaginase 5000–25,000 IU/m^2 (200–1000 IU/kg) IV or IM daily for at least two weeks.

Cytosine arabinoside, preferably 33 mg/m^2 IV eight hourly for four days, or 125 mg/m^2 IV daily for 7–10 days.

Mercaptopurine 60–70 mg/m^2/day PO.

Methotrexate 3–3·5 mg/m^2/day PO, or 90 mg/m^2 IV once every two weeks.

Cyclophosphamide 70–80 mg/m^2/day PO, or 900 mg/m^2 IV every two weeks.

Because these drugs differ in their routes of administration, modes of action, metabolism, excretion, and in their toxic effects, there are many ways in which these schedules can be modified with good effect. This is an area in which the expert in a special leukaemia centre can be particularly helpful.

Two effective modifications used in this hospital's Haematology Clinic are (*a*) *combinations* of cytosine arabinoside with L-asparaginase or cyclophosphamide, given in courses of multiple closely-spaced doses; and (*b*) *the use of a cell-cycle synchronizing dose* (see p. 112) of cytosine arabinoside given two to three days before a combination of other drugs that act in S-phase (synthesis of DNA) of the cycle. Whenever two or more cytotoxic drugs are administered concurrently, it is advisable to reduce the doses of each, usually to 10–12% less than those given above.

Meticulous attention should be paid to daily monitoring of the course of the disease and its complications, of the response to chemotherapy and its toxic effects. Full blood examination, including a platelet count, are necessary at least twice weekly during the induction phase, and serial estimations of electrolytes, uric acid and urea in the blood may be required. Though the toxic effects of drugs are fully described elsewhere (see p. 113), some are worth emphasizing. When vincristine is given, it is essential to prevent dehydration and constipation; milk of magnesia and agar preparations are useful for the latter. The alopecia caused by vincristine, daunorubicin and cyclophosphamide, can be prevented in older children by using a scalp tourniquet for five minutes from the start of the injection. Oral cyclophosphamide should always be given in the morning and never at night, to minimize the risk of haemorrhagic cystitis. The mouth should be inspected for ulcers daily in children receiving methotrexate, especially if renal function is in doubt. When L-asparaginase therapy is continued for more than a week, each injection may possibly precipitate anaphylaxis, so adrenalin, hydrocortisone and oxygen should be readily available. Great care must be taken when injecting vincristine and daunorubicin to avoid extravasation, which causes a very painful chemical cellulitis lasting several weeks.

Response to induction therapy is shown first, as a rule, by a reduction in the size of spleen and lymph nodes and in the number of blasts in the peripheral blood. The latter disappear within seven to ten days when the response is favourable, but the pancytopenia may not improve until the second or third week. Remission of symptoms commonly occurs within a week, and a complete remission with normal bone marrow within a month. As soon as a remission is clearly developing, usually by the second week, the dose of steroid should be tapered down because in excess it predisposes to unnecessary and sometimes fulminating infections, bacterial, viral or fungal.

In AML the optimal plan for inducing a remission has not yet been determined. The most effective drugs and their rate of complete remission when given singly, are: daunorubicin, 35–50%; cytosine arabinoside, more than 40%; vincristine, 20–25%. Other drugs which can be used, though with less promise of success, include mercaptopurine, thioguanine, cyclophosphamide, methotrexate, methylglyoxal-bis-guanylhydrazone (methyl GAG) and L-asparaginase. For reasons unknown, remission in AML is more difficult to induce and to maintain than in ALL. Hence, in AML a combination of drugs should always be used, and a variety of regimens are currently under trial. Steroids are often indicated for bleeding or thrombocytopenia, but several authorities consider that they are otherwise contraindicated in AML.

3. Consolidation and maintenance of remission

It has been calculated from researches in cell kinetics that when acute leukaemia is first diagnosed or in relapse, the total population of malignant cells in the body is of the order of 1×10^{12} or a million million. In addition, experimental studies indicate that any given dose or course of doses of a drug kills only a certain constant proportion of whatever leukaemic cells are present at the time. If, for example, the proportion is 99% (i.e. the 'fractional cell kill'), the leukaemic cell population is reduced from 10^{12} to 10^{10}. When induction therapy has produced a clinical remission with disappearance of leukaemic symptoms and signs, the remaining population of malignant cells is in the range 10^{10} to 10^{11}, and when a complete remission with normal bone marrow has been produced, the total leukaemic cell population is still at least 10^{9} or a thousand million cells.

Therefore if treatment is stopped when remission is 'complete' (as defined above), relapse occurs within a few weeks or months, and if maintenance therapy is limited to the simple single-drug regimens commonly used in the past twenty years, relapse almost always eventuates, though it may be delayed for one to two years or more. The long-term remissions and potential cures of ALL which can be, and are being obtained today, are the result of treatment which produces significant reductions in the population of leukaemic cells.

Chemotherapy continued after a complete remission, has been variously called consolidation, complementary, cytoreduction, reinduction or maintenance therapy. It would be inappropriate in this book even to summarize the numerous regimens which have been used for this purpose, especially as many of them will, no doubt, have been superseded by the time this is being read. It is important to observe certain general principles which are now well established.

The regimen should, as a rule, include at least two or three drugs, and some of the most successful have included four or five, e.g., vincristine, prednisolone, mercaptopurine and methotrexate (POMP). As far as possible, the drugs given in combination should differ in their modes of action and in the pattern of their toxicity, e.g. daunorubicin, cyclophosphamide and methotrexate are not an ideal combination because each acts in the S-phase of the cell cycle, each is quite myelotoxic and each tends to cause alopecia, whereas vincristine, prednisolone, L-asparaginase and daunorubicin or mercaptopurine differ widely in most respects, as do vincristine, cytosine arabinoside and L-asparaginase, so these drugs form suitable combinations. Some of the most promising reported results of consolidation therapy have been with methotrexate plus periodic doses of vincristine and prednisolone (used by Acute Leukemia Group B) and with mercaptopurine, methotrexate and cyclophosphamide following vincristine-prednisolone induction (used by the St. Jude Hospital group).

High doses given in intermittent 'pulses' are now widely accepted as more effective than lower doses administered daily. For most drugs, the optimal interval between doses or courses is two to three weeks, which is long enough to permit recovery from most of their immunosuppressive effects. The question of whether the administration of drugs, or courses of different drugs, in recurrent cycles is more effective than serial repetition of one drug or group of drugs, has not been finally settled although a national Australian Study and one in Glasgow tend to favour cyclic administration.

Considerable knowledge of the drugs available, their therapeutic potential, administration, and toxicity, are necessary to obtain the best results. While the chemotherapy of remission induction, at least in ALL, is now fairly clearly established, the management of consolidation and maintenance is made very complex by the range of permutations and combinations of the many drugs now available. It is in this area, perhaps more than any other, that the opinion of some one specializing in chemotherapy may become essential, bearing in mind that the prospect of cure may depend on how this phase of the treatment is handled.

Immunotherapy is a new form of treatment which may soon become an important factor in converting a remission into a cure. Although it has not yet progressed beyond the experimental stage, two points already seem to be clear. It is unlikely to achieve a significant effect unless the total leukaemic cell population has first been reduced by chemotherapy to 10^5–10^6 cells or lower. Preliminary reports suggest that both specific immunotherapy (with injections of modified leukaemic blast cells) and non-specific immunostimulation (with BCG) may be beneficial, but that passive immunotherapy is impracticable, and the possibility of a specific anti-leukaemic vaccine is remote.

Radiotherapy

There is reason to believe that effective treatment may so prolong survival that it will become realistic to use the term 'cure' in leukaemia. Cytotoxic agents currently in use are highly effective in children with lymphoblastic leukaemia, but relapses often occur as deposits in the central nervous system.

Most chemotherapeutic agents do not penetrate the blood-brain barrier adequately, but radiotherapy to the CNS, when given before evidence of its involvement, appears to greatly reduce the incidence of such involvement; in the case of established disease in this area, it brings about marked prolongation of remission.

A combination of 1600–2400 *rads* to the brain with *intrathecal methotrexate*, or craniospinal radiotherapy to 2000–2500 rads (given as two courses separated by four weeks), are two alternative methods in use at present. It is yet not possible to state which is preferable, but 'whole craniospinal' radiation (see Radiotherapy of the Neuraxis, p. 283) dispenses with the lumbar punctures required for intrathecal chemotherapy, and may not be attended by significantly increased depression of the marrow. The disadvantages of other side effects, e.g. temporary epilation, brief periods of nausea after treatment, and a syndrome of lassitude and hypersomnolence six weeks later, are outweighed by the benefit of fewer relapses. In infants, the greater risk of damaging effects warrants major reduction in dosage, or reliance on intrathecal therapy with no irradiation. Prophylactic 'sanctuary radiation' which includes the gonads and liver as well as the CNS, has proved to be more toxic without greater benefit.

Irradiation produces rapid improvement in those with established leukaemic infiltrates in areas which appear to have become 'sanctuaries': the brain, spinal cord, gonads, kidneys, bones, 'chloromas', eyes, etc. Even enlargement of the spleen, liver or lymph nodes which persists in a patient on chemotherapy, may respond rapidly to radiotherapy. Irradiation is also valuable in providing prompt relief of pain due to infiltration in patients with leukaemia which is becoming drug-resistant.

4. Supportive and general treatment

Supportive medical measures include transfusions of whole blood, packed cells, platelets or leukocytes; prevention and treatment of infection; allopurinol and other measures for preventing hyperuricaemia and dehydration. Each has already been discussed in earlier sections (pp. 153–159).

The clinician should also be on the alert for signs of serious electrolyte disturbances, e.g. hyponatraemia, hyperpotassaemia, hypercalcaemia, hypoglycaemia. These may develop insidiously, especially in acutely ill infants on anti-leukaemic drugs, and call for careful monitoring and remedial therapy.

Surgical complications are not uncommon, especially in terminal cases overtreated with steroids or with drugs toxic to the gastrointestinal tract. They include appendicitis, typhlitis, intussusception, perforations and peritonitis, without associated leukaemic infiltration in most cases. Consultation with a surgeon at an early stage is advisable, though experience shows that if the bone marrow is in relapse, the prognosis is so bad that it is usually wisest not to operate.

The general welfare of a child who has such a serious disease must be given special consideration. Analgesics should not be withheld, but aspirin is contra-indicated when there is a risk of haemorrhage. Papaveretum with hyoscine is usually required as premedication for punctures and other procedures, and sedatives and tranquillizers are often justifiable, especially during early hospitalization. Special efforts must be made whenever feasible to prevent distressing developments such as painful haematomas, epistaxis, pressure sores, perivenous cellulitis and alopecia. A particularly high standard of nursing care is required for leukaemic children, including attention to their considerable emotional needs.

The impact of any malignant disease on the child, and on his family, is discussed elsewhere (p. 127). Leukaemia generally has an even greater impact than a solid tumour, and because it usually involves more physical distress from injections, punctures and other procedures, there may be more emotional upset from isolation, hospitalization, intravenous therapy and bleeding, and the treatment is invariably more prolonged. This impact must be effectively countered to prevent the child becoming extremely depressed and to enable the parents to 'cope' by developing patterns of adjustment and later of anticipatory mourning.

Clinicians, nurses, medical social worker, occupational therapist, chaplains, pastors, and others all have important parts to play, in collaboration, in helping to solve the enormous emotional and social problems of the leukaemic child and his family.

The diagnosis should be discussed with the parents when the setting is appropriate and time is not rushed. The clinician and the nursing staff should be readily available to answer questions and to explain the treatment and the prognosis. False hopes must never be raised, but it is equally wrong to create feelings of despair by giving an unduly hopeless prognosis. With ALL a cautiously optimistic approach has become justified by the increasing numbers of children now going into complete remission for five to ten years or longer. To the question of what to tell the patient, there can be no general answer. Most children are satisfied to be told that they have an unusual kind of anaemia and that continuous treatment may keep them well. Those who have reached puberty or adolescence usually discover the diagnosis eventually; they should be encouraged to ask questions but many of them clearly show that they do not want to discuss the leukaemia.

The clinician's personal experience and outlook are important in influencing his ability to support the child and his family. As expressed by Carl Smith (1972): 'The physician who treats children with leukaemia, and whose aim is to provide optimal total care, must find a compromise between these two extremes . . . , emotional over-involvement and emotional withdrawal'.

PROGNOSIS

The prospects for the child with acute leukaemia depend first on the induction therapy. In ALL, this succeeds in producing a complete remission in about 90% of cases, and a partial one in another 5%. In AML, the results are less satisfactory; complete remission can be obtained in 60%, but this figure is improving with modern intensive therapy. Of those who fail to remit, the great majority are less than two or more than ten years of age.

The duration of the first complete remission varies greatly, from a few months to more than five years. During a complete remission the child is as fit for school and other comparable activities as any normal child, though regular attendances as an outpatient are usually required. Remissions have continued without interruption for over five years so far in 12 of our patients.

Survival time has been increasing steadily as better therapeutic methods have been developed; it is closely related to the length of the first remission. Until antileukaemic drugs became available, the median survival time was less than 2 months without broad-spectrum antibiotics, and 3–4 months with them. By 1960, with three drugs available, the median survival time was about 12 months; by 1966 it was 18 months; by 1972, with better planned regimens as well as more drugs, it had risen to between 2½ and 3 years for ALL in many centres. For AML the median survival time has improved from one month to almost a year, but it has not been changed much by the more potent drug combinations which have recently boosted the remission induction rate.

Long-term survival is another important measure of prognosis; 26 of our patients have survived for at least 5 years (an incidence of 15% in recent years); two American groups have claimed disease-free 5-year survival in about 20% of patients with ALL, and better results are expected now that CNS leukaemia can usually be prevented. Twelve of our leukaemic children have survived for more than 7 years to date, and six of them (four with acute, two with chronic leukaemia) for more than 10 years; all but four of these twelve survivors are free from disease. Overseas centres now have records of a number of children who have survived for 15–20 years. It should be clearly recognized that such improved prognoses have been reported from special leukaemia clinics or centres, but it is progress of this kind which justifies the 'cautiously optimistic approach' referred to above.

UNCOMMON FORMS OF CHILDHOOD LEUKAEMIA

CONGENITAL LEUKAEMIA

This appears by the age of 4–5 weeks, with infiltration of nonhaemopoietic tissues. Only three examples occurred in 505 cases of leukaemia in the Index Series, and their characteristics are of special interest.

1. *It develops in the perinatal period*, usually in the first three weeks of life, but several cases have been reported in stillborn infants.
2. *It is very commonly associated with malformations* in structures normally formed between the fifth and the ninth week of fetal life, e.g. atrial and ventricular septal defects, dextrocardia, deformities of the upper limb, and mongolism. It is probably never familial, and in no case has the mother had leukaemia.
3. In addition to *purpura* and *hepatosplenomegaly*, there is fever and in most cases bluish-red, mobile nodules in the skin due to infiltration, but little or no lymphadenomegaly.
4. *The haemoglobin is normal at birth* but falls rapidly, and numerous nucleated red cells appear in the blood; the white cell count is high; the cell

type is almost always myeloid or monocytic, and the pattern more like a chronic than an acute leukaemia.

5. *The course is rapidly downhill*, unresponsive to treatment, and the median survival time is about two weeks.

The differential diagnosis includes septicaemia, viraemia, congenital syphilis and other infections, erythroblastosis foetalis and congenital thrombocytopenic purpura. Infiltration of non-haemopoietic tissues and the absence of jaundice are useful pointers.

CHRONIC MYELOID LEUKAEMIA

Chronic forms make up only 2·7% of all our cases of childhood leukaemia; 2% were chronic myeloid leukaemia, and there were exceedingly rare examples of chronic monocytic leukaemia, reticulosarcoma or myelofibrosis with leukaemia, and other myeloproliferative diseases. Chronic lymphatic leukaemia in a child appears to have been reported in only two cases in the English literature, and even a subacute form of it is rare.

Two forms of chronic myeloid leukaemia occur in roughly equal proportions in childhood:

1 The adult type; and
2 The juvenile type.

1. *The adult type*, occurring mainly in older children, is essentially the same as in adults, with the Philadelphia chromosome in marrow cells, a leukocyte count usually greater than 100,000/cmm, a good response to busulphan or to irradiation of the spleen, and a course often exceeding five years.

2. *The juvenile type* is very different. It usually develops in the first three years of life with a clinical picture which commonly includes recurrent infections, a facial eczematoid rash, early thrombocytopenia, and a leukocyte count which is often normal or low, and rarely reaches 100,000/cmm. The Philadelphia chromosome is absent (though other chromosomal defects occur) and the fetal haemoglobin is high (15–50%).

Chronic granulomatous disease of childhood must be considered in the differential diagnosis.

Treatment with busulphan, in a dosage of 1·5 mg/m^2/day by mouth, usually succeeds in decreasing the number of white cells in the blood, particularly myelocytes, and in reducing the splenomegaly to a size which is impalpable. The dose should be reduced before a normal white cell count is reached and the drug may be stopped a few weeks later. Irradiation of the spleen is perhaps equally effective but more damaging to growing tissues. The juvenile form responds less well to busulphan, but desacetmethylcolchicine (2·5–5 mg/m^2/day) and mercaptopurine are often effective. Monitoring by means of frequent blood counts is essential with all forms of therapy (p. 116). Blastic transformation is likely to develop in both types of this disease.

RARE FORMS OF LEUKAEMIA

Erythroleukaemia occurs in 1–2% of childhood leukaemias, usually in an acute form. Characteristically it starts as erythraemic myelosis or di Guglielmo's syndrome, in which erythroblastic proliferation predominates and the leukocyte count is usually normal. Often the patient is first seen in the second phase, for which the term 'erythroleukaemia' is most appropriate for both erythroblasts and myeloblasts are then prominent and leukocytosis is common. Patients who survive long enough develop a final phase of predominantly myeloblastic proliferation, as in acute myeloid leukaemia.

Erythropoiesis is ineffective in all stages; there are many abnormal erythroblasts with multinuclearity and megaloblastic changes, but a disproportionately small reticulocytosis. Strongly PAS-positive erythroblasts and a low neutrophil alkaline phosphatase help to differentiate erythroleukaemia from chronic myeloid leukaemia and from leukaemoid reactions respectively.

Cytosine arabinoside (p. 106) has some therapeutic effect.

Myelofibrosis with myeloid metaplasia occurred in three of our younger patients, with unrelenting progression. Rare childhood cases have been reported of eosinophilic and plasma cell leukaemia, and of a familial myeloproliferative disease simulating chronic myeloid leukaemia, but no examples have been seen in the Index Series.

REFERENCES

AMROMIN, G.D. (1968). *Pathology of Leukemia*. Harper and Row, New York.

DAMESHEK, W. & GUNZ, F. (1964). *Leukemia*, 2nd ed. p. 14. Grune & Stratton. New York.

GREENWALD, E.S. (1973). *Cancer Chemotherapy*, 2nd ed. Medical Examination Publishing Company, Flushing, New York.

HAGHBIN, M., TAN, C.T.C., CLARKSON, B.D. *et al.* (1975). Treatment of acute lymphoblastic leukaemia in children with 'prophylactic' intrathecal methotrexate and intensive systemic chemotherapy. *Cancer Res.*, **35** ; 807.

HAYHOE, F.G.J., QUAGLINO, D. & DOLL, R. (1964). *The Cytology and Cytochemistry of Acute Leukaemias*. H.M.S.O. London.

MAUER, A. M. (1969). *Pediatric Hematology*. McGraw-Hill, Inc., New York.

OPITZ, H. (1954). Das Leukamieproblem. *Monatschr. Kinderh.*, **102** : 120.

SCHROEDER, T.M. & KURTH, R. (1971). Spontaneous chromosomal breakage and high incidence of leukemia in inherited disease. *Blood*, **37** : 1.

SMITH, C.H. (1972). *Blood Diseases of Infancy and Childhood*, 3rd ed., p. 584. C.V. Mosby Coy, St. Louis.

WHANG-PENG, J., FREIREICH, E.J., OPPENHEIM, J.J., FREI III, E., & TJIO, J.H. (1969). Cytogenetic studies in 45 patients with acute lymphocytic leukemia. *J. Nat. Cancer Inst.*, **42**,

Chapter 10. The malignant lymphomas

At present, the classification of malignant tumours of the reticulo-endothelial system, and the most appropriate nomenclature for them are in a state of change. In this chapter the traditional classification into lymphosarcoma, reticulum cell sarcoma and Hodgkin's disease has been retained, not because these categories are considered to be finite, nor a better classification than that proposed by Rappaport (1966), but because the great majority of malignant lymphomas in childhood can be readily allocated to one of the three groups (Table 10.1) on histological evidence in sections stained by standard methods such as haematoxylin-eosin, reticulin and Masson's stains.

Table 10.1. Malignant lymphomas. Classification of the types and sites of origin in 120 cases in the Index Series (RCH, 1950–1972)

	L. node	Mediast.	Bowel	'Burkitt's'	Other	Total
Hodgkin's disease	33	0	0	0	0	33
Lymphosarcoma	29	16	13	3	7	68
Reticulum-cell sarcoma	9	2	1	0	5	17
'Giant follicular lymphoma'	2	0	0	0	0	2
					Total	120

Some of the lymphoreticular proliferations in childhood present diagnostic difficulties, but they can be allocated to the group they most closely resemble, or reported as unclassified. Additional methods of investigation, already employed in research, will probably make it possible to reclassify the latter group on the basis of their etiology, cellular morphology or their immunological characteristics. However, these methods are not yet available for routine use in most laboratories.

A further reservation concerning Rappaport's nomenclature is the use of the term 'histiocytic' to specify some reticulum cell sarcomas, a usage which would cause confusion among clinicians and pathologists familiar with the histiocytoses of childhood (see Chapter 11) which are histologically distinct from their more malignant cousins, the malignant lymphomas.

For these reasons their classification in this chapter is as follows:

I Lymphosarcoma;
II Reticulum cell sarcoma; and
III Hodgkin's disease.

The place of Burkitt's 'lymphoma', or tumour, in non-endemic areas is to some extent uncertain. Re-examination of all specimens in the Index Series suggested that six tumours could be considered as histologically consistent with a diagnosis of Burkitt's tumour, but the clinical and serological findings were confirmatory in only three cases in which the tumour arose in the ovary, the retroperitoneal tissues and the jaw respectively (p. 328).

I. LYMPHOSARCOMA

AGE : SEX

Lymphosarcoma occurs at any age, although infrequently in children less than three years of age (Fig. 10.1). The ratio of males to females in the Index Series was 2·6 : 1 and in some series the male predominance is even greater. It appears to be more common in tropical than in temperate climates.

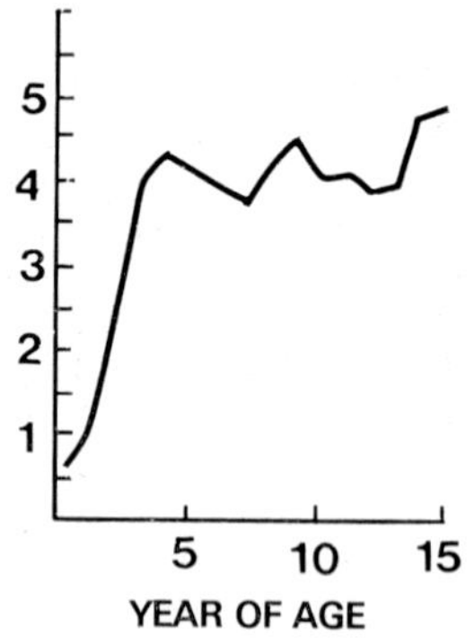

Figure 10.1. LYMPHOSARCOMA; the incidence according to age, showing a peak in the second quinquennium. (For source of figures see Fig. 2.2, p. 48.)

SITES

Lymphosarcoma occurs in several characteristic sites in childhood, in the following order of frequency.

1. *The alimentary canal*, chiefly the ileum (p. 631), possibly in Peyer's patches, causing abdominal symptoms, a palpable abdominal mass (p. 633), an intussusception, and only occasionally complete intestinal obstruction.
2. *The anterior mediastinum* (p. 446) probably arising in lymphoid tissue or in the thymus.
3. *Peripheral lymph nodes*, e.g. in the neck (p. 225), and somewhat less commonly in other superficial groups of nodes.
4. *The nasopharynx*, in one of the lymphoid components of 'Waldeyer's ring' (p. 343).

MICROSCOPIC FINDINGS

Two varieties of lymphosarcoma occur in children:
(*a*) Lymphoblastic, and
(*b*) Lymphocytic lymphosarcoma.

(*a*) *Lymphoblastic lymphosarcoma* is by far the more common. The distinctive cell is a large lymphocyte or lymphoblast with a characteristic spherical nucleus and a small or medium-sized rim of cytoplasm (Fig. 10.2a). The nucleus is often somewhat vesicular in appearance and in some cells there is a prominent, dark, eccentrically placed nucleolus. Mitotic figures are common. Most of these tumours contain a variable number of medium sized lymphoblasts (Fig. 10.2b), and prominent phagocytic reticulum cells which at low

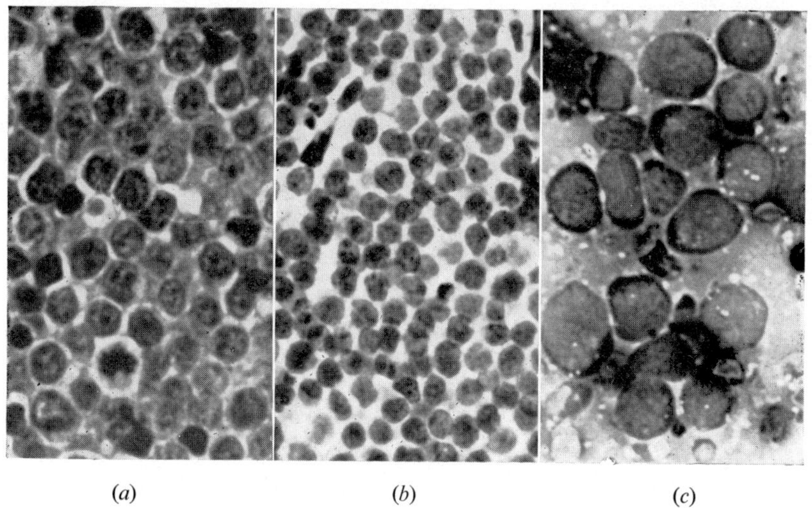

(*a*) (*b*) (*c*)

Figure 10.2. LYMPHOBLASTIC LYMPHOSARCOMA; (*a*) and (*b*) large and medium-sized lymphoblasts; the magnification in these two photographs is the same (× 38 objective). (*a*) The cells are larger with coarse chromatin, one to three nucleoli and moderate amounts of cytoplasm; those in (*b*) have a smaller nucleus, the chromatin is finer, the nucleoli inconspicuous, and there is slightly less cytoplasm; (*c*) imprint cytology of (*a*) with Leishman stain.

magnification appear as clear spaces scattered throughout the tumour (Fig. 10.3a), referred to as a 'starry-sky' appearance and first clearly described in lymphomas in children in Africa. It is now regarded as evidence of rapid growth, not confined to Burkitt's lymphoma, or lymphosarcoma, but seen in many rapidly growing tumours.

The tumour cells are usually arranged in diffuse sheets, the only variations being the presence of the phagocytic cells or infiltrated tissue planes. When a lymphosarcoma infiltrates adipose tissue, the lymphoblasts may become arranged around individual fat cells, and this may be misinterpreted as 'rosette' formation. When the tumour infiltrates tissue planes, parallel cords of tumour cells (Fig. 10.3b) growing between bundles of collagen can simulate an infiltrating carcinoma.

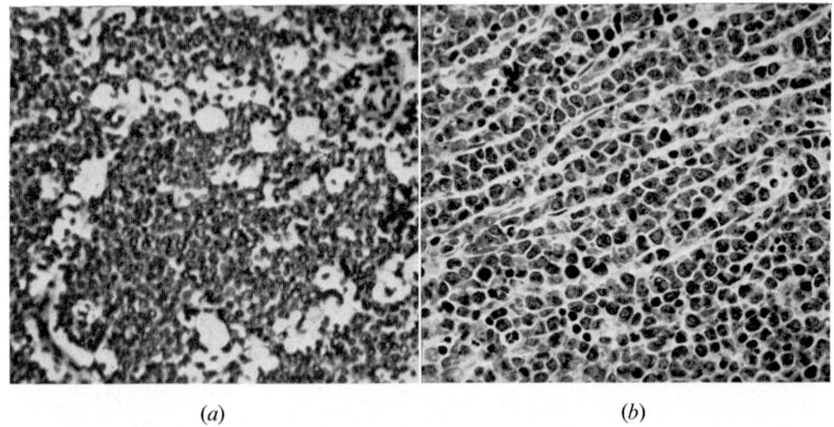

(*a*) (*b*)

Figure 10.3. Lymphoblastic lymphosarcoma; (*a*) 'starry sky' appearance caused by non-neoplastic phagocytic reticulum cells scattered among lymphoblasts. (b) Parallel cords of lymphosarcoma cells infiltrating between strands of collagen, mimicking the pattern of a carcinoma.

Reticulum formation is usually scanty or absent, except in infiltrated tissue planes and then the reticulin pattern is prominent, coarse and probably derived from the infiltrated connective tissue.

The PAS stain demonstrates very small, PAS-positive granules of glycogen in the cytoplasm of the lymphoblasts. Glycogen is rapidly degraded after removal from the body and unless fixation is very rapid and complete, the PAS stain may fail to reveal these granules. They are best seen in imprint preparations (Fig. 10.2c) in which fat droplets in the cytoplasm of the lymphoblasts can also be shown, on occasions, by appropriate stains.

(*b*) *Lymphocytic lymphosarcomas* are rare in children. They show diffuse infiltration and replacement of lymph nodes by small, round, lymphocyte-like cells averaging 12μ or less. The cells are extremely uniform, and phagocytic reticulum cells are not present. Occasionally a pseudo-follicular pattern is found in this type of lymphosarcoma in childhood, but it is uncommon. Almost all the lymphocytic lymphosarcomas in the Index Series arose in the bowel wall (p. 631) or in lymph nodes.

SPREAD

Infiltration of the bone marrow is present in some cases at the time of diagnosis, and develops at some stage in at least 40% of cases, usually accompanied by a blood picture virtually identical with that of lymphatic leukaemia.

The frequency of spread to the marrow varies with the site of the primary; it develops with about 10% of tumours arising in the alimentary tract, 40% of those arising in peripheral lymph nodes and 80–90% of those in the mediastinum, if the patient survives long enough (Webster, 1961; Sonley, 1972/73).

MODES OF PRESENTATION

The clinical picture varies according to the site and stage of the tumour. A large series from multiple reports analysed by Sonley (1972/1973) showed that the four most common forms of presentation were:

1. *A primary tumour in the alimentary canal;*
2. *Extensive intra-abdominal disease* of uncertain origin;
3. *A large mediastinal mass;* and
4. *Regional or generalized enlargement of peripheral lymph nodes.*

These four occurred with approximately equal frequency, and together accounted for 80–85% of all cases; a tumour in Waldeyer's ring (p. 343) or in the mandible provided another 11%. Children develop extranodal disease more often, but a primary in the stomach more rarely, than adults. Typical Burkitt's lymphoma is uncommon in non-endemic areas (see p. 328).

CLINICAL FEATURES

The symptoms and signs arising in tumours in the various sites are described in the relevant chapters. Certain syndromes are of particular importance because of the diagnostic or therapeutic problems they pose:

(*a*) *Abdominal pain* and distension, nausea, vomiting and fever, in which the underlying intra-abdominal mass may be masked by guarding;

(*b*) *A pleural or pericardial effusion* with pleocytosis, in which the cells may not be clearly identifiable as malignant;

(*c*) *Oedema and congestion of the upper half of the body*, eventually with dyspnoea, as the result of compression of the superior vena cava and eventually the trachea;

(*d*) *Malabsorption*, steatorrhoea and failure to thrive, which may be due to infiltration of the small bowel.

As lymphosarcoma may arise in any organ or tissue containing lymphoid cells, there are many other diseases which it may simulate.

The stage of the disease

The stage of the disease (see below) naturally influences the clinical picture, as well as the prognosis; for example, in Stage I there may be only a visible or palpable lump, or a tumour in the wall of the small bowel which presents as an intussusception (p. 633); whereas systemic symptoms (B) such as 'malignant malaise' (p. 549), loss of weight, fever, etc., are unusual except in Stage IV in which there is often extensive disease, the liver is often enlarged even without infiltration, and the marrow is commonly leukaemic.

INVESTIGATIONS

1. A full blood examination and platelet count, and aspiration of bone marrow are essential in every case. Sections of bone marrow are more effective than aspiration smears in detecting involvement, except in Burkitt's lymphoma (Vinciguerra & Silver, 1973).
2. X-rays of the chest are essential and a skeletal survey is usually carried out, though it is almost always negative (Schey *et al.*, 1973).
3. Intravenous pyelography and/or other forms of contrast radiography of the abdomen are desirable in most cases.
4. Lymphangiography via the lymphatics at the ankle is theoretically required for staging when the patient presents with lymphoid swellings in the upper half of the body, but in younger children this is often not feasible.
5. Laparotomy and splenectomy for staging are seldom justifiable in lymphosarcoma in childhood.
6. Liver function tests are useful as a guide to possible hepatic involvement, and a liver scan may also be informative.
7. When the marrow is infiltrated or when there is any indication of involvement of the CNS, a lumbar puncture is required.
8. The level of serum uric acid and blood urea should be measured before commencing treatment. The level of serum copper can be very useful as an indicator of disease status in all forms of malignant lymphoma; the level is raised before treatment and in relapse, it is higher with generalized than with local tumour, and it returns to normal during complete remission (Hrgovcic *et al.*, 1973; Tessmer *et al.*, 1973), but it may sometimes be raised in other conditions, e.g. viral infection.

STAGING

The following system of staging, introduced by Peters *et al.* (1968), is applicable to both lymphosarcoma and reticulum cell sarcoma.

Stage I: Tumour confined to one group of lymph nodes or to two contiguous structures.

Stage II: Tumour in more than two sites, but confined to one side of the diaphragm.

Stage III: Tumour on both sides of the diaphragm, but not extending beyond lymph nodes, spleen and/or Waldeyer's ring.

Stage IV: Tumour in any of the following areas: the bone marrow, bones (on x-ray), lungs, pleura, liver, kidneys, more than one skin or subcutaneous lesion, or the alimentary tract when considered to be secondary.
In each stage, the suffix **A** is added when systemic symptoms are absent, the suffix **B** when they are present.

TREATMENT

The intensity of treatment varies with the prognosis, and this is related to the site, the stage and the histology. In patients in Stages I and II, especially those with localized extranodal disease (e.g. in bowel and pharynx) treatment should definitely aim at cure. This generally includes surgical excision of the tumour, or as much of it as is practicable, always radiotherapy to the site of the primary, and chemotherapy, at least to 'cover' the operation (p. 109).

The recurrence or relapse rate without chemotherapy is very high in Stage I and approaches 100% in Stage II, so it is rational to act on the assumption that microscopic metastasis has already occurred. This means that an extended programme of chemotherapy should be given to every patient, for at least two years, with the possible exception of a patient in Stage I in whom 'spillage' or dissemination can be excluded with reasonable certainty.

Patients in Stage III differ only in that surgical removal, or even subtotal excision, is less often feasible, so chemotherapy should be more intensive and prolonged, and more irradiation may be indicated. Until the last few years, the long term prognosis for children in Stage III, and even more so for those in Stage IV, was so unfavourable that treatment was often limited to palliative chemotherapy, low-dosage radiotherapy (e.g. to a mediastinal mass) and symptomatic treatment. It was found in 1969 that the survival time in those patients in the Index Series with lymphosarcoma and who also developed leukaemia, was more than twice as long as in patients without leukaemia, and this can be attributed to the effectiveness of the antileukaemic drugs. Since then intensive combination chemotherapy, using modern drugs, has improved the short-term outlook to such an extent that patients in Stage III and even some in Stage IV may now merit full-scale multi-disciplinary treatment, with cure as the objective.

Surgery

Surgery is required mainly for biopsy and for removal of reasonably localized lesions in the alimentary canal (p. 630), the skin and occasionally elsewhere, and for abdominal complications.

Radiotherapy

Lymphosarcomas are notably radiosensitive, although the usefulness of irradiation is somewhat limited because the disease is not truly 'localized' in the great majority of patients. Radiotherapy to local lymph node masses in doses of 3000–3500 rads causes very rapid regression, and dramatic results can be obtained in patients with mediastinal masses of lymphosarcoma causing compression (p. 445). Hyperuricaemia is likely to occur when large masses or nodes are destroyed rapidly, but renal complications can be minimized or prevented by allopurinol and a high fluid intake.

Chemotherapy

Some form of chemotherapy is indicated for every patient with apparently localized disease (Stage I); radiotherapy, with or without surgery, may be combined with vincristine (weekly for four to six weeks) and prednisolone for the first week, followed by oral drugs for maintenance therapy (Aur *et al.*, 1971). When the disease is known or suspected to be disseminated, several drugs should be given in combination, for no single agent is as effective in the long run.

Vincristine combined with an alkylating agent and corticosteroids have produced overall complete remission rates approaching 50%. The best long-term results known seem to come from regimens used for acute lymphatic leukaemia (see p. 159), which is not surprising as the marrow is so often involved in both conditions.

For both induction and maintenance of remission, intermittent therapy with three-weekly 'pulses' of vincristine (1·8–2·0 mg/m^2 IV, once), cyclophosphamide (400 mg/m^2 IV, once) and prednisolone (50 mg/m^2/day for five days) is one regime which has proved to be effective. Acute Leukaemia Group B have reported that the results are better without cyclophosphamide—a finding which, if true, may be due to the immunosuppressive effect of alkylating agents.

'MOPP' (nitrogen mustard, vincristine, prednisolone and procarbazine), which has produced very good results in Hodgkin's disease, is less often effective for lymphosarcoma, probably because nitrogen mustard and procarbazine are less suitable for combating the bone marrow infiltration. When resistance to the combination of cyclophosphamide, vincristine and prednisolone (referred to as 'COP' or 'CVP') develops, remissions may still be obtained from the use of other antineoplastic drugs, e.g. daunorubicin, methotrexate, cytosine arabinoside, l-asparaginase, mercaptopurine or bleomycin. For maintenance of remission, methotrexate, cyclophosphamide and mercaptopurine are favoured in several major centres.

It is not yet clear how long chemotherapy should be continued when remission in lymphosarcoma has been achieved. We have not so far felt justified in ceasing treatment within the first three years, and at one large centre (Sonley, 1972/73) the policy is to continue chemotherapy for five years.

Some forms of lymphosarcoma have a particularly bad prognosis not greatly improved by the usual drug regimes, e.g. MOPP and CVP. In such cases investigations to identify subpopulations of lymphocytes by immunological markers on their cell membranes (Browne *et al.*, 1974; Borella & Sen, 1975) commonly show an increased proportion of T (thymus-derived) circulating lymphocytes. Recognition of this may be helpful by pointing to an urgent need for intensive and prolonged chemotherapy, and probably radiotherapy.

B-type lymphocytes predominate in some other forms, e.g. so-called 'nodular' lymphoma (Jaffe *et al.*, 1974).

Immunotherapy, combined with chemotherapy, is currently under trial for patients in remission. As the average survival time becomes longer, there is an increasing incidence of involvement of the CNS; this calls for prophylaxis and treatment as in acute lymphatic leukaemia (p. 159).

PROGNOSIS

The overall prognosis, which is steadily improving, is influenced by:

(*a*) *the site*, to some extent; those arising in the small bowel or the tonsil often respond well; massive retroperitoneal and mediastinal lymphosarcomas respond poorly;

(*b*) *the stage*, to a greater extent; most five-year survivors presented initially in Stage I (Kim and Dorfman, 1974); and

(*c*) *the treatment*, to a marked degree.

Until a decade ago, treatment relied mainly on radiotherapy and at most a single antimetabolite, which resulted in a median survival time of five months for forty patients in the Index Series, and only 10% survived for five years. The use of combinations of three or more potent drugs is extending the median survival time towards two years, but whether it will increase the five-year survival rate beyond 20–25% (as some predict) remains to be seen.

The outlook is greatly affected by the success of treatment in preventing complications—leukaemia, infiltration of the CNS, hyperuricaemia, hyperkalaemia and infections. Leukaemic transformation occurs in 75–90% of mediastinal or thymic tumours (Webster, 1961; Sonley, 1972/1973), and in some 30% of those arising in other sites, so its prevention, or at least its control, by treatment is paramount. Infiltration of the CNS may develop in as many as a third of the patients if prophylaxis as used in acute leukaemia (p. 163) is not given.

GIANT FOLLICULAR LYMPHOMA

This unusual histological type of lymphoma is best thought of as a variant of lymphosarcoma, with a particularly well-developed follicular pattern. The lymph nodes are replaced by large irregular follicles with ill-defined margins, extending throughout the cortex and medulla of the node, without any of the phagocytic reticulum cells normally seen in hyperplastic germinal centres. There were only two patients with this type amongst 120 lymphomas in the Index Series; both are alive and well four and fifteen years after commencing treatment.

II. RETICULUM CELL SARCOMA

This tumour is also referred to as reticulosarcoma, lymphoreticular sarcoma, and in the Rappaport classification as 'malignant lymphoma, histiocytic type'. Some authorities consider it to be a variant of lymphosarcoma, and a few seem to deny its existence as an entity at all. It is considered separately from lymphosarcoma in this chapter because of significant differences in macroscopic and microscopic pathology, clinical features, course and therapy.

An especially interesting feature of this tumour's etiology is that it is probably the commonest type of neoplasm to develop as a complication of immunodeficiency, e.g. in transplantation patients on prolonged immunosuppressive therapy, and in certain congenital disorders of the immune system (Gatti & Good, 1971). There have recently been reports of two patients, each of whom developed a reticulum cell sarcoma at the site of an antilymphocyte-globulin injection (Cotton *et al.*, 1973).

AGE : SEX

Only a minority of reticulum cell sarcomas estimated as less than 10% occur in the paediatric age group, in which there is generally an increase in incidence with age (Fig. 10.4). There are significant increments in each of the second and third quinquennia, and most of the patients in the Index Series were six to eight years of age or older at the time of diagnosis.

Males are affected slightly more frequently than females in childhood, in a ratio of approximately 3 : 2.

SITES

Reticulum cell sarcoma most commonly arises in:

(i) Superficial or deep peripheral lymph nodes (p. 225); but also in
(ii) The anterior mediastinum (p. 452);
(iii) The distal ileum and ileocaecal region (p. 638);
(iv) In bone (p. 764); and in
(v) Subcutaneous tissues, and very occasionally elsewhere.

There is still some controversy as to whether the tumour arising in extralymphoid tissues (e.g. in bone) is basically the same as the more common lymphoid forms.

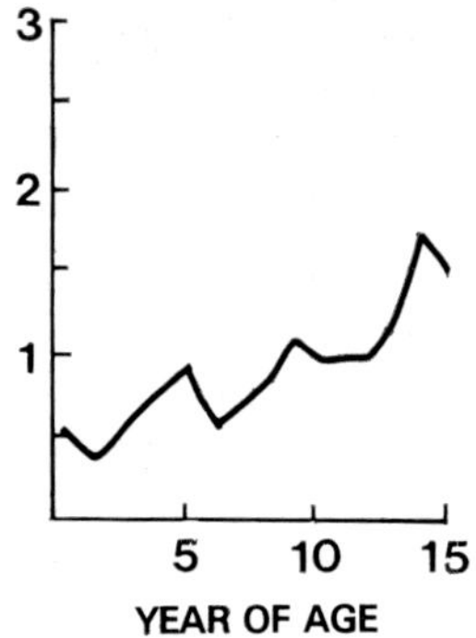

Figure 10.4. RETICULUM CELL SARCOMA; the incidence according to age, showing an increase in each quinquennium of the paediatric age group. The peak incidence occurs at thirty years of age (for source of figures see Fig. 2.2, p. 48).

Subcutaneous reticulum cell sarcoma

This separate group arising in subcutaneous tissues lie beneath the skin, but often involve the epithelium (Kim *et al.*, 1963). Microscopically they differ from those described below; the nuclei are smaller, the cytoplasm less, and variation in the size of individual nuclei much less striking. Reticulin formation is present, but in small amounts. There are four cases in the Index Series and all but one of them responded well to treatment, in striking contrast to the poor prognosis of some of those arising in other sites.

The lesions are mostly small, and as there are no characteristic clinical features, the diagnosis is usually made on biopsy. Whenever possible 'total biopsy', which includes a safe margin of the adjoining skin and subcutaneous tissues, is desirable.

Differentiation of this lesion from cutaneous lymphoid hyperplasia (Caro & Helwig, 1969) can present difficulties.

MACROSCOPIC APPEARANCES

The appearances of the tumour vary considerably according to the site of origin, and these are described in the chapters devoted to those areas.

MICROSCOPIC FINDINGS

In lymph nodes the tumour results in either complete replacement of the normal architecture of the node by diffusely proliferating reticulum cells, or partial replacement by a discrete mass of tumour cells (Fig. 10.5a), with a distinct advancing edge suggestive of a metastasis. The hallmarks of this tumour are the pleomorphism of the nuclei and great variation in the size of individual cells, which range from 12μ to 30μ in diameter (Fig. 10.5b). Mitoses are numerous and often bizarre; the cells commonly have abundant cytoplasm which is sometimes well-defined, at other times indistinct with a syncytial appearance.

One criterion for a diagnosis of reticulum cell sarcoma is the demonstration of increased amounts of reticulin formed by individual tumour cells (Fig. 10.5c). A feature which can be of particular assistance in differentiating reticulum cell sarcoma from certain other tumours is that its cells (like those of neuroblastoma, some of the histiocytoses, and acute myeloid leukaemia) are PAS-negative, while those of rhabdomyosarcoma, Ewing's tumour and acute lymphatic leukaemia are PAS-positive (see colour plate, following p. 140).

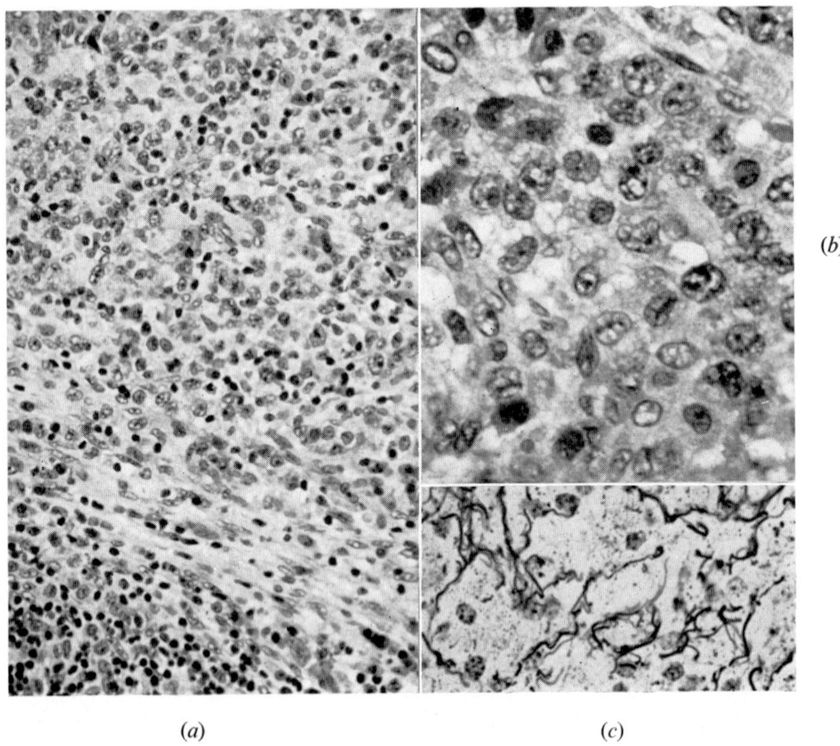

(*a*) (*b*) (*c*)

Figure 10.5. Reticulum cell sarcoma; (*a*) low power view showing partial replacement of a lymph node; (*b*) high power of cellular detail; and (*c*) reticulin fibres demonstrated by selective staining. The cells of this tumour have more open nuclei and more cytoplasm than in some reticulum cell sarcomas in childhood.

TREATMENT

For reticulum cell sarcoma, the staging, investigation and treatment follow the same general pattern as described for lymphosarcoma (p. 174). There are some differences, however, related to the tumour site, to the lesser risk of leukaemic transformation and to different drug-sensitivities.

Surgery

When a primary tumour in subcutaneous tissue is shown by full investigation to be localized (Stage I) and the diagnosis has already been established by biopsy, radical excision covered by chemotherapy (usually vincristine) is the first line of treatment, followed by skin grafts if necessary.

When the regional lymph nodes are also involved and no distant metastases are demonstrable or suspected (Stage II), complete excision of the regional nodes may also be performed, either at the same operation or at a later stage if they are then enlarged.

When the primary tumour is in bone, the situation is rather similar to Ewing's tumour (p. 766) in that radical surgery has little if any more—and possibly less—to offer than irradiation of the primary tumour combined with a full chemotherapy programme.

Chemotherapy

Recent advances in drug therapy have shown reticulum cell sarcoma to be one of the most responsive of solid tumours to modern regimens of combination chemotherapy. It should not be inferred that an advanced Stage IV tumour can be expected to be cured by drugs alone, though even this does seem to have occurred on occasions. Of a large list of agents which cause regression of this tumour, among the most effective are: the antibiotics, adriamycin, daunorubicin and actinomycin D; drugs with an alkylating action, e.g. cyclophosphamide, procarbazine, chlorambucil and nitrogen mustard; the alkaloids, vincristine and vinblastine; corticosteroids; and in high dosage the antimetabolites, methotrexate and cytosine arabinoside.

To cover the biopsy, and the initial operation (if any), a suitable course is vincristine (1·8–2·0 mg/m^2 IV weekly for four to six weeks) combined with prednisolone for at least two weeks. If radiotherapy follows, vincristine should be continued, given weekly, till the end of the course. If the tumour is in Stage III or IV or rapidly advancing, at least one additional drug should be combined with the above, e.g. adriamycin (30–35 mg/m^2) or actinomycin D (0·5 mg/m^2) or cyclophosphamide (400 mg/m^2 IV weekly); alternatively, 50 mg/m^2 of adriamycin or 750 mg/m^2 of cyclophosphamide given every two weeks.

As soon as the initial phase of remission induction and irradiation has been completed, usually by the seventh or eighth week, a regimen of recurrent 'pulses' of chemotherapy at regular intervals, preferably every three weeks, should begin. For this, several drug combinations have proved to be suitable, e.g. cycles of actinomycin D, vincristine and cyclophosphamide, or of 'MOPP', i.e. nitrogen mustard (M), vincristine (Oncovin®), procarbazine (P) and prednisolone (P).

These recurrent courses should be continued for at least two years, and in most of our survivors they have been continued for a further year or so longer. Any evidence or strong suspicion of recurrence, even a significant rise in the level of serum copper (see p. 174), warrants a further one year or more of chemotherapy.

PROGNOSIS

A fatal outcome was almost the rule until a decade ago, although the mortality was less than with lymphosarcoma. Many of the exceptions were children with a tumour arising in subcutaneous tissue, in an isolated lymph node or in bone, presumably because tumours in these sites are more likely to present while in Stage I.

Modern chemotherapy, usually combined with more radical surgery and radiotherapy, has raised the median survival time to about one year, and the chances of surviving five years are now at least 30%. Leukaemic marrow infiltration (with monocytoid cells prominent) develops in only 5–10% of cases, in marked contrast to the higher incidence in lymphosarcoma (p. 177), and infiltration of the CNS is correspondingly less frequent, except for the occurrence of intracranial reticulum cell sarcoma in transplantation patients on immunosuppressants.

Index series

An improvement in prognosis since vincristine and cytotoxic agents of the antibiotic type became available can be seen in the Index Series. Of twelve consecutive patients who began treatment in 1962–1968, five are alive and apparently free of disease 6–11 years later. The mode of presentation was with fever plus enlargement of the liver, spleen and/or lymph nodes in three patients (marrow positive in one), a chain of enlarged pectoral axillary lymph nodes in one, and a subcutaneous tumour in one. Chemotherapy was the only form of treatment used in three of these cases. Analyses of large series show that recurrence is extremely rare after 3 years (Lemerle *et al.*, 1973) and the five long term survivors in the Index Series can reasonably be considered to be cures.

III. HODGKIN'S DISEASE

This condition is less clearly defined than lymphosarcoma and reticulum cell sarcoma, but most authorities regard it as a malignant disease, with proliferation of both lymphoid and reticulo-endothelial tissues and with the multi-nucleated Sternberg-Reed cell as its chief histological characteristic. The evidence that it is truly neoplastic is far from strong and recently some workers have questioned whether Sternberg-Reed cells are essential to the diagnosis. For practical purposes, however, the description which follows is generally applicable.

Hodgkin's disease has a very great deal in common with the other malignant lymphomas, but differs materially both in its epidemiology, macroscopic and microscopic pathology and also in its clinical behaviour, course and prognosis.

AGE : SEX

Hodgkin's disease represented some 25% of 120 lymphomas in the Index Series (Table 10.1), and it is less common in children than in adults; some 8–20% of reported cases occur in patients less than 15 years of age. It is extremely rare in infancy (a boy aged 22 months in the Index Series was unique, but since the Series closed three other boys presented with Hodgkin's disease before 4 years of age). Only 2·5% of affected children are less than 4 years of age at diagnosis. The incidence increases progressively with age (Fig. 10.6) to reach a childhood peak which occurs before puberty in boys, but not until late adolescence in girls (Fraumeni & Li, 1969). This leads on to the first major peak which is in the third decade.

Boys are affected 3–4 times as commonly as girls. In the Index Series there were 33 cases of Hodgkin's disease, of which 27 were boys and 6 girls.

ETIOLOGY

The cause is still unknown although many clues have been discovered in the past decade.

Genetic factors

There is probably a genetic factor involved, as suggested by a highly significant association with certain HL-A antigens, notably A11 and W5, by a

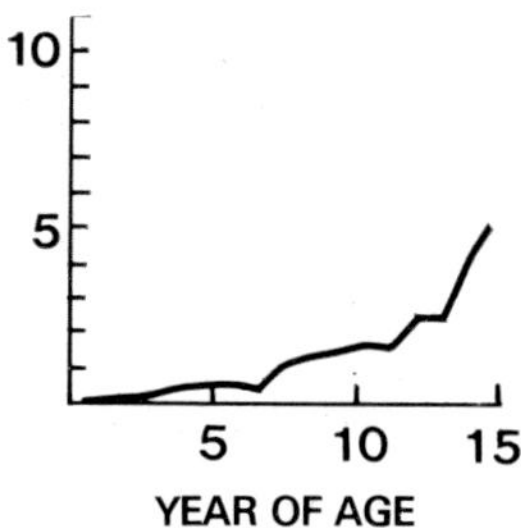

Figure 10.6. HODGKIN'S DISEASE; the incidence according to age, showing a marked increase in the third quinquennium (for source of figures see Fig. 2.2, p. 48).

positive family history of Hodgkin's or closely related neoplasms in some cases, by its association with hereditary immunological defects, and by sex differences in the incidence and age distribution.

Environmental factors

Evidence is accumulating that these may also be involved. Socio-economic status was found, in Colombia, to influence the incidence in children, which fell as the standard of living rose. Hodgkin's disease in Japan is disproportionately uncommon in youths compared with older adults, and in the U.S.A. the geographical distribution is uneven.

An infective agent

Affected children, even when in remission, are more susceptible to infections, especially viral infections, than those with other lymphomas. Some 5% of patients of all ages with Hodgkin's disease develop a second malignancy, and children with congenital immunological deficiencies are susceptible to Hodgkin's and other malignant lymphoreticular diseases. These indications of the role of the immune system in Hodgkin's disease are compatible with the view that the etiology may involve an infective agent. There have been enough reports of cases in siblings, in both conjugal partners, and in time-place clusters based on schools, to provoke a recent editorial entitled 'Is Hodgkin's Disease Contagious?' (MacMahon, 1973). The answer was: most probably not, and if there is any risk from exposure to a case, 'it must be of a very low magnitude'.

With these observations, Hodgkin's disease has naturally become the object of much current virological research. The Epstein-Barr virus (EBV) is under consideration because of its role in Burkitt's lymphoma and because two independent groups have recently shown that it induces in primates a disease resembling the closely related reticulum cell sarcoma. A high proportion of Hodgkin's disease cases have been reported to follow infectious mononucleosis (believed to be caused by the EBV). On the other hand, some Hodgkin's patients have no detectable antibodies to EBV.

The theory of the natural history of the disease has been that it commences in a lymph node or a group of nodes, spreads to involve the next contiguous group, then to distant groups and thence to the liver and spleen, with a progressively increasing likelihood of haematogenous spread, and the eventual development of discrete or diffuse visceral infiltrations. There are, however, a number of patients in whom the disease seems to have spread from cervical nodes (usually on the left side) to the abdomen without involvement of the mediastinum. Such cases, together with Rappaport's observation of vascular invasion by tumour, suggest haematogenous spread, while the evidence of a role for an infective agent would favour a multicentric origin for the disease.

In summary, the etiology seems likely to be a combination of factors in the environment and the host. Further research is required to determine whether there is an infective agent and whether the disease may be multicentric in origin, at least in some cases. The conclusions ultimately reached may prove to be applicable also to reticulum cell sarcoma, and possibly lymphosarcoma.

MICROSCOPIC FINDINGS

The microscopic pathology is described before the macroscopic appearances because the histology is of paramount importance. There may be great difficulty in distinguishing Hodgkin's disease from non-specific chronic lymphadenitis, and also in classifying its various types (Dorfman & Warnke, 1974). However, an attempt should always be made to place each patient in one of the four histological groups because this is a major factor in determining the prognosis and in choosing the most appropriate plan of treatment.

Good material for histological study is essential. Previous radiotherapy or chemotherapy may so alter the histology that it is impossible to make a definite diagnosis of Hodgkin's disease, or of its histological type, so biopsy must precede treatment. The node for biopsy should always be a prominent one, preferably taken from near the centre of the group affected; a satellite node may show only reactive hyperplasia while a more centrally placed node contains diagnostic material.

Imprints of the cut surface of the node (p. 82) before it is fixed are particularly helpful in demonstrating the large binucleate Sternberg-Reed cells which are the major criterion for the diagnosis of all histological types.

There are four main histological types of Hodgkin's disease (Figs. 10.7, 10.8) using the modification of the Lukes-Butler classification adopted at Rye (Lukes *et al.*, 1966), and all four types are encountered in childhood. They are:

Type 1: The nodular sclerosing type;
Type 2: The lymphocyte-predominant type;
Type 3: Those of 'mixed cellularity'; and
Type 4: The lymphocyte-depleted type.

The 'paragranuloma' of the earlier Jackson-Parker classification is the same as type 2, and the 'granuloma' of that classification includes types 1 and 3. The distribution of the histological types in the thirty-three cases in the Index Series is shown in Table 10.2.

1. The nodular sclerosing type

This is characterized by the formation of much fibrous tissue which surrounds nodules of abnormal lymphoid tissue (Fig. 10.7a). The collagen is mature (i.e. birefringent) and in the early stages may only be found in some areas of the specimen. The characteristic of the abnormal lymphoid tissue

Table 10.2. Hodgkin's disease. The histological types in 33 patients in the Index Series (R.C.H. 1950–1972)

Mixed cellularity	15
Lymphocyte-predominant	10
Lymphocyte-depleted	4
Nodular sclerosing	4
Total	33

is the presence of large, multilobed variants of the Sternberg-Reed cell which are more prominent because each appears to lie in a lacuna. The diagnostic Sternberg-Reed cells are often difficult to find but always present (Fig. 10.8d inset). Lymphocytes are numerous in 'young' nodules, but with the passage of time they disappear and are replaced by fibrous tissue. At this stage, or before it, the tissue becomes infiltrated with eosinophils and granulocytes.

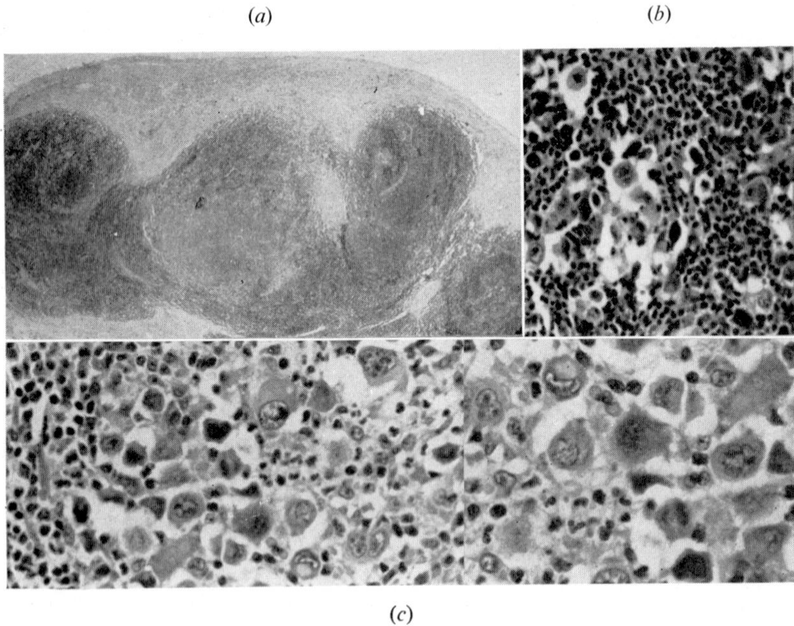

Figure 10.7. HODGKIN'S DISEASE; the nodular sclerosing type showing (*a*) nodules of Hodgkin's tissue surrounded by collagen; (*b*) early lesion consisting of 'lacunar cells' and lymphocytes; and (*c*) 'lacunar cells' with large nuclei and abundant fleshy cytoplasm.

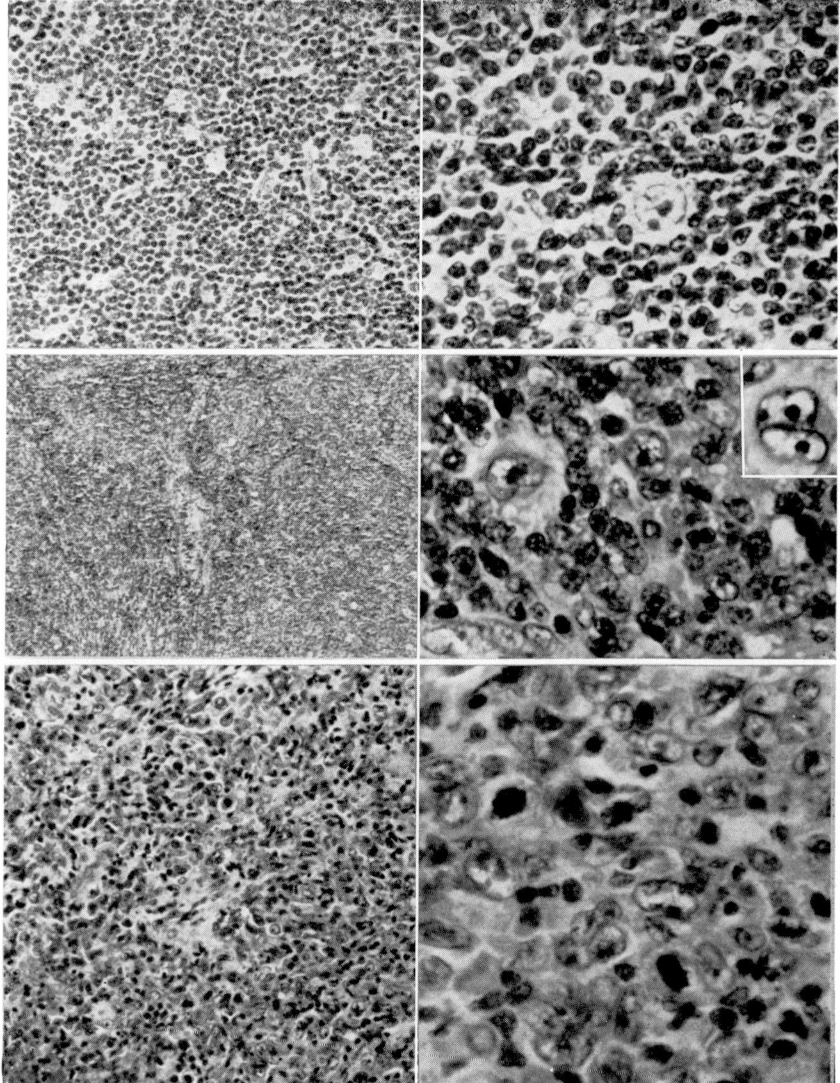

Figure 10.8. HODGKIN'S DISEASE: the histological types: (*a*) and (*b*) *the lymphocyte-predominant type* showing (*a*) medium sized lymphocytes and occasional reticulum cells; and (*b*) a small Reed-Sternberg cell near its centre; (*c*) and (*d*) *the mixed cell type* showing (*c*) the background cellular pattern—a very important diagnostic feature of Hodgkin's disease—and (*d*) lymphocytes, histiocytes, eosinophils and neoplastic reticulum cells; a typical Reed-Sternberg cell is inset; (*e*) & (*f*) *the lymphocyte-depleted type;* (*e*) many neoplastic reticulum cells, few lymphocytes; (*f*) irregular malignant reticulum cells, some of which are binucleate.

[(*a*) *Top left*. (*b*) *Top right*. (*c*) *Centre left*. (*d*) *Centre right*. (*e*) *Bottom left*. (*f*) *Bottom right*.]

Total sclerosis often occurs in the terminal stages. In any given specimen it is usually possible to find nodules of each of the various stages of development and senescence.

2. The lymphocyte predominant type

The histological pattern in this type may be so uniform that it mimics a lymphosarcoma. The affected node is replaced by a sheet of lymphocytes in which are scattered cells with a lobate nucleus and a clear halo of pale cytoplasm (Fig. 10.8a, b) which are similar to (and may be related to) the phagocytic reticulum cells seen in some lymphoblastic lymphosarcomas (p. 171). In Hodgkin's disease, however, these cells are often clustered; they have an enlarged nucleus with large nucleoli, characteristic of neoplasia.

Sternberg-Reed cells occur, but are often scanty; the typical cell has a large 'mirror-image' nucleus, a thick nuclear membrane, and a large spherical or oval eosinophilic nucleolus, often with a clear perinucleolar halo. The cytoplasm is abundant and eosinophilic or amphophilic (Fig. 10.8d, inset).

Eosinophils are rare in this type and fibrosis does not occur. The affected lymph node may be only partly replaced, and it is not uncommon to find surviving follicles at the periphery. The sheet of abnormal lymphoid tissue may be nodular rather than uniform, but the diagnosis rests on the predominance of the lymphocytes, which can usually be recognized without difficulty.

3. Mixed cellularity

This is the 'classical' pattern, i.e. with great variation in tissue pattern, cell type and cellular morphology (Fig. 10.8c, d). There are many Sternberg-Reed cells, numerous eosinophils, irregular fibrosis, areas of necrosis, and the whole range of mononuclear cells—those resembling large lymphocytes, larger cells resembling histiocytes, and small reticulum cells with some of the cytological features of Sternberg-Reed cells. A nodular distribution is usual, and the pattern and appearance varies greatly from field to field.

4. The lymphocyte depleted type

This variant is rare in childhood, at least at the time when the patient first presents, although biopsies and post mortem material from cases of other types are characteristically devoid of lymphocytes (Fig. 10.8e, f). This type has been separated histologically from the others; absence of a lymphocytic response by the host is believed to indicate a severe immunological deficiency, and a correspondingly poor prognosis. The pattern is one of a diffuse fibrous replacement of the node with few, if any, lymphocytes, but increased numbers of Sternberg-Reed cells.

In the past, the type in which there are very many Sternberg-Reed cells and great pleomorphism was referred to as 'Hodgkin's sarcoma'; this is rare in childhood and no such case was encountered in the Index Series.

MACROSCOPIC APPEARANCES

The lymphocyte-predominant type usually presents as a group of non-adherent nodes, or a single node with a firm texture. The cut surface bulges, is usually homogeneous (Fig. 10.9a) and pale yellow-tan in colour.

The nodular sclerosing type usually arises in the mediastinum (p. 196) and involves the adjacent scalene, lower cervical and axillary nodes, more often on the right side than the left. The nodes are usually firm and matted to each other, but separate from adjacent tissues.

The mixed cellularity type resembles the lymphocyte-predominant type and the node may be soft or hard, depending on the amount of fibrous tissue.

The lymphocyte-depleted type is white and usually soft, and again the texture depends on the amount of fibrosis.

SPREAD

Viscera and other tissues become involved as the disease progresses. In the spleen, diffuse involvement causes enlargement and the Hodgkin's tissue appears as nodules, seen on the cut surface as yellowish areas irregular in size, shape and distribution (Fig. 10.9b), contrasting with the more regular and whitish Malpighian corpuscles. Microscopically these deposits may be difficult to diagnose in the early stages, and a helpful point is the presence of a rim of macrophages containing haemosiderin at the margin of the deposit.

Focal infiltration can produce solitary masses of Hodgkin's tissue, occasionally in the spleen, but more frequently in the lung, liver, lymph nodes, and in the mediastinum where they probably originate in lymphoid tissue.

Bone marrow involvement is macroscopically inconspicuous, but obvious microscopically if present, and a trephine biopsy of bone marrow is necessary to confirm the diagnosis.

STAGING

Accurate staging is helpful, and to some extent indispensable, in determining the extent of the disease, in assessing the prognosis, in choosing the most appropriate regime of therapy and in comparing the effects of different therapeutic programmes. Extensive clinical investigation has steadily increased its practical importance, although as Rosenberg (1972) observed, in a critical review, there have been alternating periods of 'enthusiasm and then reservation'.

Clinical staging can be established, up to a certain point, on the basis of (*a*) a full history and clinical examination, especially the findings relating to the liver, spleen, and abdominal and peripheral lymph nodes; (*b*) biopsy of

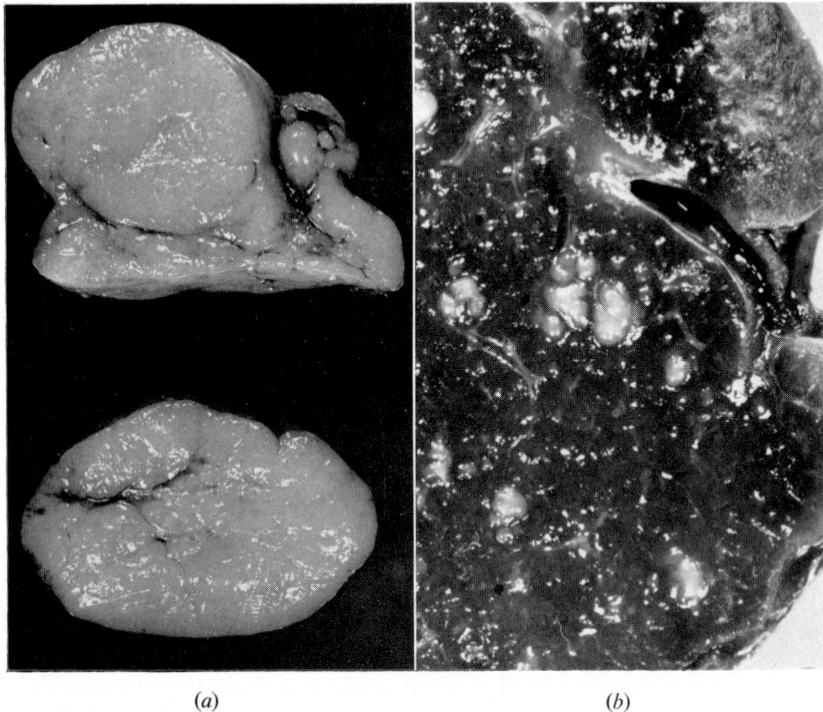

(*a*) (*b*)

Figure 10.9. HODGKIN'S DISEASE; (*a*) in a lymph node, showing typical fleshy, uniform, 'bulging' cut surface, characteristically pale tan-buff in colour; (*b*) nodules of Hodgkin's tissue in a spleen removed at staging laparotomy (p. 194). The nodules are irregular and bulging, and can usually be distinguished from Malpighian corpuscles.

one or more representative peripheral nodes; (*c*) x-rays of the chest, and when indicated, the skeleton, nasopharynx, alimentary tract, kidneys, etc; (*d*) liver function tests, the level of serum copper (p. 197), a full blood examination, sedimentation rate, bone marrow aspiration and if indicated, marrow biopsy; (*e*) lymphangiography and cavography, aortography or other special techniques as indicated.

The system of clinical staging adopted at Rye in 1965 (Rosenberg, 1966) introduced lymphangiography as a regular procedure. After injecting iodized oil via lymphatics in the foot or ankle, serial x-rays are taken to determine whether the iliac, lumbar and para-aortic nodes are involved. This procedure may be technically difficult, more so in children in whom small lymphatics are responsible for a high failure rate. Even when successful, the value of lymphangiography is limited because of failure to demonstrate malignant involvement of the para-aortic nodes above the second lumbar vertebra, in the porta hepatis, the splenic pedicle, the coeliac group and the mesentery. Nevertheless, the Rye system is still widely used, and is as follows:

Stage I: Disease limited to one anatomical region (I_1), or to two contiguous regions (I_2), on the same side of the diaphragm.

Stage II: Disease in more than two anatomical regions or in two non-contiguous regions on the same side of the diaphragm.

Stage III: Disease on both sides of the diaphragm, but not extending beyond lymph nodes, spleen and/or Waldeyer's ring.

Stage IV: Disseminated disease involving bone marrow, lung, pleura, liver, bone, skin, kidney, alimentary tract or any tissue or organ in addition to lymph nodes, spleen or Waldeyer's ring.

Sub-classification **A** and **B** are used to indicate the absence (A) or presence (B) of systemic symptoms, e.g. fever, night sweats.

Defects in the Rye system became apparent and led to its revision in 1970, at Ann Arbor (Carbone *et al.*, 1971). The major change was the realization that the abdomen is a 'blind spot' which cannot be reliably assessed by clinical and radiological methods alone. Upper abdominal nodes are usually missed on lymphangiography, the spleen and liver often contain Hodgkin's tissue when clinically and biochemically normal, and they are not infrequently free from Hodgkin's disease even when enlarged (Gamble *et al.*, 1975).

Laparotomy for staging purposes was therefore introduced, by the Stanford University group in 1969. Its objects are (*a*) to obtain for biopsy nodes suspected of malignancy or those usually missed on lymphangiography; (*b*) to detect involvement of the liver; (*c*) to remove the spleen for biopsy (the secondary advantages and disadvantages of this are discussed below); and (*d*) to relocate the ovaries in anticipation of radiotherapy to the pelvis.

The new classification (Fig. 10.10), which resulted from the Ann Arbor conference (Carbone *et al.*, 1971), is a combination of clinical staging (CS) and pathological staging (PS), defined as follows:

Clinical staging:

CS I: Disease limited to one lymph node region.

CS I_E: Disease limited to a single extralymphatic site, e.g. lung, liver, kidney, intestine.

CS II: Disease in two or more lymph node regions on the same side of the diaphragm. (A subscript $_n$ may indicate the number of regions involved, e.g. CS II_3.)

CS II_E: Localized disease in a single extralymphatic site and in one or more lymph node regions on the same side of the diaphragm.

CS III: Disease in lymph nodes on both sides of the diaphragm.

Additional disease in a single extralymphatic site is classified as CS III_E, additional disease in the spleen as CSIII_S, and when both are present, as CSIII_{SE}.

CS IV: Diffuse or disseminated disease in one or more extralymphatic sites, with or without lymph node involvement. The sites are identified by subscripts, e.g. PS IV_{H+M+}, where H+ indicates involvement of the liver, and M the marrow.

Subclassifications **A** and **B** are used for the presence or absence of systemic symptoms, as in the Rye system of staging.

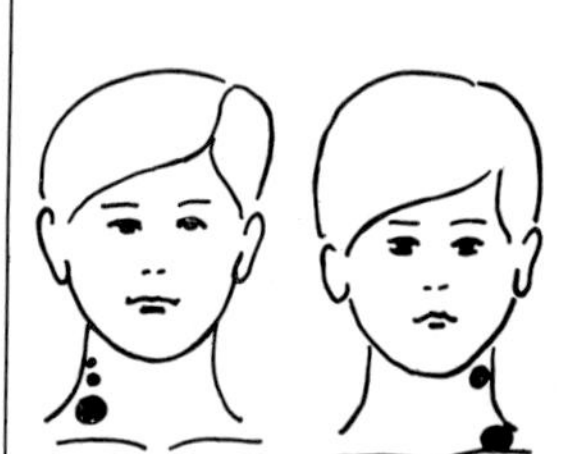

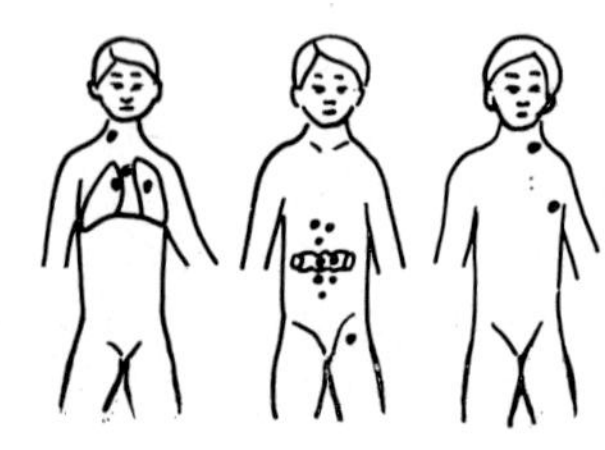

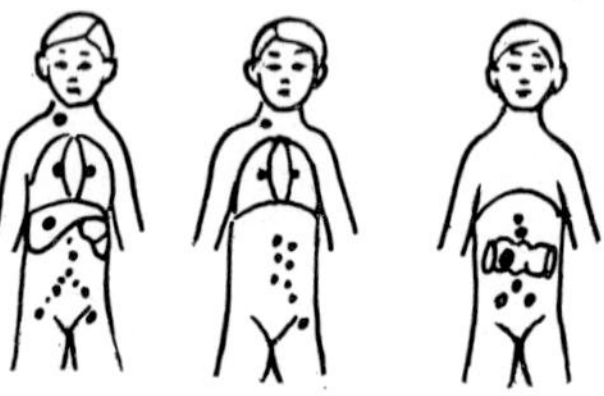

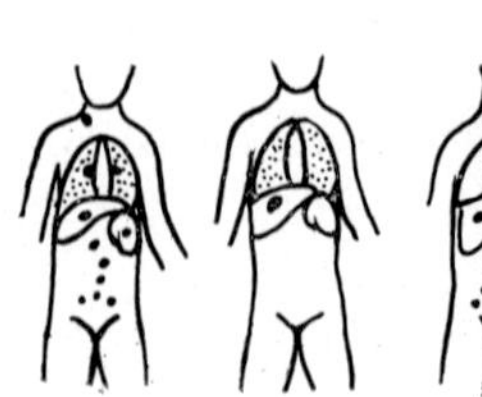

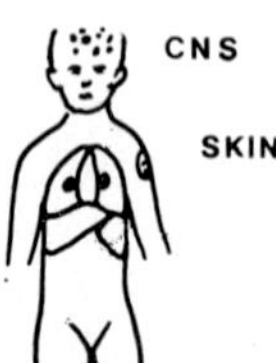

Figure 10.10. HODGKIN'S DISEASE; diagram of a system of staging based on the Ann Arbor revision, indicating the major stages, and the variations which may be encountered in each.

Pathological staging

This complements clinical staging and describes the findings in biopsies of tissues taken after the initial diagnostic node biopsy. The notation for the tissues is: N for an additional lymph node, H for hepatic tissue or liver, S for spleen, L for lung, M for bone marrow, O for osseous tissue, D for skin and P for pleura; a plus sign (+) after the letter indicates that cancer cells were detected in the biopsy, while a minus (−) sign indicates that they were not. Thus CS IA, PS $I_{S-H-N-M-}$ indicates clinical stage I without general symptoms, and pathological stage I with negative biopsies of spleen, liver, additional node tissue and bone marrow.

This clinicopathological system of staging is a major forward step in the management of the disease for it provides a more accurate record of the extent of disease and the prognosis, and better planning of therapy. There is also some evidence that splenectomy increases the patient's tolerance to radiotherapy and chemotherapy (Di Bella *et al.*, 1973; Roysten *et al.*, 1974).

On the other hand the extensive abdominal operation and splenectomy cause significant morbidity and specific complications, especially in children (Singer, 1973). Fulminating meningitis and/or septicaemia following 'staging splenectomy' has been reported in at least eleven patients; all but one of these were more than six years old; five of the eleven died, and four were found to be quite free of evident Hodgkin's disease at autopsy. A pneumococcus was the infiltrating organism in eight of the children, and in three it was *H. influenzae*. Herpes zoster also occurs more frequently when the spleen has been removed, and wound dehiscence or other complications within the first month occur in 12%.

Exploratory laparotomy with splenectomy therefore should not be performed as a routine in children (nor in adults), and is warranted only when identification of occult abdominal disease would alter the programme of treatment (Rosenberg, 1972). The presence of systemic symptoms in a child with Hodgkin's disease otherwise in Stage I or II, or possibly III, is a strong indication for laparotomy, as is hyper-splenism whatever the patient's age and stage. However, in a female with the 'nodular sclerosing' type and with no significant enlargement of the liver, spleen or left cervical lymph nodes, and little or no rise in serum copper, abdominal disease is so very rare that laparotomy or at least splenectomy is seldom justified. Between these extremes there are many children in whom the hazards of the operation may be outweighed by its potential advantages, including relocation of the ovaries in females with a prospect of cure (Rosenstock *et al.*, 1974). When abdominal disease has already been demonstrated by lymphangiography, or when it is strongly suspected on other grounds (e.g. systemic symptoms, enlarged lower left cervical nodes, a spleen estimated to weigh more than 500 g, the 'mixed cellularity' type, a very high level of serum copper, etc.), there may be little to be gained from laparotomy, for whatever the findings such cases are best treated in the same way as those with wide-spread abdominal disease.

Protocol for laparotomy

(i) All other appropriate investigations should have been performed first. The presence of pulmonary or skeletal infiltrations, any proven visceral involvement, or a positive marrow biopsy, are indicative of Stage IV, and that laparotomy is not required.

(ii) Generous access to both the upper and lower regions of the abdomen is necessary because of the several separate procedures required.

(iii) Unless contraindicated on the grounds of age, immune function, etc., the spleen is removed; wedge biopsy and even multiple needle biopsies may fail to detect focal patches of infiltration.

(iv) The liver: multiple biopsies are required, so a wedge biopsy is taken from each of the right and left lobes, and in addition needle biopsies of the deeper areas.

(v) Lymph nodes are sampled, removing as a routine one from each of the coeliac, superior mesenteric and iliac groups, and also a specimen node from any group which appears to be enlarged or indurated, or has been implicated by lymphangiography. The retroperitoneal tissues are fully explored, incising the posterior peritoneum. The removal of any suspect node seen in the lymphangiogram can be confirmed by further films taken during operation.

(vi) In girls, the ovaries are translocated by dividing the lateral ovarian pedicles, placing one in front of and one behind the uterus, or both together in the midline in the pouch of Douglas, where they lie caudal to the lower margin of the usual field of abdominal irradiation. Lateral translocation of the ovaries out of the pelvis is an acceptable alternative.

(vii) Penicillin prophylaxis should be given because most of the serious infections which have been reported in splenectomized children have been sensitive to penicillin. As in the prevention of recurrent rheumatic fever, it is given orally two or three times a day, and should be continued throughout childhood in the younger patients, and in the adolescents for at least two years after splenectomy.

Interpretation of multiple biopsies

The task of making a histological diagnosis of Hodgkin's disease in its early stages arises more frequently now that such emphasis is placed on early diagnosis, and with the increased use of laparotomy for staging. Making a histological diagnosis can be very difficult in the early stages, and particularly so when anticancer therapy has already been commenced. Hodgkin's tissue is highly susceptible both to radiotherapy and to chemotherapy, and their use before abdominal biopsies have been obtained causes small foci of Hodgkin's tissue to disappear, leading to false-negative reports. Chemotherapy should not be given to 'cover' biopsy or as treatment until the diagnosis has been firmly established and the stage of the disease determined.

Lymph nodes may show a granulomatous reaction provoked by the contrast material used in lymphangiography, although the lesions of Hodgkin's disease do not take up the lipiodol and hence are not involved in the granulomatosis.

Liver biopsy. Interpretation can be complicated by a mild nonspecific hepatitis causing an inflammatory infiltrate in the portal tracts, which may mimic Hodgkin's lesions. In this situation the infiltration should be reported as Hodgkin's disease only when Sternberg-Reed cells are identified.

The spleen. Extremely hyperplastic follicles and/or some degree of splenic fibrosis can occur in a normal spleen, and this too presents some difficulties, but one of the important findings is the presence of haemosiderin in macrophages at the margin of a tumour deposit which helps to identify such an infiltration as Hodgkin's disease.

MODES OF PRESENTATION

1. *Peripheral lymphadenopathy.* Children with Hodgkin's disease are often asymptomatic, although an enlarged lymph node, most commonly in the cervical region, has usually been noticed.
2. *General systemic symptoms*, such as fever, night sweats, anorexia, weight loss and pruritus are responsible for the presentation in about one third of the cases, and in these the disease is usually in Stage III or IV.
3. *Pressure on or infiltration* in adjacent structures, such as periosteum, spine, pleura, etc., may produce symptoms which are usually mild. Of greater importance however, are those caused by pressure of enlarged lymph nodes on tubular viscera, and two forms, seen in 5–10% of cases, require attention urgently:

(*a*) *The mediastinal syndrome* with compression of the superior vena cava and trachea, and

(*b*) *The spinal theca and cord*, where compression causes backache, weakness, sensory loss below the site, and even paralysis.

(*c*) Other effects of compression occasionally seen include hydronephrosis, from nodes adjacent to the ureter, jaundice due to obstruction of enlarged nodes in the region of the porta hepatis, malabsorption with or without bowel obstruction, from mesenteric and para-intestinal nodes, and cavitation in the lungs, caused by enlargement of parabronchial nodes.

Some fever is present at or soon after presentation in most cases, varying from a transient, asymptomatic temperature of 38°–39°C, to a persistent fever of 40°C or more in an obviously sick anorexic child with shivers, sweating and marked loss of weight. The latter is more characteristic of advanced disease and this is often supported by radiographic evidence of parenchymal infiltration of the lungs. On the other hand, immunological deficiencies, especially of the cell-mediated type, are common in children with Hodgkin's disease and lead to heightened susceptibility to herpes zoster, to other viral infections, and to many other opportunistic fungal, protozoal and bacterial infections. Fever in Hodgkin's disease may therefore be due more often to infection than is apparent. Tuberculosis should also be considered, especially in patients treated with immunosuppressives, but the Mantoux test is not likely to be positive in such cases; in the Index Series one of the long-term survivors died with miliary tuberculosis. The supposedly classical Pel-Ebstein recurrent fever is seldom seen in children.

CLINICAL SIGNS

Enlarged lymph nodes in one or more cervical regions are present in 80% of cases. They are usually discrete and shotty in the earliest stages, but by the time of presentation there is commonly an impression that they are matted together, although discrete nodes may still be found at the periphery. When the right cervical nodes are affected, the mediastinal or hilar nodes tend to be involved also (Fig. 10.11), as found at presentation in 25% of cases. When the left cervical nodes are affected, however, the abdominal nodes are more commonly involved while the mediastinum may be clear. Experience has shown that the lower left cervical nodes are affected in 95% of patients with abdominal Hodgkin's disease.

The liver and spleen are frequently enlarged, but this does not necessarily mean that they are infiltrated with Hodgkin's disease (see p. 190).

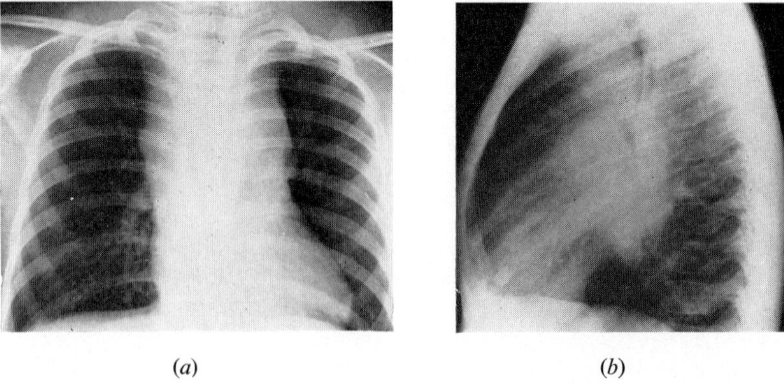

(*a*) (*b*)

Figure 10.11. HODGKIN'S DISEASE; mediastinal involvement at presentation, in an eleven-year-old boy with enlarged cervical nodes. X-rays show (*a*) bilateral hilar nodes and median periaortic nodes, causing widening of the upper mediastinum; (*b*) typical appearance of hilar nodes in the 'mid-mediastinum' (see p. 444).

Jaundice, whether due to obstruction or to haemolytic anaemia, is rare in children, and pruritus is almost as uncommon.

Leukocytosis, sometimes in excess of 30,000/cmm is frequently found on presentation, and is predominantly neutrophilic, though eosinophilia occurs in 15–20% of cases. The number of lymphocytes in the blood may be normal, but is more often reduced, sometimes markedly so.

Elevation of the serum copper occurs in proportion to the extent of the disease, and this test is useful in assessing activity of the disease and in signalling relapse (Tessmer *et al.*, 1973), as in other lymphomas (see p. 174).

Increased bromosulphthalein retention and serum alkaline phosphatase may be of significance, but the other liver function tests are of no clinical value.

Involvement of vertebrae, ribs, pelvis or other bones as shown radiologically occurs in 10–15%, but pain often precedes the appearance of x-ray changes.

Immunological competence

At the time of diagnosis, tests of immunological functions show a general tendency to depression, especially of cell-mediated immunity. Evidence so far suggests that this is the result rather than the cause of the disease; the more advanced the disease, the greater the depression of the immune system, while in a complete remission, immunocompetence usually returns to normal. Immunological defects may bear a relationship to the associated nephrosis without renal infiltration which has been reported in a number of cases.

TREATMENT

Surgery

The role of surgery in primary treatment is usually limited to excision biopsy of one or more superficial lymph nodes, and to laparotomy for staging when this is indicated (p. 194). Occasionally it is necessary to consider excision of tumour tissue compressing vital structures such as the spinal cord, trachea and superior vena cava.

Recent experiences suggest that corticosteroids and cytotoxic agents given promptly, in combination with irradiation, may be more beneficial than laminectomy or other comparable decompressive operations.

Resection of a Hodgkin's tumour in the lung or involving the gut, and splenectomy for acquired haemolytic anaemia or thrombocytopenia, are required only rarely in children.

Radiotherapy

There is no doubt that for localized Hodgkin's disease radiotherapy is the mainstay of treatment, while chemotherapy is of prime importance in generalized disease. Protocols developed in major centres in the 1960s relied predominantly on radiotherapy for patients in Stages I and II and usually for Stage IIIA, and on chemotherapy for Stages IIIB and IV. However, radiotherapy alone in children in Stages I and IIA is followed by local recurrence or dissemination in 20% (Young *et al.*, 1973), and adjuvant chemotherapy is now combined with the radiotherapy for those in the early stages. At the other end of the scale, in Stage IV, the encouraging incidence of prolonged remissions from multiple-drug chemotherapy has prompted the use of adjuvant radiotherapy in combination with the chemotherapy in an attempt to achieve permanent control of the disease.

An adequate dose-range for radiotherapy in children is a total dose of 3000–3500 rads over three to four weeks. When lymph node areas are irradiated, uninvolved adjacent tissues such as the larynx, lungs, liver, kidneys, gonads and growing bone, should be shielded as far as possible. Radiotherapy to a dose as high as 4000 rads delivered to the whole length of the spinal column and pelvis may produce (in addition to severe marrow depression) an unacceptable degree of growth defect, and a dose exceeding 3000 rads may cause radiation nephritis, hepatitis, pericarditis etc.

The plan of radiotherapy and the fields most often used are as follows:

(*a*) '*Upper mantle*' indicates a vertical field covering most of the nodes above the diaphragm, i.e., cervical, axillary and mediastinal nodes.

(*b*) '*Lower mantle*' is used to describe a field shaped like an inverted Y covering the para-aortic nodes from the diaphragm downwards, extending on each side to the iliac, inguinal and femoral nodes.

(*c*) *Total nodal irradiation* involves a combination of (*a*) and (*b*), with a rest period of one to two months between them.

In special circumstances the fields are varied, e.g. a 'modified mantle' may include a median field extending downwards to cover the upper abdominal nodes. All the fields mentioned are developments of the 'extended field' idea, i.e. irradiation of the group or groups of nodes known to be involved, extended to cover contiguous or other groups of nodes which may be the site of occult disease.

Chemotherapy

Hodgkin's disease is almost as highly sensitive to chemotherapy as reticulum cell sarcoma (McElwain, 1974). Of the long list of drugs that can cause regression of this neoplasm, the most effective, when given singly, are as follows.

(1) *Alkylating agents:* nitrogen mustard, cyclophosphamide and chlorambucil. The Southwest Cancer Chemotherapy Study Group considers cyclophosphamide the best, but this has yet to be confirmed.

(2) *Alkaloids:* vinblastine and vincristine; vinblastine is at least equal to the alkylating agents; vincristine may be as good, but trials have been less extensive because of toxicity.

(3) *Drugs acting partly by alkylation*: procarbazine, and 1·3-Bis (2- chloroethyl)-1-nitrosourea (BCNU); both are almost as effective as (1) and (2) above.

(4) *Miscellaneous*: adriamycin (responses in 80% of one European series), bleomycin (responses in 50%), and corticosteroids.

Single drug therapy has been superseded by combinations of three or more of these drugs, which can produce not just 'responses', but a complete remission in 70–85% of cases, compared with 20–30% with the best of the single agents. Various promising combinations have not yet been adequately compared, but one most widely tested in adults is 'MOPP', in pulses, repeated every 28 days, with each cycle including nitrogen mustard 6 mg/m^2 IV and vincristine (Oncovin®) 1·4 mg/m^2 IV, both on days one and eight; procarbazine 50 increasing to 100 mg/m^2/day orally on days one to ten; prednisone 40 mg/m^2/day on days one to ten, tapering to nil by day fourteen.

The disadvantages of MOPP include the degree of marrow depression which commonly develops, probably more so if the spleen is still present; the severity of nausea, vomiting and other toxic effects, especially in patients with systemic symptoms (B Stages); and the degree of immunosuppression, possibly contributing to fatal infection or a second neoplasm in some patients. It is too toxic a regimen for use by inexperienced clinicians, and it fails to produce a complete remission in up to 50% of patients in Stage IIIB or IV (Young *et al.*, 1973).

A number of modifications have been, or are, under trial, and these include smaller doses of nitrogen mustard, and/or of procarbazine; substitution of cyclophosphamide 650 mg/m^2 IV on days one and eight for nitrogen mustard ('C-MOPP'), substitution of vinblastine for vincristine, and omitting the prednisone from two of every four cycles.

Another combination of drugs which gives results comparable with those of MOPP, at least in Stage IIIB and Stage IV, is COP (or CVP) i.e. cyclophosphamide, vincristine (or vinblastine) and prednisolone, in dosages similar to those above, or 'COP' plus procarbazine (COPP) (Goldsmith & Carter, 1974).

An NCI group has used this trio combined with procarbazine and nitrosourea (BCNU) 'without undue toxicity'; one large paediatric centre in U.S.A. currently uses the trio combined with procarbazine and adriamycin, followed by vinblastine; and another is using vincristine, adriamycin, prednisolone, bleomycin and diethyl-triazeno-imidazole-carboxamide (DTIC).

Chemotherapy for Hodgkin's disease has clearly been in a state of rapid evolution ever since four-drug combinations were introduced in 1964, and it has recently almost become a revolution. Dogmatic rules cannot be given at this stage, but certain generalizations and principles can be offered as guidelines, to be considered in conjunction with Table 10.3.

Widespread or disseminated disease (Stages III and IV), or associated with systemic symptoms (subclass B), call for potent combination chemotherapy which should start without delay and take priority over radiotherapy. The initial chemotherapy should include at least one alkylating agent, an alkaloid (vincristine or vinblastine) and prednisolone, possibly with the addition of adriamycin or procarbazine.

Table 10.3. Hodgkin's disease; Outline of the plan of treatment currently recommended, according to Clinical Stage (CS)

CS I or I_E	Radiotherapy (mantle or equivalent field), combination chemotherapy (COP, MOPP or other) for 12 weeks
CS II or II_E	Radiotherapy (modified mantle or equivalent), combination chemotherapy for 12 months, as for CS I, modified after 12 weeks
CS IIIA	Radiotherapy (total nodal field), combination chemotherapy for 18 months, as for CS I, modified after 12 weeks
CS IIIB	Combination chemotherapy for 2 years (at least four drugs), modified after 12 weeks, radiotherapy (total nodal field)
CS IVA or IVB	Combination chemotherapy for at least 2 years (using four to five drugs), modified after 6 months, radiotherapy (total nodal field) commencing 6–12 weeks after starting chemotherapy

Because immunological deficiency is common in Hodgkin's disease, and since both chemotherapy and radiotherapy are immunosuppressive, it is very important to protect the immune system as much as possible by giving the drugs intermittently, i.e. in recurring pulses or cycles at intervals of three to five weeks.

Pressure by tumour tissue on a vital airway, vena cava or spinal cord calls urgently for a single dose of nitrogen mustard, cyclophosphamide or hydrocortisone, before irradiation. If a massive mediastinal tumour is to be irradiated, it should first be reduced in size by chemotherapy so as to minimize radiation pneumonitis. In stages IA or IIA as determined after laparotomy, the initial treatment should be irradiation of an appropriate extended field, but if no other treatment is given, dissemination or multicentric lesions often develop later; chemotherapy is therefore given in such cases (except those with the lymphocyte-predominant type), although it takes second place to radiotherapy.

The optimum duration of chemotherapy in different situations has yet to be determined. In Stages III and IV, a policy widely adopted is to continue intermittent drug therapy for about two years, in Stage II for twelve months, and in Stage I for twelve weeks, as first proposed by the group at St. Jude Hospital (Smith *et al.*, 1974).

Immunotherapy is still in the experimental stage, but it may well have a place in the future.

PROGNOSIS AND RESULTS

The prognostic factors in Hodgkin's disease have been studied extensively, notably by Tubiana *et al.* (1971) in a review of 454 cases.

The clinical stage is by far the most important factor; in the past not many children in Stages III and IV survived beyond five years whereas in Stages I and II even the median survival time is longer than this.

The pathological stage comes next; the nodular sclerosing type is the most favourable, followed by the lymphocyte predominant type, then the mixed cellularity and least favourable is the lymphocyte depleted type.

The presence of systemic symptoms, especially fever and loss of weight, has a significantly unfavourable influence.

The erythrocyte sedimentation rate and serum copper level seem to be useful indicators of the amount of active disease present. Various measures of immune function are also of significant prognostic value, e.g. the number of circulating lymphocytes, the Mantoux test and other delayed hypersensitivity reactions, and the leukocyte response to PHA stimulation; immunological defects worsen the prognosis.

The quality of treatment and the total management are possibly more important than any of the above. A good, immediate clinical response is easily obtained; complete remission with no evidence of disease has occurred in as many as 47 of 49 children (96%) treated with cyclophosphamide, vincristine and radiotherapy, although the small proportion of Stage IV patients in the series quoted may have influenced the result (Smith *et al.*, 1974).

For prolonged remission and survival, however, the standard of treatment is most important. In three recent publications, eighty patients (mainly children) in the favourable Stages I, II and IIIA, were treated with intensive irradiation alone, and 30% of them died within three years. Other recent reports, from both Europe and America, provide evidence that alkaloids and alkylating agents combined with expert radiotherapy improve the results in these early stages as well as in Stage IV.

For advanced disease, a large number of variations on the MOPP theme are currently under trial. In a succinct yet comprehensive review of these, Goldsmith & Carter (1974) have listed trials involving four, five or six different drugs in combinations, with early results at least as good as those reported with the standard MOPP regime.

In the Index Series, between 1954 (when chemotherapy began to be included in the routine treatment) and 1968, there were 23 patients of whom twelve (52%) survived more than 5 years, and 3 so far have become 10-year survivors. Of the twelve 5-year survivors, three were over eleven years of age at the start of treatment, in contrast with the rarity of long-term survival in children at this age with acute leukaemia. None of the Hodgkin's survivors received the intensive radiotherapy and chemotherapy that are part of today's routine, and two leading authorities have pointed out that it remains to be shown whether current intensive therapy, which gives higher response rates and prevents extension to abdominal nodes, also improves the overall long-term survival rates (Aisenberg, 1973; Carbone, 1973).

The prognosis according to Stage to be expected when children are treated with modern combined therapy is given by two recent studies with a total of 87 patients followed for from 6 months to 5 years (Young *et al.*, 1973; Smith *et al.*, 1974). The survival rate for children in Stage I was approximately 94%, Stage II 78%, in Stage III 69%, and in Stage IV 40%. The median survival time was not less than 4 years in Stages I and II, approximately 3 years in Stage III, and just over 2 years in Stage IV. In only one of these studies was chemotherapy used for all stages.

REFERENCES

Aisenberg, A.C. (1973). Malignant lymphoma. *New Engl. J. Med.*, **288** : 883 and 935.

Aur, R.J.A., Hustu, H.O., Simone, J.V., Pratt, C.B. & Pinkel, D. (1971). Therapy of localized and regional lymphosarcoma of childhood. *Cancer*, **27** : 1328.

Borella, L. & Sen, L. (1975). E receptors on blasts from untreated acute lymphocytic leukaemia (ALL): Comparison of temperature dependence of E-rosettes formed by normal and leukaemic lymphoid cells. *J. Immunol.*, **114** : 187.

Brown, G., Greaves, M.F., Lister, T.A. *et al.* (1974). Expression of tumour T and B lymphocyte cell surface markers on leukaemic cells. *Lancet*, **2** ; 753.

Carbone, P.P. (1973). Management with combination therapy. *J.A.M.A.*, **223** : 165.

Carbone, P.P., Kaplan, H.S., Musshoff, K., Smithers, D.W. & Tubiana, M. (1971). Report of the committee on Hodgkin's disease staging classification. *Cancer Res.*, **31** : 1860.

Caro, W.A. & Helwig, E.B. (1969). Cutaneous lymphoid hyperplasia. *Cancer*, **24** : 487.

Cotton, J.R., Sarles, H.E., Remmers, A.R., Lindley, J.D., Beathard, G.A., Cottom, D.L., Fish, J.C., Townsend, C.M. & Ritzmann, S.E. (1973). The appearance of reticulum cell sarcoma at the site of antilymphocytic globulin injection. *Transplantation*, **16** : 154.

DeVita, V.T. & Canellos, G.P. (1972). Treatment of the lymphomas. *Semin. Hematol.*, **9** : 193.

Di Bella, N.J., Blom, J. & Slawson, R.G. (1973). Splenectomy and hematologic tolerance to irradiation in Hodgkin's disease. *Radiology*, **107** : 195.

Dorfman, R.F. (1974). Classification of non-Hodgkin's lymphomas. *Lancet*, **1** : 1295.

Dorfman, R.F. & Warnke, R. (1974). Lymphadenopathy simulating the malignant lymphomas. *Human. Path.*, **5** : 519.

Fraumeni, J.F. & Li, F.P. (1969). Hodgkin's disease in childhood: an epidemiological study. *J. Nat. Cancer Inst.*, **42** : 681.

Gamble, R.J. (1975). Influence of staging celiotomy in localized presentations of Hodgkin's disease. *Cancer*, **35** : 3.

Gatti, R.A. & Good, R.A. (1971). Occurrence of malignancy in immunodeficiency disease. A literature review. *Cancer*, **28** : 89.

Goldsmith, M.A. & Carter, S.K. (1974). Combination chemotherapy of advanced Hodgkin's disease. *Cancer*, **33** : 1.

Hays, D.M., Hittle, R.E., Isaacs, H. & Karon, M.R. (1972). Laparotomy for the staging of Hodgkin's disease in children. *J. Pediat. Surg.*, **7** : 517.

HRGOVCIC, M., TESSMER, C.F., THOMAS, F.B., ONG, P.S., GAMBLE, J.F. & SHULLENBERGER, C.C. (1973). Serum copper observations in patients with malignant lymphoma. *Cancer*, **32** : 1512.

JAFFE, E.S., SHEVACH, E.M., FRANK, M.M. *et al.* (1974). Nodular lymphoma—evidence for origin from follicular B lymphocytes. *New Eng. J. Med.*, **290** : 813.

KIM, H. & DORFMAN, R.F. (1974). Morphological studies of 84 untreated patients subjected to laparotomy for the staging of non-Hodgkin's lymphoma. *Cancer*, **33** : 657.

KIM, R.A., WINKELMAN, R.K. & DOCKERTY, M. (1963). Reticulum-cell sarcoma of the skin. *Cancer*, **16** : 646.

LEMERLE, M., GERARD-MARCHANT, R., SARRAZIN, D., SANCHO, H., TCHERNIA, G., FLAMANT, F., LEMERLE, J. & SCHWEISGUTH, O. (1973). Lymphosarcoma and reticulum cell sarcoma in children: a retrospective study of 172 cases. *Cancer*, **32** : 1499.

LUKES, R.J., CRAVER, L.F., HALL, T.C., RAPPAPORT, H. & RUBEN, P. (1966). Report of the nomenclature committee. *Cancer Res.*, **26** : 1311.

MCELWAIN, T.J. (1974). Chemotherapy of the lymphomas. *Seminars Hematol.*, **11** : 59.

MACMAHON, B. (1973). Is Hodgkin's disease contagious? *New Engl. J. Med.*, **289** : 532.

PETERS, M.V., HASSELBACK, R. & BROWN, T.C. (1968). The natural history of the lymphomas related to clinical classification. In *Proceedings of the International Conference on Leukaemia and Lymphoma* (Zanaforetis, C.J.D. ed.), p. 357. Lea & Febiger, Philadelphia.

RAPPAPORT, H. (1966). Tumors of the hemopoietic system. In *Atlas of Tumor Pathology*, Section III, Fascicle 8. Armed Forces Institute of Pathology, Washington, D.C.

ROSENBERG, S.A. (1966). Report of the committee on the staging of Hodgkin's disease. *Cancer Res.*, **26** : 1310.

ROSENBERG, S.A. (1972). Splenectomy in the management of Hodgkin's disease. (Annotation.) *Brit. J. Haemat.*, **23** : 371.

ROSENSTOCK, J.G., D'ANGIO, G.J. & KIESEWETTER, W.B. (1974). The incidence of complications following staging laparotomy for Hodgkin's disease in children. *Am. J. Roentgenol.*, **120** : 531.

ROYSTER, R.L. Jr., WASSUM, J.A. & KINGS, E.R. (1974). An evaluation of the effects of splenectomy in Hodgkin's disease in patients undergoing extended field or total lymph node irradiation. *Am. J. Roentgenol.*, **120** : 521.

SCHEY, W.L., WHITE, H., CONWAY, J.J. & KIDD, J.M. (1973). Lymphosarcoma in children: roentgenologic and clinical evaluation of 60 children. *Am. J. Roentgenol.*, **117** : 59.

SCHNITZER, B., NISHIYAMA, R.H., HEIDELBERGER, K.P. & WEAVER, D.K. (1973). Hodgkin's disease in children. *Cancer*, **31** : 560.

SINGER, D.B. (1973). Postsplenectomy sepsis. In *Perspectives in Pediatric Pathology*, Vol. 1, p. 285. Year Book Medical Publishers, Chicago.

SMITH, K.L., JOHNSON, D., HUSTU, O., PRATT, C., FLEMING, I. & HOLTON, C. (1974). Concurrent chemotherapy and radiation therapy in the treatment of childhood and adolescent Hodgkin's disease. *Cancer*, **33** : 38.

SONLEY, M.J. (1972/1973). Lymphosarcoma in childhood. *Paediatrician*, **1** : 249.

TESSMER, C.F., HRGOVCIC, M. & WILBUR, J. (1973). Serum copper in Hodgkin's disease in children. *Cancer*, **31** : 303.

TUBIANA, M., ATTIÉ, E., FLAMANT, R., GÉRARD-MARCHANT, R. & HAYAT, M. (1971). Prognostic factors in 454 cases of Hodgkin's disease. *Cancer Res.*, **31** : 1801.

VINCIGUERRA, V. & SILVER, R.T. (1973). The importance of bone marrow biopsy in the staging of patients with lymphosarcoma. *Blood*, **41** : 913.

WEBSTER, R. (1961). Lymphosarcoma of the thymus: its relation to acute lymphatic leukaemia. *Med. J. Aust.*, **48** (1) : 582.

YOUNG, R.C., DEVITA, V.T. & JOHNSON, R.E. (1973). Hodgkin's disease in childhood. *Blood*, **42** : 163.

Chapter 11. The histiocytoses

Tumours of the lymphoreticular system other than malignant lymphomas have in the past been referred to as 'reticuloses', an imprecise term with various connotations. It would seem better to discard it in favour of the 'histiocytoses' or 'histiocytic proliferations', terms which indicate the predominant cell type, even if the nature of the various conditions, their cause and even their homogeneity as a group, are still open to question.

A definition of the histiocytoses is almost one of exclusion: '... forms of proliferation of histiocytic cells that have neoplastic or quasi-neoplastic features and which do not fall into any of the well-recognized groups of lymphoreticular neoplastic proliferations', that is, lymphosarcoma, reticulum cell sarcoma and Hodgkin's disease (see Chapter 10).

When confronted with a miscellaneous yet related group of conditions, their classification can be simplified by extracting those recognizable as clinico-pathological entities. This leaves a relatively small residuum which has so far defied categorization.

The definable histiocytoses are partly morphological and partly clinical entities, and a histogenetic classification is not possible in the present state of knowledge. Some may be abnormal responses by lymphoreticular tissues to viruses or other infective agents, while others may be true neoplasms. The histiocytoses straddle a borderland between neoplastic and reactive inflammatory conditions, and between benign and malignant neoplasms.

The most important group is now more commonly called 'histiocytosis X', as proposed by Lichtenstein (1953) and clarified as a group of clinical entities by Oberman (1961).

CLASSIFICATION

The types of histiocytosis are classified as follows:

I. Eosinophilic granuloma of bone
II. Hand-Schüller-Christian syndrome
III. Letterer-Siwe disease
} Together known as histiocytosis X
IV. Familial haemophagocytic histiocytosis;
V. Sinus histiocytosis;
VI. Unclassified histiocytoses.

Experience has shown that most patients with histiocytosis X (Table 11.1) fall into one of the following clinical categories:

1. *Lesions* (*usually single*) *confined to bone* (eosinophilic granuloma of bone),

Table 11.1. Histiocytoses, Index Series R.C.H. (1950–1972)

	No.
Eosinophilic granuloma	25
Letterer-Siwe disease	11
Unclassified malignant reticuloses	10
Hand-Schüller-Christian syndrome	5
Haemophagic reticulosis	4
Sinus histiocytosis	3
Total	58

most of which eventually heal, but in a small proportion of cases multiple lesions in bones and in soft tissues subsequently appear.

2. *Lesions* (*usually multiple*) *in both bones and soft tissues* initially; in some, visceral lesions develop later (i.e. Hand-Schüller-Christian syndrome, perhaps more justifiably 'Kays' triad' (Kay, 1905) as pointed out by Cunningham, 1970).

3. *Lesions* (*usually multiple*) *confined to soft tissues*, in particular skin and lymph nodes, almost always in infants (Letterer-Siwe disease), and sometimes present at birth.

It is often difficult to decide in which category an individual case belongs. It may be useful to stage patients according to the number of systems infiltrated, e.g. bone, skin and liver, as well as assessing whether there is dysfunction in an organ system, e.g. in bone marrow or liver. In general, the fewer systems involved and the less dysfunction in them, the better the prognosis (see Table 11.2, p. 216).

I. EOSINOPHILIC GRANULOMA OF BONE

The inclusion of this condition in this chapter rather than in the chapter on bone tumours indicates a bias toward the concept suggested by Wallgren and elaborated by Lichtenstein (1953), that eosinophilic granuloma, Hand-Schüller-Christian and Letterer-Siwe disease are all manifestations of the same disease. In the Index Series there are examples of eosinophilic granulomas of bone which progressed to the Hand-Schüller-Christian syndrome, but it is nevertheless possible to identify, on the basis of the clinical course, a fairly precise and distinctive picture (Schajowicz & Slullitel, 1973).

MACROSCOPIC APPEARANCES

The lesions are soft, yellowish-grey, with a rather ill-defined margin which is surprising in view of the usually discrete x-ray appearance (Fig. 11.1a).

Spread of the lesion through the overlying periosteum into the adjacent soft tissues is seen in some lesions, and is a sign of a poor prognosis.

MICROSCOPIC FINDINGS

The dominant cell is a fairly uniform histiocyte with an oval or indented vesicular nucleus, a small nucleolus and a large amount of amphophilic cytoplasm which is characteristically well demarcated. This demarcation is a feature of all the histiocytoses; the margins of the cells appear to be separate and discrete, even when they form diffuse cell masses.

Eosinophil leucocytes, singly and in clumps between the histiocytic cells, are invariably present (Fig. 11.1b, c). Large areas of necrosis are very common and the picture is often obscured by a secondary inflammatory reaction with polymorphs, lymphocytes, plasma cells and fibroblasts, which may incorrectly suggest osteomyelitis. In these cases a search should be made for areas of relatively undisturbed histiocytes on which the correct diagnosis can be made.

Most lesions contain osteoclastic giant cells and these may be very numerous, especially at the margins of the lesions. Occasionally lipid accumulates

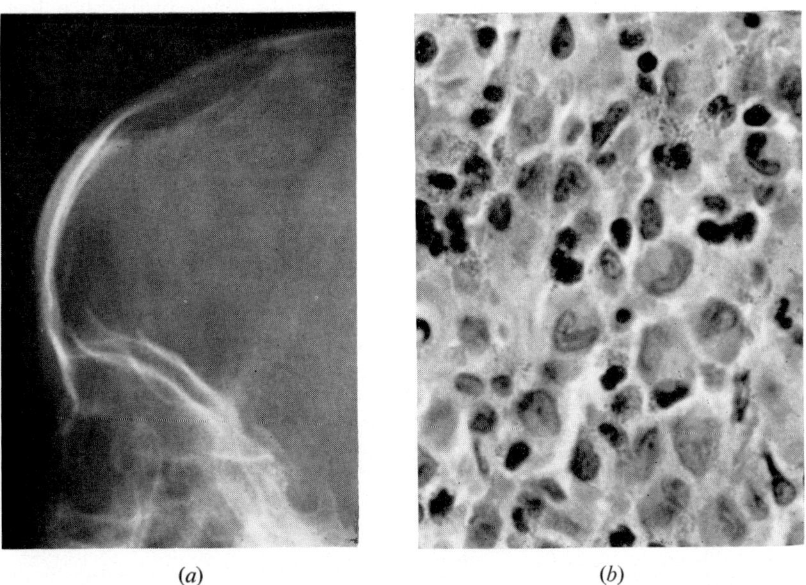

(*a*) (*b*)

Figure 11.1. EOSINOPHILIC GRANULOMA; (*a*) x-ray of the frontal region; the punched out defect has clear-cut margins and there is no bone reaction; (*b*) large, plump histiocytes with open, pale nuclei and abundant cytoplasm, infiltrated with numerous eosinophil leucocytes (note granules) (H & E. ×494); (*c*) see Fig. 11.1c, colour plate, following p. 140.

in the cytoplasm of some of the histiocytes, giving them a foamy, xanthomatous appearance, but this is rare in uncomplicated, untreated new cases in which the cytoplasm of most of the histiocytes is homogenous and lipid material is lacking.

In a few patients the disease becomes disseminated to involve other bones and soft tissues, e.g. the liver, spleen, lungs and lymph nodes, and some authors have correlated this malignant course with a particular histological picture typified by nuclear anaplasia, mitotic figures, and invasion of the soft tissues (Newton, 1973). With the possible exception of the last feature, it has not been possible to make such a correlation in the Index Series, and in the three disseminated cases, the histology was identical with those which remained localized, and resolved.

Since the Index Series was closed there has been one example of the malignant form of histocytosis X.

An 11-year old boy presented with a swelling on the skull. X-rays showed a punched-out bone lesion with an overlying soft tissue shadow. The lesion was excised and microscopy showed it was composed of histiocytes with large nuclei, some coarseness of chromatin, scattered mitoses, and few eosinophils.

Local radiotherapy was given and 4 months later a swelling appeared at the junction of the sternum and rectus abdominis, accompanied by malaise and fever. The mass arose in the anterior mediastinum and extended forwards to the region of the xiphisternum. Biopsy showed findings similar to the calvarial lesion but with more anaplasia of histiocytes and virtual absence of eosinophils, as in Fig. 11.2.

Chemotherapy with vinblastine, prednisolone and 6-mercaptopurine was commenced and the mass resolved. After 18 months treatment there was no evidence of disease, and chemotherapy was discontinued. Six months later fever, malaise and the mass in the rectus recurred. Chemotherapy (vinblastine, methotrexate, cyclophosphamide and prednisolone) was recommenced, and 5 months later he is again well with no evidence of disease.

Eosinophilic granuloma is the commonest of several lesions in children which cause localized destruction of bone. The incidence is indicated by the

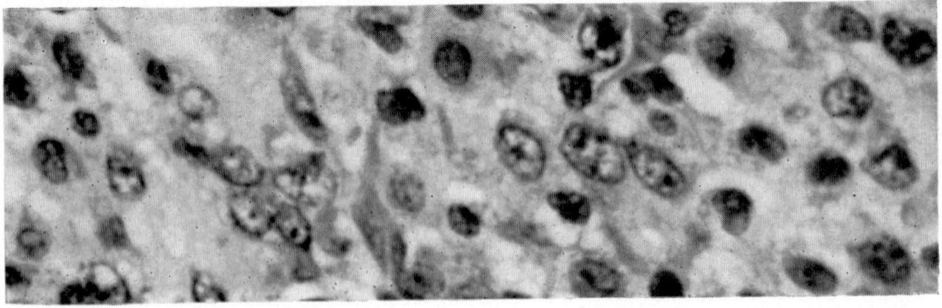

Figure 11.2. EOSINOPHILIC GRANULOMA; a more 'malignant' anaplastic type The histiocytes are large and the nuclei hyperchromatic; in places they appear almost syncitial. There are no eosinophils, but lymphocytes, neutrophils and occasional plasma cells are present (H & E. × 520).

occurrence of approximately 30 cases in the Index Series, and in the same period there were 150 cases of Wilms' tumour.

AGE : SEX

The cases are spread fairly evenly through the paediatric age group, and the sexes are affected with equal frequency.

SITE

While any bone may be affected, except those in the hands and feet, the skull and the pelvis are most often involved, followed in order of diminishing frequency by the femur, the vertebrae, humerus, ribs and the mandible.

MODES OF PRESENTATION

1. *Pain* in the affected area, with or without a swelling, mostly in accessible sites such as the calvarium, is the commonest presenting symptom.
2. *A limp* associated with aching or pain is common when the lesion arises in the pelvis or the lower limb.
3. Rarely the patient presents with cord signs when the lesion arises in a vertebra and causes vertebra plana of Calvé (Compere, Johnson & Coventry, 1954) with compression of the spinal cord (Fig. 11.3).

INVESTIGATIONS

Those required are the same as for other bone tumours (p. 739) including a skeletal survey to determine whether there are other lesions present, and in approximately 25% of patients with eosinophilic granuloma, a second bone is affected.

The radiographic picture (Fig. 11.1a) typically shows a unilocular punched out appearance, without any reaction in the surrounding bone, and in some cases involvement of adjacent soft tissues is indicated by a shadow cast by the lesion (Ennis, Whitehouse *et al.*, 1973).

DIFFERENTIAL DIAGNOSIS FROM OTHER BONE LESIONS

The various conditions described in the section on bone tumours (p. 725) should be considered, but those most likely to be misinterpreted on radiographic findings are fibrosarcoma of bone (p. 761) and Ewing's tumour (p. 741), especially when the femur is involved. These can usually be distinguished when the radiographic findings are typical, but chronic osteomyelitis may be difficult to differentiate, even on histological grounds.

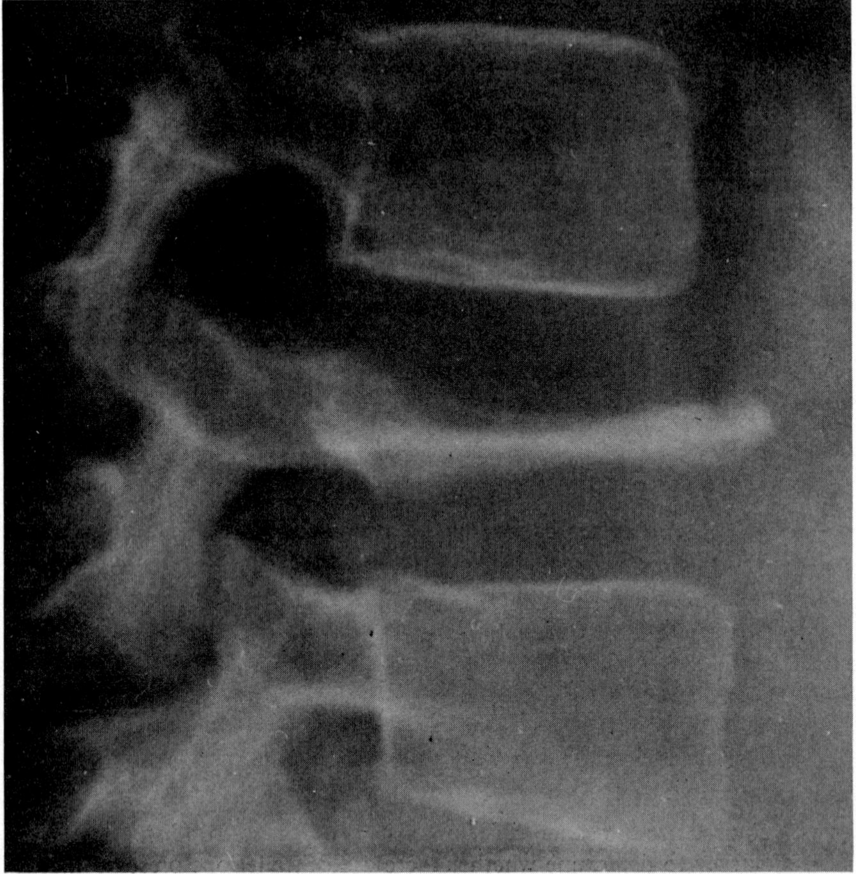

Figure 11.3. Eosinophilic granuloma of a vertebral body causing 'vertebra plana' of Calvé.

Biopsy is required for confirmation of the diagnosis in all cases of eosinophilic granuloma, and when suspected, subtotal removal of the lesion may be advantageous (see treatment). A drill biopsy is acceptable when the site is inaccessible, e.g. in some lesions in the pelvis, but an open biopsy is preferable in most cases.

HISTOLOGICAL DIFFERENTIATION OF EOSINOPHILIC GRANULOMA

Chronic osteomyelitis is the only condition in childhood likely to be mistaken for an eosinophilic granuloma. In osteomyelitis there is occasionally a pronounced histiocytic response which is more likely to occur in those with long-standing, low grade infection. However, in osteomyelitis the histiocytes are mixed with other types of inflammatory cells; there is a great deal of fibrosis; endothelial hyperplasia of vessels is pronounced, and there is usually some necrotic bone.

TREATMENT

The natural history can only be determined by the passage of time; in some lesions regression and healing occur spontaneously. Of those with a single lesion initially, some 5–6% develop multiple lesions in other bones and/or in soft tissues, leading to a fatal outcome.

Excision is desirable, and can be effected by thorough and careful curettage of most of the lesion at the time of the biopsy, e.g. in those arising in the calvarium or mandible. When the lesion is in a weight-bearing bone or unusually large, bone grafting of the cavity may improve the rate of healing.

Radiotherapy, in a dose of 500–1000 rads, may be used if the site is inaccessible and when there are no vulnerable nearby structures such as an epiphysis (Smith *et al.*, 1973).

It is generally agreed that cytotoxic drugs are not indicated when there is a single bone lesion, and are reserved for those with multiple lesions or dissemination (see below).

PROGNOSIS

The outlook for the bone lesion is good, except in vertebra plana (p. 210) which presents particular difficulties when there are neurological complications.

Of 147 cases collected from various reviews in the literature (Oberman, 1961; MacGavran & Spady, 1960; Fowles & Bobechko, 1970; etc.) only seven went on to develop other lesions, as did only 3 of 25 cases in the Index Series.

II. HAND-SCHÜLLER-CHRISTIAN SYNDROME

The triad of multiple rarefying lesions in membrane bone, exophthalmos, and diabetes insipidus, first defined by Kay (1905) and Schüller in 1915, is essentially a clinical syndrome not a pathological entity, and the term has come to be used loosely to describe disseminated histiocytosis of bone and soft tissues, with or without exophthalmos or diabetes insipidus.

MACROSCOPIC FINDINGS

The bone lesions are very similar to those of eosinophilic granuloma of bone

(Ennis, Whitehouse *et al.*, 1973), and in disseminated cases there is involvement of any or all of the spleen, lymph nodes, liver, lung, thymus, skin, bowel and bone marrow.

MICROSCOPIC FINDINGS

The typical cell in the lesions occurring in the Hand-Schüller-Christian syndrome is a mononuclear type of histiocyte with discrete cell boundaries and a certain 'separateness' of each cell so characteristic of all the histiocytoses. The histiocytes, as in eosinophilic granuloma, are well differentiated and do not appear to be truly neoplastic; eosinophils may or may not be present. The lesions often have a granulomatous appearance, including a considerable amount of central necrosis in some cases.

It is difficult to give a complete account of the histopathology except as it affects lymph nodes, liver, skin and bone marrow (all of which are accessible for biopsy) because the condition is not always fatal, and not all cases come to necropsy. Even when they do, the lesions have often been greatly altered by treatment or secondary infection, and can be very difficult to interpret. In material from the three autopsies in the Index Series, foamy cells with a relatively non-neoplastic appearance were dominant in the various tissues studied (Fig. 11.4).

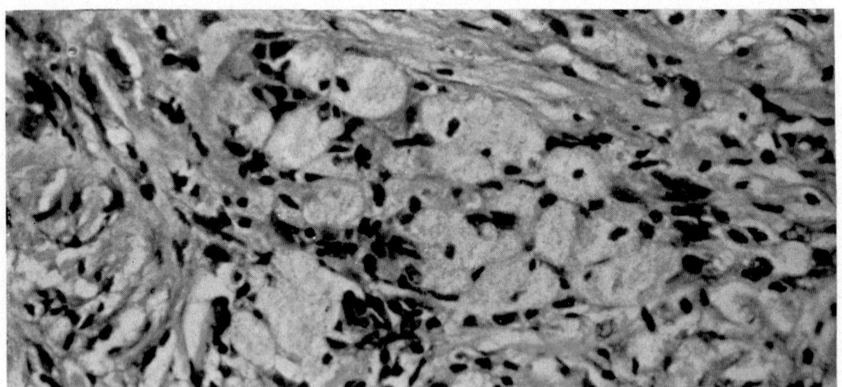

Figure 11.4. HAND-SCHÜLLER-CHRISTIAN SYNDROME; a differentiated type of histiocytosis with large, foamy histiocytes containing a dark nucleus, occurring either singly or in clusters in a dense fibrous stroma (H & E. × 520).

MODES OF PRESENTATION

1. The patient most often presents with a *persistent discharge from the external auditory meatus*, seborrhoeic lesions of the body and scalp, en-

largement of related lymph nodes, and erosions in membranous bones, chiefly in the calvarium (Fig. 11.1).
2. Less frequently the patient presents with *diabetes insipidus* and/or a *visual field defect.*

Clinical features
The skull is most frequently affected but other membranous bones may be involved too, and there may be swelling of both soft tissue and adjacent bone, with or without enlargement of the regional lymph nodes.

In the late stages, the disease may spread, causing visceral lesion in the liver, spleen, kidneys or thymus, and dissemination to these areas with organ dysfunction is an indication of a poor prognosis.

DIFFERENTIAL DIAGNOSIS

In the early stages, before there is involvement of the posterior pituitary or a visual field defect, the most frequent problem is to distinguish this condition from a *chronic ear infection.* The presence of erosions in the calvarium (p. 298) and the histological findings after biopsy excision of enlarged lymph nodes, usually establish the diagnosis.

On the rare occasions in which the patient presents with *diabetes insipidus*, other causes of this condition should be excluded, e.g. a craniopharyngioma (p. 267) or fractures of the base of the skull. The radiographic evidence is usually diagnostic, but biopsy of a superficial lesion may be required.

Distinguishing this syndrome from an eosinophilic granuloma depends upon presence of multiple lesions in x-rays of the calvarium, but especially by extension of these bony lesions into the adjacent soft tissues or to adjacent lymph nodes.

TREATMENT

This form of histiocytosis does not resolve spontaneously and active treatment is required. In patients without visceral involvement the prognosis and response to treatment appear better than when only the liver and spleen are involved. The best results have been obtained with chemotherapy (see p. 220), although symptomatic bone lesions often respond better to radiotherapy. Diabetes insipidus requires symptomatic treatment with Vasopressin®.

Chemotherapy
Prednisolone, vinblastine together with methotrexate and cyclophosphamide, or 6-mercaptopurine and vinblastine, have been used extensively, but an appreciable number of children with visceral dysfunction fail to respond. The results of combination therapy are more promising, and a recommended regime can be found at the end of this chapter.

III. LETTERER-SIWE DISEASE

This is a disease of infancy characterized by widespread infiltration by histiocytic cells with cytological features suggestive of malignancy. There is typically a diffuse, brown, papular, scaly rash covering the skin of the trunk, and sometimes the limbs (Fig. 11.5a). The rash may wax and wane, or even disappear completely in some areas only to reappear in others. Hepatosplenomegaly due to histiocytic infiltration also occurs, and lymph nodes may also be involved. Fever, anorexia and loss of weight are fairly constant features.

MICROSCOPIC FINDINGS

The skin lesions are characteristic; the epidermis is thinned out and loses its rete ridges; there is hyperkeratosis and sometimes ulceration. Collections of histiocytic cells with bean-shaped nuclei and relatively inconspicuous cytoplasm infiltrate the superficial layers of the epidermis (Fig. 11.5b).

Similar cells may extend down into the dermis and around the adnexae and blood vessels, but rarely into the subcutaneous fat. The nuclei of these cells are usually pleomorphic and mitotic figures are sometimes seen. The nuclear-cytoplasmic ratio is much higher than in the other two forms of histiocytosis X already described above, and this ratio serves to distinguish them from Letterer-Siwe disease in which another distinguishing feature is the absence of eosinophils.

MODES OF PRESENTATION

The disease is most commonly seen in infants and usually presents as *failure to thrive, with fever and an extensive rash*, often accompanied by a diffuse lymphadenopathy and hepatosplenomegaly.

Blood examination typically shows a normochromic anaemia, often associated with neutropenia, thrombocytopenia and a raised ESR.

CLINICAL FEATURES

The age of onset (the first two years of life), the extensive rash, the absence of bone lesions, and the usually fatal clinical course, all suggest that this is a distinctive entity. However, there are occasional instances in infants and young children in which there is a diffuse histiocytosis without a rash but with a similar infiltration of viscera (including infiltration of the skin without a rash); some of these remit spontaneously and completely, but most cases of this type too, are fatal.

The differential diagnosis includes the whole spectrum of viral infections in the newborn and, much less commonly, acute monocytic leukaemia (p. 166). In almost all cases the diagnosis can be established beyond doubt by skin biopsy, but staging of the disease requires histological confirmation of organ infiltration and assessment of whether there is dysfunction of the viscera affected.

TREATMENT

Responses to prednisolone and vinblastine, and to vincristine and methotrexate, have been reported. Recently, combination therapy as for Hand-Schüller-Christian syndrome (p. 220) has been used successfully, even in children with organ dysfunction.

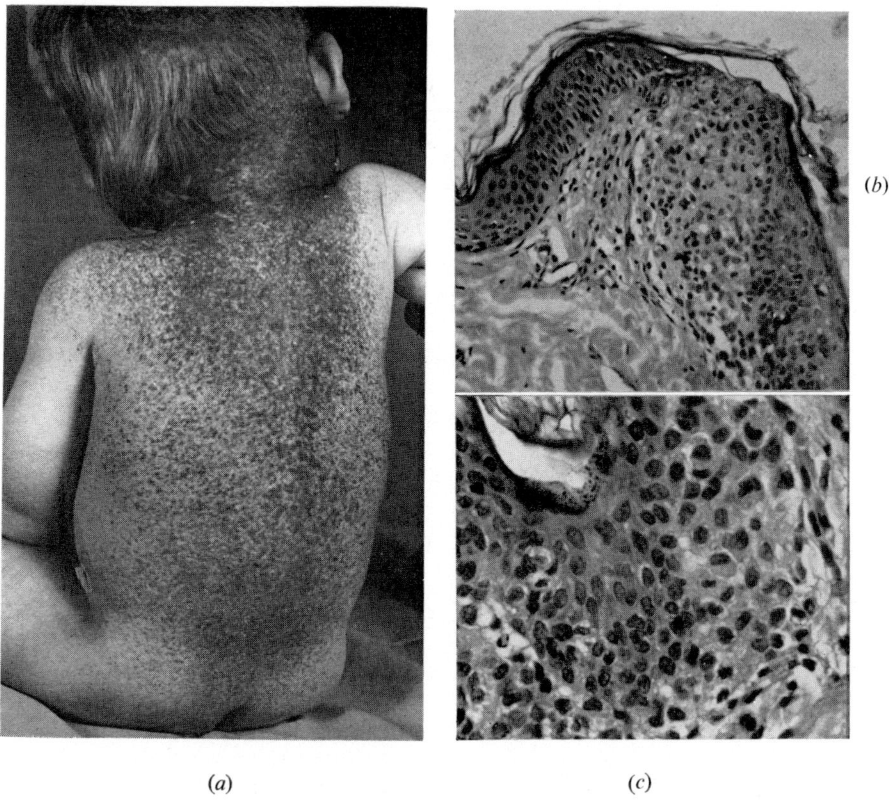

(b)

(a) (c)

Figure 11.5. Letterer-Siwe disease; (*a*) the characteristic extensive haemorrhagic rash; (*b*) biopsy of the skin lesion showing the commencement of a blister (above) in an area of epidermis infiltrated with histiocytes (H & E. × 200); (*c*) bean-shaped histiocytes infiltrating the epidermis (H & E. × 520).

The 'benign form' of Letterer-Siwe disease. There are a few reports in the literature of infants with the typical rash who without treatment, run a course of some months and ultimately recover completely. There was one such example in the Index Series.

It seems probable that a disease so difficult to define must at times be confused with benign conditions, possibly viral in origin, in which a monocytic leucocytosis and histiocytic infiltrations are prominent features.

PROGNOSIS OF HISTIOCYTOSIS X

For the purposes of comparison with other series, all cases of all three conditions in the Index Series have been classified according to the extent of the tissues involved at the time of presentation, as suggested by Oberman (1961). In the present state of knowledge this is perhaps the simplest and most useful way of planning treatment and assessing the prognosis, although a more detailed schema incorporating infiltration of tissues and organ dysfunction, suggested by Lahey (1970), is shown in Table 11.2.

The simple classification is as follows:

Group A (only bone involved); prognosis is good with recovery in 90–95%.
Group B (bone and soft tissues); a mortality of 50%.
Group C (soft tissues only); very poor prognosis.

Table 11.2. Histiocytosis X. Assessment of prognosis

Tissues/ organs involved	Good prognosis		Average prognosis		Poor prognosis	
	Infiltration	Dysfunction	Infiltration	Dysfunction	Infiltration	Dysfunction
Bones	+	—	+	—	+	—
Bone marrow	none	none	+	+	+	+
Lymph glands	+	—	+	—	+	—
Skin	+	—	+	—	+	—
Liver	none	none	+	none	+	+
Spleen	none	—	+	—	+	—
Pituitary	+	+	+	+	+	+
Lung	none	none	none	none	+	+

IV. FAMILIAL HAEMOPHAGIC HISTIOCYTOSIS

This, too, is a disease of the newborn and very young infants, characterized by large numbers of lymphocytes, and the proliferation of histiocytic cells which are erythrophagocytic (McMahon, Bedizel & Ellis, 1963).

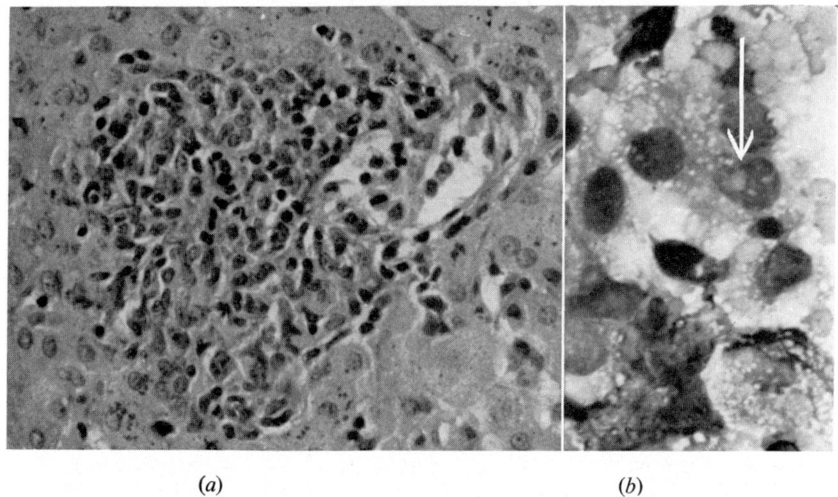

(*a*) (*b*)

Figure 11.6. FAMILIAL HAEMOPHAGIC RETICULOSIS; (*a*) liver (needle biopsy): a relatively non-specific infiltrate fills the portal tract. Numerous histiocytes with bean-shaped nuclei are present, but no eosinophils; note the clump of histiocytes in the portal venous radicle (H & E. × 300); (*b*) bone marrow; haemophagocytosis (arrow) is visible in this clump of cells composed entirely of histiocytes (Leishman, × 100). (See also Fig. 9.9, colour plate, following p. 140.)

The presenting features are fever and anaemia, and the diagnosis is suggested by finding erythrophagocytosis by histiocytes in material aspirated from the bone marrow.

The characteristic microscopic findings are histiocytic infiltration of the liver and spleen (Fig. 11.6); the lungs and skin are not involved, although peripheral lymph nodes may be. The histiocytic cells are very well differentiated and appear to be reactive rather than neoplastic. The agent responsible or the genetic basis for this condition is quite unknown.

Although this condition has been reported to be almost invariably fatal, Fullerton, Ekert *et al.* (1975) have recently reported successful treatment with a combination of vinblastine, prednisolone and 6-mercaptopurine.

V. SINUS HISTIOCYTOSIS

This is a clinically benign but long drawn out illness characterized by persistent enlargement of cervical lymph nodes, sometimes accompanied by a low fever (Lober *et al.*, 1973). The mediastinal or hilar nodes are occasionally involved (Rosai & Dorfman, 1972), and may remain enlarged for many months before returning to normal. Hepatosplenomegaly is not unusual.

MICROSCOPIC FINDINGS

These are extremely characteristic and readily recognized. The sinuses of involved lymph nodes are choked with very large histiocytic cells containing a small, compact nucleus and abundant, pink, glassy cytoplasm (Fig. 11.7). There are some variations in nuclear morphology, but mitoses are absent. The proliferation or accumulation of these cells is so extreme that the surviving lymphoid tissue in the node is much reduced and may be completely surrounded by them. However, there is neither infiltration of the capsule of the node nor invasion of the germinal centres, which may be the only lymphoid tissue remaining.

The etiology is quite unknown, and complete resolution eventually occurs without treatment.

(*a*)

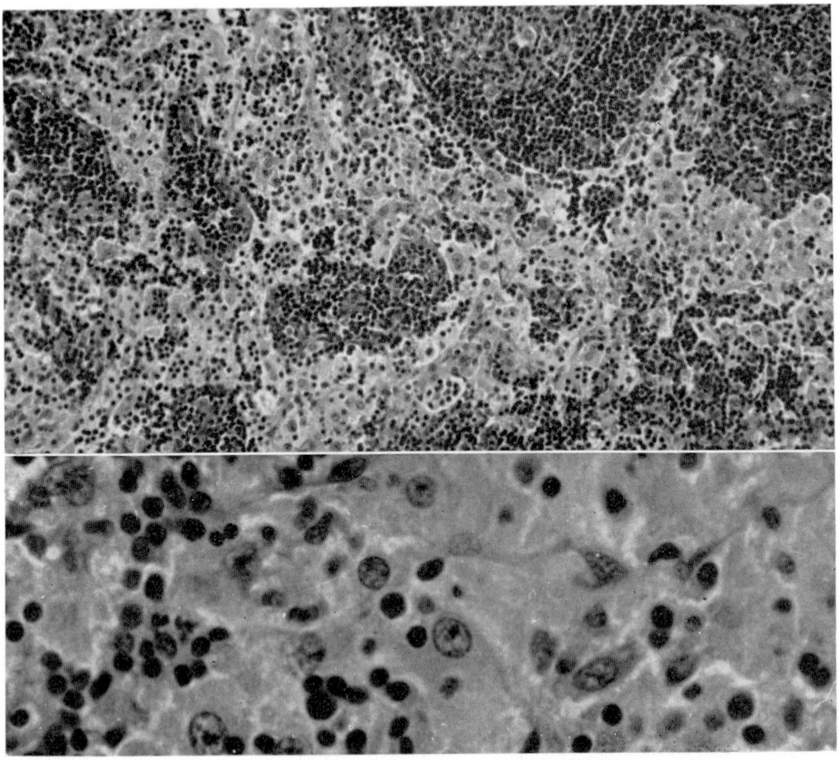

(*b*)

Figure 11.7. SINUS HISTIOCYTOSIS; (*a*) large, fleshy histiocytes filling the sinuses of a lymph node; the follicular pattern is distorted but still identifiable (H & E. × 200); (*b*) some nuclear pleomorphism of the histiocytes is common, but is not indicative of malignancy (H & E. × 520).

VI. UNCLASSIFIED HISTIOCYTOSES

These are few in number but their clinical and microscopic features vary greatly (Kauffman & Stout, 1961; Soule & Enriquez, 1973). In the current state of knowledge of the differentiation and function of the histiocyte-monocyte system, various conditions will have to be placed in this category until more precise classification of these cells is possible, on the basis of not only their microscopic morphology, but also by ultrastructure, phagocytic function, glass adherence, immuno-receptor sites, interaction with lymphocytes and enzyme content (Cline & Golde, 1973).

In childhood, there are occasional cases characterized by lymphadenopathy and fever (e.g. Lober *et al.*, 1973), with or without hepatosplenomegaly, and infiltration of various tissues and viscera is found in fatal cases; their response to cytotoxic agents is variable. Some may be examples of monocytic leukaemia, or well differentiated reticulum cell sarcoma, but the findings are not sufficiently certain or characteristic to categorize these as such.

Others follow a more benign course, and may not be neoplastic conditions at all, but rather unusual responses to unidentified infective agents.

Several other conditions in which proliferation of histiocytes is a feature have been tentatively identified, such as histiocytic medullary reticulosis (Warnke *et al.*, 1975), sex-linked reticulohistiocytosis with hyperglobulinaemia (Falleta *et al.*, 1973), familial reticulo-endotheliosis with eosinophilia (Omenn, 1965) and lymphohistiocytosis of the central nervous system.

Localized histiocytoma (syn. fibrous histiocytoma)

Some would favour including these tumour-like proliferations of histiocytes as variations of diffuse histiocytoses. It is not always clear whether the basic cell is a histiocyte or a fibroblast (Soule & Enriquez, 1972), and we have chosen to describe these lesions according to their site (see skin, p. 853; omentum, p. 676, soft tissues, p. 796).

HISTOLOGICAL DIFFERENTIATION OF GENERALIZED HISTIOCYTOSES

Several ill-defined conditions present some of the features of the histiocytoses.

Chronic non-specific lymphadenitis with pronounced sinus hyperplasia is the most common of these, and can be extremely difficult to distinguish from other forms of histiocytosis X because of the quasi-neoplastic hyperplasia which can occur in a variety of conditions. In most cases no definite etiological agent can be identified.

Specific infections or conditions which can lead to diagnostic difficulties by provoking a histiocytic response, have been recognized and these are as follows.

—Rubella
—Histoplasmosis
—Toxoplasmosis
—Cytomegalovirus infections
—Rheumatoid arthritis

In both specific and non-specific reactive histiocytoses it is most important that a malignant lymphoma or histiocytosis should not be diagnosed in error. The hallmark of a malignant histiocytosis is obliteration of the follicular pattern of the lymph node; if the follicles persist, even though there are numerous and often bizarre histiocytic cells in the sinuses and in the capsule of the node, malignancy is unlikely.

TREATMENT OF HISTIOCYTOSIS X

Treatment is considered under one heading, emphasizing the possibility of a uniform pathogenesis, and recognizing that there may be transformations from one form of the disease to another, e.g. patients with clinical features partly those of eosinophilic granuloma and Hand-Schüller-Christian disease, or partly those of Hand-Schüller-Christian disease and Letterer-Siwe disease.

There is general agreement that solitary or multiple bone lesions without involvement of soft tissue, lymph node or viscera have a very good prognosis. There is also agreement that those with widespread lesions in skin, lymph nodes and viscera with organ dysfunction, have a poor prognosis. In assessing the prognosis the system devised by Lahey (1970), summarized in Table 11.2, can be very useful. Patients with a good prognosis may have infiltration of bone, lymph nodes, skin and pituitary, but usually have no organ dysfunction or only pituitary dysfunction. Those with an average prognosis may have infiltration of all systems but dysfunction only in the marrow and pituitary. Patients with a poor prognosis usually have dysfunction of the marrow and liver.

Solitary bone lesions are best treated by excision, by curettage if they are accessible, and in most lesions a thorough curettage can be performed at the time of biopsy, e.g. in lesions arising in the calvarium or mandible. When the lesion is in a weight-bearing bone, or unusually large, bone grafting of the cavity may improve the rate of healing.

If the site is inaccessible or close to vulnerable nearby structures, radiotherapy can be used. In the case of multiple bone lesions, those which interfere with function may be treated with radiotherapy, while the others can be kept under surveillance.

In patients with multiple bone lesions cytotoxic drugs have frequently been reported to accelerate healing. In patients with lesions in bone as well as soft tissue, active treatment is required. Dysfunction in certain organ systems is particularly critical in assessing the patient's prognosis, for example disturbances in the liver (in the form of jaundice, ascites and/or hypoproteinaemia), in the lung (dyspnoea, cough, pneumothorax, effusion), or of the haemopoietic system (anaemia, leucopenia, thrombocytopenia or pancytopenia).

A preliminary analysis of the results of chemotherapy in histiocytosis X undertaken by Cancer Chemotherapy Group A indicates that in patients *without* visceral dysfunction, complete remission can be produced in at least 64% while in those *with* visceral dysfunction, a complete remission is produced in only 33%.

The most extensive studies of chemotherapy have been performed with a combination of vinblastine, vinblastine and prednisolone, or prednisone and 6-mercaptopurine. The results indicate that the combination of *vinblastine and prednisone* is associated with the best results to date.

At the Royal Children's Hospital, patients with histiocytosis X have recently been treated according to a protocol suggested by Lahey (1974). Patients eligible for chemotherapy are given oral chlorambucil (5 mg/m^2 daily) for 6 to 12 weeks. If the patient fails to respond or if the disease progresses, vinblastine (6·5 mg/m^2) is given weekly for 8 weeks. Methotrexate (20 mg/m^2) is given orally one day after each vinblastine injection, and cyclophosphamide (250 mg/m^2) orally 2 days after the vinblastine. Methotrexate and cyclophosphamide are maintained for at least 6 months, with monthly booster doses of vinblastine, given 1 week apart for 2 injections, and prednisolone. This regime has been used in 10 new patients with histiocytosis X, and so far only one has failed to respond.

REFERENCES

Cline, M.J. & Golde, D.W. (1973). A review and re-examination of the histiocytic disorders. *Amer. J. Med.*, **55** : 49.

Compere, E.L., Johnson, W.E. & Coventry, M.B. (1954). Vertebra plana (Calvé's disease) due to eosinophilic granuloma. *J. Bone Joint Surg.*, **36A** : 969.

Cunningham, J. (1970). Hand-Schüller-Christian disease and Kay's triad. *New Engl. J. Med.*, **282** : 1325.

Ennis, J.T., Whitehouse, G. Ross, F.G.M. & Middlemiss, J.H. (1973). The radiology of the bone changes in histiocytosis X. *Clin. Radiol.*, **24** : 212.

Falletta, J.M. & Fernbach, D.J. *et al.* (1973). A fatal x-linked recessive reticulo-endothelial syndrome with hyperglobulinemia. *J. Pediat.*, **83** : 549.

Fowles, J.V. & Bobechko, W.P.(1970). Solitary eosinophilic granuloma of bone. *J. Bone & Joint Surg.*, **52B** : 238.

Fullerton, P., Ekert, H., Hosking, C., & Tauro, G.P. (1975). Haemophagocytic reticulosis: A case report with investigations of immune and white cell function. *Cancer*, (in press).

Kauffman, S.L. & Stout, A.P. (1961). Histiocytic tumours (fibrous xanthoma and histiocytoma) in children. *Cancer*, **14** : 469.

KAY, T.W. (1905/06). Acquired hydrocephalus with atrophic bone changes, exopthalmos and polyuria (with presentation of the patient). *Pa. Med. J.*, 520.

LAHEY, M.E. (1970). Comparison of three treatment regimens in histiocytosis X in children. *Proc. Internation. Cancer Congress, Houston, Texas.*

LAHEY, M.E. (1974). Personal communication.

LICHTENSTEIN, L. (1953). Histiocytosis X. Integration of eosinophilic granuloma of bone, Letterer-Siwe disease and Schüller-Christian disease as related manifestations of a single nosologic entity. *Arch. Pathol.*, **56** : 84.

LOBER, M. & RAWLINGS, W. *et al.* (1973). Sinus histiocytosis with massive lymphadenopathy: report of a case associated with elevated EBV antibody titers. *Cancer*, **32** : 421.

MCGAVRAN, M.H. & SPADY, H.A. (1960). Eosinophilic granuloma of bone: a study of 28 cases. *J. Bone & J. Surg.*, **42A** : 979.

MCMAHON, H.E., BEDIZEL, M. & ELLIS, C.A. (1963). Familial erythrophagocytic lymphohistiocytosis. *Pediatrics*, **32** : 868.

NEWTON, W.A.Jr. & HAMOUDI, A.B. (1973). Histiocytosis: a histologic classification with clinical correlation. In *Perspectives in Pediatric Pathology*, Vol. 1, p. 251. Year Book Medical Publishers, Chicago.

OBERMAN, H.A. (1961) Idiopathic histiocytosis: a clinicopathologic study of 40 cases and review of the literature on eosinophilic granuloma of bone, Hand-Schüller-Christian disease and Letterer-Siwe disease. *Pediatrics*, **28** : 307.

OMENN, G.S. (1965). Familial reticulo–endotheliosis with eosinophilia. *New Eng. J. Med.*, **273** : 427.

ROSAI, J. & DORFMAN, R.F. (1972). Sinus histiocytosis with massive lymphadenopathy: a pseudolymphomatous benign disorder. *Cancer*, **30** : 1174.

SCHAJOWICZ, F. & SLULLITEL, J. (1973). Eosinophilic granuloma of bone and its relationship to Hand-Schüller-Christian and Letterer-Siwe syndromes. *J. Bone & Surg.*, **55B** : 545.

SMITH, D.G., NESBIT, M.E.Jr., D'ANGIO, G.J. & LEVITT, S.H. (1973). Histiocytosis X: role of radiation therapy in management with special reference to dose levels employed. *Radiology*, **106** : 419.

SOULE, E.H. & ENRIQUEZ, P. (1972). Atypical fibrous histiocytoma, malignant fibrous histiocytoma, malignant histiocytoma and epithelioid sarcoma. *Cancer*, **30** : 128.

WARNKE, R.A., KIM, H. & DORFMAN, R.F. (1975). Malignant histiocytosis (histiocytic medullary reticulosis). *Cancer*, **35** : 215.

Chapter 12. Lymphadenopathy of superficial nodes

In children, as in adults, enlargement of one or more superficial lymph nodes may be the earliest, and sometimes the sole clinical evidence of a malignancy —either as a primary arising in a lymph node or a metastasis from a tumour arising in the related drainage area or at a more distant site.

Regional metastatic deposits in children are less frequently seen than in adults because sarcomas are much more common than carcinomas, although some sarcomas, e.g. synovial sarcoma (p. 802) and lymphosarcoma, have a particular tendency to spread via lymphatics.

Peripheral lymphadenopathy of this kind will be described as it occurs, in order of frequency, in:
The cervical nodes;
The axilla;
The inguinal region; and
The popliteal fossa.

CERVICAL LYMPHADENOPATHY

An almost universal feature of early childhood, especially between the ages of two and six years, is non-specific reactive hyperplasia of the cervical nodes, the result of repeated encounters with the many viruses and bacteria which gain entry through the mucous membrane of the mouth and upper respiratory tract. In many children, multiple, small, firm, mobile nodes can be palpated in the anterior and posterior triangles, quite frequently on both sides.

Occasionally one of these nodes may reach a size greater than 3 or 3·5 cm in its largest dimension, and this raises the possibility of a more serious form of lymphadenopathy which requires investigation.

INVESTIGATION OF A LYMPHADENOPATHY

In the assessment of a cervical swelling which appears on clinical grounds to be arising in a lymph node, the following initial investigations are usually required.

1. *Full blood examination* including total and differential white cell count, with special stains of smears when leukaemia is a possibility.
2. *X-rays of the thorax and abdomen;* when a neuroblastoma is a possibility,

a skeletal survey and x-rays of the skull (especially the calvarium) are also indicated.

3. *Serological or other specific tests*, including a multiple Mantoux, to identify or exclude

—local specific infections, e.g. anonymous mycobacterial or cat scratch disease, or

—general infections, e.g. infectious mononucleosis.

4. *Biopsy*. Where the results of the above investigations are negative or equivocal, further investigations will be required, but foremost among them an 'excision biopsy' (see p. 945) of the maximally affected node is usually the most expeditious and informative.

CLINICAL DIFFERENTIATION OF OTHER BENIGN CONDITIONS

1. *Coccal infections*, acute or subacute, are the commonest cause of rapid enlargement of the cervical nodes. In most cases, fever, general toxaemia and local signs of acute inflammation, tenderness, reddening of the overlying skin or a brawny oedema, and a polymorphonuclear leucocytosis, leave no doubt as to the diagnosis.

Partial response to chemotherapy, especially following inadequate treatment with antibiotics, can cause a lesion containing sterile pus; when this persists and appears to be cystic, the signs can be confusing.

2. *Cysts of embryological remnants* are also common cervical conditions in childhood, but a thyroglossal cyst even when infected rarely causes diagnostic difficulties.

3. *Tuberculous cervical adenitis* also has distinctive features, but atypical signs are now rather more common since the anonymous mycobacteria have become the most usual type of tuberculous cervical adenitis in communities in which the human and bovine strains have been largely eliminated by public health measures. In the hypertrophic form of tuberculous infection due to an anonymous mycobacteria, caseation is minimal, even microscopic in its extent. Multiple Mantoux tests using material (PPD) from the human strain, the Battey strain, and from those known to occur in the particular community are helpful in making the correct pre-operative diagnosis.

4. *Cat scratch disease*. Although uncommon, the causal agent debatable and the course of the disease variable, the extent and duration of the accompanying lymphadenomegaly may arouse suspicion of a malignant condition. A history of a contact and/or a scratch is often absent, and there are no diagnostic investigations other than the appropriate skin test, with material which can be difficult to obtain or of doubtful reliability. In almost all cases the diagnosis is only made with certainty on biopsy, and even then an auramine-rhodamine stain should also be performed to exclude anonymous mycobacteria.

DIFFERENTIATION OF TUMOURS ARISING IN THE NECK

The following tumours, benign and malignant (primary and metastatic), can present as swellings in the cervical region.

Benign

Neurofibroma (of the deep cervical triangle and thoracic inlet, p. 465).

Malignant

Primary Tumours:
1. Hodgkin's lymphoma (p. 132) ⎫ arising in
2. Lymphosarcoma (p. 170) ⎬ the cervical
3. Reticulum cell sarcoma (p. 178) ⎭ lymph nodes.
4. Histiocytosis X (Letterer-Siwe disease (p. 214)).
5. Malignant neurilemmoma (p. 825).

Secondary deposits in cervical nodes

These may occur in the following conditions:

1. Neuroblastoma metastasis (e.g. from a primary in the abdomen or mediastinum, see p. 552).
2. Leukaemic deposits (p. 141).
3. Adenocarcinoma of the thyroid (p. 373).
4. Metastases from latent primary tumours in the oro- or nasopharynx (see p. 356) e.g. sarcoma or carcinoma (p. 360), lymphosarcoma of the tonsil (p. 343).
5. Metastases from tumours arising in skin or subcutaneous tissues of the face e.g. reticulum cell sarcoma (see p. 179).

When metastases develop late in the course of a malignancy arising outside the head and neck the diagnosis of the primary tumour has usually been made, and the problem is then chiefly concerned with modification of the programme of treatment already in hand. However, when the cervical metastasis is the *mode of presentation*, the results of preliminary investigations such as a full blood examination, Mantoux tests, and even x-rays of the chest and abdomen are often negative or inconclusive.

The diagnosis is in most cases made on the results of biopsy of the node or nodes most obviously involved.

It cannot be stated too strongly that any enlarged node which exceeds 3·5 cm in its greatest dimension should be excised as soon as can be conveniently arranged, and submitted to histological examination.

From the point of view of the pathologist, when the cells of a metastasis are morphologically very similar to lymphocytes, their diagnosis in a lymph node can present considerable difficulties, but the pattern and the cellular morphology can be interpreted accurately in the majority of cases (p. 171). The following clinical points may be helpful, particularly when the histological findings are difficult to interpret.

Neurofibroma
In childhood this can take the form of a peculiar tubular or 'parsnip'-shaped benign tumour deep in the neck presenting as a swelling in the supraclavicular region, and occupying part of the inlet of the thorax (p. 465). X-rays of the chest may show a contiguous intrathoracic mass, as may also occur in the cervico-thoracic type of cystic hygroma (p. 448). The density of the radiographic shadow may be helpful in distinguishing these two entities, a hygroma being the less dense.

Hodgkin's disease
This condition is so uncommon in the first two years of life that it can almost be excluded in this age group. Radiographs of the chest may show enlarged hilar glands, and complete assessment of the extent of Hodgkin's lymphoma may involve an extensive laparotomy (see p. 194).

Histiocytosis X
In infants with Letterer-Siwe disease, the presence of a typical rash and areas of erosion in the skull (see p. 297) in other forms of the disease will confirm the diagnosis and the cause of the lymphadenopathy.

Neurilemmoma (syn. Schwannoma)
One of the sites of this rare tumour appears to be in the upper cervical sympathetic ganglia, deep in the neck, often near the base of the skull, presenting as an extensive, fixed mass near the angle of the jaw, between the mastoid process and the ramus of the mandible. Apart from these clinical findings, the diagnosis can only be made by biopsy.

Metastatic neuroblastoma
Biopsy of an affected cervical node may be the first indication of a latent primary which should then be sought in the mediastinum and the abdomen (p. 543). Two of the unusual features of this source of metastasis is that the prognosis is not necessarily bad, e.g. in Stage IV S (see p. 558), and that lymphatic metastases are known to be able to evolve into benign and non-progressive ganglioneuromatous tissue (p. 464).

Leukaemic deposits
In a full blood examination, the number and morphology of the leucocytes is usually diagnostic (p. 144).

Adenocarcinoma of the thyroid gland
The ability of this tumour to produce highly differentiated metastatic thyroid tissue as small discrete metastases in cervical lymph nodes is well known (p. 373) and gave rise to terms, now superseded, such as 'lateral aberrant

thyroid' (von Haller) and 'benign metastasizing struma'. This form of adenocarcinoma and its treatment are described on p. 377.

Malignant tumours of the oro- and nasopharynx

These possible sources of metastases in the cervical lymph nodes indicate the importance of seeking a history or clinical signs of a latent primary in the recesses of the nose and throat. Even after the histological diagnosis has been made there may be nothing to find clinically, and endoscopy under anaesthesia may be required to locate and obtain a biopsy from the primary tumour (p. 361).

Malignant tumours arising on the face

Involvement of the cervical nodes may be present when the diagnosis is made, but more commonly appears after treatment has commenced. Biopsy is usually required if only to determine whether lymphadenopathy is indeed due to metastatic involvement or the result of infection following a biopsy, or the aftermath of treatment of the primary.

AXILLARY LYMPHADENOPATHY

Malignant enlargement of the lymph nodes is, except in the leukaemias, much less common in the axilla than in the cervical region, but most of the malignant conditions arising in lymph nodes listed on p. 224 may alternatively present as axillary swellings.

CLINICAL DIFFERENTIATION OF BENIGN CONDITIONS

A BCG inoculation in the arm may lead to a tuberculous axillary adenitis in the two or three months following the injection.

Apart from this and coccal adenitis, there are very few benign swellings of the axillary nodes. Simple reactive hyperplasia is much less common, and the upper limit of a normal node can be taken as 1·5–2 cm.

In the axilla, reticulum cell sarcoma and lymphosarcoma are more common than Hodgkin's disease. Investigation and management are along the same lines as in cervical lesions.

INGUINAL LYMPHADENOPATHY

Much the same can be said of primary or secondary malignant involvement of inguinal as of the cervical and axillary nodes.

CLINICAL DIFFERENTIATION OF BENIGN CONDITIONS IN THE INGUINAL REGION

Reactive hyperplasia
The usual minor infections, blisters, abrasions and lacerations in the lower limb and the perineum in childhood, often lead to enlargement of the superficial inguinal nodes, which resemble the similar process found in the cervical nodes.

Several shotty mobile inguinal nodes are normally palpable in each groin. In children less than five years of age, there is quite commonly an outlying superficial inguinal node which is situated cranial to Poupart's ligament; subacute or chronic coccal infection in this outlying node can be particularly misleading, and may resemble a complication of an inguinal hernia, particularly when the portal of entry, e.g. in the foot, has already healed and totally disappeared.

Anonymous mycobacterial adenitis occasionally occurs in the inguinal nodes, and has the same characteristics as in the cervical region (p. 224).

Investigation and initial management are the same as in the neck (p. 223).

POPLITEAL LYMPHADENOPATHY

The popliteal nodes are much more deeply situated than the other groups mentioned above, and they lie beneath the fascia at the back of the knee. They are thus less accessible than any other regional nodes, and fortunately least commonly involved.

DIFFERENTIATION OF BENIGN CONDITIONS

The semimembranous bursa, a cystic collection of crystal clear, viscid fluid, is by far the commonest swelling in the popliteal fossa. The clinical features are so characteristic that the diagnosis is rarely in doubt, but even minor departures from the typical features are important, and should lead to exploration, for a neoplasm, e.g. a synovial sarcoma, arising near the knee joint, has a particular tendency to arise in the popliteal fossa or, less commonly, a rhabdomyosarcoma or clear cell sarcoma; all three tumours were found in the popliteal fossa in the Index Series.

Popliteal coccal lymphadenitis is very uncommon, and the diagnosis is rarely immediately obvious. Deep pain, induration and tenderness, and no obvious current portal of entry, are the usual signs. Fever and polymorphonuclear leucocytosis are helpful in the differential diagnosis, but fluctuation due to abscess formation is rarely detectable because of the depth of the loculus of pus. Exploration and drainage, even before fluctuation is clinically apparent, may be necessary.

The numbers are small, but a primary sarcoma arising in the muscles bordering the popliteal space is probably more common than either a primary malignancy in the popliteal nodes or popliteal metastases.

Chapter 13. Intracranial and spinal tumours

Table 13.1. Intracranial and spinal tumours

Introduction

- Modes of presentation
- Raised intracranial pressure
- Focal neurological signs
- Cranial nerve palsies
- Endocrine disturbances
- Difficulties in prognosis
- Differentiation from other paediatric conditions
- The danger of lumbar puncture
- Classification of intracranial tumours

Intracranial tumours

A. *Tumours of the posterior fossa*

I. Astrocytoma
II. Medulloblastoma
III. Ependymoma of the fourth ventricle
IV. Glioma of the brain stem
V. Intracranial dermoids
VI. Haemangioblastoma of the cerebellum

B. *Tumours in the region of the third ventricle*

I. Tumours of the optic nerve and chiasm
II. Craniopharyngioma
III. Pineal tumours
IV. Tumours of the wall and floor of the third ventricle

C. *Superficial tumours of the cerebral hemispheres*

I. Cerebral astrocytoma
II. Glioblastoma multiforme
III. Giant cell astrocytoma
IV. Supratentorial ependymoma
V. Oligodendroglioma
VI. Papilloma of the choroid plexus
VII. Meningioma

Rarer intracranial tumours

I. Astroblastoma
II. Spongioblastoma
III. Polymorphic cell sarcoma
IV. Cerebellar sarcoma
V. Fibrosarcoma
VI. Rhabdomyosarcoma
VII. Microglioma and microgliomatosis
VIII. Neurocytoma (syn. ganglioglioma)
IX. Melanoma of the meninges (syn. neurocutaneous melanosis, lepto-meningeal melanomatosis)
X. Metastatic tumours

Spinal tumours

1. Primary tumours of the vertebrae
2. Metastatic tumours of the spine
3. Paraspinal tumours
4. Tumours of the spinal cord
5. Developmental anomalies affecting the spinal cord

INTRACRANIAL TUMOURS

The diverse origins, protean manifestations and the varied nature of the threat to function and survival, all combine to place tumours of the central nervous system in a unique position. The difficulties in eradicating them are especially challenging because of their situation or their pathological characteristics. There is little practical difference between the behaviour of a tumour with a benign histological appearance and an obviously malignant tumour when the site of the benign tumour precludes complete surgical removal.

Some 'tumours' can be regarded as disturbances of development, e.g. teratomas in the pineal region, while others are related to hereditary and generalized disorders, e.g., the various intracranial manifestations of von Recklinghausen's disease (p. 828).

Each of the wide range of pathological types has its own distinctive age group and predilection for a particular site, and when the symptoms and signs are correlated with the pathology and topography, there is generally a characteristic mode of presentation for each group of tumours.

Throughout this chapter the frequency of symptoms, tumours and other findings are expressed as percentages, and these are derived from a series of 430 consecutive children with an intracranial tumour, most of whom were treated at the Royal Children's Hospital, Melbourne. In general, the figures are very similar to those reported in other series (Tables 13.2, 13.3, 13.4), and when there are any significant differences these will be noted.

Modes of presentation of intracranial tumours

Their manifestations are extremely varied, but there are certain fairly defined and distinctive groups of symptoms and signs by which they may be recognized.

1. Headaches, vomiting and papilloedema, due to raised intracranial pressure.
2. Focal neurological signs, due to involvement of the cerebrum, cerebellum or the brain stem.
3. Cranial nerve palsies.
4. Pituitary dysfunction or disorders of the adjacent and closely related hypothalamic centres.

In the early stages only one of these patterns is usually present, but as the tumour enlarges it produces additional features likely to cause confusion unless the basic pattern is identified.

1. RAISED INTRACRANIAL PRESSURE

This is a major factor in producing symptoms, and may result from:

(*a*) Progressive expansion of a space-occupying tumour; or
(*b*) Obstruction of the CSF pathways.

(*a*) *Expansion of the tumour* is so often masked by adaptation and compensatory changes in adjacent neural tissues that focal localizing signs, e.g. motor or sensory deficits, may only become apparent in the late stages. In the early stages the changes are often insidious in onset and subtle in their effects; it is the combination of these which becomes significant and which makes their recognition important.

Headache is an unusual symptom in childhood, and is always significant, especially when it occurs in the early morning, recurs on consecutive days, and is followed by sudden vomiting with little or no nausea. Typically, in the early stages the child complains of headache soon after rising, may vomit at breakfast time, but go off to school without difficulty. A few weeks later, the headaches will be more severe and there will be reluctance to leave.

Changes in personality are all too frequently recognized only in retrospect; the good child becomes irritable and cranky; the energetic child slows down, and the thriving toddler loses his appetite. There is often a change in the child's facial appearance which expresses this alteration in mood.

Regression of motor skills, especially in children less than two years of age, is often most apparent as reversal of motor development; having learnt to walk he then becomes unsteady again; later the ability to stand is lost, and finally he is unable to sit up or hold up his head. In older children performance at school is affected; there is increasing difficulty in concentrating, loss of motivation and his results are progressively worse. Specific involvement of the language centres in the left hemisphere causes difficulties in verbal expression. These may have been present for weeks before organic involvement is suspected.

L.C., aged 12 years, had always obtained good marks at school. These deteriorated badly during one term. He was in danger of being diagnosed as a problem of early adolescence when headache and vomiting necessitated medical investigation. Later a large cyst, 7 cm in diameter, was found in the left hemisphere.

(*b*) *Obstruction of the CSF.* Even a small tumour may obstruct the flow of CSF and produce the 'midline syndrome' (Van Bogaert & Martin, 1928; Raimondi *et al.*, 1967), a clinical picture characterized by the following.

Enlargement of the head in infants, separation of the cranial sutures (in radiographs) in older children, and a characteristic 'cracked pot note' on percussion of the head.

Alterations in the level of consciousness which may be transient, but often sudden and profound.

Morning headache and vomiting, daily for a few weeks then diminishing or disappearing, only to reappear in a more severe degree.

Visual disturbances, an obvious squint is sometimes present, but deterioration of vision is more serious and often insidious and when detected it may already be irreversible. Papilloedema, often severe, is common.

Optic atrophy is usual when the tumour involves the optic chiasm (p. 265).

Ataxia, of the trunk rather than fine movements, often accompanied by a rhythmic tremor.

In the late stages, bilateral hypertonia, extensor rigidity, neck stiffness and opisthotonos appear, and finally sudden respiratory arrest may terminate the midline syndrome.

2. FOCAL NEUROGENIC SIGNS

Signs indicative of local involvement usually appear late, except in gliomas of the brain stem in which cranial nerve palsies are frequently the first overt signs and occur long before the development of raised intracranial pressure. Motor and sensory deficits also occur in brain stem tumours, rather more commonly than in tumours involving the cerebral cortex.

Epilepsy is common (27%), usually Jacksonian, and of localizing value in superficial cortical gliomas, but it can also occur as a result of ventricular obstruction. The appearance of epilepsy in a child after the age of two years should always be investigated fully.

3. CRANIAL NERVE PALSIES

Cranial nerve palsies are of the utmost importance. Signs of deterioration in vision are an indication for neurological examination and radiographs of the skull to exclude a tumour affecting the visual pathways.

A squint (CN. VI), appearing in a child over three years of age, changes in the voice or difficulty in swallowing (CN. IX and XI), and facial weakness producing a characteristic 'woebegone' appearance, may be the first signs of a glioma of the brain stem (Fig. 13.1).

4. ENDOCRINE DISTURBANCE

The effects of pituitary deficiency are usually subtle and insidious, and often precede the detection of a tumour by many years. Delayed growth and development, polyuria, and loss of energy are most often seen with suprasellar tumours; precocious skeletal and sexual development are less common, and not always pituitary in origin (e.g. p. 577).

DELAY IN DIAGNOSIS

This is common, and mainly due to the following factors:

(*a*) The rarity of intracranial neoplasms, although as a group they are the commonest of all tumours in childhood. The family doctor sees only one in an average five-year period.

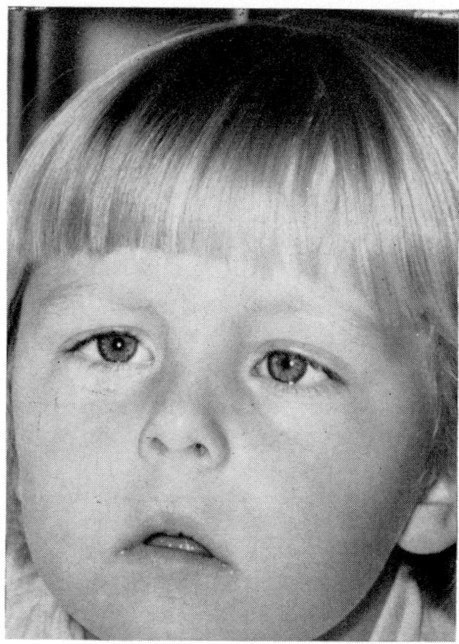

Figure 13.1. GLIOMA OF THE BRAIN STEM: the typical woebegone expression, partial facial palsy and strabismus.

(*b*) The obscurity and variety of the presenting symptoms.

(*c*) The slow and insidious onset, followed by rapid and catastrophic terminal deterioration.

DIFFICULTIES IN PROGNOSIS

It is particularly difficult to forecast the outcome of any child with a brain tumour and the following factors should be taken into account.

The rate of growth of any tumour is difficult to assess. The glioblastoma multiforme is the least difficult, for it is the most malignant and survival beyond twelve months is uncommon. At present there are no histological or clinical standards which permit an accurate prognosis in the individual patient. The medulloblastoma has a fairly uniform histological appearance, but it has been said (Bloom *et al.*, 1969) that with adequate treatment 40% of children with this tumour may survive five years, and 30% for ten years, but there are no reliable indications as to which children will survive longest.

Complete macroscopic removal has only a moderate influence on prognosis; in general the more complete the removal the better the prognosis, but survival for more than 25 years has followed incomplete removal of a fibrillary astrocytoma.

The area affected can also be important. The removal of a benign or low-grade tumour, even in an accessible site, may cause such an unacceptable neurological deficit that the tumour can be considered malignant by virtue of its situation rather than its biological behaviour.

DIFFERENTIAL DIAGNOSIS OF INTRACRANIAL TUMOURS

The clinical features of the child with an intracranial tumour may closely resemble other more common conditions which should be excluded before reaching a diagnosis. The chief presenting features will be considered in turn.

1. *Enlargement of the head* in the first years of life, often accompanied by separation of the cranial sutures and 'silver beaten' calvarium in radiographs. In infants this is more likely to be due to one of the other causes of hydrocephalus, such as stenosis of the aqueduct, than to an intracranial tumour, but when cranial enlargement is accompanied by papilloedema, it is almost always due to a tumour.

A subdural haematoma should also be excluded by subdural taps or a brain scan (p. 75).

2. *Headache* due to extracranial causes is not common in young children, and the daily early morning headache of an intracranial tumour is distinctive.
3. *Vomiting*, often unaccompanied by any complaint of headache, is still common enough with intracranial tumours, and when vomiting or abdominal pain dominates the clinical picture, some abnormality of the gastro-intestinal tract may be suspected. Investigations are instituted, are found to be negative, and further delay in diagnosis occurs.
4. *Papilloedema and visual deterioration* may be due to 'benign' intracranial hypertension (pseudo-tumour cerebri syndrome). Headache, visual loss and double vision occur. The cause is unknown and the course is long but apparently self-limiting (Hagberg & Sillanpää, 1970). It is less common than a tumour, which can only be excluded with certainty by ventriculography which demonstrates small symmetrical and undisplaced ventricles (Rose & Matson, 1967; Grant, 1971).
5. *Ataxia, sensory motor deficits or cranial nerve palsies* due to encephalitis may arise as a complication of the more common viral diseases (mumps or measles), and also in late stages of meningitis. Tuberculous meningitis with its insidious onset, is not infrequently mistaken for a cerebral tumour. Indeed, in some communities a tuberculoma is still the commonest intracranial space-occupying lesion in children.

Conversely, neck rigidity and even opisthotonus may be caused by a tumour in the posterior fossa and suggest meningitis (see Fig. 13.8).

6. *Failure to thrive* occurs in the diencephalic syndrome so often seen in children with a tumour near the hypothalamus, but also in infants with a

subdural haematoma. A malabsorption syndrome, renal tract infections or congenital heart disease may be suspected initially.

7. *Proptosis*, e.g. due to a glioma of the optic nerve, occurs in a variety of conditions arising in the orbit, such as metastatic neuroblastoma (p. 408), primary soft tissue tumours of the orbit (p. 402), congenital buphthalmos, and in arteriovenous malformations (p. 401).

8. *Space-occupying lesions other than brain tumours* should always be considered when signs of a space lesion occur in certain contexts. A hydatid cyst may be the cause in areas where such infestation is common. Tuberculomas are still frequently seen in developing countries. Chronic brain abscess following a forgotten ear or nasal sinus infection still occurs. The unusual chronic subdural haematoma in the older child is usually first diagnosed as a tumour.

9. *Lead poisoning*, in children commonly caused by ingestion of flakes of paint containing lead fillers, causes severe papilloedema as part of a hypertensive encephalopathy.

THE DANGER OF LUMBAR PUNCTURE

Lumbar puncture may be considered when investigating some of the conditions mentioned above, and it should be emphasized that this is always fraught with danger in a patient with raised intracranial pressure due to a tumour. Every year in every large hospital a death occurs from this misadventure.

Even when only a small amount of CSF is withdrawn for testing, leakage continues for some time at the site of the dural puncture, causing progressive loss of fluid and decreasing pressure in the spinal theca; the movement of the brain in adapting to these alterations in pressure may force the cerebellar tonsils downwards into the foramen magnum, where they compress the medulla. causing respiratory and cardiac arrest.

This 'coning' of structures through the foramen magnum is a life-threatening situation which may respond to urgent decompression, by needling the cerebral ventricles and/or enlarging the foramen magnum and thereby decompressing the posterior fossa.

CLASSIFICATION OF INTRACRANIAL TUMOURS

Nearly all examples can be readily classified on a topographical basis into the following three groups.

A. Tumours arising in the posterior fossa.
B. Tumours in the region of the third ventricle.
C. Superficial tumours of the cerebral hemispheres.

A systematic classification is shown in Table 13.5, which lists the various tumours arising from the various tissues of the central nervous system, including its coverings and blood vessels. For the purposes of this chapter, a topographic schema has been superimposed on the pathological classification, for we believe this is more appropriate in considering tumours of the central nervous system in childhood. The terminology used is the same as in Table 13.5 (p. 286).

Before describing the main groups some of the rarer types will be mentioned briefly.

Meningioma of the sellar region in childhood usually involves the optic nerve sheath and presents with loss of vision without any other manifestations (p. 265). It may be confused with an optic glioma (p. 262).

Chordomas arise in the basiphenoid region and spread slowly but irresistibly from the base of the skull; occasionally such a tumour protrudes into the nasopharynx (p. 264).

Teratomas are uncommon outside the pineal region, and when this group is excluded, the remainder consistute only 0·5 % of all intracranial tumours.

Hydatid cysts are rare; there were four in the Index Series, two were single cysts and two patients had multiple cysts.

Arachnoid cysts are mainly associated with disturbances in the circulation of the CSF and are more appropriately discussed with hydrocephalus (p. 233).

A. TUMOURS OF THE POSTERIOR CRANIAL FOSSA

This is the commonest site (51 %) of intracranial tumours in childhood (Fig. 13.2), a markedly different incidence from tumours in adults.

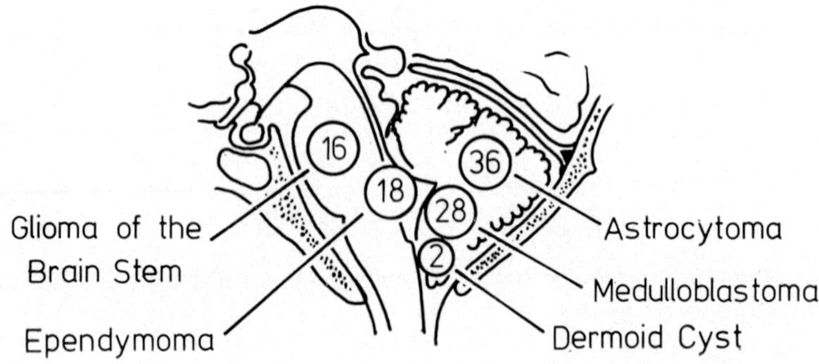

Figure 13.2. TUMOURS OF THE POSTERIOR FOSSA; the distribution and relative incidence (expressed in percentages) of the main groups in the author's series of cases.

The tumours which arose in this area were as follows.

I. Astrocytomas, 36%.
II. Medulloblastomas, 28%.
III. Ependymomas of the 4th ventricle, 18%.
IV. Gliomas of the brain stem, 16%.
V. Miscellaneous, 2%.

Table 13.2. Tumours of the posterior fossa. Relative incidence of various types of tumour, as reported from Boston (Matson, 1969), Vienna (Koos & Miller, 1971), Tokyo (Katsura *et al.*, 1959) and Melbourne (author's personal series, comprizing the Index Series of intracranial tumours, and additional cases)

	Boston	Vienna	Tokyo	Melbourne
Total	418	350	225	260
	%	%	%	%
Astrocytoma	32	33	35	36
Medulloblastoma	30	33	36	29
Ependymoma	8	8	9	18
Brain stem glioma	18	13	—	16

CUSHING'S COMPOSITE HISTORY

There is no better introduction to a description of tumours of the posterior fossa in childhood than the classic account of the mode of onset, which Cushing (1931) built up from a careful survey of the histories of a large number of children with a cerebellar tumour.

'A child between five and ten years of age and apparently normal in all respects begins, possibly after a fall or an attack of whooping cough, to have early morning headaches with vomiting. Nothing much is to be found on examination; the child subsequently feels perfectly well, and has his breakfast and wants to go out and play. This almost daily performance may continue for a considerable time, the child even going to school meanwhile. There may then be a remission for weeks or perhaps months and the episodes may be almost forgotten until they recur; the symptoms are likely to be more pronounced, and are apt to be ascribed to some gastro-intestinal upset. This appears to be the more probable since the child finds that straining at stool brings on a headache and there is a tendency to constipation. Moreover, a mild daily laxative usually serves to completely mask the symptoms.

'This story continues, off and on, until it becomes evident that the child is a little clumsy at play and gets knocked over easily. Very possibly, the periodic headache will have ceased completely or at least occurs at much longer intervals; if the parents are observant they may notice that the child's head has increased more rapidly than it should. This, however, is usually discounted for the child is now free of complaints and appears to be alert and well.

'After a further period of weeks or months possibly with some increase in clumsiness or with no noticeable changes whatever, it suddenly becomes apparent, perhaps at school, that the child's sight is poor. Glasses are usually prescribed; but even when an ophthalmoscope is used, the retina is less easily examined in a child than in an adult and, because of the decompressive effects of the enlarging head, the optic papillae often show no measurable swelling; the fact that they are pale and the margins blurred may easily pass unrecognized.'

I. ASTROCYTOMA

AGE : SEX

In most reported series the peak incidence is close to 10 years of age, but in the Index Series it lay between 3 and 5 years; these 2 years accounted for 50% of the affected children; the number of cases in the 5–10 year age group was significantly lower (Fig. 13.3). Matson (1969) and Gol & McKissock (1959) found that the proportion of cases between 5 and 10 years old was 45–50%. No satisfactory explanation for this difference can be found.

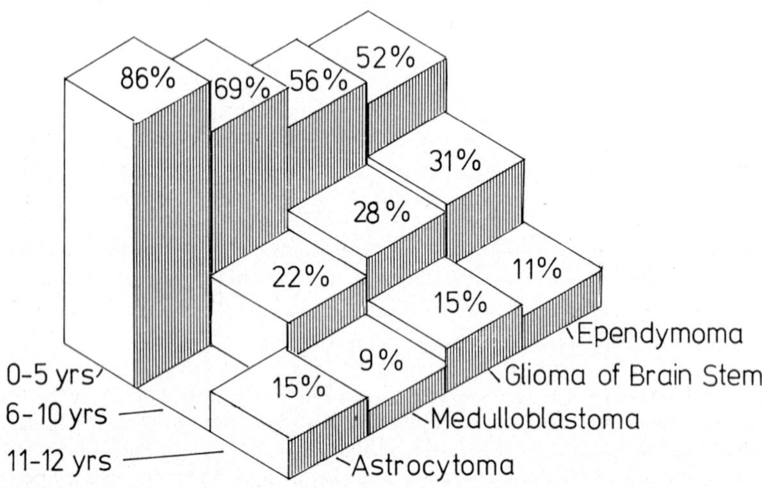

Figure 13.3. RELATIVE INCIDENCE OF VARIOUS TUMOURS ACCORDING TO AGE, showing the proportion of each the major tumours in each of the three quinquennia of childhood.

In some published series a female preponderance has been reported, but in the Index Series males and females were affected equally.

The age incidence of astrocytoma determined from a study of white children in U.S.A. is shown in Fig. 13.4.

MACROSCOPIC APPEARANCES

Most astrocytomas of the cerebellum are located in one or other lobe, and only involve the midline as the result of growth and expansion. However, some solid tumours may arise in the midline and grow laterally towards the cerebellar peduncle. Less frequently they expand into the fourth ventricle and even spill out through the foramen of Magendie.

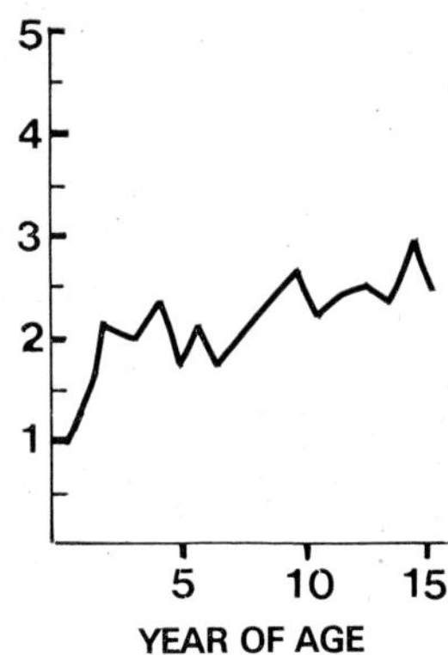

Figure 13.4. ASTROCYTOMA; the incidence according to age (for source of figures see Fig. 2.2, p. 48).

Cystic forms are common, and mostly found in the lateral lobes. The cysts may be multiple and attain a very large size; solid tumour tissue may be found between the cysts or as a nodule projecting into a cyst.

The texture of the solid tumour is variable; some are soft and mucoid, while others are firm, and there is often a clear demarcation from cerebellar tissue. Soft tumours are not always cellular (i.e. malignant) nor are firm tumours necessarily well differentiated; texture as a guide to cellularity can be very misleading.

The least frequent form is a large single cyst lined by one or two layers of astrocytic cells; complete removal of the thin wall is so difficult that it is impractical.

MICROSCOPIC APPEARANCES

To avoid repetition, the following description of the histological structure may be taken to apply to astrocytomas generally.

Tumours of astrocytic glial origin present a wide variety of histological appearances (Fig. 13.5). The most common pattern is the so-called *juvenile fibrillary astrocytoma* in which the cells have a regular oval nucleus, delicate, dust-like chromatin and prominent fibrillary cytoplasm. Cytoplasmic processes from groups of adjacent cells form compact bundles of fibrils, the so-called 'piloid' or 'hair-like' structures. Microcystic degeneration is very common and vacuoles form between individual cells. The vacuoles may coalesce, and the juvenile astrocytoma is the commonest type presenting as a mural nodule in a cyst. Nuclear anaplasia and mitotic activity are rare.

The protoplasmic pattern is another variant; the nuclei are small with a stellate vacuolated cytoplasm and form an open meshwork of cells. Larger cysts containing fluid with a high protein content form between the tumour cells, as in the piloid variety. Both these patterns are very common in cerebellar astrocytomas.

The diffuse fibrillary astrocytoma of the so-called 'adult' type is less commonly seen in children. In this form the astrocytes are evenly distributed and the amount of glial fibre formation is considerable and uniform. Anaplasia and nuclear variability is much more common in this type, which is probably the commonest histological type of glioma of the brain stem (see p. 254).

Rosenthal fibres are common in astrocytomas generally, and in particular in the piloid variety. In their most florid form Rosenthal fibres appear as swollen and brightly eosinophilic astrocytic processes. Electron microscopy shows that these consist of amorphous masses of electron-dense material occupying the astrocytic process, and apparently condensing out of glial filaments which surround them. Rosenthal fibres are not confined to tumours, and are commonly found in the pineal gland and also in areas of reactive gliosis.

Malignant astrocytoma

Nuclear anaplasia, mitotic activity, giant forms and focal areas of increased cellularity are found in approximately 15% of cerebellar astrocytomas. Vascular endothelial hyperplasia is usual and may be florid, the proliferated endothelial cells obliterating the vascular lumen.

Other histological patterns are described in astrocytomas of the cerebellum. Gemistocytic astrocytes with plump, brightly eosinophilic swollen cytoplasm are very occasionally seen, but rare in children. Some authors consider subependymal gliomas to be a form of astrocytoma, but it is our belief that they are variants of ependymoma and are considered in that section (p. 253).

Histological grading

Formal grading of childhood astrocytomas (Grade I to Grade IV, Kernohan & Sayre, 1952) is difficult in practice and can be misleading because cellularity, and hence the degree of malignancy, varies from place to place. Grading has not been employed in the Index Series, but an attempt has been made in the description to convey the degree of cellularity, the number of mitoses and whether the picture varies from one part to another.

Those tumours with obviously malignant features (including glioblastoma multiforme, a useful term since the histological picture is easily recognizable,

p. 277) should be placed in a special category and designated as 'malignant astrocytomas' for this is of help to the surgeon. The remainder are best unclassified and diagnosed simply as astrocytomas.

CLINICAL FEATURES

The synthesized case history on p. 239 is typical, and in atrocytomas the duration of symptoms before presentation was the longest of any tumour arising in the posterior fossa; 24% presented after three months, and 34% after six months of symptoms.

The child with an astrocytoma is often in good health when first seen, and in 80% of cases in the Index Series the predominant complaint was recurrent early morning headache and vomiting. Only occasionally had vomiting and anorexia progressed to a stage of severe emaciation.

Ataxia of gait and incoordination of hand movement were present in 60%, but were much later in appearance, often only just before admission to hospital.

Change in temperament was not as obvious as in other types of intracranial tumour and developed insidiously so that its onset could not be readily determined.

An obvious squint or a complaint of double vision (Fig. 13.5) was the initial reason for seeking medical advice in many patients, and in most cases this was only a week or two before admission. Nystagmus was present in 33%. Papilloedema was a fairly constant finding (over 90% on presentation). Marked enlargement of the head is not common, but a less obvious increase was found in 24%, associated with separation of sutures and a raised pitch in the percussion note, all indicative of raised pressure of some duration in the older child.

Investigations will indicate the presence of a tumour, but a firm diagnosis of an astrocytoma before operation is unusual.

Radiography will often show separation of the sutures, and rarely calcification is seen; if this is in the lateral lobe of the cerebellum an astrocytoma is probable.

Radionucleide scans (p. 75) yield variable results; cystic astrocytomas often show a high take-up.

Angiography may show a tumour circulation in the florid growths, and large avascular areas are caused by cysts.

Contrast studies are the most accurate, and a large space-occupying lesion which obstructs and displaces the fourth ventricle laterally is characteristic.

RESULTS

Generally this is the most favourable group (see p. 260).

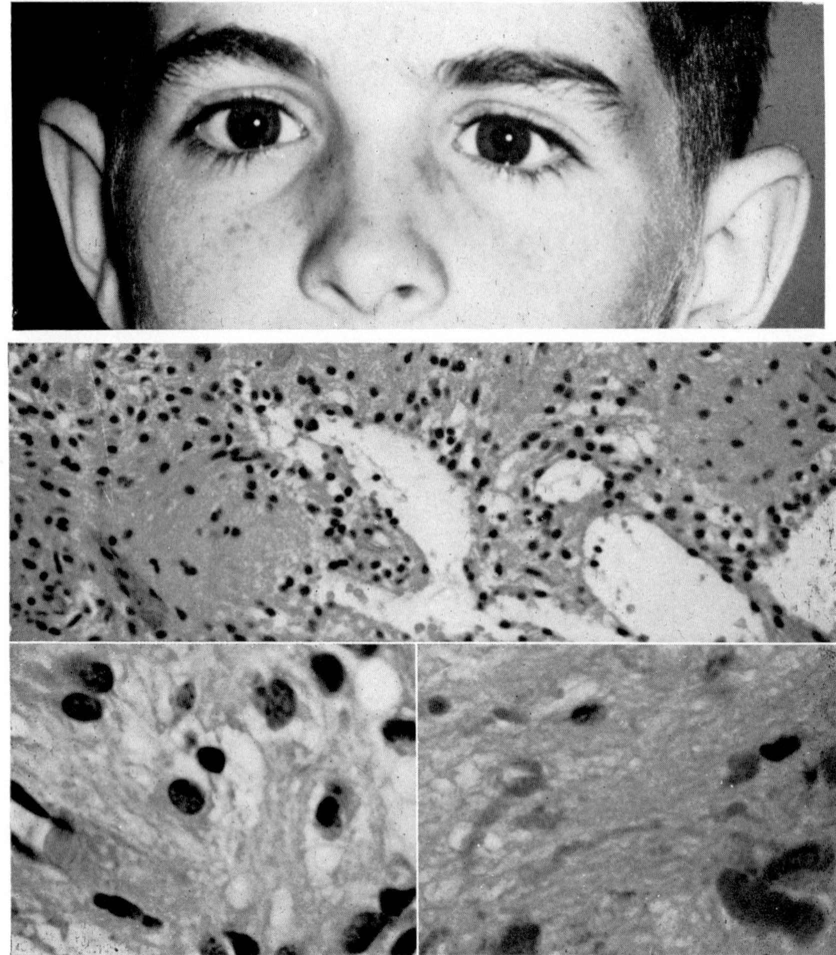

Figure 13.5. ASTROCYTOMA OF THE CEREBELLUM; (*a*) a boy presenting at seven years of age complaining of diplopia, with a squint of recent onset; (*b*) a juvenile (pilocytic) astrocytoma with abundant glial fibres like tresses of hair (hence 'piloid'), and areas of cystic degeneration ('microcystic change') which often contain neutral fat (H & E. × 130); (*c*) nuclear and cytoplasmic detail (H & E. × 430); (*d*) Rosenthal fibres, i.e. eosinophilic material, within the glial processes of the astrocytes (H & E. × 430).

[(*a*) *Top.* (*b*) *Centre.* (*c*) *Bottom left.* (*d*) *Bottom right.*]

II. MEDULLOBLASTOMA

AGE : SEX

More than half of the children (59%) were less than five years of age at the time of diagnosis (Fig. 13.3; 13.6); four babies presented in the first few months of life and had undoubtedly developed their tumour *in utero*.

This is one of the intracranial tumours with a marked sex difference (Crue, 1958; Matson, 1969; Koos & Miller, 1970). Males (64%) were affected twice as commonly as females (36%) in the Index Series.

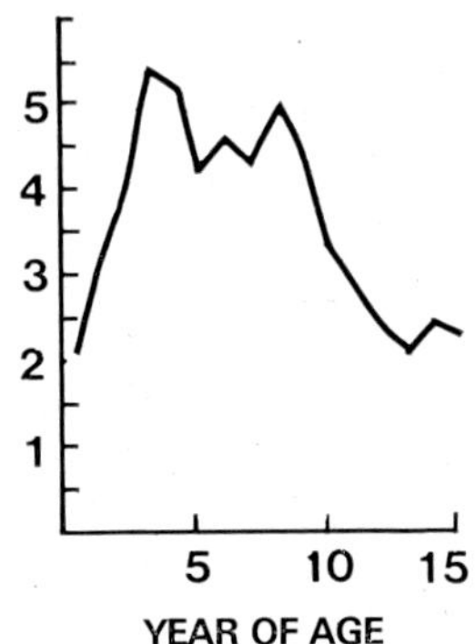

Figure 13.6. MEDULLOBLASTOMA; the incidence according to age (for source of figures see Fig. 2.2, p. 48).

HISTOGENESIS

Medulloblastomas are believed to arise from primitive cells in the roof of the developing fourth ventricle, which migrate upwards and laterally to form the external granular layer of the cerebellum. The tumour may arise anywhere along the path taken by these cells, and while most occur in the midline, in the region of the vermis and cerebellar velum (a structure which disappears early in embryogenesis), this theory also accounts for the rare medulloblastoma arising in one of the lateral lobes of the cerebellum, mostly in older children or adults.

MACROSCOPIC APPEARANCES

The tumour presents as a large, soft, pinkish-grey midline mass which distends and finally blocks the fourth ventricle. A prolongation of the tumour may pass through the foramen of Magendie to overlie the upper portion of the spinal cord or spill out into the lateral recesses.

MICROSCOPIC FINDINGS

The usual histological appearance is a cellular tumour composed of cells with hyperchromatic oat- or carrot-shaped nuclei and scanty, ill-defined cytoplasm, arranged diffusely in a delicate vascular stroma. The vessels are usually very thin-walled with no endothelial hyperplasia. The number of mitotic figures is variable, and in some tumours they are numerous; necrosis and haemorrhage are prominent in some examples. Medulloblastomas may show a degree of differentiation (Fig. 13.7) which takes one of the following forms:

1. *Pseudorosette formation* occurs in approximately 30% of tumours; the rosettes consist of radially-arranged medulloblasts around a central mass of pink neurofibrillary material resembling, in some respects, that seen in neuroblastoma. On other occasions a false appearance of rosettes is due to medulloblasts radially arranged around a delicate blood vessel (13.7c).
2. *A streaming appearance* is seen when medulloblasts are arranged in whorls or long parallel rows; in this form the medulloblasts are often elongated and appear to be polar.
3. *Pockets of astroglia* within medulloblastoma are not uncommon, and were seen in approximately 20% of the Index Series. These areas of astroglial differentiation are often sharply demarcated from the medulloblastoma cells, and may be separated by a delicate glial capsule. The astroglial cells are similar in nuclear structure to medulloblasts, but they are distributed unevenly in a loose fibrillary glial network, an appearance reminiscent of neuroblastoma.
4. *Neuronal differentiation* is very occasionally seen.
5. *A pseudopallisading* of tumour cells around an area of necrosis, resembling a glioblastoma multiforme is seen infrequently.
6. *Oligodendroglial differentiation* has been described (Bodian & Lawson, 1953); the nuclei are enclosed in the centre of rectangular cells with clear cytoplasm.
7. *A sarcomatous appearance.* When medulloblastoma cells infiltrate the dura, they provoke in it a pronounced fibroblastic reaction; the tumour cells are arranged in parallel rows similar to the appearance in an infiltrating lymphosarcoma in soft tissue. At times there is an extreme degree of fibroblastic proliferation, and in these cases differentiation from cerebellar sarcoma may be extremely difficult (13.7f).
8. *Pigmented cells* are seen in the variant described by Bodian & Lawson (1953) and Fowler & Simpson (1962), the pigmented cells being arranged in tubules and papillae, with some of the features of a neuroectodermal tumour of infancy (melanotic progonoma, see p. 334). However, it is malignant and behaves as a medulloblastoma and not as a neuroectodermal tumour of infancy.

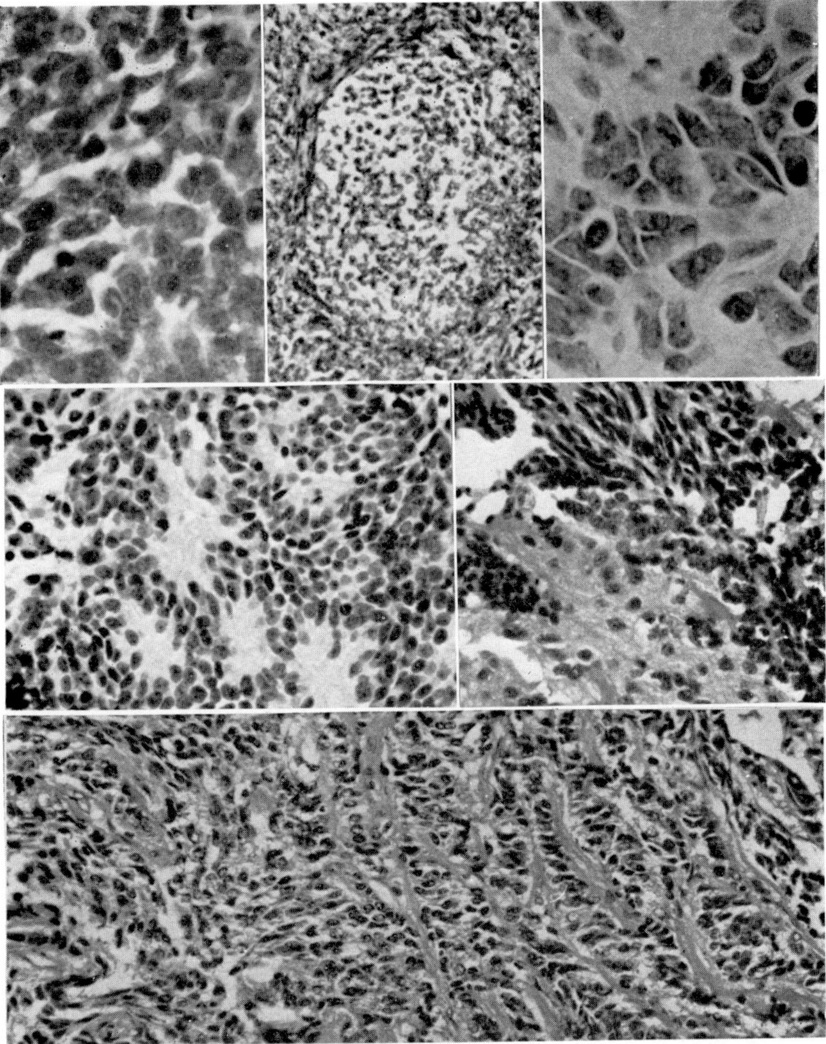

Figure 13.7. MEDULLOBLASTOMA; (*a*) typical dense cellularity, no differentiation and scanty cytoplasm (H & E. × 520); (*b*) areas of astrocytic differentiation (centre) are common (× 130); (*c*) pseudo-rosette formation; when pronounced this closely resembles ependymoma (× 520); (*d*) distinct rosette formation (× 130); (*e*) astrocytic area (below) in otherwise densely cellular medulloblastoma (× 130); (*f*) infiltration of meningeal layers provokes a dense stromal reaction which may lead to a misdiagnosis of meningeal sarcoma (H & E. × 130).

[(*a*) *Top left*. (*b*) *Top centre*. (*c*) *Top right*. (*d*) *Centre left*. (*e*) *Centre right*. (*f*) *Bottom*.]

SPREAD

Spread within the CSF is a special feature of medulloblastomas and may be observed at the primary operation as nodules or plaques of creamy tissue on the surface of the cerebellum. Metastases in the spinal theca are common, producing compression of the spinal cord and paraplegia. In rare instances this is the mode of presentation.

CLINICAL FEATURES

The duration of symptoms before admission to hospital is short in this group; in 19% it was less than one month, and in 54% less than three months; the younger the child the shorter the history.

Headache (61%) and *vomiting* (82%) were the commonest presenting symptoms. Because of the higher proportion of the very young children, headache is statistically less prominent because of the easier expansion of the skull, and because infants cannot communicate their symptoms.

Ataxia of the trunkal type (55%) was frequently observed; an unsteady gait was followed by inability to stand or walk alone, then by inability to sit unsupported, and finally inability to hold the head up. In spite of these profound changes, co-ordination of hand movement is often well maintained until the later stages when a tremor may be seen, and at that stage perhaps unsteady and clumsy hand movements.

Change in personality (45%) was almost always seen at some stage. Most were good-looking, well-nourished attractive children, but with a wan facial appearance, as if forewarned of their fate (Fig. 13.8). Later, some degree of mental dullness, irritability and emaciation appeared.

Squint and double vision (37%) occurred when the tumour filled the fourth ventricle.

Neck stiffness and head tilting (22%) were seen at a later stage and correlated with extension out of the fourth ventricle downwards below the cervico-medullary junction. Occasionally neck stiffness simulated a chronic form of meningitis, e.g. tuberculous meningitis. Tumour cells were often found free in the CSF in these children, and care is necessary in interpreting the cellular reaction in the CSF.

Papilloedema (72%) was found fairly constantly in the older children, but might not be seen early in the infants when the head could enlarge readily. Some presented as hydrocephalus. The percussion note of the skull was almost always raised. This 'boxy', high-pitched note on percussion of the skull is one of the simplest and reliable indices of raised intracranial pressure, but is still one of the least frequently recorded.

Ataxia of gait (63%) was seen twice as frequently as incoordination of hand movement (34%) and nystagmus (34%). This finding is an indication of the predominant involvement of the midline structures of the cerebellum.

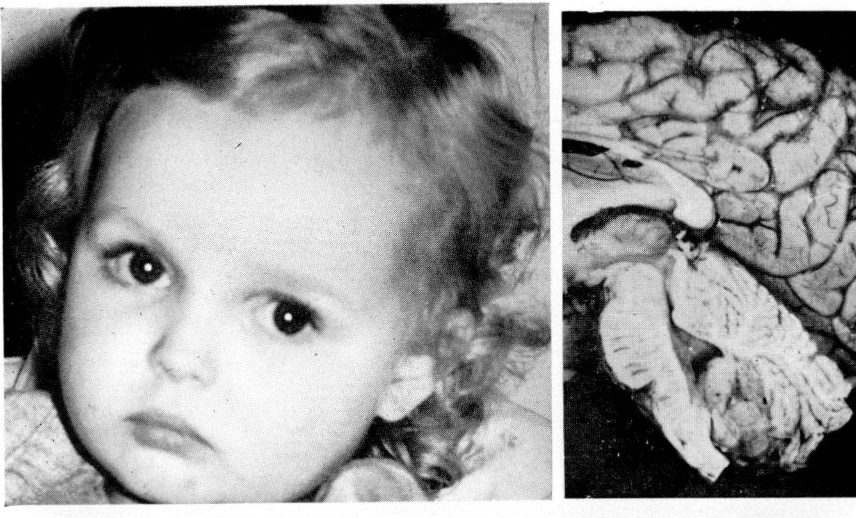

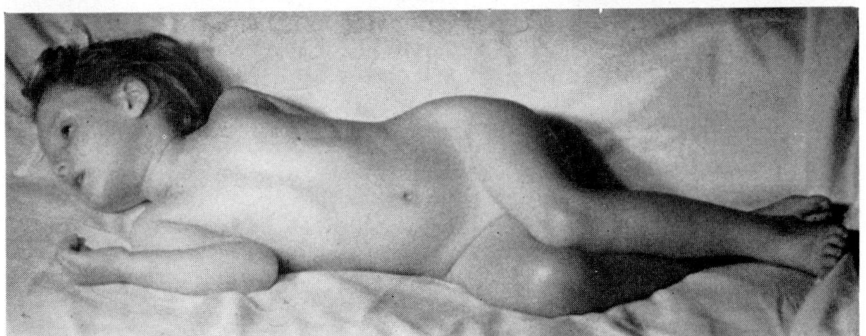

Figure 13.8. MEDULLOBLASTOMA; (*a*) a wan little girl with sad eyes and a tilted head; (*b*) sagittal section of a tumour arising in the vermis, partly filling the fourth ventricle and causing mild hydrocephalus; (*c*) a typical position adopted, with neck stiffness, opisthotonus and semicoma caused by a tumour with seeding of metastases in the CSF pathways.

[(*a*) *Top left*. (*b*) *Top right*. (*c*) *Bottom*.]

Internal strabismus (CN. VI) (32%), may be due to direct pressure on the sixth nerve nucleus or to ventricular obstruction.

DIAGNOSIS

The value of an ophthalmoscope cannot be over-emphasized; in more than 75% of patients with this tumour papilloedema is severe and easily recognizable.

INVESTIGATIONS

At the initial presentation, separation of the sutures is seen in the skull radiographs in 50%. Lumbar puncture is unwarranted and dangerous, as it may induce coning (p. 237).

Tumour cells are often found in the CSF at operation. Scanning (p. 75) is not as easily performed in these younger children, and a negative result is usually obtained.

Angiography has not been used routinely, but a well-defined tumour circulation has been observed on only one occasion.

Ventricular contrast studies are definitive tests in this tumour, and except in the earlier cases Myodil® has been most frequently used. Instillation and radiography are carried out in the operating theatre immediately prior to operation. The use of the neurosurgical wheel (Fig. 13.9), which by allowing this

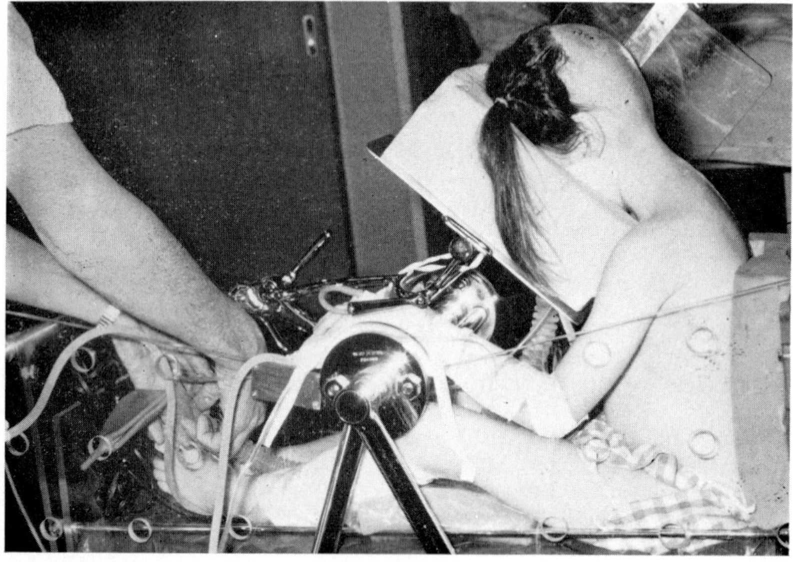

Figure 13.9. NEUROSURGICAL WHEEL; the hemispherical cradle can be rotated around a central axis to obtain any required position, from vertical to horizontal with the face downwards.

investigation and the subsequent operation to be carried out without changing the position of the patient, has made it possible to perform a much more extensive removal, with less morbidity and negligible operative mortality.

Operative treatment and results are described on p. 259.

III. EPENDYMOMAS OF THE FOURTH VENTRICLE

AGE : SEX

This tumour is similar in many ways to the medulloblastoma. There is a slight male predominance (58 %), and the younger age groups are predominantly affected; the peak incidence is in the second year of life, and 60 % occur in the first five years.

Most if not all ependymomas in children run a malignant course. Even the subependymal type belies its frequent bland histological appearance by behaving in a malignant fashion. In childhood, ependymomas appear to be true embryonal tumours, sharing their site, macroscopic appearance and high cellularity with the medulloblastomas, from which they may be difficult to distinguish histologically. It is noteworthy that three babies in the Index Series showed evidence of this tumour at birth.

MICROSCOPIC FINDINGS

A particular feature of ependymomas is their tendency to differentiation which may take two forms:

(*a*) The formation of ependymal spaces,
(*b*) The formation of perivascular pseudorosettes.

(*a*) *Ependymal spaces* appear as small clefts lined by a single layer of tumour cells (Fig. 13.10) which may be ciliated and contain blepharoplasts (cytoplasmic organelles concerned with ciliary motility, demonstrable at the luminal border of the cell by PTAH stain), and the lumen may contain proteinaceous fluid. This tubular form of differentiation appears to be a simulation of the normal canal forming function of the ependymal cell.

(*b*) *Perivascular pseudorosettes*, also described as glio-vascular systems, are dense collections of ependymal cells around a vessel, separated from it by a nuclear-free zone. Under low power magnification this has a characteristic patchy appearance with Zülch (1971) likened to a 'leopard skin' (Fig. 13.10a).

Ependymoma cells have an oval nucleus with dense chromatin and a sharp nuclear membrane. Cytoplasm is variable (Fig. 13.10) and may be either scanty or quite prominent. Poorly differentiated tumours have large nuclei and appear fleshy and epithelial; tumours with glial differentiation have more compact nuclei, and elongated polar cytoplasm.

Other features are glycogen in the cytoplasm of tumour cells related to ependymal clefts or to pseudorosettes, and affinity for acid phosphatase activity. In the Index Series ependymomas showed strong acid phosphatase activity, particularly around ependymal spaces, in contrast to medulloblastomas which were PAS negative (containing no glycogen) and showed a weak or negative acid phosphatase reaction.

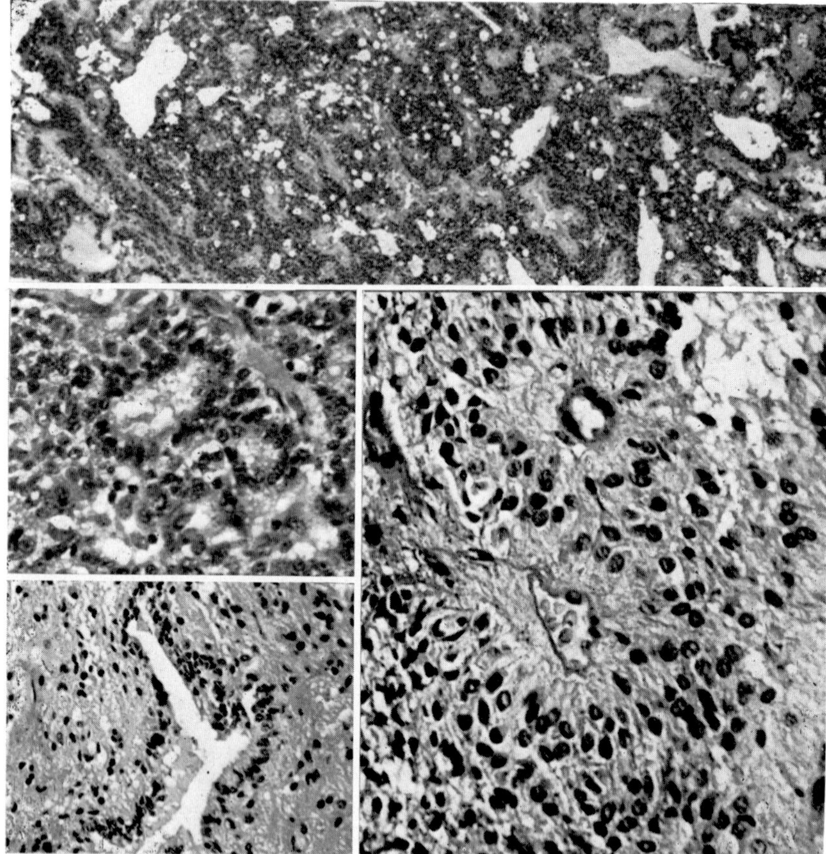

Figure 13.10. MALIGNANT EPENDYMOMA; (*a*) 'leopard-skin' pattern due to sparing of perivascular tissue surrounded by tumour cells (H & E. × 30). (*b*) (*b*) tubule formation in the tumour illustrated in (*a*) (H & E. × 260); (*c*) gliovascular systems centred on blood vessels (H & E. × 300); (*d*) ependymal spaces forming in a predominantly astrocytic area (H & E. × 100).

[(*a*) *Top.* (*b*) *Centre left.* (*c*) *Right.* (*d*) *Bottom left.*]

Ependymomas often assume a papillary form, especially when they project into a ventricle and may be confused with papillomas of the choroid plexus. However, the latter always have a collagenous core, whereas the papillae of an ependymoma form on stalks of glial tissue.

The cellularity of ependymomas varies greatly and some of the very cellular examples have been referred to as ependymoblastomas (Rubinstein, 1973).

'Subependymoma' type

This term, introduced by Scheinker (1945) to describe a particular type of tumour previously classified as an astrocytoma, is applied to those with very cellular areas containing glio-vascular systems. Glial differentiation is the chief feature, and may make up the bulk of the tumour. In some of the more cellular variants, contrasting areas of sparse cellularity and stromal oedema, described as areas of 'impoverishment' by Zülch (1971), and thought to be the result of partial ischaemia, may be seen. Hyperplasia of the endothelial lining of vessels occurs in about 20% of these tumours, and may be the cause of this appearance.

Myxopapillary ependymomas

These are rare variants usually found in the filum terminale region of the spinal cord. They consist of ependymal tubules in a myxomatous ground substance, are usually very slow growing and very rare in childhood.

CLINICAL FEATURES

The history is short, less than three months in 65%, and in general, those with a history of less than one month rarely survive for more than a year. The initial symptoms and signs are similar to those seen with the medulloblastoma (p. 248). Vomiting (85%), a clumsy gait (67%) and headache (61%) were frequent complaints. The parents noted a change in the child's personality at an early stage in 45%.

The clinical signs first observed were papilloedema (85%), ataxia (70%), and incoordination in the hands (42%). An unusual finding was the high incidence of pyramidal signs (49%) which could not be fully accounted for by the tendency of the tumour to invade structures in the floor of the fourth ventricle (Houtteville, 1970).

There is no satisfactory way of distinguishing this tumour from medulloblastoma before operation, and even the appearance at operation is very similar.

PROGNOSIS

The survival rate is poor; of the 38 patients in whom follow-up is complete, only five survive. The histological characteristics appear to have little influence on survival; of those classified as 'malignant ependymoma', five survived an average period of 4–5 months, while fifteen survived an average period of six months. In the smaller group classified as ependymoma, five children with an average age of 6·5 years survived an average period of 40 months, while eight children with an average age of 3·5 years survived 10 months. The two oldest children are still surviving (200 and 80 months). Once more there are few guidelines to indicate the prognosis (Fig. 13.12).

Thus although the tumours can be graded in order of malignancy, in each group there are few factors from which one can predict survival. Comparison with results from other centres is difficult because of the variations in histological diagnosis.

IV. GLIOMA OF THE BRAIN STEM

This tumour differs markedly from others arising in the posterior fossa because it produces obvious and often severe neurologic signs before there is a general rise in intracranial pressure.

AGE : SEX

The tumour occurs more frequently in the younger child; more than half were found in the 0–5-year age group and the average age was 5 years. The sexes were equally affected.

MACROSCOPIC APPEARANCES

There is usually uniform expansion of the brain stem (Fig. 13.11), but localized asymmetrical distortion sometimes occurs; on occasions a tumour producing uniform expansion of the pons may develop an area which grows more rapidly and asymmetrically. The tumour may produce 'cauliflower' nodulation on the external surface of the brain stem.

Eventually, the tumour involves the whole of the brain stem, often spreading upwards to involve the basal ganglia and downwards into the upper spinal cord.

MICROSCOPIC FINDINGS

The situation of the tumour tends to preclude biopsy during life, but a firm diagnosis can usually be made on the clinical features, contrast studies and a nucleide scan (p. 75). Material from little more than half of our patients is available for histological studies, and this was mainly obtained in the terminal stages.

At one end of the spectrum are the low grade astrocytomas composed of mature astrocytes with abundant astroglial fibres, which infiltrate diffusely through the brain stem, separating but not destroying neurons.

In some 65% the pattern of the tumour is the fibrillary type of astrocytoma (p. 241) with pronounced glial fibres but with plump and obviously neoplastic astrocytes which may show nuclear anaplasia and mitotic activity. In approxi-

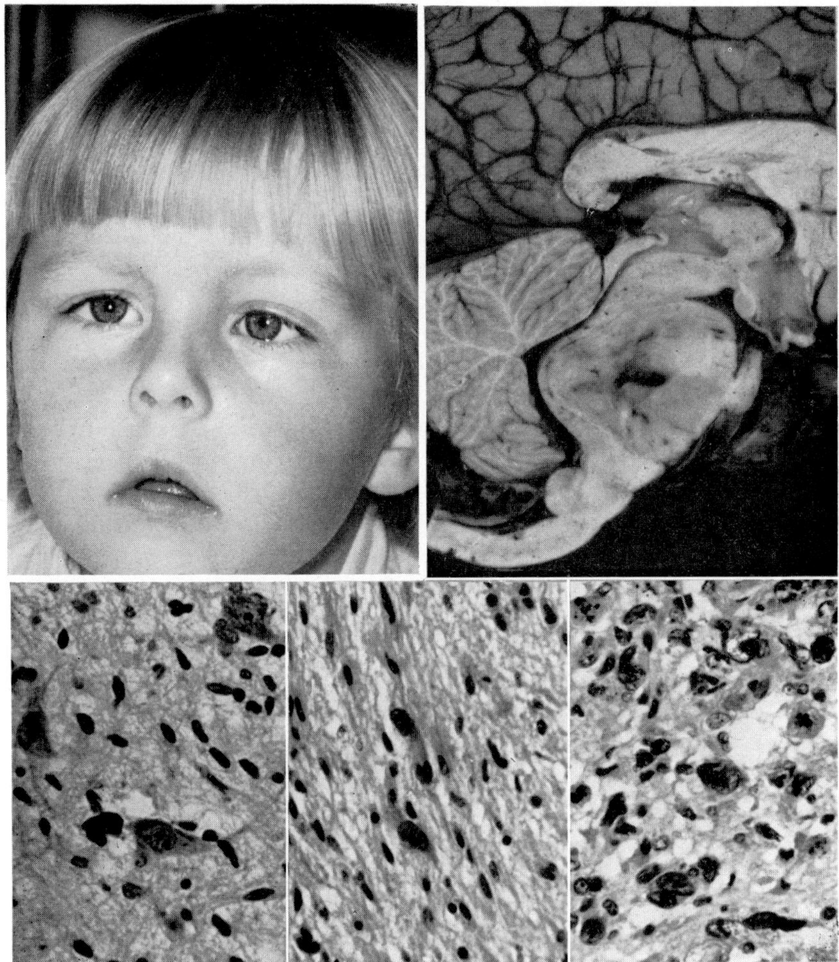

Figure 13.11. GLIOMA OF THE BRAIN STEM; (*a*) appearance at presentation, with strabismus, facial weakness and wan expression; (*b*) sagittal section of a glioma expanding and partially replacing the pons. This example is more clearly demarcated than usual, and contains areas of haemorrhage and necrosis; (*c*) (*d*) and (*e*) illustrate three grades (all H & E. × 300); (*c*) diffuse gliomatosis, infiltration by well differentiated astrocytes surrounding but not destroying neurones; (*d*) a more malignant tumour with nuclear anaplasia and marked production of glial fibres; (*e*) a highly malignant, anaplastic pleomorphic glioma.

[(*a*) *Top left.* (*b*) *Top right.* (*c*) *Bottom left.* (*d*) *Bottom centre.* (*e*) *Bottom right.*]

mately 20% of cases the histology is that of a malignant astrocytoma which may be histologically identical with glioblastoma multiforme (p. 277), or slightly less anaplastic and corresponding to a Grade III astrocytoma.

In two cases in the Index Series the tumour was thought to be a glioma of the brain stem, but proved to be a malignant ependymoma in the floor of the fourth ventricle, with diffuse spread into the brain stem.

MODES OF PRESENTATION

The duration of symptoms and signs is short, and usually less than two months. Excluding two patients whose admission was so long delayed that they were moribund, the duration of manifestations was longest in the younger age groups, 2·5 months in those in the first quinquennium and 1·7 months and 1·5 months for the second and third quinquennia. In 20% of the Index Series, symptoms had been present for less than two weeks before admission, and in 35% less than four weeks.

The neurological signs depend upon the level at which the tumour arises; ocular palsies occur in high lesions, facial and sixth nerve palsies at the pontine level, and difficulties in swallowing and speech in the lower lesions.

The cerebellar pathways are always affected causing ataxia, incoordination and nystagmus. The pyramidal tracts are involved early in about 30%, causing weakness in the limbs or frank hemiplegia. Papilloedema is uncommon and usually late.

In the Index Series, the first manifestation was most frequently ataxia and incoordination (25%); squint or a complaint of double vision was found first in 17·5%; change in personality antedated all other signs in 15%, and headache was the initial complaint in the same proportion. Facial weakness and hemiparesis were infrequent first signs (6%), but were common in the fully-developed clinical picture.

DIAGNOSIS

In a high proportion of the children the diagnosis can be made on the history obtained and the signs elicited at the first clinical examination.

The woebegone expression is the result of bilateral facial weakness, which flattens emotional expression (Fig. 13.11a). There is an internal squint, and saliva dribbles from the corner of a partially paralysed mouth because swallowing is infrequent and the face weak. Movements are clumsy and weak, and the gait is staggering.

In the final stages swallowing is impossible and urinary retention is common. Death is usually due to aspiration of food or fluid, producing terminal bronchopneumonia; urinary infection is often superimposed.

The downhill course is often rapid, but can be halted by radiotherapy, and return to normal function is often achieved, but in the smaller child relapse and rapid decline occurs within twelve months. In older children, long survivals can be achieved by radiotherapy (Fig. 13.12).

Diagnosis is most effectively confirmed by pneumo-encephalography which demonstrates posterior displacement of the aqueduct and fourth ventricle by the expanded brain stem. Myodil introduced into the lateral ventricle was used in a small number of patients.

V. MISCELLANEOUS TUMOURS

1. Intracranial dermoid cysts

A dermoid cyst in the posterior fossa is usually but not always connected to the scalp by an epithelial track. The cyst contains sebaceous material and hair, some of which may protrude through an external sinus in the occipital region. The internal part of this anomaly may lie at any level, just beneath the dura, in the cerebellum, in the fourth ventricle or in the cisterna magna.

The communication with the exterior allows the entry of infection, causing attacks of meningitis or a cerebellar abscess. If the external sinus and the small rounded defect in the occipital bone are not identified, repeated infections and even death may occur.

The cyst and the sinus can be simply excised, but when complicated by infection, the morbidity and mortality are predictably somewhat increased.

2. Haemangioblastoma of the cerebellum

This tumour is almost confined to the cerebellum, but occasionally arises in the spinal cord in childhood.

Microscopically it has a very characteristic structure, being essentially a capillary haemangioma, composed of tight curlicues of cells surrounding tiny vascular lumina. A delicate network of cells like astrocytes mingles with the endothelial cells of the capillaries. Sometimes there are foamy stromal cells containing neutral fat and these may dominate the histological picture. Their origin is uncertain (Jeffreys, 1975).

Haemangioblastomas have a very organoid structure, and, in spite of occasional mitotic figures, appear to be benign, indeed, they may be basically hamartomas rather than true tumours. This tumour of the cerebellum may be one of the manifestations of the von Hippel-Lindau syndrome (p. 832), but it appears that only between 10 and 20% of affected children have this syndrome, the remaining cases being sporadic. There may occasionally be difficulty in distinguishing a haemangioblastoma from an angioblastic meningioma, but the site of the tumour, in the cerebellum, is very characteristic.

This tumour is often associated with a cyst, and the clinical picture is then similar to that of a cystic astrocytoma. The lesion is usually on the postero-lateral surface of the cerebellum, and its distinguishing feature is the abnormally brisk uptake of radionucleides on scanning (p. 75). In spite of their tremendous blood supply, removal is usually possible and the end results are excellent.

HISTOLOGICAL DIFFERENTIATION OF TUMOURS OF THE POSTERIOR FOSSA AND BRAIN STEM

The common entities have been described above, but there are several rare tumours which enter the differential diagnosis in biopsy material. These are:

1. Medullo-epithelioma;
2. Neuroblastoma;
3. Ganglioglioma;
4. Cerebellar sarcoma;

1. *Medullo-epitheliomas* are rare and rapidly growing tumours, usually in the posterior fossa although some have been recorded in the cerebral hemispheres (Fowler, 1968).

Macroscopically they resemble medulloblastomas. Microscopically, as originally described by Bailey and Cushing, their structure mimics the primitive developing medullary plate and neural tube, and there is a papillary arrangement with occasional tubules lined by tall columnar cells with large, oval, vesicular nuclei, separated by a loose vascular stroma containing undifferentiated cells. Mitoses are numerous and the tumour grows rapidly. There is no case in the Index Series.

2. *Neuroblastoma* very occasionally arises in the posterior fossa although some dispute its existence in this site.

Macroscopically these tumours, too, are similar to medulloblastomas. Microscopically, however, they have the 'scattered wheat' appearance typical of neuroblastomas with neuroglial differentiation and sometimes rosette formation. The chief distinguishing feature of a neuroblastoma is the presence of reticulin between the tumour cells, and absent from medulloblastomas, but their differentiation can be extremely difficult.

In the Index Series one tumour was classified as a neuroblastoma of the cerebellum. The tumour occurred in a three-year old child, and was treated by excision followed by chemotherapy and radiotherapy as for neuroblastoma (p. 558). The patient is alive and free of symptoms four years later.

3. *Gangliogliomas* are extremely rare tumours which, in our experience, are commoner in the spinal cord than in the cerebellum. They are essentially hamartomatous lesions composed of a mixed astrocytic cells and neurones.

4. *Cerebellar sarcomas* are very rare tumours, usually in young children or infants, arising near the surface of the cerebellum, presumably from meningial tissues. They are composed of small dark cells with scanty cytoplasm, and although they characteristically produce reticulin, undifferentiated examples may show little or none, in which case they may be difficult or impossible to

distinguish from medulloblastomas. We believe that most of the tumours reported as cerebellar sarcomas are medulloblastomas which have evoked a pronounced stromal reaction by the invaded meningial coverings of the brain; the distinction is mainly of academic interest since they behave in much the same way as medulloblastomas. There is no example in the Index Series.

MANAGEMENT OF CHILDREN WITH A TUMOUR IN THE POSTERIOR FOSSA

Severe papilloedema indicating a high intracranial pressure is usually present and lumbar puncture should *not* be performed because of the risk of medullary coning (p. 237) leading to respiratory arrest.

Investigations

Investigations should be arranged without delay and are usually performed in the following order:

Radiographs of the skull to show separation of the sutures.

A brain scan (p. 75) using radionucleides can be readily performed in older children with a fair degree of accuracy.

Vertebrobasilar arteriography can be helpful, but is only required in a few patients, e.g. when there is an intense uptake in the scan suggestive of a haemangioblastoma.

Ventriculography; air of Myodil® is usually used, but gliomas of the brain stem can be demonstrated most clearly by pneumo-encephalography.

Treatment

Surgical excision is indicated for all cerebellar tumours, but rarely for brain stem tumours, usually only those causing obstruction of the CSF pathways. When this occurs relief of the high intracranial pressure is the first priority; a ventriculo-atrial shunt is performed, and investigation and the definitive operation can then be carried out two to three days later. In an acute crisis, one of the lateral ventricles can be drained externally for 48 to 72 hours by a fine catheter.

Surgery

The posterior fossa is exposed by a suboccipital incision, and bone is removed down to the foramen magnum. Most cerebellar tumours can be readily identified from the surface and removal proceeds. Experience has shown that complete extirpation has a lower morbidity and mortality than incomplete removal, but part of the tumour infiltrating the brain stem may have to be left behind.

The only serious complication after operation is gastro-intestinal haemorrhage (haematemesis or melaena), caused by neurogenic peptic ulceration (Cushing, 1932). This is uncommon and usually occurs in a sick child in whom complete removal of the tumour has not been possible. Energetic management including laparotomy and operative haemostasis has been successful in almost all cases (Lewis, 1973).

Chemotherapy

In two types of tumour, medulloblastoma and ependymoma, cytotoxic agents have been given after operation. The period of survival may be lengthened, but the overall mortality appears to be unchanged.

Radiotherapy

This is usually commenced some three weeks after operation, and because of the tendency of medulloblastomas and ependymomas to metastasise in the CSF pathway, the whole of the CNS is irradiated, i.e. the cranium and the spinal canal down to the mid-sacral segment.

In the other types of tumour, irradiation to a total dose of 4500 rads is confined to the posterior fossa. Radiation is not necessary in fibrillary astrocytomas or in haemangioblastomas when complete removal has been effected.

PROGNOSIS

Children with an astrocytoma have the best prognosis; 43 out of 66 children (65 %) are alive and well after follow-up averaging 8 years. In the 23 who died, the average length of survival was 4·7 years (Fig. 13.12a).

The prognosis for medulloblastomas or ependymomas has been variously reported and, in general, survival after surgery alone is unlikely to exceed 6 months; after surgery and irradiation the average survival is about 24 months but there are occasional long term survivors (Fig. 13.12b, c).

In gliomas of the brain stem the prognosis depends largely on the age at the time of diagnosis and is better in older children. In this group there are four children with an average age of 11 years who have survived for more than 5 years. Twenty-five children (an average of 7 years) survived for only 4·5 months (Fig. 13.12d).

B. TUMOURS IN THE REGION OF THE THIRD VENTRICLE

This is a convenient category for a variety of tumours (Table 13.3; Fig. 13.13) which may be briefly classified as:

I. Tumours of the optic nerve and chiasm
II. Craniopharyngiomas

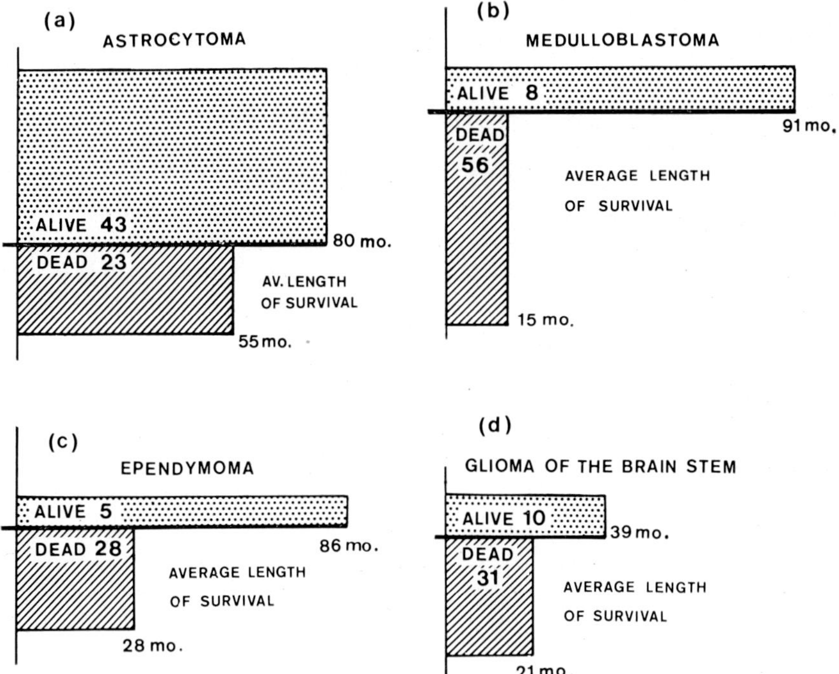

Figure 13.12. PROGNOSIS IN TUMOURS OF THE POSTERIOR FOSSA, as indicated by results. Histograms of the four common tumours illustrating individual patterns of length of survival: (*a*) astrocytomas, (*b*) medulloblastomas, (*c*) ependymomas and (*d*) gliomas of the brain stem.

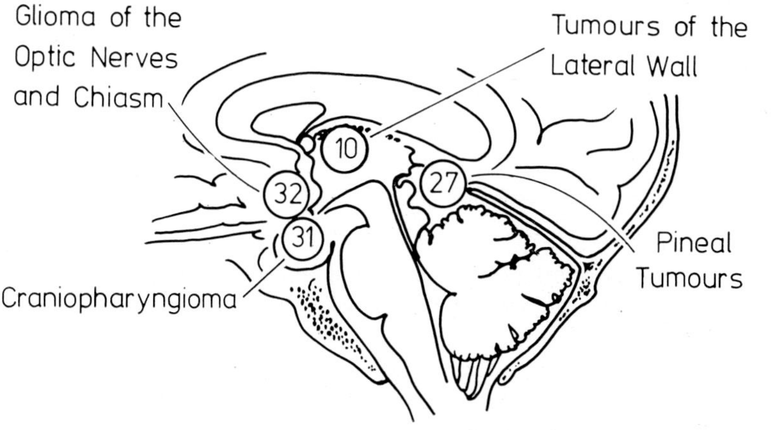

Figure 13.13. TUMOURS OF THE THIRD VENTRICLE. The distribution and relative incidence (expressed as percentages) of the main groups of tumours arising in the region of the third ventricle.

III. Pineal tumours

IV. Tumours of the wall and the floor of the third ventricle

For the most part these tumours have insidious effects with little of localizing value in the early stages; later they may evoke the 'midline syndrome' already described (p. 233).

The obstruction to the flow of CSF by the expansion of the tumour into the third ventricle produces headache, vomiting and changes in the level of consciousness. Children are often brought for examination at this stage and severe deterioration of vision due to defects in visual fields and papilloedema or optic atrophy may be found. Localizing signs are often present when the patient is first seen, but they are not always recognized.

Table 13.3. Tumours of the third ventricle. Relative incidence in four reported series (see legend for Table 13.1)

Total	Boston (125) %	Vienna 154 %	Tokyo (120) %	Melbourne 92 %
Optic glioma	21	10	—	32
Craniopharyngioma	40	30	70	31
Pineal tumour	1	19	29	27

I. TUMOURS OF THE OPTIC NERVES AND OPTIC CHIASM

This group represents 5% of all intracranial tumours in the Index Series, a higher proportion than in others published, e.g. Matson reported only 27 in 750 children (0·36%). The disparity is probably related to the high proportion of children with von Recklinghausen's disease (neurofibromatosis) in this series; 13 of the 24 children in the Index Series had obvious *café-au-lait* patches.

PATHOLOGY

Most of these tumours are benign and it has been estimated that 25% or more may undergo spontaneous arrest of growth. Some authors claim that most if not all will eventually cease growing, and that they are not true tumours but hamartomas of the optic nerve sheath. Certainly the histology of some of the examples in the Index Series shows a very low grade of activity, but in the same series there are seven children in whom the tumour extended beyond the nerve and the chiasm, to infiltrate the base of the brain and cause death by invading vital centres.

Involvement of one optic nerve by a glioma is less common than involvement of one nerve and the chiasm, or of both optic nerves. (Fig. 13.14).

MACROSCOPIC APPEARANCE

At operation there is diffuse enlargement of the nerve and/or the chiasm, less commonly a focal fusiform swelling along the course of one nerve. The pathologist occasionally receives a segment of the nerve containing tumour (Fig. 15.10c).

CLINICO-PATHOLOGICAL TYPES

There are several different patterns.

1. *A spindle-shaped swelling* limited to the intraorbital portion of one optic nerve (Fig. 13.14a) but nevertheless expanding the optic canal; four children presented in this way. A squint or proptosis, due to expansion and lengthening of the intraorbital segment of the optic nerve, develops before the child complains of loss of vision. Visual deterioration is usually noted only a week or two before admission to hospital.
2. *A dumbbell-shaped tumour* of the optic nerve (Fig. 13.14b); the constriction corresponds to the optic canal which may be two or three times the normal size on radiography. This type is also unilateral and in the young child loss of vision is well advanced at the time of presentation.
3. *Glial proliferation* in the tumour involves both optic nerves and the optic chiasm (Fig. 13.14c). These structures become rounded and enlarged, and the optic nerves are constricted at the optic foramina. Vision is grossly reduced, but in young children this is not readily apparent until a late stage. Lack of macular fixation may lead to nystagmus, a prelude to severe visual failure.
4. *More extensive involvement of the optic chiasm*, with spread into adjacent structures (Fig. 13.14d). In infancy, involvement of the hypothalamus may cause the 'diencephalic syndrome' (p. 267), i.e. failure to thrive, wasting and anorexia, together with regression in motor development. The child is thin, the skin wrinkled, and the eyes prominent.

   Alternatively involvement of the hypothalamus may produce precocious skeletal and sexual maturation, seen in 50% of older children with this tumour. Sometimes those presenting with the diencephalic syndrome in infancy go on to develop precocious puberty later.
5. *The 'midline syndrome'* (p. 233) may be the first manifestation when the effects of the tumour are so insidious that the first obvious manifestations are those of obstruction of the third ventricle at the level of the foramina of Munro (Fig. 13.14e). Four children were first found to have an optic glioma during investigation for hydrocephalus.

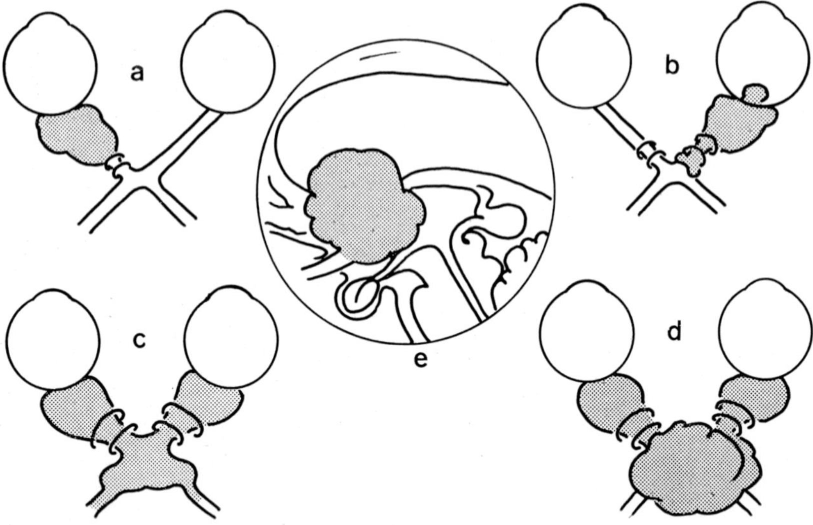

Figure 13.14. GLIOMAS OF THE OPTIC NERVE, a diagram of the various types which occur, (*a*) confined to the nerve in the orbit; (*b*) extending into the globe and proximally to the chiasm; (*c*) diffuse involvement of both optic nerves and the chiasm; (*d*) further extension of tumour tissue arising from the major mass around the chiasm and extending into the adjacent cerebral substance, or (*e*) obstructing the third ventricle.

MICROSCOPIC FINDINGS

The tumour is composed of astrocytes (Fig. 13.15) associated with plentiful glial fibres and foci of calcification are not uncommon. Sometimes the pattern is loose in texture with microcystic change similar to that found in cerebellar astrocytomas (p. 244). The astrocytes are usually well differentiated but in some tumours there is slight nuclear anaplasia. Reactive hyperplasia of epineural cells, which closely resemble fibroblasts, is a common finding adjacent to the tumour, and can be mistaken for tumour. This is of particular importance in determining whether excision of an intra-orbital tumour has been adequate.

There is a characteristic pattern to the tumour and although the cells are obviously astrocytes, there are areas which may mimic a meningioma or even a schwannoma. The former may present some difficulty in histological diagnosis, for a meningioma may arise from the optic nerve sheath and produces a clinical picture very similar to a glioma of the optic nerve. There were only two such meningiomas in the Index Series; one arose in a girl of 12 years and the other in a girl of 15 years; both contained plump fibroblastic cells with prominent psammoma bodies (Fig. 13.16). In a third example, originally classified as a meningioma, the bulk of the biopsy showed

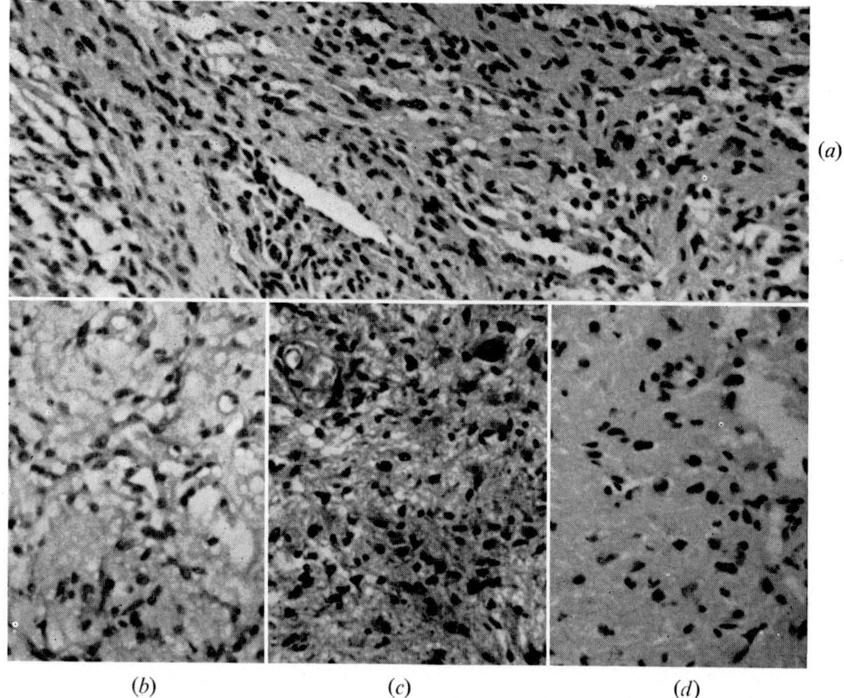

Figure 13.15. GLIOMA OF THE OPTIC NERVE; (*a*) a moderately cellular tumour with marked production of glial fibres and an interlacing 'sheath' pattern, with some microcystic changes. Other patterns encountered are (*b*): that of a juvenile astrocytoma, also with microcystic changes; (*c*) a recurrence of the tumour in (*b*) showing increased cellularity and slight nuclear polymorphism; (*d*): the pattern of a low grade astrocytoma; in spite of the benign appearance this tumour recurred locally and invaded the brain causing death.

areas containing astrocytes, but in other fields there were masses of plump rounded cells with a whorled pattern suggestive of meningioma; no psammoma bodies were present, and the diagnosis of glioma was made.

MODES OF PRESENTATION

1. *Proptosis* is the first presenting sign when there is involvement of the optic nerve alone (Fig. 13.17). The globe is displaced forwards and later downwards and outwards.
2. *Loss of vision* is severe and as a rule only recently discovered. Fundoscopy reveals a pale optic disc and sometimes glial tissue can be seen presenting at the nerve head. The visual fields show bizarre defects which are often markedly different in the two eyes.
3. *Strabismus* often occurs early (Fig. 13.17a). A rotatory type of nystagmus is sometimes seen in the infant when there is loss of central vision.

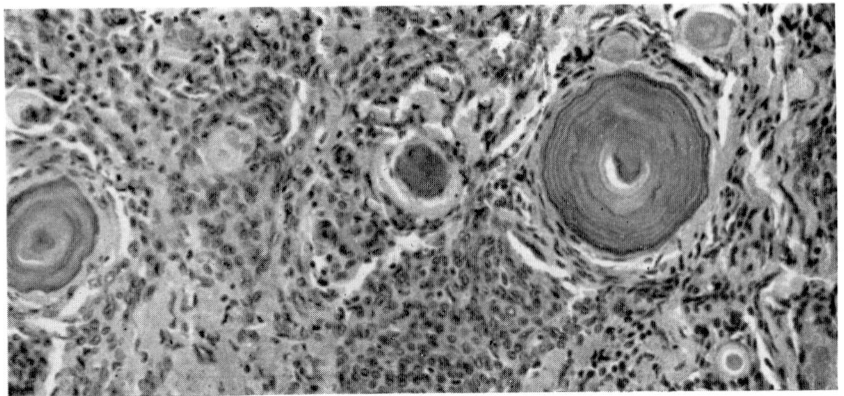

Figure 13.16. MENINGIOMA OF THE OPTIC NERVE; plump meningioma cells, set in a sparsely cellular stroma as characteristic as the accompanying psammoma bodies (H & E. × 130).

4. *Constitutional manifestations* (e.g. the diencephalic syndrome, loss of weight and delayed skeletal growth) are common when the condition develops in a young child (Fig. 13.17b). Precocious growth and skeletal development may occur at a later stage. Diabetes insipidus was the first symptom in two patients.
5. *Câfé-au-lait patches*, manifestation of von Recklinghausen's disease, were seen in more than half of these patients, so frequently that a complete examination of the skin is an important part of the examination.

DIAGNOSIS

Investigation of the clinical features by radiography of the optic foramina will show enlargement of foramina, and often a 'J' or pear-shaped sella. Pneumo-encephalography will define masses in the region of the chiasma and often suggestive but less definitive expansion of the optic nerves. A brain scan (p. 75) may indicate tumour masses in the sella region.

TREATMENT

A glioma confined to one optic nerve can usually be excised, sparing the globe in front and the chiasm behind. Exposure can be obtained by a frontal osteoplastic flap and transfrontal removal of the orbital roof in order to display the whole field in a one-stage procedure. Four children submitted to this operation are well and show no evidence of extension of the disease.

When the chiasm and both nerves are involved, resection is not possible. Strangulation of the nerve occurs as it lies in the optic canal, but vision can

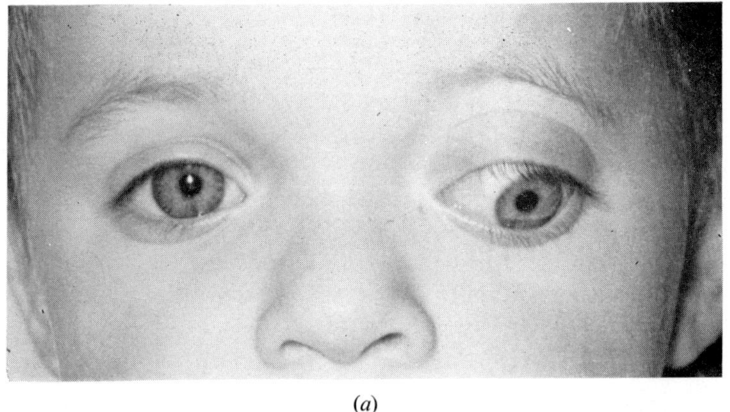

(*a*)

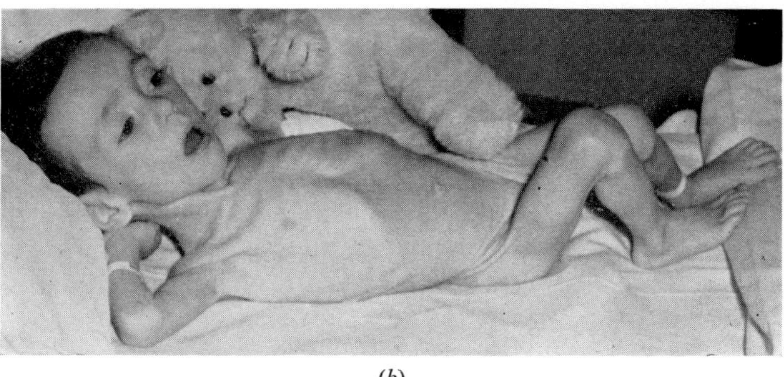

(*b*)

Figure 13.17. Glioma of the optic nerve; (*a*) presenting with proptosis and strabismus; (*b*) chiasmal glioma causing the 'diencephalic syndrome' of marasmus, hypotonia and apathy.

be preserved and sometimes improved, for some months or even years, by decompressing the nerve, removing the roof of the optic canal via a transfrontal approach.

In the Index Series, 8 of the 21 patients with bilateral involvement had a decompression operation. Local complete excision of chiasmal lesions as advocated by Matson (1969), has not been feasible in this series.

II. CRANIOPHARYNGIOMA

These accounted for 5% of intracranial tumours in the Index Series; a higher figure is quoted in some series (Matson 9%, Koos 8·2%), but these probably reflect a special interest which attracts such patients. A craniopharyngioma is technically one of the most difficult of all tumours and

Cushing described them as 'the most baffling problem which confronts the neurosurgeon'. Great changes have taken place in the past 15 years, and the outlook is no longer as gloomy as it was (Banna *et al.*, 1973). Complete excision is now often possible and followed by a near-normal development. The factors responsible for this change are considered under treatment (p. 271).

The tumour was erroneously termed craniopharyngioma by Cushing, and in spite of more accurate terminology suggested since, the term is now accepted. It has always been considered to arise from remnants of Rathke's pouch—a diverticulum of the primitive stomodaeum—and is found within or above the sella, or rarely within the third ventricle.

MACROSCOPIC APPEARANCES

The tumour usually contains both solid and cystic areas; the solid areas are firm, pale and sometimes gritty with calcification. The cystic areas are filled with straw-coloured, green or brown fluid, which characteristically has a shimmering appearance due to the cholesterol crystals it contains. Calcification in the tumour is present in more than 50%, usually in friable masses, but in two children it was a dense, hard mass, and in one, material resembling coral surrounded the optic nerves and internal carotid arteries.

The tumour extends progressively, usually upwards and backwards, to involve the optic chiasm and the third ventricle, and finally causes complete obstruction of the CSF pathway.

Extension into the pituitary fossa is common; the gland is compressed and later replaced.

Extension into the posterior fossa and beyond is said to be rare, but three children in the Index Series had large extensions in this direction; in one it reached the mid-cervical portion of the spinal canal!

MICROSCOPIC APPEARANCES

Many examples consist of dense fibrous and glial tissue surrounding clefts containing dissolved lipid, giant cells and small masses of keratin. The degenerative and reactive changes are due to the presence of keratin; 'younger' tumours usually have areas resembling the pattern of an adamantinoma, with or without squamous epithelial nests. Cords of columnar epithelial cells surround small cystic spaces containing protein-rich fluid, and blend on their deep aspect with a stroma of stellate or spindle-shaped cells set in loose myxoid ground substance. Clusters of foamy macrophages filled with lipid are common in the stroma. Islands of epithelium become surrounded by reactive gliosis and fibrosis, which may nip off small buds of epithelium, simulating malignant infiltration. However, there is no evidence that any of

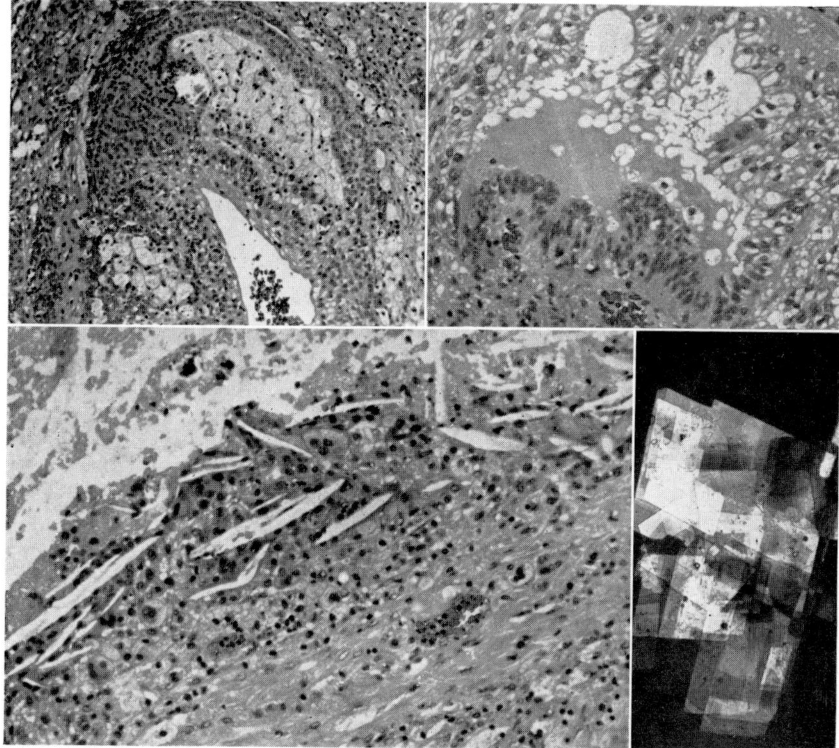

Figure 13.18. CRANIOPHARYNGIOMA; (*a*) and (*b*) epithelial masses forming cysts in a dense fibrous stroma; the resemblance to dental anlage is apparent in (*a*) (H & E. (*a*) × 30; (*b*) × 45); (*c*) edge of a cavity containing cholesterol, showing spaces left by dissolved lipid, which provokes an extreme fibroblastic reaction and giant cell formation (× 130); (*d*) cholesterol crystals from the cystic fluid (polarized light, × 130).
[(*a*) *Top left.* (*b*) *Top right.* (*c*) *Bottom left.* (*d*) *Bottom right.*]

these tumours ever become malignant, although they show a great tendency to invade locally probably due to the irritant effect of the keratin which acts as a foreign body (Fig. 13.18).

Squamous metaplasia in the lining of the cyst is very common, and the keratin it produces initiates the characteristic, dense fibroblastic and gliotic reaction. Gliosis and calcification also occur in the adjacent brain tissue, and Rosenthal fibres are very commonly seen.

MODES OF PRESENTATION

The tumour rarely presents in infancy. Although Cuneo and Rand (1952) described a child with hydrocephalus at birth due to this tumour, patients rarely present before the age of three years, and from this age onwards, there is a fairly uniform incidence extending into middle age.

Headache is the commonest early symptom; it is the first manifestation in 50% in the Index Series and was a prominent complaint in 80%, often associated with vomiting.

Loss of vision was the first complaint in only three patients, but as so often happens in childhood, the loss was severe when first detected in 15 of the 23 children. In retrospect the patients' sight had been defective for months or years.

Other subtle and insidious abnormalities are seldom complaints but emerge as enquiry and investigations proceed. Most of these result from disturbance of the hypophyseal or hypothalamic functions and are related to the hormones normally produced in this area.

(*a*) *Growth;* skeletal growth lags behind, as indicated by the radiographic bone age which can be years behind. Dwarfism may occur.

(*b*) *Lack of energy;* the child tires easily and cannot keep up with his peers.

(*c*) *Diabetes insipidus* is uncommon before operation.

(*d*) *The general appearance* can be characteristic; the child is small, delicate and immature, and there is a lack of body hair in older children. Skin texture and hair is fine, as is the hair itself.

The following typical history illustrates these points

G.L. had an x-ray of the skull because he had been hit in the face by an air-gun pellet. The radiographs revealed not only the pellet but a large sella turcica with intrasellar calcification. On questioning, it emerged that he had difficulty in seeing all of the blackboard at school, that he was smaller than his younger brother, and could not keep up with his peers in the games children play.

Other manifestations occur, depending on the direction in which the tumour extends.

Papilloedema when CSF pathway is obstructed before distortion and compression of the optic nerves.

Cranial nerve palsies (C II, III, VI and VII) are the result of lateral and posterior extensions.

Epilepsy, said to be uncommon with the craniopharyngioma, was found in four children (17%) in the Index Series.

INVESTIGATIONS

Radiography of the skull confirms the diagnosis in a high proportion. Calcification, varying from a few flecks to massive deposits, was seen in 55% of children. The sella turcica is enlarged and there is usually erosion of the posterior clinoid processes.

Separation of cranial sutures and digital impressions are frequent.

DIFFERENTIAL DIAGNOSIS

The other common tumour, the glioma of the optic chiasm, can usually be distinguished easily, but rarer tumours can usually only be identified at operation, e.g.:
Chordomas (p. 288), arising from the upper portion of the clivus (two patients);
Germinomas, either single or associated with a second tumour in the pineal region (six patients).
Dermoid cysts (three patients); and
Meningiomas arising in the region of the anterior clinoids and extending along the optic nerve sheath (one patient).

TREATMENT

It is necessary to determine the size and the extensions of the tumour before operation and this is best achieved by pneumo-encephalography, but if the pressure is high, a ventriculogram is preferable. Angiography may be necessary to establish the relationship of the tumour to the major vessels.

The administration of steroids before and after operation has decreased morbidity and mortality to an extraordinary degree.

Earlier diagnosis, microsurgical techniques, hypothermia, and a more optimistic attitude have increased the proportion of totally excised tumours.

After operation, diabetes insipidus is common, but can be controlled by Vasopressin®, given by injection or nasal spray. Failure of growth can now be remedied by the administration of growth hormone.

Diabetes insipidus can now be controlled by a variety of oral preparations, e.g. chlorpropamide (Diabetase®).

III. PINEAL TUMOURS

These can be divided into three clinico-pathological types: germinomas, pinealomas and teratomas.

1. GERMINOMA

The early controversy surrounding these tumours has been well summarized by Rubinstein (1972), and they are now considered to be derived from primitive germ cells (Fig. 13.19). Most occur in the pineal region, less frequently in the suprasellar region.

Their growth potential is very variable; they can rarely be removed completely, and many of them infiltrate and disseminate widely, although in some of the cases in the Index Series there was a long period of regression following radiotherapy.

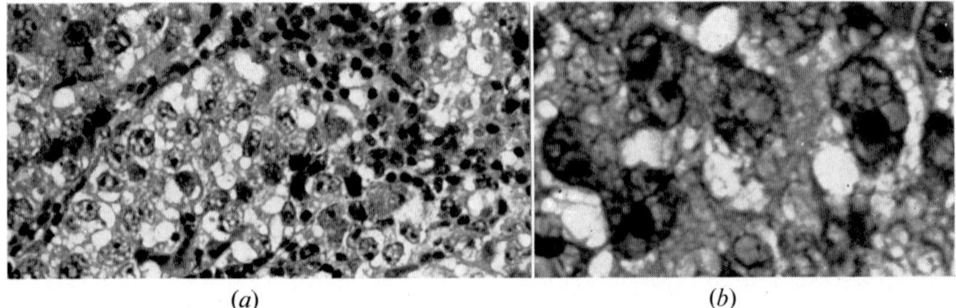

(*a*) (*b*)

Figure 13.19. CEREBRAL GERMINOMA (atypical teratoma of Russell); (*a*) groups of large cells separated by delicate fibrous septa infiltrated by lymphocytes (H & E. × 200). At times the septa are very prominent; (*b*) prominent nucleoli and 'bubbly' cytoplasm containing abundant glycogen (× 520).

MACROSCOPIC APPEARANCES

Germinomas are locally expanding tumours and usually soft, grey-pink and friable, but sometimes firm. Firm examples contain a considerable amount of fibrous tissue in the stroma, probably a form of reactive fibrosis.

MICROSCOPIC FINDINGS

There are two types of cell present:
(*a*) Large cells with a round nucleus, a single prominent nucleolus, and a good deal of rather feathery, indistinct cytoplasm containing glycogen. These cells tend to be collected in clumps surrounded by a delicate vascular network.
(*b*) Lymphocytes infiltrate the supporting stromal tissues, and small granulomas are occasionally described. The tumour cells and the lymphocytes seem to be quite distinct and no transitional cell types are found.

SPREAD

Apart from local invasion, metastasis along CSF pathways to the spinal theca is not uncommon, and an occasional example of distant metastasis has been reported (Tompkins *et al.*, 1950).

2. PINEALOMAS

True pinealomas, arising from the pineal parenchyma, are of two main types:
(*a*) *The pineocytoma* (syn. pinealocytoma) grows slowly, has a good prognosis, and is composed of cells with a compact, round, moderately dense

nucleus and a variable amount of somewhat polygonally-shaped cytoplasm, growing in clusters separated by fibro-vascular stroma. These cells may superficially resemble the cells of a germinoma, but there are no infiltrating lymphocytes in the stroma, the cells are smaller, and the cytoplasm does not usually contain glycogen. Occasionally the cells of a pineocytoma have polar cytoplasm with the processes radiating around the blood vessels.
(*b*) *A malignant variety* has been described and the differential diagnosis from other small-cell tumours in the region may be extremely difficult. In such cases one of the main factors in the diagnosis is the precise site of origin.

HISTOLOGICAL DIFFERENTIATION OF SMALL-CELL TUMOURS IN THE PINEAL AND PITUITARY REGIONS

As well as germinomas and pineocytomas, other small-cell tumours can arise in the pineal and pituitary regions.

Reticulum cell sarcoma
This is also called a 'microglioma' and may arise in this region and cause confusion, but both are extraordinarily rare in childhood.

Endodermal sinus tumours (p. 692)
These tumours can arise in a pineal teratoma, and could be confusing, although their histological structure is different.

In the Index Series there were two unusual tumours.

One arose in the pituitary region and was composed of cells with a delicate, oval, vesicular nucleus and small amounts of amphophilic cytoplasm. The cells tended to form cords and columns, but were mostly undifferentiated. The pituitary could not be identified as a separate entity, and the tumour was considered to be malignant, possibly an adeno-carcinoma of the pituitary.

In another child a tumour arising in the pineal region was composed basically of astrocytic cells. At the time of diagnosis it had already spread forward towards the infundibulum of the pituitary, and the exact site of origin was uncertain. Histologically it had a very loose pattern of spindle-shaped, astrocytic cells in a loose stroma. In this case, an origin from glial tissue adjacent to the pineal cannot be ruled out.

3. TERATOMAS

Most cerebral teratomas are well differentiated and occur in the region of the pineal, or less frequently in the suprasellar area. Macroscopically they contain solid and cystic areas and microscopically they are found to contain a variety of tissues.

In the Index Series three tumours, all in young children, contained very cellular areas of immature retinoblastic and medulloblastoma-like tissue; three others in older children contained bone, cartilage, respiratory and alimentary epithelia, and areas of pigmented epithelium resembling the retina.

There are also reports in the literature of associated teratomas and endodermal sinus tumours, but none was seen in the Index Series.

AGE : SEX

Of the twenty tumours arising in the pineal region, five were found in the first year of life, and six were between 12 and 15 years of age. The sexes were equally distributed. A wide range of tumours was found in the pineal region; four were gliomas of different types, six were pinealomas (three benign and three malignant); four were teratomas; two were germinomas; two tumours could not be classified, and no biopsy material was obtained in another two.

MODE OF PRESENTATION

Almost all patients presented with features of the 'midline syndrome', i.e. headache, vomiting, drowsiness and/or personality change, which had usually been present for some weeks.

Loss of upward gaze, is the classic sign of a pineal tumour, due to involvement of the uppermost oculomotor nuclei and can usually be demonstrated.

A large head and a raised percussion note were found in the younger children.

INVESTIGATIONS

Radiography usually shows calcification in both teratomas and pinealomas, and calcification in the pineal region in a child is almost diagnostic of this type of tumour. Separation of sutures is frequently found. Brain scans are useful in indicating the site of the tumour, but contrast studies are required to delineate the tumour clearly before operation.

MANAGEMENT

Radiography is followed by a brain scan (p. 75) which is useful in determining the next step; if the radionucleide is taken up, contrast studies are then obtained. As the aqueduct is usually obstructed, a ventriculo-atrial shunt is indicated.

Angiography is then performed and sufficient information is then available to approach the tumour, usually beside the falx or above the tentorium.

Teratomas can usually be removed completely, and the greater part of a pinealoma can be resected. A biopsy is obtained from tumours which cannot be resected.

Radiotherapy is usually indicated in children with a malignant pinealoma, glioma, and germinoma.

PROGNOSIS

The outlook is good in typical teratomas and in calcified pinealomas, but in the more malignant tumours, especially those occurring in infants, the prognosis is poor and much the same as in medulloblastoma and malignant ependymoma. In the Index Series nine of the twenty children with a tumour in the pineal region have survived.

IV. TUMOURS OF THE WALL AND FLOOR OF THE THIRD VENTRICLE

Tumours of the lateral wall of the ventricle (Fig. 13.13) include those arising in the basal ganglia. Females predominate, but the number is small. All eight of the tumours in the Index Series were glial in origin; six were astrocytomas and two were ependymomas. Their growth was usually rapid and the tumour massive.

These tumours have two main effects:

(*a*) Ventricular obstruction; and

(*b*) Local involvement of the basal ganglia, the long tracts, or the upper brain stem.

Obstruction to the flow of CSF through the third ventricle produces the 'midline syndrome' (p. 233) with headache, vomiting, papilloedema and ataxia. Superimposed on these are the effects of unilateral involvement of adjacent structures, e.g. hemiparesis (75%), unilateral tremor, unilateral sensory deficits and in posteriorly placed tumours, hemianopia. When the tumour extends downwards into the brain stem, disturbances of the oculomotor nuclei and changes in muscle tone and co-ordination may be seen.

DIAGNOSIS

A brain scan (p. 75) is the first step in diagnosis, followed by angiography and ventriculography.

MANAGEMENT

Total excision is impossible, and when there is ventricular obstruction a palliative shunt followed by an aspiration biopsy, is a prelude to radiotherapy.

PROGNOSIS

Only two children in this small series of eight patients survived for more than five years. In general, there is some correlation between the microscopic appearance of the tumour and survival.

The floor of the third ventricle is an uncommon site for primary tumours, and only four children (1%) had a tumour limited to this area; two developed precocious puberty at an early age (18 months and 2 years), and in the other two there was delay in growth and maturation.

A number of children have been reported to have a hamartoma in the floor of the third ventricle, and this was found in two patients, both of whom had precocious puberty and marked behavioural disturbances.

Macroscopically these lesions are firm and white. Microscopically their structure is that of a low-grade astrocytoma containing prominent glial fibres. In one case there were a few somewhat immature neurones within the tumour, and the term 'ganglioglioma' (p. 285) could be justified.

C. SUPERFICIAL TUMOURS OF THE CEREBRAL HEMISPHERES

These account for some 10% of all intracranial tumours in children, and in the Index Series 69% were astrocytic in type (Table 13.4).

AGE : SEX

The tumours are distributed fairly equally in each of the three quinquennia of childhood, and males are involved slightly more frequently than females.

Most of these tumours are highly malignant, but in the few relatively benign types such as fibrillary astrocytoma or haemangioma (often associated with a cyst), growth is slow and the prognosis and survival rate are excellent. Ependymomas with a superficial cyst are also found, and these have a moderately good prognosis, whereas very actively growing gliomas, e.g. glioblastoma multiforme (Fig. 13.20) have a bad outlook and very few survive for as long as a year. Meningiomas are rare, often spread widely and are difficult to eradicate.

SITE

The distribution in the Index Series is in accord with other reported series, and was as follows:

Parietal 45%;
Frontal 35%;
Temporal 10%;
Occipital 4%;
Multiple tumours 6%

Table 13.4. Tumours of the cerebral hemispheres. The relative incidence in four series (see legend for Table 13.1)

	Boston	Vienna	Tokyo	Melbourne
Total	118	196	174	60
	%	%	%	%
Glial Series:				
Astrocytic	69	42	67	69
Ependymal	20	15	16	13
Meningioma	2	9	18	8

The histological types of tumour in the cerebral hemispheres are as follows:

I. Astrocytomas;
II. Glioblastoma multiforme;
III. Giant cell astrocytoma (of tuberous sclerosis);
IV. Supratentorial ependymoma;
V. Oligodendroglioma;
VI. Papillomas of the choroid plexus;
VII. Meningioma.

I. CEREBRAL ASTROCYTOMAS

Astrocytomas arising above the tentorium in children usually have the cytological features of malignancy, i.e. Grade III or IV in the Kernohan classification. The piloid pattern seen in the cerebellum is uncommon in the cerebrum.

Cerebral astrocytomas are composed of cells with a variable amount of cytoplasm, variable production of fibres, moderate nuclear anaplasia and usually considerable vascular endothelial hyperplasia. Foci of calcification are common and as in glial tumours elsewhere, variation in cellularity from one part of the tumour to another is typical. Reactive gliosis and the formation of Rosenthal fibres is very commonly found in the adjacent invaded brain tissue.

II. GLIOBLASTOMA MULTIFORME

The validity of placing these malignant astrocytomas in a separate category may be questioned, but as a group they have a characteristic histological picture and a uniformity of behaviour. The majority of tumours of this type arise above the tentorium.

In the Index Series there were 19 examples.

Macroscopically the tumour often appears to be reasonably well defined, and the cut section shows areas of haemorrhage, necrosis, and sometimes cyst formation, producing a variegated appearance.

Microscopically the histological picture is pleomorphic, and although the cells are recognizable as astrocytic in type, they show hyperchromatism, variations in size, giant forms, multinucleate types, and some have relatively little cytoplasm or cytoplasmic processes. Mitoses are usually frequent and sometimes bizarre (Fig. 13.20).

Two important histological features common to glioblastomas are:

(*a*) *Small stellate areas of necrosis*, edged by tumour cells arranged at right angles to the surface producing pseudo-palisades; and

(*b*) *Vascular endothelial hyperplasia*, at times so extreme that it resembles an angiomatous malformation.

Sometimes clumps of swollen endothelial cells on a stalk project into the

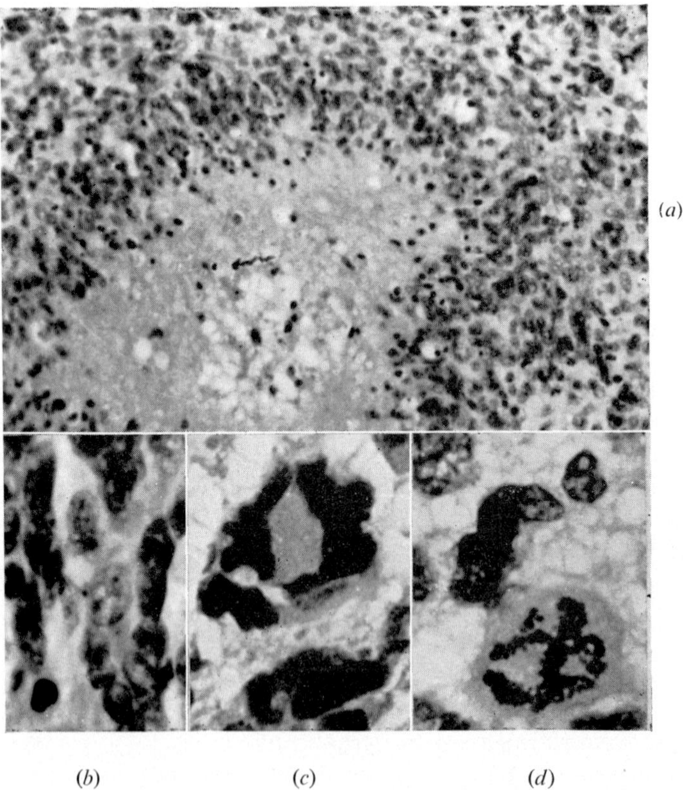

Figure 13.20. GLIOBLASTOMA MULTIFORME; (*a*) characteristic area of necrosis with pallisading of nuclei at the periphery (H & E. × 130); (*b*) (*c*) and (*d*) three areas of extreme cellular polymorphism i.e. 'multiforme' (× 520).

vessel lumen mimicking a glomerulus, and in some tumours neoplastic transformation seems to have involved the endothelial cells as well. Sinusoidal vessels are also seen and these are frequently thrombosed.

Invasion of the meninges occasionally provokes an unusual form of metaplasia in the tumour which can assume a fibrosarcomatous appearance (p. 285). Indeed, a glioblastoma which reaches the surface of the brain may feel hard and resemble a meningioma.

SPREAD

Glioblastomas invade locally and sometimes spread in the CSF. Rare examples of spread outside the central nervous system have been described, and are usually the result of invasion of systemic venous channels in the leptomeninges.

III. GIANT CELL ASTROCYTOMA
(syn. Subependymal giant cell astrocytoma)

Almost invariably subependymal in origin and confined to the lateral ventricles, these tumours are usually associated with the syndrome of tuberous sclerosis (p. 826) and the presence of other manifestations should be suspected whenever this type of astrocytoma is found.

The tumour tissue may be hard and gritty, or soft and vascular, depending on the content of glial tissue and the amount of calcification.

Microscopically the giant astrocytes which give the tumour its name are of glial origin, although they may resemble neurons, and may comprise most of the tumour or only part of it. They are arranged in swathes with elongated often strap-like cytoplasmic process. These large cells may be superficially suggestive of malignancy, but they have regular, relatively small nuclei, mitoses are rare and most examples behave in a benign fashion.

IV. SUPRATENTORIAL EPENDYMOMAS

Ependymomas can be recognized by their differentiation to form ependymal spaces or perivascular pseudorosettes (p. 252).

In the Index Series, 17% of the supratentorial tumours were ependymomas. These varied in cellularity and in their situation; in most cases it is possible to identify their origin from the lining of one of the ventricles, but when they extend to reach the surface of the brain, they may appear to arise from the cortex. Some ependymomas develop pronounced cystic changes and in general this type has a better prognosis. Histologically they are predominantly astrocytic and 'subependymal' in type (see p. 253). Less well differentiated tumours are also found, and these are structurally similar to the papillary and tubular varieties (p. 252) seen in the fourth ventricle.

V. OLIGODENDROGLIOMA

While foci of oligodendrogliomatous differentiation are occasionally found in astrocytomas arising anywhere in the neuraxis, pure oligodendrogliomas in childhood are extremely rare. They grow slowly and macroscopically they are well defined, firm and often cystic.

The only example in the Index Series was in the fourth ventricle in a ten-month old boy, and even this tumour was not a pure oligodendroglioma, for it contained some areas of astrocytoma. This site of origin seems unusual, since most reported cases arise in the cerebral hemispheres.

Microscopically they have a very typical histological appearance described as 'honeycomb-like'. The nucleus is round, dark staining and compact, and lies in the centre of a cell with vacuolated cytoplasm and sharply defined cytoplasmic margins. As in many other central nervous tumours of glial type, vascular endothelial proliferation is sometimes seen.

VI. PAPILLOMAS OF THE CHOROID PLEXUS

These unique tumours present most frequently in early life, usually as a child with a large head in whom hydrocephalus is suspected.

Macroscopically, the papilloma is a cauliflower-like mass arising from the attachment of the choroid plexus, most frequently in the fourth ventricles, or, rarely, in the third ventricle.

Microscopically, the tumour may closely resemble the structure of the choroid plexus, but in some examples there are multiple layers of cells suggesting a more active growth potential. In the Index Series one papilloma recurred following excision, and this is not an infrequent occurrence with this tumour, which sometimes implants in other sites in the ventricles.

The smaller benign tumours can escape detection, but if they are identified they can be removed satisfactorily. Massive tumours and those with malignant change are practically inoperable.

Choroid plexus carcinoma

This is also called malignant choroid plexus papilloma and is an even rarer tumour, usually arising in one of the lateral ventricles, invading the adjacent brain and seeding widely throughout the meninges.

In the Index Series there were eight benign papillomas of the choroid plexus and one which was interpreted as carcinoma; in four of them excision was possible and they are longterm survivors.

VII. MENINGIOMA

These are rare in childhood, and a few of them are associated with von Recklinghausen's disease (p. 827), usually those occurring in older children. Most are benign, but malignant meningiomas can arise *de novo* in early childhood, and these appear to be unassociated with von Recklinghausen's disease.

Macroscopically meningiomas present in childhood as sessile or rounded tumours intimately attached to the dura.

Microscopically all the histological patterns encountered in meningiomas in adults may be seen, but the commonest in childhood is the meningotheliomatous type which sometimes contains psammoma bodies. This type is often seen in meningiomas arising in the region of the optic nerve (Fig. 13.16).

The malignant meningiomas

These are rare, spread widely and are difficult to eradicate. The diagnosis may be difficult unless areas with typical meningiomatous differentiation can be identified in what is otherwise a fibrosarcoma-like tumour. The site of origin, from the meninges, can usually be determined and usually diagnostic.

In the Index Series there were two examples of cortical malignant meningiomas, both in boys, aged 3 and 5 years; both were fatal. Benign meningiomas occurred in an older age group, 10–12 years, and the results were good.

CLINICAL FEATURES OF CEREBRAL TUMOURS

There are no particularly characteristic clinical features in cerebral tumours in children and localizing or even lateralizing signs occur in no more than 30%. In more than 50% of cases, the tumour arises in a 'silent' area of the cortex. The onset of symptoms is so often insidious and unremarkable that signs of increased intracranial pressure appear suddenly and soon dominate the picture.

Headache (69%), *vomiting* (55%) and *apathy* (37%) are all indications of increasing intracranial pressure. Other non-focal signs such as diplopia (10%), incoordination (4%) and ataxia (4%), are much less common.

Convulsions occur occasionally with tumours elsewhere, but are most common when there is direct involvement of the cortex, and they occurred in 26% of the Index Series of cortical tumours. Weakness of the limbs on the contralateral side was present in approximately 30% of patients.

The signs present at the first examination emphasize the generalized nature of involvement; 53% had well-marked papilloedema while only 18% had acute motor paresis. A 'cracked-pot note' on percussion was found in 15%. Pyramidal signs could, however, be detected in over 50%, while a localizing visual field defect was seen in 16%.

INVESTIGATIONS

Electroencephalograms showed a high proportion (66%) of localizing abnormalities.

Radionucleide scanning (p. 75) provides positive evidence in a high proportion of cases and is now used routinely in later cases. Plain x-rays of the skull were of little localizing value, showing calcification, in only 4%, but separation of sutures was seen in more than 25%.

Ventriculography provides a definitive localization, but in the last ten years has been superseded by angiography (p. 69).

MANAGEMENT

Complete excision of the tumour is possible in about a third of these patients; in most cases partial or subtotal resection is performed and is followed by irradiation. The situation was so bad in this group that in 15% no definitive treatment was offered.

In summary, superficial tumours of the cerebral hemispheres are fairly equally distributed in all age groups. The duration of symptoms before presentation was about three months. Signs of increased pressure led to the diagnosis in most cases, and epilepsy or lateralizing motor and sensory signs were less evident.

Most tumours belonged to the astrocytoma group, and most of these—glioblastoma multiforme and the anaplastic type—were highly malignant and the survival was short. Only eight have survived for more than five years.

Ependymomas, although originating at the ventricular level, usually spread to the surface or had a more superficial cyst. Their prognosis is less good than the cystic type of astrocytoma.

CHEMOTHERAPY OF INTRACRANIAL TUMOURS

Cytotoxic agents have been shown to be of some value in the treatment of a number of brain tumours and it may be that further trials will widen their role. Because the cells of the central nervous system do not synthesize DNA, cytotoxic agents acting in the replicating (DNA-synthesis) cycle can attack tumour cells in the brain much more selectively than in other parts of the body. To do this the drug must, of course, reach the tumour in sufficient concentration, and this is limited by the protective barriers, the blood-brain barrier in peri-capillary glial tissues, the blood-CSF barrier in the choroidal plexus, and the CSF-brain barrier in the ependyma. These can evidently be overcome sufficiently to produce responses when potent agents are used in adequate dosage, as has been shown in the treatment of medulloblastoma, astrocytoma and some other types of intracranial tumours.

Methotrexate is administered intrathecally (Newton *et al.*, 1968), and as in other centres, our practice has been to give the drug daily (0·25 mg/kg) for 5 to 7 days, although the optimum regime is still not known. It has had its major application in medulloblastoma, and the results in recent patients in the Index Series, compared with those not so treated, are shown in Fig. 13.21, which indicates that with treatment more patients may survive longer.

BCNU (1,3-bis, 2 chloroethyl-1-nitrosourea) given intravenously, or the less toxic CCNU given orally, are the most promising drugs for brain tumours to date. Being lipid soluble they can penetrate the blood-brain barrier, and they act as alkylating agents. Given in 3 day courses or in a single dose, they may be more effective when combined with other cytotoxic agents such as vincristine (Fewer *et al.*, 1972).

Two collaborative groups in U.S.A. and in Europe are currently studying the response to combinations of vincristine, CCNU, ± dexamethasone. Experience with tumours other than those arising in the CNS suggests that chemotherapy used in planned conjunction with surgery and radiotherapy (see below) may give the best results.

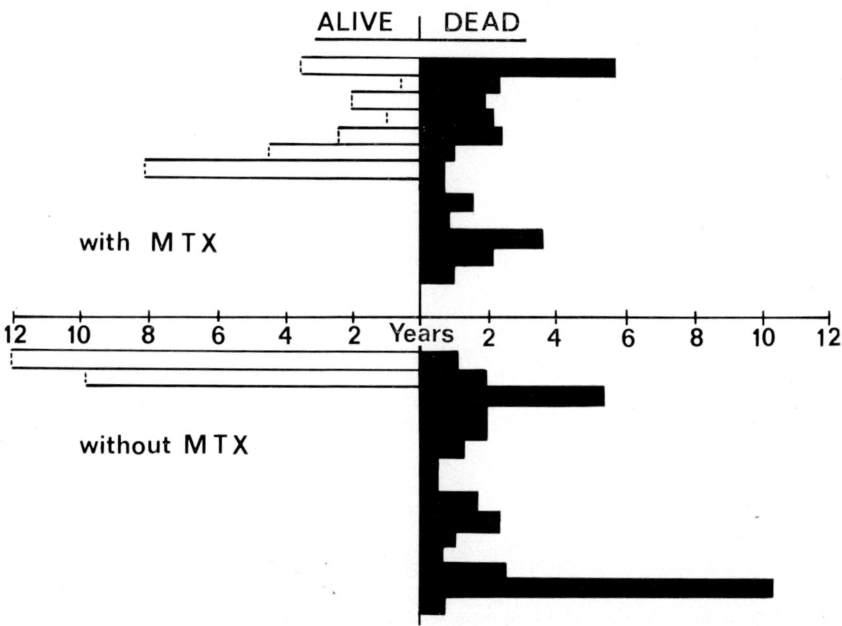

Figure 13.21. MEDULLOBLASTOMA. Histogram showing length of survival with and without intrathecal methotrexate (MTX), in a group of 37 patients, indicating that more patients are surviving and may survive longer.

RADIOTHERAPY OF THE NEURAXIS

Treatment of patients with medulloblastoma, ependymomas, intracranial deposits in leukaemia and the malignant lymphomas, and retinoblastomas which have extended to involve the CSF (p. 429), may include irradiation of the whole of the intracranial cavities and the spinal theca.

The total dose delivered varies in different circumstances, but in childhood some 3000–4000 rads is usually given via:

(*a*) Bilateral portals to the cranium; and

(*b*) A linear area extending from the posterior fossa to the filum terminale, so as to include all of the spinal theca as far as the mid-sacral region.

Various techniques can be used to avoid radiating the thyroid (e.g. by angling the beam 15° behind the vertical in a prone patient), and to prevent overlap is segmental fields. As radiotherapy to the spine causes depression of the marrow in the vertebrae, the effects on the blood picture are closely monitored and the increments are given at longer intervals when indicated.

RARER TUMOURS OF THE CENTRAL NERVOUS SYSTEM

Under this heading the following tumours are briefly described:

I. Astroblastoma;
II. Spongioblastoma (syn. polar spongioblastoma);
III. Polymorphic cell sarcoma;
IV. Cerebellar sarcoma;
V. Fibrosarcoma;
VII. Microglioma and microgliomatosis;
VIII. Neurocytoma (syn. ganglioglioma);
IX. Melanoma of the meninges (syn. neurocutaneous melanosis);
X. Metastatic tumours.

I. Astroblastoma

This term is used by some authorities (Russell & Rubinstein 1971; Zülch, 1971) to describe a variant of astrocytoma in which tumour cells are arranged in a pseudorosette around a blood vessel. The cells are loosely arranged, with scanty cytoplasm, and resemble the cellular type of subependymal glioma; the validity of separating them, especially in childhood, is questionable. There was no example of this tumour in the Index Series.

II. Spongioblastoma (syn. polar spongioblastoma)

This term has been used by different authors to describe different tumours.

(*a*) Rubinstein (1972) confined the term to a very rare medulloblastoma-like tumour of young children, composed of cells thought to resemble the spongioblasts of the developing embryonic cortex. The cells are arranged in 'pallisades' and have very long, delicate cell processes which occasionally contain neuroglial fibres.

(*b*) Zülch (1971) uses 'spongioblastoma' as an alternative for astrocytomas of the juvenile or piloid type. Because of this confusion we agree with Marsden & Steward's comment (1968) that although an attempt to separate off the piloid types of astrocytoma is useful, the term spongioblastoma is inappropriate.

III. Polymorphic cell sarcoma

This is a rare, highly malignant, small-celled tumour of infancy, usually arising in the posterior fossa, and composed of cells with round, wrinkled nuclei showing moderate pleomorphism, and scanty wispy cytoplasm. The nuclei are more vesicular than those of medulloblastomas and this serves to distinguish them, although a confident diagnosis may be very difficult because of the lack of specific histological evidence. Their differentiation from microgliomas is also difficult.

IV. Cerebellar sarcoma

This is probably not an entity but rather a form of vigorous stromal reaction to a cerebellar medulloblastoma when it infiltrates the leptomeninges.

V. Fibrosarcomas

Fibrosarcomas occasionally involve the meninges, but are rare in childhood. They are usually easy to recognize microscopically because of their characteristic herring-bone pattern (p. 795).

VI. Rhabdomyosarcoma

Rhabdomyosarcoma rarely arises in the brain, usually in the posterior fossa, either as a 'pure' tumour or as part of a malignant mesenchymal neoplasm containing a variety of embryonal tissue patterns (e.g. osteosarcoma, spindle cell sarcoma, rhabdomyosarcoma).

VII. Microglioma and microgliomatosis

Very rarely in childhood a reticulum cell sarcoma arises in the brain, and it has been termed a microglioma. Perivascular infiltration of a diffuse distribution, without involvement of the intervening brain tissue, is very characteristic. Distinguishing a sarcoma from medulloblastoma (p. 246), polymorphic cell sarcoma (q.v.), oligodendroglioma (p. 280) and from germinoma (p. 271), may be difficult.

In contrast to the rarity of primary malignant lymphomas in the brain, secondary involvement of the neuraxis occurs often and takes the form of diffuse infiltration of nerve roots or direct invasion of the brain (commonly the temporal and frontal lobes) by tumour tissue spreading from the extradural and subdural spaces in the anterior and middle cranial fossae.

VIII. Neurocytoma (syn. ganglioglioma)

A rare, slowly growing, circumscribed tumour occurring in the floor of the third ventricle, pons, crebellum or temporal lobe, a neurocytoma sometimes occurs as part of tuberous sclerosis (p. 826). Macroscopically, they are grey, firm and circumscribed; microscopically they consist of neoplastic neurones in a glial (astrocytic) stroma.

In the Index Series one such tumour occurred in the brain stem of a boy who had symptoms of vomiting dating from the age of 18 months. A diagnosis of bulbar palsy due to poliomyelitis was made when he was 3 years of age. He finally died at the age of 6 years and was found to have a circumscribed neurocytoma in the brain stem lateral to the fourth ventricle.

IX. Melanoma of the meninges

This may arise *de novo* or as part of the syndrome of neurocutaneous melanosis (p. 860). The leptomeninges normally contain melanocytes among their connective tissue cells, and primary intracranial melanomas presumably arise from these cells.

The tumour infiltrates diffusely through the meninges and may give rise to localized masses in the brain substance. The tumour cells are heavily pigmented and polygonal in shape with round nucleus; pleomorphic forms are common.

An extracranial primary should be very carefully excluded before accepting the diagnosis of an intracranial melanoma, for an occult cutaneous or ocular melanoma can produce a similar picture by metastasis.

The Index Series contains two cases, both boys, aged $2\frac{1}{2}$ years and 3 years. One presented with nausea, vomiting and ataxia, thought to be due to a brain stem glioma, and was treated with radiotherapy. Death occurred 6 months later, after an initial remission, and at autopsy there was diffuse infiltration of the meninges by a melanoma, and several large intracerebral deposits.

The second boy presented with 'shaky turns' and a shrill cry, and had a midline cerebellar lesion obstructing the fourth ventricle which caused coma and death; autopsy showed diffuse melanomatosis of the meninges and a mass in the cerebellum. In each case the tumour cells were those of a malignant melanoma and many were heavily pigmented.

Table 13.5. Classification of tumours of the central Nervous system. Based on the classification of Rubinstein (Rubinstein, L.J. (1970), in *Tumours of the Central Nervous System*, Armed Forces Institute of Pathology, Washington, D.C.), slightly modified for paediatric practice

1. Tumours showing glial differentiation

ASTROCYTOMA
- Well differentiated
  - (*a*) Piloid type (juvenile)
  - (*b*) Fibrillary (adult type)
  - (*c*) Giant cell astrocytoma
- With anaplasia
  - Glioblastoma multiforme

EPENDYMOMA
- Papillary
- Non-papillary (subependymal glioma)
- Poorly differentiated (ependymoblastoma)

OLIGODENDROGLIOMA

2. Tumours of primitive embryonal or undifferentiated cells

MEDULLOBLASTOMA
MEDULLO-EPITHELIOMA

3. Tumours of neuronal cells

NEUROCYTOMA
GANGLIOMA

4. Tumours of the meninges

MENINGIOMA
MENINGIOSARCOMA

5. Tumours of doubtful cell type

CEREBELLAR SARCOMA
NEUROBLASTOMA
PINEOCYTOMA

6. Tumours of nerves

NEUROFIBROMA
NEURILEMMOMA
OPTIC NERVE 'GLIOMA'

Table 13.5. continued

7. Tumours of vascular tissue
HAEMANGIOBLASTOMA (OF CEREBELLUM)
HAEMANGIOMA
HAEMANGIOSARCOMA

8. Teratomas (intracranial)

9. Germ cell tumours
GERMINOMA (PINEALOBLASTOMA)

10. Tumours of choroid plexus
PAPILLOMA
CARCINOMA

11. CRANIOPHARYNGIOMA

12. Epidermoid cysts

13. Metastatic tumours

X. Metastatic tumours

Theoretically any malignant tumour may metastasize to the brain, but in childhood this is extremely rare. In the Index Series there were example in cases of Wilms' tumour, rhabdomyosarcoma, Ewing's tumour and osteosarcoma (one of each), and all occurred in the terminal stages of the disease.

Malignant lymphomas occasionally produce deposits in the brain, but these are usually extradural.

Leukaemia frequently leads to infiltration of the meninges and brain via the Virchow-Rubin spaces, as a distinct type of metastasis (see Chapter 9).

SPINAL TUMOURS

Tumours involving the spine are rare in the first two decades of life. In adults, metastatic tumours involving the vertebrae and spinal canal are common, but if these are excluded, primary tumours of the spine are uncommon at any age.

In children, a wide range of tumours may affect the spinal cord directly or indirectly, and diagnosis at an early stage may be difficult. In discussing the effects and management of spinal tumours, non-neoplastic conditions which may produce the same signs and symptoms, such as congenital malformations, infections or infestations, should also be considered.

In spite of the variety of lesions, the modes of presentation show many similarities. Investigations are neither complicated nor difficult, and with few exceptions the indications for operation and the programme of management can be stated simply.

CLASSIFICATION OF SPINAL TUMOURS

The etiological and topographic categories are as follows:

1. Primary tumours of the vertebrae;
2. Metastatic tumours of the spine;
3. Paraspinal tumours;
4. Tumours of the spinal canal—
 (i) Intramedullary;
 (ii) Extramedullary;
5. Developmental anomalies.

1. Tumours of the vertebrae

Primary tumours of the vertebrae are rare in childhood, but the Index Series contains four examples of Ewing's tumour, one aneurysmal bone cyst and one reticulum cell sarcoma. All presented with signs of spinal cord compression and radiological evidence of local bone destruction.

Operative removal followed by radiotherapy has resulted in long periods of survival, in contrast to the two essentially non-malignant conditions, hydatid disease and chordoma, both of which have been impossible to eradicate.

A girl aged 10 years developed pulmonary metastases 3 years after primary Ewing's tumour of the vertebra had been controlled by surgery, chemotherapy and irradiation. The pulmonary metastases were irradiated and subsequently two small nodules were resected. She remains well and free of disease 5 years after segmental pulmonary resections.

Histological diagnosis

In our experience the two perispinal tumours which present difficulties in differential diagnosis are neuroblastoma and Ewing's tumour. The cytological features and histochemical techniques by which these two tumours can be distinguished are described on p. 736.

Hydatid disease of the spinal cord may develop as a complication of an intrathoracic cyst, but in the two cases in the Index Series there was no other evidence of the disease which presumably arose from primary lodgement in one of the vertebra. The involvement was widespread at the time of presentation, with daughter cysts scattered throughout the cancellous bone of the vertebrae, making complete removal impossible. Multiple operations may halt the onset of complete paraplegia for years, but the process is inexorable.

Chordomas (Fig. 13.22) are reported to be less frequent in the spinal column than in the sphenoid region at the base of the skull, but in the two cases in the Index Series the tumour arose in the upper cervical and sacral regions respectively. Again, complete removal has been impossible, but multiple operations have so far prevented the development of paraplegia.

2. Metastatic tumours of the spine

These are much less common in children than in adults. In children they

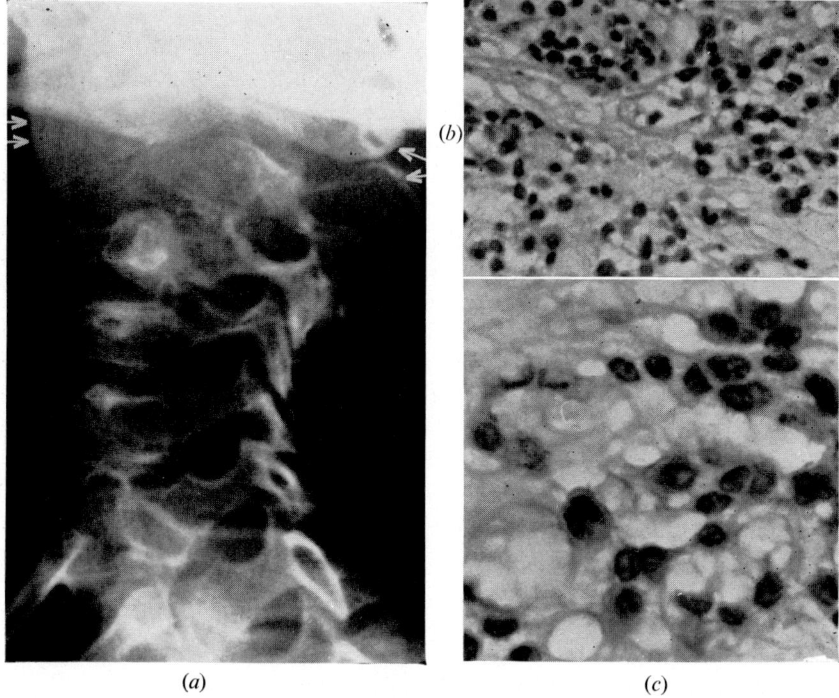

Figure 13.22. CHORDOMA; (*a*) x-ray of a chordoma arising in the odontoid process of C2 extending into C_2 and C_3; the vertebrae are greatly enlarged and have a 'soap-bubble' texture; (*b*) lobulated mucoid pattern (H & E. × 130); (*c*) physaliferous cells with a large, clearly defined nucleus and abundant bubbly cytoplasm in which glycogen can usually be demonstrated histochemically (H & E. × 520).

include metastatic infiltration of the vertebra in neuroblastoma, Hodgkin's disease, lymphosarcoma and leukaemia. In almost all cases these develop as a complication in a patient already receiving treatment for the primary condition, and not as a mode of presentation of the tumour.

3. Paraspinal tumours

The important members of this group are primary neuroblastoma and ganglioneuroma, both of which may arise from paraspinal neural tissues.

Ganglioneuromas are slowly growing tumours which usually reach a massive size before causing signs or symptoms. In the three cases in the Index Series, the tumour was in the upper thoracic region and in one case the brachial plexus was involved before compression of the spinal cord. Removal was incomplete in each case, but the residual disability is not severe and the survival time appears to be indefinite.

Neuroblastoma

Involvement of the spinal cord usually occurs as an extension in continuity from a thoracic or abdominal neuroblastoma, and is usually diagnosed in the first five years of life; a few have evidence of spinal involvement when they are born, and one case in the Index Series had a complete flaccid paraplegia at birth. Signs of spinal compression are progressive and in almost every case a paraspinal mass can be seen or felt.

The rapid development of paraplegia in a child less than five years of age should be assumed on statistical grounds to be due to a neuroblastoma until proven otherwise, and treatment should be instituted as soon as possible. The appropriate investigations (p. 461) include myelography to determine whether there is encroachment upon the spinal canal, and a laminectomy or hemilaminectomy is required as a matter of urgency, for *the extent of recovery after decompression is directly related to the duration of the compression before it is relieved.*

Chemotherapy (p. 463) is commenced before operation, and as much of the neuroblastoma as possible is removed as far as, and out into, the intervertebral foramina when necessary.

When the primary is a paraspinal or paravertebral mass, for example in the posterior mediastinum, it is usually removed at a subsequent operation, following which the full programme of radiotherapy and chemotherapy for neuroblastoma (p. 463) is completed.

Maturation of the neuroblastoma to a ganglioneuroma (p. 539) occurs in a small number of these children and in several in the Index Series who have required re-operation, biopsies have shown progressive changes in the histological picture towards ganglioneuromatous cells.

A.S. presented at the age of 2 years with progressive loss of power in the lower limbs. A large mass was visible and palpable in the erector spinae in the lumbar region. In the course of the next 19 years, three operations have been performed, during which the histological picture changed from a frank neuroblastoma to mature ganglioneuroma. There is still some radiological evidence of a static paraspinal tumour, but the young woman is free of all signs and symptoms, and is fully and gainfully employed.

4. (i) Intramedullary tumours

Neoplasms within the spinal canal arise in the spinal cord (i.e. intramedullary) or outside the cord but within the dura (intrathecal but extramedullary).

Intramedullary tumours are uncommon in childhood; an ependymoma is the tumour most frequently encountered, while an astrocytoma is rare.

Ependymomas arise in the centre of the cord and produce symmetrical signs in the lower trunk and lower limbs. In the early stages at least, it is a well-defined tumour which may be removable through a longitudinal incision in the cord. Occasionally there is extensive longitudinal involvement, making resection difficult or impossible. Resection when possible, followed by radiotherapy, will often effect a cure.

Astrocytomas are less common, usually infiltrate widely, and are not amenable to surgical excision. Some regression and improvement may be obtained by radiotherapy.

Intraspinal 'cysts'. A cystic cavity occasionally develops within the spinal cord and causes compression. It may follow trauma, e.g. a fracture dislocation of the vertebrae, and lead to an increase in the neural deficit weeks or months after the injury; in other cases the condition may be a true syringomyelia, and in yet others an astrocytomatous cyst; all three lesions are uncommon in childhood.

4. (ii) Extramedullary tumours

These tumours lie outside the cord but compress it, are most frequently found to be secondary deposits from an intracranial tumour such as a medulloblastoma or an ependymoma. They may also develop in patients with leukaemia, in which deposits within the substance of the cord may also develop (p. 157).

A solitary neurofibroma arising in a nerve root is not very uncommon; occasionally they are multiple and represent one facet of generalized von Recklinghausen's disease (p. 827). The mode of presentation is usually pain of root distribution, followed by progressive motor and sensory changes, often limited to one side, producing a Brown-Séquard type of neurological syndrome.

Epidermoid cysts usually occur among the roots of the cauda equina and may communicate with the skin by a dermal sinus; meningitis is the mode of onset when infection supervenes.

An uninfected dermoid cyst may grow slowly, due to the accumulation of its secretions, and act as an expanding lesion producing pressure on the roots of the cauda equina with signs of spinal compression. The clinical features include root pain, loss of sphincteric control and/or loss of power in the lower limbs. Investigations, including a myelogram will lead to identification of the cyst, and it can usually be removed satisfactorily.

Spinal teratoma

The spine is a very rare site for a teratoma. There were three in the Index Series of which one was a well differentiated teratoma in the cauda equina of an eight-year old boy.

A teratoma may also occur in association with an overt or occult spina bifida, apart from a sacrococcygeal teratoma. Sacrococcygeal teratomas are present at birth as a large rounded mass, sometimes of extraordinary size, and may be associated with a deformity of the sacrum (p. 713). Their treatment is described on p. 715.

5. Developmental anomalies affecting the spinal cord

A group of abnormalities within the general category of spinal dysraphism includes a variety of lesions ranging from the clinically very obvious to the completely latent. It is the latter which enter the differential diagnosis of spinal tumours, but the external markers of their existence are as follows:

1. Cutaneous and subcutaneous abnormalities; hairy patches, dermal sinus or dimple.
2. Vascular and lipomatous swellings; haemangiomas, fibrolipomas.
3. Spina bifida, varying from a narrow cleft in a lamina to the total absence of a lamina and its related spinous process.
4. Various anomalies of the cord, nerve roots and spinal canal.

Some children have only one anomaly, while others may have complex combinations of several. They may occur at any point on the spine but the most common site, and the area with the greatest variety of lesions, is the lumbo-sacral region.

Clinical features

Some signs of neural deficits may be detectable in early life, and these may become more marked as growth proceeds when the cord remains tethered to the bifid spine.

Deformities of the feet or sphincteric disturbances developing during the prepubertal or pubertal growth spurt strongly suggest the presence of this type of abnormality.

Lipomas and lipomeningoceles

These are common, and also mostly in the lumbosacral region. In most cases they overlie a bifid spinous process and cause little more than a cosmetic defect. In others the bony defect is larger and in some a protrusion of the spinal dura (a meningocele) may extend through the bony defect to join with the lipoma (Rogers *et al.*, 1971).

The term 'lipomeningocele' (Lemire *et al.*, 1971) has been suggested for an important type in which the lipoma extends into the spinal canal, and may be attached to the spinal cord. Although this fatty tissue has an abnormal texture and is readily recognizable, complete removal is often impossible because the fatty tissue merges with the neural tissue of the conus.

REFERENCES

Banna, M., Hoa, R. D., Stanley, P. & Till, K. (1973). Craniopharyngioma in children. *J. Pediat.*, **83** : 781.

Bloom, H.J.G., Wallace, E.N.K. & Henk, J.H. (1969). The treatment and prognosis of medulloblastoma in children. *Am. J. Roentg. Rad. Th. & Nucl. Med.*, **105** : 43.

Bodian, M. & Lawson, D. (1953). The intracranial neoplastic diseases of childhood. *Brit. J. Surg.*, **40** : 368.

Cuneo, H.M. & Rand, C.W. (1952). *Brain Tumours in Childhood*, p. 52. Charles C. Thomas, Springfield.

Crue, B.L. (1958). *Medulloblastoma.* Charles C. Thomas, Springfield.

Cushing, H. (1931). Experiences with the cerebellar astrocytomas. *Surg. Gynec. & Obstet.*, **52** : 129.

Cushing, H. (1932). Peptic ulcers and interbrain (Balfour Lecture). *Surg. Gynec. & Obstet.*, **55** : 1.

Fewer, D., Wilson, C.B., Boldrey E.B., Enot, K.J. & Powell, M.R. (1972). Chemotherapy of brain tumors: Clinical experience with Carmustine (BCNU) and vincristine. *J. Am. med. Assoc.* **222** : 549.

Fowler, M. (1968). Embryonic ependymoma arising in a cerebral hemisphere. *Cancer* **21** : 1150.

Fowler, M. & Simpson, D.A. (1962). A malignant melanin forming tumour of the cerebellum. *J. Path. Bact.*, **84** : 307.

Gol, A. & McKissock, A. (1959). The cerebellar astrocytomas: a report on 98 verified cases. *J. Neurosurg.*, **16** : 287.

Grant, D.N. (1971). Benign intracranial hypertension: a review of 79 cases in infancy and childhood. *Arch. Dis. Childh.*, **46** : 651.

Hagberg, B., Sillanpää, M. (1970). Benign intracranial hypertension (pseudotumor cerebri): a review and report of 18 cases. *Act. paediat. Scandinav.* **59** : 328.

Houtteville, J.P. (1970). Les épendymomes du IVieme ventricule: étude anatomique et chirurgicale. *Neurochirurgia, Stuttgart.* **12** : 101.

Jeffreys, R. (1975). Pathological and haematological aspects of posterior fossa haemangioblastoma. *J. Neurol. Neurosurg. Psych.*, **38** : 112.

Katsura, S., Suzuki, J. & Wada, T. (1959). Statistical study of brain tumours in the neurosurgical clinics in Japan. *J. Neurosurg.*, **16** : 570.

Kernohan, J.W. & Sayre, C.P. (1952). Tumors of the central nervous system. Fascicle 35. *Atlas of Tumor Pathology.* Armed Forces Institute of Pathology, Washington.

Koos, W.T. & Miller, M.H. (1971). *Intracranial Tumours in Infants and Children.* Thieme Verlag, Stuttgart; Churchill, London.

Lemire, R.J., Graham, C.B. & Beckwith, J.B. (1971). Skin covered sacrococcygeal masses in infants and children. *J. Pediat*, **79** : 948.

Lewis, E.A. (1973). Gastroduodenal ulceration and haemorrhage of neurogenic origin. *Brit. J. Surg*, **60** : 279.

Matson, D.D. (1969). *Neurosurgery of Infancy and Childhood.* Charles C. Thomas, Springfield.

Newton, W.A.H., Sayers, M.P. & Samuels, L.D. (1968). Intrathecal methotrexate for brain tumors in children. *Cancer Chemother. Rep.*, **52** : 257.

Raimondi, A.J., Yashon, D., Mutsumato, S. & Reyes, C.A. (1967). Increased intracranial pressure without lateralizing signs: the midline syndrome *Neurochirurgia*, **10** : 197.

Rogers, H.M., Long, D.M. & Chou, S.N. *et al.* (1971). Lipomas of the spinal cord and cauda equina. *J. Neurosurg.*, **34** : 349.

Rose, A. & Matson, D.D. (1967). Benign intracranial hypertension in children. *Pediatrics*, **39** : 227.

Rubinstein, L.J. (1972). *Atlas of Tumor Pathology: Tumors of the Central Nervous System*, 2nd ed.. Armed Forces Institute of Pathology, Washington, D.C.

Russell, D.S. & Rubinstein, L.J. (1971). *Pathology of Tumours of the Nervous System*, 3rd ed. Edward Arnold, London.

SCHEINKER, I.M. (1945). Subependymoma: newly recognized tumour of subependymal derivation. *J. Neurosurg.*, **2** : 232.

TOLA, J.S. (1951). The histopathology and biological characteristics of primary neoplasms of the cerebellum and fourth ventricle. *Act. Chir. Scandinav. Supp. No.* 164.

TOMPKINS, V.N., HAYMAKER, W. & CAMPBELL, E.H. (1950). Metastatic pineal tumors: clinicopathologic report of 2 cases. *J. Neurosurg.*, **7** : 159.

VAN BOGAERT, T. & MARTIN, P. (1928). Les tumeurs du quatriéme ventricule et le syndrome cérébelleux de la ligne médiane. *Rev. Neurol.*, **2** : 431.

ZÜLCH, K.J. (1965). *Brain Tumours, their Biology and Pathology.* Springer Verlag, New York.

ZÜLCH, K.J. (1971). *Atlas of the Histology of Brain Tumours*, p. 44. Springer Verlag, Berlin, Heidelberg, New York.

Chapter 14. Tumours of the head and neck

Table 14.1. Swellings of the scalp and erosions of the calvarium

Benign conditions	Malignant tumours
Epidermoid cyst*	Histiocytosis X
(syn. external angular dermoid)	Eosinophilic granuloma‖
Haemangioma	Hand-Schüller-Christian syndrome
Lymphangioma	Metastases from:
Osteoma	neuroblastoma (bone)
Encephalocele	malignant lymphoma (scalp)
Osteomyelitis	leukaemia
Fibro-osseous dysplasia	Sarcomas of soft tissues (scalp) (p. 781)
Bone defects and erosions	
Subgaleal epidermoid cyst*	
Interparietal foramina†	Neuroblastoma
Encephalocele	
Congenital generalized fibromatosis‡	Histiocytosis X (as above)
Melanotic progonoma§	

* Maybe subcutaneous, intra-osseous or extradural
† Normal variant, bilateral, symmetrical
‡ In neonates, almost invariably fatal
§ More often in jaws, occasionally in calvarium
‖ Usually 'benign'

Although the head and neck comprise a relatively small part of the body, they are the commonest site of malignant tumours in childhood, chiefly because of the high incidence of intracranial tumours (Chapter 13). Tumours of the brain and eye together represent some 15–20% of all malignant tumours in children. Even when these two categories are excluded, other tumours of the head and neck account for another 5–10% of the total.

An unusual aspect of malignant tumours in this region in childhood is a departure from the general predominance of sarcomas. It has been estimated (Keynes, 1959) that of all tumours in childhood, there are nine sarcomas for every carcinoma, whereas in adults there are twenty carcinomas for every sarcoma; when only the head and neck are considered, the ratio of sarcomas to carcinomas in childhood is about one to one (Rush *et al.*, 1963).

Intracranial tumours are described in Chapter 13, and neoplasms of the eye and orbit in Chapter 15. All other tumours of the head and neck are described in this chapter, and arranged in sections according to their site of origin and the nature of the diagnostic problems they present; the sections are as follows:

A. Swellings of the scalp and erosions of the calvarium (Table 14.1).
B. Tumours of the face (the parotid gland and external aspects of the jaws).
C. Swellings in the mouth.
D. Tumours of the oropharynx.
E. Tumours of the nasopharynx.
F. Tumours of the ear.
G. Cervical tumours.

A. SWELLINGS OF THE SCALP AND CALVARIUM

In children benign lesions, as elsewhere, are far more common than malignant tumours in this area, and the most usual mode of presentation is simply a swelling, with or without some tenderness. A thorough general examination and radiographs of the skull are the minimal requirements. As a general rule, the presence of more than one area of bone erosion is of serious significance.

BENIGN CONDITIONS

1. *Angiomas* rarely cause any diagnostic difficulty. One variety takes the form of a subcutaneous cavernous venous lake, usually but not always with the 'sign of emptying' when compressed, but they are spongy or cystic and can usually be identified correctly even when there is little or no bluish discolouration of the overlying skin.

2. *Subgaleal epidermoid cysts* are not spherical like other inclusion dermoids, and can arise as a firm discoid swelling anywhere beneath the scalp, most often in the temporal, frontal or patietal regions. Despite their pultaceous content they can erode the outer table of the calvarium and lie in the diploic space. Even when there is no intracranial extension, the inner table may also be eroded and the radiological appearance of the defect (Fig. 14.3b) may be mistaken for a malignant erosion or a small encephalocele.

3. *Superficial epidermal inclusion cysts* (external angular 'dermoids') sometimes occur in the frontal region, well above their classical site beneath the eyebrow. Their benign nature is indicated by their typical clinical features and very slow rate of growth. Haemorrhage into the central cavity, possibly following minor trauma, is a rare complication, but dramatically alters the

appearance; there is a sudden increase in size, a purplish discolouration, and hyperaemia of the overlying skin, signs which may suggest a malignant lesion. In any event it should be excised, and the benign nature confirmed by the histology.

4. *A localized compact* (*'ivory'*) *osteoma* is a great rarity and usually occurs in older children as a hard, sessile lesion with typical radiographic features of a dense plaque of bone of uniform texture.

5. Other benign lesions of bone (p. 725), or the scalp may rarely occur in the calvarium, e.g. the giant hairy naevus in infants (p. 842), and the hamartomatous sebaceous naevus (p. 852) in older children.

MALIGNANT CONDITIONS

These are very few and most arise primarily in the calvarium, e.g. the histiocytoses (p. 206) or multiple metastases, most commonly from a neuroblastoma (p. 300). The scalp is occasionally the first site of metastatic deposits in malignant lymphoma.

1. *The histiocytoses.* The general clinical features of this group of conditions are described in Chapter 11 (p. 205), but as each of the various clinical forms may cause erosions in the calvarium, these lesions are described here.

(*a*) *Eosinophilic granuloma of bone.* The calvarium is one of the common sites of this condition; there is only one lesion as a rule, and it is usually a palpable swelling. X-rays reveal an underlying erosion and the absence of sclerosis of the margin or any periosteal reaction (see p. 209), is a distinguishing radiological feature (Fig. 14.1a). Biopsy is required to confirm the diagnosis.

(*b*) *Hand-Schüller-Christian disease.* The onset is insidious, and usually after the age of two years; the bone lesions are multiple (Fig. 14.1b) and the findings on biopsy are usually diagnostic (see p. 212).

(*c*) *Letterer-Siwe disease* confined to those less than two years of age, only occasionally causes localized areas of bone destruction in the skull; the age group, the involvement of lymph nodes, the rash, and the histological findings (p. 215) are distinctive (Fig. 14.1c).

2. *Metastatic neuroblastoma.* This development in the skull usually occurs late in the course of the disease, but in a significant proportion of cases it is the mode of presentation (p. 552). In such cases there is clinical or radiographic evidence of the primary tumour (in the abdomen or thorax) or other evidence of metastases, in the marrow smears, long bones, or peripheral lymph nodes.

3. *Other sources of metastatic deposits* in the calvarium or scalp are more rare, but occur in leukaemia (p. 152), and very rarely as a complication of other tumours, e.g. carcinoma of the thyroid (p. 373).

4. *Malignant lymphomas* occasionally present as nodules in the skin and

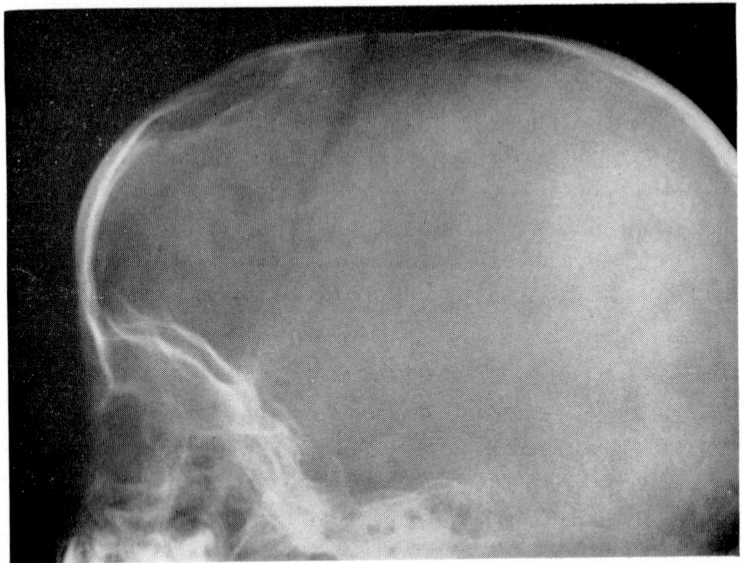

(a)

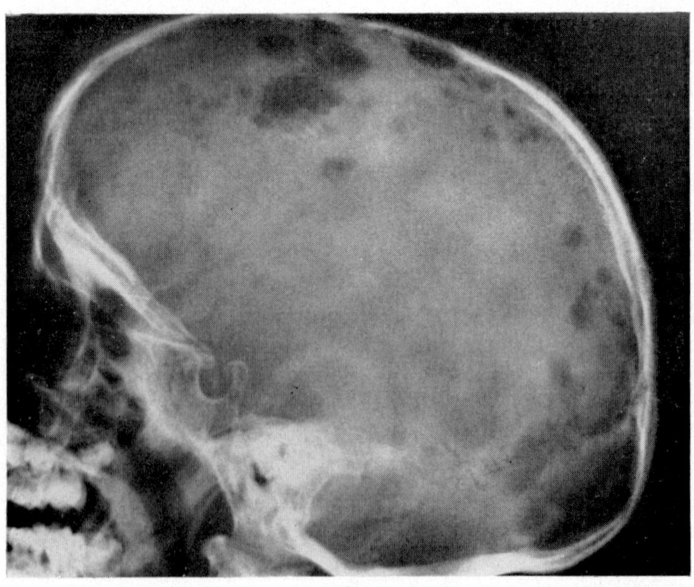

(b)

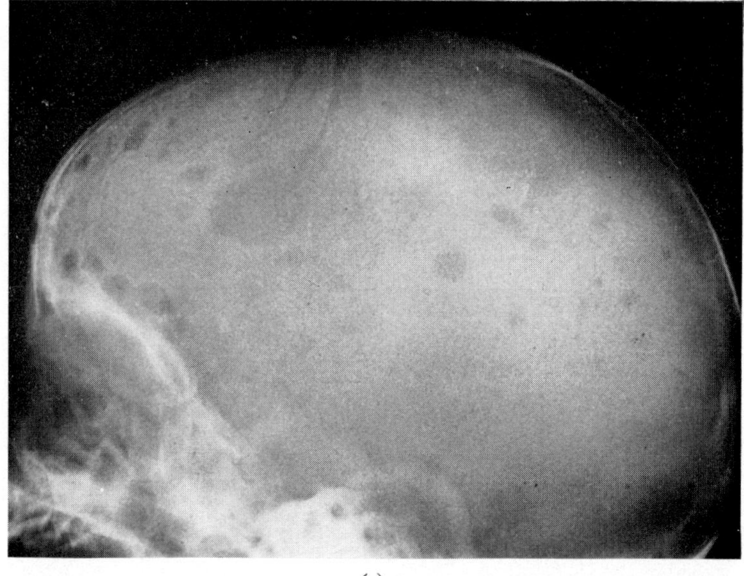

(*c*)

Figure 14.1. (*a*) EOSINOPHILIC GRANULOMA; x-ray of a clear cut defect in the frontal region with no bony reaction (see p. 209); (*b*) HAND-SCHÜLLER-CHRISTIAN SYNDROME; typical multiple punched out defects (see p. 212); (*c*) LETTERER-SIWE DISEASE; small radiolucent defects in the calvarium in infancy (see page 215).

subcutaneous tissues, and in the scalp this may lead to diagnostic difficulties until biopsy reveals their source.

In the Index Series this occurred in two cases; one was a lymphoblastic lymphosarcoma, and in the other the nodules were metastases from a reticulum cell sarcoma.

5. *The melanotic progonoma* is one of the rarest bone lesions in the skull in childhood, and sometimes affects the frontal or occipital bone, but more commonly it arises in the maxilla, and the lesion is described in the section on the jaw (p. 334).

RADIOLOGICAL DIFFERENTIATION OF EROSIONS OF THE CALVARIUM

As well as the conditions mentioned above, erosions are also found in various conditions ranging from developmental anomalies to infections. They can be subdivided according to whether they provoke a periosteal reaction detectable radiographically.

The group with periosteal reaction includes the following:

1. *Osteomyelitis*. The frontal bone is the commonest cranial site of osteomyelitis, but uncommon when compared with long bones. The local signs such as marked tenderness, oedema and hyperaemia as a rule leave little doubt as to the diagnosis, although radiographic findings are here as elsewhere usually absent until ten to fourteen days after the onset of symptoms. Extensive irregular destruction of bone, laminae of periosteal new bone and sequestra (Fig. 14.2a) are typical later findings.

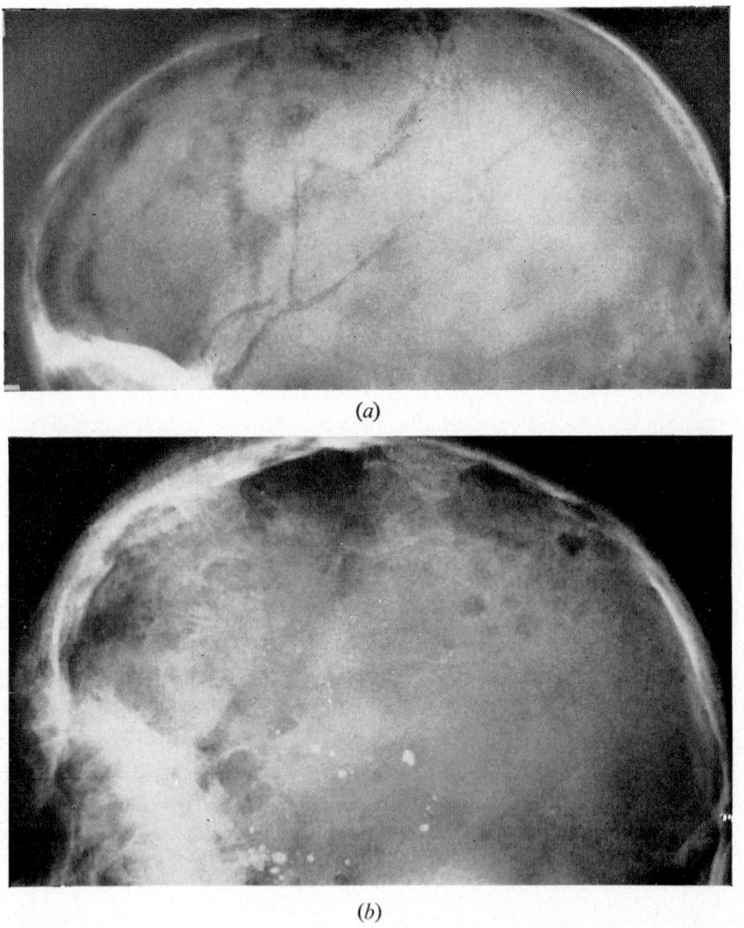

(*a*)

(*b*)

Figure 14.2. (*a*) OSTEOMYELITIS OF THE CALVARIUM; destructive changes predominate, but there is also periosteal new bone, and early evidence of sequestra; (*b*) METASTATIC NEUROBLASTOMA, with extensive destruction and new bone formation; the sutures may also be separated when there are accompanying intracranial metastases.

In chronic osteomyelitis on the other hand, the radiological findings are often equivocal; biopsy is usually required for diagnosis, and the histology may be difficult to interpret (see p. 212).

2. *Metastatic neuroblastoma* also causes much destruction and new bone formation; in this case radiographic changes are present when local symptoms first become apparent, and there are usually multiple small erosions (Fig. 14.2b.).

3. *Interparietal foramina* rarely cause any diagnostic difficulties if the existence of this entity is known. The paired, symmetrical defects (Fig.14.3a) are diagnostic and of no further importance in themselves.

4. *A subgaleal 'dermoid'* (epidermoid cyst) usually causes a fine line of sclerosis around its margin (Fig. 14.3b); the long history and the single discrete swelling are typical.

The nonreactive group contains the following:

5. *The histiocytoses*, whether single or multiple deposits are present, characteristically cause little or no periosteal reaction; the single lesion of an eosinophilic granuloma (Fig. 14.1a) separates it from Hand-Schüller-Christian disease (Fig. 14.1b). The age of the patient (under three years) is helpful in identifying Letterer-Siwe disease, in which bone changes are less common. These three entities are not distinguishable on the minutiae of the radiological appearance alone.

6. *A fibrosarcoma* (See Fig. 22.19) typically causes little or no bony reaction, and can arise in membrane bones, e.g. the clavicle or the mandible, but is exceptionally rare in the skull, and more common in the mandible.

7. *Congenital generalized fibromatosis* (Condon & Allen, 1961) is a very rare

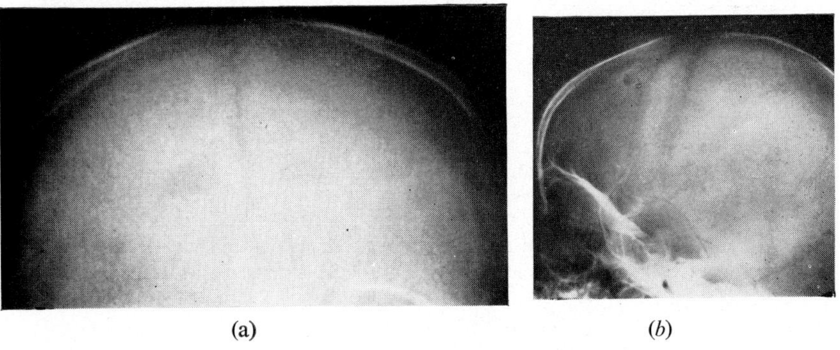

(a) (*b*)

Figure 14.3. (*a*) INTERPARIETAL FORAMINA; inconstant but normally occurring 'defects', usually bilateral when present at all, and of no significance; (*b*) SUBGALEAL EPIDERMOID CYST with a fine line of sclerosis at its margin. In some instances the defect involves both inner and outer tables and the cyst lies in contact with the dura. True intracranial extensions of epidermal remnants are more common in the occipital region.

condition with bone changes in the calvarium (Fig. 14.4) indistinguishable from those of Letterer-Siwe disease. However, in the latter, radiographic changes are rarely present at birth, and in fibromatosis there are multiple, firm spherical swellings in the subcutaneous tissue and muscles throughout the body, e.g. in multiple viscera, including the bowel wall.

8. *Calcification of Pacchionian bodies* rarely occurs before the age of ten years and hence after the age when calvarial metastases from neuroblastoma (less commonly rhabdomyosarcoma, hepatoblastoma, etc.) most commonly arise. Each area of calcification lies in a lacuna of rarefaction, and although typically parasagittal, in some cases, their site, size and number may suggest osteolytic metastases. However, the clearcut margins of the lacuna, and the mature texture of the calcified area within it, are usually distinctive.

9. *Melanotic progonoma*, one of the rarest of calvarial lesions, develops in early infancy and may occur in any of the bones of the vault, or the face (Grave & Mills, 1972), but most commonly in the alveolus (p. 334). Radiologically there is little or no bone reaction, at exploration the tissue is grey to black in colour, and complete excision together with a margin of uninvolved bone is curative.

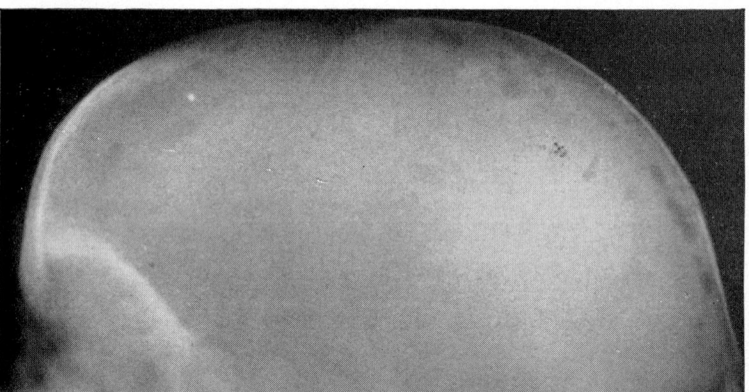

Figure 14.4. CONGENITAL GENERALIZED FIBROMATOSIS; multiple minute defects in the newborn often associated with immune deficiency and death from opportunistic infection; if the infant survives, the lesions may regress (see also Fig. 22.7e, p. 732).

BIOPSY

Even when clinical and radiographic findings are strongly suggestive, the final diagnosis often depends upon histological evidence. The calvarium is a suitable area for aspiration or drill biopsy (see p. 89) and smear techniques

(p. 87), but an open biopsy is often an advantage for it can be combined with curative excision of simple lesions.

The microscopic features of bone lesions are described on p. 736, and the histiocytoses on pp. 207–215.

TREATMENT

The treatment of the histiocytoses is described in Chapter 11 (p. 220), neuroblastoma on p. 558, and fibrosarcoma on p. 764.

B. TUMOURS OF THE FACE

Those arising in the skin are described in Chapter 24, in the eyelid on p. 420, and in lymph nodes in Chapter 12. Other than these, the commonest swellings on the face are those related to the salivary glands or the outer aspects of the jaws (Table 14.2).

THE SALIVARY GLANDS

These are divided into a major group comprising the parotid, submandibular and sublingual gland, and a minor group including all the salivary secreting cells found in the mucous membranes lining the mouth, the lips, alveolus, palate and tongue, any of which may be the site of any of the same benign or malignant tumours as arise in the major salivary glands (Kauffman & Stout, 1963). For practical purposes, this very rarely occurs, except for a mixed salivary tumour arising in the mucoperiosteum of the hard palate (Byars *et al.*, 1957, 1973).

The parotid and submandibular glands differ in their origin and their structure, and even more widely in the relative incidence of conditions affecting them, for example calculi are not uncommon in the submandibular salivary gland but almost unknown in the parotid, at least in children. Both benign and malignant salivary neoplasms are very much more common in the parotid than in the submandibular gland (Rafla, 1970; Castro *et al.*, 1972, Table 14.3).

When considering causes of 'parotid' swellings, conditions affecting the preauricular lymph nodes should also be included, for these nodes are normally situated on the surface of the parotid fascia and may actually lie in indentations in the surface of the gland. Lesions developing in such nodes can be readily misinterpreted as arising in the parotid. A similar intimate anatomical relationship also applies to the submandibular salivary gland and the submandibular group of lymph nodes.

A peculiarity of the parotid gland is the occurrence of nearby but separate small islands of ectopic parotid tissue, for example at the base or tip of the mastoid process, or even further afield in the anterior triangle of the neck.

Table 14.2. Swellings of the face

Benign conditions	Malignant tumours
Parotid tumours	
Parotitis (recurrent)	Carcinoma
Preauricular adenopathies	muco-epidermoid
Haemangioma (of parotid)	acinic cell
Lymphangioma (cystic hygroma)	adenoid cystic
Lobular lymphocytic sialadenosis	
Lympho-epithelial lesions	Malignant lymphoma
Mikulicz's syndrome	(lymphosarcoma)
Benign salivary tumours	
pleomorphic adenoma	
Warthin's tumour	
Soft tissue swellings	
Haemangioma	Sarcomas of soft tissue (p. 781)
Cystic hygroma	rhabdomyosarcoma
Teratoma (of face)	fibrosarcoma
Orbital tumours (p. 401)	
Swellings of the jaws (p. 318)	
Facial skin (p. 837)	
Pyogenic granuloma	Carcinoma
Epidermoid cyst	squamous ⎫ in xeroderma
Pilomatrixoma	basal cell ⎭ pigmentosum
Naevi	Reticulum cell sarcoma (subcutaneous)
junctional	Malignant schwannoma
intradermal	Haemangiopericytoma
compound	Malignant melanoma
Spindle/epithelial cell naevus	
Blue naevus	
Pigmentosa giganthus	
Other benign lesions of skin (p. 845)	

Table 14.3. Tumours of the major salivary glands (all ages) (Castro *et al.*, 1972)

Site	Benign	Malignant	Total	%
Parotid	1227	632	1859	88
Submandibular	104	133	237	11
Sublingual	0	4	4	0·3
Totals	1331	769	2100*	

* 35 additional patients with bilateral or multifocal tumours.

In two patients in the Index Series a pleomorphic salivary adenoma appeared to arise outside the parotid gland, in ectopic parotid tissue in the post-auricular region. Their origin is difficult to document with certainty, particularly as Nicholson (1922) reported salivary ducts and acini in lymph nodes outside the capsule of the parotid.

BENIGN SWELLINGS OF THE PAROTID GLAND

Recurrent parotitis associated with radiological evidence of sialectasis is, after mumps, the commonest cause of parotid swelling in childhood. Repeated episodes lasting five to seven days are followed by complete resolution and rarely cause any diagnostic difficulty.

Congenital superficial haemangiomas or lymphangiomas (cystic hygromas) involving soft tissues in the preauricular area are not uncommon and it is usually obvious that they do not primarily involve the parotid.

A haemangioma, however, can present as a swelling confined to and within the parotid gland, almost always in infancy; it lies beneath the parotid fascia, hence the characteristic spongy texture and the vascular discolouration are usually absent. An intraparotid haemangioma may contain areas with any or all of the histological types: capillary, cavernous and solid, as arise elsewhere (see p. 818), but from the clinical point of view the diagnosis in the parotid is usually only made on biopsy, either an 'open' or, less desirably, a drill biopsy. The latter may cause considerable bleeding, but this can usually be controlled by a firm pressure dressing.

Treatment should be conservative for the natural history is usually the same as in haemangiomas elsewhere: a phase of rapid growth during infancy, followed by considerable regression in the following two to four years. Surgical excision of any residuum may be necessary on cosmetic grounds, assessed after a period of observation, for example at three to four years of age, before the child goes to school. Other benign conditions may arise in or near the parotid and these will be considered in the differential diagnosis of parotid tumours.

TUMOURS OF THE PAROTID GLAND

Compared with other neoplasms in childhood, both benign and malignant parotid tumours (Howard, Rawson *et al.*, 1950) are rare. Only 5% of all parotid tumours occur during childhood, and malignant salivary tumours account for less than 5% of all tumours of the parotid in children (Krolls *et al.*, 1972). This is in accord with the figure of less than 1% for parotid tumours in the Index Series and the figure of 2% for all salivary tumours.

Although larger than the submandibular glands, the relatively much higher incidence of tumours in the parotids cannot be explained on size alone. Benign neoplasms account for more than half of the parotid tumours of childhood (Fig. 14.5) and are therefore considered in the differential diagnosis of malignant tumours (p. 310).

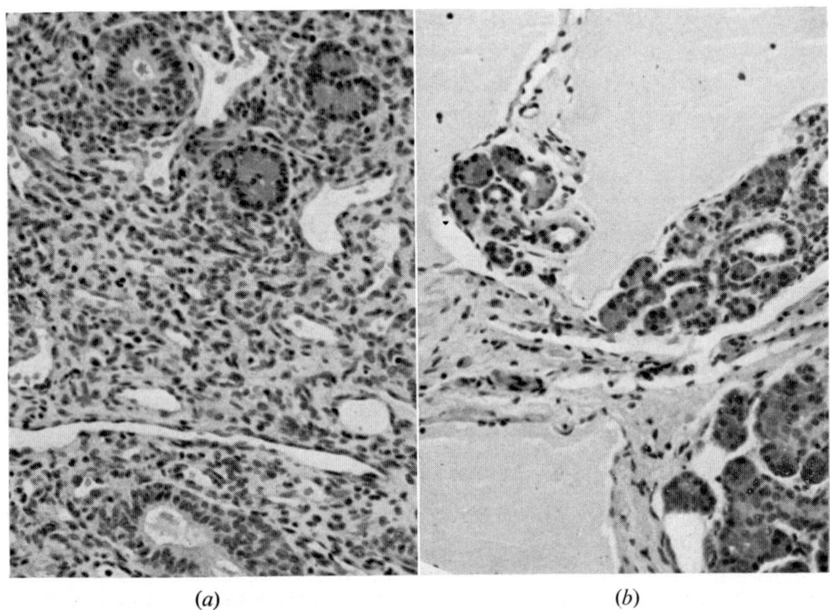

Figure 14.5. BENIGN PAROTID SWELLINGS; (*a*) CAPILLARY HAEMANGIOMA composed of nests of plump endothelial cells displacing individual acini and ducts (H & E. × 130); (*b*) LYMPHANGIOMA containing lymph-filled spaces between islands of acini (H & E. × 130).

ECTOPIC PAROTID TISSUE

A possible source of confusion is parotid tumours is that islets of ectopic salivary tissue are not infrequently found in lymph nodes in the upper cervical region, close to but separate from the parotid (Thackray & Lucas, 1974). A salivary tumour arising in ectopic tissue of this kind can lead to the incorrect conclusion that (i) as the tumour is separate from the gland clinically, it cannot be of salivary origin, or that (ii) benign tumour tissue in a lymph node represents a malignant metastasis.

Ectopic parotid tissue not associated with lymphoid folicles can also occur in the neck (Rothner, 1973) from the angle of the mandible as far caudally as the clavicle (Youngs & Scofield, 1967) and this, too, may be the site of a salivary tumour.

Malignant tumours of the parotid gland are as follows.

I. MUCO-EPIDERMOID CARCINOMA

This is the commonest type of malignant salivary gland tumour and is thought to arise from duct cells (Foote & Frazell, 1953; Healey *et al.*, 1970) (Fig. 14.6). The tumour contains both mucus-secreting and epidermoid cells, and in most examples there is a third type of cell intermediate between the mucus-

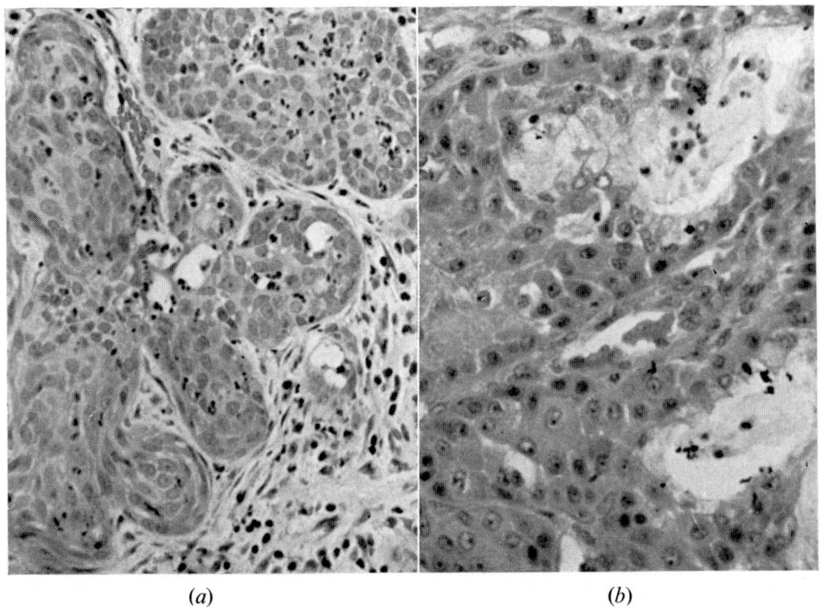

(*a*) (*b*)

Figure 14.6. MUCO-EPIDERMOID CARCINOMA; (*a*) groups of cells with squamous differentiation (H & E. × 200); (*b*) 'intermediate' cells, also showing squamous differentiation (centre), and forming two glandular spaces (to the right) containing mucus staining positively with alcian blue (H & E. × 500).

secreting columnar cells and the squamous cells; in a few tumours this intermediate type dominates the histological picture and may lead to difficulties in histological diagnosis.

In the literature, over 90% of muco-epidermoid tumours are found in the parotid, and in the Index Series all arose there.

MACROSCOPIC APPEARANCES

The tumour is 2–3 cm in diameter and often mistaken for a benign mixed salivary tumour because it has usually been present for some months and has a slow rate of growth. It is usually oval, unencapsulated, and contains cystic areas filled with clear or blood-stained mucus. The solid portions of the tumour are usually yellowish pink, and may be lobulated.

In the Index Series, two of these tumours appeared to arise outside the capsule of the parotid; one had no capsule and infiltrated the adjacent muscle and dermis.

MICROSCOPIC FINDINGS

Characteristically the tumour is pleomorphic and composed or irregular glandular structures enclosing lakes of mucus, alternating with sheets of 'intermediate' cells in which there are nests of squamous epithelial cells. All of the tumours in the Index Series were well differentiated, but there is a group in which the intermediate cell is dominant and this can be correlated with a more malignant clinical course.

Multiple sections and special stains for mucus are required to demonstrate the mucus-containing cells on which the correct diagnosis of muco-epidermoid carcinoma depends. Histochemical stains confirm the ductular origin of the tumour, for as well as cytological similarities, the pattern of acid and alkaline phosphatase activity in duct cells and in the glandular portion of the tumour are almost identical.

The pleomorphism of these tumours is exemplified by one case in the Index Series, a tumour initially thought to be a tuberculous lymph node in the capsule of the parotid gland and incompletely excised. When the histological diagnosis was established, a further excision was carried out. In the original specimen, intermediate and mucus-secreting cells predominated, while material from the second excision contained extensive sheets of squamous epithelial cells, as well as the other cell types.

SPREAD

The rate of growth tends to be slow, and this tumour is noted for local recurrence and relative radio-insensitivity. The more malignant tumours may recur rapidly and metastasize, but these are the minority. Spread to the regional lymph nodes occurs, but distant metastases are rare.

II. ACINIC CELL CARCINOMA
(syn. adenocarcinoma; carcinoma adenomatosum)

This is extremely rare, but in the series reported by Krolls *et al.* (1972), one third were classified as this type. Usually thought to be a pleomorphic salivary adenoma before operation, the true diagnosis is not made until the histology has been studied.

Microscopically there are irregular glandular formations composed of cells with a finely granular or water-clear cytoplasm, resembling the acinic or secreting cells of the salivary gland. Their malignant potential is low. None was recognized in the Index Series.

III. ADENOID CYSTIC AND OTHER CARCINOMAS

In most large series a few unclassifiable tumours are found. They appear to be adenocarcinomas, and may be anaplastic adenoid cystic carcinomas or possibly malignant pleomorphic salivary adenomas. None was identified in the Index Series.

IV. MALIGNANT MESENCHYMAL SALIVARY TUMOURS

These, like carcinomas, are almost confined to the parotid gland in children and their pathological features are the same as mesenchymal tumours arising elsewhere (see Chapter 23).

In the Index Series two rhabdomyosarcomas and one fibrosarcoma arose in the parotid gland (Fig. 14.7d).

V. MALIGNANT LYMPHOMAS OF THE PAROTID

These occasionally arise in the parotid (Johnson & Samuel, 1966), and only rarely in the submandibular glands. Most are lymphosarcomas, and in children the lymphoblastic type predominates. Their differentiation from benign lympho-epithelial lesions (p. 314) and from benign lobular lymphocytic infiltration (p. 314) is of great importance (Fig. 14.8).

The Index Series. One child had an enlargement of the parotid for some months and the gland was partially excised. The histology was at first interpreted as a lymphocytic lymphosarcoma of the follicular type, and treated by radiation. Review of the sections showed diffuse lymphocytic infiltration of lobules of parotid tissues, and in some parts almost complete replacement of the normal glandular elements. Ill-defined follicles were present in the lymphoid collections, but nowhere did the cells transgress the connective tissue boundaries of the lobules; the lymphocytes were regular and showed no cytological features of malignancy. There is no doubt in retrospect, that this lesion is benign.

Lymphoblastic lymphosarcoma can be readily identified (see p. 171), but a reticulum cell sarcoma may be more difficult, especially if the reticulum pattern is relied upon for the diagnosis.

Hodgkin's disease very rarely affects the salivary glands primarily.

Leukaemia can cause diffuse enlargement of one or more of the salivary glands and, rarely, this is the presenting manifestation of the disease. In the Index Series, Mikulicz's syndrome with involvement of the parotid and lacrymal glands was the mode of presentation of acute lymphatic leukaemia in two children; in other cases leukaemic deposits in the testicle and the orbit occurred.

With the possible exception of leukaemia, a neuroblastoma is the only tumour in childhood likely to present with metastases in a salivary gland, but both are extremely rare.

MODE OF PRESENTATION OF PAROTID TUMOURS

The patient is nearly always more than five years old, with a history of a swelling for some weeks or even months; the swelling is painless and often appears to be quite superficial, localized, and smooth or slightly lobulated. Not infrequently it is initially thought to be an enlarged preauricular lymph node, but its attachment to the parotid and slow but steady increase in size belie this. There are usually no other clinical findings.

INVESTIGATIONS

The role of sialography in the diagnosis of intraparotid swellings is increasing, and distortion of the subsidiary ducts by and around a tumour can be readily demonstrated. It is still debatable whether there are any sialographic findings which can be taken as definite indications of invasion and so distinguish malignant from benign lesions. Radiosialography (Gates, 1972) may provide additional information.

CLINICAL DIFFERENTIATION OF BENIGN AND MALIGNANT TUMOURS OF THE PAROTID

As a general rule, malignant tumours grow more rapidly than benign tumours, but this is rarely helpful in differentiating them in children, who usually present with a small swelling, 'just noticed'.

Although invasion of the facial nerve causing palsy is a classic sign of malignancy in adults, it almost never occurs in malignant tumours in children.

Non-parotid swellings

Apart from diseases affecting the preauricular nodes, few other conditions can be mistaken for a parotid tumour when the lesion is small and well-defined.

1. *Tuberculosis of the preauricular nodes.* This group of nodes is one of the two most commonly infected with anonymous mycobacteria (see p. 224), and implicates the conjuctiva as a possible portal of entry. In the early proliferative phase, this type of tuberculosis can be difficult to exclude from other causes of enlarged, tender, fixed nodes.

Multiple Mantoux tests using PPD (Human) and at least one other antigen, preferably from the locally prevalent strain, can be helpful; otherwise differentiation may only be possible at exploration and biopsy.

2. *Metastases in cervical nodes.* Very rarely there may be metastatic involvement of the parotid nodes, e.g. from an advanced retinoblastoma, but the primary is usually diagnosed before metastasis occurs, except in malignant tumours of the nasopharynx (p. 356).

3. *Rhabdomyosarcoma* of soft tissues adjacent to the parotid occur rarely, for example in masseter muscle, and the diagnosis usually depends on exploration and biopsy.

4. *Fibro-osseous dysplasia* of the facial bones (p. 331) occasionally resembles a parotid tumour.

Non-salivary tumours in the parotid

5. *Intraparotid haemangioma.* Most cases occur in the first year of life, when salivary tumours are extremely rare. In an older child a haemangioma could cause difficulties only resolved by exploration (Fig. 14.5a). This also applies to other rare mesenchymal lesions such as an intraparotid lipoma, neurofibroma, neurilemmona or xanthoma.

6. *Mikulicz's syndrome* is rarely confined to one parotid; it may be possible to determine clinically that the whole of the gland is uniformly enlarged. Among the possible causes are leukaemia and Hodgkin's disease.

7. *Sarcomas* arising in the parotid, e.g. rhabdomyosarcoma or fibrosarcoma, are extremely rare and seldom distinguished before exploration.

BIOPSY OF PAROTID TUMOURS

The lack of distinctive clinical findings by which benign and malignant parotid tumours can be distinguished might suggest the need for preliminary incision biopsy, but the majority of parotid tumours, whether benign or malignant, are adequately treated by total removal, together with a reasonable margin of normal surrounding tissue. Partial excision carries the general disadvantage of interfering with tissue planes to be entered during any subsequent operation, and the specific risk of dispersing tumour cells leading to local recurrence, which can occur by implantation even in benign tumours such as a pleomorphic adenoma.

Incision biopsy should be reserved for conditions which (i) appear at operation to affect the greater part or all of the parotid, or, rarely, (ii) when there is obviously extensive malignant disease and histological diagnosis is required primarily to determine the most appropriate method of treatment (Thackray & Lucas, 1974).

Excision biopsy

The principles are the same as those observed in all operations on the parotid (Anderson & Byars, 1965):

1. An incision planned to provide adequate exposure, i.e. a vertical incision closely following the anterior attachment of the pinna, curving beneath and behind the lobe of the ear, and then forward caudal to the subcutaneous border of the mandible.
2. Identification of the trunk of the facial nerve, tracing the subdivisions forwards or upwards into the parotid and towards the tumour.
3. Removal of the tumour and also an adequate margin of adjacent normal gland tissue, without spillage, from between the cleared and retracted branches of the nerve (Byars *et al.*, 1957).

Almost every benign tumour displaces some branch of the nerve; a nerve-stimulator may be helpful, but may stimulate too much of the nerve; gentle mechanical stimulation, e.g. with a pair of fine non-tooth forceps, can be equally effective.

HISTOLOGICAL DIFFERENTIATION OF BENIGN PAROTID LESIONS

1. *The pleormorphic salivary adenoma* (syn. mixed salivary tumour) is the commonest benign epithelial neoplasm of the parotid in childhood. Most occur in older children (Fig 14.7) (as do muco-epidermoid carcinomas).

Macroscopically they are grey, firm to hard, lobulated, and apparently encapsulated, with a somewhat slimy cut surface.

Microscopically the typical findings are strands of polygonal epitheloid cells streaming off and fading out into rather mucoid stromal tissue containing islands of tissue resembling cartilage.

Occasionally this tumour has a malignant potential, but in the Index Series there has been no instance of local recurrence after excision and, as pre-

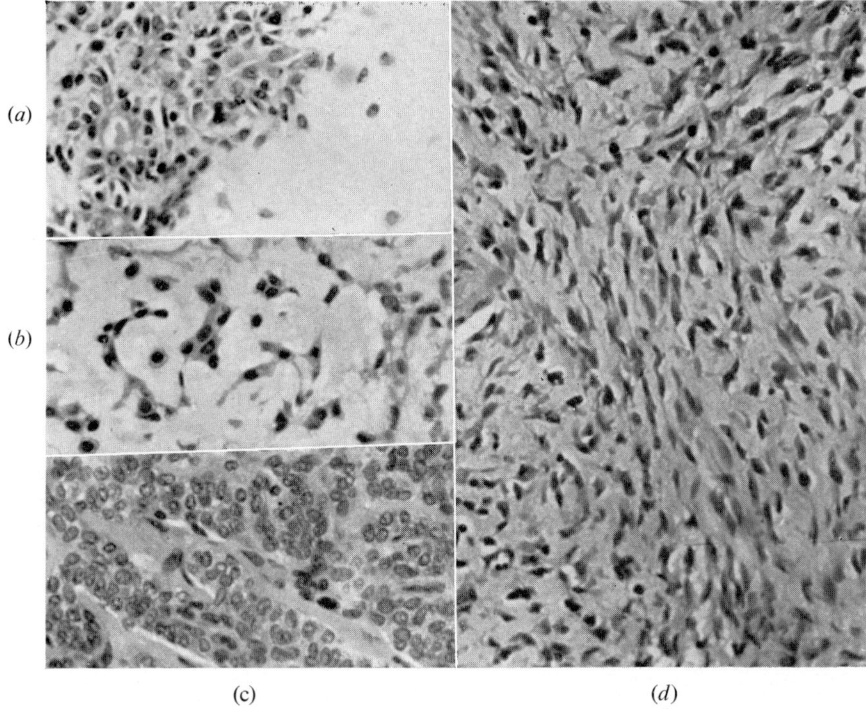

Figure 14.7. PLEOMORPHIC SALIVARY ADENOMA; (*a*) cells streaming (to the right) into areas of 'chondroid' mucus; (*b*) mucoid matrix between compressed stellate cells; (*c*) more rounded nuclei, in cells arranged in linear tubular pattern (all H & E. × 200); (*d*) FIBROSARCOMA OF THE PAROTID for comparison, with typical interlacing pattern of spindle cells (H & E. × 200).

dicted from their histological appearance, they have all followed a benign course.

2. *Warthin's tumour* (syn. adenolymphoma, papillary cystic adenoma, adenoma lymphomatosum). This is composed of papillary epithelial formations intermingled with lymphoid cells usually containing germinal centres. They are very rare in childhood and in Kroll's extensive series there were only two typical examples; surgical excision is curative.

None was seen in the Index Series.

3. *Benign mesenchymal tumours.*

(*a*) *A haemangioma* of the parotid is probably the most common and the most important intraparotid lesion. It is confined beneath the parotid capsule and may affect only some of the lobules of the gland (Fig. 14.5a).

In some cases the diagnosis can only be made by excision, particularly when the lesion is extremely cellular and relatively avascular. In this type the clinical findings are not suggestive of an angioma, and even the macroscopic appearance at operation may suggest a tumour, since the affected lobules are firm, pink, fleshy and solid (Howard, Rawson *et al.*, 1950).

Microscopically there is extensive disruption of individual lobules by infiltrating, capillary angiomatous vessels with plump lining cells. The occasionally alarming histological appearance in infancy of haemangio-endotheliomas is noted elsewhere (p. 819), but invariably benign in children.

(*b*) *Lymphangiomas*, of the parotid and very occasionally the submandibular gland, are much less common than haemangiomas. They are usually more obviously cystic, and microscopically this is borne out by ectatic lymph-angiomatous spaces of varying size, filled with lymph and displacing normal parotid tissue (Fig. 14.5b). Infiltration or involvement of adjacent soft tissues outside the capsule of a gland may also occur.

(*c*) *Other hamartomas* such as mesenchymal tissues composed of fat, fibrous tissue or muscle can occur in the parotid. They are quite benign and of no particular histological importance.

4. *Lobular lymphocytic infiltration of the parotid.* This appears to be a definite entity which presents clinically as a unilateral, diffuse, painless enlargement of the gland, and is to be distinguished from a deeply situated or diffuse malignant tumour (Fig. 14.8). The chief importance of these lesions is their differentiation from lymphosarcoma (p. 171).

Macroscopically the gland is firm and white, and the lobular pattern is usually preserved.

Microscopically the individual lobules are disrupted and replaced by sheets of lymphocytes containing germinal centres. Here and there ducts and acini may survive in a sea of lymphocytes, but often they are completely replaced. Characteristically, while some lobules may be completely replaced by lymphoid tissue, immediately adjacent lobules are almost completely normal or at most contain only a few islands of lymphoid cells.

The nature of this lesion is unclear and may be a type of inflammatory response, but it has recently been suggested that it may be a hamartoma of lymphoid tissue. In one case in the Index Series, an obvious lymphangioma of the parotid, several lobules were replaced by lymphoid tissue with the same appearance as lobular lymphocytic infiltration.

5. *Benign lympho-epithelial lesion.* This entity, described by Foote & Frazell (1953), consists of diffuse lymphocytic infiltration associated with proliferation of ductal and periductal cells in irregular masses scattered among the lymphoid tissue. It is apparently rare in childhood and none was seen in the Index Series. The histogenesis is obscure, and again it may represent an inflammatory process, possibly viral in origin.

SUMMARY

Tumours of the salivary glands in children are almost entirely confined to the

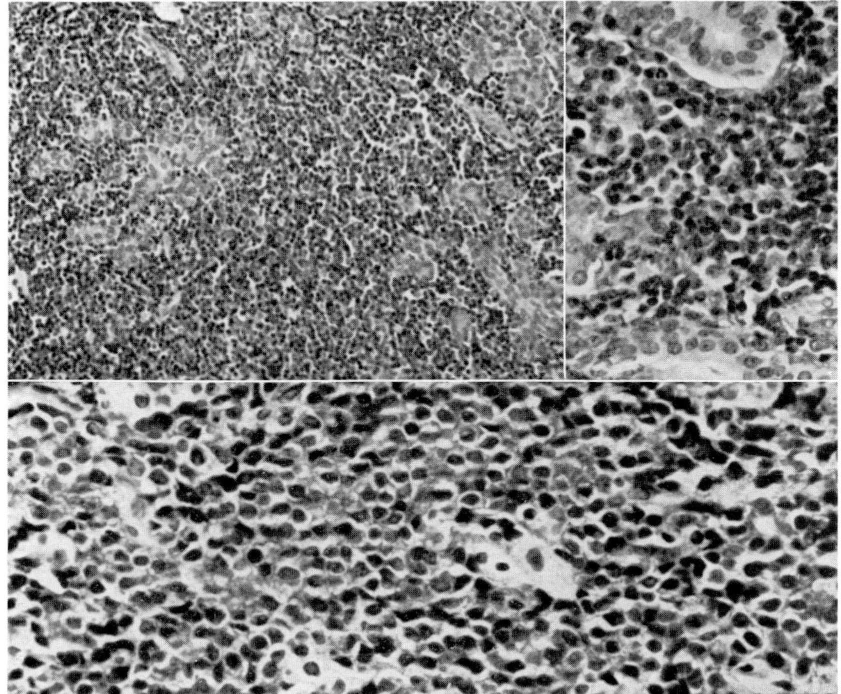

Figure 14.8. BENIGN LYMPHOCYTIC INFILTRATION (PAROTID); (*a*) the dense infiltrate of mature lymphocytes is confined by lobular septa (H & E. × 30); and (*b*) displaces, without destroying, the acini and ducts (H & E. × 300) and, for comparison (*c*) lymphosarcoma of the parotid, which replaces the gland with a sheet of lymphoblasts (H & E. × 300).

[(*a*) *Top left*. (*b*) *Top right*. (*c*) *Bottom*.

parotid, and the great majority are benign. Hamartomas of vascular, lymphatic, and possibly lymphoid types occur.

Pleomorphic salivary adenomas are the commonest true tumours, and muco-epidermoid carcinoma heads the list of malignant neoplasms.

Malignant lymphomas and other malignant mesenchymal tumours such as rhabdomyosarcoma and fibrosarcoma are rare, but should be considered in the differential diagnosis of enlargement of any of the major salivary glands.

All types of salivary tumours accounted for a little less than 2% of all the tumours in the Index Series; malignant salivary neoplasms accounting for much less than 1% of the total. However, in spite of their rarity, it is important to realize that malignant neoplasms of the parotid can occur in children; most arise in early adolescence, but a few cases occur in toddlers.

TREATMENT

Because of the mode of presentation, the tendency for parotid tumours to recur after excision (in at least 25% of muco-epidermoid carcinoma), and the fact that some malignant tumours may falsely appear to be encapsulated, the details of the excision biopsy are of particular importance.

A generous margin of macroscopically uninvolved parotid tissue should be excised when a tumour is to be removed, and the principles of exposure and excision have been described by Anderson & Byars (1965).

If subsequent histological studies show that the tumour is a carcinoma, radiation may be required.

Radiotherapy plays an important part in the treatment of malignant parotid tumours, after excision; a dose of 2500 to 3000 rads in approximately three weeks is usually given.

Chemotherapy. At present chemotherapy plays little or no part in the treatment of tumours of the parotid.

PROGNOSIS

With reasonably early diagnosis, complete excision of the tumour and no evidence of metastasis in the relevant lymph nodes (Stage I), five-year survival rates of 90% are to be expected.

When lymph node metastases are present (Stage II), the survival rates are lower, but may be as high as 75–80%.

TERATOMA OF THE FACE

The common sites of teratomas are shown in Fig. 2.1 but a teratoma can arise almost anywhere in the body, in the nasopharynx (Crook, 1965), the orbit (Jensen, 1969), the tongue (Grier *et al.*, 1967), and the palate (Willis, 1962).

A series of five children with a teratoma of the face and very similar clinical features has been reported by Gifford and MacCollum (1972). In each case the mass was 5 to 12 cm in size, and present at or shortly after birth. All were on the side of the face, in the cheek, extending from above the zygomatic arch to the lower border of the mandible. They were varied in consistency, ranging from softly cystic to rubbery, and four of the five tumours showed transillumination. All were excised, three of them completely; in the two incompletely removed the tumour recurred, in one case causing pulmonary metastases, and in both children the tumour proved to be unresponsive to radiotherapy and fatal.

Microscopically all five were teratomas containing a preponderance of neural tissues, with areas resembling choroid plexus, and two of the five contained areas of calcification.

TREATMENT

Early and complete excision is apparently as important in achieving a permanent cure as in teratomas of the sacrococcygeal region (p. 718). When excision is incomplete, the appearance of a malignant recurrence is likely, and in both facial and sacrococcygeal teratomas, the malignant tissue is usually an endodermal sinus tumour (p. 692) in the terminology suggested by Teilum (1959).

OTHER SWELLINGS OF THE FACE

Rhabdomyosarcoma can arise in the cheek (Donaldson *et al.*, 1973), in the region of masseter muscle, or in the orbit (p. 402).

Metastatic neuroblastoma of the orbital bones (p. 408) or primary Ewing's tumour (p. 735) can cause painless localized swellings of the upper part of the face.

Osteosarcoma or fibrosarcoma. The facial bones are among the rarest sites for these tumours; the clinical features and differential diagnosis is mentioned on p. 326, and the principles of treatment are described in the chapters on sarcomas of bone (p. 723) and soft tissues (p. 776).

Fibro-osseous dysplasia (syn. osteofibroma, leontiasis ossea etc.) predominantly affect the bones of the jaws, chiefly their external aspect (p. 332), but occasionally the inner surfaces, e.g. of the maxilla (p. 343) or the nose (p. 363).

C. SWELLINGS IN THE MOUTH

The mouth lends itself so well to direct inspection and palpation that a topographic classification of swellings based on the exact anatomical situation is practical (Table 14.4).

In many cases the site of the lesion together with the age of the patient, the history and the macroscopic appearance of the swelling, point to the probable diagnosis (Bhaskar, 1963; Jones, 1965, 1966; Conley, 1970; Jaffe, 1972).

THE TONGUE

Most enlargements of the tongue are benign hamartomas, and choristomas are probably the commonest type of lesion if haemangiomas and lymphangiomas are excluded.

1. *Idiopathic macroglossia* causes symmetrical enlargement present at birth, and is not likely to be mistaken for a tumour. Choristomas are usually present at birth and are sometimes referred to as teratomas, for they may contain tissues several types of tissue, mostly of mesodermal origin, e.g. cartilage, bone, blood vessels, occasionally glandular acini, nerves and glial tissue. The granular cell 'myoblastoma' (p. 857) is also found in the tongue and is probably a form of hamartoma. True teratomas of the tongue also occur (Grier & MacNerland, 1967).

2. *Haemangiomas of the tongue* present the same range of types as those found elsewhere (p. 818). The larger examples may cause difficulties in swallowing and breathing, which can be life-threatening, particularly in early infancy; tracheostomy and/or gastrostomy may be required. Those of lesser size can be expected to regress spontaneously, at least partially, and in the absence of symptoms they should be left to do so when they present in the first year of life.

3. *Lymphangiomas* are relatively common (Koop & Moschakis, 1961) and those confined to the tongue often cause asymmetric enlargement and some degree of ankyloglossia. More extensive lesions may be only part of a more generalized cystic hygroma (see below).

The typical features of a lymphangioma of the tongue are the presence of small translucent cysts resembling blisters on the surface of the tongue, the

Table 14.4. Swellings in the mouth and oropharynx

Benign lesions	Malignant tumours
Tongue	
Macroglossia	Rhabdomyosarcoma
(Beckwith or other syndromes)	Fibrosarcoma
Hamartoma or choristoma	
Lymphangioma	Other sarcomas of soft tissues (p. 776)
Haemangioma	
Papilloma	Squamous carcinoma
Pyogenic granuloma	
Granular cell tumour	
Teratoma	
Cystic hygroma	
Cretinism	
Neurofibroma	
Thyroid cyst	
Thyroglossal duct cyst	
Lingual thyroid	
Multiple neurinomas	

Table 14.4 continued

The jaws	
'Epulis'	Histiocytosis X
congenital (granular cell tumour)	eosinophilic granuloma
vascular (haemangioma)	Ewing's tumour
fibrous (pyogenic granuloma)	Rhabdomyosarcoma
giant cell (reparative giant cell granuloma)	Burkitt's tumour
Gingival hypertrophy	Chondrosarcoma
Paradental abscess	Carcinoma of minor salivary glands
Osteomyelitis	muco-epidermoid
Osteochondroma	undifferentiated
Aneurysmal bone cyst	Squamous carcinoma
Fibrous dysplasia	Metastatic deposits from:
cherubism	neuroblastoma
osteofibroma	leukaemias
benign osteoblastoma	lymphomas
Odontogenic cysts and swellings	retinoblastoma
	Wilms' tumour
	Fibrosarcoma
	Osteosarcoma
	Malignant odontogenic tumours

Mucous membrane	
Retention cyst of mucous gland	Lymphosarcoma
Salivary tumours	Reticulum cell sarcoma
pleomorphic adenoma	Salivary carcinoma
Cystic hygroma	mucoepidermoid
Ranula	undifferentiated
Submandibular calculus	Squamous carcinoma
Multiple mucosal neurinomas (p. 563)	

Oropharyngeal isthmus and tonsil	
Enlarged tonsils	Lymphosarcoma
Quinsy	Rhabdomyosarcoma
Haemangioma	Fibrosarcoma
Lateral pharyngeal abscess	Reticulum cell sarcoma
Osteomyelitis of cervical vertebrae	
coccal	
tuberculous	
Juvenile angiofibroma	

'woody' texture on palpation, and its restricted malleability. Microscopically the superficial location is obvious, the thin-walled lymphatic vessels lying immediately beneath the squamous epithelium stretching it to form blebs.

4. *Cystic hygromas* involving the tongue rarely present any diagnostic difficulties for there is usually diffuse involvement of the floor of the mouth and

the submandibular region, often continuous with an extensive and sometimes enormous anterior and lateral cervical mass causing opisthotonus and life-threatening respiratory distress. Attempts at surgical excision can be effective, but are often followed by considerable post-operative oedema which, at least temporarily, results in an even more extensive swelling. Haemorrhage into a cystic space, or superadded infection may occur spontaneously, or after operation, and cause additional swelling.

Other rare swellings involving the tongue are as follows.

5. *Plexiform neurofibroma* (p. 823), either localized or diffuse.

6. *Lingual ectopic thyroid*, typically a more or less spherical swelling on the dorsum of the tongue in the region of the foramen caecum (Neinas *et al.*, 1973), usually producing distortion of speech and 'snorting' or snoring during sleep. Its importance lies in the fact that in most cases the lingual thyroid is the only thyroid tissue the patient possesses. The absence of normotopic thyroid tissue can be established by radionucleide uptake scintillography (Al-Hindawi *et al.*, 1969), or by exploration. Removal of the lingual thyroid and autotransplantation into a suitable muscle has been performed successfully (Jones, 1961).

7. *A cyst of thyroid origin* in the same position, and producing the same clinical symptoms and signs, is probably more common than true total lingual ectopia.

8. *Ludwig's angina* (infective cellulitis of the floor of the mouth) in its fully established form has the appearance of enlargement of the tongue accompanied by ankyloglossia, and with extensive oedema of the floor of the mouth and the submental region. Death has been ascribed to oedema of the glottis, but this is probably a terminal event, and the immediate cause of obstructive asphyxia is the pressure of the oedema forcing the tongue posteriorly against the posterior pharyngeal wall, thus cutting off the airway (Donald, 1948). Although the primary condition may be extensive cellulitis, this should not be assumed to be the only element present until the space between the genioglossus and genihyoid muscles has been explored for a loculus of pus, often under great tension. This loculus can be approached in the midline in the submental region, under local anaesthesia if necessary, passing a pair of forceps through the mylohyoid raphe into the region of the genial tubercles. When pus under pressure is discovered there is usually immediate improvement; if not, tracheostomy may be required.

9. *Macroglossia* as an isolated congenital abnormality is rare, and more likely to occur as part of a group of conditions, e.g. in Beckwith's syndrome with visceromegaly, exomphalos and hypoglycaemia (Beckwith, 1969), in the mucopolysaccharidoses (Types I, II and III), or as focal or regional giantism due to diffuse plexiform neurofibromatosis (p. 419) or lymphangiomatosis.

10. *Localized tumours and cysts* in the tongue are rarities, mostly in the posterior third of the tongue, and may cause respiratory obstruction. Lofgren

(1963) reviewed fourteen cases in infants, and noted that in eight of them the diagnosis had been made at autopsy. Cystic lesions outnumber solid lesions, and of the latter a lingual thyroid appears to be the commonest. A cystic swelling may be a dermoid, a retention cyst of a mucous gland or a cyst of a lingual duct. Symptoms begin in early infancy, chiefly as feeding difficulties. An important feature of these cystic lesions is that they fluctuate in size and may enlarge very rapidly, e.g. during respiratory infections, and cause acute respiratory distress.

The cyst can usually be seen and palpated, delineated in lateral radiographs, and can be aspirated in an emergency, followed by marsupialization or excision.

11. *Multiple submucosal 'neurinomas'*, of the tongue, oral mucous membrane and lip ('bumpy lip' syndrome) are part of a rare group of conditions, Sipple's syndrome, (p. 563).

MALIGNANT TUMOURS OF THE TONGUE

RHABDOMYOSARCOMA

This is the commonest primary malignant tumour of the tongue, but the tongue is a less common site for this tumour than the cheek, the soft palate, the wall of the pharynx, and the recesses of the nasopharynx (Dito & Batsakis, 1963; Donaldson *et al.*, 1973).

Rapid asymmetric enlargement of the tongue, usually developing within the first five years of life, should suggest the possibility of an embryonic rhabdomyosarcoma. These lesions also occasionally present as a polyp which ulcerates and bleeds.

A biopsy is required for confirmation of the diagnosis (O'Day *et al.*, 1965) and the prognosis has been improved considerably in recent years by the integration of partial excision, followed by radiotherapy and recurring courses of chemotherapy with cytotoxic agents (Donaldson *et al.*, 1973). When possible the tumour and a generous margin of uninvolved tissue should be excised, and even when the tongue is considerably reduced in size, it can prove to be remarkably effective in performing its functions. Treatment of rhabdomyosarcoma is described on p. 789.

THE JAWS

Most swellings of the jaws are benign lesions, chiefly hamartomas, benign neoplasms, reactive inflammatory lesions, or dysplasias and cysts; the latter two are remarkable for their diversity of types (p. 336). Malignant tumours of bone or mucous membrane are extremely rare in children.

Swellings arising in the mouth, excluding the tongue, can be classified according to the four types of tissue from which they arise:

1. *The mucous membrane*, including mucous and salivary gland epithelium which covers the palate, the buccal and lingual aspects of the jaws, and the inner aspect of the cheeks.
2. *The alveolus and the basal bone* forming the maxilla, mandible and palate.
3. *Connective tissues* and muscles attached to the jaws.
4. *The odontogenic epithelium* (also ectodermal in origin) which has the capacity to induce metaplasia in adjacent mesoderm, normally leading to the formation of the tooth buds. This inductive force is retained by cells derived from the odontogenic epithelium and accounts for the broad spectrum of tumour types which may arise, e.g. odontomas (p. 341), ameloblastomas (p. 340), dentinomas and cementomas (p. 341).

The torus palatinus is remarkably well developed in some individuals and may be a hemispherical sessile swelling up to 1 cm in height and 2–3 cm in diameter. When such a swelling on the palate is suddenly found by the patient or first noted during examination of the mouth, it may be mistaken for a tumour, for example a pleomorphic adenoma of salivary gland origin (p. 312), which occasionally arises in the mucoperiosteum covering the hard palate. The strictly median position of the swelling provides a clue to the diagnosis; when small, it will probably be identified correctly, but in large examples biopsy may be required to confirm its inconsequential nature.

1. THE MUCOUS MEMBRANE

The mucous membrane, composed of modified squamous epithelium, salivary and mucous glands, is rarely the site of a true tumour, the commonest lesion being a retention cyst in the form of a pearly white, almost translucent, cystic swelling, rarely more than 1 cm in diameter.

Papillomas, filiform or sessile, are probably viral in origin but seldom associated with verruca of the hands; they are not uncommon and can be readily removed.

Malignant tumours are exceptionally rare, and these are as follows:

SQUAMOUS CARCINOMA

Squamous carcinoma is very uncommon in childhood, but 40 of the 48 cases of squamous carcinoma in childhood, collected from the world literature by Moore (1958), arose in the mouth or pharynx. Willis (1962) reviewed four cases in children, and Jones (1966) added another, an alveolar tumour in a four-year old girl, who survived despite a local recurrence and metastasis in a submandibular lymph node. In this case there was some evidence suggesting that the primary may have arisen from ameloblastic epithelium.

SALIVARY CARCINOMA

All types of salivary tumours arising from mucous membrane or muco-periosteum in the mouth are exceptionally rare in childhood. Benign pleomorphic adenomas (p. 312) are more common. Muco-epithelial carcinoma is probably the commonest type of carcinoma, but the only one in a series of 161 oral tumours reported by Jones (1966) was undifferentiated, and in the series of 60 tumours of the jaws reviewed by Dehner (1973) there were no salivary tumours, benign or malignant.

2. THE ALVEOLAR AND BASAL BONES

Tumours arising in or from the bone forming the alveolus, the jaws or the overlying soft tissues in childhood, are classified as follows:

Benign swellings:
Hypertrophic gingivitis
Fibromatosis gingivae
Pyogenic granuloma
(syn. fibrous/vascular epulis)
Granular cell tumour
(syn. congenital epulis)
Giant cell (reparative) granuloma
Aneurysmal bone cyst
Eosinophilic granuloma
Chondroma
Fibrous dysplasias
Teratoma (of face see p. 316)
Benign odontogenic tumours or
cysts (p. 340)
Melanotic progonoma (p. 334)

Malignant tumours:
Osteosarcoma (p. 326)
Ewing's tumour (p. 734)
Fibrosarcoma (p. 794)
Burkitt's tumour (p. 328)
Chondrosarcoma

Metastatic tumours:
neuroblastoma
lymphomas
leukaemic infiltrations
Wilms' tumour
retinoblastoma
Malignant odontogenic tumours
(p. 342)

Precise terminology for swellings in the alveolar region is hampered by the persistence of two antiquated topographical terms, neither of which has a universally accepted definition, and each has been applied to a group of pathological entities: (i) 'epignathus': any mass present at birth and attached to the jaw (and/or the hard palate), and (ii) an 'epulis': traditionally applied to a lesion attached to the maxillary or mandibular alveolus, and originally confined to lesions arising from soft tissues.

(i) **'Epignathus'**

Pathological conditions under this heading may be:

(*a*) *hamartomas, choristomas and teratomas* present at birth, believed to be 'monozygotic' in origin (Krafka, 1936); or (*b*) *examples of incomplete dizygotic twinning* (palatopagus parasiticus) as interpreted by Ehrich (1945).

The former are closely related anatomically and histologically to congenital 'pedunculated teratomas' or 'dermoid cysts' of the nasopharynx (see p. 348) as described by Loeb & Smith (1967).

(ii) **'Epulis'**

This is a potentially confusing term, further complicated by subdivision into 'congenital', 'vascular', 'fibrous', and 'giant cell' epulides; outside the field of dentistry, one or other term has been applied, at one time or another, to almost any excresence on the alveolus, arising from mucous membrane, soft tissues or bone. The term 'congenital epulis' has a claim to preservation for it is applied to a definite clinical entity with almost constant histological features, as shown in a review of the literature by Langley and Davson (1950).

CONGENITAL 'EPULIS'

AGE : SEX

A congenital epulis is practically confined to females and to the newborn (Hankey, 1955; Fuhr & Krogh, 1972).

SITE

The maxilla is affected at least twice as often as the mandible, and in either case the alveolar ridge in the region of the central incisors is the usual site of attachment. Rarely is there more than one mass, and occasionally the lesion is attached to the premolar or molar region.

MACROSCOPIC APPEARANCES

The swelling is sessile or partially pedunculated, unencapsulated and usually the same colour as the gingiva. Most are 2 to 5 cm in greatest dimension, but a few are much larger; even those of moderate size may interfere with feeding. The surface is generally smooth or partially lobulated like a fetal kidney, and covered with intact epithelium. Rarely a large example has an ulcerated surface, especially when it protrudes outside the lips.

MICROSCOPIC FINDINGS

The histological findings are those of a granular cell tumour (p. 857) which is most often found in childhood, and most commonly in the tongue and the jaw (Strong *et al.*, 1970). In a congenital epulis the component cells are quite large, very tightly packed and extend right up to the thinned out covering of squamous epithelial mucous membrane. The histogenesis of this form is even less certain than that of other granular cell tumours elsewhere. In the Index Series a congenital epulis in a newborn infant was proven by biopsy, then spontaneously regressed over a period of six months and finally disappeared. Cussen & McMahon (1972) have reported a similar experience. Granular cell tumour ('myoblastoma') is a benign lesion in infancy (Colberg, 1962), but its attachment to the gingiva is often ill-defined or irregular. It may extend into the alveolus beyond the margin visible to the naked eye, but in view of the probability of spontaneous remission, this is unimportant.

DIFFERENTIAL DIAGNOSIS OF SWELLINGS IN THE ALVEOLAR REGION

1. 'Epignathus'

There are no specific clinical features by which an epignathus can be distinguished from a congenital epulis of the maxilla, except perhaps the extent of its attachment. Strictly, the attachment of an epulis is confined to the alveolus; an epignathus may be, too, but some extend on to the hard palate or even to the basisphenoid ('episphenoid' or 'encrania'; Ehrich, 1945).

Histologically, the epignathus group contain no tissue resembling granular cell myoblastoma, but are composed mainly of dermal elements or teratomatous derivatives of all three germ layers.

One type of epignathus has been described as a 'hairy dermoid' (Wynn *et al.*, 1956) with a peduncular attachment to the nasal surface of the palate, and is thus indistinguishable from the pedunculated nasopharyngeal hamartoma (Loeb & Smith, 1967) described in the section on the nasopharynx (p. 348).

Theoretically a congenital sarcoma of the alveolus could produce a similar clinical picture to an epignathus, but none appears to have been reported.

Conditions occurring in older children with erupted teeth (Eversole & Rovin, 1973) and also loosely described as 'epulides', are as follows.

2. Hypertrophic gingivitis

Generalized enlargement of the mucosa of the interdental papillae and gingivae occurs in a number of conditions, for example in scurvy and leukaemia, or as a side effect of anticonvulsive drugs such as Dilantin®. Poor oral hygiene is the commonest cause, and cyclic neutropenia also causes generalized gingivitis.

In scurvy and leukaemia there is increase in vascularity, oedema and purplish discolouration; the 'swollen' papillae are spongy and bleed readily. Diagnosis depends upon the dietary history and other stigmata of scurvy such as radiological changes in the epiphyses, or a leukaemic blood picture.

Dilantin 'gingivitis' is due to hyperkeratosis and proliferation of the epithelium extending deeply into the dental equivalent of the corium. Increase in collagen and a moderate chronic inflammatory infiltrate also occur.

Chronic gingivitis due to dental caries or gross oral sepsis occasionally causes focal enlargement of the interdental papillae, especially when there is periodontitis. Subacute inflammatory infiltration and hyperaemia are typical findings.

Fibromatosis gingivae is a very rare form of fibromatosis in childhood, and causes a keloid type of alveolar excrescence composed of dense collagenous tissue of variable vascularity.

TREATMENT OF 'CONGENITAL EPULIS'

Removal is always desirable, either as a biopsy to confirm the diagnosis, or in some cases as a matter of urgency because of interference with breathing, sucking or swallowing.

Simple conservative excision is all that is required; even when abnormal tissue is found up to the margin of the excised specimen no further removal is indicated. Recurrence of a granular cell tumour is unknown, even when some of the lesion has obviously been left *in situ.*

Cussen & McMahon (1972), in reporting their experience of four cases noted absence of any detectable enlargement of this lesion after birth (also noted by O'Brien & Pielou, 1971), suggested that the condition may be a hamartoma, and that it may be associated with high levels of oestrogens in the mother.

MALIGNANT TUMOURS OF THE JAWS

I. OSTEOSARCOMA

The jaw is one of the least common sites of this tumour, and is said to have a particularly poor prognosis because of the difficulty in eradicating the tumour surgically. The general histological aspects and the principles of treatment are described on p. 748 *et seq.*

The clinical features are those of a rapidly progressive and usually painful swelling of the affected bone, initially with intact mucosa, which produces multicystic osteolytic areas on radiography. The clinical and radiological findings are not clearly distinctive, and in all cases the diagnosis is only made by biopsy and histological examination.

DIFFERENTIAL DIAGNOSIS

1. *Ewing's tumour* (p. 734), *fibrosarcoma* of bone (p. 761), *metastatic lesions*

such as neuroblastoma, and in particular the whole group of fibro-osseous dysplasias (Schmaman *et al.*, 1970), in which some cases may be extremely difficult to distinguish from osteosarcoma on histological grounds; misinterpretation may account for the long term survivors reported in some series of osteosarcomas of the jaw (Garrington *et al.*, 1967).

2. *Fibrous dysplasias* with painless asymmetrical enlargement of one side of the face due to thickening of the underlying mandible or maxilla (Schmaman *et al.*, 1970), or in the nasal cavity (p. 363). Occasionally the enlargement is symmetrical, and when all four quadrants of the jaws are involved, the condition is referred to as cherubism (Hamner & Ketcham, 1969), i.e. a symmetrically rounded chubby face which may be a syndrome rather than a pathological entity (von Wowern, 1972) except in the familial type described by Talley (1952).

TREATMENT

As diagnosis depends on accurate histological diagnosis, this is of the utmost importance.

Surgical excision, either wide local resection or maxillectomy may be indicated, but are undesirably mutilating in childhood.

Chemotherapy (p. 753) and radiotherapy would probably be indicated, regardless of the extent (or omission) of surgical excision.

PROGNOSIS

There is a strong possibility that at least some of the patients reported as long term survivors may have been examples of a hypercellular form of dysplasia. Because of the rarity of osteosarcoma of the facial bones, there are few guidelines to the best regime of treatment.

II. FIBROSARCOMA

In the jaw, this tumour occasionally arises as a periosteal or parosteal tumour in children and young adults (Thoma, 1960), most frequently in the region of the chin or the angle of the mandible. They tend to be more malignant than truly intra-oral fibrosarcomas which occur more frequently in older children. In the patient described by Jones (1966), a three-year old girl, the tumour was in the submandibular region and was successfully treated by excision and radiotherapy.

Fibrosarcomas arising in the jaw vary greatly in their degree of malignancy and their histological differentiation includes the fibrous dysplasias and other lesions described above.

Other conditions causing rarefactive lesion in radiographs of the jaws include aneurysmal bone cyst (p. 730) and the various forms of histiocytosis X (p. 205), in particular eosinophilic granuloma (p. 206). In this group, too, diagnosis depends on biopsy findings.

III. BURKITT'S TUMOUR

The typical feature of this tumour in tropical parts of Africa (Burkitt & Wright, 1970) is the development in children more than one year old of rapidly growing tumours of the jaws, not infrequently multiple, usually bilateral, and sometimes affecting both maxilla and mandible (Burkitt & Kyalwazi, 1969; Osunkoya & Ajayi, 1972/73).

In Australia, as in other temperate climates, the incidence is low, in marked contrast to the figures for New Guinea where climate and incidence resemble those in tropical parts of Africa, specifically regions less than 5000 ft above sea level, with a rainfall of more than 20 inches a year, and a mean minimum temperature above 15°C.

Children of dissimilar African tribes but living in similar climatic circumstances have the same incidence. Children born to European or Asian parents are also susceptible, and to quote Burkitt (1969), it is not a 'tumour of African children', but a 'tumour of children in Africa'.

AGE : SEX

Even in areas with a high incidence, the tumour is unknown in children less than one year old, rare under two years, chiefly seen between four and eight years, with a peak at six to seven years. Boys are affected slightly more often than girls.

SITES

The rank order of frequency of individual sites varies from one endemic area to another, and is even more varied in non-endemic areas.

The jaw, particularly the maxilla, is the commonest site in Africa (Fig. 14.9).

The abdomen, more specifically bilateral renal or bilateral ovarian tumours, are next in frequency.

Spinal (extradural) tumours are next, followed by bones other than the jaws, then in descending order of frequency, the salivary glands, testicles and subcutaneous tissues.

In non-endemic areas the incidence is so much less that the proportion in each site is not well documented. The most common is probably retroperitoneal tissues, followed by lymph nodes.

MACROSCOPIC APPEARANCES

The tumour is usually soft, white and friable, except where it is infiltrating other tissues which impart a somewhat firmer texture and yellowish colour. In the jaw, the tumour expands the alveolus and loosens the teeth; when one is extracted, portion of the friable tumour is usually adherent to the root (Fig. 14.9a).

MICROSCOPIC FINDINGS

The histological features are best seen in imprints of the freshly cut surface (see p. 82). The typical Burkitt cell is 12–25μ in diameter, with a round or oval nucleus, in a delicate but clear-cut nuclear membrane, containing one to three nucleoli. The cytoplasm is plentiful, deeply basophilic, and contains numerous large fat droplets which distend the cell membrane and overlie the nucleus (Fig. 14.9b).

In paraffin sections the tumour is composed of sheets of lymphoblasts with a moderate amount of cytoplasm, containing a rounded or sometimes polygonal nucleus (Fig. 14.9c). The nuclear chromatin is evenly dispersed, and the nucleoli are less conspicuous than in imprint preparations. Phagocytic

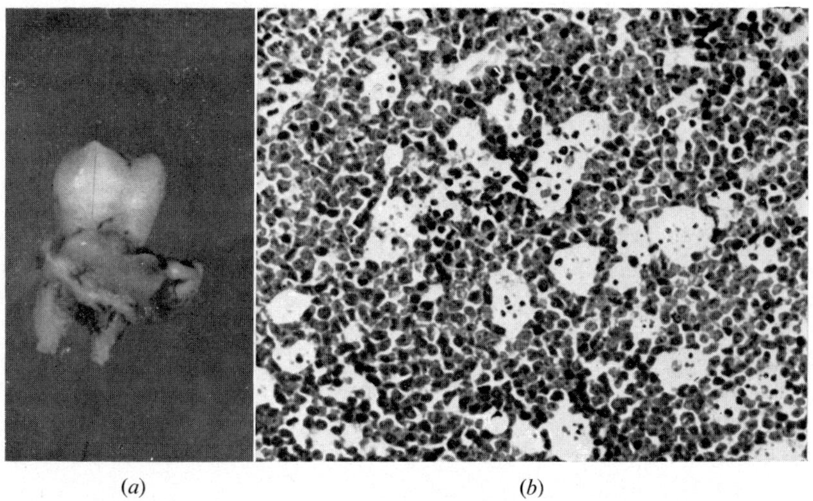

(*a*) (*b*)

Figure 14.9. Burkitt's tumour, arising in the jaw; (*a*) tumour adherent to the root of removed, loosened tooth; (*b*) phagocytic reticulum cells as prominent, clear, rounded spaces between the tumour cells which resemble large, immature lymphoblastic cells, with a moderate rim of basophilic cytoplasm (H & E. × 200); (*c*) colour plate following p. 140.

reticulum cells are evenly scattered between the lymphoblasts and produce a marked 'starry sky' appearance (p. 171). Although typical of Burkitt's lymphoma, this is also seen in other rapidly growing tumours, for example, non-Burkitt lymphosarcoma, and also in reticulum cell sarcoma (p. 180) rhabdomyosarcoma (p. 783), and in some of the histiocytoses (p. 205).

SPREAD

Rapid infiltration and extensive local spread are typical features, as is metastasis by lymphatics to regional nodes, and by the bloodstream to almost any part of the body, with a preference for the kidney, ovaries or testes.

MODES OF PRESENTATION

Apart from tumours of the jaws, there are the following:
1. *An abdominal mass*, e.g. tumours of both kidneys, often involving the adrenal glands and occasionally the liver. In girls, bilateral ovarian masses are not uncommon in endemic areas.
2. *Paraplegia;* the rapid development of flaccid paraplegia and double incontinence usually occurs without radiological evidence of destruction of vertebrae.
3. *Other sites* are numerous and include bones other than the jaws, salivary glands, the thyroid, testis, subcutaneous tissues and the breast.

DIAGNOSIS

A typical swelling in the jaw is almost diagnostic and can quickly be confirmed by histological examination of tumour tissue adherent to a loosened and readily removable tooth. However, even in communities with a high incidence, nearly half of all children with *a facial swelling have a lesion other than Burkitt's tumour.*

The conditions which may stimulate it are as follows:
Giant cell reparative granuloma (p. 333);
Metastatic neuroblastoma (p. 552);
Ewing's tumour (p. 734);
Histiocytosis X (p. 209);
Leukaemic deposits in the facial bones.

BIOPSY

In all cases the final diagnosis rests on the histological findings, and in many cases this is the only means of distinguishing other lesions.

HISTOLOGICAL DIFFERENTIATION

Preparations of the highest quality are essential, and additional techniques such as imprint cytology (p. 82), tissue cultures (p. 86) and multiple sections, are sometimes required.

Non-Burkitt type of lymphosarcoma. The distinction is partly clinical and partly histological. Imprints of a non-Burkitt lymphoblastic lymphosarcoma show cells with a round nucleus, up to three nucleoli and coarsely clumped chromatin, compared with fine, evenly stippled chromatin in Burkitt's lymphoma.

The main difference is in nuclear morphology, and in the slate blue-grey cytoplasm, instead of the deeply basophilic cytoplasm of the Burkitt cells which has been shown to be due to intensely active synthesis of immunoglobulin, in keeping with rising titres of EB virus antibody.

Histological differentiation is more difficult in temperate climates where Burkitt's tumour is a rarity and there is no preponderance of lesions in the jaws. In temperate climates other abnominal tumours in childhood (Wilms' tumour p. 516, and neuroblastoma p. 538) are so predominant that a Burkitt's tumour arising in the abdomen is likely to be mistaken for one or other of them.

TREATMENT

Chemotherapy has proved to be effective and a satisfactory remission is the usual result of treatment although the relapse rate is high, and the five-year survival rate 30–35%. The tumour has been shown to be sensitive to a wide variety of cytotoxic agents such as methotrexate, actinomycin D and particularly cyclophosphamide. Each has been used successfully in combinations of two drugs, usually given in two courses, each spread over 3–7 days, with an interval of 10–14 days. Methotrexate (1 mg/kg IV) and cyclophosphamide (30–40 mg/kg) intravenously or orally, is the combination considered to produce the best results.

Radiotherapy (3000–3500 rads in three weeks) may also be given when the tumour is localized and relatively accessible.

The prognosis is best in younger children (less than five years), when the diagnosis has been made at an early stage, when there are no lymph node metastases, and when the response to treatment is rapid and the tumour undergoes complete remission within 2–3 weeks of commencing treatment (Burkitt & Kyalwazi, 1969).

BENIGN TUMOURS OF THE JAWS

FIBROUS DYSPLASIAS

In most children with fibrous dysplasia of the jaw, no other bone is involved; in some it is part of a polyostotic dysplasia involving many bones, or a component of Gardner's syndrome with polyposis of the bowel (p. 656), or related to hyperparathyroidism (p. 384).

Whether monostotic or polyostotic, the lesions of fibro-osseous dysplasia have essentially the same microscopic appearances, consisting of proliferation of a fibroblastic stroma containing trabeculae of immature woven bone. The stroma varies greatly in cellularity; in general, the younger the patient the more cellular the stroma. The fibroblasts tend to be interlaced and interwoven, while the osteoid and woven bone are intimately related to and derived from the stromal cells. The amount of osteoid formed varies greatly; in some examples there is little or none, and these have been described as 'non-ossifying fibromas' or 'desmoplastic fibromas' (Dehner, 1973).

Three other fibroblastic lesions arising in the jaws in children may have somewhat similar histological appearances to fibro-osseous dysplasia; these are:

(i) Ossifying fibroma;
(ii) Benign osteoblastoma; and
(iii) Cementifying fibroma.

(i) *Ossifying fibromas* are distinguished from fibrous dysplasia by a looseness and relative hypocellularity of the stroma, and a more mature appearance of the bony trabeculae which may have a lamellar appearance with osteoblasts aligned along the margins of the trabeculae.

(ii) *Osteoblastomas* are very rare lesions occasionally encountered in the jaw (Byers, 1968) and their particular features are that they are painful and extremely tender, have a moderately cellular stroma and very prominent, almost confluent, masses of osteoid surrounded by prominent osteoblasts. Osteoclastic activity in the form of giant cells, is often present as well. The initial diagnosis is usually a sarcoma, and the lesion can only be identified on histological examination (see p. 728).

(iii) *A cementifying fibroma* is also basically a fibroblastic lesion, and calcification within it is characteristic, consisting of rounded spherules of strongly basophilic material, often with concentric lamellar structures which are strongly PAS (p. 85) positive. The surrounding fibroblasts tend to be arranged in curlicues reminiscent of meningioma. Another finding typical of a cementifying fibroma is that it is attached to the root of a tooth.

RADIOGRAPHIC APPEARANCES OF FIBROUS DYSPLASIAS

In fibrous dysplasia causing an erosion, there is a ground glass appearance with a sharp margin, and the outer table of the jaw is sometimes involved. Non-ossifying fibromas and osteoblastomas may produce an area of rarefaction resembling a simple bone cyst, while a cementifying fibroma is usually more radio-opaque.

TREATMENT OF FIBROUS LESIONS OF THE JAWS

Curettage is usually adequate in most instances, and recurrence is uncommon but not unknown. The most troublesome lesions in this regard are the fibrous dysplasias, and it is possible that 'recurrences' may be in reality new areas of dysplasia appearing in adjacent or contiguous areas of the mandible or maxilla.

GIANT CELL (REPARATIVE) GRANULOMA

This lesion (Jaffe, 1953) may develop peripherally, i.e. on the surface of the alveolus (syn. giant-cell 'epulis'), or centrally within the substance of the jaw.

AGE : SITE : SIZE

In the thirteen children reviewed by Dehner (1973a), their ages ranged from 3–14 years, and seven were between 10 and 14 years of age. There were six girls and seven boys.

The mandible and maxilla were affected with equal frequency. The mandible and ipsilateral maxilla were both involved in one girl, and one boy had bilateral mandibular and maxillary lesions with the appearance of cherubism (p. 327).

The swelling was chiefly located in the nasal fossa in one child, and in five children the palate was also involved. A history of recent extraction of a tooth was obtained in only one case. In the mandible the lesions were from 1·7–7 cm in diameter, with a mean of 4·5 cm.

The mode of presentation was a painless swelling in all but one patient who presented with repeated epistaxis. The swelling produced asymmetry in those with unilateral lesions.

Occasionally the overlying mucosa is ulcerated, and necrotic material is extruded into the mouth.

The radiographic findings in maxillary lesions included opacification of the antrum and stippled calcification; destruction of the adjacent bone was present in some cases. In the mandible the typical appearance is a well circumscribed osteolytic lesion with fine trabeculation into multiple compartments. A fine rim of calcified 'cortex' was preserved in all cases.

Microscopically the lesion is composed of cellular granulation tissue containing plump fibroblastic cells interspersed with large numbers of giant cells containing many nuclei (Jaffe, 1953). The nuclei are very similar to those in the fibroblasts of the stroma, and mitotic figures are occasionally present, but the granulomatous nature of the lesion is usually readily discerned. A rim of reactive new bone around the periphery of the lesion is characteristic, and there may be haemosiderin due to associated haemorrhage.

DIFFERENTIAL DIAGNOSIS

Eosinophilic granuloma (p. 206) is the condition most likely to be confused with giant cell reparative granuloma, but sheets of histiocytes together with clumps of infiltrating eosinophils distinguish this entity.

PROGNOSIS

Only two of the thirteen patients reviewed by Dehner showed any radiographic evidence of residual lesions after curettage and a follow-up averaging eight years.

In the Index Series there were three children with a reparative granuloma of this type and all responded to simple curettage without any recurrence.

MELANOTIC PROGONOMA

(syn. retinal anlage tumour, neuro-ectodermal tumour of infancy, melanotic adamantinoma, pigmented ameloblastoma)

The histogenesis of this benign tumour is disputed and a universally acceptable name has yet to be suggested. Evidence is accumulating that it arises in cells derived from the neural crest (Borello & Gorlin, 1966; Koudstaal *et al.*, 1966). Although the origin of the cells is uncertain, their histological features are quite distinctive.

SITES : AGE : SEX

Characteristically the tumour arises in the skull, often in or near the midline and most commonly in the maxilla (Jones & Williams, 1960), but occasionally a morphologically identical tumour arises in other sites, e.g. the epididymis (Eaton & Ferguson, 1956), the mediastinum (Misugi *et al.*, 1965), or in soft tissues elsewhere.

The great majority are confined to infancy, especially the first six months of life, and more commonly in females.

Microscopically the characteristic picture can be alarming; the tumour contains two types of cells, set in a very dense fibrous stroma:

(i) Heavily pigmented cells, apparently lining irregular cleft-like spaces; and

(ii) Masses of smaller cells resembling neuroblasts, usually without any definite neurological tissues. The smaller cells may occur alone, in groups in the fibrous stroma, or closely related to the melanotic epithelium, appearing at times to merge with it. Occasionally there are groups of the smaller cells lying in the centre of spaces lined by the pigmented cells, somewhat suggestive of a glomerular pattern. 'String cell artefacts' are very prominent and related to the difficulty of cutting sections of delicate cells in a very dense fibrous stroma.

Mitoses may occasionally be seen in the neural type of cells, but all reported cases have ultimately behaved in a benign fashion without distant metastases, although they have a marked tendency to recur locally if inadequately excised.

TREATMENT

All visibly pigmented tissue should be excised, together with a generous margin of macroscopically normal tissue, ideally 1 cm beyond the pigmented area. It is particularly important that a misdiagnosis of malignancy should not be made, for many of the cases reported in the literature appear to have been over-treated. Radiation and chemotherapy are not required, and simple rather than radical excision is all that is necessary. Local recurrences are not uncommon and further conservative excision is required, sometimes on more than one occasion, but this is preferable to primary radical excision which could be unnecessarily mutilating.

The ultimate prognosis for life is good in infants, even when there have been several local recurrences, but there is always some local dental deformity. Some of the similar tumours in older children or adults have been reported to behave in a malignant fashion, but it is probable that these are not 'progonomas'.

3. SARCOMAS ARISING IN CONNECTIVE TISSUES ATTACHED TO THE JAWS

These are chiefly rhabdomyosarcoma which is described, in general, on p. 783, those arising in the face on p. 317, and those in the oropharynx or tonsillar regions on p. 345. Fibrosarcoma of soft tissues (p. 794) and bone (p. 761) are mentioned in sections dealing with the regions in which they arise; those in the jaw are described on p. 327.

4. TUMOURS DERIVED FROM ODONTOGENIC EPITHELIUM

According to Bhaskar (1963) this group accounts for approximately 15% of all tumours of the jaws and together with the 12% of tumours arising from non-odontogenic tissues, they contribute 27% of all tumours arising in the mouth.

The capacity of odontogenic derivatives to induce metaplasia in adjacent mesenchymal tissues explains the wide variety of cysts and tumours which may result; these are classified in Table 14.5, which follows the general schema proposed by Pindborg, Kramer & Torloni (1971), with slight modification to accord with paediatric practice.

Table 14.5. Neoplasms arising from odontogenic epithelium

Benign tumours	Malignant tumours
Ameloblastoma and its variants	Odontogenic carcinoma and sarcoma
Odontogenic cysts	
Fibroma (odontogenic fibroma)	
Myxoma (odontogenic myxoma)	
Complex and compound odontomas	
Cementoma and dentinoma	
Melanotic progonoma (syn. neuro-ectodermal tumour of infancy)	

GENERAL FEATURES

Most tumours of odontogenic tissues arise centrally, within the maxilla or mandible. In general the presenting clinical features of both benign and malignant odontogenic tumours are essentially the same, although differing in their rate of growth (Pizer & Hamner, 1967).

MODES OF PRESENTATION

Apart from a swelling of the jaw, and often preceding this sign are the following:
1. *Malposition* or lack of eruption of teeth, indicating disturbed development of the tooth bud, and the need for radiological examination.
2. *Migration and loosening* of teeth in infants and children is particularly suggestive of a malignant lesion, especially when accompanied by pain, which may be referred to the face or the ear.
3. *Ulceration* of tissues, with or without bleeding, may also occur, but is more typical of non-odontogenic lesions of the jaws (p. 338).
4. *Expansion of the cortical plates* of the jaws, resulting in a swelling presenting beneath the cheek or lips, is a relatively late finding in tumours. *Asymmetry* of the face or jaws may be the presenting complaint, but in the absence of the other signs listed above, it is most likely to be due to a benign lesion.

DIAGNOSIS

A detailed history, including the history of the dental lesion, and a general as well as a local examination, together with a full blood examination, and possibly a selective skeletal survey, are essential.

In relatively few cases, mainly those with a swelling arising in soft tissues or the mucosa (p. 322), it may be possible to make the diagnosis on the clinical findings alone, but more usually both radiographic examination and biopsy are necessary.

Enlargement of regional nodes is most often caused by infection and is rarely significant in the differential diagnosis of tumours of the jaws.

RADIOLOGICAL EXAMINATION

The first evidence of any abnormality in the bone of the jaws is often the failure of a deciduous or permanent tooth to erupt at the normal time, and this is always an indication for radiography using extra- or intra-oral or panoramic techniques (Worth, 1963), supervised by a paedodontist or oral surgeon.

Cystic lesions are as a rule unilocular and have smooth, curved margins; in the mandible the outer (buccal) plate usually shows more expansion than the lingual plate.

Trabeculated or multilocular lesions are more likely to be due to a tumour than a cyst.

Perforation of the cortical plate may occur in both benign and malignant lesions, and appears as an area of greater radiolucency within the shadow of the 'cyst'. When the margin of the perforation is irregulaı, the lesion is more likely to be malignant.

The shape of the lesion is also some guide to the cause. Cysts and benign lesions are usually regular and more or less circular in outline, and only irregular when anatomic structures impede the path of expansion.

The typical radiographic findings of various simple cysts are as follows:

(*a*) *Dental cysts;* these involve the apex of the root of a tooth, although the related tooth, and root, may have been removed.

(*b*) *Dentigerous cysts;* the crown is usually within the cavity of the cyst.

(*c*) *A primordial cyst* (keratocyst) is related to a tooth, or occurs in place of a tooth, usually in the region from the last molar to the angle of the mandible. Primordial cysts may be multiple and bilateral.

(*d*) *A solitary bone cyst* ('traumatic' or 'haemorrhagic cyst') usually occurs in the cuspid, bicuspid or molar regions.

(*e*) *Ameloblastoma;* a cyst-like space situated at the angle of the mandible is one of the features of this lesion (p. 340).

Resorption of the root of a tooth is typical of a benign tumour, whereas a cyst is more prone to displace the tooth, and malignant tumours usually do not cause root resorption.

Vascular lesions arising in the jaws are uncommon but particularly dangerous because surgical procedures may lead to uncontrollable haemorrhage; when suspected, selective angiography of the external carotid artery should be performed.

BIOPSY

The optimum method depends on the clinical and radiographic findings, and the following techniques are appropriate to different types of lesions.

1. *Exfoliative cytology*. A smear on a slide is of limited value, but has the advantage that it can be readily performed at the initial examination.
2. *Incision-biopsy* is the method of choice when a tumour is suspected. A wedge of tissue is excised, in older children under local or regional anaesthesia injected at a distance from the tissue to be removed. Frozen sections may be obtained if excision is to follow immediately, otherwise paraffin sections are preferable.
3. *Punch biopsy* is an alternative to incision biopsy, but little or no tissue may be obtained in cystic lesions.
4. *Excision-biopsy* is the method of choice when a benign lesion is suspected, but should not be employed if there is any clinical indication of malignancy.
5. *Aspiration* of the centre of a lesion is indicated when a haemangioma is suspected. Haemorrhage may occur into a cyst when its wall has involved the inferior dental vessels by expansion.

Odontogenic lesions and non-neoplastic dental cysts are described below. In general, dental cysts of various kinds in childhood are not uncommon, benign tumours are rare, and malignant tumours are almost unknown. The relative incidence of these lesions is indicated in Table 14.6.

NON-NEOPLASTIC DENTAL CYSTS

In the differential diagnosis of swellings of the maxilla or mandible, a cyst of the jaw is the commonest expanding lesion, and the most important type is the dentigerous cyst (syn. cyst of the enamel; follicular cyst) which is developmental in origin and presents as a localized swelling often associated with non-eruption of the related tooth. Most arise in close relation to the primordium of an unerupted tooth.

Macroscopically the wall of the cyst may be thick or thin; secondary infection is common and may make it impossible to determine the exact origin of the cyst.

Microscopically there is a fibrous capsule lined by squamous or, occasionally, ciliated epithelium. Considerable chronic inflammatory changes are common, and occasionally there are ameloblastic elements in the wall, in the form of small tubules of columnar cells which may appear to be infiltrating, and this can lead to an erroneous diagnosis of ameloblastoma.

When there is marked secondary infection, a neoplastic cyst may also be difficult to distinguish from a dental cyst. The latter is simply an epithelialized abscess cavity at the apex of the root of an infected and usually carious tooth. Histologically these may be similar to follicular cysts, but there is usually a

Table 14.6. Relative incidence of swellings of the jaw in children; biopsy diagnoses from 93 cases (Royal Dental Hospital, Melbourne, 1968–1972)

Gingival (alveolar) lesions		
Fibrous epulis	34	62
Papilloma (not verrucal)	8	
Giant cell reparative granuloma	8	
Viral papilloma	6	
Pyogenic granuloma	5	
Vascular hamartoma	1	
Palatal lesions		
Pleomorphic salivary adenoma	1	2
Neurofibroma	1	
Buccal mucosa		
Lipoma	1	1
Mucosal excrescences (irritational hyperplasia, including polyps, excluding alveolar lesions)	16	16
Central lesions (either jaw)		
Giant cell reparative granuloma	6	8
Cementoma	1	
Odontogenic fibroma	1	
Malignant tumours		
Burkitt's lymphoma (from Papua-New Guinea)	2	4
Reticulum cell sarcoma	1	
Embryonal rhabdomyosarcoma	1	
Total		93

history of caries or a preceding abscess, and as a rule there is no missing tooth.

Fissural cysts

Developmental cysts in the midline of the jaws occasionally occur. These are almost invariably in the maxilla and are interpreted by some as ‘fusion’ cysts (fissural cysts) formed by the inclusion of remnants of squamous epithelium at the time of closure of the embryonic processes of the facial bones. Their situation in the midline is typical and suggestive of their true nature.

BENIGN TUMOURS OF THE ODONTOGENIC EPITHELIUM

AMELOBLASTOMA (syn. adamantinoma) AND ITS VARIANTS

These are rare lesions in children in temperate climates, but more common in tropical areas. In a recently studied series of patients from New Guinea the incidence was six times greater than in Melbourne.

Ameloblastomas usually present as unilateral swellings of the face, sometimes with displacement of teeth and occasionally with pain. When very large, the buccal plate of the mandible may be perforated and the tumour presents as a soft swelling inside the mouth.

Radiologically the lesions are expansile, multilocular and osteolytic, but the outer plate of the jaw is usually preserved. Characteristically the areas of bone destruction have smooth curved margins, and are subdivided by disordered coarse trabeculae, often radiating from a central core. Some examples, especially when they are small, may be indistinguishable from other rarefactive lesions and cysts.

Macroscopically they contain cystic and solid areas. The solid component is grey-white, spongy or firm; the cystic areas contain yellow or brown fluid.

Microscopically they consist of a fibrous stroma containing nests of odontogenic epithelium composed of stellate or polygonal cells resembling stellate reticulum, merging on one side with the fibrous stroma and lined on the other side by a layer of odontogenic epithelium. Cystic change commonly occurs in the stellate areas; the connective tissue becomes hyalinized in some tumours and on occasions cords of epithelium may form a network of strands with a plexiform appearance. Rarely, squamous or granular metaplasia of the epithelial cells occurs.

Spread occurs by expansion and local invasion of bone.

Treatment

Radical local excision, as far as normal tissue, is required, if possible without destroying the continuity of the bone. The inner wall of the cavity is treated with coagulation diathermy. When the tumour is extensive, resection of the mandible beyond the lesion is advocated, and a bone graft may be required.

The recurrence rate of these tumours is high and careful follow-up is required.

ODONTOGENIC CYST

A variety of cystic lesions lined by epithelium of the dental lamina and containing a variety of tissues of dental types are encountered in children. While cystic degeneration sometimes occurs in soild tumours of the jaws in childhood, most cysts appear to be developmental in origin and are considered in the differential diagnosis below. Thus apart from cystic change in ameloblastomas, the only lesion that may be properly considered here is the calcifying odontogenic cyst, described by Pindborg, Kramer & Torloni (1971) as a non-neoplastic cystic lesion with an epithelial lining consisting of columnar cells, covered by a layer of spindle cells resembling stellate reticulum. Masses of ghost epithelial cells, somewhat resembling those seen in pilomatrixoma (p. 851), desquamate into the cavity. It is doubtful whether odontogenic cysts are neoplasms, and they are most likely to be a type of developmental cyst (see below).

MYXOMA (ODONTOGENIC MYXOMA)

This arises centrally, i.e. within the bone of the maxilla or mandible, and is often associated with a missing tooth.

Radiologically it is similar in appearance to an ameloblastoma, i.e. a rarified area with a 'soap bubble' appearance due to trabeculation. It expands the cortex of the bone but does not destroy it.

Macroscopically the material is mucoid and its boundaries often ill-defined; *microscopically* the lesion is very characteristic: the definitive cells are fibroblasts but with extremely elongated, wispy cytoplasmic processes and an abundance of intercellular mucin. The nuclei of the cells may be irregular, but they show no atypia nor mitotic figures. The lesion is essentially benign, although on occasions local recurrence follows incomplete excision.

ODONTOMA

This is a benign lesion, probably hamartomatous in nature, composed of a mixture of cementum, dentine and connective tissue, usually with ameloblastic epithelium. They are commonly encapsulated, slowly growing, arise in the region of the tooth follicle, and are associated with absence of the corresponding tooth. They are subdivided into *complex odontomas* in which all dental tissues are represented but completely disordered; and *compound odontomas* in which a more orderly pattern of growth leads to the formation of many tooth-like structures.

Radiologically the lesion commences as a radiolucent area containing small masses of calcified material representing the forming teeth. Their growth potential is limited and simple excision is curative.

CEMENTOMAS AND DENTINOMAS

These are extremely rare lesions, particularly in childhood. There are at least four types of cementoma and their classification is still open to dispute.

Basically they consist of deposits of cementum around the apex of a tooth root, to form a tumour-like mass.

Microscopically the cementum is laid down in a haphazard fashion and may provoke a foreign-body giant-cell reaction. Some authorities regard cementifying fibroma and cementoma as the same lesion. They do not recur following excision and their neoplastic nature is open to question.

Dentinomas are extremely uncommon and consist of odontogenic epithelium in slender strands related to immature connective tissue in which poorly organized dentine is laid down.

MALIGNANT TUMOURS OF THE ODONTOGENIC EPITHELIUM

Primary malignant neoplasms of the jaws arise much more commonly in non-dental tissue than from odontogenic epithelium (Schilli & Eschler, 1966).

Odontogenic carcinoma and odontogenic sarcoma have both been described, and Pindborg, Kramer & Torloni (1971) suggest that they should be classified according to which element, epithelial or stromal, predominates. In the past they have been referred to as 'malignant ameloblastomas', but their occurrence in childhood is almost unknown.

TREATMENT OF MALIGNANT TUMOURS OF THE JAWS

As with malignant tumours elsewhere, surgery, radiotherapy and chemotherapy should be carefully co-ordinated, the sequence and dosages etc. being determined by appropriate consultations (p. 24).

Surgical excision should be only as radical as determined by the extent of the lesion, although hemi-mandibulectomy or maxillectomy may occasionally be required for some malignant tumours because of their particular tendency to spread along the inferior dental canal. In the maxilla, partial resection rather than complete disarticulation (maxillectomy) is always preferable, especially in childhood.

A cast silver splint should be constructed and cemented in place before excision to control or prevent fracture of the mandible after operation.

Radiotherapy is usually employed for malignant tumours, and also possibly for benign central cavernous haemangiomas. The jaws are vulnerable to radiation in doses exceeding 1500 rads, and maximum effects are produced by doses of 2500 rads. Subsequent dental infection and the trauma of extraction may lead to radiation-necrosis, sequestra, diffuse osteomyelitis and pathological fracture.

Effects of irradiation

Radiographic changes may not appear until six to twelve months after irradiation, although changes in developing teeth may be identifiable earlier.

Disintegration of erupted teeth occurs two to three years after 'heavy' radiation (more than 2000 rads).

Asymmetric growth of the whole mandible occurs when the condylar growth centre has been damaged by irradiation, and deformity resulting from arrest of growth is particularly severe when the child is less than five years old at the time the jaw is irradiated.

All carious or infected teeth, and those with periodontal disease, should be removed before commencing radiotherapy.

Cytotoxic chemotherapy is indicated for Ewing's tumour (see p. 745) and for Burkitt's lymphoma (p. 328), for osteosarcoma (p. 753) and other malignant tumours arising in bone. The treatment of rhabdomyosarcoma (p. 790), malignant lymphomas (p. 175) and metastatic lesions such as neuroblastoma (p. 558) is described in the appropriate chapters.

D. TUMOURS OF THE OROPHARYNX

For clinical purposes, the oropharynx contains the tonsil, the pillars of the fauces, the hard and soft palate, and the adjacent pharyngeal wall. Swellings and tumours of this region fall into two groups.

(*a*) *Those extending outwards* to involve adjacent structures, but which usually cause some bulging inwards. This group includes a number of parapharyngeal inflammatory conditions in which the diagnosis, and the exclusion of a tumour, may be difficult (see oropharyngeal rhabdomyosarcoma, p. 345).

(*b*) *Those projecting into the cavity* of the oropharynx. This group includes benign tumours such as pleomorphic salivary adenoma of the palate, fibro-osseous dysplasias (usually of the maxilla, p. 331), and some cystic or solid dental lesions arising in the maxilla (p. 335).

Malignant tumours of the maxilla arising in bone (p. 326), in soft tissues (p. 335), or in derivatives of the odontogenic membrane, may also appear at or near the upper pole of the tonsil, or in the adjacent hard palate.

Three malignant tumours of childhood may develop in this region; all are rarities, but they tend to arise in or near the tonsillar fossa, and they are as follows:

I. Lymphosarcoma of the tonsil.
II. Rhabdomyosarcoma of the oropharyngeal wall.
III. Fibrosarcoma of the wall of the pharynx.

I. LYMPHOSARCOMA OF THE TONSIL

The histological features are the same as in lymphosarcomas elsewhere

(p. 171), and in childhood the modes of presentation, usually in children between five and ten years of age, are as follows:

(*a*) *Symptoms related to the oropharynx:* discomfort or difficulty in swallowing, alterations in the voice, or 'snoring' due to distortion and narrowing of the airway.

(*b*) *Enlargement of cervical lymph nodes*, typically the jugulo-digastric node, due to metastasis.

(*c*) *The incidental finding* of considerable enlargement of one tonsil; there may be a loss of the normal pitted, reticular appearance, and its replacement by ulceration, or a haemorrhagic or cauliflower-like surface.

In the early stages there may be nothing obviously abnormal except disparity in the size of the two tonsils. Minor degrees of asymmetry in normal children are not unusual, but as a general rule, if one tonsil is noted to be more than half as large again as the other, biopsy, in form of tonsillectomy, is indicated to determine as early as possible whether the enlargement is due to a tumour.

DIFFERENTIAL DIAGNOSIS

1 *Chronic or recurrent subacute tonsillitis* is far more likely to be the cause of such an enlargement; both tonsils are usually affected, but if one is significantly larger than the other, excision and histological examination are required.

2 *Other rare malignant tumours* arising in the tissues in the tonsillar fossa or the pillars of the fauces (see below).

DIAGNOSIS

The diagnosis of the primary tumour or of metastases in cervical nodes can only be made with certainty on histological grounds. The identification of a lymphosarcoma *in situ* in lymphoid tissue may be difficult; paraffin sections are preferred, but touch prints (p. 82) of the cut surface, before the excised tonsil is fixed, may be helpful. The distinguishing points are the replacement of the normal follicular pattern by a diffuse sheet of lymphoblasts, and phagocytic reticulum cells producing a 'starry sky' pattern (p. 172).

TREATMENT

Treatment is conducted on three lines. Total excision of the enlarged tonsil is desirable, or diathermy loop excision when it is fixed and infiltrating.

Radiotherapy to the tonsillar fossa, with portals selected so as to include the jugulo-digastric nodes, is given in a dose of 3000–3500 rads in approximately three weeks (Sagerman *et al.*, 1966; Parker, 1968).

Combination chemotherapy has become an important aspect of treatment and because of the incidence of conversion to lymphatic leukaemia in children with lymphosarcoma, regimes as for leukaemia have been introduced (p. 176), including prophylactic radiotherapy to the neuraxis.

PROGNOSIS

The prognosis is uncertain and the numbers treated by modern methods (p. 175) are as yet too small to obtain specific figures; the three cases in the Index Series, including one presenting with metastasis in cervical lymph nodes, responded well to the treatment outlined; two children are surviving without evidence of residual disease, 10 and 14 years after treatment.

II. RHABDOMYOSARCOMA OF THE OROPHARYNX

AGE : SEX

In one of the most recently published reports of rhabdomyosarcomas of the head and neck in childhood, a series of 19 cases reviewed by Donaldson, Castro *et al.* (1973), the age range was from 2–15 years with an average of nearly 9 years, and a median of 7 years.

The sex incidence was approximately equal (eight males, eleven females) and in 6 of the 19 children the tumour arose in the cheek or the adjacent maxillary, retromolar or tonsillar regions.

In 13 of the 19 rhabdomyosarcomas the histological pattern was embryonal in type (p. 785).

MODES OF PRESENTATION

In the Index Series some presented as a swelling beneath the tonsil, with local findings somewhat similar to those of a lymphosarcoma (p. 344), but with more extensive involvement of one of the pillars of the fauces, the adjoining retromolar part of the maxilla, or the hard palate. The tonsil tends to be displaced and more prominent, and may therefore appear to be enlarged.

DIFFERENTIAL DIAGNOSIS

In some cases the tumour arises more deeply, in the wall of the oropharynx, and causes an ill-defined swelling bulging into the oropharynx, for example in the recess between the posterior pillar of the fauces and the posterior wall of the pharynx.

This raises the possibility of a number of extrapharyngeal conditions which, apart from fibrosarcoma (p. 346), are mostly inflammatory in nature.

1. *A paratonsillar abscess* ('quinsy') is usually an acute illness accompanied

by local and general signs and symptoms of acute inflammation. Incision is indicated, but if no pus is evacuated, aspiration or excision biopsy may be required to obtain material for histological examination.

2. *A lateral pharyngeal abscess* is a sinister and much rarer condition which presents as a paratonsillar swelling, with trismus, an accompanying swelling beneath the angle of the mandible and sometimes bleeding from the ear. Selective external carotid angiography may show an accompanying mycotic erosion of one of the terminal branches of the maxillary artery or internal carotid artery (Shipley, Winslow & Walmer, 1937; Harrison, 1954).

3. *A retropharyngeal inflammatory swelling* may be due to tuberculous or pyogenic osteitis of the cervical vertebra. Plain films of the cervical vertebrae usually show bony erosion by the time such an abscess has formed; alternatively, a characteristic prevertebral soft tissue shadow may be seen at an earlier stage, especially in lateral films centred on the oropharyngeal air column (Fig. 14.10).

4. *Tumours arising primarily in the nasopharynx* may extend below the level of the soft palate and appear in the nasopharynx. This group includes the rare pedunculated teratoma or 'glioma' of the newborn (p. 348), nasopharyngeal angiofibroma (p. 352) or a basi-occipital chordoma (see also nasal polyps p. 351).

Examination under anaesthesia and biopsy are necessary for diagnosis.

TREATMENT OF OROPHARYNGEAL RHABDOMYOSARCOMA

From the literature, and the experience of two cases in the Index Series, the tumour is often vascular, firmly fixed to adjacent structures, and usually embryonal in type (p. 785).

The plan of treatment is much the same as in rhabdomyosarcomas arising in other comparable sites (p. 358). Total excision, although desirable, is not feasible in the oropharynx, and is not essential to effect a cure. Because of inevitably incomplete excision, *combination chemotherapy* is indicated (e.g. vincristine, actinomycin D and cyclophosphamide, p. 359), and followed by *radiotherapy* in doses of 3000–4000 in four weeks (see p. 359).

Aggressive co-ordinated treatment of this kind has improved the prognosis to as high as 75% of two-year survivals (p. 359) as reported by Donaldson *et al.* (1973).

III. FIBROSARCOMA

The oropharynx is an uncommon site for a fibrosarcoma in childhood, and the diagnosis is only made by biopsy of a tumour with much the same clinical findings as a rhabdomyosarcoma of the oropharynx (see above).

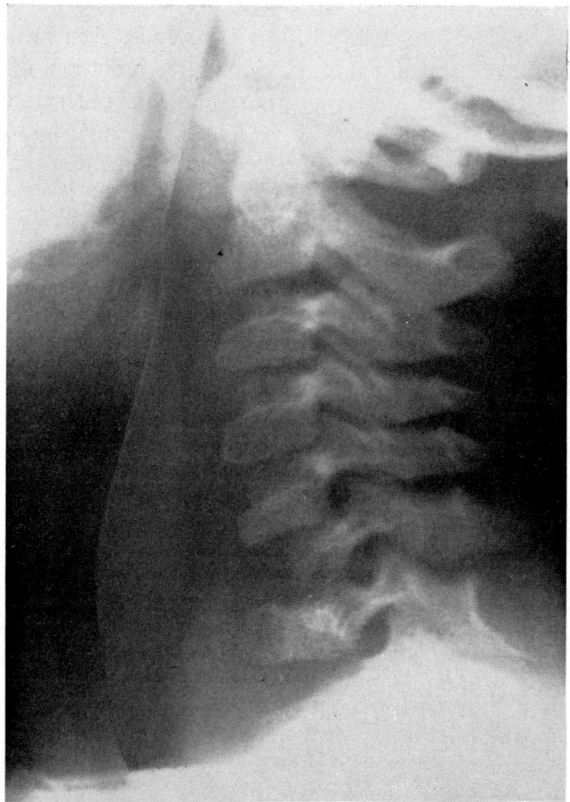

Figure 14.10. A RETROPHARYNGEAL INFLAMMATORY SWELLING showing characteristic prevertebral soft tissue shadow of a tuberculous abscess due to cervical caries.

TREATMENT

Total surgical excision is important in the treatment of this lesion, but in a confined area such as the oropharynx, excision is almost always incomplete. In such cases it would be useful to rely on chemotherapy and radiotherapy, but neither method has as yet a well established role in the treatment of fibrosarcoma.

Chemotherapy

Because of the rarity of this tumour, the effects of chemotherapy are difficult to assess; most fibrosarcomas appear to be relatively resistant, and combination chemotherapy (p. 802) is required.

Radiotherapy
Because of the tendency to delayed local recurrence, even in fibrosarcomas with a highly differentiated histological picture, radiation of the tumour should be considered, although fibrosarcomas in general are relatively radioresistant.

When the operative or histological evidence indicates that excision is incomplete, radiotherapy can be given, in a dose of 3000 for younger children (less than five years of age) and 4000 rads for older children.

In the Index Series one fibrosarcoma arose in the posterior pillar of the fauces and extended downwards as a finger-like process below the lower pole of the tonsil. The diagnosis was made on partial excision, ('incision') biopsy, and treatment initially was with radiotherapy (4000 rads in 5 weeks) and chemotherapy (vincristine and methotrexate). One month later the residual tumour had shown no response, and chemotherapy was changed to adriamycin (40 mg/m^2), given at intervals of 2 weeks. Within 10 weeks there was complete remission. Maintenance therapy with adriamycin was discontinued after 18 months, and she is well with no evidence of disease 2 years after commencing treatment.

E. TUMOURS OF THE NASOPHARYNX

BENIGN SWELLINGS (Table 14.7)

PEDUNCULATED NASOPHARYNGEAL HAMARTOMA
(syn. nasopharyngeal teratoma, epignathus, dermoid cyst, 'nasal glioma')

This rare, 'benign' but nevertheless life-threatening condition can present very early in life as an emergency, and prompt action is often required to prevent death from sudden asphyxiation. It is a clearly defined clinical entity due to hamartoma or choristoma (p. 39) causing respiratory obstruction (Crook, 1965; Loeb & Smith, 1967; Jover *et al.*, 1972).

AGE : SEX

Symptoms usually occur immediately after delivery or in the first few hours of life.

Females are much more commonly affected than males, in a ratio of at least 6 : 1 (Boeckman, 1968).

SITE

The mass is typically attached to the wall of the nasopharynx above the level of the soft palate (Brown-Kelly, 1918).

Table 14.7. Tumours of the nasopharynx and ear

Benign conditions	Malignant tumours
	Nasopharynx
Allergic/inflammatory polyp	Rhabdomyosarcoma
Adenomatous polyp	Lymphosarcoma
Haemangioma	Fibrosarcoma
Pedunculated hamartoma (glioma)	Metastatic deposits
Fibrous dysplasia (facial bones)	Hodgkin's disease
Fibroxanthoma	leukaemias
Neurofibroma	lymphosarcoma
Schwannoma	Carcinoma
Meningioma	squamous
Granular cell tumour	lympho-epithelial
'Epignathus'	undifferentiated
Tumours or cyst of Rathke's pouch	
Juvenile angiofibroma	Chordoma
	Olfactory neuroblastoma
	Craniopharyngioma
	The ear
Inflammatory aural polyp	Rhabdomyosarcoma
Cholesteatoma	Lymphosarcoma
Chemodectoma	Ewing's tumour
	Histiocytosis X
	eosinophilic granuloma
	Hand-Schüller-Christian syndrome

MACROSCOPIC APPEARANCES

There is usually a narrow stalk 5–10 mm in diameter, to which is attached a somewhat rounded, nodular or polypoid mass 2–4 cm in diameter. The mass is firm, whitish and covered by intact epithelium. The cut surface is usually a uniform grey colour, and sometimes shows cystic spaces.

MICROSCOPIC FINDINGS

The covering epithelium is almost always squamous, and the mass contains a variety of structures without any organized plan, including sebaceous glands, fat, muscle cartilage and occasionally disorganized glial tissue.

MODE OF PRESENTATION

Typically the newborn infant breathes well and respiration is satisfactorily established, for a few minutes or hours, until obstruction of the upper airways suddenly occurs, followed by vigorous attempts at inspiration with no audible intake of air. This sudden obstruction may be precipitated by a minor change in posture, and another sudden change, e.g. during attempts to resuscitate the infant, may dislodge the pedunculated mass from the choanal ring and bring instant relief. The problem of maintaining an airway with this lesion is accentuated by blockage of the nasal route at an age when nasal breathing is compulsive and obligatory.

The sudden onset and relief of obstruction following a change in position or posture should suggest the diagnosis, and it is usual to find that in a particular position, e.g. with the head lower than the thorax and the neck hyperextended, respiration is unhampered.

INVESTIGATIONS

The diagnosis can be confirmed by the absence of stridor, normal air entry in the lungs in the interval between obstructive attacks, no accumulation of mucus, and absence of a hyper-resonant percussion note which would suggest a pneumothorax.

X-rays of the chest are normal; lateral films of the head and neck indicate a mass in the upper air shadows (Fig. 14.11).

TREATMENT

Treatment can be carried out without anaesthesia if the situation is urgent, but preferably removal of the mass is performed under intratracheal anaesthesia.

The region above and behind the soft palate is explored by palpation with the little finger; the mass is grasped with forceps, retracting the soft palate as necessary. Traction usually brings to light the pedicle which can then be ligated and transected, and the mass removed.

ENCEPHALOCELES

Removal of a swelling resembling the lesion described above is occasionally followed by a leak of CSF indicating that the 'tumour' was associated with an anterior encephalocele, which may also contain dysplastic brain tissue resembling a 'nasal glioma'. Although 'rhinorrhoea' may occur, in a supine infant leaking CSF tends to accumulate in the oropharynx causing respiratory obstruction, and repeated clearing of the airways by suction is required. When this follows removal of a nasopharyngeal tumour, it should suggest the source of the fluid, and when confirmed by air studies, repair of the defect in the dura, and the floor of the anterior cranial fossa, should be performed without delay to prevent dehydration and the development of meningitis.

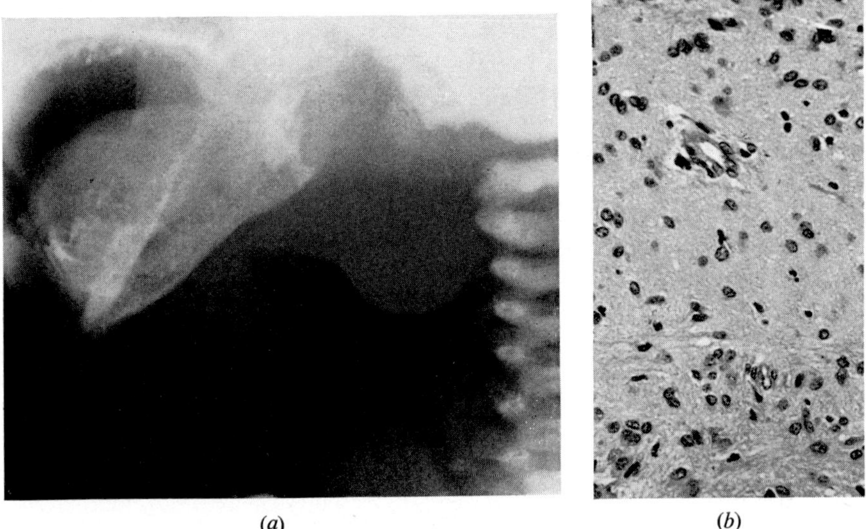

(*a*) (*b*)

Figure 14.11. NASAL 'GLIOMA'; (*a*) x-ray of a mass in the nasopharynx in a neonate, encroaching on the nasopharyngeal air shadow and containing an area of calcification; (*b*) the mass is composed of well differentiated glial tissue, without any neurones (H & E. × 150).

DIFFERENTIATION OF NASAL POLYPS

The great majority of polyps (Table 14.8) arising from the nasal cavity or nasopharynx in childhood are allergic or 'vasomotor' in origin, but a polyp can also develop in both benign and malignant lesions, and every polyp removed should be submitted to histological examination which will show one of the following:

1. **Simple nasal polyp** (Fig. 14.12a)

The only important aspect of these lesions is that they are by far the commonest type of nasal polyp in childhood and should not be confused with the polypoid neoplasms, in particular with rhabdomyosarcoma (p. 358) and neuroblastoma (p. 362). Simple polyps arise from the turbinates and present in the nasal cavity. They are often associated with an allergic diathesis, are probably inflammatory in origin and not true neoplasms.

Macroscopically they are smooth, grey or pink, with a mucoid texture on section.

Microscopically there is a loose mucoid stroma of stellate fibroblastic cells, covered by respiratory epithelium. Scattered throughout the polyp are glandular structures similar to the mucous glands lining the respiratory

Table 14.8. Polypoid lesions of the nasal cavity

Benign conditions	Malignant tumours
Simple (inflammatory, allergic) polyp	Rhabdomyosarcoma
Adenomatous polyp	Olfactory neuroblastoma
Nasal glioma (syn. choristoma, glial ectopia)	Lymphosarcoma
Fibrous dysplasia of nasal bones	Carcinoma (lympho-epithelial)
Anterior ethmoidal encephalocele	Ewing's tumour (of nasal or ethmoid bones)
Juvenile angiofibroma	
Neurofibroma	
Meningioma	

tract. Infiltrations of inflammatory cells are the rule, and numerous plasma cells are also found in the stroma. Most are quite obviously non-neoplastic, but on occasions there is evidence of more active growth such as a more intricate epithelial component, often associated with multi-layered surface epithelium.

2. **Nasal 'glioma'** (syn. nasopharyngeal hamartoma, p. 348)
This is not a true tumour but a form of glial ectopia or choristoma, with intimate mingling of glial and fibroblastic tissue. Pleomorphism of the fibroblasts may occasionally pose a problem in diagnosis.

Microscopically nasal gliomas contain islands of neuroglial tissue resembling disordered white matter of the brain; neurons are very rarely present, although swollen astrocytes may closely resemble them. There are variable amounts of fibroblastic tissue; the nuclei of the fibroblasts are occasionally irregular, bizarre and suggestive of malignancy, and resemble the cells found in the more aggressive examples of fibromatosis in infancy (p. 798). However, no malignant nasal glioma has ever been recorded, and they are considered to be choristomas, i.e. tumour-like malformations composed of tissues not normally found in the particular area.

3. **Fibrous dysplasia** of the nasal bones (Fu & Perzin, 1974b), see p. 331.

4. **Anterior nasal encephalocele:** see p. 350.

5. **Juvenile angiofibroma** (syn. nasopharyngeal fibroma). This uncommon condition is found predominantly in boys and most often during puberty; it is variously interpreted as a vascular fibroma or an aggressive type of haemangioma (Apostol & Frazell, 1965) and most recently as a glomus tumour (see p. 366) of the terminal branches of the maxillary artery (Girgis & Fahmy, 1973), arising from the periosteum of the basisphenoid.

The mode of presentation is severe epistaxis or a bleeding nasal polyp in a boy more than twelve years old (MacComb, 1963).

Macroscopically the lesion presents as a fleshy, reddish, polypoid mass, usually non-ulcerated and extremely vascular, arising from the vault of the nasopharynx (Tapia Acuña, 1973).

Microscopically the lesions consist of a loose mucoid fibroblastic stroma containing numerous vascular channels (Fu and Perzin, 1974a), many of them dilated and sinusoidal, with delicate walls which appear to be formed by stromal cells; there are also vessels typical of capillary haemangiomas (Fig. 14.12b).

With the passage of time, the stroma becomes more collagenous and sclerotic, and the smaller vessels atrophy or disappear, leaving only the larger vessels in which the walls are much thickened. The histological picture holds little that is alarming, but their clinical behaviour has some of the attributes of a neoplasm for they may extend into every available recess and

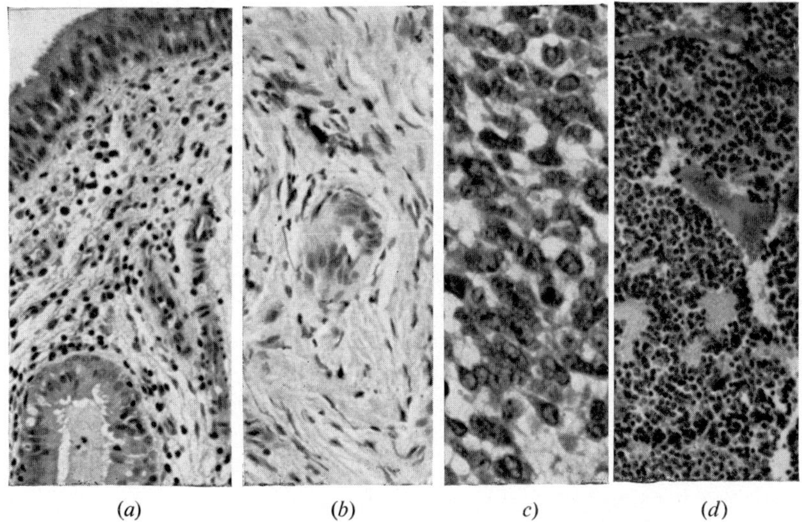

(*a*) (*b*) c) (*d*)

Figure 14.12. NASAL POLYPS. Various nasopharyngeal lesions present as a polyp to be distinguished histologically from (*a*) A SIMPLE INFLAMMATORY POLYP, covered with respiratory epithelium and containing islets of mucous glands in an oedematous stroma infiltrated by many inflammatory cells; (*b*) JUVENILE ANGIOFIBROMA composed of many small blood vessels in a loose fibroblastic stroma; (*c*) RHABDOMYOSARCOMA (usually embryonal, p. 785) composed of cells with hyperchromatic nuclei and strap-like cytoplasmic processes; (*d*) OLFACTORY NEUROBLASTOMA with typical small cells, some of which are arranged in rosettes, and containing fragments of bone from the floor of the olfactory groove.

orifice, e.g. into sinuses via their ostia, and may recur locally after attempts to excize them.

Biopsy is somewhat hazardous because of the torrential haemorrhage which may follow. The diagnosis can be confirmed, and the anatomy of the feeding vessels determined by angiography (Rosen *et al.*, 1966; Williams & Chisolm, 1973).

There was only one case in the *Index Series*, but the actual incidence may be higher than this indicates, as the age of presentation tends to be just outside the paediatric age range, and biopsy is rarely performed.

TREATMENT

Total excision is difficult but not impossible, and hazardous because of the risk of haemorrhage.

Radiotherapy in small doses causes shrinkage of the lesion and facilitates subsequent surgical removal.

Cryotherapy in staged applications has also been used successfully, and oestrogens have recently been advocated, both for their reported sclerozing effects on the tumour, and to minimize blood loss during operation.

Several recent reports have discussed the merits of the various forms of treatment available (Neel, Whicker *et al.*, 1973; Tapia Acuña, 1973; Williams & Chisolm, 1973).

6. Neurofibroma

A solitary neurofibroma of the nose or throat is virtually unknown in children, but a plexiform neurofibroma occasionally involves the submucosa of the nose, or the larynx, either primarily or by extension from a deeply placed parapharyngeal lesion or in the thoracic inlet (p. 465), almost always as part of generalized neurofibromatosis (p. 827), which also includes various types of meningioma (p. 416) found in childhood.

A neurofibroma of the base of the skull may present as a nasal polyp, usually attached to the mucosa in the region of the turbinates. Alternatively, it may form a diffuse submucosal or mural mass which tends to infiltrate and deform the nasopharynx and adjacent tissues.

Microscopically it has the same features as neurofibromas and related lesions elsewhere (p. 823), but Schwannomas with pallisading or Verocay bodies (p. 822) do not occur in the upper respiratory tract in children.

7. Meningioma

This may also present in the nasal cavity, more rarely in the maxillary or ethmoid sinus. It is almost always an extension of an intracranial meningioma arising in the floor of the anterior or middle cranial fossa, and most are an expression of von Recklinghausen's disease (p. 827).

MALIGNANT TUMOURS OF THE NASOPHARYNX

Tumours arising in this region account for approximately 1% of all malignant tumours in childhood but they may pose particular problems in diagnosis and in treatment (Table 14.7).

Difficulty in diagnosis is not uncommon and delay is usually due to one or a combination of the following factors.

1. Most of the varied symptoms of malignant tumours in the upper respiratory tract are the same as those produced by chronic infections which are so much more common in childhood.
2. The nasopharynx is inaccessible to simple direct inspection, and there is an understandable reluctance to resort to examination under anaesthesia, although this is required for thorough examination of this area in a child, and in many cases it is an essential step in clarifying the diagnosis.
3. Malignant tumours of this area tend to infiltrate for some time before they cause definite symptoms or signs.

Difficulties in treatment are attributable to the following:

1. Malignant tumours of the nasopharynx or its recesses tend to be highly invasive and involve nearby vital structures relatively early.
2. There is virtually no scope for radical excision in such a confined space with difficult access, great vascularity, and adjacent structures which cannot be sacrificed.
3. Radiotherapy has limitations in lesions which are often ulcerated, usually infected, where the normal structures tolerate irradiation poorly and the long-term effects may be undesirable, including radiation induced tumours.

Malignant tumours arise in the lining or the wall of the nasopharynx close to the base of the skull (Fig. 14.13), in an area bounded by the basisphenoid-basi-occiput, the cribiform plate of the ethmoid, the ethmoid and maxillary sinuses, the choanal ring, the palate and the muscular posterior wall of the nasopharynx. Although some tumours may have a predilection for one of these structures, this is often obscured by their subsequent extension and infiltration.

None produces a specific pattern of symptoms; in most cases the diagnosis is based on examination under anaesthesia and confirmed by biopsy.

Malignant nasopharyngeal tumours grow and spread in the following directions:

1. *Infiltration in the submucous plane* to involve progressively more of the mucosa.
2. *Polypoid protrusions* into the cavity of the nasopharynx, or its openings and recesses, especially the posterior nares and nasal passages, often predominantly into one of them. Some eventually appear below the level of the soft palate in the oropharynx; others occlude the inner orifice of the Eustachian tube, causing a serous effusion into the middle ear (p. 356), but only rarely extend along it.

3. *Ulceration and infiltration*, together cause erosion of the underlying bone and involvement of nearby structures such as the paranasal sinuses, cranial nerves and blood vessels (Fig. 14.13).
4. *Lymphatic metastases* in cervical nodes, sometimes bilateral, may be the first clinical evidence that nasopharyngeal symptoms are not due to chronic infection.

MODES OF PRESENTATION

The variety of symptoms and signs of malignant tumours of the nasopharynx is formidable, and they are grouped according to the common patterns encountered.
1. *Pain or headache* referred to the forehead, the nose, the ear or the face; the pain is often ill-defined and poorly localized, even by articulate older children.
2. *Persistent blockage of one or both nasal passages*, usually accompanied by catarrhal rhinorrhoea. Streaks of blood in a nasal discharge, or epistaxis not coming from Little's area, are particularly significant.
3. *The discovery of a polyp* in a patient with either of the above is an indication for biopsy of the 'polyp' (p. 351).
4. *Significant enlargement of the cervical lymph nodes* due to metastases, particularly in the jugulo-digastric group of deep cervical nodes.
5. *Earache, deafness or tinnitus* will direct attention to the ear; when there is a 'serous' otitis media (due to obstruction of the medial end of the Eustachian tube) this is stated to be so suggestive of a neoplasm, at least in adults, that the patient should be considered to have a tumour affecting the ear until proven otherwise (Straka & Bluestone, 1972).
6. *Cranial nerve palsies*, associated with 1 and 2 above, develop when the tumour infiltrates beyond the nasopharynx (see Fig. 14.13). The incidence of palsies in tumours of the nasopharynx is between 20 and 40% in various reported series. The clinical effects of palsies vary according to the nerve(s) affected:
(*a*) *Diplopia*, transient at first, followed by strabismus (CN. III, IV, VI).
(*b*) *Ptosis*, occurs following involvement of the facial nerve in the middle ear (CN. VII).
(*c*) *Hyperaesthesia* of the face or forehead (CN. V).

CLINICAL EXAMINATION

The usual examination of the ear, nose and throat may yield no positive findings; when the signs and symptoms are persistent, severe, or in any way unusual, a thorough examination by an otorhinolaryngologist is indicated, including examination under anaesthesia, and biopsy of any suspicious lesion such as a polyp (see p. 351).

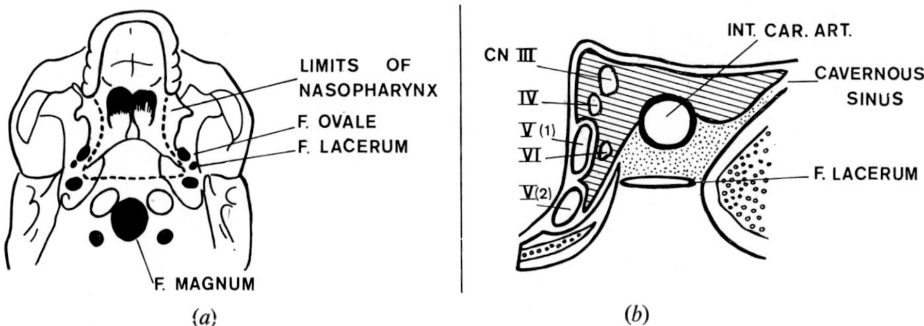

Figure 14.13. ANATOMY OF THE NASOPHARYNX; (*a*) diagram of the base of the skull showing site of attachment of the nasopharynx (interrupted line); (*b*) sagital section through foramen lacerum showing proximity of nasopharynx to intra-cranial structures, cavernous sinus and cranial nerves.

Attention should also be directed to any enlargement of the cervical nodes, and any node more than 3 cm in its maximal dimension should be biopsied (see p. 225).

INVESTIGATIONS

1. *X-rays* of the paranasal sinuses, the mastoid cells, and lateral penetrating views of the nasopharyngeal region may yield important information. A nasopharyngeal tumour is strongly indicated by:
(*a*) an irregular or atypical filling defect in the nasopharyngeal air shadow, or outlined by barium instillation, is more likely to be due to a neoplasm than to benign enlargement of the adenoids;
(*b*) erosion of bone, e.g. the basi-occiput or sphenoid.
2. *Carotid angiography* will usually show highly vascular lesions not otherwise easy to demonstrate, and is practically diagnostic in the highly vascular juvenile angiofibroma (p. 352), in which biopsy is contra-indicated by the likelihood of massive haemorrhage.

DIFFERENTIAL DIAGNOSIS

Most of the early symptoms of a tumour are the same as those caused by chronic infection in the upper respiratory tract. The age of the child is a helpful point, for most tumours arise in an age group somewhat older than those maximally affected by the common nasal ills. *Persistent and troublesome nasal symptoms commencing at ten to twelve years of age in a child not asthmatic and not previously prone to chronic nasal infections, should arouse suspicion of a neoplasm.*

The tumours which may arise in the nasopharynx are as follows:

I. Rhabdomyosarcoma;
II. Carcinoma (lympho-epithelial);
III. Malignant lymphoma (usually lymphosarcoma);
IV. Olfactory neuroblastoma;
V. Chordoma;
VI. Tumours and cysts of Rathke's pouch.

I. RHABDOMYOSARCOMA OF THE NASOPHARYNX

Of the several tumours which may arise in the nasopharynx, the commonest in childhood is the rhabdomyosarcoma (Fig. 14.12c), most if not all of which are histologically embryonal in type (p. 785). The macroscopic form known as 'sarcoma botryoides' can present as a polypoid mass in the nose, or rhabdomyosarcoma may arise in the maxillary or ethmoidal sinuses and occasionally, in the middle ear (p. 364) or the pharynx (p. 345).

The Index Series contains five cases of rhabdomyosarcoma in this area, one in each of the tonsil, the soft palate and the middle ear, while the exact site of origin was difficult to determine in two, but was probably the vault of the nasopharynx at its attachment to the base of the skull.

TREATMENT OF RHABDOMYOSARCOMAS OF THE NASOPHARYNX

Their site and inaccessibility preclude extensive surgical excision, and treatment therefore rests on radiotherapy or chemotherapy. The prognosis has been hopeful since Edland (1967) reported good results in some patients treated with combined radiotherapy and chemotherapy and results have been further improved in recent reports (p. 359), although the longterm effects of irradiation of the nasopharynx in children may be serious.

In two recent reviews, with a total of 47 rhabdomyosarcomas arising in the head and neck in children (Donaldson *et al.*, 1973; Jaffe *et al.*, 1973), the nasopharynx and nasal cavity were the commonest sites; ten arose in the orbit (see p. 402), and other sites affected were the tonsil, the alveolar and buccal region, maxillary antrum, the forehead and the temple. The histological pattern was embryonal in 13 of the 19 patients in the first of these reviews, and the system of staging used in that review is as follows:

T1 Tumour localized to one 'region' or site (one zone of lymphatic drainage).
T Tumour involving two or more 'regions' (e.g. tonsil and palate).
T3 Radiographic evidence of bone destruction, or clinical involvement of cranial nerves (Fig. 14.13b).
N0 No clinical evidence of lymph node metastases.

N1 A single node clinically involved, but less than 3 cm in diameter.
N3 Fixed unilateral nodes, or bilateral significantly enlarged nodes.

Surgical excision

To remove as much of the tumour as possible is a principle of management in rhabdomyosarcoma, but is rarely practicable in the nasopharynx, and in Donaldson's series partial excision was feasible in only 3 of 19 cases.

Radiotherapy

This is an integral part of the treatment of nasopharyngeal rhabdomyosarcoma, to a total dose of 4000 rads in 4–5 weeks. Both the primary tumour and the related lymph nodes should whenever possible be included in the area treated. Because of the frequency of lymph node metastases, elective irradiation is indicated when they lie at some distance from the primary tumour.

Chemotherapy

Combination chemotherapy is justified by the hitherto poor prognosis of rhabdomyosarcomas; three cytotoxic agents, viz. vincristine, actinomycin D and cyclophosphamide, in the following regime are recommended by Donaldson *et al.* (1973).

Vincristine (2 mg/m^2 IV) weekly for 12 weeks; later doses may be omitted when indicated; subsequent courses (four injections at weekly intervals for 4 weeks) are repeated every 3 or 4 months.

Actinomycin D (0·075 mg/kg IV) is given over 5–8 days, and repeated every 3 months for five courses (i.e. for 15 months).

Cyclophosphamide, in a longterm course of 2·5 mg/kg daily, is given for 2 years.

The regime used for most of the recent cases of rhabdomyosarcoma in the Index Series (p. 791) is basically similar, though it differs in several details. In Jaffe's series, with ten head and neck cases surviving more than 2½ years, the major drug used was actinomycin D, and others included vincristine and methotrexate. Adriamycin has recently been added.

RESULTS

With this plan of treatment, Donaldson *et al.* (1973) obtained 75% of 2-year survivals (14 out of 19); local control of the primary was unsuccessful in only 2 of the 19 cases, i.e. a local control rate of 89% assessed at least 2 years after commencing treatment. This represents a considerable improvement when compared with reports of earlier series yielding 10–30% of 2-year survivals.

The best results are obtained in patients in Stage T1, N0, and the worst in Stage T3, N3.

Optimism should be tempered by the fact that rhabdomyosarcomas of the nasopharynx had until recently had one of the worst prognoses of all sites. However, more than half of Donaldson's and Jaffe's patients have survived free of disease for 2–2½ years, and sohave 3 of the 5 cases in the Index Series, who are well 4–7 years after starting treatment.

OTHER SARCOMAS

Fibrosarcoma, liposarcoma, fibroxanthoma (p. 470), chondrosarcoma and osteosarcoma have all been reported in the nasopharynx, and in general there are no special clinical features which would distinguish them from each other or from rhabdomyosarcomas. The definitive diagnosis is almost invariably made on biopsy, and the prognosis is determined by the degree of malignancy of each type of tumour.

II. CARCINOMA OF THE NASOPHARYNX
(syn. lympho-epithelioma, transitional cell carcinoma)

These are chiefly tumours of adults, especially in Asia (p. 6) and some parts of Africa (p. 6), and occur only occasionally in childhood. In some races and communities, notably in Chinese communities, it is extremely rare until after the age of 20 years (Straka & Bluestone, 1972). A viral agent (Epstein-Barr virus) has been implicated by the high incidence of positive reactors in affected populations, and by the continued high incidence in those who emigrate, but this may not prove to be of etiological significance.

Nasopharyngeal carcinomas are much less common in Europeans and very rare in Australia; no case has been seen in the Index Series.

Macroscopically they are described as soft, grey tumours often containing areas of haemorrhage and necrosis.

Microscopically they are squamous cell carcinomas with lymphoid tissue forming focal collections between the neoplastic epithelial cells, or infiltrating diffusely among them, leading to the descriptive term 'lympho epithelial' carcinoma. In almost all cases the squamous nature of the epithelial cells can be identified, but some are relatively undifferentiated.

The tumour cells have oval vesicular nuclei, a prominent nucleolus, and peripheral clumping of their chromatin. The cytoplasm is variable in amount, usually scanty, and with ill-defined edges. Differentiation towards a frankly squamoid appearance with intercellular bridges and even keratin formation is occasionally seen.

Their differentiation from reticulum cell sarcoma may be extremely difficult and when there are no epithelial or squamoid areas, it may be impossible.

In an extensive review of squamous carcinoma in children, Moore (1958) collected 47 cases, of which 24 arose in and around the mouth, 16 in the nasopharynx, and 7 elsewhere, mainly in the genital region.

Boys were affected twice as often as girls (2 : 1), and the peak age was between 10 and 15 years (Nishiyama *et al.*, 1967).

In general, the histological appearance was relatively undifferentiated and 'lympho-epitheliomatous', although several authors have recommended that the term be abandoned as the 'lymphoid' element is not neoplastic.

MODE OF PRESENTATION

Painless enlargement of the regional cervical lymph nodes, due to metastasis and not infrequently bilateral, is the commonest clinical finding, and typically occurs before any symptoms caused by the primary.

The site of the primary tumour may be difficult to identify and sometimes repeated re-examination under anaesthesia and biopsy are required to locate an inaccessible lesion.

TREATMENT

Pick *et al.* (1974) recently reported a series of 9 children with lympho-epithelioma. In 7 the tumour arose in the nasopharynx and the commonest mode of presentation was tender enlargement of cervical nodes, due to metastasis, causing torticollis and marked trismus. Repeated epistaxis and downward displacement of the soft palate were findings which pointed to a lesion in the nasopharynx. Surgical excision was limited to biopsy in most cases, but radiotherapy (4000 to 6000 rads) and chemotherapy (chiefly cyclophosphamide) led to satisfactory remission in 7 of the 9 cases.

III. LYMPHOSARCOMA

A malignant lymphoma may arise at any point in Waldeyer's ring, e.g. in the tonsil, but also in less obvious sites above the level of the soft palate. The histological types are described on p. 171, general clinical features of nasopharyngeal tumours on p. 355, and differential diagnosis on p. 351.

The Index Series contains two cases of lymphosarcoma of the tonsil, both lymphoblastic in type with numerous phagocytic reticulum cells scattered among the lymphoma cells (p. 171). However, leukaemic infiltration of the nasal mucosa is more common than primary lymphosarcoma in the nasopharynx.

Treatment of lymphosarcoma is described on p. 175.

IV. OLFACTORY NEUROBLASTOMA
(syn. neuro-aesthesiocytoma, olfactory neuro-epithelioma)

AGE : SEX : SITE

This tumour may occur at any age, but in contrast to other neuroblastomas, it is extremely uncommon in children less than ten years of age, and occurs with equal frequency in both sexes. It appears to arise from sympathetic nerve tissue or primitive cells in the olfactory bulb, and presents with epistaxis and/or nasal obstruction. The history may be quite short, a matter of weeks, but several cases have been reported in which the tumour apparently grew more slowly and caused symptoms for several months before the diagnosis was made. Infiltration of the nasal bones does not usually occur until late, and most cases present as a nasal polyp (p. 351); local invasion is the rule, but metastasis is rare.

Macroscopically the tumour is grey or white, with areas of necrosis, and calcification is occasionally present.

Microscopically the findings are very similar to neuroblastomas elsewhere (p. 544). The histological diagnosis may be very difficult or even impossible unless there is some differentiation to form neurofibrillary tissue (Fig. 14.12d).

Ewing's tumour of the frontal or ethmoid bones, and reticulum cell sarcoma may also be difficult to distinguish without special staining techniques (p. 83). In adults an anaplastic carcinoma may enter the differential diagnosis, but this unknown in children, apart from the rare lympho-epitheliomatous tumours mentioned above.

TREATMENT

Olfactory neuroblastomas are reported to be very radiosensitive and radiotherapy may achieve a prolonged remission. Their treatment is along the same lines as in neuroblastomas arising in the abdomen (p. 558).

V. CHORDOMA

This slowly growing tumour arises in remnants of the notochord, characteristically in one of three sites, the pelvis, the spinal canal (p. 288) and in the region of the sphenoid or the clivus, where it may erode into the nasopharynx to form a polypoidal mass in the nasal cavity. The paranasal sinuses or retropharyngeal connective tissues may also be involved and the tumour eventually projects into the oropharynx. The microscopic findings and treatment are described on p. 289.

VI. TUMOURS AND CYSTS OF RATHKE'S POUCH
(syn. craniopharyngioma)

Rathke's pouch develops as a diverticulum of the oropharynx at approximately 6–8 weeks gestation, and grows into the base of the brain to fuse with the infundibular portion of the pituitary gland to form the anterior lobe. Normally the pouch becomes completely obliterated, but persistence of any part of it may lead to the development of a tumour, e.g. a craniopharyngioma (p. 267) or a squamous epithelial cyst which may present in the nasopharynx.

DIFFERENTIATION OF BENIGN CONDITIONS IN THE NASOPHARYNX

Those which tend to form polyps have been described on p. 351. Other benign lesions arising in the area are as follows:

1. Fibrous dysplasia of the facial bones (syn. focal or generalized ossifying fibroma; 'leontiasis ossea')
Although most often affecting the external aspect, it may involve the nasal bones maximally or solely on the deep surface, and lead to nasal obstruction (Fig. 14.14). There is sometimes an external deformity as well, and this may suggest the diagnosis. When entirely internal, the relationship to a bony lesion may not be at all apparent and diagnosis is correspondingly more difficult (Schmaman *et al.*, 1970).

In the Index Series, there were two such cases; both tumours were gritty, grey, and consisted of fairly cellular but nonmalignant fibroblastic tissue in which there were irregular

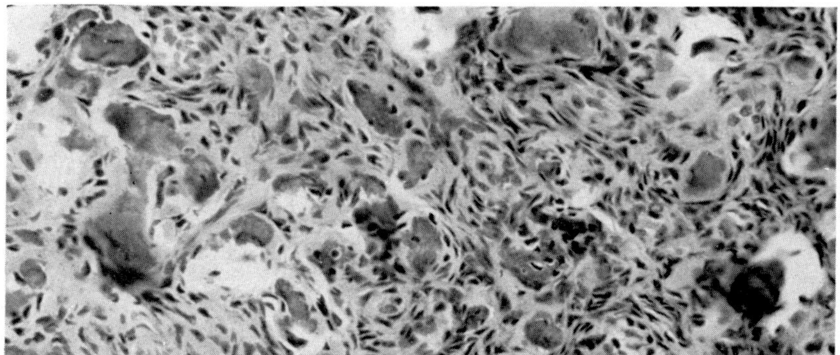

Figure 14.14. FIBROUS DYSPLASIA (NASAL BONE), predominantly fibromatous with an unusual curlicue arrangement of the collagen and an excessive amount of irregular ossification and calcification (H & E. × 300).

spicules of osteoid tissue, some of it intricately calcified, an unusual histological picture which seems to be unique to dysplasia of the facial bones.

2. Haemangiomas of the ear, nose and larynx

Apart from angiofibroma (p. 352), these are rarities in childhood. In infancy a submucosal haemangioma of the larynx at, or more commonly just below, the level of the vocal cords is a clinical entity presenting considerable problems in management (see p. 469).

Other benign neoplasms

These are very rare, but may include granular cell tumours ('myoblastoma') described on p. 858, and pleomorphic salivary adenomas ('mixed' salivary tumour) on p. 312.

F. TUMOURS OF THE EAR

There are few conditions in childhood which occur with sufficient frequency, and with symptoms, which warrant inclusion in a discussion of tumours of the nasopharynx and the ear. They are:

I Rhabdomyosarcoma;
II Cholesteatoma;
III Chemodectoma (in adolescents).

I. RHABDOMYOSARCOMA OF THE EAR

A rhabdomyosarcoma may arise in the middle ear and eventually spread through the ear drum to present as a polyp in the external auditory canal (Potter, 1966; Jaffe, Fox & Batsakis, 1971).

MODES OF PRESENTATION

1. *Deafness and/or giddiness*, as a result of infiltration of the cochlear and vestibule.
2. *A blood-stained, watery or offensive discharge* from the external auditory canal.
3. *A polyp*, with or without bleeding, at the internal orifice of the Eustachian tube.

The diagnosis is usually made on the result of biopsy of the polyp.

Microscopically it is almost always embryonal in type (p. 785), and not infrequently covered with intact surface epithelium. The cells of the tumour are irregular and pleomorphic, with a variable amount of elongated cytoplasm; cross-striations may or may not be demonstrable (p. 786). The stroma is characteristically loose and oedematous, and some areas are only sparsely cellular. Nevertheless, their irregular hyperchromatic nuclei cannot be mistaken for those of a benign condition.

DIFFERENTIAL DIAGNOSIS

This includes inflammatory polyps, the conditions causing nasal polyps (p. 351) and cholesteatoma (see below).

Parapharyngeal cellulitis is a little understood inflammatory lesion arising close to the wall of the pharynx or in the pterygopalatine fossa. This causes trismus, a swelling deep to the tonsillar fossa which sometimes erodes into the external auditory canal and also into the external carotid artery or one of its terminal branches, with massive haemorrhage from the ear. A malignant tumour is sometimes suspected, and except for arteriography is difficult or impossible to exclude without exploration.

Chemodectomas of the glomus jugulare are rare in childhood, but their age range includes adolescence; the clinical and pathological aspects of this tumour are described below.

TREATMENT

The principles of treatment of rhabdomyosarcomas of the ear are the same as those arising in the nasopharynx (p. 345). Surgical excision of the aural lesion may require radical mastoidectomy.

II. CHOLEASTEATOMA

This term is applied to a benign tumour-like mass in the middle ear, composed of fibroblastic granulation tissue, giant cells and keratin. The lesion is basically a foreign-body giant-cell reaction to keratin or squamous epithelium, and arises in chronic otitis media following squamous metaplasia of the normal cuboidal epithelium lining the cavity of the middle ear (Fig. 14.15).

Although not strictly a neoplasm, a choleasteatoma is a progressively infiltrative condition leading to destruction of the bony walls of the middle ear and the tympanic cavity, eventually eroding into the cranial cavity, introducing infection and consequently causing meningitis and/or a temporal lobe abscess.

A similar type of histological lesion, unrelated anatomically, can arise in the cranium, in a cyst of Rathke's pouch (p. 269) lined with squamous epithelium, or when a craniopharyngioma containing squamous epithelium infiltrates adjacent structures by virtue of a foreign-body giant-cell reaction to keratin.

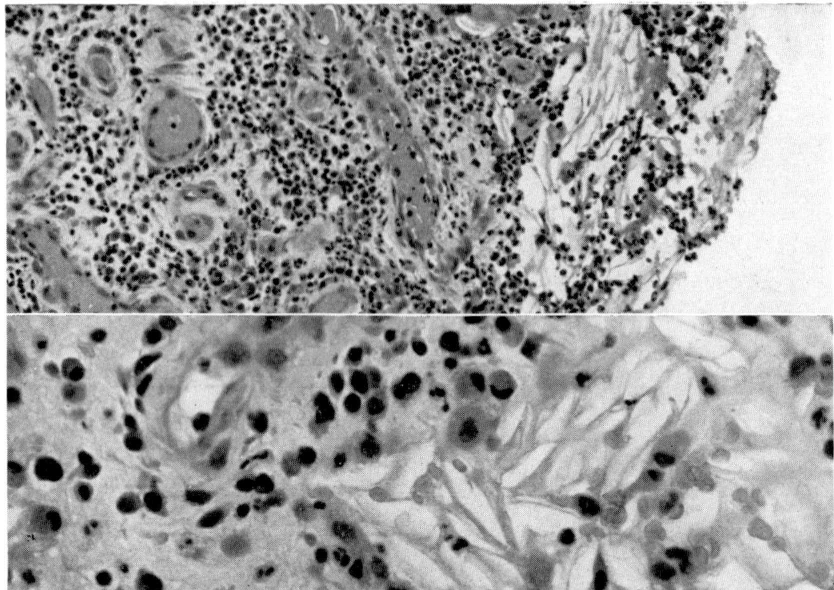

Figure 14.15. CHOLESTEATOMA OF THE EAR, presents as a mass in the middle ear or as (*a*) an aural polyp composed of markedly inflamed granulomatous tissue containing keratin squames (right) (H & E. × 130); (*b*) the stroma contains plasma cells, fibroblasts and macrophages surrounding masses of keratin that are thought to provoke the inflammatory reaction (H & E. × 520).

[(*a*) *Top.* (*b*) *Bottom.*]

Radical excision or at least curettage of the affected area is required, although hampered by important structures nearby.

Other tumours of the middle ear have been described (Tucker, 1965); squamous cell carcinoma (Moore, 1958), adenocarcinoma, and bone tumours (for example Ewing's tumour, p. 734) may occur in the ear, but all of them are rare.

III. CHEMODECTOMAS OF THE INNER EAR

Chemodectomas are derived from homologues of the 'glomus' cells, such as those forming the carotid body, and they may arise in various sites (Hewitt, 1972). In childhood they are most commonly found in the skin (p. 855), as shown in the Index Series. The histological features are described on p. 856.

Very rarely a tumour of this type arises from one of the baroreceptor and chemoreceptor cells normally present on the surface of the jugular vein in the jugular foramen (i.e. the glomus jugulare), or from cells scattered in groups along the course of Jacobson's nerve (the tympanic branch of the vagus) or Arnold's nerve (the postauricular branch of the vagus) as they run in canals in the substance of the temporal bone (Rosenwasser, 1945; Guild, 1953; Snyder, 1961; Moore, Robbins *et al.*, 1973).

Chemodectomas occur mainly in adults, only occasionally in adolescents and very rarely in children. Simpson & Dallachy (1969) reviewed case reports of vascular polypoid tumours arising in the middle ear, and accepted a diagnosis of glomus tumour in fourteen of them. The ages in reported series range from 16–69 years, and the clinical picture is determined by the site of the tumour and the direction in which it grows (Bickerstaff & Howell, 1953).

1. *The most common history is of localized aural symptoms*, unilateral deafness, tinnitus, otorrhoea or bleeding from the ear. Secondary infection often occurs and leads to an erroneous diagnosis of 'chronic suppurative otitis with polyp formation'.
2. *Neurological signs* may develop after years of aural symptoms and signs; hoarseness, palatal and pharyngeal paralysis arise from involvement of cranial nerves in the foramen lacerum (Fig. 14.13b).
3. *Aural and neurological symptoms* may develop at the same time, and even more rarely neurological signs precede aural symptoms.

The tumour usually erodes through the floor of the hypotympanum and presents as a mass in the middle ear, or as a highly vascular 'polyp' in the external auditory meatus. The diagnosis may not be suspected until removal of an aural polyp is followed by excessive bleeding, and histological examination reveals that it is a chemodectoma. This emphasizes the importance of biopsy for all aural polyps.

Treatment

A radical mastoidectomy may be required, and an important point (Hatfield *et al.*, 1972) is the high incidence of recurrence, as long as fourteen years after apparently successful removal. For this reason, radiotherapy of not less than 4500 rads following radical mastoidectomy is usually recommended in adults.

G. CERVICAL TUMOURS

For the purposes of this section, the cervical region is taken to extend from the lower border of the mandible to the clavicles. This area is one of the commonest sites of swellings in childhood because of the incidence of developmental anomalies leading to epithelial remnants, and the active state of the cervical lymph nodes busily engaged in controlling, or at least reacting to, the host of bacteria and viruses the young child first encounters by way of the oropharynx.

Table 14.9. Cervical tumours

Benign conditions	Malignant tumours
Lymph nodes	
Nonspecific hyperplasia	Lymphomas
Lymphadenitis	Hodgkin's disease
coccal } acute	lymphosarcoma
coccal } chronic	reticulum cell sarcoma
tuberculous	Metastatic deposits from:
cat scratch disease	neuroblastoma
Sinus histiocytosis (p. 217)	lymphosarcoma
	reticulum cell sarcoma
	rhabdomyosarcoma
	thyroid carcinoma
	tumours of nasopharynx
	Histiocytosis X
	(Letterer-Siwe disease)
	Burkitt's tumour
Thyroid gland	
Thyroglossal cyst	Carcinoma
Epidermoid cyst	papillary, follicular
Median ectopia	alveolar
Congenital goitre	(medullary)
Hashimoto's disease	Metastatic deposits
Thyroid adenoma	leukaemias
Cervical teratoma	lymphomas
Thyroid abscess	Other sarcomas of soft tissue (p. 781)
Submandibular salivary gland	
Submandibular calculus	Metastatic deposits
Haemangioma or lymphangioma	leukaemia
Pleomorphic adenoma	lymphoma
	Carcinoma
	muco-epidermoid
	undifferentiated
Soft tissues and cell rests	
Sternomastoid 'tumour'	Rhabdomyosarcoma
Cystic hygroma	Primary neuroblastoma
Haemangioma	Neurofibrosarcoma
Fibromatoses (p. 798)	(malignant Schwannoma)
Plexiform neuroma	Haemangiopericytoma
Ganglioneuroma	
Paraganglioma	
Phaeochromocytoma	Other sarcomas of soft tissues (p. 781)
Chemodectoma	
Teratoma	
Skin (see p. 837)	
Epidermoid cyst	Carcinoma (in xeroderma pigmentosum)
Pilomatrixoma (p. 849)	Malignant melanoma
Other benign skin lesions (p. 848)	Kaposi's sarcoma

Individual benign swellings arising in this region are generally mentioned only once, in relation to the diagnosis of a particular tumour, and are cross-referenced to avoid repetition. Tumours of the parotid gland are described on p. 306, and the conditions considered in this section (Table 14.9) are swellings in the following tissues:

(*a*) The submandibular salivary gland;
(*b*) The thyroid gland;
(*c*) The parathyroid gland;
(*d*) Tumours of soft tissues (excluding sarcomas for which see p. 781);
(*e*) The cervical lymph nodes (see Chapter 12, p. 223).

(a) TUMOURS OF THE SUBMANDIBULAR SALIVARY GLAND

Differences in the incidence of tumours in this salivary gland, in the parotid and in sublingual glands are most clearly shown in an analysis of tumours of the salivary glands (in all ages) reported by Castro *et al.* (1972) from Memorial Hospital, New York. As shown in Table 14.3, tumours of the parotid were nearly ten times more common than those in the submandibular gland, but more than 50% of the latter were malignant, whereas less than 30% of those in the parotid were malignant.

All of the few tumours which arose in the sublingual salivary gland were malignant, but none of them occurred in a child.

AGE : SEX

The third quinquennium contained all but a fraction of the 38 children with a salivary tumour in the series quoted, and girls were affected twice as frequently as boys.

Only 5 of the 38 arose in the submandibular gland and in each case a hard, mobile, nontender mass in the gland was the mode of presentation and the only clinical abnormality. In 4 of the 5 patients the tumour was what would now be described as a benign pleomorphic adenoma (p. 312). In the remaining case a malignant mixed tumour was found, apparently the only example in the English literature, up to that time, of such a tumour in the submandibular gland in childhood. The gland was excised *in toto*, but the patient died of metastases at the age of 8 years, without local recurrence. This outcome was also unusual, for the authors reported 92–94% cures in children with a 'malignant' salivary tumour, most of which were slowly growing muco-epidermoid carcinomas (see p. 307).

In the Index Series one salivary tumour, a pleomorphic adenoma, was found in the submandibular gland. All other salivary tumours both benign and malignant, were in the parotid, and none arose in the sublingual gland.

(b) TUMOURS OF THE THYROID GLAND

CARCINOMA OF THE THYROID GLAND

The thyroid gland has achieved notoriety because of the incidence of malignant tumours following irradiation of the neck (Silverman, 1966; Pincus *et al.*, 1967) which was a method of treatment in vogue in the 1940s for 'enlargement' of the thymus (p. 446), a consequence first suspected by Duffy & Fitzgerald (1950). A continuing study by Toyooka, Hempelmann *et al.* (1963) of 2878 individuals treated in this way has shown an incidence of thyroid carcinoma 700 times the natural incidence. In one group of 268 children who received a mean dose of 353 rads, 30% developed nodularity in the thyroid, and 4·3% a carcinoma. It might be expected that the incidence would eventually fall once radiation of thymus or adenoids had been discontinued, and this may yet be shown to have occurred, but Winship & Rosvoll (1961) reported a continuing increase in the number of carcinomas of the thyroid in children after 1945.

Other examples of the potential carcinogenetic effect of radiation on the thyroid are the Bikini tests in 1954, as a result of which 19 children on the island of Rongelap received 175 rads of total body radiation; 15 of them (80%) have developed nodules in the thyroid or hypothyroidism, but none has yet been reported to have developed a carcinoma.

Among 15,000 survivors of Hiroshima and Nagasaki, 21 developed a thyroid carcinoma, an incidence of 140 per 100,000 compared with 0·7 per 100,000 for the general population of Japan (Socolow *et al.*, 1963).

The cumulative long term incidence of neoplasia of the thyroid gland after irradiation has been confirmed by Refetoff *et al.* (1975) who found the highest incidence yet reported, 7%, in a series of children irradiated at 4–5 years of age and re-examined 24–25 years later.

In a small number of instances, thyroid carcinoma arises in a remnant of a thyroglossal duct, outside the thyroid gland (Latimer *et al.*, 1968; Jaques, Chambers & Oertel, 1970).

The Index Series contains four cases of carcinoma of the thyroid (Webster & Howard, 1954) and until recently only one new case had appeared in this community since 1955, a child who developed a thyroid carcinoma 9 years after radiotherapy for a cerebellar medulloblastoma.

The series of 62 carcinomas in childhood collected by Exelby and Frazell (1969) provides the basis for the figures quoted in the following account. In 13 of these 62 children (21%) the neck had been irradiated for thymic enlargement, adenoid hyperplasia, or a cerebellar tumour, etc., and the mean interval between irradiation and diagnosis of a carcinoma was 8·7 years.

AGE : SEX

Girls were affected twice as frequently as boys (40 : 22), and the mean age at the time of diagnosis is usually reported to be 9 years, somewhat earlier in boys, and closely related to the menarche in girls (Tawes & Delorimier, 1968).

MACROSCOPIC APPEARANCES

In most cases the tumour is small (1–2 cm in diameter), pink to grey in colour, appears to be discrete and encapsulated, and has a granular cut surface. The papillary carcinoma is the commonest type (Harness *et al.*, 1971), and a single lesion in most cases, less commonly multiple, and generally arises in a normal gland without any hyperplasia or nodularity. Intrathyroid metastases or multifocal origin is seen in 10% of cases.

MICROSCOPIC FINDINGS

There are several histological types, of which the two important in childhood are (i) the papillary and (ii) the follicular. The undifferentiated or anaplastic type is extremely uncommon in childhood. The medullary type is also uncommon, and only 4 of 67 medullary carcinomas reviewed by Williams *et al.* (1966) occurred in patients between 10 and 20 years of age; none was younger than 10 years.

(*i*) *The papillary type* consists of fronds of fibrovascular stroma clothed by layers of tall cells of thyroid type (Fig. 14.16b) with feathery cytoplasm and a central nucleus which may show slight anaplasia. Follicle formation is sometimes seen in solid parts of the tumour, and small cysts lined by papillary formations are numerous. Calcified foci in the stroma are seen quite frequently; their origin is unknown and their presence does not appear to have any bearing on the behaviour of the tumour.

The papillary type is the most hormone dependent and is favourably affected by suppression of TSH production in the pituitary, by giving oral thyroxine. After adequate excision, local recurrence is not a problem, and metastases may respond favourably to ^{131}I in therapeutic doses (p. 378).

(*ii*) *The follicular type* of carcinoma accounts for 10–20% of thyroid carcinomas in children. It is composed of glandular acini containing colloid; the cells are thyroid-like, but show some pleomorphism and anaplasia (Fig. 14.16c). In less well differentiated examples the diagnosis may be difficult, but can usually be made on the presence of occasional colloid-filled acini. On the other hand, a well differentiated tumour may be difficult to distinguish from a solitary adenoma, and distinguishing features relied upon in adults also apply in children, particularly the presence or absence of vascular and/or capsular invasion.

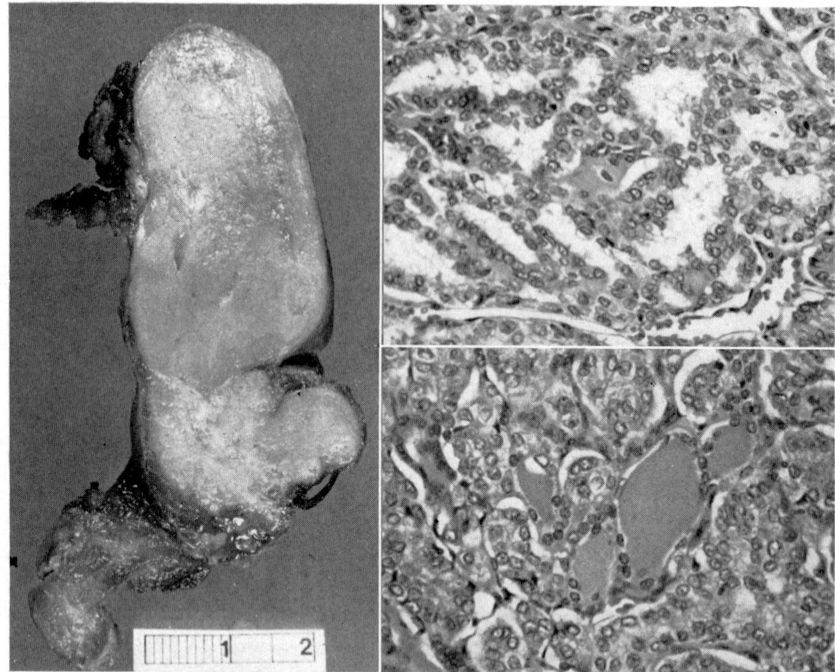

Figure 14.16. CARCINOMA OF THE THYROID; (*a*) sagittal section of the left lobe entirely replaced by uniform, tan coloured, firm tumor tissue; where the lower pole joins the isthmus the cut surface is grey, firmer and gritty; (*b*) the papillary type (H & E. × 180); (*c*) the follicular type, from tumour in (*a*), forming irregular acinar follicles (H & E. × 180).

[(*a*) *Left.* (*b*) *Top right.* (*c*) *Bottom right.*]

In the follicular type metastasis to lymph nodes is less common, but there is a greater tendency to pulmonary metastasis than in the papillary type.

(*iii*) *The medullary type* is believed to arise from parafollicular ('C') cells (Dunn *et al.*, 1973) derived originally from the ultimobranchial body, and some authors (e.g. Wade, 1972) exclude this variety from a classification of true thyroid carcinomas. It certainly differs from all other types in its secretion of thyrocalcitonin, in its familial incidence, its relationship to Sipple's syndrome (p. 562) which includes medullary carcinoma of the thyroid, phaeochromocytomas (Sipple, 1961) pancreatic adenomas, von Recklinghausen's disease and 'hyperparathyroidism' (Steiner *et al.*, 1968), and its association with multiple mucosal neuromas the 'bumpy lip' syndrome (Gorlin *et al.*, 1968; Levy, Habib *et al.*, 1970; Schimke, 1973). In the medullary type, the typical cells are relatively large, subdivided by slim fibrous septa, and many of them have amyloid in their stroma (Williams *et al.*, 1966).

Spindle-cell and giant-cell carcinomas and Hurthle cell tumours are all extremely rare in childhood and behave in a similar fashion to their adult counterparts.

Occasionally sarcomas of soft tissue appear to arise in the thyroid gland, and their behaviour varies according to their histological appearances.

SPREAD

Metastases to the juxtathyroid and lateral deep cervical nodes (middle and inferior groups) is the rule, and not infrequently bilateral. It is more common in the papillary type in which cervical metastases are the commonest mode of presentation (see below). Papillary tumours are also remarkable for the tendency of their metastases to appear over long periods of time, up to twenty years, and for their slow rate of growth.

Metastases to the lungs are more common in the follicular type, and there, too, their rate of growth may be extremely slow. Widespread dissemination rarely occurs and metastases in bone, though classical, are only seen in advanced cases.

Even in the presence of lymph node metastases the prognosis is good.

MODES OF PRESENTATION

In the 62 children reported by Exelby & Frazell (1969), a swelling in the neck was the mode of presentation in every case.

1. *A lymph node* enlarged by thyroid metastasis was the commonest swelling (47, 75%), and in 13 of the 62 children (25%) bilateral lymph node metastases were present at the time of diagnosis.
2. *A nodule in the thyroid gland* itself was the presenting sign in the other 15 patients (25%); the proportion of these two modes varies somewhat from one reported series to another, but taken together the two account for nearly all cases.

In many of the children the swelling in the neck, whether metastatic or primary and intrathyroid, had been present for a considerable period, with an average of two years.

INVESTIGATION

The general condition of the patient is determined by the usual investigations, including the blood picture, and further investigations are necessary to determine the extent of spread.

1. *X-rays of the lung fields* for pulmonary metastases. These are less common in children than in adults; they were present in 7 (11%) at the time of diagnosis, and developed later in another 6, a total of 20%.
2. *Scanning with* ^{99m}Tc has become a standard method of investigating nodules in the thyroid gland in adults (p. 78), the nodule being classified as 'hot' or 'cold' according to its ability to take up the radionucleide. Theoretically a 'cold' nodule can be taken as an indication that it may be a neoplasm (Messaris *et al.*, 1973), but some colloid cysts and adenomas fail to take up the nucleide, and some well differentiated carcinomas may concentrate ^{99m}Tc, giving rise to a small proportion of both false positive and false negative results.
3. *Estimation of protein-bound iodine* and other tests of thyroid function are performed.

DIAGNOSIS

Exploration, biopsy, and definitive excision when indicated, may all be combined as one operation, but when the diagnosis has not been established this places a considerable responsibility on the histopathologist in interpreting frozen sections of a malignant tumour renowned for its ability to reach a high degree of differentiation approaching normal thyroid morphology.

The identification of thyroid metastases in lymph nodes, on the other hand, is an easy task and will establish the diagnosis in those presenting with cervical lymph node metastases.

There is much to be said for a preliminary biopsy and for time to examine paraffin sections before proceeding to definitive operation.

DIFFERENTIAL DIAGNOSIS

Two groups of conditions are to be distinguished, depending on the mode of presentation:
(a) Enlargement of cervical lymph nodes due to benign or malignant causes;
(b) Non-malignant nodules in the thyroid gland.

(a) (i) Benign lymphadenopathies

These are discussed in some detail in the section on peripheral lymphadenopathies (p. 224), but the important conditions *vis-à-vis* carcinoma of the thyroid are as follows.
1. *Non-specific reactive hyperplasia* of the cervical nodes is so common as to be virtually normal in children less than ten years of age, and the general rule is that there are no grounds for concern or biopsy unless an individual node exceeds 3 cm in its maximum dimension. However, it should be noted that in the series reported by Exelby & Frazell, the average size of

the metastatic nodes was 2·5 cm, and this could account for delay averaging two years before the diagnosis of thyroid carcinoma was made.

2. *Tuberculous cervical adenitis* most commonly involves the submandibular and jugulo-digastric nodes, whereas thyroid metastases occur mostly in the middle and lower groups of lateral deep cervical nodes, along the internal jugular chain. Multiple Mantoux tests using PPD (Human) plus antigenic material from one or more of the geographically appropriate anonymous strains will, in most cases, indicate whether tuberculosis is the cause of the enlargement and may also suggest which strain is responsible.

3. *Cat scratch disease* as a cause of cervical lymphadenopathy may be diagnosed on the history or evidence of scratches, the rapid enlargement of the nodes, the specific skin test when available, or the histological findings in a biopsied lymph node.

(a) (ii) Malignant lymphadenopathies

These can rarely be identified without a biopsy, unless they arise late in the course of a disease already diagnosed. In almost all other instances the diagnosis rests on histological evidence (pp. 225–7).

(b) Non-neoplastic swellings in the thyroid gland

These enter into the differential diagnosis when the patient presents with a swelling in the thyroid gland, and they are as follows:

1. Hashimoto's disease.
2. Thyroid adenoma.
3. Nodular goitre.
4. Epidermoid cyst of the thyroid gland.
5. Median ectopia of the thyroid gland.
6. Cervical teratoma.

1. *Hashimoto's disease*

Hashimoto's disease (lymphocytic thyroiditis) is now diagnosed more frequently than in the past (Leboeuf & Ducharme, 1966), and is currently the commonest cause of what appears to be, clinically, a single nodule in the thyroid gland, despite statements that in this condition the gland is usually diffusely and symmetrically enlarged. Hashimoto's disease is probably more common than either a single adenoma or a nodular goitre in girls between five and fifteen years of age living in areas where goitre is not endemic. The condition also arises in the sex and age group most likely to present with a carcinoma of the thyroid.

In all three conditions the patient is euthyroid, although hypothyroidism usually develops subsequently in children with lymphocytic thyroiditis.

In all children with what appears to be a single nodule in the thyroid gland, biopsy should be undertaken without delay because approximately 20% *of* '*single*' *nodules in the thyroid in children are malignant* (Winship & Rosvoll, 1961).

At operation it is not unusual to find that more than one nodule is present in the thyroid gland (i.e. in Hashimoto's disease), and biopsy of more than one nodule is usually required.

2. *Adenomas*

The commonest histological type has a follicular pattern, and the more cellular examples can be difficult to distinguish from a well-differentiated carcinoma. Fetal, embryonal, oxyphil and papillary adenomas have also been described.

3. *Nodular goitre*

The acini are usually large and colloid in type; the epithelium is low and inactive, but more cellular nodules may occur, as well as degenerate areas. Theoretically the multiplicity of nodules makes it easy to distinguish clinically a nodular goitre from a true tumour.

4. *An epidermoid cyst*

This is a rare lesion sometimes found beneath the thyroid fascia and in or on the isthmus of the gland. It is one of the operative findings when exploring what appears to be a swelling in the thyroid gland.

5. *Median ectopia*

This is an even greater rarity, and may be at the normal level of the isthmus or somewhat higher in the midline of the neck. Although occasionally suspected before operation, and provable by scanning, it can be recognized macroscopically at operation and readily confirmed by absence of normotopic thyroid tissue. In almost all cases the ectopic thyroid is the only thyroid tissue the patient possesses, and it should be preserved when possible, moving it laterally to one side of the larynx for cosmetic reasons.

6. *Cervical teratoma*

This is a rare lesion in the newborn which may occupy the site of the thyroid gland (p. 388).

TREATMENT OF CARCINOMA OF THE THYROID

Although total thyroidectomy offers the best prospect of curative surgery, there are some reservations regarding its application in children: (*a*) in this age group most carcinomas of the thyroid are highly differentiated (Roeher *et al.*, 1972), (*b*) with a remarkably slow rate of growth, and (*c*) the prognosis is, relatively, very good (Crile, 1971). Even in the best of hands, total thyroidectomy carries a significant complication rate, (*d*) with approximately 5% of permanent laryngeal paralysis, and (*e*) the same figure for permanent hypoparathyroidism (Thompson & Harness, 1970). Finally, there is the need for lifelong substitution therapy with thyroid preparations, and possibly parathormone as well.

On the other hand, these disadvantages must be weighed against the mortality rate of thyroid carcinoma in childhood, and in the 62 cases reviewed by Winship & Rosvoll (1961), 10·5% of the affected children died within five years of diagnosis (Winship & Rosvoll, 1969).

If alternatives to total thyroidectomy are preferred, less radical operative procedures, soundly based and with acceptable results, are available (Buckwalter & Thomas, 1972) depending on the extent of the disease, as determined by operative findings:

1. *A nodule of carcinoma confined to one lobe*, with no metastasis; total unilateral lobectomy, including removal of the isthmus, is recommended.
2. *If the primary tumour arises in the isthmus*, or when the primary is confined to one lobe but extensive, unilateral total lobectomy plus excision of the isthmus, and subtotal removal of the contralateral lobe are indicated.

Prophylactic 'modified' block dissection is not usually indicated in the absence of lymph node metastases.

3. *When there are unilateral metastases in regional nodes*, ipsilateral total lobectomy and excision of the isthmus are required. Also a formal block dissection of the neck may be performed, but in childhood an acceptable alternative is a 'modified' block resection of the nodes, preserving the jugular-vein, the accessory nerve and the sternomastoid muscle, while meticulously clearing all nodes and connective tissue from the jugular vein. This is preferable in childhood, particularly when there are bilateral metastases, as occur in 20–25% of patients.
4. *When there are bilateral lymph node metastases*, total lobectomy on one side, including the isthmus, and subtotal lobectomy on the other side is the plan recommended; a modified dissection of the nodes on one or both sides can be performed at the same operation, but the removal of the nodes on the second side may be deferred and performed at a later stage.

Examination of both biopsy and operative material in Exelby & Frazell's series showed lymph node metastases in 87% of cases, such a high incidence that a 'prophylactic' modified dissection of the nodes, at least on one side, could be justified, but this has not apparently become standard practice in childhood. The evaluation of various methods of surgical management is made more difficult by the extraordinarily slow rate of growth of the tumour and its metastases, and the good prognosis in 90% of cases, without prophylactic excision of lymph nodes.

SUBSEQUENT TREATMENT

Administration of thyroxine for an indefinite period, is considered to be an important adjuvant, not merely to replace thyroid function after operation, but to depress the amount of TSH produced by the pituitary, and hence to prevent stimulation of any residual tumour tissue, particularly the hormone-dependant papillary type.

Radioactive iodine in therapeutic doses is now reserved for inoperable patients, including those with demonstrable pulmonary metastases shown to be capable of taking up ^{131}I (by tracer test doses); ^{131}I is then given in therapeutic doses. In eight patients treated in this way (Exelby & Frazell, 1969) the metastases completely cleared in four, and were controlled for long periods of time in the others. With regard to the latter group, it is not uncommon for proven pulmonary metastases of papillary thyroid carcinoma to remain static for many years when TSH production is suppressed by thyroid feeding (Crile, 1971).

Although ^{131}I in therapeutic doses has a place in the treatment of thyroid carcinoma in adults, especially in those with well-differentiated metastases shown to be capable of 'take-up', its disadvantages contra-indicate its use in childhood; total thyroidectomy is a necessary prerequisite to obtain the full effect of ^{131}I on metastatic deposits, and the long term effects of radiation, when the nucleide is concentrated in metastases, may also be undesirable, e.g. pulmonary fibrosis with metastases in the lung, or radiation-induced sarcoma in any site.

Chemotherapy

Reports are accumulating of the effectiveness of adriamycin in carcinoma of the thyroid in adults (e.g. Gottlieb & Hill, 1974), but as yet there have been no opportunities for evaluating the long term benefits in children.

Long term follow-up is required because of the extremely slow evolution of the disease, in which metastases can appear as late as 20 to 40 years after apparent cure. In the course of time further removal of cervical lymph node metastases, and possibly contralateral subtotal lobectomy, may become necessary.

In the Index Series (Webster and Howard, 1954) there were three cases of papillary carcinoma all seen between 1946 and 1957; two were girls and both were 10 years old when swellings (bilateral in one) were detected in cervical lymph nodes, shown on biopsy to contain thyroid metastases. In each case total thyroidectomy was performed in two stages, with bilateral clearance of lymph node metastases, and in one a huge mass of retrosternal lymph node metastases was also removed. Both girls were well, free of disease, and maintained on oral thyroid extract, several years after operation.

The third patient, a boy aged 9 years, was found to have miliary nodules throughout both lung fields, and two enlarged nodes in the right cervical region. The pulmonary lesions were at first thought to be tuberculous, then due to sarcoidosis, and 2 years later biopsy of one of the cervical nodes led to the diagnosis of thyroid carcinoma, with multiple pulmonary metastases which had slowly increased a little in size; 10 years after he presented (8 years after diagnosis) he was alive but restricted in his activities by pulmonary insufficiency due to progressively enlarging pulmonary metastases.

There has been only one additional case in the subsequent 20 years, a child in whom a carcinoma of the thyroid gland developed 9 years after radiotherapy for a medulloblastoma of the cerebellum. In the most recent case encountered, after the *Index Series* closed, treatment was along the lines indicated above.

A girl aged 8 years was referred with the history of a swelling in the left side of the neck for 6 months before a biopsy of a left jugular lymph node revealed adenocarcinoma of the thyroid gland. There was no history of exposure to radiation at any time (including *in utero*).

On examination there was a swelling in the left lobe of the thyroid, shown to be a 'cold' area on scanning with ^{99m}Tc (Fig. 14.17a). Tests of thyroid function were normal and there was no evidence of metastasis, except for a second palpable node near the site of the previous biopsy.

At operation, covered by a dose of adriamycin (see below), the tumour was found to have largely replaced the left lobe which was totally removed, identifying and preserving two left parathyroid glands and the recurrent laryngeal nerve. The isthmus was obviously involved and was removed in continuity with the left lobe. The tumour could be clearly seen infiltrating the adjacent part of the right lobe, which was subtotally removed, leaving the posterior third *in situ*.

The middle group of the lateral deep cervical nodes was cleared from the left jugular vein and histological examination showed that the palpable node in this group was the only site of metastasis. Examination of the primary tumour (Fig. 14.16a) showed it to be not papillary but a follicular adenocarcinoma (Fig. 14.16c), with some less well-differentiated areas, and invasion of lymphatic or vascular spaces.

Subsequent scans with ^{129}Cs (Fig. 14.17b) showed no thyroid tissue remaining on the left side, and normal uptake of ^{131}I (Fig. 14.17c) in the residuum of the right lobe.

Adriamycin (45 mg/m^2) was given in two equal doses of 30 mg, on the day of operation and 10 days later. It is planned to continue adriamycin, at intervals of 6–12 weeks, to a total cumulative dose short of myocardial toxicity.

PROGNOSIS

There is accumulating evidence that the outlook in young patients is particularly favourable in a tumour which has a relatively good prognosis at any age (Crile, 1971; Wade, 1972).

The factors influencing the prognosis have been identified as follows:

1. The age of onset; the younger the better the prognosis.
2. Absence of lymph node and pulmonary metastases.
3. The type of carcinoma; children tend to have a high proportion of the more favourable papillary and follicular types.

The rare medullary carcinoma (Levin *et al.*, 1973) has had a particularly evil reputation, but a recent review by Chong, Beahrs *et al.* (1975) indicates that with early diagnosis and aggressive surgical treatment of both the primary and cervical metastases, the results may not be as poor as previously reported.

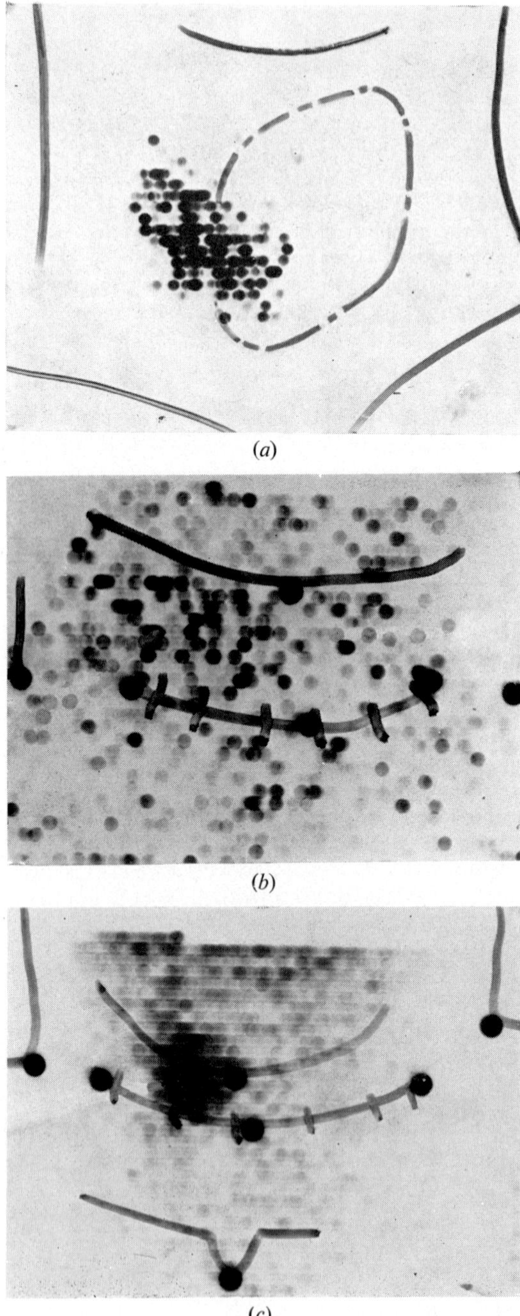

(*a*)

(*b*)

(*c*)

Figure 14.17. THYROID CARCINOMA; (*a*) preoperative scan with ^{99m}Tc showing the 'cold' tumour, and normal uptake in the right lobe. Postoperative scans using (*b*) Cesium and (*c*) ^{125}I, show no residual uptake at the site of the tumor, and normal uptake in the remaining posterior portion of the right lobe (subtotal right lobectomy).

RESULTS

The good prognosis of the more usual types is borne out by the results in the series of 62 patients reported by Exelby & Frazell (1969); 47 (76%) were alive and free of disease when reviewed at least 5 years after definitive treatment (8 after 20 or more years, and 35 after at least 10 years).

Of the 12 deaths in the series, only 3 died from the effects of the tumour; one was an operative death, 8 died of other causes but 3 of these 8 were found to have residual tumour at autopsy.

(c) TUMOURS OF THE PARATHYROID GLANDS

Benign adenomas and hyperplasia of the parathyroid glands are exceptionally uncommon, and apparently only one case of parathyroid carcinoma has yet been reported in childhood (Schantz & Castleman, 1973). Despite the presence of three different types of cell, the parathyroid has so far only been demonstrated to elaborate one hormone, the complex polypeptide parathormone, which exerts its effects reciprocally with calcitonin secreted by the parafollicular cells of the thyroid gland. This relationship also occurs in Sipple's syndrome (p. 562) in which a medullary carcinoma of the thyroid arising in the 'parafollicular' cells (p. 372) is associated with hyperparathyroidism and hyperplasia of the chief cells.

The 'chief' cells found in the parathyroid are normally of two kinds: (i) dark cells with secretory granules which elaborate parathormone, and (ii) clear cells containing less RNA, much glycogen and some lipid. When enlarged and vacuolated these cells are the 'waterclear' or 'wasserhelle' cells found in parathyroid adenomas.

Oxyphil cells also occur in the parathyroid gland, only appearing a year or two before puberty, and they may be derived from chief cells.

The clinical effects of hyperparathyroidism vary to some degree from patient to patient, as expressed in a variety of clinical manifestations, which can be caused by either an adenoma or hyperplasia of the gland.

PARATHYROID ADENOMA

Since the first adenoma was identified and removed from an adult in 1926, there have been two extensive reviews of adenomas arising in children. Nolan *et al.* (1960) collected 22 cases from the world literature up to 1960, and added another of their own. Bjernulf *et al.* (1970) brought the total to 35 cases up to 1970.

The etiology of parathyroid adenomas is unknown, but in a small proportion of cases there is a familial factor, an adenoma developing in (usually one) of the progeny of an affected parent. In another familial entity, Sipple's syndrome (p. 562) there is a genetically determined condition with a distinctive facies resembling scaphocephaly, distinctively thickened everted lips, multiple submucosal neurinomas of the tongue (p. 563), hyperplasia of the parathyroid glands with hyperparathyroidism, and phaeochromocytoma (Levin *et al.*, 1973).

The clinical and physiological effects of hyperparathyroidism due to hypertrophy or adenoma have been reviewed in detail, in 140 patients in all age groups, by Woolner *et al.* (1952). In another review, Bjernulf *et al.* (1970) indicated the relative incidence of these two lesions in children: 35 cases of adenoma to 7 cases of hyperplasia.

AGE : SEX

In the series of 35 cases quoted, the age of children with an adenoma was from 3–15 years, most cases arising after the age of 10 years. The sex incidence was approximately equal (also noted by Nolan *et al.*, 1960) in contrast to adenomas in adults, of whom 70% were females.

MACROSCOPIC APPEARANCES

The size of the adenoma varies from 1–5 cm, and cannot always be correlated with the amount of parathormone detectable in the blood. An adenoma is usually yellowish brown and somewhat darker in colour than a normal gland. The cut surface is typically uniform, but some contain small cystic spaces, and areas of haemorrhage can occur.

MICROSCOPIC FINDINGS

An adenoma is composed of nodular masses of either chief or oxyphil cells, separated by fibrous septa from the cells of the adjacent normal gland, which may appear atrophic. Some of the cells in the adenoma are large and contain bizarre nuclei, but they are not indicative of malignancy (cf. adrenal cortical adenoma, p. 581). Occasionally the acini contain colloid and resemble thyroid tissue (Castleman, 1952). It may be impossible to distinguish between an adenoma and hyperplasia affecting chief cells on histological criteria alone, because of the identical structure and arrangement of the component cells (Roth, 1971).

HISTOLOGY OF PRIMARY PARATHYROID HYPERPLASIA

As a rule all four glands are enlarged, and each is tan or brown in colour. Two forms of hyperplasia occur depending on which of the component cells are involved.

Clear-cell hyperplasia

The hyperplastic gland consists of sheets of uniform cells 10–15 μ in diameter, with clear cytoplasm and a small central nucleus. This may form cords or acini, and electron microscopy reveals multiple vacuoles in the cytoplasm, consisting of structures 0·2–2 μ in diameter, derived from Golgi tubules and surrounding a limiting membrane. Some secretory granules can usually be seen.

Chief-cell hyperplasia

The chief cells are arranged in uniform sheets, may also form glandular structures; their nucleus is also central, but slightly larger than that of the clear-cell, with amphophilic cytoplasm which varies from light to dark staining depending on the degree of granularity. Oxyphil cells may also be present. Electron microscopy shows that the granularity appears to reflect hypertrophy of a rough endoplasmic reticulum indicative of protein synthesis, and there are also numerous secretory cells.

ENDOCRINE EFFECTS OF HYPERPARATHYROIDISM

Normally the concentration of serum calcium is controlled within a narrow range 9–10·5 mg/dl (2·20–2·70 mmol/l), of which a little more than half is ionized and freely diffusible; the remainder is bound to protein, mainly albumin. The level of ionized calcium is controlled by parathormone, and increased by hypersecretion which acts in three ways: (*a*) by a direct effect on the bone, activating osteoblasts to mobilize calcium; (*b*) by increasing the amount of calcium reabsorbed by the renal tubules; and (*c*) by increasing the amount of calcium absorbed from the intestinal contents, although parathormone is less important in this regard than vitamin D.

The balance between secretion of parathormone and calcitonin is not controlled by tropic hormones but by the concentration of calcium ion in the extracellular fluid.

Hyperparathyroidism, by mobilizing calcium, causes osteoporosis, the formation of bone cysts, and an elevated level of serum calcium. A high level of serum calcium leads to:

(i) Increased excretion of calcium in the urine (in spite of some increase in the amount of calcium reabsorbed in the renal tubules);

(ii) Decrease in serum phosphorus, and increased excretion of phosphorus in the urine;

(iii) Increased urinary excretion of water, sodium, potassium and chloride; and

(iv) Deposition of calcium in soft tissues, especially in the kidney causing nephrocalcinosis.

MODES OF PRESENTATION

1. *Nonspecific symptoms;* early signs and symptoms of hyperparathyroidism are largely nonspecific, and Nolan *et al.* noted that the average duration of symptoms before diagnosis was nearly two years.

The general effects are weakness, lassitude, anorexia and irritability and in some cases, somewhat more specific features: abdominal distension, constipation, thirst and polyuria.

2. *Disordered calcium metabolism;* manifestations may be due to the disordered metabolism in skeletal or soft tissue and the signs and symptoms in either may predominate.

(i) Skeletal symptoms such as bone pain, a pathological fracture or progressive collapse and deformity due to softening, were noted in 21 of the 35 cases reviewed by Bjernulf *et al.* (1970).

(ii) Renal disease, causing urinary calculi and renal colic, was less common and occurred in 6 of the 23 cases reviewed by Nolan *et al.* (1960), and 11 of the 35 by Bjernulf *et al.* (1970).

(iii) Even less common modes of presentation are secondary hypomagnesaemia (causing myoclonic spasms), peptic ulceration (Tsumori *et al.*, 1952), pancreatitis or, very rarely, acute parathyroid crisis involving mental disturbances, drowsiness, severe hypercalcaemia, and incipient renal failure.

INVESTIGATIONS

1. *Serum electrolytes*, particularly serum calcium and inorganic phosphorus, are usually diagnostic of hyperparathyroidism in which there is a high level of calcium and a correspondingly low level of inorganic phosphate. (Normal levels in children : serum phosphorus 3·5–4·5 mg/dl; serum calcium 9–10·5 mg/dl.)
2. *Urinary calcium and phosphorus;* there is increased excretion of phosphorus in the urine; the level of calcium in the urine is less predictable and usually decreased, but it may be increased if the serum calcium is greatly elevated and vice versa (see below).
3. *Skeletal radiological survey.* The earliest radiographic changes are seen as resorption of bone in the phalanges and in the lamina dura of the teeth; generalized decalcification, or single or multiple focal (cystic) areas of resorption, are also typical.
4. *Plain films of the abdomen* may show renal calculi, or streaks of calcification in the renal areas indicating nephrocalcinosis. Pyelography may show secondary effects of the calculi.
5. *Radio-immuno-assay* now makes it possible to measure the level of parathormone in the blood and, estimations in blood obtained by transcardiac

venous sampling, are sufficiently sensitive to use as a probe to determine which of the cervical veins have the highest level of parathormone and hence identify the precise site of an actively secreting adenoma (O'Riordan *et al.*, 1971; Monchik *et al.*, 1973).

DIFFERENTIAL DIAGNOSIS

The delay averaging nearly two years is an indication of the difficulty in diagnosis, partly due to the extreme rarity of an adenoma, but also because of the variety of the presenting symptoms which may be suggestive of other conditions, for example polyostotic fibrous dysplasia, or renal disease.

1. '*Malignant malaise*', described in relation to neuroblastomas (p. 549), closely resembles the early nonspecific symptoms caused by a parathyroid adenoma, and focal radiological changes in bone may be misinterpreted as due to metastatic neuroblastoma. Negative results of screening tests for neuroblastoma (p. 551), and multiple bone lesions in hyperparathyroidism, should lead to estimation of the serum calcium, and specific tests to determine the level of serum parathormone will confirm the diagnosis.
2. *Rheumatic fever* may be suggestive by the early symptoms, but can be excluded by positive findings in a skeletal survey and abnormal serum calcium and phosphorus.
3. *In idiopathic hypercalcaemia*, or in vitamin D intoxication, the level of serum calcium is high but the inorganic phosphorus is usually normal.
4. *Primary renal disease*, for example renal calculi causing colic, or tubular abnormalities causing polyuria, are also possible causes of abnormally elevated serum calcium, but the serum phosphorus is normal, and in some cases the serum calcium may also be low, because of large amounts excreted in the urine.
5. *Chronic renal failure* from other causes can lead to accumulation of phosphorus with high levels in the serum; this in turn stimulates the parathyroid gland, causing secondary hyperplasia, increased serum calcium, and many of the clinical features of primary hyperplasia. However the serum phosphorus is actually elevated or normal, and this is usually found to be a reliable guide as to whether parathyroid hyperplasia is primary or secondary. The late effects of hyperparathyroidism itself can cause severe renal damage and failure, leading to reduced clearance of phosphorus and the level of serum phosphorus then rises; and in such cases the only means of distinguishing primary and secondary hyperplasia may be a radio-immuno-assay to determine the level of serum parathormone.
6. *Primary hyperplasia* may be impossible to distinguish before operation (Hey & Seim, 1972) and in a small number of cases exploration is required to make the diagnosis. However, Bjernulf *et al.* noted that in the seven cases of parathyroid hyperplasia in their series, all were male, and four of the

seven were less than two years of age; thus hyperplasia tends to occur in a younger age group than an adenoma.

7. *Secondary hyperparathyroidism.* Reliable demonstration of hypercalcaemia may require repeated estimations of the serum calcium, and levels consistently above 10·5 mg/dl are considered to be diagnostic. True primary hypercalcaemia may be due to 'idiopathic' parathyroid hyperplasia or to a parathyroid adenoma; these are also to be distinguished from other causes of hypercalcaemia.

(i) *Bone metastases;* secondary hyperparathyroidism may occur when any malignant tumour gives rise to bony metastases, for these may lead to extremely high levels of serum calcium, with normal or elevated levels of serum phosphorus. In rare instances tumours other than those arising in the parathyroids secrete parathormone, as demonstrated by immuno-assay of tumour tissue (Lafferty, 1966).

(ii) '*Pseudohyperparathyroidism*' is rare in adults and unknown in children; the findings include hypercalcaemia, hypophosphataemia, and no evidence of skeletal metastases. The cause is unknown.

(iii) *Various conditions* such as leukaemia, myeloma and sarcoidosis can cause hypercalcaemia which may also occur in chronic hypervitaminosis D (possibly a factor in idiopathic hypercalcaemia in infants).

(iv) *Chronic renal disease* (see above).

TREATMENT

In most cases the presence of the symptoms which led to the diagnosis, supported by persistently elevated levels of serum calcium, diminished serum phosphorus and increased excretion of calcium in the urine, establish the need for exploration. This can be further confirmed by a radio-immunoassay to demonstrate increased levels of circulating parathormone, a technique which can also be used in sampling blood from individual cervical veins (Bilezikian *et al.*, 1973) in order to localize the source of parathormone in complicated cases (Bradley & McGarity, 1973). Selective arteriography has also been used to demonstrate a parathyroid adenoma (Doppman *et al.*, 1973).

Morris *et al.* (1974) recommended exploration of the parathyroid glands in all cases (with or without symptoms) in which the serum calcium is 11 mg/dl or more (average of 6 estimations), and also in patients with a serum calcium of 10·5 mg/dl when accompanied by symptoms.

In children, parathyroid adenomas are virtually confined to the neck, although one has been described as arising in the mediastinum. The progressive steps in exploration, commencing in the cervical region, have been set out by Cady (1973).

The current treatment of the rare parathyroid 'crisis' and the more common post operative hypocalcaemia have recently been described by Newmark and Himathongkam (1974).

Because of the possibility of a second adenoma at the time of presentation or developing subsequently, all four parathyroid glands should be identified and a biopsy obtained from each. When one is found to contain an adenoma, the gland and the adenoma are excised, and there is an increasing support for removing all but approximately 50 mg of normal parathyroid tissue (Morris *et al.*, 1974), i.e. all but $\frac{1}{2}$ to $\frac{1}{4}$ of one parathyroid gland.

Recurrent hyperparathyroidism may result from accidental autotransplantation of some of the cells of an adenoma during removal.

The Index Series

In the period covered by the Series there was one case of parathyroid adenoma (Myers, 1963), and a second was encountered more recently. There were remarkable similarities in the two patients as to age of onset of symptoms (11 years in each case), presentation as renal colic due to calculus, an adenoma in one of the left parathyroid glands, and a nodule of thymus at or near the site of the inferior parathyroid glands.

In the second case, not previously reported, the findings were as follows.

A girl aged 11 years presented with a history of recurrent abdominal colic for 8 months, and haematuria for 2 months. Excretory pyelography suggested a calculus in the left ureter and this was confirmed by retrograde studies, which excluded an anatomical basis for calculus formation. The possibility of a metabolic cause was investigated and the serum calcium was 12·8 mg/dl ('normal' in our laboratory: 8·5–10·5 mg/dl) with a low serum phosphorus, 2·1 mg/dl (normal 4–5·5 mg/dl). Excretion of calcium in the urine was increased, the calcium/creatinine excretion ratio being 0·484 (upper limit of normal 0·25).

Renal function tests showed no evidence of disease, e.g. normal excretory pyelogram, blood urea 25 mg/dl, and creatinine clearance 81 ml/min/1·73m². There were no radiological signs of primary hyperparathyroidism. The calculus was removed by extra-peritoneal ureterolithotomy so that it could be excluded as a cause of any symptoms which might occur after removal of a parathyroid adenoma.

Two days later the neck was explored and an adenoma 1·3 × 0·5 × 0·5 cm weighing 200 mg was removed, together with a left (?superior) parathyroid gland. The adenoma was confirmed by frozen sections during operation, and paraffin sections later showed that it was composed of 'chief' cells with some variation in size and staining properties, surrounded by a rim of normal parathyroid gland. Two parathyroid glands on the right side were identified at operation, shown to be normal on biopsy, with neither hyperplasia nor hypoplasia, and were left *in situ*. A nodule of tissue below the lower pole of the left lobe of the thyroid was biopsied and found to be thymus tissue.

In the 12 hours following removal of the adenoma the serum calcium fell from 12·9 to 11·5 mg/dl, and 24 hours later to 8·9 mg/dl; intravenous calcium gluconate was given prophylactically for the next 48 hours, and the serum calcium thereafter was maintained spontaneously between 8·8 and 9·2 mg/dl. Recovery was uneventful and she remains free of symptoms.

This patient has a large café-au-lait patch on the right thigh; a sibling, the mother, and the maternal grandmother all have similar patches, but there is no evidence or history of neurofibromatosis or endocrine adenomas in the family.

(d) TUMOURS OF CERVICAL SOFT TISSUES

CERVICAL TERATOMA

AGE: SEX

Teratomas in the neck (Stone, Henderson & Guidio, 1967) are uncommon, and almost always found in the newborn, also in the fetus and in stillborn infants. There does not appear to be a preponderance in either sex.

SITE

The thyroid region is by far the commonest site (Keynes, 1959) and many, perhaps most of them, may be teratomas of the thyroid gland itself (Silberman & Mendelson, 1959).

MACROSCOPIC APPEARANCES

They are cystic or semisolid, and are large enough to cause acute respiratory obstruction in the newborn.

MICROSCOPIC FINDINGS

Most are benign, but a few have proved to be malignant. They contain a wide variety of tissues representing derivatives of all the germinal layers; the presence of thyroid tissue is not unusual but is not found in every case.

CLINICAL FINDINGS

The modes of presentation include obstructed labour; the mass in the neck is present at birth, and often causes severe respiratory embarrassment. Most teratomas in this region are 5–15 cm in diameter, with a clearly defined edge, and are situated anteriorly or to one side of the neck, extending from the level of the mastoid process to the clavicle.

The tumour is lobulated, feels cystic, is usually mobile, and the skin moves freely over it. It does not transilluminate.

Difficulties in respiration are present in all but a few cases and radiographs usually show displacement and obstruction of the trachea.

Difficulties in swallowing due to oesophageal and pharyngeal obstruction are also fairly common at birth and this may explain an association with hydramnios noted in a few cases.

DIAGNOSIS

The diagnosis is readily apparent in the newborn, and rarely poses any problem in older children. Of the many other swellings found in the region only three are likely to resemble a cervical teratoma : a *facial teratoma* (p. 316), *a cystic hygroma*, or a *congenital goitre*, especially the latter when a teratoma chiefly occupies the region of the thyroid gland.

A cystic hygroma, although similar in site, size and age incidence, is usually lax, has poorly defined boundaries, and is easily transilluminated.

Distinction from a huge congenital goitre is largely academic when there is life-threatening respiratory obstruction, for urgent operation is required in both conditions.

Calcification is present in most cervical teratomas, and is almost unknown in the other two cervical conditions. Malignant cervical teratomas are almost confined to those presenting in adults, and both sarcomas and embryonic neural tumours (possibly endodermal sinus tumours, p. 692) have been described; 4 of the 60 cases reviewed by Silberman and Mendelson were malignant, but only one of the 4 presented during childhood.

TREATMENT

In children, removal of the teratomatous mass is all that is required, often as a matter of great urgency in neonates. The mass can usually be enucleated easily, but the thyroid gland and the superior laryngeal nerve may require careful attention. Tracheostomy may occasionally be necessary if respiration is still embarrassed after excision of a teratoma (McGoon, 1952), for example, if the larynx or trachea remains misshapen.

REFERENCES

A. Scalp and Calvarium

GRAVE, G.F. & MILLS, A.E. (1972). Retinal anlage tumors. *J. Pediat. Surg.*, **7** : 36.

B. Tumours of the face

ANDERSON, R., & BYARS, L.T. (1965). *Surgery of the Parotid Gland.* C.V. Mosby, St. Louis.

BYARS, L.T., ACKERMAN, L.V. & PEACOCK, E. (1957). Tumors of salivary gland origin in children: a clinical pathologic appraisal of 24 cases. *Ann. Surg.*, **146** : 40.

BYARS, R.M. & JESSE, R.H. *et al.* (1973). Malignant tumors of the submaxillary gland.

BYERS, P.D. (1968). Solitary benign osteoblastic lesions of bone. Osteoid osteoma and benign osteoblastoma. *Cancer*, **22** : 43.

Amer. J. Surg., **126** : 458.

CASTRO, E.B., HUVOS, A.G., STRONG, E.W. & FOOTE, F.W.Jr. (1972) Tumors of the major salivary glands in children. *Cancer*, **29** : 312.

CONDON, V.R. & ALLEN, R.P. (1961). Congenital generalized fibromatosis case report with roentgen manifestations. *Radiol.*, **76** : 444.

FOOTE, F.W. & FRAZELL, E.L. (1953). Tumors of the major salivary glands. *Cancer*, **6** : 1065.

GATES, G. (1972). Radiosialographic aspects of salivary gland disorder. *Laryngoscope*, **82** : 115.

Gifford, G.H. & MacCollum, D.W. (1972) Facial teratomas in the newborn. *J. Plastic & Reconstr Surg.*, **49** : 616.

Healey, W.V., Perzin, K.H. & Lorne Smith. 1970). Muco-epidermoid carcinoma of salivary gland origin. Classification, clinicopathological correlation and results of treatment. *Cancer*, **26** : 368.

Howard, J.M. & Rawson, A.S. *et al.* (1950). Parotid tumors in children. *Surg. Gynec. & Obstet.*, **90** : 307.

Johnson, D.G. & Samuel, S.K. (1966). Primary lymphosarcoma of the parotid glands in a child. *J. Pediat. Surg.*, **1** : 170.

Kauffman, S.L. & Stout, A.P. (1963). Tumors of the salivary glands in children. *Cancer*, **16** : 1317.

Keynes, W.M. (1959). Teratomas of the neck in relation to the thyroid gland. *Brit. J. Surg.*, **46** : 466.

Krolls, S.O., Trodahl, J.N. & Boyers, R.C. (1972). Salivary gland lesions in children : a survey of 430 cases. *Cancer*, **30** : 459.

Nicholson, G.W. (1922). Studies on tumour formation; anomalies of position and blending. *Guy's Hosp. Rep.*, **72** :

Rafla, S. (1970). Submaxillary gland tumors. *Cancer*, **26** : 821.

Rothner, A.D. (1973). Aberrant salivary fistulas. *J. Pediat Surg.*, **8** : 931.

Rush, B.F.Jr., Chambers, R.G. & Ravitch, M.M. (1963). Cancer of the head and neck in children. *Surgery*, **53** : 270.

Thackray, A.C. & Lucas, A.B. (1974). Tumors of the major salivary glands, Second series. Fascicle 10. *Atlas of Tumor Pathology*. Armed Forces Institute of Pathology, Washington D.C.

Youngs, L.A. & Scofield, H.H. (1967). Heterotopic salivary gland tissue in the lower neck. *Arch. Pathol.* **83** : 550.

C. Tumours of the mouth, jaws and pharynx

Al-Hindawi, A.Y. *et al.* (1969). The clinical presentation of ectopic thyroid with radio-iodine studies. *Brit. J. Clin. Prac.*, **23** : 372.

Bhaskar, S.N. (1963). Oral tumors of infancy and childhood : a survey of 293 cases. *J. Pediat.*, **63** : 195.

Beckwith, J.B. (1969). Macroglossia, omphalocele, adrenal cytomegaly, gigantism and hyperplastic visceromegaly. *Birth Defects*, **V** : 2 : 188.

Borello, E.D. & Gorlin, R.J. (1966). Melanotic neuroectodermal tumor of infancy : a neoplasm of neural crest origin. *Cancer*, **19** : 196.

Burkitt, D.P. & Wright, D.H. (1970). *Burkitt's Lymphoma.* Livingstone, Edinburgh and London.

Burkitt, D.P. & Kyalwazi, S.K. (1969). In *Neoplasia in Childhood.* Year Book Medical Publishers Inc., Chicago.

Colberg, J.E. (1962). Granular cell myoblastoma: collective review. *Intl. Abst. Surg.* **115**: 205.

Conley, J. (1970). Tumors or the head and neck in children. In *Concepts in Head and Neck Surgery.* Thieme-Verlag, Stuttgart; Grune & Stratton, New York.

Cussen, L.J. & MacMahon, R.A. (1972). Congenital epulis. *Aust. paediat. J.*, **8** : 209.

Dehner, L.P. (1973a). Tumors of the mandible and maxilla in children. I. Clinicopathological study of 46 histologically benign lesions. *Cancer*, **31** : 364.

Dehner, L.P. (1973b). Tumors of the mandible and maxilla in children. II. A study of 14 primary and secondary malignant tumors. *Cancer*, **32** : 112.

Dito, W.R. & Batsakis, J.G. (1963). Intra-oral, pharyngeal and nasopharyngeal rhabdomyosarcoma. *Arch. Otolaryngol.*, **77** : 123.

DONALD, C. (1948). Clinical pictures: cellulitis. In *British Surgical Practice*, vol. 3, p. 20. Butterworth, London.

DONALDSON, S.S., CASTRO, J.R., WILBUR, S.R. & JESSE, R.H. (1973). Rhabdomyosarcoma of head and neck in children: Combination treatment by surgery, irradiation and chemotherapy. *Cancer*, **31** : 26.

EATON, W.L. & FERGUSON, J.P. (1956). Retinoblastic teratoma of epididymis: case report. *Cancer*, **9** : 718.

EHRICH, W.E. (1945). Teratoid parasites of the mouth (episphenoids, epipalati, epignathi). *Am. J. Orthodontics.*, **31** : 650.

EVERSOLE, L.R. & ROVIN, S. (1973). Diagnosis of gingival tumefactions. *J. Periodont.*, **44** : 429.

FUHR, A.H. & KROGH, P.H.J. (1972). Congenital epulis of the newborn: centennial review of the literature and a report of a case. *J. Oral Surg.*, **30** : 30.

GARRINGTON, G.E. & SCOFIELD, H.H. *et al.* (1967). Osteosarcoma of the jaws: analysis of 56 cases. *Cancer*, **20** : 377.

GRIER, E.A. & MACNERLAND, R.H. (1967). Benign teratoma of the tongue. *Ill. Med. J.*, **132** : 43.

HAMNER, J.E. & KETCHAM, A.S. (1969). Cherubism: an analysis of treatment. *Cancer*, **23** : 1133.

HANKEY, G.T. (1955). Congenital epulis (granular cell myoblastoma or fibroblastoma) in a 10 weeks premature infant. *Proc. Roy. Soc. Med.*, **48** : 1015.

HARRISON, D.F.N. (1954). Two cases of bleeding from the ear from carotid aneurysm. *Guy's Hospital. Rep.*, 103, 207.

JAFFE, B.F. (1972). Neck masses and malignant tumors of the head and neck. In *Pediatric Otolaryngology*. Saunders, Philadelphia.

JAFFE, H.L. (1953). Giant cell reparative granuloma, traumatic bone cyst and fibrous (fibro-osseous) dysplasia of the jaw bones. *Oral Surg.*, **6** : 159.

JONES, J.H. (1965). Non-odontogenic oral tumours in childhood. *Brit. dent. J.*, **119** : 439.

JONES, J.H. (1966). Soft tissue oral tumours in children: their structure, histogenesis and behaviour. *Proc. Roy. Soc. Med.*, **59** : 673.

JONES, P.G. (1961). Autotransplantation in lingual ectopia of the thyroid gland: review of the literature and report of a successful case. *Arch. Dis. Childh.*, **36** : 164.

JONES, P.G. & WILLIAMS, A.L. (1960). A case of multicentric melanotic adamantinoma. *Brit. J. Surg.*, **48** : 282.

KOOP, C.E. & MOSCHAKIS, E.A. (1961). Capillary lymphangioma of the tongue complicated by glossitis. *Pediatrics*, **27** : 800.

KOUDSTAAL, J., OLDHOFF, J., PONDERS, A.K. & HARDONK, M.J. (1966). Melanotic neuro-ectodermal tumors of infancy. *Cancer*, **22** : 151.

KRAFKA, J.Jr. (1936). Teratomas. *Arch. Path.*, **21** : 756.

LANGLEY, F.A. & DAVSON, J. (1950). Epulis in the newborn. *Arch. Dis. Childh.*, **25** : 89.

LOEB, W.J. & SMITH, E.E. (1967). Airway obstruction in a newborn by pedunculated pharyngeal dermoid. *Pediatrics*, **40** : 20.

LOFGREN, R.H. (1963). Respiratory distress from congenital lingual cysts. *Am. J. Dis. Child.*, **106** : 610.

MOORE, C. (1958). Visceral squamous cancer in childhood. *Pediatrics*, **21** : 573.

MISUGI, K. & OKAJIMA. *et al.* (1965). Mediastinal origin of a melanotic progonoma or retinal anlage tumor. *Cancer*, **18** : 477.

NEINAS, F.W. & GORMAN, C.A. *et al.* (1973). Lingual thyroid. *Ann. Int. Med.*, **79** : 205.

O'BRIEN, F.V. & PIELOU, W.D. (1971). Congenital epulis: its natural history. *Arch. Dis. Childh.*, **46** : 559.

O'DAY, R.A., SOULE, E.H. *et al.* (1965). Embryonal rhabdomyosarcoma of oral soft tissues. *Oral Surg.*, **20** : 85.

OSUNKOYA, B.O. & AJAYI, O.O. (1972/73). Burkitt's lymphoma: a clinicopathological review of Ibadan cases. *Paediatrician*, **1** : 261.

PARKER, R.G. (1968). Radical radiotherapy of lymphomas. *Rad. Clin. North Amer.*, **6** : 71.

PINBORG, S.S., KRAMER, I.R.M. & TORLONI, H. (1971). Histological Typing of Odontogenic Tumours, Jaw Cysts and Allied Lesions. *International Histological Classification of Tumours No.* **5**. World Health Organization, Geneva.

PIZER, M.E. & HAMNER, J.E. (1967). Odontogenic Tumors. A survey of their manifestations in childhood. *Clin. Paediat.* **6** : 593.

SAGERMAN, R.H., WOLFF, J.A. *et al.* (1966). Radiation therapy for lymphoma in children. *Radiology*, **86** : 1096.

SAPP, J.P. (1972). Ultrastructure and histogenesis of peripheral giant-cell reparative granuloma of the jaws. *Cancer*, **30** : 1119.

SCHMAMAN, A., SMITH, I. & ACKERMAN, L.V. (1970). Benign fibro-osseous lesions of the mandible and maxilla: a review of 35 cases. *Cancer*, **26** : 303.

SCHILLI, W. & ESCHLER, J. (1969). Malignant jaw tumours in children and adolescents. *Deutsch Zahnaerztl. Z.*, **24** : 280.

SHIPLEY, A.M., WINSLOW, N. & WALKER, W.W. (1937). Aneurysm in the cervical portion of the internal carotid artery. *Ann. Surg.*, **105** : 673.

STRONG, E.W., MCDIVITT, R.W. & BRASFIELD, R.D. (1970). Granular cell myoblastoma. *Cancer*, **25** : 415.

TALLEY, D.B. (1952). Familial fibrous dysplasia of the jaws. *Oral Surg.*, **5** : 1012.

THOMA, K. H. (1970). *Oral Pathology*, 6th ed. Ed. Gorlin, J.R. & GOLDMAN, H.M. Mosby, St. Louis.

VON WOWERN N. (1972). Cherubism. *Int. J. Oral Surg.*, **1** : 240.

WILLIS, R.A. (1962). *Pathology of Tumors in Childhood.* Charles C. Thomas, Springfield.

WORTH, H.M. (1963). *Principles and Practice of Oral Radiologic Interpretation.* Year Book Medical Publishers Inc., Chicago.

WYNN, S.K., WAXMAN, S. RITCHIE, G. & ASKOTZKY, M. (1956). Epignathus. *A.M.A. J. Dis. Child.*, **91** : 495.

E. The nasopharynx

APOSTOL, J.V. & FRAZELL, E.L. (1965). Juvenile nasopharyngeal angiofibroma. *Cancer*, **18** : 869.

BROWN-KELLY, A. (1918). Hairy or dermoid polypi of the pharynx and nasopharynx. *J. Laryng.*, **23** : 65.

CROOK, J.P. (1965). Nasopharyngeal teratoma. *J. Tennessee Med. Assoc.*, **58** : 372.

DONALDSON, S.S., CASTRO, J.R., WILBUR, J.R. & JESSE, R.H. (1973). Rhabdomyosarcoma of head and neck in children. *Cancer*, **31** : 26.

FU, Y-S & PERZIN, K.H. (1974a). Nonepithelial tumours of the nasal cavity, paranasal sinuses and nasopharynx: a clinicopathologic study. I. General features and vascular tumours. *Cancer*, **33** : 1275.

FU, Y-S. & PERZIN, K.H. (1974b). Nonepithelial tumours of the nasal cavity paranasal sinuses and nasopharynx: a clinicopathologic study. II. Osseous and fibro-osseous lesions, including osteoma, fibrous dysplasia, ossifying fibroma, osteoblastoma, giant-cell tumour and osteosarcoma. *Cancer*, **33** : 1289.

GIRGIS, I.H. & FAHMY, S.A. (1973). Nasopharyngeal fibroma: its histopathological nature. *J. Laryng. Otol.*, **87** : 1107.

JAFFE, B.F. & JAFFE, N. (1973). Head and neck tumors in children. *Pediatrics*, **51** : 731.

JOVER, P., LASSALETTA, L. & TOVAR, J. (1972). Nasopharyngeal teratoma. *Ann. Clin. Inf.*, **13** : 95.

LOEB, W.J. & SMITH, E.E. (1967). Airway obstruction in a newborn by pedunculated pharyngeal dermoid. *Pediatrics*, **40** : 20.

MACCOMB, W.S. (1963). Juvenile nasopharyngeal fibroma. *Am. J. Surg.*, **106** : 754.

MARSDEN, H.B. & STEWARD, J.K. (eds). (1968). *Tumours in Childhood.* Springer Verlag, New York.

MOORE, C. (1958). Visceral squamous cancer in children. *Pediatrics*, **21** : 573.

NEEL, H.B., WHICKER, J.H. *et al.*, (1973). Juvenile angiofibroma: a review of 120 cases. *Amer. J. Surg.*, **126** : 547.

NISHIYAMA, R.H., BATSAKIS, J.G. & WEAVER, D.K. (1967). Nasopharyngeal carcinoma in children. *Arch. Surg.*, **94** : 214.

PICK, T., MAURER, H.M. & MCWILLIAMS, N.B. (1974). Lymphoepithelioma in childhood. *J. Pediat.*, **84** : 96.

ROSEN, L., HANAFEE, W. & NANUM, W. (1966). Nasopharyngeal angiofibroma, an angiographic evaluation. *Radiol.*, **86** : 103.

SCHMAMAN, A., SMITH, I. & ACKERMAN, L.Y. (1970). Benign fibro-osseous lesions of the mandible and maxilla: a review of 35 cases. *Cancer*, **26** : 303.

STRAKA, J.A. & BLUESTONE, C.D. (1972). Nasopharyngeal malignancies in children. *Laryngoscope*, **82** : 807.

TAPIA ACUNA, R. (1973). Nasopharyngeal fibroma. *Acta Otolaryngol.*, **75** : 119.

WILLIAMS, J.D. & CHISOLM, D. (1973). Internal maxillary artery ligation for the removal of juvenile nasopharyngeal angiofibroma. *J. Laryng. Otol.*, **87** : 1153.

F. Tumours of the ear

BICKERSTAFF, E.R. & HOWELL, J.S. (1953). Neurological importance of glomus jugulare tumours: a review of 90 cases. *Brain*, **76** : 576.

GUILD, S.R. (1953). The glomus jugulare, non-chromaffin paraganglion in man. *Ann. Otol. Rhinol. Laryngol.*, **62** : 1045.

HATFIELD, P.M., JAMES, A.E. & SCHULZ, M.D. (1972). Chemodectomas of the glomus jugulare. *Cancer*, **30** : 1164.

HEWITT, R.L. *et al.* (1972). Chemodectomas. *Surgery*, **71** : 275.

JAFFE, B.F., FOX, J.E. & BATSAKIS, J.G. (1971), Rhabdomyosarcoma of the middle ear and mastoid. *Cancer*, **27** : 29.

MOORE, C. (1958). Visceral squamous cancer in children. *Pediatrics*, **21** : 573.

MOORE, G.R., ROBBINS, J.P. *et al.* (1973). Chemodectomas of the middle ear. *Arch. Otolaryngol.*, **98** : 330.

POTTER, G.D. (1966). Embryonal rhabdomyosarcoma of the middle ear in children. *Cancer*, **19** : 221.

ROSENWASSER, H. (1945). Carotid body tumor of the middle ear and mastoid. *Arch. Otolaryngol.*, **41** : 64.

SIMPSON, I.E. & DALLACHY, R. (1969). Glomus jugulare tumors. *J. Laryngol. Otolaryngol.*, **72** : 103.

SNYDER, G.G. (1961). Paraganglioma of the middle ear and mastoid. *A.M.A. Arch. Otolaryngol.*, **73** : 54.

TUCKER, W.N. (1965). Cancer of the middle ear: a review of 89 cases. *Cancer*, **18** : 642.

G. Cervical Tumours

BUCKWALTER, J.A. & THOMAS, C.G.Jr. (1972). Selection of surgical treatment for well differentiated thyroid carcinoma. *Ann. Surg.*, **176** : 565.

CHONG, G.C., BEAHRS, O.H. *et al.* (1975). Medullary carcinoma of the thyroid gland. *Cancer*, **35** : 695.

CRILE, G.Jr. (1971). Changing end results in patients with papillary carcinoma of the thyroid *Surg. Gynec. & Obstet.*, **132** : 460.

DUFFY, B.J. & FITZGERALD, P.J. (1950). Cancer of the thyroid in children: a report of 28 cases. *J. Clin. Endocrin. Metab.*, **10** : 1296.

DUNN, E.L., NISHIYAMA, R.M. & THOMPSON, N.W. (1973). Medullary carcinoma of the thyroid gland. *Surgery*, **73** : 848.

EXELBY, P.E. & FRAZELL, E.L. (1969). Carcinoma of the thyroid in children. *Surg. Clin. North Amer.*, **49** : 249.

GORLIN, R., SEDANO, M., VICKERS, R. & CERVENKA, J. (1968). Multiple mucosal neuromas, phaeochromocytoma and medullary carcinoma of the thyroid : a syndrome. *Cancer*, **22** : 293.

GOTTLIEB, J.A. & HILL, C.S.Jr. (1974). Chemotherapy of thyroid cancer with adriamycin: experience with 30 patients. *New Eng. J. Med.*, **290** : 193.

HARNESS, J.K., THOMPSON, N.W. & NISHIYAMA, T.H. (1971). Childhood thyroid carconoma *Arch. Surg.*, **102** : 278.

JACQUES, D.A., CHAMBERS, R.G. & OERTEL, J.E. (1970). Thyroglossal tract carcinoma: a review of the literature and addition of 18 cases. *Am. J. Surg.*, **120** : 439.

LATIMER, R.G., SNOW, E. & HICKS, H.G. (1968). Papillary adenocarcinoma arising in a thyroglossal duct remnant. *Arch. Surg.*, **97** : 161.

LEBOEUF, G. & DUCHARME, J.R. (1966). Thyroiditis in children. *Pediat. Clin. N. Amer.*, **13** : 19.

LEVIN, D.L. PERLIA, C. & TASHJIAN, A.H.Jr. (1973). Medullary carcinoma of the thyroid gland: the complete syndrome. *Pediatrics*, **52** : 192.

LEVY, M., HABIB, R. & LYON, G. *et al.* (1970). Neuromatose et epithelioma à stroma amyloide de la thyroide chez l'enfant. *Arch. Franç Péd.*, **27** : 561.

MESSARIS, G., EVANGELON, G.N. & TOUNTAS, C. (1973). Incidence of carcinoma in cold nodules of the thyroid gland. *Surgery*, **74** : 447.

PINCUS, R.A., REICHLIN, S. & HEMPELMANN, L.H. (1967). Thyroid abnormalities after radiation exposure in infancy. *Ann. Int. Med.*, **66** : 1154.

REFETOFF, S., HARRISON, J. *et al.* (1975). Continuing occurrence of thyroid carcinoma after irradiation to the neck in infancy and childhood. *New Eng. J. Med.*, **292** : 171.

ROEHER, H.D., DAUM, R., PIEPER, M. & RUDOLPH, H. (1972). Juvenile thyroid cancer. *J. Pediat. Surg.*, **7** : 27.

SCHUMKE, R.N. (1973). Phenotype of malignancy; the mucosal neuroma syndrome. *Pediatrics*, **52** : 284.

SILVERMAN, F.N. (1966). Thyroid carcinoma and x-irradiation. *Pediatrics*, **38** : 943.

SIPPLE, J. (1961). The association of pheochromocytoma with carcinoma of the thyroid gland. *Amer. J. Med.*, **31** : 163.

SOCOLOW, E.L., HASHIZUMI, A., NERIISHI, S. & NIITANI, R. (1963). Thyroid cancer in man after exposure to ionizing radiation. A summary of findings in Hiroshima and Nagasaki. *New Engl. J. Med.*, **268** : 406.

STEINER, A.L., GOODMAN, A.D. & POWERS, S.R. (1968). Study of a kindred with phaeochromocytoma, medullary thyroid carcinoma, hyperparathyroidism and Cushing's disease: multiple endocrine neoplasia Type 2. Medicine 47 : 371.

TAWES, R. & DE LORIMIER, A.A. (1968). Thyroid carcinoma during youth. *J. Ped. Surg.*, **3** : 210.

THOMPSON, N.W. & HARNESS, J.K. (1970). Complications of total thyroidectomy for carcinoma. *Surg. Gynec. Obstet.*, **131** : 861.

TOYOOKA, E.T., PIFER, J.W. & HEMPELMANN, L.H. (1963). Neoplasms in children treated with X-rays for thymic enlargement. III. Clinical description of cases. *J. Nat. Cancer Inst.*, **31** : 1379.

WADE, J.S.H. (1972). Clinical research in thyroid surgery. *Ann. Roy. Coll. Surg. Engl.*, **50** : 112.

WEBSTER, R. & HOWARD, R.N. (1954). Papillary adenocarcinoma of the thyroid: so-called 'lateral' aberrant thyroid'. *Aust. N.Z. J. Surg.*, **24** : 1.

WILLIAMS, E.D., BROWN, C.L. & DONIACH, I. (1966). Pathological and clinical findings in a series of 67 cases of medullary carcinoma of the thyroid. *J. Clin. Pathl.*, **19** : 103.

WINSHIP, T. & ROSVOLL, R.V. (1961). Childhood thyroid carcinoma. *Cancer*, **14** : 734.

WINSHIP, T. & ROSVOLL, R.V. (1969). Cancer of the thyroid in children. *U.I.C.C. Monograph.*, **12** : 75.

Parathyroid Glands

BILEZIKIAN, J.P. *et al.* (1973). Preoperative localization of abnormal parathyroid tissue—cumulative experience with venous sampling and arteriography. *Amer. J. Med.*, **55** : 505.

BJERNULF, A., HALL, K., SJÖGREN, I. & WERMER, I. (1970). Primary hyperparathyroidism in children: a brief review of the literature and a case report. *Acta paediat. Scandinav.*, **59** : 249.

BRADLEY, E.L. & MCGARITY, W.C. (1973). Surgical evaluation of parathyroid arteriography. *Am. J. Surg.*, **126** : 67.

CADY, B. (1973). Neck exploration for hyperparathyroidism. *Surg. Clin. N. Amer.*, **53** : 301.

CASTLEMAN, B. (1952). Tumors of the parathyroid gland. *Atlas of Tumour Pathology*, Fascicle 15. Armed Forces Institute of Pathology, Washington D.C.

DOPPMAN, J.L., WELLS, S.A. *et al.* (1973). Parathyroid localization by angiographic techniques in patients with previous neck surgery. *Brit. J. Radiol.*, **46** : 403.

HEY, D. & SEIM, K. (1972). Primary hyperparathyroidism in childhood. *Klin. Paediat.*, **184** : 200.

LAFFERTY, F.W. (1966). Pseudohyperparathyroidism. *Medicine* (*Baltimore*), **45** : 247.

MONCHICK, J.M., NELSON, T.G. & POWELL, D.A. (1973). Adenoma of a fifth parathyroid : the role of selective venous catheterization. *Surgery*, **73** : 782.

MORRIS, W.D., WESTBROOK, K.C. *et al.* (1974). Hyperparathyroidism: surgical problems. *Amer. J. Surg.*, **128** : 767.

MYERS, N.A. (1963). Parathyroid adenoma. *Med. J. Aust.*, **1** : 735.

NEWMARK, S.R. & HIMATHONGKAM, T. (1974). Hypercalcemic and hypocalcemic crises. *J. Amer. Med. Assoc.*, **230** : 1438.

NOLAN, R.B., HAYLES, A.B. & WOOLNER, L.B. (1960). Adenoma of the parathyroid gland in children. *Am. J. Dis. Child.*, **99** : 622.

O'RIORDAN, J.L.M., KENDALL, B.E. & WOODHEAD, J.S. (1971). Preoperative localization of parathyroid tumours. *Lancet*, **2** : 1172.

ROTH, S.I. (1971). Recent advances in parathyroid gland pathology. *Am. J. Med.*, **50** : 612.

SCHANTZ, A & CASTLEMAN, B. (1973). Parathyroid carcinoma: a study of 70 cases. *Cancer*, **31** : 600.

TSUMORI, H., JENSEN, E., HUNNICUTT, A.J. *et al.* (1955). Juvenile hyperparathyroidism associated with peptic ulcer. *J. Clin. Endocrin.*, **15** : 1141.

WOOLNER, L.B., KEATING, F.R. & BLACK, B.M. (1952). Tumors and hyperplasia of the parathyroid glands: a review of the pathologic findings in 140 cases of primary hyperparathyroidism. *Cancer*, **5** : 1069.

Cervical Teratomas

KEYNES, W.M. (1959). Teratoma of the neck in relation to the thyroid gland. *Brit. J. Surg.*, **46** : 466.

McGoon, D.C. (1952). Teratomas in the neck; In Symposium on Pediatric Surgery. *Surg. Clin. N. Amer.*, **32** : 1389.

Rickham, P.P. (1972). Cervical teratomas in the newborn. *Helv. Paediatr. Acta.*, **27** : 459.

Silberman, R. & Mendelson, I.R. (1960). Teratoma of the neck: a report of two cases and review of the literature. *Arch. Dis. Childh.*, **35** : 159.

Stone, H.H., Henderson, W.D. & Guidio, F.A. (1967). Teratomas of the neck. *Am. J. Dis. Child.*, **113** : 222.

Chapter 15. Tumours of the eye and orbit

Table 15.1. Benign swellings and malignant tumours of the eye and orbit

Benign conditions	Malignant tumours
	Orbit
Haemangioma	Glioma of the optic nerve
Lymphangioma	Primary sarcoma of orbital soft tissues
Epidermoid cyst	rhabdomyosarcoma
Orbital cellulitis	round-cell sarcoma
Osteomyelitis of maxilla	lymphosarcoma
Haematoma (intraorbital)	Ewing's tumour (of orbital bones)
Neurofibromatosis	Metastatic tumours
Arteriovenous fistula	neuroblastoma
Osteoma	leukaemias
Mucocele, pyocele (ethmoid)	lymphomas
Fibrous dysplasias	Histiocytosis X
Dysostosis (cranial bones)	eosinophilic granuloma
Infantile cortical hyperostosis	Hand-Schüller-Christian syndrome
Craniostenosis	Letterer-Siwe disease
Pseudotumour	Nasopharyngeal tumours (extensions)
Exophthalmic thyrotoxicosis	rhabdomyosarcoma
Retrobulbar cyst	angiofibroma
Unilateral progressive myopia	neuro-epithelioma
	adenocarcinoma
Myxoma of the paranasal sinuses	Radiation induced sarcoma
	Eye lids
Haemangioma	Malignant melanoma
Lymphangioma	Reticulum cell sarcoma
Epidermoid cyst	Other sarcomas of soft tissues
Naevus (pigmented)	Squamous } carcinoma in xeroderma
Neurofibroma (plexiform)	Basal cell } pigmentosum
Papilloma cornucutaneum	
Xanthoma	
Adenoma	
Chalazion	
	Conjunctivae
Haemangioma	Soft tissue sarcomas
Epidermoid cyst	Metastatic deposits
Dermolipoma	leukaemias
Papilloma	lymphomas

Table 15.1. continued

Benign conditions	Malignant tumours
	Retina
Pseudoglioma	Retinoblastoma
Phakomas	
angiomatous	
neurofibromatous	
tuberous sclerosis	
Sturge-Weber syndrome	
	Choroid
Haemangioma	Malignant melanoma
Pigmented naevus	
	Iris
Haemangioma	Malignant melanoma
Pigmented naevus	
Clear cyst	
Neurofibroma	
Juvenile xanthogranuloma	
Congenital abnormalities:	
muscular atrophy	
bands	
	Ciliary body
	Diktyoma
	Lacrimal gland
Haemangioma	Muco-epidermoid carcinoma
Pleomorphic adenoma	Lymphosarcoma (primary or metastatic)
	Leukaemic deposits (Mikulicz's syndrome)

Primary malignant tumours in this region are rare even among tumours in childhood. Benign tumours and non-neoplastic swellings are much more common, and not infrequently their signs and symptoms mimic a malignant tumour (Table 15.1).

It is difficult to obtain representative figures of the relative incidence of various ocular tumours because practically all reported series have an inbuilt bias determined by the particular interests of the staff or the facilities of the centre from which the report comes. However, data from centres where children are treated show that the frequency and types of malignant tumours of the eye and orbit in childhood differ significantly from those found in adults; for example the two most common malignant tumours in children, rhabdomyosarcoma and retinoblastoma, rarely occur beyond the age of ten years, and for practical purposes these two tumours are not seen in adults. In contrast, carcinoma and malignant melanoma, the common tumours of adult life, are almost never seen in children.

In infancy benign tumours are common and malignant tumours, with the exception of retinoblastoma, are rare. In older children benign tumours are still the more common, but there is a greater likelihood of a malignant tumour than in infants.

OCULAR SYMPTOMS AND SIGNS IN CHILDHOOD

One of the important aspects of intraocular tumours developing in very young children is that although they lead to progressive failure of vision, this is almost never a complaint voiced by the patient, at least until quite late. Loss of vision is extremely difficult to detect clinically in children less than three years of age, and gross defects may go unsuspected even by normally observant parents.

Tumours arising in the orbit or in the eye present with one or more of the following effects:

(*i*) *Disturbances of vision*, resulting from interference, at any point, with transmission of impulses along the visual pathway from the eye. If structural damage is profound, it will prevent the transmission of a clear image from the affected eye, which may result in searching movements, with or without nystagmus, or inability to align the eye correctly (strabismus).

Functional loss of vision may be caused by failure to receive a clear image on the retina, for example, due to a congenital bulky lesion of the eyelid which blocks the view.

Space occupying lesions arising in the orbit can distort the globe and deform it so that changes in refraction occur.

(*ii*) *Proptosis* is the commonest evidence of an expanding lesion in the orbit, and is best appreciated by looking downward over the patient's forehead. The direction taken by the protrusion depends on whether the causal swelling arises within or outside the muscle cone (see Fig. 15.1).

Rhabdomyosarcoma produces rapidly progressive proptosis in the course of a few weeks; the tumour commonly arises *outside* the cone, in the upper inner quadrant of the orbit, and displaces the eyeball downwards and laterally.

On the other hand, the proptosis caused by an optic glioma or a haemangioma, both of which typically arise *within* the muscle cone, is axial (i.e. directly forwards) and develops much more slowly.

Proptosis which is pulsating, intermittent or reducible by pressure is more likely to be caused by a benign condition, e.g. a bony or vascular

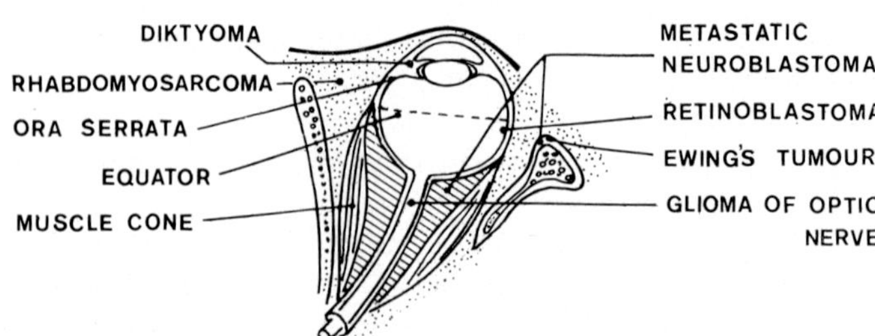

Figure 15.1. DIAGRAM OF THE ORBIT; the connective tissues are divided into two concentric compartments by the rectus muscles and the fascial condensations which unite them to form a 'cone'. The sites of the various types of tumours of the eye and orbit are indicated.

abnormality, whereas inflammatory masses and malignant tumours are firm and not compressible.

Inconsequential asymmetry of the orbits is common, even at birth, and may cause nonprogressive proptosis of up to 3–4 mm.

(*iii*) *Strabismus* can be primarily the result of poor vision in one eye, or alternatively due to interference with movement of the ocular muscles either by pressure on or invasion of the muscles or the motor nerves which supply them. When movements of the eye are impaired, secondary loss of vision may occur (i.e. amblyopia).

(*iv*) *Buphthalmos* ('ox's eye') is the term used to describe enlargement of the globe of the eye (Fig. 15.2), e.g. in infantile glaucoma in which the intra-ocular pressure is raised due to obstruction of the outflow of aqueous humor; the iris and cornea are larger than normal, and usually accompanied by a watering eye (epiphora) and photophobia.

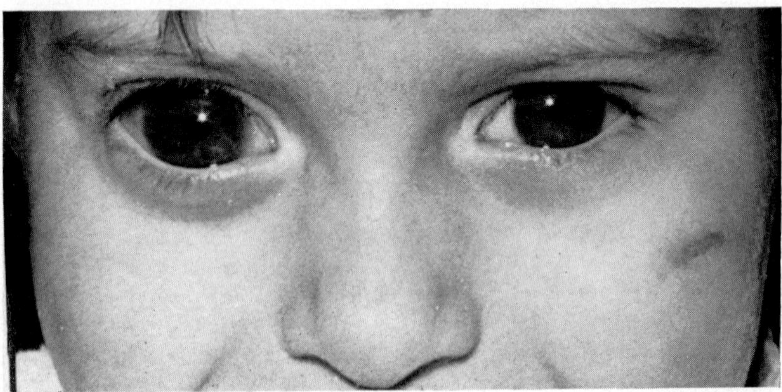

Figure 15.2. BUPHTHALMOS; both the globe and the cornea are enlarged, producing an appearance resembling proptosis.

DIAGNOSIS OF OCULAR TUMOURS

(*i*) *The age of the patient.* Although the ultimate diagnosis of a swelling in the orbit or the eye depends upon histological evidence, a decision to perform a biopsy should be based on a knowledge of the probability and likelihood of certain tumours in particular age groups. For example, increasing proptosis in infancy is most likely to be due to a congenital tumour, such as haemangio-endothelioma; the vast majority of tumours of this type occur in the first year of life, and if biopsy of this tumour is attempted, serious haemorrhage may result.

(*ii*) *Evidence of systemic disease* or other clues to the diagnosis are important and should be carefully sought for; the presence of *câfé-au-lait* patches in the skin suggests that a lesion in the eye or the orbit may be one of the manifestations of generalized neurofibromatosis, such as glioma of the optic nerve (see phakomatoses, p. 825). Latent thyrotoxicosis causing proptosis is also a possibility, though extremely rare in childhood.

An abdominal mass on the other hand, is suggestive of neuroblastoma, a tumour with a well known tendency to produce orbital metastases (Fig. 15.7). In other cases haematological investigations may reveal leukaemia which not infrequently produces leukaemic deposits in the orbit.

(*iii*) *Radiological examination* of the cranium is often helpful in children with ocular signs, for example it may show absence of the greater wing of the sphenoid or enlargement of the optic canal, both of which are associated with neurofibromatosis.

Orbital venography (Trokel, 1972) (Vignaud *et al.*, 1974) is useful in confirming or excluding vascular abnormalities (Fig. 15.3), and ultrasonography (Karlin, 1972) is also finding a useful role in depicting the density and extent of orbital and intraocular lesions.

Clearly, proper management of the child requires close team work and co-operation between the family doctor, the paediatrician, the neurologist, radiologist, haematologist and histopathologist.

Malignant tumours of the orbit and the eye are classified as follows:

A. Tumours of the orbital tissues and adnexae.
B. Tumours of the eyelids, conjunctivae and caruncle.
C. Intraocular tumours.

A. TUMOURS OF THE ORBIT

These include tumours of the bones forming the orbit, as well as the soft tissue it contains, such as the connective tissue, the ocular muscles and the lachrymal gland.

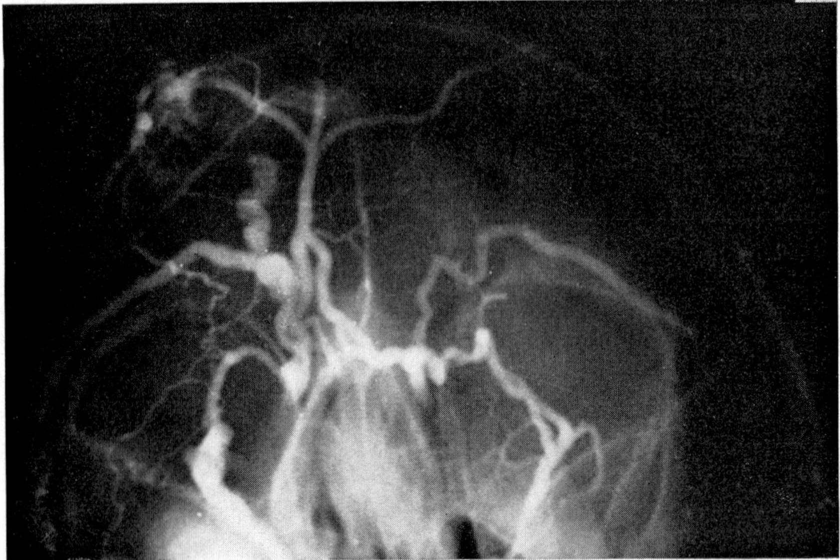

Figure 15.3. ANGIOMATOUS MALFORMATION; an orbital venogram showing multiple anomalous vessels responsible for proptosis.

Benign swellings in the orbit are much more common than malignant tumours at any age, but in childhood a number of important malignant conditions arise in the orbit (Trokel, 1974).

These can be divided into two groups according to their rate of growth, which may be (a) *very rapid*; in some cases with signs suggestive of an acute inflammatory condition; or (b) *much more slowly growing* but steadily progressive lesions, which present undramatically, often at a late stage in their development.

(a) **Tumours which tend to present dramatically with a short history:**
I. Rhabdomyosarcoma of the orbit;
II. Teratoma (p. 406);
III. Metastatic deposits in the orbit.

(b) **Tumours which grow more slowly:**
IV. Gliomas of the optic nerve and chiasm.

I. RHABDOMYOSARCOMA OF THE ORBIT

This is the most important malignant tumour of the orbit in childhood. (Greer, 1966; Jones, Reese & Krout, 1965).

AGE : SITE

The tumour occurs predominantly in the first ten years of life, chiefly in children less than five years old, and may be present at birth.

It arises more commonly in unspecialized connective tissue than in the ocular muscles, and most often in the upper medial quadrant of the orbit.

MACROSCOPIC APPEARANCE

The tumour is soft, fleshy and infiltrating, and it is often impossible to determine the exact site of origin. Many are extremely vascular and resemble an acute inflammatory lesion (Fig. 15.4a).

MICROSCOPIC FINDINGS

In the orbit the embryonal type (p. 785) is the commonest variety, and the typical findings are marked nuclear polymorphism, giant forms, variable amounts of cytoplasm and, infrequently, cross striations (p. 786). Glycogen can usually be demonstrated in the cytoplasm of the tumour cells. Some tumours have a loose myxomatous structure, and the so-called 'myxosarcoma' of the orbit in childhood is very probably a variant of embryonal rhabdomyosarcoma.

In the Index Series one example contained areas with large, polygonal epithelial-looking cells; in other fields there were more typical irregular spindle shaped cells, on which the diagnosis was made. Definite cross-striations were not demonstrated, but longitudinal myofibrils could be seen with PTAH stains.

SPREAD

Despite the reputation of rhabdomyosarcomas to spread at an early stage to lymph nodes and by the bloodstream to the lungs, this is not commonly found in those arising in the orbit; in most cases there is no evidence of spread beyond the orbit tissues at the time of diagnosis.

MODE OF PRESENTATION

The three clinical features of this tumour are closely inter-related and often develop with great rapidity;

1. *Proptosis* with displacement of the eye downwards and outwards;
2. *Diplopia*, due to interference with the action of the ocular muscles, is a complaint made by older children;
3. *Signs suggestive of acute inflammation*, e.g. rapidly developing hyperaemia and oedema of the peri-orbital skin and orbital tissues.

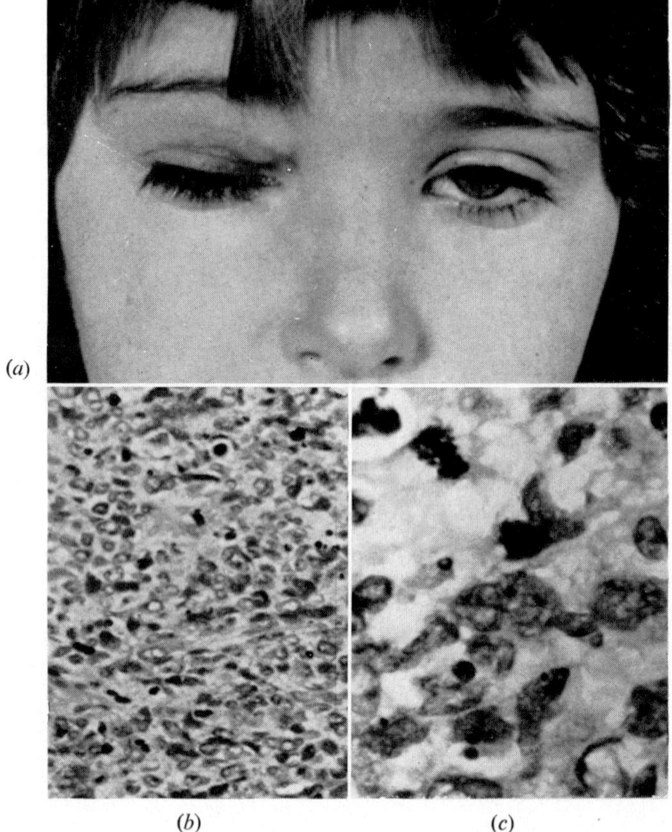

(*a*) (*b*) (*c*)

Figure 15.4. RHABDOMYOSARCOMA arising in the orbital soft tissues; (*a*) causing hyperaemia and ptosis of the upper eyelid; (*b*) irregular pleomorphic cells with elongated cytoplasm, (H & E. × 130); (*c*) hyperchromatic nuclei, mitotic activity and broad cytoplasmic streams (H & E. × 520).

INVESTIGATIONS

1. X-rays of the skull and the lungs are required to exclude the presence of metastases before deciding on the regime of treatment.
2. A full blood examination is necessary to exclude inflammatory conditions, and to establish a baseline for monitoring the effects of chemotherapy (p. 116) and radiotherapy.
3. Biopsy is often required to confirm the diagnosis and to exclude inflammatory lesions or metastatic tumours; histological confirmation is mandatory before commencing chemotherapy or radiotherapy.
4. Endoscopy to detect extension of the tumour into the nasal cavity or sinuses.

DIFFERENTIAL DIAGNOSIS FROM BENIGN LESIONS

1. **Cellulitis**

Because of its rapidity of onset a rhabdomyosarcoma is not infrequently mistaken for orbital cellulitis or an abscess. The distinction is all the more difficult because the ethmoid sinus, which forms part of the medial wall of the orbit, is the commonest paranasal sinus to be involved in acute infections in infants, and ethmoid sinusitis is not infrequently complicated by spread of infection to the orbit.

2. **Osteomyelitis of the maxilla**

This is due to staphylococcal bacteraemia and is another potential source of confusion, particularly in the first few months of life when neonatal osteomyelitis is most common; a subperiosteal abscess points on the surface through inferomedial quadrant of the orbit. However, osteomyelitis almost never causes proptosis, and bone destruction due to infection can usually be demonstrated in x-rays when the signs of infection are first noted.

3. **Pseudotumour of the orbit**

Although by definition not neoplastic, the clinical features are often suggestive of an orbital tumour, for it is usually subacute in onset and commences with painful proptosis developing over a period of some weeks. Vision may be diminished, ocular palsies may occur, and there may also be changes in the visual fields. Investigations are often uninformative, except for biopsy; the condition is usually self-limiting, and the cause is unknown.

4. **A haematoma of the orbit** (Fig. 15.5)

This is usually clearly related to an identifiable episode of trauma, but may also occur as the result of a haemorrhage into a tumour, or a blood dyscrazia

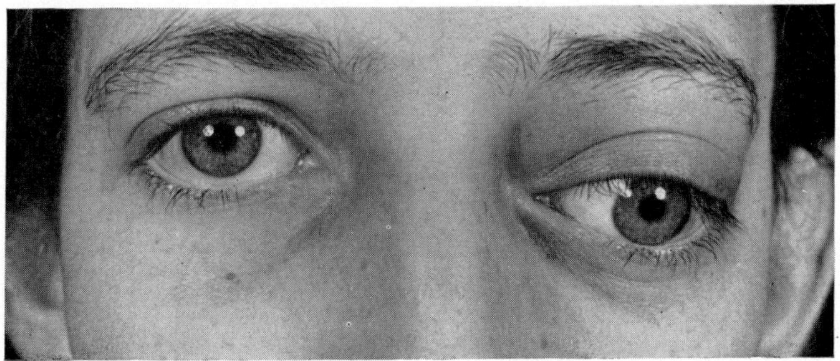

Figure 15.5. HAEMATOMA of the orbit, causing marked proptosis and strabismus which resolved in the course of several weeks, without treatment.

causing a haemorrhagic diathesis. Ecchymoses in the peri-orbital tissues are also a typical feature accompanying orbital metastases from a neuroblastoma (see below).

5. **Swellings in the upper inner quadrant of the orbit**

As well as an internal angular 'dermoid' (inclusion epidermoid cyst) and the rare fronto-nasal encephalocele, a swelling in this region may be a mucocele of the ethmoid or frontal sinus in childhood, especially in association with cystic fibrosis (Robertson & Henderson, 1969).

Exophthalmic thyrotoxicosis is produced by oedema and leucocytic infiltration of the ocular muscles which become greatly enlarged, leading to proptosis and/or ophthalmoplegia.

DIFFERENTIATION OF OTHER MALIGNANT CONDITIONS IN THE ORBIT

1. **Teratoma of the orbit**

This is a particularly rare tumour usually present at birth (Jensen, 1969), and which grows rapidly, resulting in death. The tumour contains benign tissues representing all three embryological elements, but the rare highly malignant examples contain poorly differentiated embryonal carcinoma.

Virtually no survivors have been reported until recently (Barber, Barber *et al.*, 1974). Diagnosis depends upon biopsy, and benign cystic lesions can be aspirated initially and later excised.

No case occurred in the Index Series.

2. **Ewing's tumour**

This is one of the commest primary tumours arising in the bones forming the orbit, but these are uncommon in infancy and childhood. Early involvement of the adjacent soft tissues in the orbit depends upon the site of origin; in some cases the tumour arises at the margin of the orbit and extends chiefly posteriorly or laterally, producing a mass situated in the temporal region rather than in the orbit. A biopsy is required to make the diagnosis, and the histochemistry of the tumour cells is important (p. 736), particularly in distinguishing Ewing's tumour from metastatic neuroblastoma, either of which may involve the tissues of the orbit.

In the Index Series, there were three examples of Ewing's tumour arising in the bones of the orbital margin; the radiological findings were strongly suggestive, and drill biopsy was found to be a particularly suitable technique in this area. All three patients are alive and free of tumour two years after diagnosis following treatment with radiotherapy and chemotherapy as described in the section on Ewing's tumour (p. 745).

3. **Metastatic deposits**

These deposits in the orbital tissues, from a variety of malignant conditions, are individually uncommon but together constitute a group in which the primary condition may be latent and orbital signs and symptoms the first signs of their presence. These are discussed in the section on metastatic tumours of the orbit.

TREATMENT OF RHABDOMYOSARCOMA

Rhabdomyosarcoma arising in the orbit appears to have a better prognosis than in other sites, possibly because the effects are obvious and the diagnosis may be made at an early stage. The methods of treatment available are surgery, chemotherapy and radiotherapy.

Exenteration of the orbit has long been the standard method of treatment until recently, as it produced the best results (Porterfield & Zimmerman, 1962).

Radiotherapy. A recent report from Columbia Presbyterian Center reviewed the results in 17 cases, of which five were treated by biopsy and radiotherapy alone. All 17 patients were alive and well 15 months to 5 years later (Cassady *et al.*, 1969).

Chemotherapy. Recent trends in the treatment of rhabdomyosarcoma in general are towards less radical ablative surgery, for cures are now being reported with increasing frequency following minimal excision or biopsy alone, followed by chemotherapy and/or radiotherapy (Kilman, Clatworthy *et al.*, 1973).

Management of rhabdomyosarcoma today emphasizes intensive combination chemotherapy (Heyn, 1971) and radiotherapy (Hyman, Ellsworth *et al.*, 1968). The chemotherapy of rhabdomyosarcoma is described in the section on soft tissue sarcomas (p. 789). Radiotherapy is usually given as 3500–4000 rads over three to four weeks.

PROGNOSIS

Survival rates of up to 40–50% were reported before current methods of treatment were introduced, and it seems possible that figures as high as 75–80% may now be obtainable (Sutow *et al.*, 1970: Donaldson *et al.*, 1973), by integrated therapy (Sagerman *et al.*, 1972).

In the Index Series there is an example of the favourable results which can be obtained.

A 4-year old girl presented with a seven-week history of a swelling above the right eye and 'drooping' of the right upper eyelid (Fig. 15.4). The eyelid was hyperaemic and oedematous with local signs suggesting an inflammatory lesion, except for displacement of the globe downwards and laterally. Biopsy revealed an embryonal rhabdomyosarcoma, and as there were no demonstrable metastases, exenteration was advised but rejected by the parents.

Combination chemotherapy with vincristine (1.35 mg IV) and rubidomycin (25 mg IV) at weekly intervals was commenced. One week later (after two injections of each cytotoxic agent) the swelling was detectably smaller, and a very satisfactory remission was apparent within three weeks.

Concurrent radiotherapy was commenced one week after the first doses of chemotherapy and the tumour received 4000 rads in 20 fractions over 60 days. Treatment was complicated by florid chickenpox. Two months after diagnosis the tumour had shrunk to a small indurated nodule, palpable through the upper eyelid.

She is alive and well five years later, with no evidence of tumour and normal sight in both eyes. The only sequela is slight enophthalmos, probably due to some shrinkage and fibrosis in the soft tissues of the orbit. There are early signs of a post-irradiation cataract which is not unexpected following the dose employed.

III. METASTATIC AND OTHER TUMOURS INVOLVING THE ORBIT

In childhood there are a variety of tumours which have a tendency to produce metastases either in the bones or the soft tissue or the orbit. Also included in this category are tumours arising close to the orbit and which may extend into it by direct infiltration rather than blood-borne metastasis. Radiation-induced sarcomas arising in the orbit are also mentioned in this section as they may arise as a complication following radiotherapy of primary tumours in or near the orbit.

The malignant conditions to be described in this section are as follows:

1. Metastatic neuroblastoma;
2. Orbital deposits in leukaemias and malignant lymphomas;
3. Extension of nasopharyngeal tumours;
4. Radiation-induced sarcomas of the orbit;
5. Extension of a retinoblastoma.

1. **Metastatic neuroblastoma** (Blake & Fitzpatrick, 1972)

Dissemination from a primary neuroblastoma, usually arising in the abdomen and less commonly in the thorax, should be suspected when a child less than five years of age develops proptosis, particularly when it is bilateral and accompanied by peri-orbital ecchymoses (Fig. 15.6). In 3–5% of cases of neuroblastoma this is the mode of presentation (p. 552), and orbital metastases are found at some stage in the clinical course of approximately 40% of cases of neuroblastoma.

The primary tumour in the abdomen may or may not be palpable; biopsy of the orbit tissues is not always required when appropriate investigations (see neuroblastoma, p. 554) demonstrate the site of the primary and confirm the diagnosis. In a number of cases the source of orbital metastasis can be quickly confirmed by plain films of the abdomen, showing speckled calcification in the suprarenal area, or by a spot test for catecholamines in the urine (p. 551). Metastases from a neuroblastoma are almost never deposited

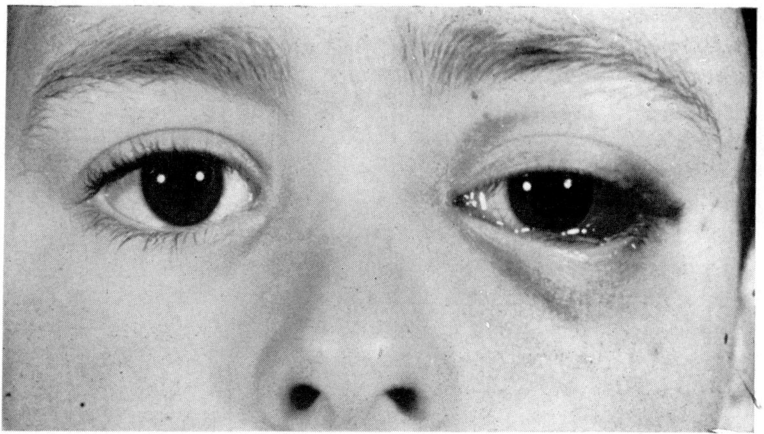

Figure 15.6. NEUROBLASTOMA; orbital metastases causing proptosis, with subconjuctival and palpebral ecchmoses.

directly in the soft tissues of the orbit, but more usually in one of the bones forming the wall of the orbit before invading the soft tissues.

Interpretation of an orbital biopsy may be difficult, for metastatic neuroblastoma cells are usually poorly differentiated and difficult to identify. However, the initial bony metastases can often be demonstrated radiologically, and the nature of the primary tumour can be identified by appropriate investigations (p. 554) (Ferman & Apt, 1972).

Olfactory neuroblastoma (p. 362) is a rare tumour which occasionally involves the orbit by direct invasion, causing proptosis.

2. Orbital deposits in leukaemia and malignant lymphomas

Metastatic deposits in these two conditions are among the commonest forms of orbital malignancy in childhood. Proptosis is usually the first ocular sign, and while it may be the first evidence of the underlying disease, in most cases the deposits occur relatively late when the diagnosis has already been established.

The orbital bones and soft tissues are diffusely infiltrated, and a biopsy may be difficult to interpret unless taken in conjunction with the findings in peripheral blood, marrow, lymph nodes or other biopsies.

Leukaemia. The diagnosis may not be apparent when leukaemia is not suspected; the leukaemic cells are closely packed, slightly irregular, hyperchromatic, contain very little cytoplasm, and may closely resemble those of a lymphoma, neuroblastoma or even rhabdomyosarcoma. However, the origin of leukaemic cells can be clarified by the presence of typical cells in the blood or in the marrow.

Lymphomas. Occasionally a lymphosarcoma, less commonly a reticulum cell sarcoma, presents as infiltration of the orbit. This is seen more frequently in tropical areas where Burkitt's lymphoma (p. 328) is endemic, for example, in central Africa and New Guinea, approximately 10% of children with Burkitt's lymphoma present with an orbital tumour, and the orbit is involved at some stage in a further 20% of cases.

3. Extension from nasopharyngeal tumours

(a) *Rhabdomyosarcoma* of the nasopharynx (see p. 358) in childhood, on rare occasions invades the orbit, usually via the foramen lacerum.

Pain referred to the orbit, or proptosis (Fig. 15.7) may occur before signs or symptoms direct attention to the nasopharynx; and the facial nerve may also be involved causing facial palsy, followed by loss of oculomotor movements when CN III and VI become involved (Fig. 14.12).

Careful examination of the nose and throat including endoscopy is required, usually under anaesthesia in infants and young children. The diagnosis and treatment of rhabdomyosarcoma of the nasopharynx are described on p. 359.

(b) *Juvenile angiofibroma.* The clinical aspects of this tumour are described on p. 352, and its propensity to extend into every recess and ostium is responsible for occasional involvement of the orbit, usually at a late stage of the disease.

4. Radiation-induced sarcomas

Nasopharyngeal tumours (p. 355), retinoblastoma (p. 432) and medulloblastoma (p. 260) are all commonly treated with radiotherapy, and one of

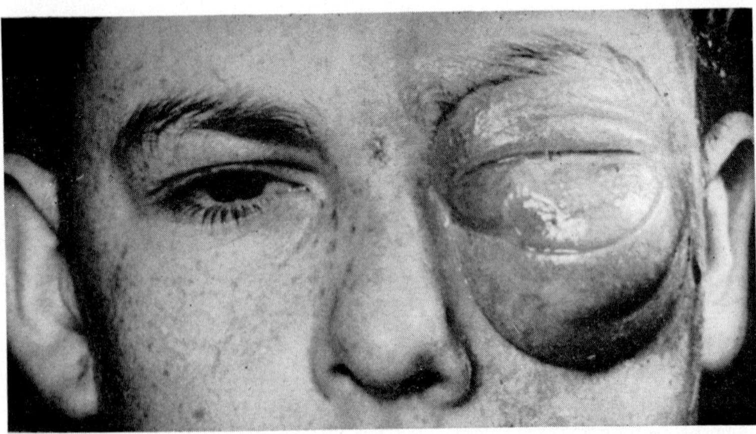

Figure 15.7. NASOPHARYNGEAL RHABDOMYOSARCOMA invading the orbit causing gross proptosis and chemosis.

the recognized hazards is the development of a bone sarcoma, (Yoneyama & Greenlaw, 1969), less commonly a soft tissue sarcoma (p. 433) in the area irradiated, as a rule some eight to ten years later (p. 526).

Sarcomas of this type are usually resistant to treatment and rapidly fatal.

In contrast to the malignant tumours described above, other neoplasms in the orbit are much more slowly growing, and symptoms and signs develop over the course of months or even years rather than weeks.

(b) SLOWLY GROWING ORBITAL TUMOURS

IV. GLIOMA OF THE OPTIC NERVE

This tumour is described in this chapter and also in the section concerning intracranial tumours (p. 262), for it occupies a borderland where neurosurgery and ophthalmology meet. Those examples with disturbances of vision present as ocular problems, whereas patients tend to be referred to a neurosurgeon when the tumour chiefly affects the chiasm or more posterior structures. Each contributor has been encouraged to describe the condition as he sees it.

SITE : AGE

Gliomas of the optic nerve form an important group of neoplasms in childhood (Davis, 1940), and although only one third of them affect the intra-orbital portion of the optic nerve, all are associated with ocular signs.

The age groups maximally affected extend throughout the first and second quinquennia with a peak at three years of age (Chutorian, Schwartz *et al.*, 1964).

From the pathological point of view, the natural history of the condition is still debatable, and to some extent unpredictable (Udvarhelyi *et al.*, 1965). While some examples continue to grow indefinitely like true neoplasms, to the extent of infiltrating the tissues of the central nervous system (p. 265) with a fatal outcome, others eventually cease to grow and are interpreted by some authorities as hamartomas (Hoyt, 1969). Uncertainty is bound up with the ill-defined nature of the group of conditions comprising neurofibromatosis (which includes gliomas of the optic nerve), and also the broader category, even less well understood, referred to as the phakomatoses (Tasman, 1971).

In the 23-year period covered by the Index Series, there were 18 patients with an optic glioma, of whom eight had stigmata of von Recklinghausen's disease at the time of diagnosis (Table 15.2).

Most gliomas are benign, and while some authorities have reported that 25% or more will undergo spontaneous arrest, others believe that this occurs in most if not all cases.

Table 15.2. Tumours of the optic nerve (Index Series, RCH, 1950–1972)

Age at diagnosis	Sex	Site of tumour	Clinical evidence of associated von Recklinghausen's disease	
1 year	F	nerve	Yes	Survivor
7 years	F	nerve	Yes	Survivor
2 years	F	chiasm	Yes	Death*
13 years	M	chiasm	No	Survivor
4 months	M	chiasm	No	Death*
4 months	M	chiasm	?	Survivor
8 years	F	nerve	No	Death*
11 years	F	nerve	No	Death*
7 years	F	chiasm	No	Survivor
2 years	F	chiasm	Yes	Death*
4 years	M	nerve	Yes	Survivor
3 days	M	nerve	No	Death*
9 days	F	nerve	No	Survivor
7 days	M	nerve	No	Survivor
11 months	F	chiasm	Yes	Death*
? months	M	chiasm	Yes	Survivor
2 years	F	nerve	Yes	Survivor
4 months	F	nerve	No	Survivor
		Meningioma		
15 years	F	nerve sheath	Unknown	Survivor
12 years	F	nerve sheath	No	Survivor

In the Index Series the histological picture in some of the optic gliomas showed a very low grade of activity, but on the other hand the same series contains seven children with a glioma which infiltrated the base of the brain and ended fatally (Table 15.2).

MACROSCOPIC APPEARANCES

The typical finding at operation is diffuse (cylindrical) enlargement of the optic nerve and/or the chiasm, and less commonly a focal (fusiform) swelling of one nerve. In the majority one nerve and the chiasm, or both optic nerves, are involved; only a minority are confined to one optic nerve (Spencer, 1972).

The pathologist occasionally receives a segment of the nerve containing the tumour (Fig. 15.9c) but more often the material submitted consists of fragments of pink to grey, firm tumour.

The meninges are greatly thickened by reactive meningeal proliferation, one of the characteristic features which can lead to confusion with a meningioma (p. 264, and Fig. 13.16, p. 266).

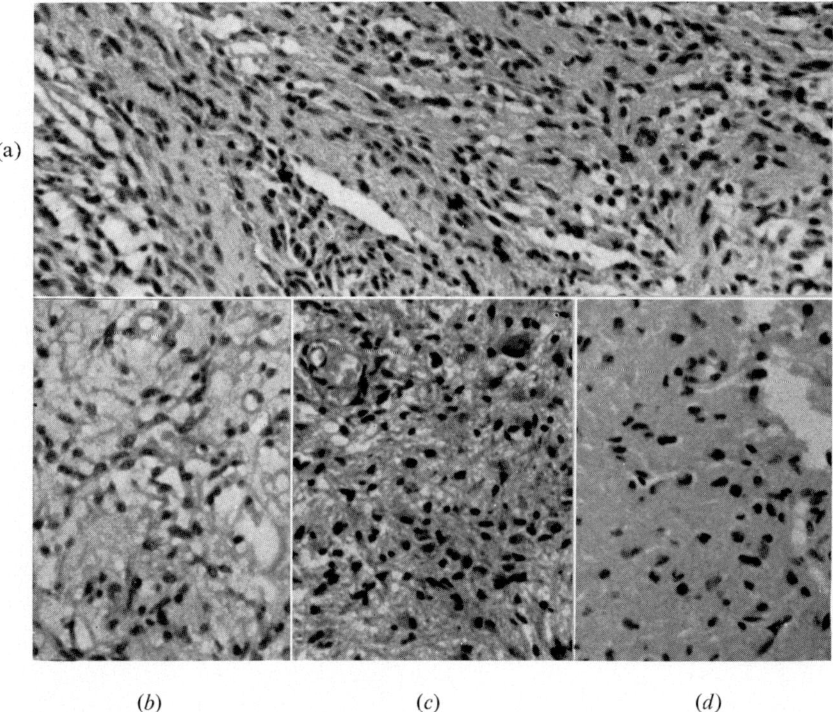

(a)

(*b*) (*c*) (*d*)

Figure 15.8. Glioma of the optic nerve; (*a*) a moderately cellular tumour with marked production of glial fibres and an interlacing 'sheath' pattern, with some microcystic changes. Other patterns encountered are (*b*) that of a juvenile astrocytoma, also with microcystic changes; (*c*) a recurrence of the tumour in (*b*) showing increased cellularity and slight nuclear polymorphism; (*d*) the pattern of a low grade astrocytoma; in spite of the benign appearance this tumour recurred locally and invaded the brain causing death.

MICROSCOPIC FINDINGS

The tumour is composed of astrocytes, plentiful glial fibres (Fig. 15.8a), and foci of calcification are not uncommon. In some examples there may be microcystic changes as seen in cerebellar astrocytomas (p. 244). The astrocytes are usually well differentiated, but in some examples there is slight nuclear anaplasia (Fig 15.8c).

Reactive hyperplasia of epineural cells closely resembling fibroblasts is found adjacent to the tumour, and may be mistaken for tumour, an important point in determining whether an intra-orbital tumour has been completely excised (Fig. 15.9c).

The characteristic cells are obviously astrocytes, but some gliomas contain areas which mimic a schwannoma or a meningioma.

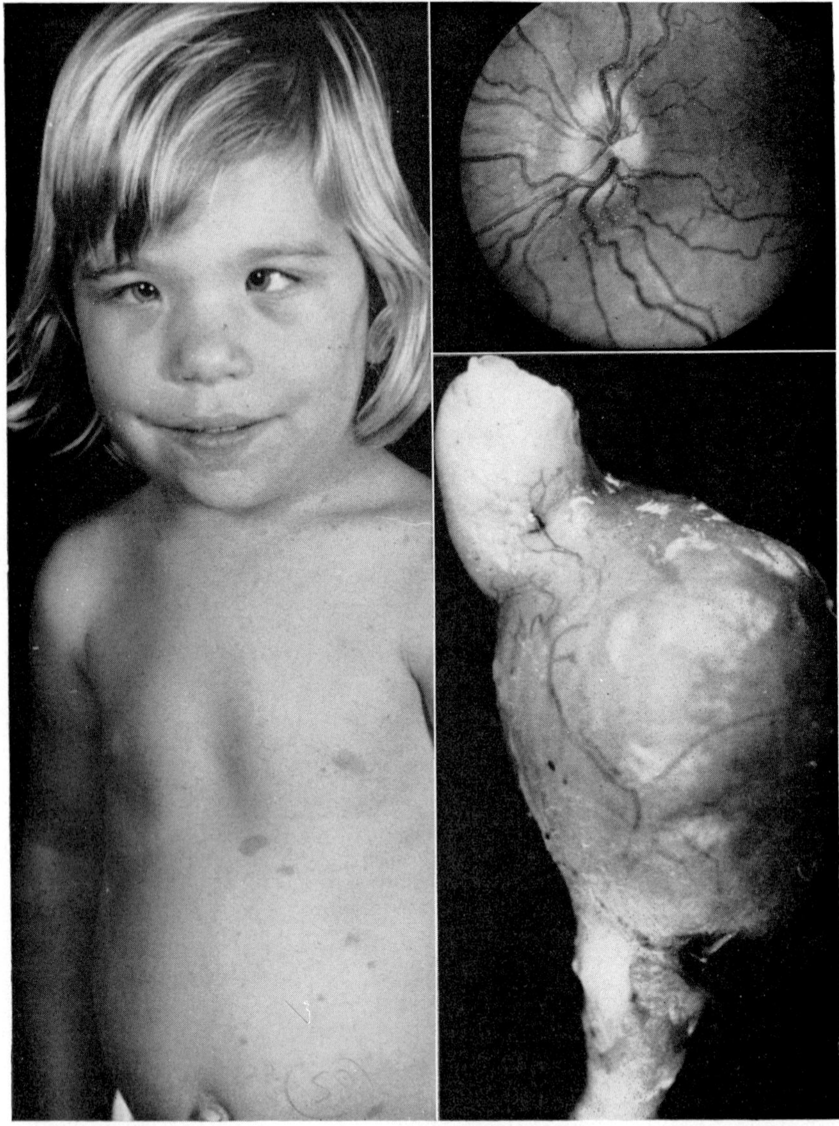

Figure 15.9. GLIOMA OF THE OPTIC NERVE; (*a*) in a retarded girl with telecanthus, mild proptosis, strabismus and the câfé-au-lait patches of generalized neurofibromatosis; (*b*) the accompanying papilloedema and (*c*) the fusiform tumour in the optic nerve, which histologically had an astrocytomatous pattern (see Fig. 15.8b).

[(*a*) *Left*. (*b*) *Top right*. (*c*) *Bottom right*.]

MODE OF PRESENTATION

The symptoms and signs vary to some extent according to the age at which the tumour develops. In twenty cases analysed, the clinical features can be divided into two groups according to the age at which the patient presented (Table 15.3). The modes observed were as follows:

1. *Proptosis* is the most common sign; it is axial in type, and there is no impairment of ocular motility until a late stage (Fig. 15.9a). Abnormalities of the optic disc are present in nearly every case (Fig. 15.9b).

The diagnosis can be made on these findings together with radiographic evidence of enlargement of the optic canal, and other features of von Recklinghausen's disease such as *câfé-au-lait* patches or precocious puberty.

Proptosis has been looked upon as a favourable prognostic sign as evidence that the tumour probably does not involve the chiasm, but this is not always the case in the very young. In the Index Series two patients presented in the first year of life with proptosis (at 3 days and 11 months respectively); the chiasm was extensively involved and both subsequently died of their tumour.

2. *Strabismus* can be due to either severe loss of vision (and hence lack of fixation) or, less commonly in optic gliomas, to direct interference with the action of the ocular muscles.

3. *'Infantile' nystagmus* is common when a glioma involves the chiasm; occasionally the nystagmus is 'see-saw', but most are 'fixational' in type with searching movements and strongly suggest a glioma, particularly when there

Table 15.3. Glioma of the optic nerve; modes of presentation according to age (Index Series. RCH, 1950–1972)

	No.
Less than 5 *years old* (14)	
Infantile nystagmus Unilateral 2, Bilateral 6	8
Proptosis	4
Strabismus	2
Patients more than 5 *years old* (6)	
Visual defects (school tests)	4
Proptosis	2
Total	20
Other abnormalities present	
Hydrocephalus	7
Failure to thrive	5
Precocious puberty	5
Câfé-au-lait patches	5
Mental deficiency and epilepsy	4

is a family history of von Recklinghausen's disease, or any of the associated findings listed in Table 23.6 (p. 829).

Hereditary congenital nystagmus (the cause of which is unknown) is a benign condition to be distinguished (by exclusion) from infantile nystagmus, usually by negative findings in all the standard investigations employed for a glioma of the optic nerve. In hereditary congenital nystagmus, vision is usually unaffected.

INVESTIGATIONS

Precise radiological investigations, including views of the optic canals (Fig. 15.10), and pneumo-encephalography and tomography, not only confirm the diagnosis but also indicate the extent of involvement of intracranial structures, e.g. of the optic nerves, chiasm or the ventricles. If the situation is still in doubt after these investigations, orbitotomy and/or craniotomy may be required to determine the nature and extent of the lesion.

DIFFERENTIAL DIAGNOSIS OF OPTIC GLIOMAS

This includes other conditions causing slowly progressive proptosis, which are as follows.

1. *A meningioma* arising in the sheath of the optic nerve is rare in children, but important in relation to gliomas of the optic nerve, for both are associated with von Recklinghausen's disease. A glioma can be mistaken for a meningioma if reactive meningeal proliferation, common in gliomas, is misinterpreted histologically.

In the Index Series there were two meningiomas in older children (Table 15.2); both tumours contained plump fibroblastic cells with prominent psammoma bodies (Fig. 13.16, p. 266). In a third patient biopsy showed areas of astrocytes, but in other fields there were masses of plump rounded cells with a whorled pattern suggestive of meningioma; no psammoma bodies were present, and the diagnosis of glioma was made.

Meningiomas are more aggressive and life-threatening than gliomas, and tend to cause proptosis before visual failure, in contrast to optic nerve gliomas in which the reverse order is more usual. If the diagnosis is uncertain and a meningioma is still a possibility after careful radiological investigation and direct observation at operation, the lesion should be excised, along with the optic nerve if necessary (Karp *et al.*, 1974).

2. *A haemangioma or a vascular abnormality* is one of the commonest tumours of the orbit in infancy and childhood, but may escape detection until puberty when located in the depths of the orbit. It is occasionally associated with capillary or cavernous haemangiomas elsewhere, particularly in the eyelid, the skin and sometimes on the face.

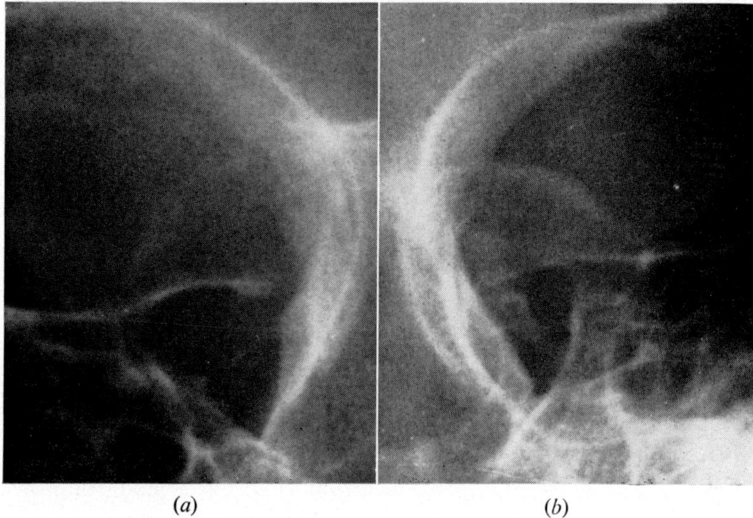

Figure 15.10. GLIOMA OF THE OPTIC NERVE; x-rays of the optic foramina showing marked enlargement of the canal in (*a*) compared with the normal (*b*).

The clinical features depend to a large extent on the site (whether inside or outside the muscle cone) and on the size of the vessels of which it is composed. In infants and young children, haemangiomas are most often diffuse, and from the practical point of view inoperable; a few examples are localized, encapsulated and removable. Systemic corticosteriods may have a place in treatment, particularly if visual function is threatened (Hiles & Pilchard, 1971).

3. *Swellings of the lachrymal gland* are uncommon in childhood; the most common is probably atypical mumps, in which only one lachrymal gland may be transiently enlarged. This produces a swelling beneath the upper lid which may be large enough to cause some displacement of the eye. If neither parotid gland is swollen, the cause is not immediately apparent.

Tumours of the lachrymal gland are extremely uncommon at any age, and the following have been described as rare causes of an intra-orbital mass.

(i) *A haemangioma* of the lachrymal gland has many similarities to those occurring in the parotid (p. 305), and is usually the capillary type. Rarely the lachrymal gland is involved in a more extensive angioma arising in the eyelid, or in orbital soft tissues.

(ii) *Pleomorphic adenoma* (p. 312) (McPherson, 1960) or muco-epidermoid carcinoma (p. 307) (Sanders *et al.*, 1962) are very rare in children, and similar to those occurring in the parotid. Proptosis with displacement of the globe downwards and medially, and a swelling in the region of the lachrymal gland, are practically diagnostic.

(iii) *Mikulicz's syndrome*, involving parotid, lachrymal and sometimes other salivary glands, is most often due to leukaemic deposits in childhood, and when leukaemia has not previously been recognized, diagnosis rests on biopsy.

4. *Histiocytosis X.* The closely related syndromes comprizing the histiocytoses are described in Chapter 11 (p. 205).

(i) *The Hand-Schüller-Christian* syndrome occasionally involves the wall of the orbit, causing proptosis, in children five to ten years of age, although the classic triad of exophthalmos, diabetes insipidus and radiological defects in membrane bones (Fig. 14.1b) is extremely rare.

(ii) *Eosinophilic granuloma* occasionally arises in one of the bones forming the orbit, as a rule in older children, in the third quinquennium.

In both these conditions the diagnosis is usually suggested by the radiographic appearances in the calvarium (Fig. 14.1), and confirmed by biopsy. Treatment and prognosis are described on p. 220 *et seq.*

5. *Regional giantism* occurring as one of the manifestations of generalized neurofibromatosis (p. 829) may include hypertrophy of soft tissues, or diffuse plexiform neurofibromatosis (Fig. 15.6), causing proptosis and occasionally buphthalmos (Fig. 15.2).

The *Index Series* contains the following example of an optic glioma in a child with von Recklinghausen's disease.

A 9-month old girl (R.C.H. 273322) who presented with a pulmonary infection was found to have hypertelorism and multiple *câfé-au-lait* patches, chiefly on the chest, abdomen and limbs (Fig. 15.9). Strabismus and nystagmus were also present and radiological investigation showed normal optic canals, but obliteration of the optic recess of the third ventricle, and bilateral optic atrophy consistent with glioma of the chiasm, was also present.

Cystic enlargement of the right breast developed at the age of 18 months, at which time the plasma luteinizing hormone was 2·8 μ/ml and follicle stimulating hormone 3·0 μ/ml, levels suggestive of precocious puberty due to gonadotropic stimulation. The cystic swelling in the breast subsided over the next 12 months and no other secondary sexual changes occurred.

In the following 2 years her sight has not deteriorated; the bone age is normal, and no other stigmata of von Recklinghausen's disease or precocious puberty have appeared.

TREATMENT

The value of surgery for glioma of the optic nerve is currently in question, particularly in those who still have some useful vision remaining in the affected eye. The following procedures have been employed.

1. Excision of the glioma (and the optic nerve)

This is indicated when there are gross cosmetic deformities and no useful

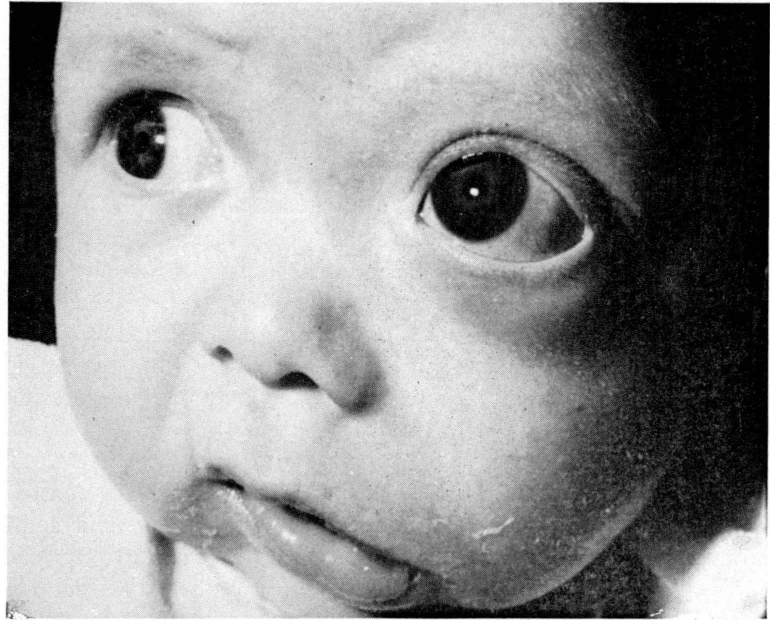

Figure 15.11. Regional fibromatosis affecting the soft tissues of the orbit, cheek and lip, causing regional giantism and proptosis. The eye was sightless, and when enucleated diffuse neurofibromatosis was seen surrounding the optic nerve.

vision in the eye. Complete excision of the glioma, leaving the globe intact, can be carried out via a lateral orbitotomy, or at craniotomy (see p. 437).

Incomplete removal of a tumour confined to the optic nerve does not appear to influence the period of survival. In cases in which involvement of the optic nerve is less marked, surgical excision is probably not justified unless there is clearly documented evidence of progressive deterioration of vision in the affected eye. The latter is rarely seen.

2. **Unroofing the optic canal**

In patients in the Index Series in whom this has been performed, the level of vision at the time of diagnosis appears to have been maintained, but this is difficult to evaluate because the children were too young for precise assessment of visual function.

3. **Radiotherapy**

There is no conclusive evidence that this was of value in any of the cases in the Index Series treated in this way, and this is in accord with the findings of Glaser *et al.* (1971).

4. **CSF shunt**

This is indicated when involvement of the chiasm causes hydrocephalus by obstructing the third ventricle (p. 264).

B. TUMOURS OF THE EYELIDS, CONJUNCTIVAE AND CARUNCLE

Any sizeable blemish on the face of a child, particularly one near the eyes, is of considerable emotional significance, to the parents initially, and later to the patient. One consequence is that parental pressures may be exerted to improve the appearance of a lesion which would be better left alone, at least for the time being. Haemangiomas of the eyelids (not obstructing vision) and aggressive examples of juvenile fibromatosis (see p. 798) are examples of such conditions.

In infants and children, primary tumours in this region are almost invariably benign, and treatment is usually conservative, in contrast to adults, in whom malignant conditions are more common and complete removal of the lesion is one of the principles of treatment. In the eyelids in children, malignant lesions are usually the result of direct extension from a sarcoma arising in the orbit, or deposits of leukaemic cells or a malignant lymphoma.

Perhaps the most important aspect of benign swellings in the eyelids is that any lesion which causes obstruction of vision (e.g. Fig. 15.13), especially during infancy and early childhood, can lead to functional blindness by interfering with fixation and the development of sight. This has been amply confirmed by animal experiments which have shown that even partial obstruction of vision for as little as three weeks has this effect (Hubel & Wiesel, 1962, 1965).

Early removal of such a lesion is essential to preserve the sight in the affected eye.

Benign tumours of the eyelids or conjunctivae are as follows:

1. Haemangioma;
2. Epidermoid cyst;
3. Dermolipoma;
4. Pigmented naevus;
5. Papilloma;
6. Neurofibroma.

1. **Haemangioma**

Two types are distinguishable both clinically and histologically: capillary and cavernous haemangiomas. Those affecting the conjunctivae are very frequently associated with haemangiomas of the lid (Fig. 15.12), the orbit or intraocular structures.

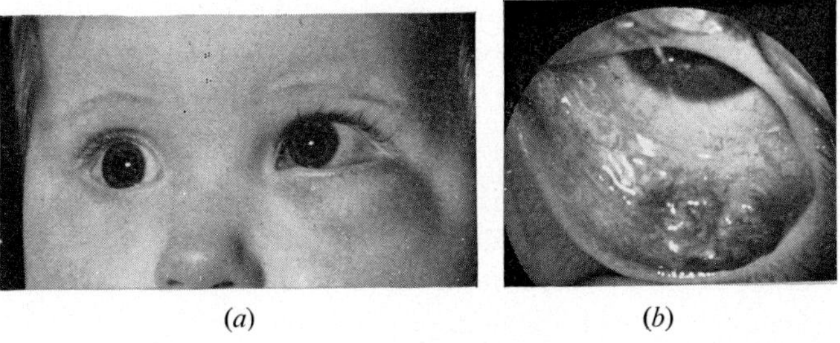

(*a*) (*b*)

Figure 15.12. HAEMANGIOMA of the orbit causing (*a*) mild strabismus and proptosis; (*b*) the same lesion, involving subjunctival and orbital tissues.

Capillary angiomas are common in the eyelid, frequently seen as a 'strawberry naevus' in the neonate, and usually disappear spontaneously in the first few years of life. The general principle of management is simply observation (p. 819). The only indication for early surgical excision is obstruction of vision and this may be a difficult decision in an infant, at an age when operation poses technical problems such as adequate excision and potential blood loss.

Cavernous haemangiomas are less common, and less inclined to spontaneous closure than capillary haemangiomas. Their appearance and behaviour are determined by the ratio of large venous sinuses to capillaries and endothelial cells, often in various proportions (p. 818). The lesion is essentially a hamartoma rather than a benign neoplasm. In children, cavernous haemangiomas are often not encapsulated, and any excision should be approached with caution.

In our experience, the eye on the affected side may also have a significant difference in refraction compared with the normal side, and this is an additional factor contributing to poor vision.

Lymphangiomas may be difficult to distinguish clinically, except for a tendency to develop small haemorrhages into the cystic spaces, producing repeated episodes of ecchymoses and temporary enlargement.

Sturge-Weber syndrome. The facial angioma is referred to as a 'naevus flammeus', a pinkish 'port wine' stain present at birth which is an important external marker associated with partly calcified angiomas in the cerebral cortex, and pyknolepsy. The typical naevus flammeus is impalpable clinically, without elevation of the skin, and often limited to the area supplied by the ophthalmic division of the trigeminal nerve.

2. **Epidermoid cyst**

By far the commonest site is the upper outer angle of the orbit, and less often in the upper nasal quadrant. It may also arise anywhere in the conjunctivae, but usually at the limbus in the lower quadrant. These may be associated with partial facial clefts and the Treacher-Collins syndrome.

3. **Dermolipoma**

This lesion is characteristically seen at the outer canthus and may only become apparent when the eye is directed towards the opposite side. It is a congenital lesion covered by epidermal epithelium in which fine hairs can be seen under magnification. Their removal is not always necessary, but requires careful technique to avoid scarring.

4. **Pigmented naevi of the lids or conjunctivae**

These are commonly found in the anterior margins of the lids as elevated areas of the same types and with the same potentialities as those elsewhere in the skin, described on p. 844.

5. **Papillomas of the lids or conjunctivae**

These are often multiple, and the typical site of those in lids is at the muco-cutaneous junction. In the very young child and in neonates, small papillomas may be overlooked as a cause of epiphora. In papillomas occurring in the region of the caruncle, chronic vernal conjunctivitis may need to be excluded; a history of seasonal exacerbations and other allergic manifestations such as asthma and eczema is typical. Vernal conjunctivitis predominantly involves the upper fornix of the conjunctiva.

6. **Neurofibroma**

A plexiform neuroma occasionally arises in the upper eyelid, and causes ptosis (Fig. 15.13). The outer half of the upper lid is usually involved first,

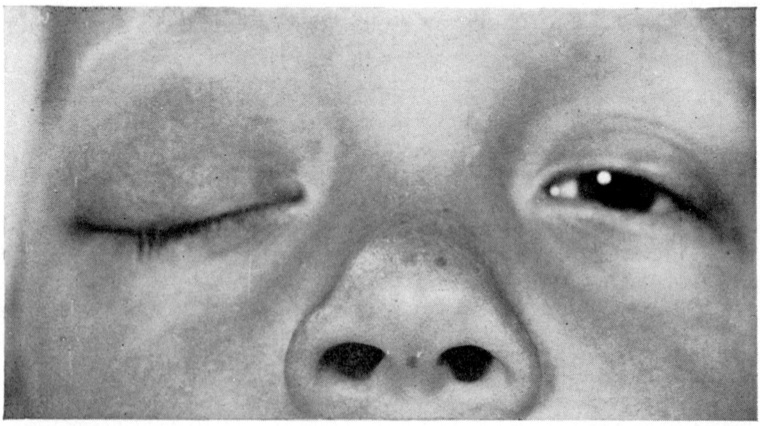

Figure 15.13. PLEXIFORM NEUROMA of the upper eyelid causing ptosis. Note the direction of the nostrils, indicating the degree of extension of the head and neck in an attempt to use the right eye.

and the convoluted strands formed by greatly enlarged nerve fibres (p. 824) are responsible for the clinical finding described as a 'bag of worms'. The adjacent conjunctiva may also be involved.

Other features associated with von Recklinghausen's disease (p. 827) are usually present and confirm the diagnosis.

C. INTRAOCULAR TUMOURS

Tumours arising in the globe of the eye can be classified according to their appearances, including the findings on fundoscopy. All malignant and benign intraocular conditions can be placed in one or other of the following categories:
(a) Those which present with a white mass of tissue which reflects light giving the appearance of a white pupil (or 'white' reflex).
(b) Pigmented lesions, often black in colour, arising in the eye.

(a) THE WHITE REFLEX

The most important but not the most common causes are malignant tumours of the retina or ciliary body, and they are:
I. Retinoblastoma.
II. Diktyoma.

I. RETINOBLASTOMA

INCIDENCE

Although the commonest malignant intra-ocular tumour in childhood, it is very rare. The incidence has been estimated as one per 21,000 to 34,000 live births; in Australia this would be equivalent to eight cases per annum, and two of these would be in Victoria, on the basis of the proportion of the total population and the current birth rate.

A review of the records of the Royal Victorian Eye and Ear Hospital reveals approximately three cases in every two years, and at the Royal Children's Hospital there have been 13 cases in the last 12 years. Taken together this represents the expected incidence of slightly more than two cases per annum in the community concerned, in accord with the estimate of the incidence above.

HEREDITY

There is a strong familial incidence in reported series; recent clarification of the genetic patterns (Knudson, 1971) has shown that inheritance of the tumour follows one of two lines, and the differences are important in genetic counselling.

(i) In the familial and bilateral form, 45% of the offspring of affected persons will develop a retinoblastoma.

(ii) Those with a unilateral sporadic retinoblastoma who survive transmit the tumour to only 5–10% of their offspring.

All children of an affected parent or sibling should be reexamined frequently, at intervals of one month until they are 3 years old and then every 3–6 months until the age of 10 years.

AGE : SEX : BILATERALITY

Retinoblastoma is practically confined to the first 10 years of life (Fig. 15.14); 66% of cases occur before the age of 3 years, and some are detectable at birth. The average age in a large series (Ellsworth, 1969) was 18 months.

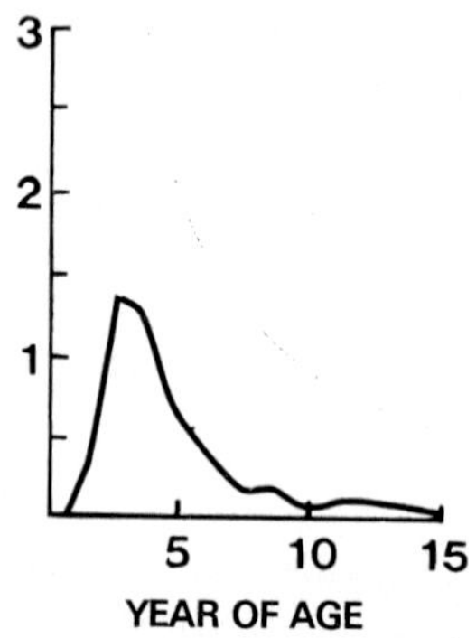

Figure 15.14. RETINOBLASTOMA; incidence according to age, showing the peak in the first quinquennium (for source of figures see Fig. 2.2, p. 48).

Girls are said to be affected slightly more commonly than boys, but in large series the incidence in the two sexes is equal (Sorsby, 1972).

Although only one eye is affected in 70% of patients, there is frequently more than one tumour in the affected retina, and in 30% of patients there is at least one tumour in each eye. Different figures reported from various centres are probably the result of unintentional selection of cases, and may also be affected by the predominant racial group in the community concerned. It has been suggested that the highest incidence is in Europeans, least in black races, and intermediate in Asians.

MACROSCOPIC APPEARANCES

Single or multiple (up to five or six) separate tumours develop as flocculent nodules, resembling cream cheese in appearance and consistency, in the posterior half of the retina. In the later stages the optic nerve is infiltrated and tumour cells permeate along the nerve itself as well as in the sleeve of subarachnoid space which surrounds it. Eventually the neoplasm bursts through the corneoscleral junction into the orbit and rapidly forms the large fungating mass occasionally seen in late cases in developing countries.

MICROSCOPIC FINDINGS

The tumour is composed of small cells with a round or oval hyperchromatic nucleus, forming festoons around vessels. Stroma is minimal or absent, and when present it is loose and fibrillary, resembling neuroglial tissue. Areas of necrosis are almost always present, and calcification often occurs in necrotic tissue. The festoons are the result of the survival of tumour cells close to afferent blood vessels (Fig. 15.15b).

In approximately 50% of tumours the cells are differentiated and form rosettes, i.e. circular collections of cells, usually in a single layer, around a central cavity (Fig. 15.15c). The cytoplasm is more obvious, and tiny structures resembling cilia may be found lining the inner surface of the cytoplasm. In a few cases differentiation is more pronounced and the cells lining the spaces and clefts resemble rod and cone cells of the retina.

It has been suggested that tumours in which rosettes have formed may be less malignant and the prognosis more favourable. This is difficult to assess because of the variable length of time between diagnosis and histological examination, during which changes may occur in response to treatment before the eye is enucleated and examined histologically.

The proximity of the origin of the tumour to the optic nerve, and the extent of its invasion by tumour cells, are the most important factors in determining the prognosis (Ramirez & de Buen, 1973), and tumours which extensively invade the optic nerve tend to have an undifferentiated histological pattern.

SPREAD

(i) *Infiltration along the optic nerve* and/or in the extension of the subarachnoid space which surrounds the nerve is the most important route (Fig. 15.15a). Death is usually due to intracranial extensions, but seeding of metastases via the CSF can occur. On the other hand, Merriam (1950) reported extracranial extension as the cause of death in approximately half of 17 fatal cases submitted to autopsy.

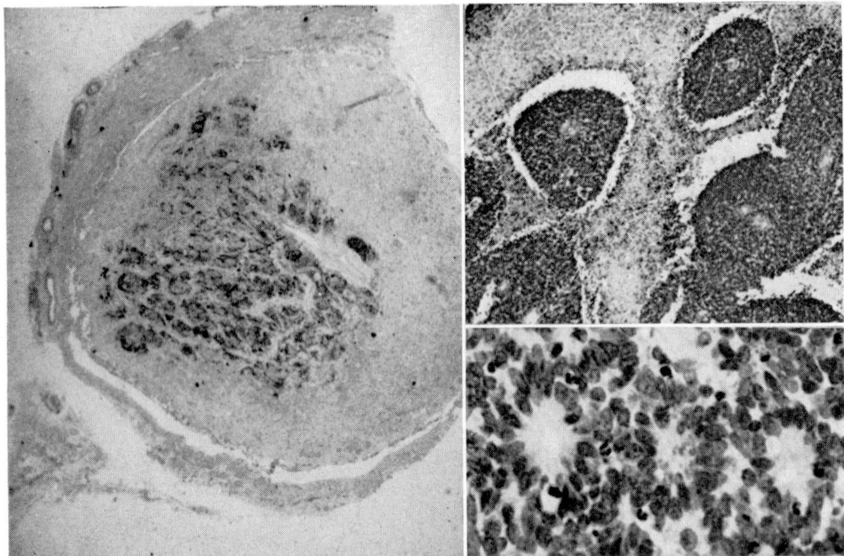

Figure 15.15. RETINOBLASTOMA; (*a*) cross section of an optic nerve infiltrated with retinoblastoma (H & E. × 13); (*b*) groups of tumour cells surviving around blood vessels (H & E. × 30), and (*c*) arranged in rosettes with a central 'lumen' (H & E. × 520); (*d*) colour plate, following p. 140.

[(*a*) *Left.* (*b*) *Top right.* (*c*) *Bottom right.*]

Exfoliated tumour cells may appear in the aqueous fluid of the anterior chamber, and in the Index Series histological confirmation of the fundoscopic diagnosis was obtained in this way (Fig. 15.15a, colour plate, following p. 140).

(ii) *Lymph node metastases* only occur following involvement of the orbital tissues; the pre-auricular and jugulodigastric groups are most frequently affected.

(iii) *Local recurrence*, in the orbit or in the bones of the skull, occurs after incomplete removal of the primary tumour (Wolter, 1973).

(iv) *Distant metastases* outside the cranium are rare and chiefly in the long bones in the limbs or in the liver.

MODES OF PRESENTATION

In the 13 cases in the Index Series, the presenting features, in order of frequency, were in general accord with those noted in other published series.

1. A 'white' reflex, i.e. amaurotic cat's eye (Fig. 15.16a);
2. Strabismus;
3. Secondary glaucoma (buphthalmos);
4. Discovery during fundoscopic surveillance of siblings at risk (p. 424);

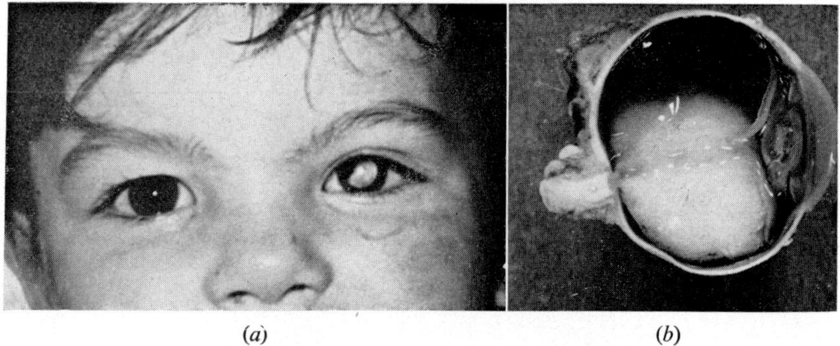

(*a*) (*b*)

Figure 15.16. RETINOBLASTOMA; (*a*) 'white reflex' in the left eye; (*b*) the bisected enucleated eye with the tumour occupying more than half the vitreous and commencing to infiltrate the head of the optic nerve.

5. Proptosis is practically confined to developing countries, where it is the commonest mode of presentation.

In some cases in the Index Series strabismus was the first indication of the presence of a tumour, but was ignored until a white pupil was noted some time later.

DIAGNOSIS

1. *A 'white' reflex, or 'amaurotic' cat's eye*, the term introduced by Beer in 1817 to describe the white pupil seen when light is reflected from a white mass behind the lens (Fig. 15.16a, 15.18) is not confined to tumours and occurs in a variety of non-neoplastic conditions. These are as follows:

(i) The phakomatoses;
(ii) Massive exudative retinitis (Coatts' disease);
(iii) Pseudogliomas (retrolental fibroplasia, toxocara canis infestation and tuberculous retinitis);
(iv) Severe choroiditis;
(v) Congenital cataract;
(vi) Persistent hyperplastic primary vitreus.

Differentiation of these non-neoplastic conditions, and of tumours other than retinoblastoma, requires a complete ophthalmological examination with the proper equipment and under ideal conditions, usually under anaesthesia, and will not be described in detail.

(i) *The phakomatoses* (Vinken & Bruyn, 1972; Font & Ferry, 1972). The ocular manifestations of this group of conditions are of particular importance (Fig. 15.17).

In von Hippel-Lindau disease ocular lesions are often the first signs of the condition, and may precede cerebral signs by more than a decade (Usher,

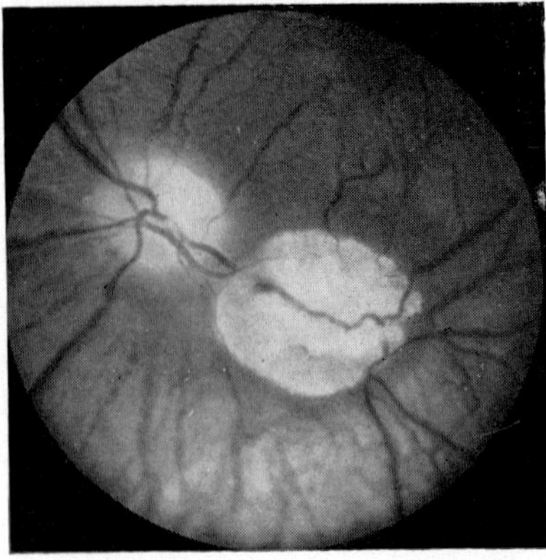

Figure 15.17. PHAKOMA OF THE RETINA; fundoscopic appearance in a child with tuberous sclerosis.

1935). The cerebellar lesions constitute 2% of all brain tumours (in all age groups), and 10% of all posterior fossa tumours (Lindau, 1957).

Tuberous sclerosis. In infants this may present as a form of epilepsy ('infantile spasms') and fundoscopy has proved to be particularly useful in identifying tuberous sclerosis as the cause by demonstrating the retinal lesions. Other features of tuberous sclerosis are described in the section on the phakomatoses (p. 826).

(ii) *Massive exudative retinitis* (Coatts' disease), although not the most common cause of a white reflex, is the most difficult to distinguish from a retinoblastoma; it may mimic exactly a retinoblastoma which has progressed to invasion of the choroid and detachment of the retina. When both retinas are affected and the diagnosis lies between retinitis and retinoblastoma, the more severely affected eye is usually enucleated to obtain histological evidence of the nature of the lesions.

2. *Strabismus and/or nystagmus.* One or other or both may occur when the process of fixation is interferred with by loss of vision very early in life, for example as the result of a retinoblastoma.

3. *Secondary glaucoma* can occur when a retinoblastoma causes a rise in intraocular pressure; the eyeball enlarges and the cornea may become hazy, i.e. producing the classic signs of infantile glaucoma (buphthalmos, Fig. 15.2), usually accompanied by photophobia. Buphthalmos may be mistaken for proptosis which it resembles to some extent.

INVESTIGATIONS

The diagnosis of retinoblastoma can be confidently made when the ocular media are clear, by direct ophthalmoscopy with appropriate equipment for magnification. If doubt exists, e.g. when obscured by the ocular media, supplementary investigations may be required.

(i) *Ultrasonic scanning* of the globe (Stern *et al.*, 1974) and fluorescein angiography (Glass, 1972) are useful in providing additional evidence for diagnosis.

(ii) *Enucleation of the more severely affected eye* in bilateral cases will provide material for exact diagnosis.

(iii) *Exfoliative cytology*. The presence of retinoblastoma cells in fluid obtained by aspirating the anterior chamber can provide histological confirmation of the diagnosis without interfering with the tumour. CSF obtained at lumbar puncture may reveal the presence of retinoblastoma cells; this is indicative of dissemination and the need for extensive treatment including systemic chemotherapy, intrathecal chemotherapy (p. 282) and radiotherapy to the neuraxis (p. 283).

TREATMENT

Ellsworth (1969) has clearly stated the central problem in the treatment of retinoblastoma: conservative management involves a calculated risk in that saving the sight may risk the life of the patient. However, the good prognosis with treatment, in most cases, justifies this risk.

The prospect of successful treatment depends upon whether the tumour is still confined within the eye at the time of the diagnosis. Extension into the orbital tissue, or evidence of metastases, are indications of a poor prognosis.

Conservative treatment, with radiotherapy to the tumour and systemic chemotherapy, is indicated in some cases (in spite of the possibility that the tumour may not be brought under control), provided the eye is not massively involved, and there are grounds for believing that vision can be salvaged. This is exemplified in the bilateral case in which a retinoblastoma develops in the opposite eye after the other has been removed. The tumour in the second eye will be recognized at an early stage if the patient is being carefully followed.

MANAGEMENT

A careful and detailed assessment of the eye and the tumour is the first requirement. Fundoscopic examination under anaesthesia is required, including photographic records and drawings for subsequent comparison. Indirect ophthalmoscopy with scleral indentation allows a wider view of the retina and clear delineation of the extent of the tumour or tumours. Other investigations required are x-rays of the orbit and cranium, and a full blood examination.

The methods of treatment chosen depends upon the extent of the lesion and whether it is confined to the eye or has spread beyond it. Treatment directed specifically to the *tumour* involves locally applied radiotherapy, coagulation or cryotherapy; treatment of *the eye as a whole* requires surgical excision (enucleation), radiotherapy and/or chemotherapy; while treatment of *metastases* may include radiotherapy of the neuraxis as well as chemotherapy.

STAGING

For the purposes of evaluating results and formulating a prognosis, the following system of clinical staging is based on the work of Reese & Ellsworth (1964) and Stallard (1955, 1964).

Stage I: Solitary or multiple tumours less than 4 dd* in diameter, at or behind the '*equator*' (Fig. 15.1).

Stage II: Solitary or multiple tumours up to 11 dd in size, at or behind the equator.

Stage III: Tumour anterior to the equator, or a solitary tumour 10 dd, behind the equator.

Stage IV: Multiple tumours of which some are *larger* than 10 dd, or any lesion involving the *ora serrata* (Fig. 15.1).

Stage V: Tumour involving more than half the retina, or a tumour of any size causing seeding of the vitreus.

The classification of cases and the treatment employed in the Index Series, is as follows.

Group I

Unilateral tumour confined to one eye and not involving the optic nerve.

The usual treatment is enucleation of the eye. However, if there is a family history of retinoblastoma, the appearance of a second tumour in the other eye is very likely (40–45% probability), and conservative measures should be seriously considered. In centres with good facilities for radiotherapy, patients in Stage I, II and III have a very favourable prognosis, but this must be weighed against the risk of radiation induced tumours (Yoneyama & Greenlaw, 1969).

Radiotherapy

Radiation of the whole retina should form part of the treatment (with or without chemotherapy) in most cases of retinoblastoma, because of the multifocal origin of the tumour. A radiation-induced cataract is a possible complication, but this can be removed and sight restored.

* dd: disc diameters.

Group II

Tumour confined to one eye but involving the optic nerve or the choroid. Additional investigations required are a radiological survey of the skeleton, a marrow biopsy and examination of CSF (obtained at lumbar puncture) for exfoliative cytology (p. 426). Further information can also be obtained from the exfoliative cytology of fluid aspirated from the anterior chamber of the eye (see below).

The treatment indicated is enucleation of the eye, followed by chemotherapy, and radiotherapy to the orbit. If the tumour extends into the optic nerve for more than 1 cm (as measured in the operation specimen), or if the central artery of the retina is involved, the CSF is likely to contain malignant cells. When these can be demonstrated, radiotherapy of the neuraxis (see p. 283) and intrathecal chemotherapy are required.

The Index Series contains one example of the value of exfoliative cytology.

A boy aged eight months presented with strabismus, initially treated conservatively elsewhere, and referred two months later with suspected uveitis. When examined under anaesthesia, the appearances of uveitis were confirmed, but the retina could not be clearly seen, and as the patient was in the age group in which retinoblastoma should be suspected, a few drops of fluid were aspirated from the anterior chamber for microscopic examination. This revealed cells arranged in the typical rosettes of retinoblastoma (Fig. 15.15d). CSF obtained at lumbar puncture also contained tumour cells.

The eye was enucleated two days later under cytotoxic cover (see p. 433). Sections of the optic nerve (Fig. 15.15a) showed that the tumour extended to a point proximal to the entry of the central artery of the retina, indicating the source of the cells in the CSF. Radiotherapy to the orbit and the neuraxis (p. 283) was combined with systemic and intrathecal chemotherapy (see p. 282). The patient is alive and free of disease 2 years later; the traditional view is that the prognosis is less than one year, but this may be revised when results obtained with modern protocols of combined chemotherapy and irradiation are available.

Group III. Bilateral tumours

The extent of the tumour is almost never the same in both eyes and is usually more advanced in one than in the other (Bedford *et al.*, 1971; Ellsworth, 1971).

(i) When neither tumour involves the optic nerve or the choroid, radiotherapy to both eyes is indicated.

(ii) When the tumour in one eye involves the choroid or the optic nerve, enucleation followed by radiotherapy to both orbits is indicated. When there is doubt as to the diagnosis because the lesion cannot be seen clearly (e.g. due to opacifation of intervening tissues or to total retinal detachment) the eye is enucleated under a cover of cytotoxic agents (see p. 433); when the diagnosis of retinoblastoma has been confirmed by histological findings, the tumour in the second eye is usually treated conservatively, e.g. by radiotherapy, and chemotherapy if indicated, in an attempt to salvage some sight.

Radiotherapy

Retinoblastomas are very radiosensitive and radiotherapy is the cornerstone of conservative management, usually to a total dose of 3500–4000 rads in three to four weeks. A supervoltage source is preferable because it affects the skin less than megavoltage irradiation and the area treated can be more sharply defined; both scatter and shielding are also subject to better control (see p. 125). In young children restraint of movement during irradiation of the neuraxis (p. 283) is required, and anaesthesia is usually necessary for safety and effective control.

Radiation of the whole retina, alone or combined with chemotherapy, should be the primary form of treatment in most cases of retinoblastoma because of the multifocal nature of the tumour.

Assessment of the tumour's response to treatment is carefully recorded, ideally by serial photographs. Tumours less than 4 dd may disappear completely; larger lesions shrink and may develop a whitish change which is a very favourable sign. In others, the tumour decreases in size but the surface remains grey, and this is a less favourable response. As long as the tumour continues to decrease in size it can be assumed that it has been brought under control.

Irradiation of the retina may be combined with local treatment, e.g. a *Cobalt applicator*, to an anterior tumour, particularly on the nasal side, where it can be placed with less risk of cataract or radionecrosis or subsequent radiation induced tumours.

Light coagulation or cryotherapy is useful for treatment of small tumours at the ora serrata for the same reasons.

Complications of radiotherapy

1. *Post-radiation necrosis*

Post-radiation necrosis in the tissues of the eye is likely to occur when the dose exceeds 5000 rads, but may occur with doses of less than 3000 rads.

2. *Radiation cataract*

With proper control of dosage, changes in the lens are mild and are not severe enough to interfere with sight; adequate fundoscopic surveillance of the effects of treatment is not affected because changes in the lens do not appear until several years after irradiation.

3. *Radiation-induced tumours*

As yet the incidence of such tumours with current methods of irradiation cannot be assessed because of the latent period of several years before they appear. However, the risk certainly is present (Yoneyama & Greenlaw, 1969), particularly with doses greater than 4000–5000 rads, and tumours of several kinds have been reported following smaller dosage (p. 526). A sarcoma of the connective tissue in the orbit (p. 410) is the commonest type of second tumour induced by radiotherapy in patients with retinoblastoma. Osteoblastoma and osteosarcoma have also been reported following irradiation.

In the present state of knowledge, a second full course of radiotherapy after an initial course of 3500–4000 rads is inadvisable because the visual results are poor, and the risks of post-irradiation necrosis or radiation-induced tumour are considerable.

Chemotherapy

Although concrete proof of the direct benefits of pre-operative chemotherapy is lacking, it is our practice to give a cytotoxic agent before biopsy or excision of a tumour where a malignancy is suspected, and vincristine, 1·75–2 mg/m^2 IV, is usually employed.

Maintenance chemotherapy

Vincristine and cyclophosphamide appear to be the most appropriate cytotoxic agents for disseminated retinoblastoma. Recurring cycles of six weeks vincristine (1·75–2 mg/m^2, at intervals of one week) followed by cyclophosphamide for nine weeks (10 mg/kg body weight, orally twice a week) are given. A two-week interval without chemotherapy is used before each cycle to allow recovery from toxic affects on the marrow. The cyclic programme is continued for 18 months to 2 years after definitive surgery.

Intrathecal chemotherapy

When the exfoliative cytology of the CSF shows that tumour cells are present, chemotherapy in the form of methotrexate can be given into the spinal theca, and integrated into the plan of radiotherapy (see p. 283).

RESULTS

The case reports from the Columbia Presbyterian Centre (Tapley, 1969a, 1969b; Ellsworth, 1969) show an improvement of 20% in the 'control' of retinoblastoma, as the result of increased experience in diagnosis and selection of the most appropriate methods of treatment and improved techniques in radiotherapy and chemotherapy.

The full potential of chemotherapy in reducing mortality has not yet been fully explored.

PROGNOSIS

Factors which influence the prognosis unfavourably are as follows:

1. A family history of retinoblastoma.

2. Extensive involvement of the choroid, the optic nerve or the central artery of the retina.
3. The presence of retinoblastoma cells in the CSF.
4. Involvement of orbital soft tissues.

II. DIKTYOMA
(syn. medulloepithelioma of the ciliary body)

This rare embryonal tumour also arises from primitive neuroepithelial cells (Andersen, 1962; Apt, Heller *et al.*, 1973), in the non-pigmented layer of the ciliary body, i.e. it is analogous with the retinoblastoma, but grows more slowly and has less tendency to metastasize.

AGE : SEX

The tumour occurs mostly in young children less than three years of age, and is invariably unilateral. No familial incidence nor evidence of genetic transmission has yet been suggested.

A diktyoma arises in the region of the ciliary body and spreads to involve the lens, the cornea and the iris. Blockage of the canal of Schlem causes glaucoma, distension of the globe and buphthalmos (p. 400). The rate of growth is slow and the clinical history may extend over many months, but invasion of extraocular orbital tissues may eventually occur.

Macroscopically a diktyoma is a firm, white mass or a flat plaque, arising in the region of the ciliary body, causing a partial white reflex when it has grown sufficiently to appear in the pupil.

Microscopically the tumour is composed of small dark cells, very similar to those of retinoblastoma, arranged in cords and tubules resembling the structure of the embryonic retina. Unlike retinoblastoma, the cells of a diktyoma orientate themselves to lie parallel to one surface, and they are set in a loose connective tissue or neuroglial stroma.

The degree of malignancy is low, and although locally destructive, metastasis outside the orbit is unknown.

TREATMENT

Because only one eye is affected, and in view of the progressively local invasive nature of the tumour, enucleation of the eye is the usual method of treatment.

There is no case of diktyoma in the Index Series.

(b) PIGMENTED INTRAOCULAR TUMOURS

This group includes both benign and malignant conditions. Malignant melanoma of the choroid (Fig. 15.18) is the most important, while the more common benign lesions are haemangioma and pigmented naevi.

MALIGNANT MELANOMA OF THE CHOROID

Although a well recognized tumour in adults, malignant melanoma of the choroid in childhood was almost unknown until recently. In a review of 3628 malignant melanomas of the choroid, Paul *et al.* (1962), found only four in childhood. Chaves & Granville (1972) have reported a case in a 2½-year old child, and another example in a 9-year old was reported in 1973 (Newman & Wolter, 1973; McBride White, 1974).

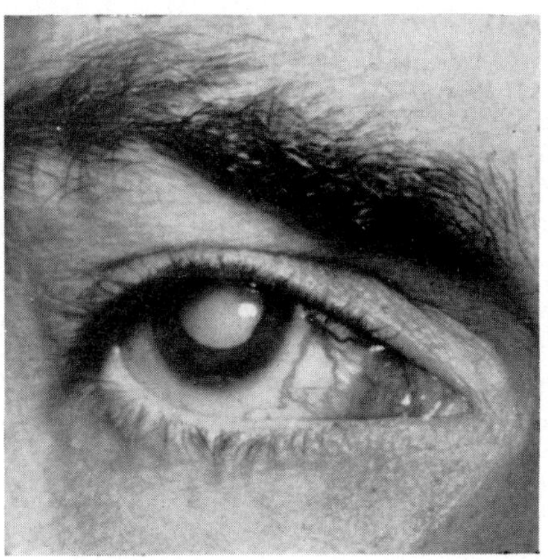

Figure 15.18. MALIGNANT MELANOMA OF THE CHOROID; as well as the 'white' reflex, there is tumour at the inner canthus, having infiltrated through the sclera into the subconjunctival tissues.

MODES OF PRESENTATION

1. *Discovery on routine ophthalmological examination* is the most common mode of presentation.
2. *Strabismus*, due to involvement of the macula region by the tumour, occasionally occurs.

DIFFERENTIAL DIAGNOSIS

1. *Haemangioma.* An isolated haemangioma of the choroid is extremely rare

and because it arises in pigmented tissue, it may be difficult or impossible to distinguish from a malignant melanoma. Sometimes pressure on the globe during fundoscopy can be seen to produce blanching of an angioma when the arterial pressure is exceeded, but this is not always observed.

Uptake studies with ^{32}P, or fluorescent angiography (Gass, 1972) may be helpful, but are sometimes inconclusive; however, when the latter fails to produce fluorescence, a haemangioma can be excluded.

2. *A pigmented naevus of the choroid* is a flat asymptomatic lesion frequently detected as an incidental finding in routine examination of the fundus; it poses no difficulty in diagnosis.
3. *Hypertrophy of retinal pigment*, a congenital lesion and hence found in children, is due to excess production of pigment which is not neoplastic in origin (Buettner, 1975).

TREATMENT

Because of the rarity of this tumour in childhood, there are no data on the advantages of various methods of treatment or the 5-year survival rate.

Starr and Zimmerman (1962) reviewed the results of ocular malignant melanoma in all age groups, and reported a mortality rate at 5 years of 33% when there was no extrascleral extension at the time of diagnosis. In the absence of more detailed reports, treatment of patients in the paediatric age group should be influenced by this information.

Local irradiation, using radon plaques, offers a method of conservative treatment if the tumour is small and does not involve the posterior segment of the eye. Absence of normal sight in the opposite eye strengthens the case for conservatism.

Enucleation of the eye is indicated when the tumour is large or the macular area involved, and when sight in the other eye is normal.

Exenteration of the orbit should be considered when the tumour has extended through the sclera to involve the soft tissues of the orbit.

MALIGNANT MELANOMA OF THE IRIS AND CILIARY BODY

A malignant melanoma in the iris is exceptionally rare in childhood, but should be included in the differential diagnosis when there is disturbance of pupillary function.

DIFFERENTIAL DIAGNOSIS

Other lesions of the iris are as follows:

1. *Haemangiomas*, which are extremely rare.

2. *Pigmented naevi* are the commonest abnormality of the iris, and appear as pigmented freckles which are often bilateral. No treatment is necessary.
3. *Juvenile xanthogranuloma.* In some reported series (e.g. Ferry, 1972), some 'haemangiomas' are found to be xanthogranulomas. These are yellowish plaques in the iris in infants and tend to cause spontaneous recurrent hyphema, which obscures the details of the underlying cause. Their recognition is important for they can be controlled by radiotherapy and vision preserved.
4. *Leiomyoma of the iris* has also been reported.

TREATMENT

Malignant melanoma of the iris or ciliary body appears to be of low grade malignancy, and when confined to the iris can be treated by simple iridectomy, or iridocyclectomy when the ciliary body is involved.

THE SURGERY OF ORBITAL AND OCULAR TUMOURS

TUMOURS OF THE ORBIT

Lateral orbitotomy. When exploration and biopsy are required to reach a diagnosis orbitotomy, with or without reflection of the lateral wall, provides excellent access for palpation, inspection, biopsy etc., and is the procedure of choice in 80–90% of tumours confined to the orbit.

A frontal approach is less frequently employed because of the small proportion of tumours arising in the medial half of the orbit.

A curved incision is made below the nasal portion of the eyebrow. The supraorbital vessels are identified. The periosteum is reflected as in an approach to remove a mucocele of the frontal and ethmoid sinus. Other palpable tumours may be approached directly.

Transfrontal (bifrontal) orbitotomy is a neurosurgical procedure required when the orbital lesion extends proximally into the region of the chiasm.

TUMOURS OF THE EYELIDS AND CONJUNCTIVAE

Excision biopsy of small lesions is the procedure most frequently performed in childhood. When an extensive lesion is to be removed, e.g. a plexiform neuroma, or a persistent vascular lesion, removal of skin and conjunctiva may require reconstructive procedures requiring the co-operative participation of the plastic surgeon.

TUMOURS OF THE ADNEXAE

Enlargement of the lachrymal gland usually requires exploration and biopsy to determine whether the lesion is a metastatic deposit (e.g. from a lymphoma) or a primary tumour of the gland. When the latter is present, excision of the adjacent periosteum is advised, to prevent local recurrence.

A primary malignant tumour of the lachrymal gland requires exenteration of the orbit and possibly radical excision of the adjacent wall of the orbit, and occasionally the dura. Operations of this extent are best performed with the close co-operation of a plastic surgeon, neurosurgeon and ophthalmic surgeon.

INTRAOCULAR TUMOURS

The type of tumour and its site determine the extent of the excision required.

Total excision of the tumour, e.g. iridectomy or iridocyclectomy, can be performed for certain tumours of the iris or the ciliary body (e.g. melanoma). Excision of the entire globe is the operation of choice in some tumours of the choroid and retina, e.g. advanced retinoblastoma or melanoma of the choroid.

Exenteration of the orbit is usually reserved for tumours involving the soft tissues of the orbit, e.g. intraocular tumours infiltrating the orbital tissues, such as a retinoblastoma which has penetrated the globe. Rhabdomyosarcoma of the orbit has traditionally been treated by exenteration, but recent developments (p. 793) may lead to re-evaluation of this policy.

REFERENCES

ANDERSEN, S.R. (1962). Medulloepithelioma of the retina. *Int. Ophthalmol. Clin.*, **2** : 483.

APT, L., HELLER, M.D. *et al.* (1973). Dictyoma (embryonal medulloepithelioma) : recent review and case report. *J. Pediat. Ophthal.*, **10** : 30.

BARBER, J.C., Barber, L.F. *et al.* (1974). Congenital orbital teratoma. *Arch. Ophthalmol.*, **91** : 45.

BEDFORD, M.A., BEDOTTO, C. & MACFAUL, P.A. (1971). Retinoblastoma : a study of 139 cases. *Brit. J. Ophthalmol.*, **55** : 19.

BLAKE, J. & FITZPATRICK, C. (1972). Eye signs in neuroblastoma. *Trans. Ophthalmol. Soc. U.K.*, **92** : 825.

BUETTNER, H. (1975). Congenital hypertrophy of the retinal pigment epithelium. *Am. J. Ophthalmol.*, **79** : 177.

CASSADY, J.R. *et al.* (1969). Radiation therapy in retinoblastoma : an analysis of 230 cases. *Radiology*, **93** : 405.

CHAVES, E. & GRANVILLE, R. (1972). Choroidal malignant melanoma in a 2½ year old girl. *Amer. J. Ophthalmol.*, **74** : 20.

CHUTORIAN, A.M., SCHWARTZ, J.F. *et al.* (1964). Optic gliomas in children. *Neurology*, **14** : 83.

DAVIS, F.A. (1940). Primary tumors of the optic nerve (a phenomenon of von Recklinghausen's disease) : a clinical and pathologic study with a report of 5 cases and a review of the literature. *Arch. Ophthal.*, **23** : 735, 957.

DONALDSON, S.S., CASTRO, J.R. *et al.* (1973). Rhabdomyosarcoma of head and neck in children : combination treatment by surgery, irradiation and chemotherapy. *Cancer*, **31** : 26.

ELLSWORTH, R.M. (1969). The practical management of retinoblastoma. *Trans. Amer. Ophth. Soc.*, **67** : 462.

ELLSWORTH, R. (1971). Tumours of the retina. In *Retinal Diseases in Children* (Tasman, W., ed.). Harper & Row, New York.

FEMAN, S.S. & APT, L. (1972). Eye findings associated with pediatric malignancy. *J. Pediat. Ophthalmol.*, **9** : 224.

FERRY, A.P. (1972). Ocular and Adnexal Tumors. *Internatl. Ophthal. Clin.*, **12** : 1.

FONT, R.L. & FERRY, A.P. (1972). The phakomatoses. *Internatl. Ophthal. Clin.*, **12** : 1.

GASS, J.D.M. (1972). Fluorescein angiography : an aid in the differential diagnosis of intraocular tumors. *Internatl. Ophthal. Clin.*, **12** : 85.

GLASER, J.S., HOYT, W.F. & CORBETT, J. (1971). Visual morbidity with chiasmal glioma : longterm studies of visual fields in untreated and irradiated cases. *Arch. Ophthalmol.*, **85** : 3.

GREER, C.H. (1966). Rhabdomyosarcoma of the head and neck with special reference to the orbit. *Trans. Ophthalmol. Soc. Aust.*, **25** : 80.

HEYN, R.M. (1971). Chemotherapy in pediatric orbital tumors. *J. Pediatr. Ophthal.*, **8** : 141.

HILES, D.A. & PILCHARD, W.A. (1971). Corticosteroid control of neonatal hemangiomas of the orbit and ocular adnexa. *Am. J. Ophthal.*, **71** : 1003.

HOYT, W.F. & BAGHDASSARIAN, S.A. (1969). Optic glioma of childhood. *Brit. J. Ophthal.*, **53** : 793.

HUBEL, D.H. & WIESEL, T.N. (1962). Receptive fields, binocular interaction and functional architecture in the cats visual cortex. *J. Physiol. (London)*, **160** : 106.

HUBEL, D.H. & WIESEL, T.N. (1965). Binocular interaction in striate cortex of kittens reared with artificial squint. *J. Neurophysiol.*, **28** : 1041.

HYMAN, G.A., ELLSWORTH, R.M., FEIND, C.R. *et al.* (1968). Combination therapy in retinoblastoma. *Arch. Ophthal.*, **80** : 744.

JENSEN, O.A. (1969). Teratoma of the orbit. *Acta Ophthal.*, **47** : 317.

JONES, I.S., REESE, A.B. & KROUT, J. (1965). Orbital rhabdomyosarcoma. *Traus. Amer. Ophthalmol. Soc.*, **63** : 233.

KARLIN, D.B. (1972). Ultrasound in the diagnosis of intraocular and retrobulbar tumours. *Internatal. Ophthal. Clin.*, **12** : 121.

KARP, L.A., ZIMMERMAN, L.E. *et al.* (1974). Primary intraorbital meningiomas. *Arch. Ophthalmol.*, **91** : 24.

KILMAN, J.W., CLATWORTHY, H.W.Jr., NEWTON, W.A. & GROSFELD, J.L. (1973). Reasonable surgery for rhabdomyosarcoma : a study of 67 cases. *Ann. Surg.*, **178** : 347.

KNUDSON, A.G.Jr. (1971). Mutation and cancer: statistical study of retinoblastoma. *Proc. Nat. Acad. Sci. U.S.A.*, **68** : 820.

LINDAU, A. (1957). Capillary angiomatosis of the central nervous system. *Acta Genet.*, **7** : 338.

MCBRIDE WHITE, J. (1975). Malignant melanoma of the choroid in young people. *Aust. J. Ophthal.*, **3** : 51.

MCPHERSON, S.D.Jr. (1966). Mixed tumor of the lacrimal gland in a 7 year old boy. *Amer. J. Ophthal.*, **61** : 561.

MERRIAM, G.R. (1950). Retinoblastoma: analysis of 17 autopsies. *Arch. Ophthalmol.*, **44** : 71.

NEWMAN, L.P. & WOLTER, J.R. (1973). Malignant melanoma of the choroid in a 9-year old girl. *J. Pediat. Ophthal.*, **10** : 44.

PAUL, E.V., PARNELL, S.L. & FRAKER, M. (1962). Prognosis of malignant melanomas of the choroid and ciliary body. *Int. Ophth. Clin.*, **2** : 387.

PORTERFIELD, J.F. & ZIMMERMAN, L.E. (1962). Rhabdomyosarcoma of the orbit: a clinicopathologic study of 55 cases. *Virchow's Arch. Path. Anat.*, **335** : 329.

RAMIREZ, L.C. & DE BUEN, S. (1973). Clinical and pathologic findings in 100 retinoblastoma patients. *J. Pediat. Ophthal.*, **10** : 12.

REESE, A.B. & ELLSWORTH, R.M. (1974). Management of retinoblastoma. *Ann. N.Y. Acad. Sci.*, **114** : 958.

ROBERTSON, D.M. & HENDERSON, J.W. (1969). Unilateral proptosis secondary to orbital mucocele in infancy. *Am. J. Ophthalmol.*, **68** : 845.

SAGERMAN, R.H., TRETTER, P. & ELLSWORTH, R.M. (1972). The treatment of orbital rhabdomyosarcoma of children with primary radiation therapy. *Am. J. Roentgenol. Rad. Ther. Nucl. Med.*, **114** : 31.

SANDERS, T.E., ACKERMAN, L.V. & ZIMMERMAN, L.E. (1962). Epithelial tumours of the lacrimal gland: a comparison of the pathologic and clinical behaviour with those of salivary glands. *Amer. J. Surg.*, **104** : 657.

SORSBY, A. (1972). Bilateral retinoblastoma: a dominantly inherited affection. *Brit. med. J.*, **2** : 580.

SPENCER, W.H. (1972). Primary neoplasms of the optic nerve and its sheaths: Clinical features and current concepts of pathologenetic mechanisms. *Trans. Am. Ophthalmol. Soc.*, **70** : 490.

STALLARD, H.B. (1955). Multiple islands of retinoblastoma: incidence rate and time span of appearance. *Brit. J. Ophth.*, **39** : 241.

STALLARD, H.B. (1964). The conservative management of retinoblastoma. In *Ocular and Adnexal Tumors.* C. V. Mosby Co., St. Louis.

STARR, H.J. & ZIMMERMAN, L.E. (1962). Extrascleral extension of malignant melanoma of the choroid and ciliary body. *Int. Ophthalmol. Clin.*, **2** : 369.

STERN, G.K., COLEMAN, D.J. & ELLSWORTH, R.M. (1974). Ultrasonographic characteristics of retinoblastoma. *Am. J. Ophthalmol.*, **78** : 606.

SUTOW, W.W., SULLIVAN, M.P. *et al.* (1970). Prognosis in childhood rhabdomyosarcomas. *Cancer*, **25** : 1384.

TAPLEY, N. DU V. (1969a). The treatment of retinoblastoma. In *Neoplasia in Childhood.* Year Book Medical Publishers Inc., Chicago.

TAPLEY, N. DU V. (1969). Treatment of retinoblastoma with radiation and chemotherapy. In *Ocular and Adnexal Tumors.* C.V. Mosby Co., St. Louis.

TASMAN, W. (ed.) (1971). The phakomatoses. In *Retinal Diseases in Children.* Harper & Row, New York.

TROKEL, S.L. (1972). Radiological techniques in the diagnosis of ocular and orbital tumors. *Internatl. Ophthal. Clin.*, **12** : 145.

TROKEL, S.L. (1974). The orbit. *Arch. Ophthalmol.*, **91** : 223.

UDVARHELYI, G.B., KHODADOUST, A.A. & WALSH, F.B. (1965). Gliomas of the optic nerve and chiasm in children: an unusual series of cases. *Clin. Neurosurg.*, **13** : 204.

USHER, C.H. (1935). Angiomatosis retinae. The Bowman Lecture. On a few hereditary eye affections. *Trans. Ophth. Soc. U.K.*, **55** : 183.

VIGNAUD, J., CLAY, C. & BILANIUK, L.T. (1974). Venography of the orbit; an analytical report of 413 cases. *Radiol.*, **110** : 373.

VINKEN, P.J. & BRUYEN, G.W. (eds.). The Phakomatoses. In *Handbook of Clinical Neurology*, vol. 14. American Elsevier, New York.

WOLTER, J.R. (1973). Extension of retinoblastoma along the optic nerve. *J. Pediat. Ophthal.*, **10** : 25.

YONEYAMA, T. & GREENLAW, R.H. (1969). Osteogenic sarcoma following radiotherapy for retinoblastoma. *Radiology*, **93** : 1185.

Chapter 16. Thoracic tumours

Primary malignant tumours of the lungs, ribs, bronchi or diaphragm are extremely rare in childhood, and the mediastinum is the commonest site of intrathoracic tumours in this age group. The mediastinum is also the commonest site of benign intrathoracic masses, which outnumber malignant tumours by 4 or 5 to 1 (Table 16.1).

Table 16.1. Benign swellings and malignant tumours

Benign conditions	Malignant tumours
A. *Mediastinal masses*	
ANTERIOR MEDIASTINUM	
Thymic hyperplasia	Lymphosarcoma
Thymic cysts	
Thymolipoma	
Thymoma	(Malignant thymoma)
Teratoma	(Malignant teratoma)
Cystic hygroma	Rhabdomyosarcoma
Lipoma	
Haemangioma	
Neurofibroma (plexiform)	
Benign lymphocytic hamartoma	
MID MEDIASTINUM	
Cardiac tumours and hamartomas	Malignant lymphoma of
Tuberculous hilar nodes	the hilar nodes
Spring-water cyst of pericardium	
POSTERIOR MEDIASTINUM	
Phaeochromocytoma	Neuroblastoma and
Ganglioneuroma	ganglioneuroblastoma
Neurofibroma	Neurofibrosarcoma
Bronchogenic cyst	Malignant mesenchymoma
Duplication (of the stomach, oesophagus)	(syn. stem cell tumour)
(enterogenous cysts)	Paraganglioma (malignant)
Neurenteric cysts	Phaeochromocytoma (malignant)
Paraganglioma	
Split notochord syndrome	

Table 16.1. continued

Benign conditions	Malignant tumours
	B. *Tumours of the trachea, bronchi or lung*
Subglottic haemangioma (larynx)	Pulmonary metastases
Papilloma (larynx, trachea, bronchus)	
Hamartoma (lung)	
Plasma cell granuloma (trachea, bronchus)	Bronchial 'adenoma' (bronchus)
Pseudotumour (syn. pseudosarcoma)	Bronchogenic carcinoma:
(bronchus, trachea)	adenocarcinoma
Neurofibroma (bronchus)	squamous cell
Leiomyoma (bronchus)	undifferentiated
	small-cell carcinoma
	Leiomyosarcoma (bronchus, lung)
Lymphangioma (lung)	Fibrosarcoma (bronchus, lung)
Haemangioma (lung)	Pulmonary blastoma
Arteriovenous fistula (lung) Chondromatous hamartoma (lung)	Papillomatosis (lung)
Bronchogenic cyst (lung)	Mesothelioma (pleura)
Hydatid cyst (lung)	
	C. *Cardiac tumours*
Rhabdomyoma	Rhabdomyosarcoma
Fibroma	
Myxoma	
Haemangioma	
Hamartoma	
Teratoma (intrapericardiac)	
	D. *Tumours of the chest wall and diaphragm*
Osteomyelitis	Chondrosarcoma
Fibrous dysplasia	Ewing's tumour
Chondroma	Eosinophilic granuloma
Aneurysmal bone cyst	Reticulum cell sarcoma
Osteoid osteoma	Fibrosarcoma
	Metastatic deposits (costal)
Chondromyxoid fibroma	neuroblastoma
Other benign bone lesions (see p. 725)	Ewing's tumour
	synoviosarcoma
Desmoma (syn. desmoid fibroma)	malignant lymphoma
	Rhabdomyosarcoma (intercostal muscle or diaphragm)
	Haemangiopericytoma (malignant)

Mediastinal masses are thus the most common and important, but the literature concerning rare tumours arising in the trachea and bronchi, the lung, the heart, the chest wall and the diaphragm is also reviewed in this chapter. The contents are divided into the following sections:

A. Mediastinal masses;
B. Tumours of the larynx, trachea and bronchi;
C. Tumours of the lung;
D. Cardiac tumours;
E. Tumours of the chest wall and diaphragm.

A. MEDIASTINAL MASSES

ANATOMY AND RADIOLOGY OF THE MEDIASTINUM

The mediastinum extends from the first rib to the diaphragm and is bounded on each side by the mediastinal pleura, in front by the sternum, and posteriorly by the vertebral bodies. The structures it contains fall into two groups. The first comprises the heart and great vessels, the oesophagus, the trachea and primary bronchi; the anatomy of this group is familiar and constant. The second group of structures, chiefly the thymus and mediastinal lymphoid tissues, show considerable variations in size and location.

In infants, the thymus is a relatively large organ which occupies the upper anterior mediastinum in front of the great vessels. Although the thymus increases steadily in size up to puberty, its size in relation to the volume of the thorax diminishes steadily from birth, to the extent that it can only rarely be demonstrated radiologically after the age of two years. A considerable amount of lymphoid tissue is present in the anterior mediastinum in young children, both within the thymus and also in adjacent areolar tissues. Lymph nodes also surround the hilum of each lung, partially fill in the angle formed by the lower margin of the carina, and contribute to the thymic shadows.

The inaccessibility of the mediastinum to clinical examination increases the importance of radiological findings, and the shadow cast by the mediastinal structures can be usefully divided into three regions, each of which is closely related to a particular group of tumours (Table 16.2).

SUBDIVISIONS OF THE MEDIASTINUM

Several schemes of subdivision have been suggested; the one illustrated in Fig. 16.1 is one of the simplest, yet of practical importance in examining lateral projections of the mediastinum.

(i) *The posterior mediastinum* is defined as the area containing the projections of the vertebral bodies, and the costovertebral or paravertebral sulcus on each side.

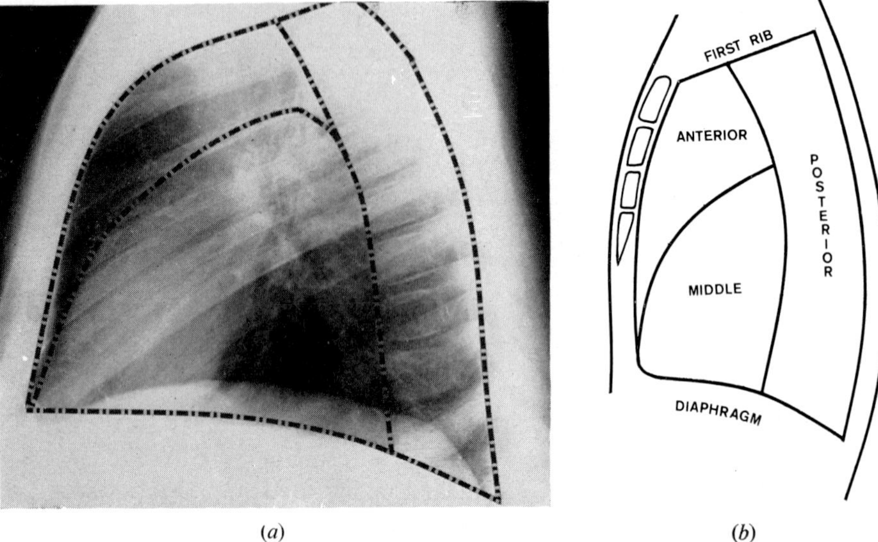

(*a*) (*b*)

Figure 16.1. THE MEDIASTINUM; (*a*) lateral x-ray of chest showing radiological subdivisions of the mediastinal shadow into anterior, posterior and mid-mediastinum (see text); and (*b*) a diagram illustrating their boundaries.

(ii) *The anterior mediastinum* is bounded above by the first rib, in front by the inner surface of the sternum, and arbitrarily by a curved line following the cardiac border and extending backwards to a line joining the anterior borders of the vertebral bodies.

(iii) *The mid-mediastinum* occupies the area between the other two subdivisions, bounded by the diaphragm below and contains little more than the hilar lymph nodes.

These subdivisions and the various mediastinal masses usually arising in each area are shown in Fig. 16.2.

MODES OF PRESENTATION OF MEDIASTINAL MASSES

The range of presenting modes is limited and less varied than tumours arising in other sites, for example in the abdomen.

(a) *Symptoms* are more common and more important than clinical signs in mediastinal masses, and the symptoms produced are the result of pressure on mediastinal structures: cough, dyspnoea or stridor.

(b) In another group of patients a mediastinal mass is first discovered *incidentally in an x-ray of the chest*, e.g. as part of a routine survey, or in x-rays taken during treatment of a respiratory infection.

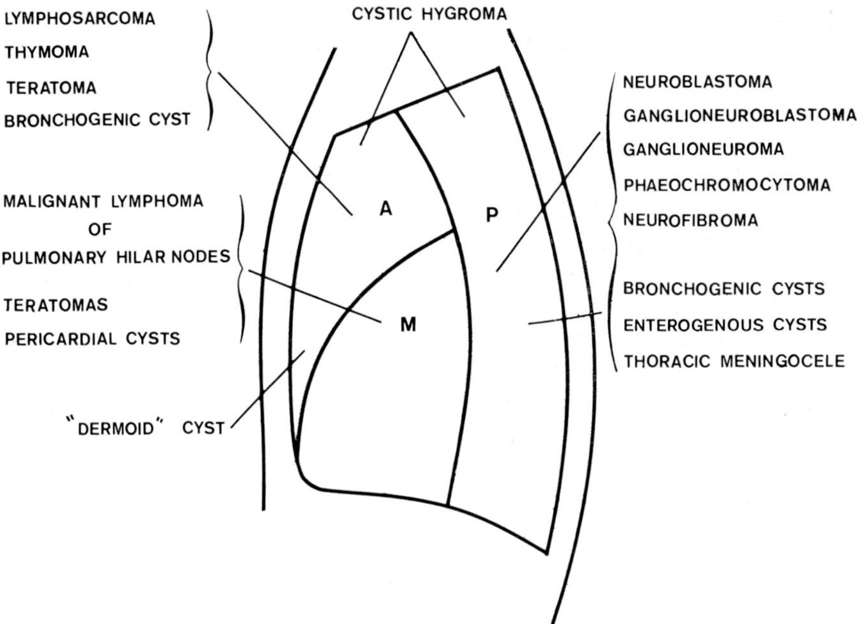

Figure 16.2. MEDIASTINAL MASSES; the subdivisions of the mediastinum, showing the tumours which typically arise in each area.

Tumours presenting with the features of mediastinal compression are usually malignant; those discovered incidentally are usually benign.

(a) **Mediastinal compression**

1. *Congestion* of veins in the head, neck and upper limbs follows compression of the superior vena cava; the skin of the face and neck has a suffused or oedematous appearance, in contrast to the trunk and the lower limbs.

2. *Respiratory obstruction* due to tracheal compression usually presents as a wheeze, initially heard only in expiration, but rapidly progresses to affect both inspiration and expiration. Gradually increasing dyspnoea and tachypnoea may become suddenly much worse with the development of infection in the respiratory tract.

A persistent cough, usually 'brassy', i.e. resonant and unproductive, is sometimes the presenting symptom, and may also be due to tracheal compression. Compression of a bronchus by enlarged hilar lymph nodes may cause 'air-trapping' and over-inflation of the corresponding portion of the lung, visible in x-rays. Narrowing of the lower airways may lead to obstruction of a bronchus by a plug of mucus, pulmonary collapse and supervening infection.

3. *Oesophageal compression* and dysphagia are uncommon and usually a late sign indicating advanced mediastinal disease, particularly when the patient cannot swallow solid foods.

4. An uncommon but important sign of a mediastinal mass in early childhood is forward protrusion of the sternum and the adjacent chest wall. This is seen most clearly when the patient is standing and unclothed, and when noticed by the parents as a recent development, it is a strong indication of a rapidly growing malignant tumour.

(b) **Incidental discovery in radiographs**

Once the mass has been demonstrated, closer enquiry often reveals that some of the symptoms described above have, in fact, been present. Very occasionally a mediastinal mass is the result of metastasis from an extrathoracic tumour already under treatment or surveillance, but in childhood mediastinal metastases in lymphoid tissue are less common than pulmonary metastases (p. 479).

The location, shape and size of such a mass may give a useful indication of the 'likely' nature of the tumour (Fig. 16.2) but further investigations are usually required to clarify the diagnosis before deciding on thoracotomy (Hope, Borns & Koop, 1963).

INVESTIGATIONS

A detailed history and a thorough examination, with particular attention to regional lymph nodes and the spleen, may provide further information.

The peripheral blood, the bone marrow, and the urine (e.g. for increased levels of catecholamines, p. 551) should also be examined. However, the most informative investigations are radiological, including oblique views and contrast studies when indicated.

RADIOLOGICAL DIFFERENTIATION OF MEDIASTINAL MASSES

The anterior mediastinum

The thymus is not uncommonly enlarged and of variable shape in the first few months of life (Fig. 16.3) and a tumour within it may be suspected. Such tumours are, in fact, extremely rare, particularly in this age group, and serial x-rays showing a gradual decrease in the size of the thymic shadow are useful evidence that the unusual shape is not due to a tumour. Screening may also be helpful (Shackelford *et al.*, 1974).

Lymphosarcoma is the commonest malignant mediastinal tumour in childhood (p. 452), usually arises in the region of the thymus, in the anterior mediastinum (Fig. 16.6), and displaces the trachea backwards. It is an expanding lesion, spreading downwards in front of the heart and eventually

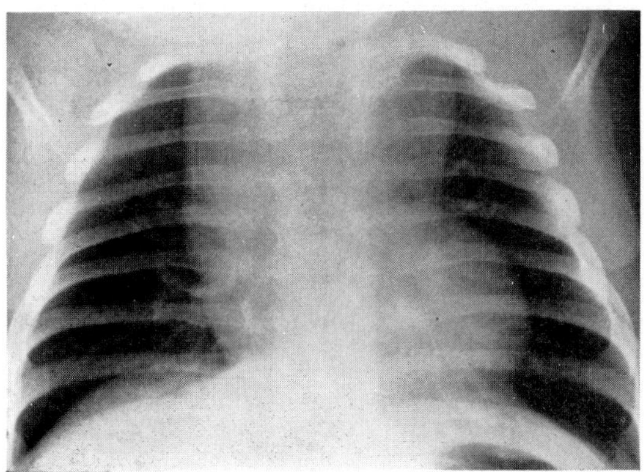

Figure 16.3. BENIGN ENLARGEMENT OF THE THYMUS; x-ray of a 3-month old infant showing the extent of 'physiological' enlargement within the 'normal' range. X-rays at 9 months of age showed no thymic shadow and a normal mediastinum.

laterally to involve the pleural cavities. The margin of its shadow is traditionally described as indistinct; the mass is often large enough to obscure most of the mediastinal structures (Fig. 16.6), and occasionally projects above the sternum into the suprasternal notch.

A pleural effusion usually indicates that the mediastinal pleura is infiltrated; a large blood-stained effusion is not unusual, and the cytology of fluid removed for symptomatic relief may provide confirmation that the tumour is a lymphosarcoma (Fig. 16.6b).

Malignant thymoma, a rare condition, may be indistinguishable radiologically from a lymphosarcoma; its growth is as a rule slower, so that the mass may be actually larger, and its margins may be more sharply defined and more distinct than lymphosarcoma.

Teratomas also arise in the anterior mediastinum (p. 456), either in the thymus, or close to the pericardium. These tumours usually have a clearly defined rounded shadow and may show calcification. In rare instances a teratoma may have a pedicle and project into one or other pleural cavity. Some are situated inside the pericardial sac (p. 483) or, in very few, in the myocardium itself. Even those outside the pericardium may mimic cardiomegaly, but this can usually be excluded by fluoroscopic screening which demonstrates that the part of the heart shadow formed by the teratoma is non-pulsatile. In rare instances angiocardiography may be required to exclude a congenital cardiac malformation (Fig. 16.8b).

In most cases the distinction between a teratoma and a true dermoid cyst can only be made by the pathologist, but in one case in the Index

Series the primary tumour and metastatic pulmonary deposits were visible in the same film, indicating that the mediastinal mass was malignant.

Benign lymphocytic hamartoma (*giant lymph node hyperplasia*)
First described by Castleman *et al.* (1956), the cause of this often exuberant form of lymphoid hyperplasia is unknown. The mediastinum is the usual site (p. 458).

The posterior mediastinum
Neuroblastomas typically arise in the costovertebral sulcus, and calcification is sometimes evident. Occasionally there is visible erosion of the posterior ends of the ribs. Enlargement of the spinal nerve root canal can rarely be demonstrated, despite the fairly common occurrence of soft fleshy tumour extending through the foramen into the spinal canal and causing compression. Myelography should always be undertaken when a mediastinal tumour is thought to be a neuroblastoma (Fig. 16.9).

Neurofibromas are rarer then neuroblastomas in infants and children, and enlargement of a nerve root canal (Fig. 16.4) typical of a 'dumb-bell' tumour (see p. 465) is even rarer. Myelography should be performed in all patients with any neural symptoms or signs.

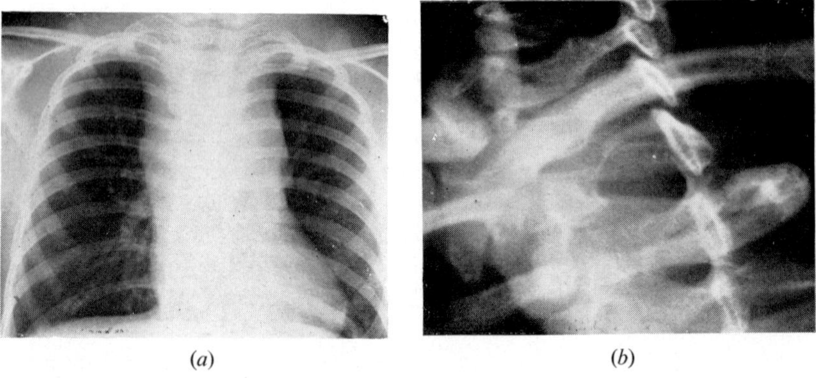

(*a*) (*b*)

Figure 16.4. Neurofibroma; (*a*) a large midline tumour in the upper part of the posterior mediastinum; (*b*) oblique view of an upper thoracic nerve root canal enlarged by a neurofibroma arising in the posterior mediastinum and extending into the vertebral canal i.e. a 'dumb-bell tumour'.

Cystic hygromas entirely confined to the mediastinum are unusual; more often they are in the 'superior' mediastinum and extend upwards into the neck, almost always on the right side (Broomhead, 1964), as a palpable mass

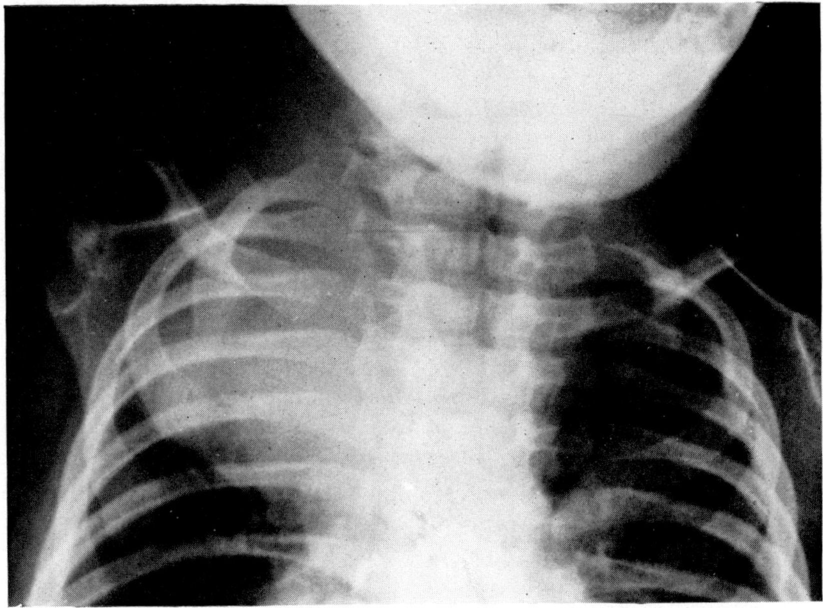

Figure 16.5. CYSTIC HYGROMA; the mediastinal shadow is continuous with a clinically palpable extension in the deep triangle of the neck on the right side.

in the deep or posterior cervical triangle (Fig. 16.8). Rarely an extensive lymphangiomatous hamartoma of the mediastinum is large enough to cause symptoms of mediastinal compression (Krieg *et al.*, 1973).

Plexiform neurofibromas of the thoracic inlet (p. 465) occupy a cervico-thoracic position (Raffensperger & Cohen, 1972) much the same as the mediastinal type of cystic hygroma described above.

NON-NEOPLASTIC CYSTIC LESIONS

The thorax is remarkable for the variety or cystic anomalies which may occur during the development of the viscera it contains. The content of the cyst may initially be fluid or air, or both once it has ruptured into the air passages. Infection in or around a cyst may occur, leading to signs and symptoms of infection which may be the mode of presentation, and contribute to difficulty in determining the nature of the initial lesion.

Classification. The various intrathoracic cystic structures can be classified as follows:

1. *Pulmonary 'cysts':*

(*a*) *Bronchogenic cysts*, derived from the primitive bronchial tree, and lined by bronchial epithelium. Those in the lung fields (as opposed to 'hilar cysts', see below) usually contain air, and may show a fluid level (Lumpkin, 1966).

(*b*) *Pulmonary sequestrations*, more complex lesions containing some pulmonary tissue, and bronchi lacking a communication with the rest of the bronchial tree; these bronchi may become dilated to form cystic structures. There is often an accompanying abnormality of the pleural reflection, and the vessels supplying the sequestrated lobe arise directly from the aorta, often below the diaphragm.

(*c*) *An abscess cavity*, most commonly due to *Staphylococcus aureus* causing focal destruction of tissue, becoming localized and difficult to distinguish from a pre-existing bronchogenic cyst.

(*d*) *A hydatid cyst;* in children a pulmonary hydatid cyst is usually an intact fluid-filled cavity, less commonly containing fluid and air as a fluid level following rupture into a bronchus. Radiographic evidence of the collapsed parasitic membrane in the fluid in cystic cavity (the 'water-lily' sign) is distinctive but seldom seen, and serological tests (Casoni and complement fixation) are both negative in 25% of proven cases in childhood.

2. *Hilar* (*mid-mediastinal*) *cysts*, usually 'bronchogenic' and typically but not invariably lacking communication with a bronchus.

3. *Posterior mediastinal cysts:*

(*a*) *Oesophageal duplication* (syn. enterogenous cyst), arising in the dorsal part of the mediastinum, may be lined by stratified squamous or respiratory epithelium, and appears to be a localized abnormality of the primitive tube from which both the trachea and oesophagus develop.

(*b*) *Dorsal enteric remnants*, more complex anomalies forming a spectrum which extends to the 'split-notochord' syndrome and 'neurenteric fistula'. This group is thought to be the result of an adhesion between ectoderm and endoderm at an early stage of embryonic development. Rarely is there a complete fistula between the alimentary canal and the skin of the back; more commonly only part of the track persists, as a cystic structure, often lined by gastric mucosa. The diagnosis is suggested by a posterior mediastinal lesion accompanied by a hemivertebra. In such cases there may be also an irregular tubular structure joining a supradiaphragmatic to an abdominal component (Kirwan *et al.*, 1973).

The differentiation, on histological grounds, of a neurenteric anomaly, typically in the posterior mediastinum, from a teratoma, which only rarely arises in this region, may present difficulties. Neurenteric lesions may contain cystic spaces lined by alimentary, respiratory and squamous epithelium (Bale, 1973), but when a wider variety of tissues is found, it may be difficult to exclude a teratoma. The latter is a neoplasm with a small but definite malignant potential, whereas a neurenteric lesion is a wholly benign malformation, and the more likely when accompanied by a closely related malformation of one or more vertebrae (Piramoon & Abbassioun, 1974).

The symptoms caused by this subgroup of anomalies are varied and include cough and dyspnoea, on rare occasions haemoptysis when a lesion erodes into a bronchus, or a gastro-intestinal haemorrhage when there is ectopic gastric mucosa in a supra- or sub-diaphragmatic duplication communicating with the alimentary canal.

DIAGNOSIS

All the cystic thoracic lesions above may have the same modes of presentation as intrathoracic tumours (p. 444), and should therefore be considered in their differential diagnosis. While some cystic lesions can be distinguished from tumours by their clinical findings, by biochemical tests such as the level of catecholamine excretion, or on specific radiographic findings, e.g. hemivertebrae, in many cases a cystic structure cannot be recognized with certainty until excised and examined histologically. Although individually rare, as a group these structures represent a significant proportion of space-occupying lesions in the thorax (see Tables 16.2 and 16.3).

Table 16.2. Mediastinal masses

Mediastinal mass (Diagnosis)		No.
Bronchogenic cyst		8
Thymic hyperplasia		6
Neuroblastoma		4
Duplication cyst		3
Lymphoid granuloma		3
Lymphangioma		3
Cystic teratoma (benign)		3
Neurofibroma		2
Ganglioneuroma		2
Hodgkin's disease		2
Ganglioneuroblastoma	1 each	6
Cavernous haemangioma		
Malignant endothelioma		
Malignant teratoma		
Rhabdomyosarcoma		
Lymphosarcoma		
Total		42

After Heimburger and Battersby (1965)

Table 16.3. Intrathoracic tumours and cysts

Type of tumour	Total no.	No. malignant	
Neurogenic	9	5	
Duplications	10	0	
Angiomatous	5	1	
Teratoid	5	1	
Lymphoid	6	3	
Other	1	1	
Total	36	11	47

From Heimburger and Battersby (1965)

TUMOURS OF THE ANTERIOR MEDIASTINUM

I. Lymphosarcoma;
II. Thymoma;
III. Teratoma;
IV. Benign lymphocytic hamartoma.

I. LYMPHOSARCOMA

Lymphosarcomas arise more commonly in the mediastinum than in any other site in childhood, the other sites being the small bowel (p. 630) and the cervical nodes (p. 225). The tumour is usually highly malignant, rapidly progressive, and until recently very few patients survived more than a year after diagnosis (Table 16.4).

The pleura is infiltrated fairly frequently, causing a large blood-stained effusion containing malignant cells (Fig. 16.6b).

Direct extension into the neck may also provide accessible material for diagnosis, as may involvement of the cervical, axillary or inguinal lymph nodes.

INVESTIGATIONS

A skeletal survey, full blood examinations, marrow biopsy and examination of the CSF are required to determine the extent of the disease, and in monitoring the patient for recurrences following the customary but often short lived, initial remission.

DIAGNOSIS

The onset of mediastinal compression is usually insidious, but may become worse very rapidly with alarming pressure effects developing in the course of two or three days. A dry cough, dyspnoea and cyanosis are often present, in addition to suffusion and congestion of the head and neck from obstruction of the superior vena cava.

Although radiological evidence of a large mediastinal mass is rarely lacking (Fig. 16.6) and a lymphosarcoma is the most likely cause of rapidly developing mediastinal compression in children, appropriate treatment depends upon the histological diagnosis, not only to exclude benign lesions such as a 'giant' lymphocytic hamartoma (p. 458), but also to determine which type of lymphoma is present, for this governs the choice of cytotoxic agents to be employed. The pressing need for biopsy in such a case is complicated by the patient's cardiorespiratory distress which, however, can be quickly relieved within two or three days by either cytotoxic chemotherapy or radiotherapy.

Material for histological diagnosis may be obtained from an enlarged lymph node (e.g. in the neck), from a marrow biopsy, from exfoliated tumour cells in an accompanying pleural effusion (Fig. 16.6b), or biopsy of an extension of the mediastinal mass into the suprasternal notch. If none of these

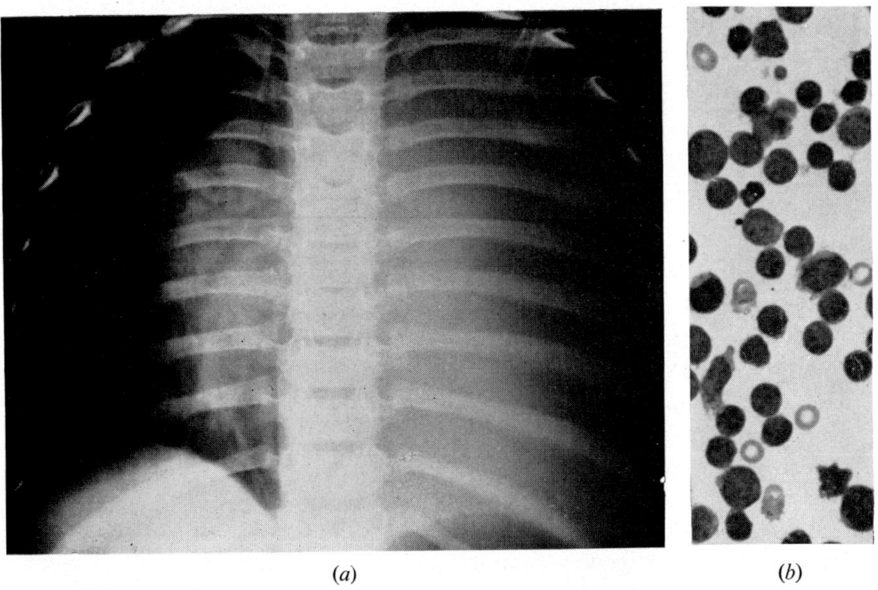

(*a*) (*b*)

Figure 16.6. Lymphosarcoma; (*a*) a large lymphoblastic lymphosarcoma arising in the thymus and extending into the left pleural cavity, displacing the carina to the right of the sternum and causing marked respiratory distress. The left margin of the tumour is poorly defined, an indication of rapid growth. There is also a left pleural effusion containing (*b*) tumour cells in fluid aspirated to relieve dyspnoea.

sources is available, thoracotomy is usually required. As thoracotomy (and most biopsy procedures) require general anaesthesia, it is highly desirable that mediastinal compression should be relieved beforehand. However, biopsy should not be delayed for more than four or five days after commencing chemotherapy or radiotherapy, because even a large lymphosarcoma can melt away in five to seven days, to such an extent that biopsy of what remains may fail to reveal malignant cells.

Cortisone, to minimize oedema in a tumour treated by either radiotherapy or cytotoxic agents, allopurinal to facilitate excretion of uric acid and prevent the development of high levels in the serum, a high fluid intake and alkalinization of the urine, are important means of preventing exacerbation of obstructive symptoms, and nephropathy due to hyperuricacidaemia, both of which may complicate treatment. These measures can be commenced as soon as the provisional diagnosis is made.

Radiotherapy can be used to obtain urgent relief of obstructive symptoms, and after biopsy may be continued to a total dose of 2000–2500 rads given in fractions over a period of two to three weeks, combined with cytotoxic agents. Alternatively, radiotherapy may be terminated after the initial 400 to 500 rads, substituting an appropriate combination of 2, 3 or 4 cytotoxic agents (i.e. the same regime as for acute lymphatic leukaemia, p. 159) which appears to be a promising regimen.

Cytotoxic agents have been demonstrated to be as capable of rapidly relieving compression as radiotherapy.

TREATMENT

Radiotherapy

The remarkably rapid response to radiotherapy is of particular value in patients presenting with severe respiratory distress, and relief can be expected within 24 hours of commencing treatment. Doses of 200 rads at each treatment seldom cause reactionary oedema or exacerbation of symptoms. However, to minimize this complication, steroids are usually commenced at the same time as irradiation.

In all cases, urgent or otherwise, a total dose of 2500 rads, in approximately ten treatments in a period of four weeks, can be expected to produce prolonged remission, and not infrequently complete disappearance of the mass.

Local recurrences or the appearance of lymphosarcomatous tissue elsewhere are unfortunately common, and call for treatment with cytotoxic agents as well as radiotherapy, both initially or in treating recurrence.

Chemotherapy

The management and chemotherapy of lymphosarcoma in general is described on p. 175.

PROGNOSIS

In view of the rapid initial response to radiotherapy, the high recurrence or relapse rate is disappointing, and the prospects of cure, or at least prolonged periods in complete remission, without the appearance of generalized dissemination (p. 172) or a leukaemic blood picture (p. 177) depend almost entirely on the response to chemotherapy.

The Index Series. The wide age range is shown in Table 16.4 the youngest infant was twelve months old. The sole long-term survivor is a boy who presented at the age of seven years with respiratory distress so severe that, as indicated above, radiotherapy was commenced without histological confirmation of the diagnosis. Response was immediate, satisfactory and typical of lymphosarcoma, but it has not been possible to confirm this histologically; in retrospect a benign lymphocytic hamartoma (p. 458) cannot be completely excluded.

The following history of a recent case is typical.

A girl aged six years presented with a history of slight puffiness of the eyelids and a mild 'brassy' cough for two weeks. Over the next three days her face, neck, shoulders and upper arms became oedematous; her face became florid, Cushingoid and slightly cyanotic, with marked elevation of the jugular venous pressure. The unproductive cough became more persistent and exhausting, and the optic discs were also found to be congested. Plain films of the chest showed a widened upper mediastinum and a large anterior mediastinal opacity, with some posterior displacement of the trachea.

Following a provisional diagnosis of lymphosarcoma, prednisolone and allopurinol were commenced immediately, followed by megavoltage radiotherapy 12 hours later. Within 48 hours, i.e. after two treatments of 200 rads each, all obstructive symptoms and signs had disappeared and the face had returned to normal. Next day thoracotomy and biopsy of the thymus, by now only slightly enlarged, revealed lymphoblastic lymphosarcoma. Treatment as for acute lymphatic leukaemia (including radiotherapy of the neuraxis, p. 157) continues, and there is no evidence of disease 12 months after diagnosis.

II. THYMOMA

Thymomas are exceedingly rare tumours in children, for example none was found in the series of 80 mediastinal masses reviewed by Haller *et al.* (1969).

Whereas in adults thymomas are often associated with myasthenia gravis, this relationship appears to be unknown in children, in whom apparently functionless thymomas are usually discovered incidentally in the anterior mediastinum in x-rays of the chest (Talerman & Amigo, 1968).

In children they are almost invariably benign (Neale & Menten, 1945) and well encapsulated, although infiltration of adjacent tissues has been reported occasionally.

MODE OF PRESENTATION

Signs and symptoms are for the most part non-existent, but in a few cases

Table 16.4. Lymphosarcoma of mediastinum; the age at onset and the outcome of 16 cases in the Index Series (RCH, 1950–1972)

Number of cases	:	16
Age at onset	:	13 months to 13 years mean : 7 years
Length of survival	:	1 day to 20 months mean : 6 months
Deaths	:	15
One long term survival	:	7 years+

general systemic effects such as fever and loss of weight occur, and when unusually large, the effects of *mediastinal compression* (p. 445) may be present, notably cough, dyspnoea and retrosternal pain (Legg & Brady, 1965).

Differential diagnosis from other masses in the mediastinum cannot be made with certainty before histological examination, although the distinctive calcification in teratomas (see below) is helpful. Treatment is confined to excision which is curative except in the exceptionally rare infiltrating malignant examples.

III. MEDIASTINAL TERATOMA

As in teratomas occurring elsewhere (p. 45), these contain by definition, tissues representative of more than one germinal layer (Rusby, 1944) and the earlier term 'dermoid cyst' should be discarded. Nevertheless most teratomas of the mediastinum are relatively simple, slowly growing, cystic structures (Fig. 16.7) containing one or two cystic loculi and predominantly ectodermal derivatives, including dental structures which when present in radiographs of the chest are helpful in indicating the diagnosis before thoracotomy (Hope *et al.*, 1963).

Teratomas are the second most common radiographic lesion in the anterior mediastinum in childhood, after non-pathological enlargement of the thymic shadow (p. 447). Rusby noted that young infants with a teratoma tended to present with signs of mediastinal compression (p. 445), including cough, dyspnoea and cyanosis, while in older children and adults, a teratoma is usually asymptomatic and found incidentally in x-rays of the chest. In a unique case (Honicky & de Papp, 1973) hypoglycaemia, due to functioning islet tissue in a thoracic teratoma, was the presenting feature.

Almost all teratomas encountered in childhood are cystic and benign (Heimburger & Battersby, 1965), but a minority are solid, or composed of multiple small cysts, and malignant, usually containing poorly differentiated

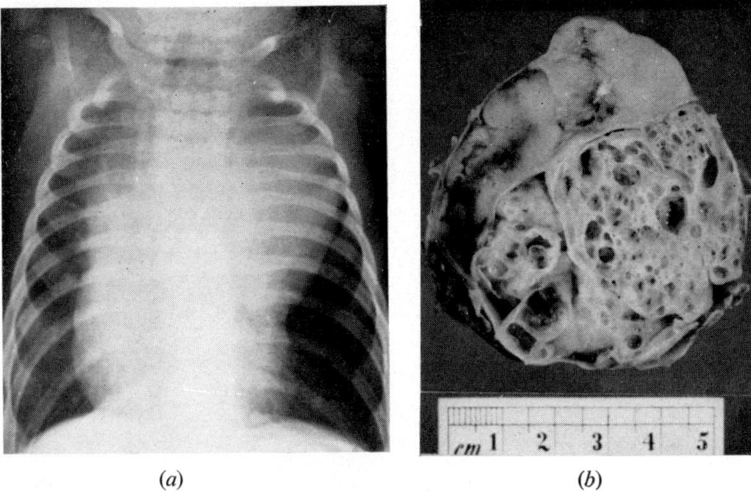

(*a*) (*b*)

Figure 16.7. BENIGN TERATOMA in the anterior mediastinum causing mediastinal compression in a 3-month old boy; (*a*) large, dense, shadow extending into the left pleural cavity; (*b*) the same teratoma, containing both multicystic spaces (right), and solid material (above) composed mainly of neuroglial tissue.

material closely resembling endodermal sinus tumours (p. 692). The very rare undifferentiated highly malignant tumours, or mesenchymomas, apparently arising *de novo* in the mediastinum, including undifferentiated 'stem cell tumours' (Haller *et al.*, 1969), may have a similar derivation.

MODES OF PRESENTATION

Clinical signs and symptoms are usually lacking; all eight children with a teratoma in the series of 80 mediastinal masses reported by Haller *et al.* (1969) were asymptomatic, as were 7 of the 10 cases in the Index Series. Very few are large enough to cause symptoms and these are chiefly found in infants, sometimes presenting as acute respiratory or cardiac distress (Reynolds *et al.*, 1969; Thompson & Moore, 1969).

DIAGNOSIS

Pre-operative diagnosis depends upon the presence of the typical calcification as an incidental finding in x-rays of the chest; teratomas are otherwise not distinguishable from other anterior mediastinal masses before exploration (Fig. 16.8). Excision is required to determine the diagnosis, to remove the potentiality of malignant change and, only rarely, to relieve symptoms.

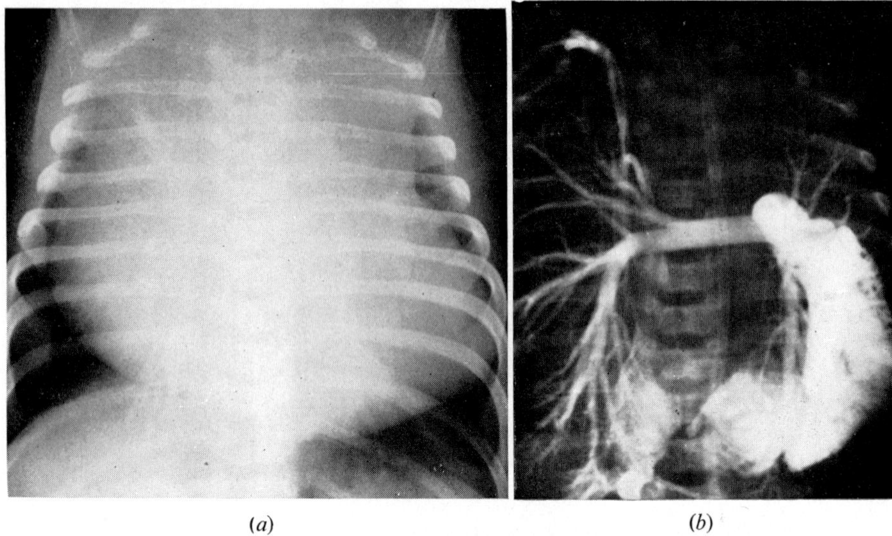

(*a*) (*b*)

Figure 16.8. MALIGNANT TERATOMA; (*a*) a very large tumour in a 4-year old child who presented with cardiac signs and symptoms; and (*b*) an angiocardiogram which excluded a primary cardiac lesion, indicating compression by an extracardiac tumour.

PROGNOSIS

In some cases their close attachment to the great vessels causes major technical difficulties, notably those arising within the pericardium (see p. 483). The result and prognosis are uniformly good in benign teratomas, which are the great majority.

IV. BENIGN LYMPHOCYTIC HAMARTOMA

(syn. giant lymph node hyperplasia, angiomatous lymphoid hamartoma, hamartomatous lymphoma)

This entity was first described by Castleman *et al.* (1956) as a localized mediastinal mass due to a form of lymph node hyperplasia. In the mediastinum, the important differential diagnosis in children is lymphosarcoma (p. 452) or Hodgkin's disease, and in adults, a thymoma. Keller *et al.* (1972) reported 61 new cases and reviewed the 20 previously reported in the literature. Most arose in the mediastinum (Lee, 1965), but single cases were encountered in the pelvis, in retroperitoneal tissues (Tung & McCormack, 1967), or in the axilla, and five arose in the cervical region.

Macroscopically this form of hamartoma is white or grey, firm, and often well defined (Fischer, Sieracki *et al.*, 1970).

Microscopically the lesion is composed of lymphoid tissue lacking the usual organized structure of a lymph node, and accompanied by proliferation of vessels which are extensively hyalinized and may mimic Hassal's corpuscles. Some examples contain numerous plasma cells.

The pathogenesis of this condition is not clear. Some appear to be hamartomas, since other than lymphoid elements, e.g. vascular tissues (Tung & McCormack, 1967), fibrous tissue, fat or smooth muscle, may share in the proliferative process. It is possible that the lesion is infective, as suggested by the chronic inflammatory nature of the histological changes, and the association with fever and systemic symptoms. However, no infective agent has yet been isolated, and the systemic effects may result from proliferation of the lymphoreticular cells of which the lesion is composed.

CLINICAL FEATURES

These vary, and some present with systemic symptoms of fever, anaemia, hyperglobulinaemia and hyperthrombocytaemia, but many of those in the mediastinum are found incidentally on radiography of the chest.

DIAGNOSIS

This can be made before excision when the patient presents with the symptoms described above, and when subsequent investigations reveal typical hyperglobulinaemia and hyperthrombocytaemia, which were also noted in a patient in the Index Series with a somewhat similar tumour in the mesocolon (p. 676).

In patients without systemic symptoms the diagnosis may only become apparent from the histological findings after removal of the tumour.

TREATMENT

Simple excision, even when incomplete, is curative, and no cases of recurrence have been reported. Systemic symptoms, when present, regress following excision.

TUMOURS OF THE POSTERIOR MEDIASTINUM

I. Neuroblastoma;
II. Neurofibroma;
III. Paraganglioma;
IV. Phaeochromocytoma.

The most common cause of a tumour in the 'posterior sulcus', or paravertebral gutter, in childhood is a neuroblastoma; much less commonly a neurofibroma arises in this area. Either of these tumours may on rare occasions form a 'dumb-bell' tumour, a macroscopic entity consisting of a narrow segment of tumour in an intervertebral foramen joining two larger portions, one in the costovertebral sulcus and the other in the spinal canal. The term has no histological implications; a dumb-bell tumour may be benign or malignant, or a mixture of both (e.g. ganglioneuroblastoma).

I. INTRATHORACIC NEUROBLASTOMA

The features of neuroblastoma are described in the chapter on abdominal tumours (p. 538) for most arise in the adrenal gland or in the adjacent retroperitoneal tissues.

In the thorax, a neuroblastoma may arise at any level along the ganglionated sympathetic chain.

A few arise at the level of the diaphragm and may extend in both directions, into retroperitoneal tissues in the abdomen and into the posterior mediastinum. Neuroblastoma arising primarily in the mediastinum can be generally grouped into three macroscopic types:

1. Large, soft, necrotic and rapidly growing tumours;
2. More slowly growing and firmer tumours which tend to infiltrate extensively and involve chiefly the mediastinum, spreading around the great vessels; and
3. Very slowly growing, rounded encapsulated tumours containing differentiated areas of ganglioneuroma, i.e. the so-called 'ganglioneuroblastoma' (see p. 550).

The size, site and rate of growth of each of these types determine to a large extent the mode of presentation, the prospects of surgical excision, and the prognosis.

MODES OF PRESENTATION

General signs and symptoms such as fever, loss of weight, appetite and energy, the syndrome referred to as 'malignant malaise' described on p. 549.

A mediastinal neuroblastoma may present in the same way as other intrathoracic tumours, i.e. with mediastinal compression or as an incidental discovery in radiographs of the chest (p. 444).

Specific modes of presentation are:

1. *Mediastinal compression* is typical in type 1 described above, a large, rapidly growing, necrotic, semifluid, undifferentiated tumour, often extending

as a mass into one pleural cavity, and attached on its medial aspect to the mediastinum (Fig. 16.9a). Progressive dyspnoea or tachypnoea, a 'brassy' cough, dysphagia and congestion of the face and neck are similar to the effects of a lymphosarcoma, described fully on p. 452.

2. *Pain in the back* and/or a visible dorsal swelling are often the first evidence of type 2, the diffuse, infiltrating tumour (Fig. 16.9b). Others are (*a*) compression of the spinal cord with paraplegia of rapid onset (p. 290) when the tumour extends into the epidural plane; or (*b*) a distant metastasis, e.g. in bone, orbit or peripheral lymph nodes (see the case report, p. 464).

3. *Incidental discovery in x-rays* of the chest, taken for intercurrent respiratory infection, corrosive ingestion or a fractured clavicle, etc. is not unusual in type 3, the well differentiated, slowly growing, encapsulated non-infiltrating type of neuroblastoma (Fig. 16.9c). Many contain extensive areas of ganglioneuroma and these may predominate, i.e. 'ganglioneuroblastoma (p. 550), but in some metastases occur, e.g. in the marrow; in the majority the tumour is entirely confined to the primary paravertebral site.

Maturation of neuroblastoma to benign ganglioneuroma, partially or completely, is statistically more likely to occur in those arising in the thorax than in any other site (Clatworthy & Newton, 1970; Filler *et al.*, 1972). This, and their tendency to present in younger children (those less than 18 months of age) chiefly account for the better prognosis in thoracic neuroblastoma (approximately 40–60% two years survivors) than in those arising in other sites, e.g. less than 10% two-year survivors in abdominal neuroblastoma (p. 561).

4. *Rare modes of onset*, such as diarrhoea etc. have also been reported and these are described in the section on abdominal neuroblastoma (p. 552).

INVESTIGATIONS

These are described in detail on p. 554. In summary they are:

(i) *Full blood examination* including Hb, white cell count and ESR;
(ii) *Marrow biopsy and smear*, for the presence of metastases;
(iii) *X-rays* of the chest, tomograms and thoracic aortography;
(iv) Skeletal survey;
(v) Estimation of total and individual catecholamines in a 24-hour specimen of urine;
(vi) *Biopsy* of any sites of metastases, e.g. in the orbit, calvarium or peripheral lymph nodes;
(vii) *Lumbar puncture, and myelography* if there is any evidence of spinal compression.

The results of these investigations permit as complete an estimate as possible (before thoracotomy) of the nature and extent of the tumour.

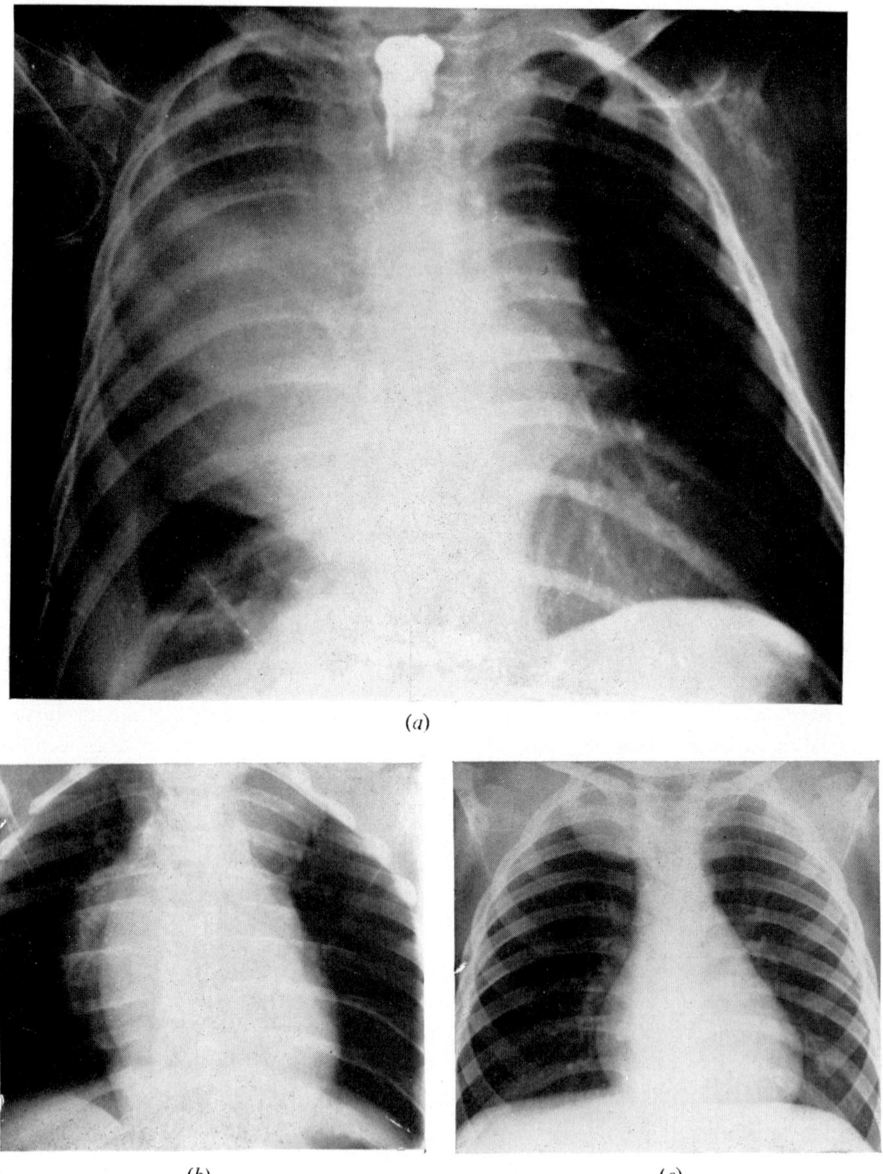

(*a*)

(*b*) (*c*)

Figure 16.9. THORACIC NEUROBLASTOMA; (*a*) rapidly growing massive lesion extending into the pleural cavity, and accompanying myelogram showing complete block at the level of the upper extent of the tumour (type 1, see text); (*b*) slowly growing posterior mediastinal tumour extending from left apex to the diaphragm (type 2, see text and case report p. 464); (*c*) spherical encapsulated tumour (type 3, see text) first discovered incidentally during a barium swallow.

DIFFERENTIAL DIAGNOSIS

The evidence in x-rays and angiographs of a posterior mediastinal tumour, the biochemical data and the histological findings in the marrow or other biopsies, is usually conclusive.

When the histological diagnosis is still uncertain, macroscopic findings at thoracotomy and frozen sections will exclude other tumours such as a neurofibroma, rhabdomyosarcoma, rarely a teratoma, or an anomaly such as a dorsal foregut cyst or 'gastric' duplication. Associated vertebral anomalies are an indication of the rare 'split-notochord syndrome' (p. 450).

TREATMENT OF THORACIC NEUROBLASTOMA

Surgical excision, as in abdominal neuroblastoma, is rarely complete except in encapsulated, differentiated tumours (type 3). However, in a number of cases an attempt should be made to remove as much of the tumour as possible. In neuroblastoma more than in any other tumour, incomplete or subtotal excision is acceptable (see p. 31) and in mediastinal neuroblastoma, 'cure' or maturation to disappearance or complete quiescence is always a possibility.

Early operation may be determined by uncertainty as to diagnosis or by the type of tumour. Localized tumours (type 3) are usually completely removable, but experience has shown that some tumours which appear to be clearly demarcated in x-rays, are found to infiltrate more than expected, with unpredicted extensions. Even a benign ganglioneuroma can be difficult to remove and densely adherent to major structures such as the aorta or vena cava.

Covered by a pre-operative dose of one or more cytotoxic agents (see p. 24), and through a wide exposure, as much as possible of the tumour is removed. In 'type 1' the 'capsule' is incomplete or ruptures readily, much of the tumour is semi-fluid in consistency and can be removed by suction. In type 2 parts of the tumour are often inaccessible or irremovable.

Chemotherapy, e.g. vincristine or vinblastine and cyclophosphamide (p. 558) is continued after operation, to the completion of the primary course, and co-ordinated with radiotherapy along the same lines as for abdominal neuroblastoma.

Deferred operation, after a full course of combination chemotherapy and radiotherapy plus an additional period of four weeks for full tumour-effect and remission, is an alternative when dissemination has occurred, or when the tumour is very large, or when respiratory function is sufficiently reduced to make early operation hazardous. In general, delayed thoracotomy and excision is resorted to less frequently than in abdominal neuroblastoma.

When there is an accompanying intraspinal extension with compression, laminectomy and removal of tumour tissue pressing on the spinal cord becomes the first priority, as a matter of urgency, to obtain the best prospect of recovery of neural function. Excision of the intrathoracic component can then be performed one to two weeks later.

The general principles and methods of treatment of patients with disseminated thoracic neuroblastoma are the same as when the primary arises in the abdomen (p. 558).

PROGNOSIS

The outlook for children with an intrathoracic neuroblastoma is better than in those arising in any other site, except, in the Index Series, a group in whom the tumour arose in or near the epidural space, without any demonstrable intrathoracic component, and those in the pelvis (p. 709).

Favourable factors associated with mediastinal neuroblastoma are that:

(i) They tend to arise in children less than 18 months to two years of age, i.e. in the most favourable age group (p. 561);

(ii) They have the highest incidence of maturation to benign ganglioneuroma;

(iii) Some remain localized (type 3) without any metastasis (Stage I); and

(iv) In those presenting with spinal compression the tumour is often small, and causes clinical effects while still at a very early stage.

In the Index Series there was an example of an extensive infiltrating neuroblastoma (type 2) with distant metastases and subsequent maturation to what appears to be static ganglioneuroma.

A baby girl was noted to have multiple discrete nodules in the left axilla and posterior cervical triangle at the age of 15 months. No investigations were performed until 3 months later, when 'malaise' (p. 549), fever and loss of energy led to biopsy of one of the swellings in the left axilla, which was found to be a lymph node largely replaced by entirely benign ganglioneuroma.

An x-ray of the chest at that time showed a large posterior mediastinal mass occupying both paravertebral sulci and extending from the clavicles to the diaphragm (Fig. 16.9b). Calcification at its lower pole appeared to be below the diaphragm. The level of MHMA in the urine was 53·7 μg/1 (upper limit of normal 2–3 μg/1), and a diagnosis of mediastinal neuroblastoma, with metastases (and maturation) in axillary and cervical nodes was made. Exploration showed an irregular subpleural tumour surrounding the aorta from the diaphragm to the thoracic inlet. Biopsy of the mass showed neuroblastoma with extensive areas of ganglioneuroma, and cells in all intervening stages of maturation (i.e. 'ganglioneuroblastoma'). Marrow smears were negative for metastases.

Radiotherapy to the mediastinum (3000 rads in 4 weeks) was given, preceded by vincristine (2 mg/m^2 at weekly intervals for 8 weeks) and followed by maintenance chemotherapy with cyclophosphamide (125 to 250 mg/week), continued in cycles for 18 months.

The mediastinal tumour slowly increased in size over the next 4 years, during which time she was symptomless, well and normally active. In the following year the tumour appeared to decrease in size, probably relatively, as she grew larger. The level of MHMA in the urine has remained elevated, and over the last 5 years has ranged from 37 to 73 to 24 μg/1. She is now 11 years old, symptomless and has grown normally.

Although they have remained unchanged for nine years so far, for cosmetic reasons it is planned to remove, at an appropriate time, the nodular masses which are taken to be 'multiple ganglioneuromas' in the cervical lymph nodes.

II. INTRATHORACIC NEUROFIBROMAS

This essentially benign lesion varies greatly in its clinical expression, from a single simple benign tumour to an extremely wide range of conditions broadly grouped together as von Recklinghausen's disease, an autosomal dominant form of neurofibromatosis with many types and sites of abnormality (p. 827).

The two forms most likely to arise in the mediastinum are:
(i) A plexiform neurofibroma in the thoracic inlet;
(ii) A posterior mediastinal mass.

(i) Neurofibroma of the thoracic inlet (Raffensperger & Cohen, 1972)
This benign but often unencapsulated tumour arises in a nerve sheath and typically forms a plexiform mass extending along and/or actually within the nerve causing considerable enlargement, with a tubular shape often described as 'radish' or 'carrot' shaped, but perhaps more accurately as a parsnip, in both colour and shape. Although a plexiform neuroma may arise in any of the cranial or peripheral nerves, it has a special predilection for the cervical region, the thoracic inlet and the adjacent superior mediastinum; approximately half of all plexiform neurofibromas arise in these sites. Plexiform neurofibromas also occur on the trunk, in the extremities (p. 829) or the eyelid (p. 422), and are recognized as one of the features of von Recklinghausen's disease (p. 822).

AGE : SEX

The sexes are almost equally affected, and more than half appear in children less than six years of age.

MODES OF PRESENTATION

1. *A symptomless swelling*, e.g. in the lateral part of the neck or in the deep cervical triangle, causing a supraclavicular swelling, is the commonest mode of presentation.
2. *Symptoms of irritation or compression* of mediastinal structures, such as a cough, dyspnoea and dysphagia arise when the oesophagus and trachea are compressed in the neck or the thoracic inlet.
3. *Cord signs* (see p. 448) e.g. muscle weakness, due to pressure on nerve trunks.
4. *The development of scoliosis* or torticollis may be the reason for seeking medical attention, and the swelling in the neck is then identified on palpation.

INVESTIGATIONS

X-rays of the neck and mediastinum demonstrate a soft tissue mass in the deep triangle of the neck, or displacement of cervical vertebrae, or a mediastinal mass. Penetrating films, to display the air column in the oesophagus and trachea, will indicate whether there is displacement or obstruction in patients with dysphagia or dyspnoea.

Lateral films may show an increase in the size of the intervertebral foramina and a myelogram is indispensible in all those in whom there is tumour adjacent to the vertebrae.

The levels of catecholamines excreted in the urine (see p. 556) are helpful in excluding neuroblastomas, ganglioneuromas and phaeochromocytomas.

DIAGNOSIS

The presence of *câfé-au-lait* patches (present in about half the patients) or a family history of neurofibromatosis is strongly suggestive (p. 830) of neurofibroma. The investigations will also help to exclude other tumours which may arise in the neck and/or mediastinum. The final diagnosis rests on the histological findings.

PROGNOSIS

Malignant degeneration into neurofibrosarcoma is extremely rare and almost unknown until after adolescence. In some series of patients followed into adult life, as many as 10% of neurofibromas have become malignant. The prognosis depends upon the completeness of removal, and on minimal delay between the development of signs of neural or spinal compression and surgical decompression.

TREATMENT

Surgical excision is sometimes relatively simple, for example those which are confined to the thoracic inlet and can be removed via a cervical approach. However, additional operations such as thoracotomy and laminectomy, in stages, may be required to remove their deeper extensions. As a general principle, in patients with a mediastinal mass and signs of spinal compression, laminectomy should be performed first. Recurrences are not unknown, and are often not true recurrences but further growth or an extension of abnormal tissue not detected at the first operation, or incomplete removal because the adjacent structures involved, e.g. the brachial plexus or the vertebrae, cannot be sacrificed.

(ii) Neurofibromas in the posterior mediastinum

These often reach a large size without causing any symptoms, and hence may be found incidentally in x-rays taken for some other condition (Fig. 16.4).

In rare cases, usually in children five to ten years of age, the first symptoms are neurological and produced by a slowly growing extension through the intervertebral foramina into the spinal cord. The differential diagnosis of this group is described on p. 556.

III. PARAGANGLIOMAS OF THE THORAX

After physiological condensations of chemoreceptor cells in the head and neck (p. 366), the thorax is the second commonest site of chemoreceptor 'organs'. Although it is probable that not all of these condensations have been completely mapped, the sites already located in the thorax are as follows:

(i) At the pulmonary end of the obliterated ductus arteriosus;
(ii) Near the origin of the left coronary artery;
(iii) At the bifurcation of the innominate artery;
(iv) On the aortic arch near the origin of the left subclavian artery.

Tumours of non-chromaffin cells are not invariably located in these precise sites (Haber, 1964; Pachter, 1963; De Buse, 1972). In a review of the literature, Barrie (1961) collected 12 cases of paraganglioma in the thorax and added two more. Of these 14 patients, only two were less than 19 years of age, and only one was a child.

A boy of seven years, previously reported by Gillis *et al.* (1956), presented with anorexia, fever, loss of weight and pallor. X-rays of the chest revealed a tumour subsequently found to be on the anterolateral surface of the lower lobe of the right lung. The tumour, 4 cm in diameter, was removed at operation but recurred locally two years later and death occurred shortly after.

As a group, paragangliomas of the thorax are extremely vascular and resemble angiomas. The cells are arranged in alveolar clumps surrounded by interwoven reticulin fibres, forming the typical 'Zellballen' pattern, found in 12 of the 14 tumours in Barrie's series. None of them showed a positive chromaffin reaction, and neither nerve cells nor intracellular glycogen could be demonstrated with special stains.

The general features of paragangliomas are described on p. 586.

B. TUMOURS OF THE LARYNX, TRACHEA AND BRONCHI

These are all rarities in children and the more common clinical entities are as follows:

I. Papillomas and papillomatosis;
II. Subglottic haemangioma;
III. Plasma cell granuloma (syn. fibroxanthoma).

I. PAPILLOMAS OF THE LARYNX, TRACHEA AND BRONCHI

Involvement of the trachea, bronchi or the lungs is an extremely rare complication of papillomatosis of the larynx, which has been demonstrated to be due to infection with the 'papova' virus (Boyle *et al.*, 1973). A review of the literature (Al-Saleem *et al.*, 1968) indicates that only 2–3% of patients who develop papillomas of the larynx during childhood go on to develop papillomas in the lower respiratory passages. The first reported case (Hitz & Oesterlin, 1932) was a three-year old girl who died of multiple papillomatosis of the larynx and upper trachea; only seven additional cases had been reported up to 1968; in four of these seven cases papillomas developed in the larynx during childhood and subsequently in the lower airways.

Malignant transformation of a papillomatosis commencing in childhood is apparently restricted to those treated with radiotherapy; by contrast, when laryngeal papillomas first appear after the age of 20 years, malignant change can be expected in some 50% of cases. On the other hand, 'benign' papillomatosis extending to involve the lower respiratory tract and lung, is much less likely to occur in adults with laryngeal papillomas than when the papillomas appear during childhood.

Papillomas first arise in areas of the pharynx lined by squamous epithelium, particularly the vocal cords and the larynx.

Clinically they present with huskiness, and laryngoscopy reveals small and usually multiple, sessile or pedunculated, pink, warty lesions on the cords, extending into the ary-epiglottic region, and occasionally downwards into the trachea.

Microscopically they are composed of delicate fibro-vascular cores clothed with a layer of exuberant and very hyperplastic stratified squamous epithelium. Inclusion bodies have recently been observed on electron microscopy (McCoy *et al.*, 1971).

Laryngeal papillomas are particularly prone to recur locally after removal (Oleske & Kushnick, 1971), but their natural history is to undergo spontaneous regression at about puberty. They are not truly malignant despite their persistence, recurrence and occasional propagation downwards.

Very rarely papillomatous tumours develop in the main bronchi or its primary subdivision, and can be demonstrated as small circular opacities in x-rays of the lung fields (Fig. 16.10).

TREATMENT

In childhood, repeated endoscopic removal of papillomas of the larynx should be persisted with indefinitely, and radiotherapy is absolutely contra-indicated.

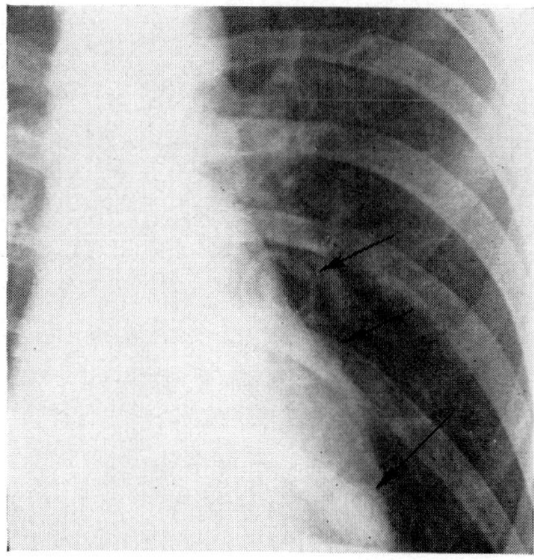

Figure 16.10. PAPILLOMATOSIS; x-ray of a 15-year old boy, who presented with laryngeal papillomas at the age of 20 months. The papillomas were removed, but recurred repeatedly, culminating in multiple 'coin' lesions in the left lower lobe; two of the papillomatous tumours have cavitated, while the lowest appears as solid (p. 473).

Bronchopulmonary papillomatosis carries a high mortality (three out of the seven cases reported), even when the lesions remain individually benign. Pulmonary resection, for example lobectomy, may be required when papillomas of the bronchus cause persistent or recurrent lobar collapse and consequent infection.

II. SUBGLOTTIC HAEMANGIOMA

In this rare hamartomatous condition, of which less than 100 cases have been reported in the literature (Williams, Phelan *et al.*, 1969), the subglottic region of the larynx is chiefly affected. The natural history of enlargement during early infancy followed by spontaneous resolution in later months, is very similar to the favourable evolution of capillary haemangiomas occurring in the skin (p. 819).

The principle clinical features are episodes of inspiratory and expiratory stridor, of variable severity, developing insidiously some weeks or months after birth. There are also episodes of respiratory obstruction, and a croupy cough. The cry is usually normal, but may be hoarse in the rare case in which the angioma involves the vocal cords.

The diagnosis is suggested by the history of recurring episodes of stridor, worse during periods of respiratory tract infection, but also present between them. The diagnosis is confirmed by laryngoscopy which will also exclude other laryngeal causes of stridor, but the appearances of the haemangioma of the larynx vary from time to time; they are not always as impressive as might be expected, and may be missed (Ferguson & Blake, 1961) unless examined by an experienced endoscopist.

Treatment

Various methods have been employed and their risks and results are to be evaluated in the light of the eventual spontaneous regression of the lesion and disappearance of symptoms which are typical of the natural history.

Irradiation is reported to have been employed successfully, but of 27 patients so treated, 18 required tracheotomy (Tefft, 1966); mild cases may become worse, at least temporarily, as a result of treatment. There is also the undoubted risk of the delayed development of carcinoma of the thyroid (p. 370) when radiotherapy is administered to this area.

Laryngotomy and partial surgical excision of the lesion has been advocated, but the operation is difficult and not without mortality.

Injections of sclerosing solutions (Christiaens *et al.*, 1965) or diathermy, have also been employed, but both are followed by reactionary swelling, often serious enough to require tracheostomy.

Conservative management, with close surveillance until the lesion resolved has been used successfully in a series of six consecutive patients (Williams, Phelan *et al.*, 1969). This may require management of some patients in hospital (for as long as eight months), and prolonged periods of nasotracheal intubation for relief of respiratory obstruction, but in all six in this series, the condition resolved satisfactorily without local treatment, without tracheostomy and without mortality.

III. PLASMA CELL GRANULOMA

(syn. xanthomatous granuloma, pseudo-sarcoma, xanthogranuloma, fibrous xanthoma, histiocytoma)

This uncommon benign lesion frequently causes alarm because the radiological features and even the operative findings may strongly suggest a malignant tumour.

AGE : SEX : SITE

In the 18 cases reviewed by Pearl and Woolley (1973), the sexes were almost equally represented (10 girls, 8 boys); all were between 3 and 16 years of age, with a peak incidence between 8 and 12 years.

Any lobe of the lung may be affected, but the right lung was affected twice as often as the left. The trachea is affected much less commonly, causing wheezing, dyspnoea and/or an exhausting cough (Taraska, 1966; Witwer & Tampas, 1973).

A few have been described as arising in the nose or the larynx.

MACROSCOPIC APPEARANCES

The granuloma is usually 2–5 cm in diameter, but a few were up to 10 cm in maximum diameter. They vary in texture from friable to rubbery or very hard, and grey to orange yellow in colour. The lesion may be embedded in the lung and densely adherent to the parenchyma, or to the chest wall or diaphragm when it arises on the surface of the lung.

MICROSCOPIC FINDINGS

The histological picture is chiefly one of chronic inflammation, and as well as a cellular fibroblastic stroma, a variety of cell types has been reported, particularly histiocytes with foamy vacuolated cytoplasm and a large amount of lipid, which give the lesion its yellowish colour. Plasma cells are prominent, and lymphocytes, foreign-body giant cells and areas of patchy necrosis are common. Plump young fibroblasts or dense lymphocytic infiltration in rows can be mistaken for sarcomatous cells (Kauffman & Stout, 1961), the basis for the synonym 'pseudo-sarcoma'.

Being a benign lesion, it does not 'spread', but satellites lobules, multiple lesions, and associated enlargement of hilar nodes have all been reported, thus adding to the impression that the lesion is malignant.

CLINICAL FEATURES

It is surprising that almost 50% of reported cases were asymptomatic and were found incidentally or unexpectedly in x-rays of the chest. In the other 50% there were signs and symptoms of pulmonary infection, e.g. fever, cough and haemoptysis, and the clinical diagnosis before the x-ray findings were known, was 'lobar collapse' or 'pneumonia'.

The radiological appearances were interpreted as a tumour in more than half of the cases reported. Calcification is a common radiological finding, and is sufficiently unusual in pulmonary tumours (other than osteosarcoma metastases) and in non-tuberculous pneumonitis, to raise the possibility of a plasma cell granuloma; in the few cases observed for some months there was no increase in the size of the lesion.

The etiology is obscure, and there appears to be no pre-existing bronchial or pulmonary disease which might explain the development of the lesion. A virus has been implicated by the presence of similar though smaller multiple lesions in some cases of measles (Young *et al.*, 1970), and also by similar appearances in pulmonary lesions due to the Yaba virus in primates (Sproul *et al.*, 1963).

TREATMENT

Exploration and surgical excision are indicated, and several authors have remarked that the macroscopic appearances are strongly suggestive of a malignant tumour (Carter *et al.*, 1968: Dubilier *et al.*, 1968; Pearl & Woolley, 1973). In such cases frozen sections may be required to make the correct diagnosis, for segmental resection, or at most lobectomy, is all that is required.

C. TUMOURS IN THE LUNGS

Although extremely rare, there are sufficient isolated case reports and small collected series of primary tumours to establish which are most likely to be encountered in children, and these are classified as follows:

(*a*) Benign lesions:
I. Hamartoma;
II. Papillomatosis;
III. Plasma cell granuloma (see above).
(*b*) Primary malignant tumours:
IV. Bronchial adenoma;
V. Bronchogenic carcinoma;
VI. Sarcoma of the trachea or bronchus:
VII. Pulmonary blastoma.
(*c*) Metastatic tumours in the lungs.

I. HAMARTOMAS

Malformations of the bronchi and lungs of a hamartomatous nature are very uncommon, and lesions such as lymphangioma, arteriovenous fistula and the rare chondromatous subpleural hamartoma sometimes found in adults, have been described (Ravitch, 1969).

Cystic adenomatoid hamartomas form a particular group (Craig *et al.*, 1956) which appear to be solid and confined to one lobe in x-rays in neonates. The related bronchus is often malformed and as the infant grows, air enters the 'cystic' portions of the hamartoma which become inflated with trapped air. This reduces effective aeration in the same way as occurs in lobar emphysema, and may culminate in respiratory distress due to compression of the remainder of the lung on the same side and of the contralateral lung as well. Lobectomy is curative.

II. PAPILLOMATOSIS

On rare occasions papilloma of the larynx is associated with or follows papillomatosis of the trachea and bronchi (p. 468) which may be numerous or large enough to cause bronchial obstruction and consequent atelectasis and/or infection and, very rarely, intrapulmonary papillomatous lesions (Fig. 16.10).

In the Index Series, there is only one case of spread of laryngeal papillomatosis beyond the larynx.

P.G., a boy, was first seen at the age of 20 months, in 1957, for noisy breathing and a hoarse cry present since 10 months of age. At laryngoscopy there were multiple papillomas on both vocal cords. These were removed for microscopic examination, which showed typical squamous papillomas, and cultures for virus which were repeatedly negative over the following years.

Within 3 months the papillomas recurred and proliferated to the point of causing stridor and cyanosis, treated by further removal of papillomas, and a tracheostomy which he had for the rest of his life. Radiotherapy to the larynx (3200 rads over 4 weeks) was given in 1958.

Crops of papillomas were removed by diathermy, cold cautery and 'shaving', and the bases painted with podophylin and nitramin, at intervals averaging 2 months for the following 15 years.

In 1968, when he was 11 years of age, a field of papillomas developed in the trachea just above the carina, and these too were removed and recurred repeatedly.

At 13 years of age he developed diabetes, and during investigation of a chest infection, x-rays showed collapse and consolidation in the left lower lobe, and three circular lesions (Fig. 16.10) all of which eventually cavitated. Response to antibiotics was satisfactory and no additional lesions developed in the lungs during the remaining 5 years of his life which was terminated by complications of diabetes at 17 years of age. By this time papillomas had grown out the tracheostomy, and lesions were spreading across the skin of the neck as far as the clavicles.

Although histological proof is lacking, the radiological findings in the left lower lobe are exactly those described as typical of pulmonary parenchymal (broncho-alveolar) papillomatosis by Rosenbaum, Alavi & Bryant (1968).

III. BRONCHIAL 'ADENOMA'
(syn. adenocarcinoma)

Although long thought to be benign, bronchial adenomas are now recognized as being, in most if not all cases, adenocarcinomas with a variable but often slow rate of growth. First defined as a clinical and pathological entity in 1932, their malignant potential gradually became apparent (Goldman, 1949) and has been emphasized by Turnbull *et al.* (1972) who reported a high proportion of early deaths from this form of malignancy.

Verska and Connolly (1968) reviewed the 21 cases reported in children between 1935 and 1966, and their data were as follows.

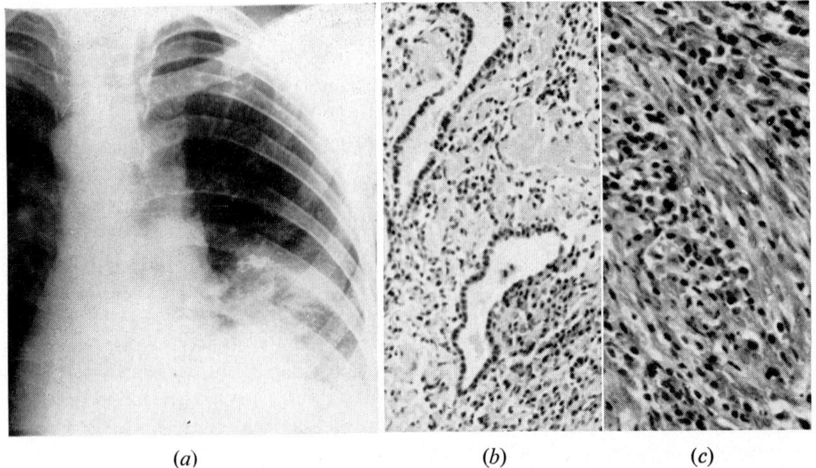

(*a*) (*b*) (*c*)

Figure 16.11. FIBROSARCOMA OF BRONCHUS; (*a*) X-ray of lesion in the left lower lobe, containing extensive patches of calcification, treated by left lower lobectomy; (*b*) sparsely cellular tissue containing irregular clefts lined by cuboidal cells, leading to an erroneous diagnosis of hamartoma (H & E. × 30); (*c*) recurrence in left lung, composed of cellular tissue, an interlacing 'herring-bone tweed' pattern of cells with slight nuclear polymorphism, and a heavy infiltrate of plasma cells and histiocytes (H & E. × 200).

AGE : SEX

Most of the children (18 out of 20) were between 9 and 15 years of age, although two were 4 years old, and seven were between 5 and 10 years of age. Males and females were almost equally represented (12 boys, 8 girls).

SITE

In the 17 cases in which the site was recorded, more were on the right side (12 : 5); all were in a large bronchus (main bronchus, 8; primary division, 9) and hence all were theoretically visible at endoscopy.

MACROSCOPIC APPEARANCES

The tumour arises in or beneath the mucous membrane and becomes a spherical swelling encroaching on the lumen. The deeper surface infiltrates the wall of the bronchus and as the tumour becomes roughly spherical, in some of them the greater part of the 'sphere' lies outside the bronchus, the so-called 'iceberg' phenomenon (de Paredes *et al.*, 1970).

O'Grady *et al.* (1970) noted in their series of 29 carcinoid adenomas that 15 were endobronchial and polypoid, without ulceration of the overlying mucosa; in eight the amounts of tumour within and outside the bronchus were about equal, and six were predominantly extrabronchial.

MICROSCOPIC APPEARANCES

Three histological types occur:

(i) *The carcinoid type* is the commonest (85–90%) and most favourable type, and arises from Kulchitsky cells in the bronchial mucosa. They are identical to carcinoid tumours of the alimentary canal (p. 639) and the carcinoid syndrome, due to excess secretion of serotonin (p. 670), has been described in bronchial carcinoids in adults (Fontana *et al.*, 1963).

(ii) *The 'cylindroma' type* (approximately 8%) has the same microscopic picture as the adenoid-cystic type of carcinoma of the salivary glands (p. 309) and arises from mucus-producing cells in the bronchial mucosa. This type is more invasive and infiltrates further into the parenchyma, but no case of metastasis has been described.

(iii) *The muco-epidermoid type* is the least common (approximately 2%), the most invasive, and has the same histological picture as its counterpart in the salivary glands (p. 307).

SPREAD

Extremely slow but steadily progressive infiltration into the adjacent parenchyma is a feature of bronchial adenomas. Local recurrence after inadequate resection is more common than metastasis, but distant metastasis has been reported (Goodner *et al.*, 1961).

MODES OF PRESENTATION

There are three typical clinical features:

1. *A cough* is by far the earliest symptom, and an accompanying wheeze is common in children. The duration of the cough is, in retrospect, remarkable for the length of time it has been present. In Verska and Connolly's series of 21 children, two had had a cough for 4 years, one for 3 years and two for 2 years.
2. *Atelectasis* and pneumonia. Encroachment of the adenoma on the lumen of a bronchus leads to retention of secretions, obstruction, atelectasis, recurrent attacks of 'pneumonia' leading to destructive inflammation and bronchiectasis; 15 of the 21 patients quoted had at least one episode of pneumonia.
3. *Haemoptysis*. Bronchial adenomas tend to be markedly vascular, and haemoptysis at some time during the course of the disease occurs in more than half of the cases; it was the presenting feature in 8 of the 21 patients quoted.

DIAGNOSIS AND DIFFERENTIAL DIAGNOSIS

Although extremely rare, early diagnosis is of considerable importance, not only because of its potential as a malignant tumour, but also to prevent progressive destruction of pulmonary tissue.

(*a*) **Cough and wheezing**

1. *Foreign body*. As Verska and Connolly pointed out this is the commonest cause of a localized obstruction of a major bronchus; cough, wheeze and diminished aeration (lobar or sublobar in distribution) are the same as the early findings in a bronchial adenoma.

Bronchoscopy reveals a fleshy tumour and, together with biopsy, offers the best prospect of making the diagnosis at an early stage. Biopsy at bronchoscopy is not without risk, and serious haemorrhage from a vascular tumour is occasionally fatal; Wilkins *et al.* (1963) reported a mortality from biopsy of 2·6%.

A sarcoma (see below) may also present as a fleshy tumour in the lumen of a main bronchus.

2. *Tuberculosis* producing a mass of hilar nodes distorting a major bronchus, may produce a clinical picture somewhat similar to a bronchial adenoma, but radiographs of the chest usually indicate the perihilar site of the nodes and an active pulmonary focus.

3. *Asthma* has been misdiagnosed in some cases because of the persistent wheeze and cough. There is a cautionary tale of a child who died in 'status asthmaticus' and who was found to have a bronchial adenoma of the trachea causing asphyxiation (Ravitch, 1969).

(*b*) **Recurrent attacks of pneumonia with incomplete resolution**

This should point to the need for further investigation, particularly when persistently confined to one lobe. General systemic conditions predisposing to pulmonary infections, such as cystic fibrosis, may also need to be excluded, but rarely cause recurrent infection confined to one lobe.

(*c*) **Haemoptysis**

This is an unusual symptom in childhood, and is always an indication for full investigation of the respiratory tract and the lungs.

TREATMENT

Once the diagnosis has been established, resection of the adenoma is indicated. Bronchoscopic removal, once considered to be the method of choice and often followed by marked improvement for many years, is now regarded as inadequate and contra-indicated by the malignant potential of this tumour. The extent of the resection required is determined by the site of the adenoma, and the distribution of irreversible changes in the bronchi and the related parenchyma. Bronchography is helpful in assessing the latter, but when the pathological changes are severe, obstruction usually prevents the entry of contrast material.

Lobectomy is usually employed (Simpson & Smith, 1974), but occasionally pneumonectomy is required when a bronchial adenoma arises at or near the carina. In suitable cases a sleeve resection of a main stem bronchus (Verska & Connolly, 1968) can be performed without resecting any of the lung.

RESULTS : PROGNOSIS

The outlook is extremely good even when the adenoma has been producing symptoms for years.

The prognosis is best with the carcinoid type which is the least invasive; the five-year survival rate is reported to be 95 %, but probably rather less for the other histological types.

V. BRONCHOGENIC CARCINOMA

It has been estimated that less than 0·2 % of all bronchogenic carcinomas arise in children. Cayley *et al.* (1951) collected 15 cases from the world literature between 1880 and 1951, and added one of their own. The following description is based on data in their review.

In a recent series of 102 cases of carcinoma of the lung in males less than 45 years of age, the 3 youngest were 12, 13 and 18 years respectively (Kyriakos & Webber, 1974).

AGE : SEX : SIDE

Of the 16 patients, 11 were more than 5 years old, and 8 children were between 10 and 15 years of age. Girls and boys were equally affected, and most of the tumours arose in the right lung (10 : 6).

MICROSCOPIC FINDINGS

An extraordinary variety of histological types were found in these cases: 'adenocarcinoma' (4), 'undifferentiated' (4), 'epitheliod' (3), squamous cell (2), oat-cell (1), small-cell (1) and 'carcinoma' (1).

MODES OF PRESENTATION

Two patterns can be extracted from the information available:

1. *Signs and symptoms related to pulmonary disease;* these were present in half of the patients, chiefly cough, dyspnoea, haemoptysis and 'asthma'.

2. *Metastases in peripheral tissues* (femur, shoulder, spine, chest wall and leg) gave rise to pain and/or swelling as the presenting symptom or sign which led to investigation and diagnosis.

DIAGNOSIS

From the few details available, x-rays of the chest or of the sites of metastases, led to the diagnosis in the majority of cases.

There was only one survivor, an 11-year old boy with an adenocarcinoma of the right lung; in the large proportion who presented with metastases, the prognosis would be little better today.

TREATMENT

In the absence of metastases, the resection required is determined by the extent of the tumour, and management is along the same lines as in adults.

VI. SARCOMAS OF THE TRACHEA, BRONCHUS OR LUNG

Leiomyosarcomas of the trachea or bronchus in children have been reported by Killingsworth *et al.* (1953) and Watson & Anlyan (1954). In four of six cases the tumour was visible in the trachea or in the main bronchus at bronchoscopy. A few have been reported in the lung (Dowell, 1974).

Fibrosarcomas of the bronchus also occur, and in a collected series of nine affected children (Holinger *et al.*, 1960), five were less than 15 years of age and four survived following pulmonary resection (3) or endoscopic removal (1).

Fibrosarcomas also arise in the parenchyma of the lung unrelated to a major bronchus (Martini *et al.*, 1971), and in children they are characteristically extremely indolent in their rate of growth, with a striking degree of plasma cell infiltration throughout the tumour. Their histological differentiation from plasma cell granuloma (p.470) may be extremely difficult.

In the Index Series there is one example.

A boy aged 10 years presented with cough and clinical signs of 'unresolved pneumonia'. X-rays showed a rounded opacity containing areas of calcification in the right lower lobe. The lesion was excised by lobectomy and classified as a hamartoma because of a dense fibrous stroma, numerous clefts lined by bronchial mucosa and dense infiltration with plasma cells. Three years later masses were again found in the lung and mediastinum and these, too, were resected. Most sections showed an appearance similar to the material previously removed, but in some there were cellular areas of spindle cells with a 'herring bone' pattern (Fig. 16.11) leading to the diagnosis of fibrosarcoma.

Further pulmonary masses appeared, but he remained well and symptomless for a further five years before dyspnoea and loss of weight appeared.

VII. PULMONARY BLASTOMA

This, the rarest of all pulmonary tumours, is composed of epithelial and mesenchymal elements, as described by Spencer (1968) who postulated its origin from primitive pulmonary mesenchymal anlage. The tumour has been variously described as an 'embryonal adenomyosarcoma', 'carcinosarcoma', and muco-epidermoid carcinoma. Histologically there are glandular structures composed of columnar or stratified nonciliated cells in a stroma of pleomorphic mesenchyme.

Only 3 of the 19 cases so far reported (Iverson & Straehley, 1973) were less than 16 years of age. There is possibly a slight predominance in males.

The mode of presentation was cough, haemoptysis or pain in the chest, in order of frequency, and radiographs usually show a large mass in one lung or involving the hilar nodes.

Treatment of reported cases has been chiefly excision of the tumour, by lobectomy or pneumonectomy. The best method of treatment is uncertain and because of rarity of the tumour, there is no evidence on which the value of radiotherapy or chemotherapy can be assessed.

The prognosis is in general poor, although some have apparently been cured by radical excision; 3 patients, one now 19 years of age, are alive with no evidence of tumour 8 years after surgical excision (Iverson & Straehley).

METASTATIC TUMOURS OF THE LUNGS

Primary tumours of the lungs are extremely rare in children, and less common than pulmonary metastases which occur in a number of tumours of childhood.

Wilms' tumour, osteosarcoma, Ewing's sarcoma and Hodgkin's disease are the tumours most likely to produce pulmonary metastases in childhood. Metastases may be demonstrable at the time of the initial presentation, but more often develop later. Their appearance is always ominous and may be the signal for a change in the objectives of treatment from an aggressive 'curative' approach to one of palliation, especially when multiple bilateral pulmonary deposits develop early, before the primary tumour has been removed or clinically controlled.

However, in some circumstances aggressive treatment, including excision, or intensive irradiation or chemotherapy, may still be worthwhile and the following factors influence selection of the plan of management.

1. *The nature of the primary tumour*, and whether it has been or can be adequately controlled, e.g. in Wilms' tumour in which metastases are sensitive to irradiation and (to a lesser degree) to cytotoxic agents. Secondaries from an osteosarcoma are, in contrast, very much more difficult, and as resistant to radiation as the primary. Strangely, neuroblastoma for all its invasiveness, rarely produces pulmonary metastases.

2. *The time interval between diagnosis of the primary tumour and the appearance of pulmonary metastases.* Deposits appearing **during** treatment of the primary tumour, i.e. only a few months after presentation, are indicative of a highly invasive tumour, or impaired immune defences, and are unlikely to be controlled by currently available means. However, metastases appearing months or years after the initial treatment may be single and resectable.
3. *The number and distribution* of the radiologically visible metastases. When few in number and confined to one lung or to one lobe, the situation is obviously more favourable, and more suitable for excision.
4. *The response of previous metastases* (in the lungs or elsewhere) to treatment. Clear evidence of susceptibility of the tumour to radiotherapy or chemotherapy is an indication for aggressive therapy.
5. *The presence of multiple metastatic deposits* elsewhere. Resection of pulmonary metastases is as a rule not justified until other sites of metastases have been excluded or adequately controlled.

TREATMENT OF PULMONARY METASTASES

The methods available are surgery, radiotherapy and chemotherapy.

Radiotherapy is usually the most useful form of treatment and pulmonary metastases from a Wilms' tumour are sensitive to irradiation; in many cases they can be eradicated by radiotherapy focused on the deposit (or deposits), augmented by radiation to both lung fields (p. 523).

Chemotherapy, e.g. with actinomycin D and vincristine, has also been shown to be effective in treating metastases of Wilms' tumour, but their response is less predictable than with radiotherapy.

Surgical removal, by local wedge excision, lobectomy, or pneumonectomy, may be required when other forms of treatment are found to have been ineffective or when resolution is incomplete. Tomography to determine the site and number of metastases is an essential prerequisite.

The plan of treatment for pulmonary metastasis depends upon the nature of the primary tumour and the extent of metastatic deposits elsewhere; in most cases the results of treatment are much less favourable with other types of tumour than Wilms' tumour, in which the lungs are frequently the only site of metastases. Aggressive treatment of pulmonary metastasis from a Wilms' tumour has proved to be worthwhile and cure rates of up to 50% have been reported (see p. 528).

D. CARDIAC TUMOURS

Tumours of the heart are exceptionally rare in infancy and childhood, but sufficient reports of collected series have appeared to describe the types of tumour encountered in this age group and their clinical findings.

Simcha *et al.* (1971) noted that a cardiac tumour was found in 0·08% of all cases of congenital heart disease investigated at Great Ormond Street, and that in an infant or child presenting with cardiomegaly, a systolic murmur and congestive failure, the possibility of a tumour as the cause would not even be considered in the differential diagnosis until angiocardiography had demonstrated an intracavitary filling defect.

Cardiac tumours can be classified as follows:

(*a*) Benign tumours:

I. Rhabdomyomas (usually multiple);

II. Fibroma (? hamartoma);

III. Myxoma.

(*b*) Malignant tumours:

IV. Rhabdomyosarcoma.

(*c*) Teratomas of the heart and pericardium.

I. RHABDOMYOMA

These are usually found at autopsy in children suffering from tuberous sclerosis (p. 826), a syndrome with a strong familial incidence which includes epilepsy, mental retardation, tumours or cysts in the kidney and multiple intramural rhabdomyomas (Lagos & Gomez, 1967).

The cardiac signs are usually confined to disturbances of conduction, presumably due to the multiple tumours, and take the form of paroxysmal atrial extrasystoles or heart block, causing cardiomegaly and congestive cardiac failure, noted in four of the six cases of rhabdomyomas collected by Van der Hauwaert (1971). Occasionally one or more of the tumours protrudes into one of the cardiac chambers and causes obstruction of the inflow or outflow (Kilman *et al.*, 1973).

In the series of eight tumours reported by Simcha *et al.*, four of the eight were rhabdomyomas; three of the four were multiple, intramural and associated with tuberous sclerosis.

In the Index Series two of the three cardiac tumours were rhabdomyomas in children with tuberous sclerosis.

II. FIBROMA

These, too, are usually intramural, but single, and most are situated in the wall of one of the ventricles or in the interventricular septum. Geha *et al.* (1967) reviewed 36 such cases, of which 31 were found in children; Keith,

Rowe & Vlad (1967) noted that in childhood most patients with a fibroma were less than 10 months of age at the time of diagnosis. This was confirmed by Van der Hauwaert's report of five cases, all males, between 5 and 8 months of age. In this group of five patients, four presented with cardiac signs; the correct diagnosis was made on angiocardiography, and in three of them the tumour was removed successfully; in the fourth the tumour was too extensive to be resected.

III. MYXOMA

Although a myxoma is the commonest intracardiac tumour in adults, accounting for 50% of all such tumours, it is exceedingly rare in childhood, and Bigelow *et al.* (1953) could find only five cases in childhood in the literature up to that time.

It is typically pedunculated and most often attached to the wall of the left atrium (75%) while the remainder are found in the right atrium. Being intracardiac rather than intramural, a myxoma directly affects the haemodynamics of the heart, and characteristically causes a cardiac murmur, chiefly the murmur typical of mitral stenosis, and when due to a tumour, the murmur can vary from time to time, and even from moment to moment with changes in position.

In the Great Ormond Street series (Simcha *et al.*, 1971), two of the eight tumours were myxomas; one was typically pedunculated and in the left atrium of a 7-year old, and one filled the cavity of the right ventricle. In both cases the heart was greatly enlarged, with a filling defect on angiocardiography. Echocardiography correctly indicated an atrial myxoma in one case, and this was subsequently removed successfully on bypass.

A family history was noted in one of three cases of myxoma reported by Van der Hauwaert (1971).

IV. RHABDOMYOSARCOMA

As a cardiac tumour, this is chiefly found in adults, and more than 125 have been reported; 80% were intramural, and only 20% were polypoid and intracavitary.

In childhood they are the rarest of all cardiac tumours; there was none in the 20 years covered by the review from Great Ormond Street, and none in Van der Hauwaert's series of 29 tumours. Engle *et al.* (1962) reported one case, in a 4-month old infant, with metastases in the lung, mediastinum and thymus, and one such case occurred in the Index Series.

MODES OF PRESENTATION

These depend to a large extent on whether the tumour remains within the septum or the wall of a cardiac chamber, or whether it encroaches on the cavity causing obstruction to its outflow or inflow, or both. The clinical signs and symptoms vary greatly from case to case, but can be assigned in general to one of two groups.

1. *Disorders of conduction*, such as extrasystoles, heart block or ventricular fibrillation and cardiac arrest, tend to occur with 'silent' intramural tumours.
2. *Congestive cardiac failure*, dyspnoea, variable cardiac murmurs and cardiac enlargement are all prone to occur in intracavitary tumours; embolism, obstruction of coronary arteries and myocardial infarction have also been reported as complications.

DIFFERENTIAL DIAGNOSIS

1. *Congenital heart disease* includes the very large range of developmental cardiac abnormalities. The general picture of incipient cardiac failure in infancy (restlessness, difficulty in feeding, cyanosis, failure to thrive) is an indication for urgent investigation, including cardiac catheterization and angiocardiography, now that cardiac surgery can be carried out effectively even in very young infants.
2. *Extracardiac conditions*, such as intrapericardial teratomas, possibly partial defects of the pericardium, pericardial or 'spring water' cysts, can be clearly distinguished from intracardiac tumours by angiocardiography, although their precise pathological nature may have to await removal at thoracotomy and subsequent histological examination.

TERATOMAS OF THE HEART AND PERICARDIUM

In Van de Hauwaert's series of 29 tumours in infancy and childhood, six were teratomas. Only one was intracardiac, in a neonate who died of a huge multilocular cyst occupying most of the right side of the heart. The remaining five were intrapericardial, and three presented with acute cardiac distress, massive enlargement of the cardiac shadow, no murmur and a low voltage ECG. Pneumopericardium, combined with paracentesis, revealed an intrapericardial mass; in all three cases the teratoma was found to be attached by a short pedicle to the root of the aorta, and each was removed successfully.

In a small number of cases, rupture of a teratoma (Thompson & Moore, 1969) or a secondary pericardial effusion (Reynolds *et al.*, 1969) causes acute cardiopulmonary distress as the first sign of the condition.

TREATMENT OF CARDIAC TUMOURS

Once the diagnosis of an intracavitary cardiac tumour has been made, there should be no delay in proceeding to its removal on cardiopulmonary bypass, for sudden deterioration may occur at any time.

The prognosis of each type of tumour is indicated in the descriptions above.

E. TUMOURS OF THE CHEST WALL AND DIAPHRAGM

Tumours arising in the ribs, costal cartilages, intercostal musculature and pleura are all extremely rare, and metastatic deposits in the ribs are, collectively, more common than all the others combined.

In the Index Series one Ewing's tumour and one eosinophilic granuloma arose in a rib, and costal metastases from neuroblastoma, Ewing's tumour, synovial sarcoma and hepatocarcinoma have also been encountered.

Ravitch (1969), in a review of the literature, noted that primary tumours of the chest wall in childhood are more likely to be malignant than benign. Of the benign lesions, chondroma and osteoid osteoma appear to be the more common. Malignant tumours reported included metastatic neuroblastoma, histiocytosis X, Ewing's tumour and chondrosarcomas (Watkins & Gerard, 1960). Osteoblastoma and osteosarcoma have been noted to occur following radiotherapy to pulmonary metastases.

Mesotheliomas of the pleura in childhood have also been described (Kauffman & Stout, 1964; Grundy & Miller, 1972).

Rhabdomyosarcoma and haemangiopericytoma arising in the diaphragm have been recorded (Wiener & Chou, 1965), but are exceptionally rare.

Treatment of malignant tumours of the chest wall should aim at resection of the full thickness including pleura, excising a safe margin of univolved tissues, and repair of the defect with prosthetic material to restore stability when the area is not sufficiently supported by more superficial muscles such as latissimus dorsi or the pectoral muscles.

Radiotherapy may be required if the excision is incomplete, and chemotherapy with cytotoxic drugs appropriate to the particular tumour would also be indicated.

TUMOURS OF THE RIBS

Primary malignant tumours of the ribs are rare in childhood, but benign tumours appear to be equally rare, or even less common in this region and age group (Joseph & Fonkalsrud, 1972).

Malignant tumours

Chondrosarcoma and osteosarcoma occur in children (Watkins & Gerard, 1960); 'round-cell' sarcoma, lymphosarcoma (p. 170), histiocytosis X (p. 209) and fibrosarcoma (p. 761) of the rib have also been reported, but Ewing's tumour (p. 734) is probably more common than any of these. Of 311 patients of all ages with Ewing's tumour reviewed by Kent and Ashburn (1948), 21 arose in a rib, mostly in patients less than 13 years of age.

It is usually possible to distinguish between a tumour and acute infections by appropriate investigations (e.g. full blood examination, blood culture, etc.), but in chronic osteomyelitis, mixed destruction and new bone formation or atypical radiological findings (common in Ewing's tumour arising in other than long bones, p. 740) may only be resolved by biopsy. The release of grey-pink diffluent material in such cases should suggest the possibility of a tumour, e.g. reticulum cell sarcoma of bone, as well as Ewing's tumour.

Ewing's tumour occasionally affects the internal aspect of a rib producing a mass presenting radiographically in the anterior or posterior mediastinum. However, radiographic changes in the structure of a rib, such as 'moth-eaten' destruction (p. 741), are unusual in mediastinal tumours other than intrathoracic neuroblastoma which is almost invariably in the posterior mediastinum.

Benign tumours

Reviews of those arising in the ribs (O'Neal & Ackerman, 1951) have shown the wide variety of benign lesions encountered. Chondroma and osteochondroma are reported to be the most common (Hochberg, 1957), followed by osteoma, osteoid osteoma (p. 728), eosinophilic granuloma (p. 209), fibrous dysplasias (p. 732), aneurysmal bone cyst (p. 730) and osteoblastoma (p. 728). The radiographic findings may suggest the diagnosis, but confirmation by excision-biopsy is almost always required.

BIOPSY

If the operative findings are informative, e.g. in osteomyelitis, material for contact imprints (p. 82) or culture and a limited biopsy are usually sufficient; when the macroscopic appearances are uncertain, a reasonably wide excision-biopsy is usually required, because of the frequency of malignant lesions and because benign lesions may recur locally unless removed completely.

TREATMENT

When biopsy reveals a malignant lesion, a more extensive excision may be indicated, e.g. removal one or more ribs, and possibly the full thickness of the chest wall, repairing the defect with prosthetic material such as Marlex® or by relocating muscle flaps, e.g. pectoralis or latissimus dorsi.

Chemotherapy and radiotherapy have been shown to play an important role in the treatment of malignant bone tumours, e.g. in Ewing's tumour (p. 743), more recently in osteosarcoma (p. 753), and also in rhabdomyosarcoma (p. 789) which on rare occasions arises in the chest wall.

DESMOMA
(syn. desmoid tumour)

AGE : SEX : SITE

Few desmomas develop in childhood, but Bolanowski & Groff (1973) collected 21 such cases and, as in adults, females predominated (15 : 6). No less than 16 of the 21 cases were in children less than five years of age, and the anterior abdominal wall was by far the commonest site, chiefly in the rectus sheath or the external oblique aponeurosis (Booker & Pack, 1951).

Only two desmomas (Keeley *et al.*, 1960; Bolanowski & Groff, 1973) involved the chest wall, and the more recent case appears to be unique in growing entirely internally, causing progressive dyspnoea by compressing the underlying lung.

Only four cases of a desmoid clearly arising from the intercostal muscles have been reported.

Microscopically the tumour is composed of well differentiated spindle-shaped fibroblasts, and the three characteristics of a desmoma are extreme hardness, relative avascularity and a strong tendency to recur locally (Musgrove & McDonald, 1948). In adults the recurrence rate of abdominal desmoids is said to be approximately 60%, and in extra-abdominal sites, 75%.

DIAGNOSIS

A desmoid is usually firm, painless, well demarcated and slowly growing.

Other conditions which may present some of these features are haemangiomas, a foreign body surrounded by a chronic fibrotic reaction, and some subcutaneous hamartomas. None, except perhaps a fibrotic mass around a foreign body, is as hard as a desmoid.

The diagnosis is usually made with certainty after excision-biopsy, and unless the lesion is widely excised, recurrence is likely.

TREATMENT

Radical excision offers the best prospect of cure, and when the diagnosis is made after a conservative excision, a further excision is usually indicated, removing a wide margin of macroscopically uninvolved tissue, beneath as well as around the site of the tumour. The same principle applies to a recurrent desmoma; removal of the full thickness of the abdominal or thoracic wall, including skin and peritoneum or pleura, may be necessary if further recurrences are to be prevented.

REFERENCES

Tumours of the Mediastinum Bronchus and Lungs

BARRIE, J.D. (1961). Intrathoracic tumours of carotid body type (chemodectoma). *Thorax*, **16** : 78.

BALE, P.M. (1973). A congenital intraspinal gastroenterogenous cysts in diastematomyelia. *J. Neurol. Neurosurg. Psych.*, **36** : 1011.

BROOMHEAD, I.W. (1964). Cystic hygroma of the neck. *Brit. J. Plastic Surg.*, **17** : 225.

CASTLEMAN, B., IVERSON, L. & MENENDEZ, V.P. (1956). Localized mediastinal lymph node hyperplasia resembling thymoma. *Cancer*, **9** : 822.

CAYLEY, C.K., CAEZ, H.J. & MERSHEIMER, W. (1951). Primary bronchogenic carcinoma of the lung in children: review of the literature and report of a case. *Amer. J. Dis. Child.*, **82** : 49.

CLATWORTHY, H.W.Jr. & NEWTON, W.A. (1970). Mediastinal ganglion cell tumours in children. *Proc. Surgical Congress, Melbourne*, **1** : 185.

CRAIG, J.M., KIRKPATRICK, J. & NEUHAUSER, E.B.D. (1956). Congenital cystic adenomatoid malformations of lung in infants. *Am. J. Roentgenol.*, **76** : 516.

DE BUSE, P. (1973). Malignant nonchromaffin paraganglioma. *Arch. Dis. Childh.*, **47** : 976.

DE PAREDES, C.G., PIERCE, W.S., GROFF, D.B. & WALDHAUSEN, J.A. (1970). Bronchogenic tumours in children. *Arch. Surg.*, **100** : 574.

DOWELL, A.R. (1974). Primary pulmonary leiomyosarcoma. *Ann. Thorac. Surg.*, **17** : 384.

FILLER, R.M., TRAGGIS, D.G., JAFFE, N. & VAWTER, G.F. (1972). Favourable outlook for children with mediastinal neuroblastoma. *J. Pediat. Surg.*, **7** : 136.

FISCHER, E.R., SIERACKI, J.C. & GOLDENBERG, D.M. (1970). Identity and nature of isolated lymphoid tumours etc. *Cancer*, **25** : 1286.

FONTANA, R.S., TYCE, G.M., FLOCK, E.V. *et al.* (1963). Serotonin and the carcinoid syndrome in patients with bronchial tumours. *Ann. Otol.*, **72** : 1024.

GILLIS, D.A., REYNOLDS, D.P. & MERRITT, J.W. (1955/56). Chemodectoma of an aortic body. *Brit. J. Surg.*, **43** : 585.

GOODNER, J.T., BERG, J.W. & WATSON, W.L. (1961). The non-benign nature of bronchial carcinoids and cylindromas. *Cancer*, **14** : 539.

HABER, S. (1964). Retroperitoneal and mediastinal chemodectoma. *Am. J. Roentgen.*, **92** : 1029.

HALLER, J.A., MAZUR, D.O. & MORGAN, W.W.Jr. (1969). Diagnosis and management of mediastinal masses in children. *J. Thorac. Cardiovasc. Surg.*, **58** : 385.

HEIMBURGER, I.L. & BATTERSBY, J.S. (1965). Primary mediastinal tumors of childhood. *J. Thorac. Cardiov. Surg.*, **50** : 92.

HOLINGER, P.H. *et al.* (1960). Primary fibrosarcoma of the bronchus. *Dis. Chest*, **37** : 137.

HONICKY, R.E. & DE PAPP, E.W. (1973). Mediastinal teratoma with endocrine function. *Amer. J. Dis. Child.*, **126** : 650.

HOPE, J.W., BORNS, P.F. & KOOP, C.E. (1963). Radiological diagnosis of mediastinal masses in infants and children. *Radiol. Clin. N. Amer.*, **1** : 17.

IVERSON, R.E. & STRAEHLEY, C.J. (1973). Pulmonary blastoma: longterm survival ot juvenile patient. *Chest*, **63** : 436.

KELLER, A.R., HOCHHOLZER, L. & CASTLEMAN, B. (1972). Hyaline vascular and plasma cell types of giant lymph node hyperplasia of the mediastinum and other locations. *Cancer*, **29** : 670.

KILLINGSWORTH, W.P., MCREYNOLDS, G.S. & HARRISON, A.W. (1953). Pulmonary leiomyosarcoma in a child. *J. Pediat.*, **42** : 466.

KIRWAN, W.O., WALBAUM, P.R. & MCCORMACK, R.J.M. (1973). Cystic intrathoracic derivatives of the pregut and their complications. *Thorax*, **28** : 424.

KRIEG, H., JUNGST, B.F. & HOFMANN, S. (1973). Lymphangioma cysticum des Mediastinums mit übergriefen auf Peri-und Epicardiums. *Z. Kinderchirurg.*, **12** : 111.

KYRIAKOS, M., & WEBBER, B. (1974). Cancer of the lung in young men. *J. Thorac. Cardiovasc. Surg.*, **67** : 634.

LEGG, M.A. & BRADY, W.J. (1965). Pathological and clinical behaviour of thymomas. *Cancer*, **18** : 1131.

LUMPKIN, S.M.M. (1966). Bronchogenic cysts: presentation of a case and review of the literature. *Arch. Otolaryngol.*, **84** : 346.

MARTINI, N., HAJDU, S.I. & BEATTIE, E.J.Jr. (1971). Primary sarcoma of the lung. *J. Thorac. Cardiov. Surg.*, **61** : 33.

NEALE, A.E. & MENTEN, M.L. (1948). Tumors of the thymus in children. *Am. J. Dis. Child.*, **76** : 102.

O'GRADY, W.P., MCDIVITT, R.W., HOLMAN, C.W. & MOORE, S.W. (1970). Bronchial adenomas. *Arch. Surg.*, **101** : 558.

PACHTER, M.R. (1963). Mediastinal nonchromaffin paraganglioma. *J. Thorac. Cardiov. Surg.*, **45** : 152.

PIRAMOON, A.M. & ABBASSIOUN, K. (1974). Mediastinal enterogenous cyst with spinal cord compression. *J. Pediat. Surg.*, **9** : 543.

RAFFENSPERGER, J. & COHEN, R. (1972). Plexiform neurofibromas in childhood. *J. Pediat. Surg.*, **7** : 145.

RAVITCH, M. (1969). Tumors of the lung. In *Pediatric Surgery*, ed. Mustard, W.T. *et al.* 2nd ed. Year Book Medical Publishers Inc., Chicago.

REYNOLDS, J.L., DONAHUE, J.K. & PEARCE, C.W. (1969). Intrapericardiac teratoma: a cause of pericardial effusion in infancy. *Pediatrics*, **43** : 71.

RUSBY, N.L. (1944). Dermoid cysts and teratomas of the mediastinum. *J. Thorac. Surg.*, **13** : 169.

SHACKELFORD, G.D. & MACALISTER, W.H. (1974). The aberrant positioned thymus. *Amer. J. Roentgenol.*, **120** : 291.

SIMPSON, J.A., SMITH, F. *et al.* (1974). Bronchial adenoma: a review of 26 cases. *Aust. N.Z. J. Surg.*, **44** : 110.

SPENCER, H. (1968). Pulmonary blastoma. In *Pathology of Lung*. Macmillan, New York.

TALERMAN, A. & AMIGO, A. (1968). Thymoma associated with regenerative and aplastic anaemia in a 5 year old child. *Cancer*, **21** : 1212.

THOMPSON, D.P. & MOORE, T.C. (1969). Acute thoracic distress in childhood due to spontaneous rupture of a large mediastinal teratoma. *J. Pediat. Surg.*, **4** : 416.

TUNG, K.S.K. & MCCORMACK, L.J. (1967). Angiomatous lymphoid hamartoma: report of 5 cases with a review of the literature. *Cancer*, **20** : 525.

TURNBULL, A.D., HUVOS, A.G., GOODNER, J.T. & BEATTIE, E.J. (1972). The malignant potential of bronchial adenoma. *Ann. Thorac. Surg.*, **14** : 453.

VERSKA, J.J. & CONNOLLY, J.E. (1968). Bronchial adenomas in children. *J. Thorac. Cardiovasc. Surg.*, **55** : 411.

WATSON, W.L. & ANLYAN, A.J. (1954). Primary leiomyosarcoma of the lung. *Cancer*, **7** : 250.

WILKINS, E.W.Jr. *et al.* (1963). A continuing clinical survey of adenomas of the trachea or bronchus in a general hospital. *J. Thorac. Cardiovasc. Surg.*, **46** : 279.

Larynx: Trachea and Bronchus (Papilloma and Papillomatosis)

AL-SALEEM, T., PEALE, A.R. & NORRIS, C.M. (1968). Multiple papillomatosis of the lower respiratory tract. Clinical and pathological study of 11 cases. *Cancer*, **22** : 1173.

BOYLE, W.F., RIGGS, V.L., OSHIRO, L.S. & LENNETTE, E.H. (1973). Electron microscopic identification of papova virus in laryngeal papilloma. *Laryngoscope*, **83** : 1102.

HITZ, H.B. & OESTERLIN, E. (1932). Case of multiple papillomata of larynx with aerial metastasis to lungs. *Amer. J. Path.*, **8** : 333.

MCCOY, E.G., BOYLE, W.F. & FOGARTY, W.A. (1971). Electron microscopic identification of virus-like particles in laryngeal papilloma. *Ann. Otol. Rhinol. Laryngol.*, **80** : 693.

OLESKE, J.M. & KUSHNICK, T. (1971). Juvenile papillomas of the larynx. *Am. J. Dis. Child.*, **121** : 417.

ROSENBAUM, H.D., ALAVI, S.M. & BRYANT, L.R. (1968). Pulmonary parenchymal spread of juvenile laryngeal papillomatosis. *Radiology*, **90** : 654.

Subblottic Haemangioma

CHRISTIAENS, L., DECROIX, G. *et al.* (1965). Les hémangiomes du larynx et de la trachée chez le nourrisson. *Arch. Franç. Pédiat.*, **22** : 513.

FERGUSON, C.F. & FLAKE, C.G. (1961). Subglottic hemangioma as a cause of respiratory obstruction in infants. *Ann. Otol. Rhin. Laryng.*, **70** : 1095.

TEFFT, M. (1966). The radiotherapeutic management of subglottic hemangioma in children. *Radiology*, **96** : 207.

WILLIAMS, H.E., PHELAN, P.D., STOCKS, J.G. & WOOD, H. (1969). Haemangioma of the larynx in infants: diagnosis, respiratory mechanics and management. *Aust. paediat. J.*, **5** : 149.

Plasma Cell Granuloma

CARTER, R., WAREHAM, E.E. & BULLOCK, W.K. (1968). Intrathoracic fibroxanthomatous pseudotumor. *Ann. Thorac. Surg.*, **5** : 97.

DUBILIER, L.D., BRYANT, L.R. & DANIELSON, G. (1968). Histiocytoma of the lung. *Am. J. Surg.*, **115** : 420.

KAUFFMAN, S.L. & STOUT, A.P. (1961). Histiocytic tumours (fibrous xanthoma and histiocytoma) in children. *Cancer*, **14** : 469.

PEARL, M. & WOOLLEY, M.W. (1973). Pulmonary xanthomatous postinflammatory pseudotumors in children. *J. Pediat. Surg.*, **8** : 255.

SPROUL, E.E., METZGAR, R.S. & GRACE, J.T. (1963). The pathogenesis of Yaba virus induced histiocytomas in primates. *Cancer Res.*, **23** : 671.

TARASKA, J.J. (1966). Case report of a postinflammatory pseudotumour of the trachea. *J. Thorac. Cardiovasc. Surg.*, **51** : 279.

WITWER, J.P. & TAMPAS, J.P. (1973). Tracheal fibroxanthoma in a child. *Post grad. Med.*, **54** : 228.

YOUNG, L.W., SMITH, D.I. & GLASGOW, L.A. (1970). Pneumonia of atypical measles: residual nodular lesions. *Am. J. Roentgen.*, **110** : 439.

Cardiac Tumours

BIGELOW, N.H., KLINGER, S. & WRIGHT, A.W. (1954). Primary tumours of the heart in infancy and early childhood. *Cancer*, **7** : 549.

ENGLE, M.A., ITO, T., EHLERS, K.H. & GOLDBERG, H.P. (1962). Rhabdomyomatosis of the heart: diagnosis during life with clinical and pathological findings. *Circulation*, **26** : 712.

GEHA, A.S., WEIDEMAN, W.H., SOULE, E.H. & MCGOON, D.C. (1967). Intramural ventricular cardiac fibroma. *Circulation*, **36** : 427.

KEITH, J.D., ROWE, R.D. & VLAD, P. (1967). Heart Disease in Infancy and Childhood, 2nd ed., p. 1171. Macmillan, New York.

KILMAN, J.W., CRAENEN, J. & HOSIER, D.M. (1973). Replacement of entire atrial wall in an infant with a cardiac rhabdomyoma. *J. Pediat. Surg.*, **8** : 317.

LAGOS, J.C. & GOMEZ, M.R. (1967). Tuberous sclerosis: reappraisal of a clinical entity. *Mayo Clin. Proc.*, **42** : 26.

SIMCHA, A., WELLS, B.G., TYNAN, M.J. & WATERSTON, D.J. (1971). Primary cardiac tumours in childhood. *Arch. Dis. Childhd.*, **46** : 508.

VAN DE HAUWAERT, L.G. (1971). Cardiac tumours in infancy and childhood. *Brit. Heart J.*, **33** : 125.

Tumours of the Thoracic Wall and Diaphragm

ANDERSON, L.S. & FORREST, J.V. (1973). Tumors of the diaphragm. *Am. J. Roentgenol.*, **119** : 259.

BOLANOWSKI, P.J.P. & GROFF, D.B. (1973). Thoracic wall desmoid tumor in a child. *Ann. Thorac. Surg.*, **15** : 632.

BOOKER, R.J. & PACK, G.T. (1951). Desmomas of the abdominal wall in childhood. *Cancer*, **4** : 1052.

GRUNDY, G.W. & MILLER, R.W. (1972). Malignant mesothelioma in childhood. Report of 13 cases. *Cancer*, **30** : 1216.

HOCHBERG, L.A. (1953). Primary tumors of the rib. *Arch. Surg.*, **67** : 566.

JOSEPH, W.L. & FONKALSRUD, W.E. (1972). Primary rib tumors in children, *The Amer. Surg.*, **38** : 338.

KAUFFMAN, S.L. & STOUT, A.P. (1964). Mesothelioma in children. *Cancer*, **17** : 539.

KEELEY, J.L., DE ROSARIO, J.L. *et al.* (1960). Desmoid tumors of the abdominal and thoracic walls in a child. *Arch. Surg.*, **80** : 144.

KENT, E.M. & ASHBURN, F.S. (1948). Ewing's sarcoma of the rib. *Amer. J. Surg.*, **75** : 845.

MUSGROVE, J.E. & MCDONALD, J.R. (1948). Extra-abdominal desmoid tumours: their differential diagnosis and treatment. *Arch. Path.*, **45** : 513.

O'NEAL, L.W. & ACKERMAN, L.V. (1951). Cartilaginous tumors of ribs and sternum. *J. Thorac. Surg.*, **21** : 71.

RAVITCH, M.M. (1969). Thoracic tumors. In *Pediatric Surgery*, 2nd ed. (Mustard, W.T., Ravitch, M.M. *et al.*, eds.) Year Book Medical Publishers Inc., Chicago.

WATKINS, E. & GERARD, F.P. (1960). Malignant tumors involving the chest wall. *J. Thorac. Cardiovasc. Surg.*, **39** : 117.

WIENER, M.F. & CHOU, W.H. (1965). Primary tumors of the diaphragm. *Arch. Surg.*, **90**: 143.

Chapter 17. Abdominal masses: tumours of the kidney

ABDOMINAL TUMOURS IN CHILDHOOD

A palpable mass in the abdomen is one of the commonest and most important clinical findings in childhood. For practical purposes abdominal tumours in this age group can be divided into those arising in the upper part of the abdomen or the loin (Table 17.1), and a smaller number typically found in the lower abdomen or the pelvis (p. 683). Tumours in the upper part of the abdomen are more numerous, for this is the site of the two commonest

Table 17.1. Malignant abdominal masses: tumours arising in the upper part of the abdomen in the paediatric age group

Site		Tumour	Page
Kidney	1.	Wilms' tumour	495
	2.	Adenocarcinoma	529
Adrenal gland	3.	Neuroblastoma	538
	4.	Ganglioneuroblastoma	549
	5.	Cortical adenocarcinoma	574
	6.	Phaeochromocytoma	562
Retroperitoneal tissues	7.	Malignant teratoma	584
	8.	Paraganglioma	586
	9.	Sarcomas	590
		Rhabdomyosarcoma	
		Liposarcoma	
		Fibrosarcoma (embryonal)	
		Haemangiopericytoma	
	10.	Burkitt's tumour	328
Liver	11.	Hepatoblastoma	598
	12.	Hepatocarcinoma	612
	13.	Hepatomegaly due to metastases	606
Bile ducts	14.	Rhabdomyosarcoma	621
	15.	Adenocarcinoma	623
Pancreas	16.	Adenocarcinoma (exocrine)	662
	17.	Non-beta cell carcinoma	667
Alimentary canal	18.	Lymphosarcoma	630
	19.	Adenocarcinoma	641

malignant tumours in childhood, neuroblastomas arising in the adrenal gland or in retroperitoneal tissues (p. 538), and Wilms' tumour (nephroblastoma) (p. 495).

A common mode of presentation of both these tumours is the unexpected discovery of a mass, for example by the mother while drying or dressing the child, or during a routine clinical examination. The reasons why such a tumour becomes so large before it is discovered are as follows:

(i) Most tumours in the upper abdomen (Table 17.1) are 'embryonal' in type (p. 37), probably present at birth, and usually found in children less than 5 years of age.

(ii) In children in this age group the contour of the abdomen is normally full and often protruberant.

(iii) The upper part of the abdominal cavity is capacious and accommodates considerable daily variations in the size of the viscera it contains.

(iv) The overhanging costal margins shelter a tumour from palpation until it has reached a considerable size.

While inspissated faeces in the colon is the commonest palpable abdominal mass in childhood, it is rarely located in the upper half of the abdomen, usually in the sigmoid colon, and most commonly palpated in the hypogastrium or the iliac fossae.

BENIGN MASSES

In children less than five years of age, benign conditions as the cause of a large palpable mass in the upper abdomen are less common than malignant tumours. These conditions can be summarized as follows:

1. Massive enlargement of the liver or spleen;
2. Renal swellings, including hydronephrosis, dysplasias of various types, mesenchymal hamartoma, and following renal vein thrombosis;
3. Choledochal cyst;
4. Duplication cyst of the alimentary canal, and occasionally a mesenteric cyst;
5. Pseudocyst of the pancreas; and
6. 'Giant cystic' meconium peritonitis (in neonates);
7. Intramuscular abscess;
8. Tropical infestations and infections.

1. *Benign enlargement of the liver or spleen.* In most cases the shape of the organ is retained, but the definitive diagnosis is usually made from the result of radiological investigations (p. 506), on the blood picture (e.g. in thalassaemia or leukaemia), on specific biochemical tests or needle biopsy in conditions such as the storage diseases, inborn errors of metabolism, etc.

A hydatid cyst can cause gross enlargement of the liver; in affected children the Casoni test and the hydatid complement fixation tests are both negative in some 25% of cases. Selective hepatic arteriography (p. 69) or scintillography (p. 76) will usually demonstrate a hydatid cyst as an avascular or 'cold' area in the substance of the liver.

Hamartomas of the liver, i.e. a multilocular mesenchymal hamartoma, or possibly derived from primitive intrahepatic bile duct epithelium (p. 609), may reach a very large size without producing any symptoms. Radiological investigations (p. 611) will exclude a retroperitoneal or a renal tumour, but the final distinction from a hepatic neoplasm may require laparotomy and biopsy.

2. *Benign enlargement of the kidney.* A giant hydronephrosis can closely resemble a renal tumour, although obstruction in the urinary tract presenting primarily as a mass in the first few years of life is less common than constitutional symptoms due to infection, such as fever, malaise and failure to thrive. Haematuria, on the other hand, is a common presenting sign in hydronephrosis, and may also occur in renal tumours.

Transillumination of the loin, using a powerful light in a completely darkened room, often demonstrates whether a mass in the loin is fluid-filled and likely to be a hydronephrotic kidney.

3. *A choledochal cyst*, during phases of distension, is palpable as a large, smooth mass extending from beneath the right lobe of the liver; however, the distension is typically episodic and the cyst may not be palpable for long. Colic, jaundice and a palpable mass form the classic triad, but this occurs in only about 30% of cases.

A barium meal showing displacement of the second part of the duodenum downwards, forwards and to the left is highly suggestive, but an excretory cholangiogram and tomography may be required to confirm the diagnosis between acute episodes.

4. *A duplication cyst* of the short 'non-communicating' type usually obstructs the lumen of the contiguous bowel causing symptoms of intestinal obstruction. A large, tense duplication cyst is occasionally found in a symptomless patient; the nature of the mass may be suggested by its extraordinary mobility within the peritoneal cavity, but the diagnosis is only made with certainty at laparotomy.

Mesenteric cyst. One form is a large mass composed of small, tense cysts of various sizes (p. 674), attached by a narrow pedicle to the mesentery of the colon, and may resemble a tumour. Aortography (p. 507) usually provides the distinction. The more common unilocular type of mesenteric cyst is often large but usually lax and resembles ascites rather than a tumour.

5. *A pseudocyst of the pancreas* following abdominal injury causes epigastric fullness, but is usually not sufficiently tense to simulate a tumour. The preceding injury is, as a rule, severe enough to be a feature of the patient's history.

6. *The 'giant cystic' form of meconium peritonitis* may present as an upper abdominal mass in a neonate, but accompanied by signs, symptoms and radiological evidence of intestinal obstruction; plain films of the abdomen may also show typical plaques of intraperitoneal (or intrascrotal) calcification.

7. *Intramuscular abscess* of the anterior abdominal wall. In young children in the tropics, a specific form of low-grade myositis (Burkitt, 1947) may be mistaken for an intra-abdominal tumour (Wong, 1973). It presents as an ill-defined induration with little or no sign of inflammation other than tenderness, and often without any general systemic evidence of sepsis. Careful palpation usually indicates that the 'mass' is more superficial than an intra-abdominal tumour.

8. *Tropical infestations and infections*, e.g. bilharzia, amoebic hepatic abscesses and ascariasis, should also be considered as possible causes of an abdominal mass in children in endemic areas.

MALIGNANT TUMOURS

While clinical findings may strongly suggest that a palpable mass is a tumour, further information as to its nature, site, and size are required, and can be obtained by investigations such as plain films of the abdomen, chest, other bones, etc., aortography and selective arteriography, scintillography (p. 76) and ultrasonography.

Specific biochemical investigations, such as measurement of urinary catecholamines may be indicated by the provisional diagnosis suggested by angiography. The scope and direction of the investigations required to confirm diagnosis, and to determine the extent of the tumour, including metastases, are described in the sections dealing with each malignant abdominal tumour.

Sonography (ultrasonic echography) has proved to be of value in distinguishing between solid and cystic masses, and is expected to become a standard method of investigation (Holder, Stuber *et al.*, 1972).

Malignant tumours which may arise in the upper part of the abdomen are listed in Table 17.1.

For the purposes of description they are grouped as follows in this and the following chapters:

Tumours of the kidney;

Tumours of the adrenal gland and retroperitoneal tissues, Chapter 18, p. 537;

Tumours of the liver and bile ducts, Chapter 19, p. 597;

Tumours of the alimentary canal, spleen, pancreas, omentum and mesenteries, Chapter 20, p. 627.

TUMOURS OF THE KIDNEY

I. WILMS' TUMOUR
(syn. nephroblastoma)

Wilms' tumour is one of the two commonest solid malignant tumours of childhood and accounts for 5–10% of all such cases. In recent years, there has been a very significant improvement in the results of treatment mainly due to the introduction of cytotoxic agents.

HISTORY

In 1899, Max Wilms, a German surgeon, published a treatise on the common renal tumour of childhood which has come to be known by his name. However, Rance (1814) almost 100 years earlier, had reported the first case of a probable renal tumour in an infant. In 1870, Catanni had recognized the sarcomatous character of the lesion, and two years later Eberth gave the first accurate description of the mixed nature of its histology. In 1875 Conheim invoked his theory of the embryonic nature of the tumour to explain the presence of muscle cells.

In 1898 Birch-Hirschfeld noted the characteristic embryonic tubules and connective tissue, and coined the term 'embryonal adenomyosarcoma', in modern terminology a nephroblastoma, but in common usage still known as Wilms' tumour, perhaps partly because of potential confusion between 'nephroblastoma' and 'neuroblastoma'. In the animal kingdom, Wilms' tumour also occurs in cows, sheep, swine, dogs, rabbits, rats and chickens.

During the 19th century, knowledge of the pathology of this tumour accumulated rapidly and a remarkably clear description was given by Bland Sutton in 1893:

> 'It is characteristic of these sarcomas that the ureter is rarely obstructed [which] explains the rarity of haematuria . . . and perhaps what is otherwise remarkable, the painlessness of these tumours in children for there is no pressure from accumulated urine. Though the ureter so constantly escapes invasion, yet the veins are always implicated; and this constitutes a most peculiar as well as a most dangerous feature of renal sarcomas in children. The tumour tissue extends into the renal vein and often projects and even runs for a long distance into the inferior vena cava; portions are detached and carried to the pulmonary circulation . . .'

The era of treatment commenced when Kocher first excised a Wilms' tumour in 1876; Jessop, frequently cited as the first surgeon to remove such a tumour, actually did in 1877. Surgical treatment has remained the cornerstone of treatment, but long-term survival was for many years relatively rare. In 1923, Bland-Sutton collected 21 'renal sarcomas' in infancy treated by nephrectomy, and reported that life was prolonged to any extent in only 10% of these patients.

With the discovery of therapeutic irradiation, radiotherapy was introduced, but was found to have little place as the sole therapeutic measure. However, it has earned its rightful role as an adjunct to surgery, and by the late 1940s surgical excision was combined with immediate post-operative irradiation, and was reported by Robert Gross to produce a survival rate of 47·5%. The introduction of cytotoxic agents in the last 15 years has brought further improvement in results, but there is still lack of uniformity as to the regime and the dosages. Perhaps the most contentious aspect is the use of pre-operative cytotoxic drug therapy.

The final chapter in the treatment of Wilms' tumour has yet to be written. From a hopeless prognosis in the 19th century, the present survival figures, approaching 90% of two-year survivals with repeated post-operative courses of chemotherapy (Wolff *et al.*, 1968), represent a remarkable development, but this figure will inevitably be further improved.

From data collected by U.I.C.C. (1973), it appears that Wilms' tumour occurs with a more regular frequency from country to country than any other tumour. Innis (1972) independently suggested that the incidence in each country might be used as a standard index with which the incidence of other tumours could be compared and computed.

A familial incidence in Wilms' tumour has not been reported often, but with the increasing number of survivors, tumours may appear in their offspring. The penetrance of the genetic factors appears to be low, but variable; in one sibship four out of five children had a Wilms' tumour and in the same kindred three successive generations were affected (Brown *et al.*, 1972).

A familial syndrome comprising multiple bilateral Wilms' tumours, visceromegaly and somatomegaly has recently been described by Perlman, Goldberg *et al.* (1973).

A review of reports of familial cases led Knudson (1975) to a hypothesis that there may be two elements in the development of a Wilms' tumour: an initial prezygotic mutation (either germinal or somatic), and a second mutation solely somatic in type; in familial cases both elements are operative (and bilateral tumours occur in 21% of cases), while in the sporadic (non-familial) cases only the second mutation occurs, and the incidence of bilateral tumours is 5–10%.

AGE : SEX

The tumour essentially arises in the first quinquennium (Fig. 17.1), more specifically between the ages of one and four years in 62% of the patients in the Index Series (Table 17.2), and this is in accord with reports of larger

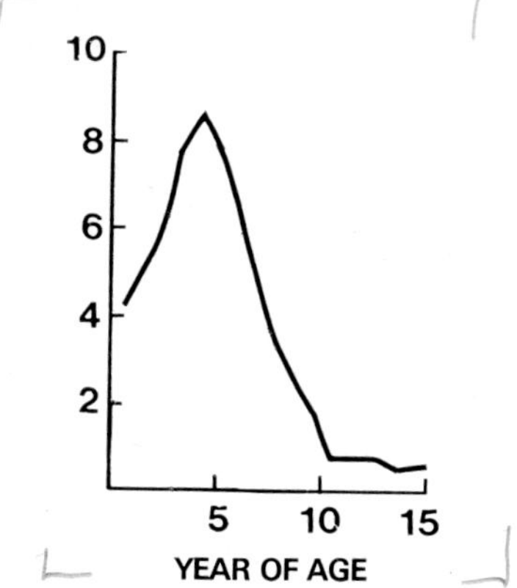

Figure 17.1. WILMS' TUMOUR; the incidence according to age, indicating the peak between three and six years of age (for source of figures see Figure 2.2, p. 48).

series. However, the range in our patients extended from two weeks to twelve years, and there are a number of reports of a Wilms' tumour present at birth.

Males are affected slightly more frequently than females in a ratio of approximately 1·25 : 1 in most reported series.

EXTRARENAL TUMOURS

On rare occasions a Wilms' tumour arises outside the kidney, presumably in ectopic nephrogenic cells, e.g. caudal to the kidney, where it may cause ureteric obstruction. There was one such case in the Index Series, and in another case the tumour arose at the upper margin of a horseshoe kidney, an association noted by Willis (1967), Thompson *et al.* (1973) and Shashikumar *et al.* (1974).

An extrarenal Wilms' tumour has been reported arising in adjacent retroperitoneal tissues (Bhajeker *et al.*, 1964; Edelstein *et al.*, 1965), the mediastinum (Moyson *et al.*, 1961), the inguinal canal (Thompson *et al.*, 1973) and in a sacrococcygeal teratoma (Tebbi *et al.*, 1974).

BILATERAL WILMS' TUMOURS

Involvement of both kidneys varies from 3% to as high as 13% in some series; in the Index Series, 4% appeared to be bilateral at the time of diagnosis. Martin & Reyes (1969) reported that as many as 40% of cases were found to be bilateral when the contralateral kidney was fully explored at the time of the initial nephrectomy. It is usually impossible to determine whether these represent metastases or multiple primaries, but in most cases, including

Table 17.2. Wilms' tumour; age at presentation of 84 patients in the Index Series (RCH, 1950–1972)

Age (years)	No.	
0–1	9	
1–2	19	52 patients (62%) 1–4 years
2–3	18	
3–4	15	
4–5	5	
5–6	5	
6–7	5	
7–8	4	
11	1	
12	3	
Total	84	

bilateral cases in the Index Series in which the contralateral kidney was involved at the time of the primary resection, there was no evidence of metastasis elsewhere. Young & Williams (1969) concluded that at least some cases were examples of multicentric origin. On reviewing the literature concerning bilateral cases, Ragab, Vietti *et al.* (1972) found an overall incidence of 4·4% (see p. 497).

It is possible that in the natural history of Wilms' tumour (i.e. unmodified by any form of treatment) primary tumours may develop simultaneously or seriatim in each kidney in a large proportion of cases; it is also possible that many are suppressed by chemotherapy, so that only a small number, perhaps 1 in 10 (cf. 40% and 4%, above), come to clinical attention, a proportion comparable with the necropsy finding of neuroblastoma-*in-situ* and the lesser incidence of clinical neuroblastoma (see p. 538).

The treatment of bilateral Wilms' tumour is described on p. 524.

MACROSCOPIC APPEARANCES

The typical Wilms' tumour is a large rounded mass, partly replacing the kidney in which it arises, and confined by a 'capsule' which is partly fibrous and partly composed of compressed renal tissue, with minimal adhesions to surrounding structures (Fig. 17.2). By the time diagnosis is made the tumour is usually at least 6 cm in diameter and many are larger, up to 20 cm or more in diameter.

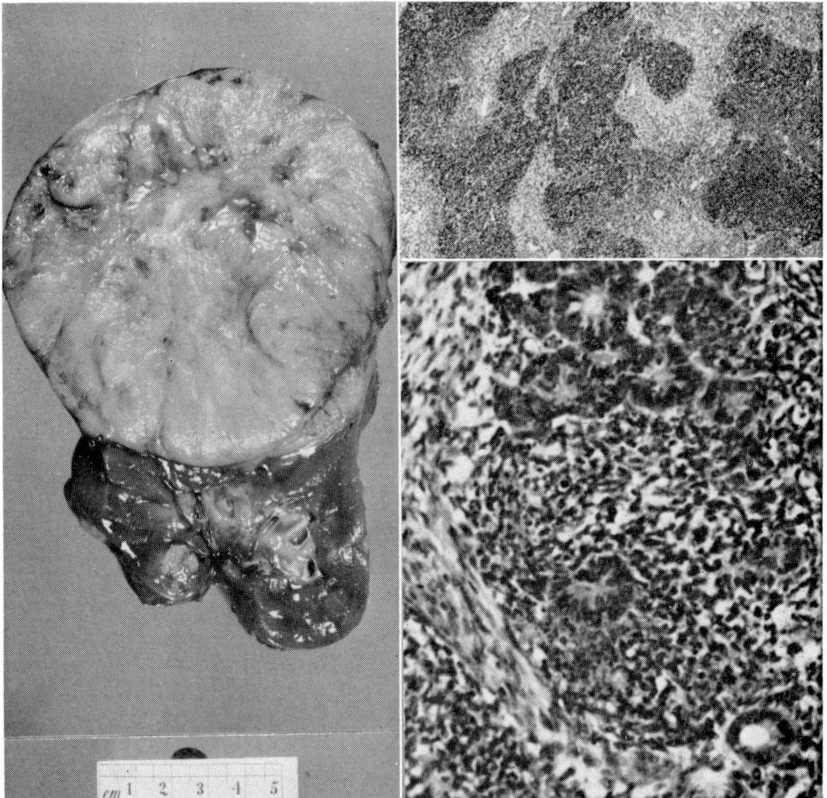

Figure 17.2. WILMS' TUMOUR; (*a*) typical tumour with a uniform cut surface, only small areas of necrosis, bulging and 'growing out' from the kidney. The clear demarcation by a compressed 'pseudocapsule' is also evident; (*b*) the usual 'geographic' or lobular pattern of epithelial islands separated by loose spindle-cell mesenchyme (H & E. × 30); (*c*) tubules and ducts of epithelial appearance, intimately related to and merging with the stromal cells (H & E. × 200).

[(*a*) *Left.* (*b*) *Top right.* (*c*) *Bottom right.*]

The cut surface is usually homogeneous, rather soft, slightly mucoid or slimy, and greyish-pink in colour. In some there are areas of haemorrhage and necrosis (Fig. 17.3a). The inner part of the pseudocapsule is composed of compressed renal tissue, and it is rare for the tumour to actually invade the kidney; rather, the growing tumour mass compresses the parenchyma, and causes distortion of the pelvicalyceal system. The extrarenal portion of the tumour is often much larger than the part within the outline of the kidney.

Invasion of the renal vein (see p. 508) is not necessarily related to the size of the tumour, and can occur when the tumour is still quite small.

VARIATIONS IN MACROSCOPIC APPEARANCES

The following have been seen in the Index Series.

1. *Small tumours*, ill-defined, haemorrhagic and invasive, tending to invade the renal pelvis causing haematuria as the presenting symptom (Fig. 17.3).
2. *Very large tumours* 15–20 cm in diameter and weighing 1250 g; when a tumour reaches this size, much of it is infarcted or haemorrhagic, or both.
3. *Pronounced cyst formation* can occur and when prominent, the tumour can be misleadingly similar to a multilocular cyst of the kidney (Fig. 17.6a).
4. *Necrotic tumours* in which almost the entire tumour is infarcted or haemorrhagic; in some this may be the result of trauma, but in others it occurs spontaneously. Angiographic studies clearly show that the blood supply of a Wilms' tumour usually arises from slender, elongated arcuate branches of the renal artery, which commonly arch over its surface before entering the tumour. In such cases infarction in the tumour is likely to occur relatively early in its growth, and arteriography often shows an apparent paucity of vessels in the area occupied by the tumour.

Calcification is found radiologically in some 5% of Wilms' tumours, (compared with 50% of neuroblastomas) and in Wilms' tumour this can be correlated with histological calcification in areas of previous necrosis, usually in the capsular region. This linear and circumferential distribution may be distinguishable from the diffuse speckled calcification characteristic of a neuroblastoma (Fig. 18.11, p. 553).

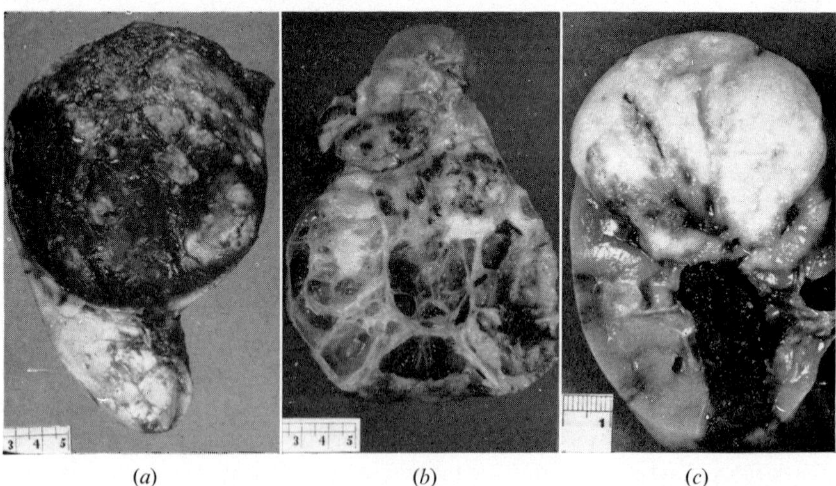

(*a*) (*b*) (*c*)

Figure 17.3. WILMS' TUMOUR; the variant macroscopic types; (*a*) massive haemorrhage and necrosis following trauma; (*b*) extensive cystic degeneration; and (*c*) a small intrarenal tumour invading the renal pelvis and presenting with massive haematuria (note clot in the pelvis).

5. *A pronounced lobulation* is present in some tumours with variable texture from one lobule to another; some are soft, white and rather diffluent, while others are firm, yellowish and tough. These differences are reflected in the microscopic appearances, the firm areas being well differentiated with a structure identical with 'fibromas' and benign mesenchymomas (see p. 510). Lobulation is occasionally due to dysplasia of the kidney in which the tumour arose.

6. *Dysplastic changes* in a kidney the site of a Wilms' tumour are not usual (15% of the 122 in Index Series), and a greater incidence would probably be found if the uninvolved parts of the kidney were sampled more thoroughly. The association with renal dysplasia is significant because of the high incidence in patients with a Wilms' tumour of various associated developmental malformations, including hemihypertrophy and aniridia (Hewitt *et al.*, 1966; Haicken & Miller, 1971), especially anomalies of the genito-urinary system, e.g. hypospadias (Miller *et al.*, 1964), horseshoe kidney (Shashikumar *et al.*, 1974) and cryptorchidism.

MICROSCOPIC FINDINGS

The classical picture (Fig. 17.4a) is a cellular tumour with two components: (i) islands of closely packed cells with an epithelial appearance, separated by (ii) a loose embryonic connective tissue stroma with areas of differentiation to form smooth or striated muscle, and occasionally bone or cartilage. However the cells in both components have a very similar nuclear structure and appear to be variants of one cell type. In the 'epithelial' areas differentiation to form tubules is usually seen (Fig. 17.4b); this may be minimal, or widespread with a papillary structure in some places (Fig. 17.4e). Collections of mesenchymal cells resembling imperfectly formed glomerular bodies (Fig. 17.4f) occur in approximately 15% of Wilms' tumours.

HISTOLOGICAL VARIATIONS

The following were encountered in the Index Series.

1. *Undifferentiated tumours* (20%), with a macroscopically homogeneous cut surface and, microscopically, uniform sheets of cells with an oval, vesicular hyperchromatic nucleus and rather scanty cytoplasm (Fig. 17.4c). Complete absence of any pattern in the tumour is unusual, and even in poorly differentiated tumours the biphasic pattern can usually still be recognized in some areas.

2. *A 'rhabdomyosarcomatous' type* (Fig. 17.4d) is also rare, with differentiation to form plump cells with eosinophilic cytoplasm containing cross striations. When only this pattern is present, a case can be made for a diagnosis of 'rhabdomyosarcoma of the kidney', but a careful search usually reveals other

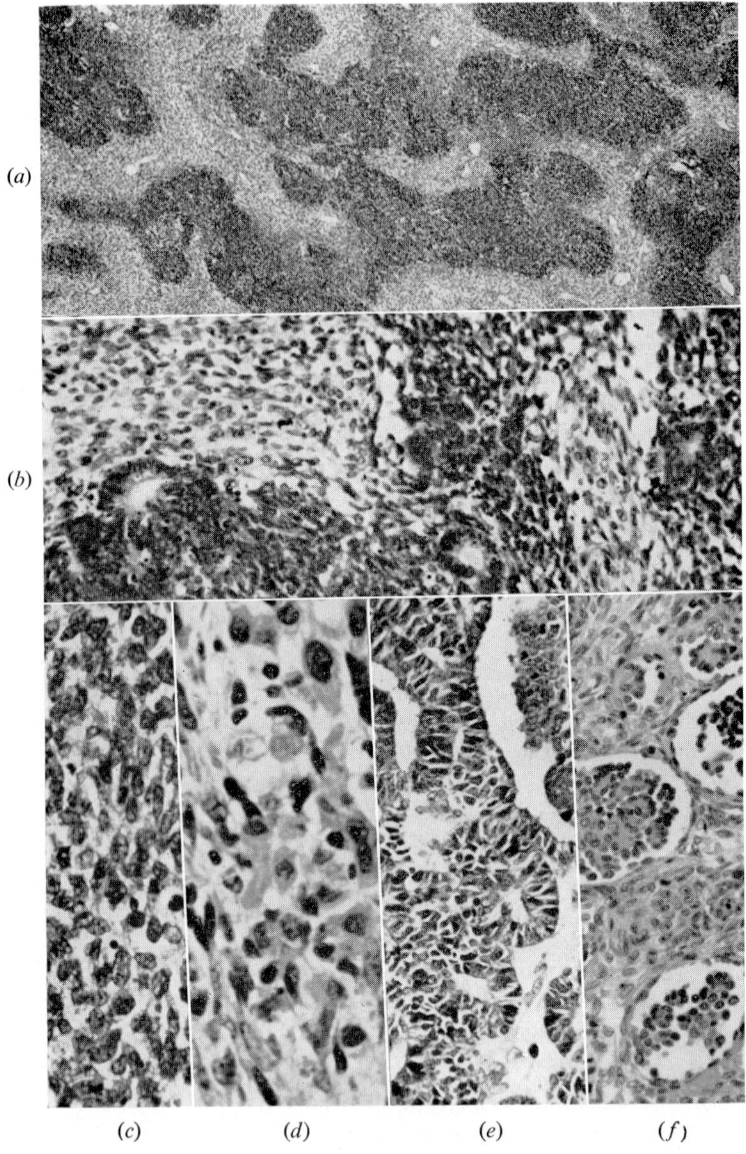

Figure 17.4. WILMS' TUMOUR; (*a*) the classical 'geographic' or 'exploded jig-saw' pattern, seen at low magnification, due to islands of epithelial cells separated by spindle-cell mesenchymal tissue (H & E. × 30); (*b*) typical picture at a higher magnification with some differentiation to tubular formation in the epithelial component (H & E. × 200); (*c*) to (*f*) variations in the histological pattern; (*c*) undifferentiated 'epithelial' cells; (*d*) rhabdomyoblastic differentiation sometimes seen in the stromal component; (*e*) marked tubular ('papillary') differentiation; and (*f*) glomeruloid bodies (all H & E. × 300).

areas typical of Wilms' tumour and this variant seems to be one in which differentiation to form striated muscle is extreme. There were two such tumours in the Index Series; both developed late metastases, in each case in bone and not in the lungs.

3. *A papillary type* largely composed of glandular tissue with an intricate, reticulated papillary pattern, often without much intervening stroma (Fig. 17.4e).

4. *A highly-differentiated form* in which glomeruloid bodies (Fig. 17.4f) are predominant but situated in tissue with the typical histological appearance of Wilms' tumour. In one such case in the Index Series there was evidence that the tumour secreted large amounts of a renin-like substance (p. 506).

HISTOLOGICAL EFFECTS OF CHEMOTHERAPY

As well as unequivocal clinical and radiological evidence, there is histological evidence that Wilms' tumour is affected by chemotherapy, and also radiotherapy. Two types of change have been observed in the primary tumour in patients who received actinomycin D and vincristine for three days before the kidney with its tumour was removed:

(i) A great increase in the number of mitotic figures after exposure to vincristine which causes mitotic arrest (see p. 25).

(ii) Diffuse and widespread necrosis in the centres of the epithelial zones, a constant finding in cases treated in recent years, and so rare in tumours resected before the introduction of pre-operative chemotherapy that it seems likely to be due to the cytotoxic agents.

In pulmonary metastases resected after chemotherapy and radiotherapy the stromal element of the tumour shows an astonishing degree of differentiation to form rhabdomyoblasts. The epithelial elements are also extremely well-differentiated, and indeed, in many cases, scarcely appear to be neoplastic. In only one case of pulmonary metastases was chemotherapy alone used; irradiation was also employed in the others, and it is therefore uncertain whether differentiation in pulmonary metastases is entirely due to chemotherapy, or mainly attributable to irradiation as suggested by Marsden & Steward (1968).

SPREAD

Local spread occurs into the perirenal fascia, retroperitoneal tissues, the adrenal gland, liver, diaphragm, and the bowel, but this occurs rather late, as shown by the small number of local recurrences after operation in the Index Series. In general, the larger the tumour the more the likelihood of local extrarenal invasion.

Extension into the renal vein cannot be predicted from the size of the tumour alone, and should always be anticipated. Pre-operative cavography

(Fig. 17.5b) is helpful in identifying extension into the renal vein or the inferior vena cava. Oedema of the lower limbs and ascites, due to massive caval and intracardiac extensions, occurred in two cases in the Index Series (see p. 507).

Spread to lymph nodes is fairly common, and extensive clearance of all the adjacent nodes is advocated by some (e.g. Martin & Reyes, 1969) because of the significant number of cases with deposits in nodes which did not appear to be involved macroscopically. Conversely, it is not uncommon to find much enlarged hyperplastic nodes which are free of metastases.

The renal hilar nodes are involved first, then the para-aortic chain; bilateral involvement of retroperitoneal lymph nodes is uncommon except as a late event, and is reported to indicate a bad prognosis.

Pulmonary metastases are typical of Wilms' tumour, in which the lungs are the commonest site of dissemination, both before and after operation, forming single or multiple spherical deposits. While pulmonary metastases develop early in a few cases, far more frequently they do not develop (or are not found radiologically) until several months after removal of the primary tumour. In a very few cases there is direct spread through the diaphragm into the lung via the pleura.

Secondary metastasis from the lung to other organs occurs in a small proportion of cases, the brain and bone being the sites most commonly involved, but usually only in the terminal stages.

Metastasis to the liver, without direct invasion, occurs in some cases and may be the result of invasion of portal vein radicles, e.g. in the mesentery of the bowel, or of secondary spread from metastases in the lungs.

MODES OF PRESENTATION (Table 17.3)

1. *A symptomless abdominal mass* is the classic mode, the mass being discovered by a parent, or less commonly by a doctor during a routine examination. Abdominal distension is often present, and even when the mass is large and fills out the flank, it is seldom tender. The textbook descriptions of a renal swelling as extending upwards to disappear under the costal margin may lead not only to confusion but to diagnostic delay; a Wilms' tumour in the left kidney can be mistaken for an enlarged spleen and observed for weeks or even months. The prognostic significance of such a delay can be serious.

A Wilms' tumour rarely crosses the midline, being more 'vertically' disposed and extending into the iliac fossa. Its extent can usually be readily defined, but palpation should be kept to a minimum because of the possibility of increasing dissemination by excessive handling.

2. *Abdominal pain.* Recurrent abdominal pain is so common in childhood and so rarely due to a tumour, that a Wilms' tumour may not be suspected,

Table 17.3. Wilms' tumour; modes of presentation (and survivals) in 59 cases in the Index Series, treated according to protocol, (RCH. 1969–1972)

Mode of presentation	No. of patients			No. surviving (2 years+)
Abdominal mass palpated	30			19
by a parent		15	6	
by a family doctor		8	6	
by a welfare nurse		1	1	
uncertain		6	6	
Haematuria	8			5
Abdominal pain	9			4
'Acute surgical abdomen'	2			2
Trauma	3			3
'Hepatomegaly and/or splenomegaly'	5			4
Hypertension	1			1
Gigantism (hemihypertrophy)	1			1
Totals	59			39 (67%)

and this possibility should be borne in mind when examining a child with abdominal pain. In a few cases pain is severe and mimics an 'acute abdomen'.

Haemoperitoneum due to rupture of the tumour, or from adjacent congested veins, occurred in three cases in the Index Series, and in two other cases simulated 'retrocaecal' appendicitis with peritonitis.

3. *Haematuria.* In the differential diagnosis of macroscopic haematuria in children, a Wilms' tumour should always be considered and the flanks carefully palpated. If the tumour is small and impalpable, and if there is a recent but irrelevent history of minor abdominal trauma, the real cause may be overlooked. The existence of a renal abnormality (including a Wilms' tumour) in cases of 'traumatic' haematuria is well known, and the pyelogram which should follow usually demonstrates the underlying tumour.

A potential cause of considerable delay in the recognition of a tumour is a provisional diagnosis of a non-surgical condition such as focal nephritis, which may lead to delay in obtaining a pyelogram.

4. *Hypertension* in patients with a Wilms' tumour is possibly more common than generally recognized; the incidence of a minor degree of hypertension, reported to be as high as 15% (Hastings & Gwinn, 1965) or 28% (Aron, 1974), depends on how intensively it is sought. In most cases it is mild and raises no particular problems in diagnosis or management. In some, however, it is extremely severe, and its effects or complications constitute the mode of presentation.

The hypertension has been variously attributed to compression of the kidney as a whole or of the renal artery alone, causing renal ischaemia and consequent production of excess renin (Sukarochana *et al.*, 1972), or to the presence of arteriovenous fistulae in the tumour (Sukarochana *et al.*, 1972); or to the production of excess renin (or angiotensin) by the cells of the tumour, as proven in one case in the Index Series (Mitchell *et al.*, 1970).

A girl of 23 months presented with failure to thrive, hypertension (220/200 mmHg), albuminuria, a renal mass, micro-angiopathic haemolytic anaemia, retinal haemorrhages and exudates, hypertensive encephalopathy and high levels of plasma renin. After intensive medical preparation a Wilms' tumour was removed and assays showed that there were very significantly increased amounts of renin in the tumour, but not in the parenchyma of the affected kidney. She made an excellent recovery and is now well, normotensive, and free of disease seven years later.

5. *Gigantism.* Hemihypertrophy or focal giantism (Fraumeni *et al.*, 1967), with or without aniridia and other anomalies (Fraumeni *et al.*, 1968) are recognized associations of Wilms' tumour (Haicken & Miller, 1971). This raises the questions of how often and how intensively investigations should be repeated in such patients in order to detect the development of a tumour as early as possible. An excretory pyelogram at intervals of six months would appear to be an acceptable and effective method of surveillance (see p. 11).

6. *Aniridia.* The association with Wilms' tumour (p. 17) has been recognized for more than a decade, and as Pilling (1975) has pointed out, this specifically concerns the congenital, sporadic (and bilateral) form of aniridia, not the familial type, in which apparently only one Wilms' tumour has been reported. A Wilms' tumour has been reported in 12 (approximately 33%) of 35 children with sporadic aniridia, an incidence which would warrant a programme of surveillance for such children, e.g. an excretory pyelogram when aniridia is first detected and, at least, palpation of the abdomen at frequent intervals until the age of 4 years (Pilling, 1975).

7. *Other unusual presentations or findings* include pyrexia (Hastings & Gwinn, 1965), polycythaemia (Murphy, Mirand *et al.*, 1967), possibly hypoglycaemia (Loutfi, Mehrez *et al.*, 1964), and Cushing's syndrome (Cummins & Cohen, 1974).

INVESTIGATIONS

The diagnosis of Wilms' tumour can usually be made correctly on the clinical findings, but investigations are required to (i) confirm the diagnosis; (ii) establish the diagnosis when the clinical findings are atypical; (iii) determine whether dissemination has occurred; and (iv) by determining the stage of the disease, help in planning treatment.

1. *Radiological investigations.* The following are required in each case:

(*a*) *Plain films of the abdomen* to show the size and shape of the tumour, the presence or absence of calcification, and displacement of the intestine.

(*b*) *Radiographs of the chest* to detect pulmonary metastases.

(*c*) *A skeletal survey* is not essential, but may be helpful when the diagnosis lies between a Wilms' tumour and a neuroblastoma; it becomes essential when there is clinical evidence of secondary deposits in bone.

(*d*) *Aortography and selective renal arteriography* (Fig. 17.5a) are the most informative (McDonald & Hiller, 1968) and lead to the correct diagnosis in more than 95% of cases. They have largely replaced excretory pyelography, for an IVP is also obtained at the conclusion of angiography. Although there may be no excretion in a few cases, the characteristic finding is pelvicalyceal distortion and dispersion (Fig. 17.5a), in contrast to displacement without calyceal distortion which is typical of a neuroblastoma (see Fig. 18.12, p. 555) and other para- or extrarenal tumours. Angiography will also demonstrate the vessels supplying the tumour and the 'tumour circulation' in the capillary phase.

Selective renal arteriograms of the contralateral kidney are also obtained to demonstrate the presence of an adequate second kidney, and to exclude any abnormality such as a contralateral tumour.

(*e*) *Inferior vena cavography* shows the degree of displacement of the cava, particularly in a large tumour arising in the right kidney, and is especially valuable in demonstrating, before operation, the presence of extension of the tumour along the renal vein into the vena cava (Fig. 17.5b). Thus forewarned, the necessary steps can be taken to remove the extension and prevent dissemination of tumour emboli. Radiological evidence of complete obstruction of the cava, usually accompanied by deflection of contrast material into the inferior hemi-azygos veins, was accepted by some authorities as an indication that the tumour was 'inoperable', but it is now realized that this is not necessarily so (p. 73). However, extensive filling of hemi-azygos collaterals, accompanied by clinical evidence of caval obstruction such as oedema of the lower limbs and/or ascites, is an indication for right heart catheterization to determine whether there is evidence of extension of the tumour via the cava into the right atrium. When present, this requires an abdominothoracic approach and pulmonary bypass to cope with intra-atrial extensions (Murphy, Rabinovitch *et al.*, 1973) which were present in two of our cases in the last two years.

(*f*) *Excretory pyelography* as an initial investigation still has its place, particularly in a child presenting with haematuria and without a palpable abdominal mass.

2. *Haematological investigations* are required:

(*a*) Grouping and cross-matching of blood to be available at operation.

(*b*) Peripheral blood counts and smears will show whether there is anaemia requiring transfusion before operation, and provide a base line for monitoring the effects of cytotoxic agents.

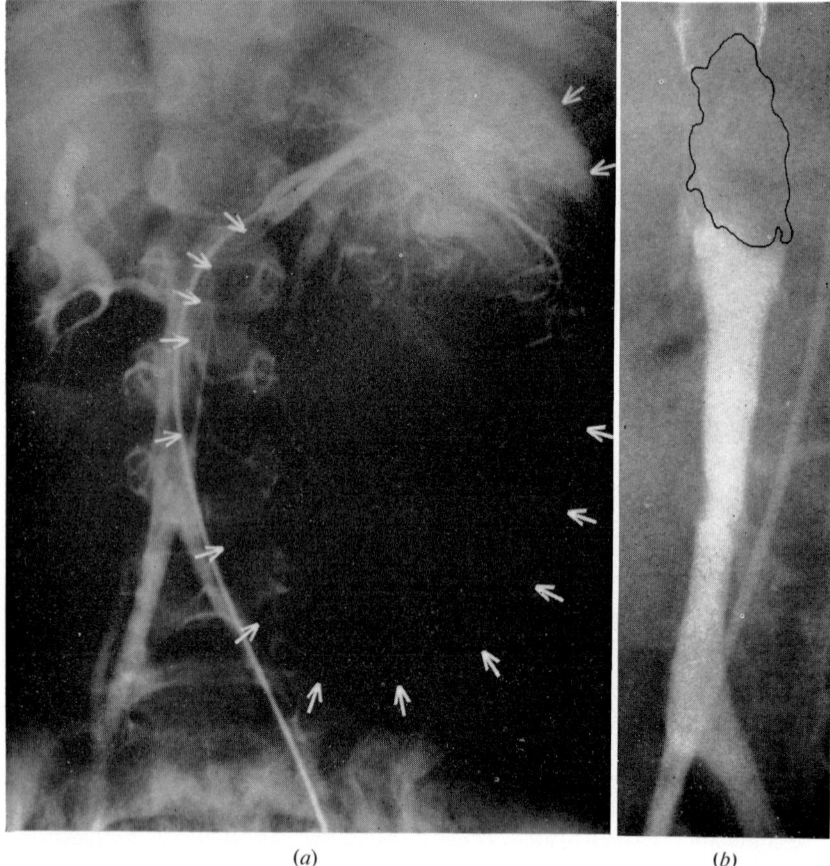

(*a*) (*b*)

Figure 17.5. WILMS' TUMOUR; (*a*) renal arteriogram of a relatively avascular but typical tumour with 'neovasculature', i.e. tortuous tumour vessels; the tumour is distorting and deforming the calyces; (*b*) inferior vena cavogram showing a filling defect due to an intracaval extension of the tumour. There is also some filling of the left inferior vena hemi-azygos, indicative of caval obstruction.

3. *Urine tests* will determine the presence and amount of haematuria and a 24-hour specimen is occasionally necessary, to estimate the urinary catecholamines (p. 539) and exclude a neuroblastoma.

Some Wilms' tumours have been shown to produce a complex protein-polysaccharide-mucin in the serum (Tomasi, Robertson *et al.*, 1966), in the urine (Morse & Nussbaum, 1972) and also demonstrable in the tumour itself (Powars, Allerton *et al.*, 1972). The latter reported a correlation between volume of tumour tissue present and the amount of mucinous substance in the serum; in one case the material had disappeared from the serum eight days after removal of a large tumour, but reappeared following recurrence. They suggested that such estimations may prove useful in pre-operative diagnosis and also in monitoring patients for evidence of recurrence.

DIFFERENTIATION OF BENIGN CONDITIONS

Several benign conditions to be excluded before treatment is commenced are as follows.

1. Hydronephrosis

This rarely presents as a large mass in early childhood, and can usually be identified by massive enlargement of the calyces and/or the renal pelvis, by poor excretion of dye, or the absence of any excretion, which is very unusual in Wilms' tumour.

Transillumination of the flank with a bright light in a darkened room can be particularly helpful in infants and young children by identifying a 'giant' hydronephrosis, for the transmission of light through a large fluid-filled hydronephrosis is diagnostic.

2. Renal dysplasia

Polycystic disease causing a renal mass in childhood, is extremely rare and essentially affects both kidneys in adults. Unilateral cystic disease of the kidney poses a greater problem (see below) and remains a potential source of error in diagnosis. Another form of dysplasia associated with an atretic ureter is mentioned in the differential diagnosis of Wilms' tumour in infancy (p. 514).

3. **Multilocular cyst of the kidney** (syn. 'cystadenoma', cystic hamartoma)

This localized cystic malformation (Fig. 17.6) usually causes moderate enlargement (Aterman *et al.*, 1973) of the kidney which is currently indistinguishable from a Wilms' tumour on clinical and radiological grounds (Johnson, Ayala *et al.*, 1973).

Fowler (1971) has suggested that the lesion is a cystic form of differentiation of a Wilms' tumour and a totally benign aftermath. It is to be distinguished from a simple polycystic kidney, in which the entire kidney is involved, whereas a multilocular cyst is a large but localized and encapsulated collection of cysts in an otherwise histologically normal kidney (Johnson, Ayala *et al.*, 1973).

Microscopically, a multilocular cyst of the kidney contains multiple cavities separated by thick, relatively acellular fibrous septa with clusters of small tubules composed of a single layer of cuboidal epithelium (Fig. 17.6b). A Wilms' tumour with pronounced cystic degeneration may closely

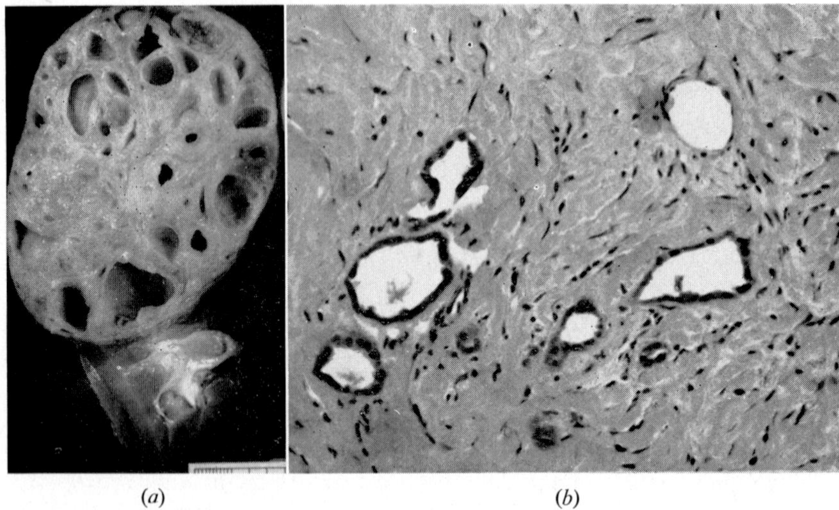

(*a*) (*b*)

Figure 17.6. MULTILOCULAR CYST OF THE KIDNEY; although externally resembling Wilms' tumour (*a*) the cut surface shows a multicystic lesion sharply demarcated from the normal part of the kidney; (*b*) multiple cystic cavities separated by thick fibrous septa containing scattered clusters of small tubules similar to those seen in dysplastic kidneys (H & E. × 130).

resemble this lesion externally, but the distinction can be suspected from examination of the cut surface (Fig. 17.6a) and proven by the distinctive microscopic findings.

4. **Mesenchymal hamartoma**
   (syn. mesoblastic nephroma, fetal mesenchymoma,
   congenital renal hamartoma, fibroma, fibrosarcoma)

This is a localized, solid and often small fibrous mass occurring in the kidney (Fig. 17.7) in infants (Richmond & Dougall, 1970; Bogdan *et al.*, 1973a, b; Bolande *et al.*, 1967, 1972, 1973, 1974; Annotation, *Brit. med. J.*, 1973). The characteristic microscopic finding is a fibromatous pattern of interlacing bundles of spindle-shaped cells (Fig. 17.7b), in some cases enclosing islands of tubules and immature glomeruli similar to those found in the nephrogenic zone of the neonatal kidney. Fowler (1971) has suggested that this condition, too, is the result of maturation of a Wilms' tumour, in this case to a predominantly solid form. Walker & Richard (1973) reported an unusual case in which a renal tumour thought to be a fetal hamartoma of the kidney, in a two-year old girl, recurred fatally. A recent report of the induction of glomerular and renal tubular structures in tissue culture of cells from a 'fetal renal hamartoma' (Crocker & Vernier, 1973) confirms the link between

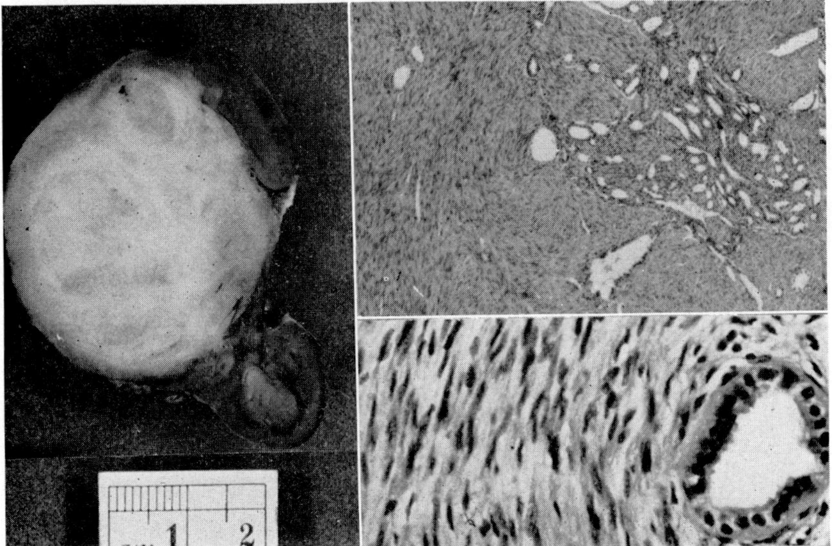

Figure 17.7. Mesenchymal hamartoma of the kidney; (*a*) whorled, whitish cut surface, and firm, fibrous texture, merging into the renal parenchyma at its margins; (*b*) islands of renal tubules surrounded by interlacing bundles of fibroblasts (H & E. × 30); (*c*) fibroblasts and a tubule at higher magnification (H & E. × 200).

[(*a*) *Left*. (*b*) *Top right*. (*c*) *Bottom right*.]

mesenchymal hamartomas and Wilms' tumours, and suggests the possibility of a common origin for both lesions from metanephrogenic blastema (Favara *et al.*, 1968).

The angiographic appearances may be exactly those of a Wilms' tumour (Fig. 17·8). It is important that these tumours, whatever their nature, be distinguished from Wilms' tumour (although this is usually possible only after excision) to avoid unnecessary chemotherapy and irradiation (Bolande *et al.*, 1967, 1972; Hilton & Keeling, 1973) (see also p. 515).

5. **Horseshoe kidney**

This rarely presents as a palpable mass, but a Wilms' tumour may arise in such a kidney (Eliason & Stevens, 1944) and may give rise to diagnostic confusion not entirely resolved by angiography (see also extrarenal Wilms' tumours and horseshoe kidneys, p. 000). In the series reported by Hardwick & Stowens (1961) no less than 6 out of 81 Wilms' tumours arose outside the kidney, and Shashikumar *et al.* (1974) collected reports of 20 cases of Wilms' tumour arising in a horseshoe kidney.

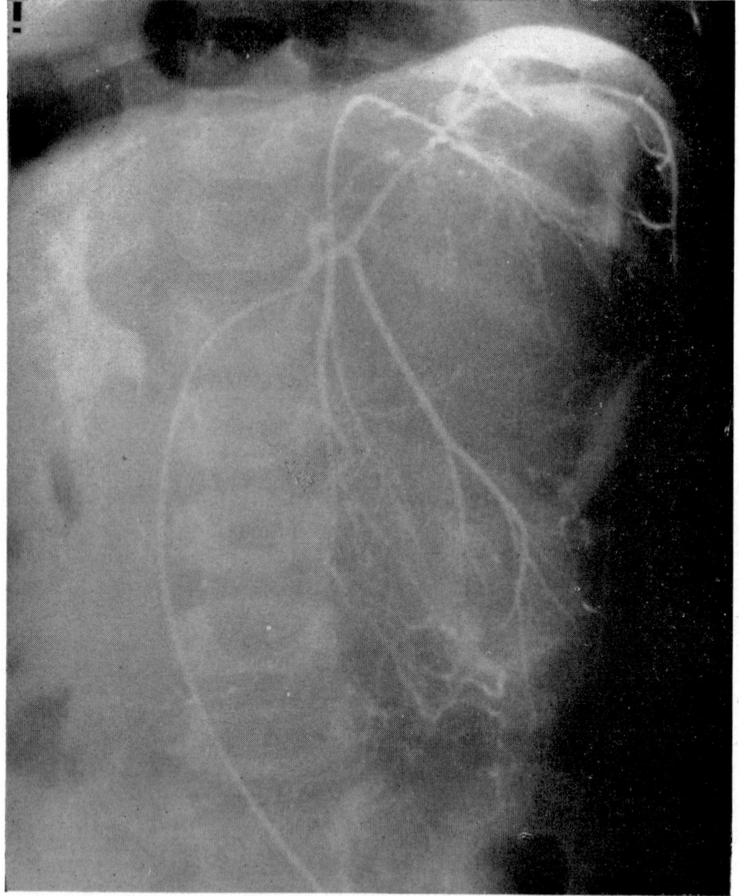

Figure 17.8. MESENCHYMAL HAMARTOMA; arteriogram showing a huge left kidney with stretched arcuate vessels and moderate distortion of the calyces.

6. Perirenal haematoma

A history of severe trauma, and haematuria or signs of blood loss, are usually apparent, and the early investigation of renal trauma by angiography which is now established practice makes it possible to identify the rare case in which trauma and a perirenal mass mimic a Wilms' tumour, or are in fact the result of traumatic rupture of such a tumour.

7. Splenomegaly

This usually presents no diagnostic difficulty, even when grossly enlarged or irregular in outline, but a Wilms' tumour in the left kidney can be mistaken for an enlarged spleen. If the cause of the 'splenomegaly' cannot be established, or if there is any uncertainty as to the nature of the mass, there should be no hesitation in obtaining a pyelogram and so avoid delay in the diagnosis of a tumour.

8. **Retroperitoneal teratoma**
This rare lesion can be shown by angiography to be extrarenal, and usually displaces the kidney and its calyces in the same way as other retroperitoneal tumours (see neuroblastoma, p. 554). Its extrarenal situation alone will exclude a Wilms' tumour, except in those rare instances (less than 1%) when a Wilms' tumour arises outside the kidney (see p. 497). On even rarer occasions a teratoma arises in the kidney itself (Scott, 1955; Dehner, 1973).

9. **Xanthogranulomatous pyelonephritis (retroperitoneal xanthogranuloma)**
This rare condition (Habib *et al.*, 1968; Graivier & Vargas, 1972; Kahn, 1973) can be mistaken for Wilms' tumour, for the commonest site of the lesion is in retroperitoneal tissues (Bissada & Fried, 1973), and it may present as a large renal mass in young children, although more commonly in an older age group (in 4 of the 19 cases reported the patient was less than six years old). Clinically the findings may be very similar to a Wilms' tumour, but the presence of urinary tract obstruction, renal calculi, overt pyobacilluria, and calyceal dilatation without gross displacement or distortion, are generally sufficient to exclude Wilms' tumour.

WILMS' TUMOUR IN INFANCY

The diagnosis of Wilms' tumour in this age group is complicated by two groups of conditions:
1. Non-neoplastic or non-renal lesions presenting in infancy, which may resemble a Wilms' tumour clinically.
2. A group of more or less distinct renal 'neoplasms' related to Wilms' tumour, but differing in their pathogenesis, morphology and/or behaviour.

1. **Non-neoplastic or non-renal lesions**
These conditions are recognized causes of a renal or peri-renal mass. Some have been mentioned above, but in approximate order of frequency in neonates or infants, they are as follows:
Dysplastic (multicystic) kidney;
Mesenchymal (fetal) hamartoma (p. 510);
Retroperitoneal lymphangiomatous (or chylous) hamartoma (p. 674);
Perirenal haematoma (p. 512);
Renal vein thrombosis;
'Pseudocyst' of the adrenal gland.

Dysplastic kidney

The most common palpable renal mass in neonates is enlargement due to 'unilateral multicystic dysplasia' associated with an atretic ureter (Griscom, 1965; Kyaw, 1974). The diagnosis can be made on the classical triad: a palpable renal mass with no excretory function on that side, absence of the ureter on retrograde pyelography, and absence or marked hypoplasia of the related renal artery as demonstrated by angiography (Kyaw, 1974).

This sporadic unilateral form of dysplasia is distinct from familial bilateral polycystic kidneys, which typically presents in adult life, and from a multilocular cyst of the kidney (p. 509). However, in sporadic 'unilateral' dysplasia, some dysplasia of lesser degree in the opposite kidney can often be demonstrated by thorough investigation.

Perirenal haematoma

In this age group, it is usually the result of the trauma of birth in a patient with a perinatal coagulopathy, and a similar cause has been suggested for the condition referred to as a 'pseudocyst of the adrenal gland', of which ten cases have been reported in the literature (Levin, Collins *et al.*, 1974). In both these conditions pyelography usually shows at least some evidence of excretion, without distortion of the calyces, while angiography can be expected to exclude those in which the site of the haemorrhage was extrarenal.

Renal vein thrombosis

This causes total absence of excretion on the affected side. Although a palpable abdominal mass and the occurrence of haematuria may suggest a tumour, aortography and vena cavography usually show not only absence of a tumour circulation, but also absence of any demonstrable renal artery and vein on the affected side (McDonald & Tarar, 1974; Lang, 1974).

Confirmatory evidence of renal vein thrombosis can usually be obtained from the history, e.g. maternal diabetes, a recent episode of severe dehydration, and from haematological evidence of haemoconcentration, leucocytosis, thrombocytopenia and fibrin degradation products (Miller, Tremman *et al.*, 1974).

Nevertheless, it may not be possible to exclude a neoplasm with certainty, in which case exploration is indicated. It is recognized that nephrectomy for unilateral cases of renal vein thrombosis is not essential; it may prove to be desirable, in at least some cases, in removing a kidney which is necrotic and a current source of toxic breakdown products, and which may become sclerotic and a cause of hypertension (Johannessen, 1974).

Some return of function in the affected kidney has been demonstrated in those treated conservatively (Belman *et al.*, 1970), but as yet there is insufficient data to determine whether this is the best treatment in infancy, nor the proportion of cases in this age group in which nephrectomy may subsequently become necessary.

Heparinization is recommended when disseminated intravascular coagulation is still present, and transfusions of platelets are also indicated.

The place of operative thrombectomy has yet to be determined, but in view of the poor overall survival rate in bilateral cases, may lead to improved results (Thompson *et al.*, 1975).

2. Neoplasms related to Wilms' tumour

It has become apparent in the last 10 years that 'congenital Wilms' tumour' comprises several tumorous conditions, recently clarified and classified by Bolande (1974) as follows:

(*i*) *Congenital mesoblastic nephroma of infancy* (syn. fetal renal hamartoma, Wigger, 1969; leiomyomatous hamartoma, Bolande, 1973)
More than 70 examples have been reported (Bogdan *et al.*, 1973). Often large, and sometimes massive, this tumour is usually diagnosed in the first few months of life, and can be distinguished from typical Wilms' tumour by its earlier presentation, the firm-to-hard homogeneous texture, and by its composition of predominantly fibrous mesenchymal stroma.

Although lacking a capsule and tending to infiltrate perihilar tissues, the great majority are benign. Nevertheless a few are more aggressive, less mature, hypercellular, recur locally after nephrectomy, and/or produce metastases (Fu & Kay, 1973; Joshi *et al.*, 1973; Walter & Richard, 1973; Bolande, 1974). Even if these few are exceptions, their existence shows that this entity cannot be considered as a simple hamartoma, and confirms the necessity for nephrectomy without delay.

Beckwith (1974) concluded that the histology ranged from a benign 'mesoblastic nephroma' to an unequivocally malignant tumour, and that the tumour is usually curable by nephrectomy alone, but when it is not certain that the tumour has been excised *in toto* together with a clear margin of uninvolved tissue, adjuvant therapy is indicated, e.g. as for Wilms' tumour.

(*ii*) *Well-differentiated epithelial nephroblastoma*
Less common than (i) above, this is composed of well-differentiated epithelial tubules or cysts, with an inconspicuous stroma. Three types are described:
(*a*) *Multilocular cystic nephroma* (syn. multilocular cyst (p. 509); polycystic nephroblastoma). Clearly encapsulated by compressed fibrotic renal tissue, this tumour is composed of closely packed cysts of various sizes (Fowler, 1970) lined by low cuboidal epithelium (Fig. 17.6b).
(*b*) *'Tubular' Wilms' tumour*, with a pattern similar to (a) but with cystic spaces lined by cells resembling those of mature renal tubules.
(*c*) *Papillary adenoma of the kidney*, resembling the 'tubular Wilms' tumour' except for the prominence of convoluted papillary projections lining the cysts.

(iii) Nodular renal blastema and diffuse nephroblastomatosis

The basic lesion is a discrete subcapsular nodule of primitive epithelium (resembling a miniscule Wilms' tumour), mostly found in young infants, sometimes unilateral but more often bilateral (Bove *et al.*, 1969). Although usually a microscopic finding at autopsy or in nephrectomy specimens, lesions large enough to be identified with the naked eye at operation were seen in the Index Series. This lesion, also called 'focal dysplasia', may account for some of the cases reported in the literature as 'bilateral' Wilms' tumour.

The nodules of renal blastema may be single, or few in number, or in some cases large, numerous and confluent, constituting 'nephroblastomatosis' which may be identified radiographically (Neuhauser, 1960), and has been described as 'diffuse bilateral Wilms' tumours' (Anderson *et al.*, 1968). This lesion has also been associated with trisomy 18 (Bove *et al.*, 1969), with agenesis of the spleen and malformations of the liver, or in a few heredo-familial cases, with visceromegaly, hypoglycaemia and nesidioblastosis.

There is a distinct possibility that a true Wilms' tumour can develop in a focus of 'nodular renal blastema', particularly in lesions which fail to differentiate or to regress and disappear in early infancy (Bolande, 1974).

It should also be clearly stated that true Wilms' tumours can occur in infancy.

DIFFERENTIATION OF WILMS' TUMOUR FROM OTHER ABDOMINAL TUMOURS (Table 17.1)

1. Neuroblastoma

Arising close to the midline, in the adrenal gland or in the adjacent retroperitoneal tissues, this is typically a 'horizontal' tumour and often crosses the midline, rather than a 'vertical' mass such as a Wilms' tumour. The angiographic findings, e.g. displacement of the calyces, rather than the dispersion and distortion typical of Wilms' tumour (Fig. 17.5a) and the arterial supply from other than the main renal artery (Fig. 18.12, p. 555) are usually diagnostic.

On the rare occasions when a neuroblastoma arises in the kidney it can only be distinguished before nephrectomy when the level of catecholamines in the urine is significantly elevated (see p. 551), or when marrow smears or biopsy of other metastatic lesions (e.g. in peripheral lymph nodes) enable the diagnosis of neuroblastoma to be made (p. 554) on other evidence.

One intrarenal neuroblastoma occurred in the Index Series, and was not identified until the tumour was examined histologically.

2. Retroperitoneal sarcoma

The extrarenal origin of such a tumour can usually be demonstrated by angiography, but the histological diagnosis is only made following exploration and biopsy.

3. **Phaeochromocytoma**

Although most phaeochromocytomas are small, rarely palpable and typically present with episodes of hypertension, sweating, etc. (p. 565), in exceptional cases it is large and malignant, and may resemble a neuroblastoma or Wilms' tumour. The extrarenal site can almost always be demonstrated by angiography, and the diagnosis can be established before operation on biochemical evidence of metabolites excreted in the urine (see p. 565).

4. **Hepatoblastoma and hepatocarcinoma**

A Wilms' tumour on the right side can closely resemble a hepatic tumour, particularly when it arises in the upper pole of the kidney and extends upwards behind the liver displacing it downwards and forwards. When this occurs the liver appears to be much enlarged and in fact it accounts for most of the mass palpable in the right hypochondrium or the epigastrium. Here again, the correct diagnosis can be made by angiography which in this case may include selective hepatic arteriography (Fig. 19.5, p. 604).

5. **Malignant renal tumours other than Wilms' tumour**

These are exceptionally rare in children and account for less than 1% of renal malignancies. A clear cell adenocarcinoma (p. 529) is one example, and at present there is no way in which this tumour can be identified with certainty before nephrectomy, except perhaps its greater tendency to cause pain and gross haematuria, both of which can occur in Wilms' tumour.

6. **Lymphosarcoma of the kidneys**

Dissemination of lymphosarcoma involving one or both kidneys usually develops in the later stages, after the appearance of hepatosplenomegaly or generalized peripheral lymphadenopathy. On rare occasions a renal tumour due to lymphosarcoma is the presenting feature and may closely simulate Wilms' tumour, sometimes bilaterally as reported by Jaffe & Tefft (1973).

Burkitt's tumour is recognized as a rare cause of a renal or perirenal retroperitoneal mass, and is not infrequently bilateral (p. 328).

In both these lymphomas biopsy of any enlarged superficial nodes should precede laparotomy, but unless angiography clearly indicates that the mass is extrarenal, the correct diagnosis can only be made when the kidney(s) is explored, or following nephrectomy.

The possibility that bilateral renal tumours may be due to metastatic or generalized lymphosarcoma (p. 173) rather than Wilms' tumour should be borne in mind.

Other malignant tumours which very rarely arise in or involve the kidney and form a renal mass include intrarenal malignant teratomas and disseminated histiocytosis (p. 220). Leukaemic infiltrations may also occur, but usually late in the course in the disease, and in such cases renal involvement is bilateral and diffuse rather than a single unilateral mass.

Summary

Experience has shown that diagnostic difficulties which occasionally arise in a patient with a Wilms' tumour are as follows:

(*a*) Errors in differentiating clinically between a Wilms' tumour of the left kidney and an enlarged spleen;

(*b*) Occasional difficulties, both clinical and radiological, in differentiating a Wilms' tumour from a neuroblastoma;

(*c*) Mistaking a polycystic or dysplastic kidney for a Wilms' tumour, and vice versa;

(*d*) Difficulty in making the correct diagnosis before operation when the tumour is unusually small, impalpable, and presents with haematuria;

(*e*) Delay in recognizing haematuria as a symptom of a Wilms' tumour, accepting it as evidence of focal nephritis, or trauma when there is a history of moderate but irrelevant injury.

STAGING

Several systems of staging have been described, and the system used in the Index Series is very similar to the schema employed in the National Wilms' Tumour Study (D'Angio, 1972).

Stage I. Tumour confined to the kidney and completely resected without rupture or spillage, without any macroscopic residual tumour left *in situ*, no metastases found in lymph nodes removed at the time of nephrectomy, and no evidence of pulmonary metastases.

Stage II. Tumour extending outside the kidney but completely removed, i.e. local extension beyond the capsule, metastases in para-aortic lymph nodes, or extension along the renal veins but removed without discernable embolism.

Stage III. Residual tumour confined to the abdomen; this category includes patients with any one or more of the following:

(i) Biopsy of the tumour performed before definitive excision;
(ii) Rupture and spillage of tumour cells during excision;
(iii) Metastasis in nodes beyond the ipsilateral para-aortic nodes;
(iv) Implanted metastases on peritoneal surfaces;
(v) Infiltration of organs or tissues not completely excised.

Stage IV. Distant metastases, i.e. blood-borne, in lung, bone or brain.

Stage V. Bilateral tumours, either at the time of presentation, or a second tumour appearing later in the remaining contralateral kidney.

The TNM classification

The system listed by the U.I.C.C. (1973) for Wilms' tumour is more elaborate and based on pre-operative clinical and radiological information, although operative findings and histological data, including the presence or absence of regional lymph node metastases are appended.

This system is as follows:

T0 No evidence of primary tumour.

T1 No enlargement of kidney; urography shows minimal calyceal abnormality.

T2 Kidney enlarged with no limitation of mobility, or urography shows gross deformity affecting one or more calyces, or displacement of the ureter.

T3 Kidney enlarged and mobility limited without complete fixation, or there is evidence of vascular compression, e.g. a varicocele.

T4 Kidney enlarged with complete fixation.

NX When it is impossible to assess regional nodes, the symbol NX is used (subsequently modified to NX+ or NX− after operation).

N0 No deformity of regional nodes on lymphangiography.

N1 Regional nodes deformed on lymphangiography.

M0 No evidence of distant metastases.

M1 Distant metastases.

TREATMENT OF WILMS' TUMOUR

The plan employed in the Index Series has been in use for some twelve years at the Royal Children's Hospital. Modifications based on our experience and on reports from other centres have been incorporated, e.g. the addition (in 1969) of recurring courses of cytotoxic agents after definitive primary treatment.

Surgery, chemotherapy and radiotherapy are usually employed, although the details have varied minimally from one case to another. The place of pre-operative chemotherapy is still debatable (see p. 109), but has been adopted because of the advantage that excision of the kidney is covered by cytotoxic agents theoretically capable of affecting tumour emboli liberated during operative handling of the tumour. The contrary view is that chemotherapy should not be commenced before the histological diagnosis has been established. However, the accuracy of pre-operative diagnosis in the Index Series, chiefly on angiographic evidence, is approximately 97%. In the other 3%, with a malformation or a benign lesion, chemotherapy was discontinued as soon as the correct diagnosis was known, with no known harm to the patient.

In the Index Series, pre-operative chemotherapy has been routinely employed and the current protocol, in use since 1971, is set out in brief in Table 17.4.

Table 17.4. Wilms' tumour; summary of the current protocol of treatment

	Actinomycin D		Vincristine
Primary course*			
Day 1	0·5 mg/m² (20 mcg/kg)	Day 1	1·75 mg/m² (0·07 mg/kg)
	Operation		
Day 3	0·5 mg/m² (20 mcg/kg)	Day 8	1·75 mg/m² (0·07 mg/kg)
Day 5	0·5 mg/m² (20 mcg/kg)	Day 15	1·75 mg/m² (0·07 mg/kg)
Day 8	0·5 mg/m² (20 mcg/kg)	Day 22	1·75 mg/m² (0·07 mg/kg)
Total	2·0 mg/m² (80 mcg/kg)	Total	7·0 mg/m² (0·28 mg/kg)
Radiotherapy	**Commencing on Day 22**		
Standard secondary course			
Day 1	0·5 mg/m² (20 mcg/kg)	Day 1	1·75 mg/m² (0·07 mg/kg)
Day 3	0·5 mg/m² (20 mcg/kg)		
Day 5	0·5 mg/m² (20 mcg/kg)		
Day 8	0·5 mg/m² (20 mcg/kg)	Day 8	1·75 mg/m² (0·07 mg/kg)
Repeated secondary courses			
At 10 weeks, 4 months; 6 months, 9 months; 12 months, 15 months	after commencing primary treatment		

* Full blood examination and platelet counts are performed on days 1, 7, 11 and 14, and before each secondary course.

The most recent amendment has been the addition of six secondary courses of chemotherapy (DTM and VCR) given at 10 weeks, 4 months, 6 months, 9 months, 12 months and 16 months after initial diagnosis and treatment. The standard secondary course is four doses of actinomycin D (DTM 20 mcg/kg) given on days 1, 3, 5 and 8, and two doses of vincristine (VCR 1·75 mg/m²) on days 1 and 8.

Specific points in treatment

Immediate consultation between the radiologist, chemotherapist and surgeon during aortography and inferior vena cavography, makes it possible to give the initial injections of chemotherapy via the Seldinger catheter while it is still in the inferior vena cava. Blood for all investigations can also be obtained at the same time, thus avoiding unnecessary physical and psychological trauma.

Administration of cytotoxic drugs in both the primary and later courses requires careful monitoring of the peripheral blood before each injection (see p. 114). Although neutropenia and thrombocytopenia are perhaps the most important toxic side-effects of these drugs, infection (which may be largely the result of reduced immunological competence) can cause considerable morbidity and even mortality. Troublesome rashes amounting to exfoliative dermatitis may develop; oral ulceration and secondary moniliasis may occur; intussusception also may occur and has been attributed to altered motility and/or enlarged Peyer's patches. There is almost always some loss of hair, but a suitable wig can be worn until it has grown again.

The treatment employed in most cases in the Index Series commences with pre-operative chemotherapy on day 1, operation on day 3, and radiotherapy commencing on day 22. Secondary courses of chemotherapy are given even in uncomplicated cases in which complete excision has apparently been performed. The calculation of doses is ideally based on surface area rather than body weight (see nomogram, p. 934).

The standard primary course of chemotherapy is shown in Table 17.4.

Modification of chemotherapy

The dosages may be modified according to the age of the patient or the stage of the disease.

Age

In patients less than 18 months of age at the time of diagnosis, the injection of vincristine on day 22 may be omitted, and secondary courses may also be omitted.

Stage of disease

In general, the plan outlined in Table 17.3 can be applied to Stages I to IV, with the addition in Stage IV of an extra dose of actinomycin D (0·5 mg/m^2 or 20 mcg/kg) on day 12, i.e. in the primary course; this extra dose is also optional for patients less than 18 months of age.

Operation

Access is important and a transabdominal transperitoneal approach is usually used, the length of the incision varying with the size of the tumour. In general, the supra-umbilical incision extends from the lateral extremity of the abdomen on the side of the tumour, across the midline to the lateral edge of the rectus on the opposite side.

Various views have been expressed regarding the position of the patient on the operating table; most advocate a normal supine position, or slight elevation of the side with the tumour to facilitate its delivery. However, elevation of the opposite side, suggested by Swenson, causes the tumour to fall away from the IVC and access to the renal vein, an important landmark in the dissection, is somewhat easier.

Occasionally an abdomino-thoracic incision maybe of some advantage, but this carries with it some slight theoretical risk of contaminating with tumour cells a previously uninvolved pleural cavity.

The renal vein should be ligated as soon as possible so as to minimize intra-operative dissemination. However, closure of the vein causes increasing congestion and some increase in the risk of rupture of the tumour. The renal artery should therefore be clamped as soon as possible after the vein has been tied.

Metal clips inserted after the nephrectomy are useful in identifying the extent of the tumour bed, and guide the radiotherapist by delineating the area to be irradiated.

Enlarged lymph nodes in or near the renal hilum, or in front of the vertebral bodies, should be resected, but regional clearance of the nodes has not been our practice. Martin's observations (1969) suggest that this should be considered in view of the high incidence of small metastases in lymph nodes in the adjacent retroperitoneal tissues.

The opposite kidney should also be inspected, but in our experience involvement of the contralateral kidney does not usually appear until several months or years after the initial nephrectomy. This could be taken as an indication that the contralateral kidney should always be carefully explored, and Martin's findings of tumour tissue in the contralateral kidney in 40% of patients would support this view (Ehrlich & Goodwin, 1973).

Radiotherapy

Megavoltage therapy is usually commenced on day 22, but may be delayed or interrupted when the patient's general condition is poor, the neutrophil count is less than 1500/cmm, or the platelet count less than 75,000/cmm.

The volume irradiated includes the tumour bed, the para-aortic lymph nodes and inferior vena cava, extending from the tenth thoracic vertebra to the iliac crest and from the flank to 2 cm on the contralateral side of the midline. Metal clips inserted at operation and skin markers are useful in planning the area to be treated.

The usual dose is 3000 rads in 20 fractions given as five doses a week, using anterior and posterior opposed fields. In children less than 18 months old the dosage is reduced, to 2000 rads for those less than 6 months old, and 2500 rads for those between 6 and 18 months of age.

When the tumour extends across the midline the whole of the abdomen is irradiated to a total of 3000 rads, shielding the contralateral kidney so that it does not receive more than 1500 rads. For bilateral tumours (see below) the whole abdomen receives 2000 rads in 13 fractions, given on five days a week. After 2000 rads the renal tissue remaining is shielded and the side on which nephrectomy was performed then receives a further 1000 rads in seven treatments.

Special care is taken to shield unaffected renal tissue, the gonads, and the ends of growing bones.

Treatment of recurrences or metastases

Local recurrence at or near the site of the primary (Soper, 1961) carries a serious prognosis, and our current plan is a course of chemotherapy, not necessarily the same cytotoxic agents as used initially, followed by exploration to determine the extent of the recurrence and to remove as much tumour as possible, and a further course of irradiation to the area affected.

Pulmonary metastases. Irradiation of the whole of both lung fields is given (usually to a total of 2000 rads) with an additional 1000 rads directed at any localized concentration of metastases. Concurrent chemotherapy is given, not necessarily those agents used initially.

Experience has shown that pulmonary metastases are not necessarily fatal and an aggressive policy is justified (Wedemeyer *et al.*, 1968; Martin & Rickham, 1970; O'Gorman Hughes, Bowring *et al.*, 1973). If they persist after radiation of the thorax and chemotherapy, they should be excised if their number, size and distribution makes this surgically feasible (Haas & Jackson, 1968). In arriving at such a decision tomography is essential.

A Wilms' tumour in the opposite kidney, appearing after treatment of the original tumour, is treated by a course of chemotherapy followed by exploration to determine the extent and to remove as much as feasible, by heminephrectomy or such modifications as the size and number of areas affected may require (see treatment of bilateral tumours p. 524).

Disseminated metastases. In some instances treatment may still be feasible and surgical excision may play a part, in general preceded by chemotherapy and followed by radiotherapy.

Follow-up

The patient is followed closely throughout the 16 months of active treatment.

1. The peripheral blood should be monitored during all courses of chemotherapy and while receiving radiotherapy, neutropenia and/or thrombocytopenia being carefully noted (see p. 116).
2. Radiographs of the chest are taken at intervals of 1 month during the first year, at intervals of 3 months during the second year, every 6 months during the third year, and then once a year for a further two years.
3. Renal function is assessed before each secondary course of chemotherapy, and at 18 months after operation.

The patient is encouraged to lead a normal life. In boys there is the problem of sport and the possibility of injury to the remaining kidney. The concensus is that 'school' football is permissible, but that boys should be encouraged to take up sports with less body contact, both at school and in later years.

BILATERAL WILMS' TUMOURS

The diagnosis of bilateral tumours is made in a variety of circumstances. Depending upon the time at which the diagnosis of bilateral tumours is made, patients can be placed into one of the following categories.

1. Bilateral tumours are suspected early, either clinically or as a result of angiographic studies (p. 507), and confirmed at operation.
2. A tumour in the contralateral kidney is not suspected until inspection of the kidneys at exploration reveals bilateral involvement, usually as one or two small nodules in the contralateral kidney.
3. A tumour in the opposite kidney only becomes apparent months or years after the initial nephrectomy. There were two such patients in the Index Series.

Although involvement of both kidneys is undoubtedly an unfavourable prognostic sign, the outlook is not necessarily hopeless. Controversy has long existed regarding the pathogenesis of bilateral Wilms' tumour; some have suggested that the condition represents multicentric origin of at least two primary tumours, while others hold that the tumour(s) in the contralateral kidney are metastatic (Scott, 1955). It is probable that each of these explanations may be valid in different patients (Leen & Williams, 1971).

In a collective review of bilateral Wilms' tumour, Ragab, Vietti *et al.* (1972) noted an incidence of 77 in 1746 cases, or 4·4%. They recommended that the contralateral kidney should be carefully inspected and palpated at the time of the initial nephrectomy, as described by Martin & Reyes (1969), and that as most contralateral tumours appear in the nine months following the first nephrectomy, an excretory pyelogram should be performed every three months during the first year after operation, and at less frequent intervals for some years thereafter.

An aggressive approach is warranted unless the clinical situation is clearly hopeless. All three methods of treatment should be employed, but modified by the extent of involvement of the second kidney, the time at which it appears, and the particular circumstances.

The following surgical procedures on the second kidney may be required:

(*a*) Partial excision, removing the portion of the kidney containing the tumour, if single;

(*b*) Heminephrectomy when one or more nodules, or a large mass of tumour, is confined to one area;

(*c*) Enucleation of the tumour or tumours, if large, multiple or scattered and beyond the scope of partial or heminephrectomy.

Chemotherapy. When the contralateral tumour first appears after the initial nephrectomy, the regular secondary courses of chemotherapy may be continued, or augmented by the addition of another cytotoxic agent.

Radiotherapy may be given in a dosage calculated to avoid fibrosis and preserve the function in the remaining kidney.

Renal transplantation. It is generally agreed that renal transplantation in Wilms' tumour (DeLorimier *et al.*, 1968) should be reserved for children with tumours in both kidneys, in whom all other forms of treatment (unilateral nephrectomy, uni- or bilateral partial or heminephrectomy, chemotherapy and radiotherapy) have been pursued as far as possible without success, before removing such renal tissue as remains (Ehrlich *et al.*, 1974). In a series of 103 cases of which 10% were bilateral (Fay *et al.*, 1973), renal transplantation (following bilateral nephrectomy) was performed in 6 children, 4 of whom died in the following 2 years.

The prognosis without transplantation is by no means hopeless and Vietti (quoted by Sullivan, Hussey & Ayala, 1973) reported 'cures' in 21 out of 52 patients with bilateral tumours.

Complications

Apart from the usual surgical complications and direct side effects of chemotherapy, there are several which have come to be recognized as particularly associated with current methods of treating children with a Wilms' tumour.

Intussusception, often jejunal, has been reported on a number of occasions, and occurred in two patient in the Index Series, possibly as the result of mucosal oedema or alteration in motility caused by chemotherapy.

Intestinal obstruction due to adhesions occurred in two patients in the Index Series in the year following nephrectomy. Both were and are free of tumour.

Hepatitis with marked hepatomegaly simulating massive hepatic metastases occurred in two patients in the Index Series; the more recent is better documented and was as follows.

A girl aged 3½ presented with a Wilms' tumour in the right kidney infiltrating the right lobe of the liver and the under surface of the diaphragm. Nephrectomy was accompanied by chemotherapy vincristine according to protocol (Table 17.4) followed by megavoltage radiotherapy to the bed of the tumour, including the liver to the right of the midline, to a dose of 3000 rads in 20 fractions over 31 days. Two weeks after radiotherapy was completed, malaise and anorexia appeared, together with enlargement of the liver to 6 cm below the costal margin in the epigastrium, a high swinging fever to 38·5°C and elevated SGOT: 182–234 U/l; (Hb 10·3 g/dl; platelets 15,000; WCC 7200).

A liver scan (^{99m}Tc) showed 'only a rim of liver . . . the rest appears to have been replaced; probably there is massive infiltration with tumour'. Selective hepatic arteriography showed poor filling of the superior and lateral areas of the right lobe, indicating 'secondary deposits, an abscess or the effects of radiotherapy'. A needle biopsy of this area of the liver was obtained at the same procedure, guided by fluoroscopic control, and the three cores of liver obtained were reported to show 'foci of fibrosis infiltrated with a small number of round cells, consistent with non-specific tissue injury'.

In the following week the liver decreased in size and a second scan two weeks later showed a decrease in the size of the 'defect'; the SGOT fell to 18 U/l during the same period; fever disappeared and appetite and general condition improved. The patient had a similar but less severe episode following a subsequent secondary course of chemotherapy, and again no pathogen was isolated from blood, stools, urine, throat swabs or rectal swabs, repeated on several occasions.

Having been made aware of misleading findings in a similar occurrence following successful hepatic lobectomy for a hepatoblastoma (Cohen, D., personal communication, 1973), needle biopsy was used to test the evidence of scanning and arteriography, and metastasis was thus excluded. As cytotoxic agents are also immunosuppressants, general or local suppression of immune mechanisms could lead to an opportunistic infection causing hepatitis, and cytomegalovirus has been incriminated in similar circumstances (Foster, Ralston *et al.*, 1972).

The most likely explanation, as demonstrated by Tefft, Mitus and Jaffe, (1971), is exacerbation of the toxic effects of actinomycin D (disproportionate to the dosage) as a result of damage to the parenchyma of the liver by irradiation; as actinomycin D is chiefly detoxified in the liver, its cytotoxic action is thus prolonged or enhanced, causing further damage to liver cells.

The possibility that apparent metastases can be simulated by some other condition should be borne in mind when enlargement of the liver occurs in a child receiving chemotherapy following excision of a malignant abdominal tumour.

Bone tumours induced by irradiation (Arlen, Shan & Higinbotham, 1972) have occurred, particularly in children with recurrent pulmonary metastases treated by radiotherapy. Osteoblastomas of the ribs and osteochondroma of the ilium have been reported, and in the one case in the Index Series the tumour was an osteosarcoma of the scapula.

A boy aged 3 years 8 months presented in 1965 with a large Wilms' tumour arising in a dysplastic right kidney. At operation, the kidney and tumour were removed, and the left kidney was found to contain several small nodules, one of which was removed and proved to be Wilms' tumour tissue. At a second operation the left kidney was explored and two further nodules of Wilms' tumour removed. Bilateral pulmonary metastases appeared 6 months later (October, 1965) and were treated with 2500 rads, of which 600 rads were deep x-ray therapy and 1900 rads megavoltage therapy (4 MeV). One month later the metastases were no longer demonstrable radiographically.

Six months later (May, 1966) a further single metastasis appeared in the right upper lobe and this was treated with 3000 rads of megavoltage irradiation (4 MeV) in six increments over 11 days, with subsequent disappearance of the metastasis and apparent cure.

Five years later (December, 1971) a swelling appeared in the right scapula and proved to be an osteosarcoma; pulmonary metastases developed and death followed within 12 months.

Tefft, Vawter & Mitus (1968) stated that a second primary tumour is likely to arise in 5% of all children who survive for more than two years after receiving radiotherapy in a dose exceeding 1000 rads. In most of the cases reported in the literature the total dose delivered was considerably higher than this figure, and in the case from the Index Series (above) the total dose to the thorax was 5500 rads.

RESULTS OF TREATMENT IN WILMS' TUMOUR

These are based on a retrospective and prospective study of the 122 patients with Wilms' tumour in the Index Series. Up to 1959, 43 patients had been treated, with 36 deaths and 7 long term survivors.

Since 1959, nearly all patients have received cytotoxic therapy before operation (p. 519). Experience has shown that patients who remain free of disease for a period of two yeaıs from the date of nephrectomy have an excellent prognosis with almost 100% survival.

From 1959 through 1971, 79 patients were treated; 68 are available for assessment of the two-year survival rate, and of these 68, 56 were treated 'according to protocol'. There are 37 survivors and 19 died. The survival rate of 66% to the end of 1969 (i.e. at least two years survival) compares more than favourably with the 1945–1955 survival; 11%, and the 1955–1959 group; 23%. Nevertheless, 66% is far from ideal, and dissatisfaction with these results was a major factor in extending the programme of treatment to include secondary courses of chemotherapy. Time will tell whether this has improved our results, but recent reports indicate that survival rates as high as 86–90% should be obtainable.

In the period 1967–1969, there were 25 'protocol' patients with 20 survivors, i.e. a current survival rate of 80%. Of the five who died, one had bilateral tumours, one died of sepsis soon after operation; the others were aged 4, 6 and 7 years respectively. In the 7-year old, local spread was present (Stage II) at the time of nephrectomy.

PROGNOSIS

The following factors appear to be important:

1. *The age at diagnosis*

The outlook is worse in those more than four years of age, and generally better in younger patients and infants (see Table 17·5).

2. *Mode of presentation*

In the Index Series the prognosis appeared to be worse when a mass was first found by the parents, and better when found during a medical examination. This may simply reflect an assumption (not supported by the next paragraph) that a doctor can identify a small renal mass whereas it has to be larger, and presumably of longer standing, to be palpated by a parent.

3. *The size of the tumour*

Although some reviews have shown a poorer prognosis in those with a large tumour, this has not been the case in the Index Series, in which the weight of the tumour somewhat surprisingly seemed to have little or no bearing on the outcome.

Table 17.5. Wilms' tumour; results in 56 patients at least two years after treatment according to the protocol in Table 17.4

Age (years)	No. of patients	Survivors Number	Survivors Rate %
0–1	6	4	66·6*
1–2	13	10	77
2–3	10	7	70
3–4	12	8	66
4–5	6	5	83
5+	9	3	33

* One post-operative death due to cytotoxic therapy.

4. *The degree of histological differentiation*

There appears to be a slightly worse prognosis when the tumour is undifferentiated, as suggested by Hardwick & Stowens (1961) who proposed a complex classification based on the degree of differentiation of both epithelial and stromal components.

The tumours in the Index Series have been divided histologically into three classes: undifferentiated, extremely well-differentiated, and average-differentiation. It is possible to show a significantly worse outcome in the undifferentiated group; the difference between the well-differentiated group and tumours of average-differentiation was not significant. It would seem that with modern methods the outcome is much more likely to be determined by the age, the stage of the disease and the plan of treatment than by the histological appearance or the size of the tumour.

5. *The stage of the disease*

Although the prognosis in Stages III and IV is naturally worse than in the early stages, the outlook is by no means hopeless. There are reports of long term (3–5 year) survival, free of disease, in patients with hepatic metastases Smith, Wara *et al.*, 1974), with pulmonary metastases (O'Gorman Hughes, Bowring *et al.*, 1973), and also in patients who develop both pulmonary *and* hepatic metastases following nephrectomy in Stage I or II (Wedemeyer, White *et al.*, 1968).

Aggressive surgical excision, including hepatic and pulmonary lobectomy when feasible, followed by radiotherapy to the site(s) of metastases, recurrent courses of combination chemotherapy, and possibly further operation ('second look' 3–6 months later) to determine whether the metastases have been controlled, offer the best prospect of cure.

6. *Histological findings in the tumour*
Recent studies at St. Jude's Hospital, Memphis, have indicated that those with microscopic invasion of the tumour capsule (or rupture before or at operation), may have a higher local recurrence rate, while those with a tumour in which intravascular invasion can be identified microscopically, appear to have a higher incidence of pulmonary metastases.

A prospective assessment of these criteria is currently being conducted on material from the American National Wilms' Tumour Study to determine whether re-staging after operation, on the basis of operative and histological findings, should be recommended.

The investigation and treatment of children with an abdominal mass, and in particular Wilms' tumour, may be modified in the future by improvements in techniques, or favourable results from trials already in progress. Some of these aspects, none of which has yet reached the stage of a firm recommendation, are as follows.

1. *Less 'invasive' methods of investigation*, replacing or augmenting percutaneous aortography and arteriography by echography, and/or tomography combined with excretory pyelography (Grossman, 1975).
2. *Preoperative radiotherapy* for 1–2 weeks in those with a very large Wilms' tumour, with the object of reducing its size, and thickening the 'capsule', in an attempt to decrease the incidence of 'spill' during operation.
3. *Omission of radiotherapy* (and perhaps chemotherapy) in Stage I Wilms' tumour in the first year of life, when all the evidence points to complete surgical excision.
4. *Incorporation of adriamycin*, from the beginning of chemotherapy, for patients in Stage II, III and IV.
5. *Cessation of recurring cycles of maintenance chemotherapy* earlier than 15 to 16 months in patients with Stage I Wilms' tumour in the younger age group, e.g. those less than 2 years of age.

The survival rates in Wilms' tumour are still improving, and these modifications could only gain acceptance if it were shown that none of them interferes with this improvement.

II. ADENOCARCINOMA OF THE KIDNEY
(syn. clear-cell carcinoma, papillary adenocarcinoma, hypernephroma, Grawitz' tumour)

AGE : SEX

This is a very rare tumour in childhood (Dehner *et al.*, 1970); most of those reported in children presented between 10 and 15 years, and the majority present in adult life (Shanberg, Srouji & Leberman, 1970). Manson *et al.*

(1970) reviewed the world literature and added three cases, making a total of 47 reported in children; Castellanos, Aron *et al.* (1974) found 150 cases, of which four were reasonably documented. Vawter (1969) provided a perspective of the incidence in a review of 434 renal tumours in children less than 14 years of age; 10 (i.e. 2·5 %) were clear cell carcinomas, in contrast to adults, in whom 80 % of renal tumours are hypernephromas. Castellanos, Aron *et al.* (1974) suggested a proportion of 6·6 % in children, while the figure for the Index Series is 0·8 %.

MACROSCOPIC APPEARANCES

The tumour is usually of moderate size, and the cut surface is fleshy pink in colour with areas of haemorrhage and necrosis. While some tumours appear to be encapsulated, others infiltrate through the renal capsule and into adjacent tissues.

MICROSCOPIC FINDINGS

In a 'clear cell' adenocarcinoma the cells are arranged diffusely in sheets, or more typically as papillary projections from delicate fibrovascular septa (Fig. 17.9). In some tumours the cells have dark nuclei and compact eosinophilic cytoplasm.

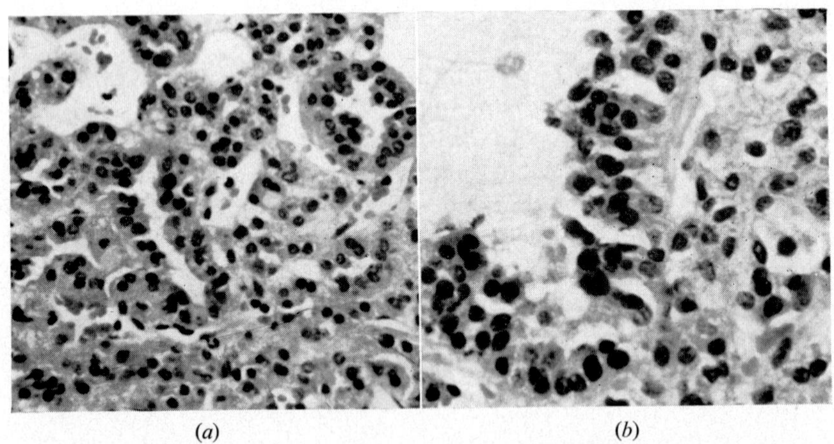

(*a*) (*b*)

Figure 17.9. CARCINOMA OF THE KIDNEY, from the only case in the Index Series; (*a*) cuboidal tumour cells with regular, round nuclei and abundant pale pink cytoplasm, arranged in tubules, sheets, and papillary formations (H & E. × 200); (*b*) a papillary glandular structure forming in a sheet of undifferentiated cells (H & E. × 300).

SPREAD

Local spread through the capsule of the tumour or into the substance of the kidney is a typical feature, and metastasis to the lungs occurs frequently. One and sometimes both forms of spread had occurred by the time of operation in 66% of the series reported by Dehner *et al.* (1970).

MODES OF PRESENTATION

1. *Gross painless haematuria* is a very typical feature and was a major part of the presenting picture in 16 (38%) of the cases reported by Manson *et al.* (1970). Dehner *et al.* (1970) found haematuria in 66% of the patients they reviewed.
2. *Pain* in the abdomen or loin occurred in 11 of 36 patients.
3. *A renal mass* was palpable in 26 of the 36 patients.
4. *General systemic symptoms* (loss of weight, anorexia, nausea and vomiting) were reported in 14 patients, and 4 were febrile.

DIAGNOSIS

Differentiation of adenocarcinoma from Wilms' tumour (p. 517) is of some importance. In childhood the latter is overwhelmingly the more common; in the Index Series the ratio of the two tumours was approximately 0·8 : 100, and in Vawter's review (1969) the figure was 2·3 : 100.

The peak age incidence is different, but there is sufficient overlap in the 5–10-year age group to make age alone an unreliable basis for differential diagnosis.

Gross haematuria occurs in a greater proportion of patients with an adenocarcinoma than those with a Wilms' tumour, but even after complete angiographic studies (p. 507) it is unlikely that these two tumours could be distinguished with certainty on radiological grounds. Adenocarcinoma thus represents an error of slightly more than 1% in the angiographic pre-operative diagnosis of Wilms' tumour.

PROGNOSIS

Although the number of cases reported is small, records date back to the time when treatment was confined to surgical excision, and even then the prognosis was not hopeless.

In the series reported by Manson *et al.*, 24 case histories were sufficiently documented for analysis; in 8 children the tumour was found at operation to be confined to the kidney and only one of these is known to have subsequently died of the disease. Of the 16 with metastasis at the time of operation, 11 died;

of the 5 survivors, only one had been followed for more than three years. The authors compared these results with a large series of adult cases and found the two groups to be very similar in prognosis, and in other respects.

Nygaard and Simon (1974) found reports of only 3 'cures' (5-year + survivors) among 43 cases in children less than 10 years of age, collected from the literature.

On the other hand, Dehner *et al.* (1970) reported a survival rate of 64% in children, and two of the four cases reported by Palma *et al.* (1970) appeared to be cures.

TREATMENT

Prompt nephrectomy is the most important step in treatment. When the tumour is confined to the kidney, and removable *in toto* without spillage, (Stage I) a survival rate of some 60–80% may be expected.

Radiotherapy does not appear to be of much benefit in adults, but has been used in some cases, and should probably be given to all patients in whom the tumour extended beyond the kidney.

Chemotherapy may be useful, but until recently (Talley, 1973) it has not been reported to be particularly effective in adults. In children it is probably desirable, but has not been shown to be essential.

In the Index Series there was only one case of adenocarcinoma of the kidney.

A 12-year old boy developed acute abdominal pain and gross haematuria after 3 months of malaise, vomiting and loss of weight. A large, smooth mass was palpable in the right loin, and excretory pyelograms showed no function in the right kidney. At operation a greatly enlarged kidney containing a well encapsulated adenocarcinoma (Fig. 17.9) 8 cm in diameter was removed. No other tumour tissue was found. One course of actinomycin D (120 mcg/kg in nine doses) was given after operation; he is well and free of disease 14 years later.

REFERENCES

Introduction

BURKITT, R.T. (1947). Tropical pyomyositis. *J. Trop. Med. Hyg.*, **50** : 71.

HOLDER, T.M., STUBER, J.L. & TEMPLETON, A.W. (1972). Sonography as a diagnostic aid in the evaluation of abdominal masses in infants and children. *J. Pediat. Surg.*, **5** : 532.

WONG, H.B. (1973). Abdominal wall abscesses. *Proc. 46th Annual General Scientific Meeting* p. 393. R.A.C.S., Singapore.

Wilms' tumour

ANDERSON, E.E., HARPER, J.M. *et al.* (1968). Bilateral diffuse Wilms' tumour: a 5-year survival. *J. Urol.*, **99** : 707.

ANNOTATION (Leading article) (1973). *Brit. Med. J.*, **4** : 627.

ARLEN, M., SHAN, I.C., HIGINBOTHAM, N. *et al.* (1972). Osteogenic sarcoma of the head and neck induced by radiation therapy. *N.Y. State J. Med.*, **72** : 929.

ARON, B.S. (1974). Wilms' tumour: a clinical study of 81 patients. *Cancer*, **33** : 637.

ATERMAN, K., BOUSTANI, P. & GILLIS, D.A. (1973). Solitary multilocular cyst of the kidney. *J. pediat. Surg.*, **8** : 505.

BECKWITH, J.B. (1974). Mesenchymal renal neoplasms of infancy revisited. *J. Pediat. Surg.*, **9** : 803.

BELMAN, A.B., SUSMANO, D.F. *et al.* (1970). Nonoperative treatment of unilateral renal vein thrombosis in the newborn. *J. Amer. Med. Assoc.*, **211** : 1165.

BHAJEKAR, A.B., Joseph, M. & BHAT, H.S. (1974). Unattached neproblastoma. *Brit. J. Urol.*, **36** : 187.

BISSADA, N.K. & FRIED, F.A. (1973). Retroperitoneal xanthogranuloma: case report and review of the literature. *J. Urol.*, **110** : 354.

BOGDAN, R., TAYLOR, D.E.M. & MOSTOFI, F.K. (1973). Leiomyomatous hamartoma of the kidney: a clinical and pathological analysis of 20 cases from the Kidney Tumour Registry. *Cancer*, **31** : 462.

BOLANDE, R.P. (1972). Discussion in *Year Book of Pediatrics*, p. 371. Year Book Publishers, Chicago.

BOLANDE, R.P., BROUGH, A.J. & IZANT, R.J. (1967). Congenital mesoblastic nephroma of infancy: a report of 8 cases and the relationship to Wilms' tumour. *Pediatrics*, **40** : 272.

BOLANDE, R.P. (1973). Congenital mesoblastic nephroma of infancy. In *Perspectives in Pediatric Pathology*, Vol. 1, p. 227. Year Book Medical Publishers, Chicago.

BOLANDE, R.P. (1974). Congenital and infantile neoplasia of the kidney. *Lancet*, **2** : 1497.

BOVE, K.E., KOTTLER, H. & MCADAMS, A.J. (1969). Nodular renal blastema. Definition and possible significance. *Cancer*, **24** : 323.

BURKITT, R.T. (1947). Tropical pyomyositis. *J. Trop. Med. and Hyg.*, **50** : 71.

CROCKER, F.S. & VERNIER, R.L. (1972). Congenital nephroma of infancy: induction of renal structures in organ culture. *J. Pediat.*, **80** : 69.

CUMMINS, G. & COHEN, D.H. (1974). Cushing's syndrome secondary to ACTH secreting Wilms' tumour. *J. Pediat. Surg.*, **9** : 535.

D'ANGIO, G.J. (1972). Management of children with Wilms' tumour. *Cancer*, **30** : 1528.

DEHNER, L.P. (1973). Intrarenal teratoma occurring in infancy: report of a case with discussion of extra-gonadal germ cell tumours in infancy. *J. pediat. Surg.*, **8** : 369.

DELORIMIER, A.A., BELZER, F.O. *et al.* (1968). Simultaneous bilateral nephrectomy and renal allotransplantation for bilateral Wilms' tumor. *Surgery*, **64** : 850.

EDELSTEIN, G., WEBB, R.S., ROMSDAHL, M.M. & ARBOIT, J.M. (1965). Extrarenal Wilms' tumor. *Am. J. Surg.*, **109** : 509.

EHRLICH, R.M. & GOODWIN, W.E. (1973). The surgical treatment of nephroblastoma (Wilms' tumor). *Cancer*, **32** : 1145.

EHRLICH, R.M., GOLDMAN, R. & KAUFMAN, J.J. (1974). Surgery of bilateral Wilms' tumors: role of renal transplantation. *J. Urol.*, **111** : 277.

ELIASON, E.L. & STEVENS, L.W. (1944). Wilms' tumour in a horseshoe kidney: case report. *Ann. Surg.*, **119** : 788.

FAVARA, B.E., JOHNSON, W. & ITO, J. (1968). Renal tumours in the neonatal period. *Cancer*, **22** : 845.

FAY, R., BROSNAN, S. & WILLIAMS, D.I. (1973). Bilateral nephroblastoma. *J. Urol.*, **110** : 119.

FLEMING, I.D. & JOHNSON, W.W. (1970). Clinical and pathologic staging as a guide to the management of Wilms' tumour. *Cancer*, **26** : 660.

FOSTER, K.M., RALSTON, M. *et al.* (1972). Primary cytomegalovirus infection and hepatitis in a renal allograft recipient. *Aust. N.Z. J. Med.*, **2** : 148.

FOWLER, M. (1971). Differentiated nephroblastoma: solid, cystic or mixed. *J. Pathol.*, **105** : 215.

FRAUMENI, J.F.Jr. & GLASS, A.G. (1968). Wilms' tumour and congenital aniridia. *J. Amer. Med. Assoc.*, **206** : 825.

FRAUMENI, J.F.Jr., GEISER, C.F. & MANNING, M.D. (1967). Wilms' tumour and congenital hemihypertrophy. *Pediatrics*, **40** : 886.

FU, Y-S. & KAY, S. (1973). Congenital mesoblastic nephroma and its recurrence. *Arch. Path.*, **96** : 66.

GRAIVIER, L. & VARGAS, M.A. (1972). Xanthogranulomatous pyelonephritis in childhood. *Amer. J. Dis. Child.*, **123** : 156.

GRISCOM, N.T. (1965). The roentgenology of neonatal abdominal masses. *Am. J. Roentgenol.*, **33** : 447.

GROSSMAN, M. (1975). The evaluation of abdominal masses in children with emphasis on non-invasive methods. *Cancer*, **35** : 884.

HAAS, L. & JACKSON, A.D.M. (1961). Wilms' tumour: lobectomy for pulmonary metastases. *Brit. J. Surg.*, **48** : 516.

HABIB, R., LEVY, M. & ROYER, P. (1968). La pyelonephrite chronique xanthogranulomateuse. *Arch. Franç. Pédiat.*, **25** : 489.

HAICKEN, B.N. & MILLER, D.R. (1971). Simultaneous occurrence of congenital aniridia, hamartoma and Wilms' tumour. *J. Pediat.*, **78** : 497.

HARDWICK, D.F. & STOWENS, D. (1961). Wilms' tumours. *J. Urol.*, **85** : 903.

HASTINGS, N. & GWINN, J.L. (1965). Retroperitoneal tumours of infants and children: treatment and prognosis. *Amer. J. Surg.*, **110** : 203.

HEWITT, D., LASHOFF, J.C. & STEWART, A.M. (1966). Childhood cancer in twins. *Cancer*, **19** : 157.

HILTON, C. & KEELING, J.W. (1974). Neonatal renal tumours. *Brit. J. Urol.*, **46** : 157.

HOLDER, T.M., STUBER, J.L. & TEMPLETON, A.W. (1972). Sonography as a diagnostic aid in the evaluation of abdominal masses in infants and children. *J. Pediat. Surg.*, **7** : 532.

INNIS, M.D. (1973). Nephroblastoma: index cancer of childhood. *Med. J. Aust.*, **2** : 322.

JAFFE, N. & TEFFT, M. (1973). Unsuspected lymphosarcoma of the kidneys diagnosed as bilateral Wilms' tumors. *J. Urol.*, **110** : 593.

JOHANNESSEN, J.V. (1974). Renal venous thrombosis: report of a case with ultrastructural findings and critical evaluation of the literature. *Arch. Path.*, **97** : 277.

JOHNSON, D.E., AYALA, A.G. *et al.* (1973). Multilocular renal cystic disease in children. *J. Urol.*, **109** : 101.

JOSHI, V.V., KAY, S. *et al.* (1973). Congenital mesoblastic nephroma of infancy: report of a case with unusual clinical behaviour. *Am. J. Clin. Path.*, **60** : 811.

KAHN, L.B. (1973). Retroperitoneal xanthogranuloma and xanthosarcoma (malignant fibrous xanthoma). *Cancer*, **31** : 411.

KNUDSON, A.G. Jr. (1975). The genetics of childhood cancer. *Cancer*, **35** : 1022.

KYAW, M.M. (1974). The radiological diagnosis of congenital multicystic kidney: a radiological triad. *Clin. Radiol.*, **25** : 45.

LANG, E.K. (1974). Contributions of arteriography in the assessment of renal lesions encountered in the neonatal period and infancy. *Radiol.*, **110** : 429.

LEEN, R.L.S. & WILLIAMS, I.G. (1971). Bilateral Wilms' tumor: seven personal cases with observations. *Cancer*, **28** : 802.

LEVIN, S.E., COLLINS, D.L. *et al.* (1974). Neonatal adrenal pseudocyst mimicking metastatic disease. *Ann. Surg.*, **179** : 186.

LOUTFI, A., MEHREZ, I., SHAHBENDER, S. & ABDINE, F.H. (1964). Hypoglycaemia with Wilms' tumour. *Arch. Dis. Childh.*, **39** : 197.

MCDONALD, P. & HILLER, H.G. (1968). Angiography in abdominal tumours in childhood with particular reference to neuroblastoma and Wilms' tumour. *Clin. Radiol.*, **19** : 1.

MCDONALD, P. & TARAR, R. (1974). Some radiologic observations in renal vein thrombosis, *Ann. J. Roentgenol.*, **120** : 368.

MARSDEN, H.B. & STEWARD, J.K. (1968). *Tumours in Childhood.* Springer Verlag, Stuttgart and New York.

MARTIN, L.W. & KLOECKER, R.J. (1961). Bilateral nephroblastomas. *Pediatrics*, **28** : 101.

MARTIN, L.W. & REYES, P.M. (1969). An evaluation of 10 years with retroperitoneal lymph node dissection for Wilms' tumor. *J. Pediat. Surg.*, **4** : 683.

MARTIN, J. & RICKHAM, P. (1970). Pulmonary metastases in Wilms' tumour: treatment and prognosis. *Arch. Dis. Childh.*, **45** : 805.

MILLER, R.A., TREMANN, J.A. & ANSELL, J.S. (1974). The conservative management of renal vein thrombosis. *J. Urol.*, **111** : 568.

MILLER, R.W., FRAUMENI, J.F. & MANNING, M.D. (1964). Association of Wilms' tumour with aniridia, hemihypertrophy and other congenital malformations. *New Engl. J. med.*, **270** : 922.

MITCHELL, J.D., BAXTER, T.J., BLAIR WEST, J.R. & MCCREDIE, D.A. (1970). Renin levels in nephroblastoma (Wilms' tumour). *Arch. Dis. Childh.*, **45** : 376.

MORSE, B.S. & NUSSBAUM, M. (1972). The detection of hyaluronic acids in the serum and urine of a patient with nephroblastoma. *Am. J. Med.*, **42** : 996.

MOYSON, F., MAURUS-DESMAREZ, R. & GOMPEL, C. (1961). Tumeur de Wilms mediastinale. *Acta Chir. Belg. Suppl.*, **2** : 118.

MURPHY, D.A., RABINOVITCH, H., CHEVALIER, L. & VIRIMANI, S. (1973). Wilms' tumour in right atrium. *Amer. J. Dis. Child.*, **126** : 210.

MURPHY, G.P. & MIRAND, E.A. *et al.* (1967). Erythropoietin release associated with Wilms' tumour. *Johns Hopk. med. J.*, **120** : 26.

NEUHAUSER, E.B.D. (1960). Case records of the Massachussetts General Hospital. Case 46372. *New Eng. J. Med.*, **263** : 557.

O'GORMAN HUGHES, D.W., BOWRING, A.C. *et al.* (1973). Wilms' tumour: increasing hopes for survival. *Med. J. Aust.*, **2** : 917.

PERLMAN, M., GOLDBERG, G.M. *et al.* (1973). Renal hamartomas and nephroblastomatosis with fetal gigantism: a familial syndrome. *J. Ped.*, **83** : 414.

PILLING, G.P. (1975). Wilms' tumour in seven children with congenital aniridia. *J. Pediat. Surg.*, **10** : 87.

POWARS, D.R., ALLERTON, S.E., BEIERLE, J. & BUTLER, B.B. (1972). Wilms' tumour clinical correlation with circulating mucin in 3 cases. *Cancer*, **29** : 1597.

RAGAB, A.H., VIETTI, T.J., CRIST, W., PEREZ, C. & MCALLISTER, W. (1972). Bilateral Wilms' tumour: a review. *Cancer*, **30** : 983.

RICHMOND, H. & DOUGALL, A.J. (1970). Neonatal renal tumours. *J. pediat. Surg.*, **5** : 413.

SCOTT, L.S. (1954). Renal tumours in childhood. *Glasgow med. J.*, **35** : 33.

SCOTT, L.S. (1955). Bilateral Wilms' tumour. *Brit. J. Surg.*, **42** : 513.

SHASHIKUMAR, V.L., SOMERS, L.A. *et al.* (1974). Wilms' tumor in the horseshoe kidney. *J. Pediat. Surg.*, **9** : 185.

SMITH, W.B., WARA, W.M. *et al.* (1974). Partial hepatectomy in metastatic Wilms' tumour. *J. Pediat.*, **84** : 259.

SOPER, R.T. (1961). Management of recurrent or metastatic Wilms' tumour. *Surgery*, **50** : 555.

SUKAROCHANA, K., TOLENTINO, W. & KIESEWETTER, W.B. (1972). Wilms' tumour and hypertension. *J. pediat. Surg.*, **7** : 573.

SULLIVAN, M.P., HUSSEY, H.H. & AYALA, A.G. (1973). Wilms' tumor. In *Clinical Pediatric Oncology*. C.V. Mosby Co., St. Louis.

TEBBI, K., RAGAB, A.H., TERNBERG, J.L. & VIETTI, T.J. (1974). An extrarenal Wilms' tumor arising from a sacral teratoma. *Clin. Pediat.*, **13** : 1019.

TEFFT, M., MITUS, A. & JAFFE, N. (1971). Irradiation of the liver in children: acute effects enhanced by concomitant chemotherapeutic administration. *Am. J. Roentgenol.*, **111** : 165.

TEFFT, M., VAWTER, G.F. & MITUS, A. (1968). Second primary neoplasms in children. *Amer. J. Roentgenol.*, **103** : 800.

THOMPSON, M.R., EMMANUEL, I.G., CAMPBELL, M.S., ZACHARY, R.B. (1973). Extrarenal Wilms' tumour. *J. pediat. Surg.*, **8** : 37.

TOMASI, T.B.Jr., ROBERTSON, W.V.B., NAEYE, R. & REICHLIN, M. (1966). Serum hyperviscosity and metabolic acidosis due to circulating hyaluronic acid. *J. Clin. Invest.*, **45** : 1080.

U.I.C.C. (1972). *Oncology for Medical Practitioners*, Geneva.

WALKER, D. & RICHARD, G.A. (1973). Fetal hamartoma of the kidney: recurrence and death of patient. *J. Urol.*, **110** : 352.

WEDEMEYER, P.P., WHITE, J.G. *et al.* (1968). Resection of metastases in Wilms' tumour: a report of three cases cured of pulmonary and hepatic metastases. *Pediatrics*, **41** : 446.

WIGGER, H.J. (1969). Fetal hamartoma of kidney. A benign symptomatic congenital tumor, not a form of Wilms' tumor. *Am. J. Clin. Path.*, **51** : 323.

WILLIS, R.A. (1967). *Pathology of Tumours*, 4th ed. Appleton Century Crofts, New York.

WILMS, M. (1899). Die Mischgeschwülste der Niere. A. Georgi, Leipzig.

WOLFF, J.A. *et al.* (1968). Single versus multiple dose dactinomycin therapy in Wilms' tumour: a controlled cooperative study conducted by the Children's Cancer Study Group A. *New Engl. J. Med.*, **279** : 290.

WONG, H.B. (1973). Abdominal wall abscesses. *Proceedings of 46th General Scientific Meeting*, p. 393. R.A.C.S., Singapore.

YOUNG, D.G. & WILLIAMS, D.I. (1969). Malignant renal tumours in infancy and children. *Brit. J. Hosp. Med.*, **2** : 744.

Carcinoma of the Kidney

CASTELLANOS, R.D., ARON, B.S. & EVANS, A.T. (1974). Renal adenocarcinoma in children: incidence, therapy and prognosis. *J. Urol.*, **111** : 534.

DEHNER, L.P., LEESTMA, J.E. & PRICE, E.B. (1970). Renal cell carcinoma in children: a clinicopathologic study of 15 cases and review of the literature. *J. Pediat.*, **76** : 358.

LYNNE, C.M. & MACHIZ, S. (1973). Renal cell carcinoma in children: a report of 4 cases and a review of the literature. *J. Pediat. Surg.*, **8** : 925.

MANSON, A.D., SOULE, H.E., MILLS, S.D. & DEWEERD, J.H. (1970). Hypernephroma in childhood. *J. Urol.*, **103** : 336.

NYGAARD, K.N., SIMON, H.B. (1974). Hypernephroma in children. *Arch. Surg.*, **108** : 97.

PALMA, L.D., KENNY, G.M. & MURPHY, G.P. (1970). Childhood renal carcinoma. *Cancer*, **26** : 1321.

SHANBERG, A.M., SROUJI, M. & LEBERMAN, P.R. (1970). Hypernephroma in the pediatric age group. *J. Urol.*, **104** : 189.

TALLEY, R.W. (1973). Chemotherapy of adenocarcinoma of the kidney. *Cancer*, **32** : 1062.

VAWTER, G.F. (1969). Review of renal tumors at the Children's Hospital Centre. *Abstracts of the Pediatric Pathology Club*.

Chapter 18. Tumours of the adrenal gland and retroperitoneum

Endocrine tumours arise in ectopic cell rests, as well as in sites where the parent cells are normally found, and this applies to adrenal tumours which may develop in ectopic cortical or 'medullary' cells in the sites illustrated in Fig. 18.1.

Tumours of the adrenal gland are classified as follows:

Tumours of the adrenal medulla:

I. Neuroblastoma (also 'ganglioneuroblastoma' and ganglioneuroma);
II. Phaeochromocytoma (syn. argentaffinoma);
III. Neurofibroma.

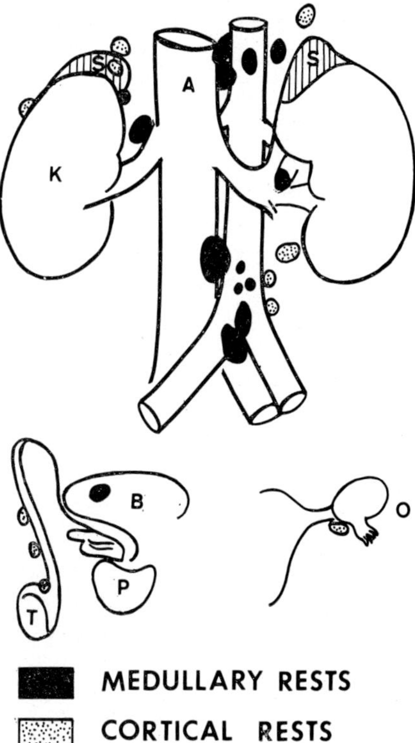

Figure 18.1. Sites of ectopic adrenal tissue; retroperitoneal and other sites of cortical and medullary cells, and where tumours derived from them may occur (after Able, 1969).

Tumours of the adrenal cortex:
IV. Adenoma;
V. Adenocarcinoma.

A. TUMOURS OF THE ADRENAL MEDULLA

I. NEUROBLASTOMA

This tumour, one of the commonest and the most malignant in childhood, arises in cells of the sympathetic nervous system derived from the embryonic neural crest. The parent cells migrate widely throughout the body and consequently neuroblastomas can develop in a variety of sites, although most frequently close to the autonomic chain, predominantly in the adrenal gland and the adjoining perivertebral tissues in the abdomen and, next in order of frequency, in the thorax (p. 543).

Ganglioneuromas also arise from the same precursors (Fig. 18.2) and are entirely benign, but they have a special relationship with neuroblastomas, many of which contain differentiated ganglion cells, the so-called 'ganglioneuroblastoma'.

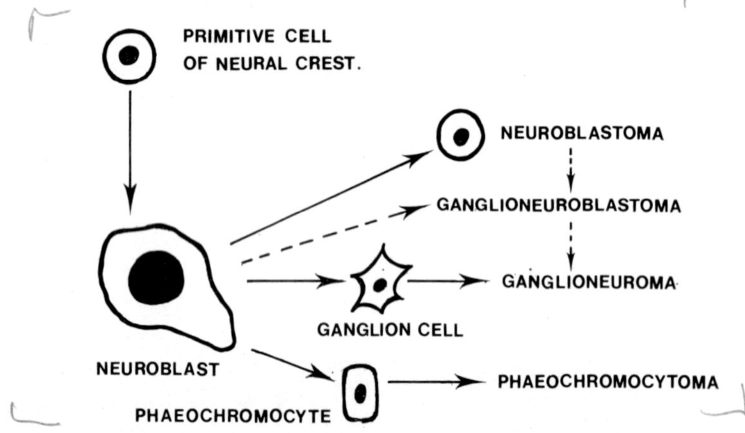

Figure 18.2. TUMOURS OF THE NEURAL CREST; a schematic diagram of the evolution of neuroblastoma, 'ganglioneuroblastoma' and ganglioneuroma; via another cell line, phaeochromocytomas are also derived from neuro-ectodermal tissues.

NEUROBLASTOMA-IN-SITU

The embryonic nature of neuroblastomas is indicated by their occurrence extremely early in life, and there are several reports of metabolites from a tumour in a fetus *in utero* crossing the placenta to cause symptoms in the mother (Joute *et al.*, 1970). In such cases the tumour can be well established and even disseminated at birth.

The presence of small groups of neuroblastoma cells in the adrenal gland (neuroblastoma-*in-situ*) can be demonstrated at autopsy in some infants dying of unrelated illnesses (Beckwith and Perrin, 1963; Beckwith and Martin, 1968). This finding is estimated to be 14 to 40 times more common than a neuroblastoma tumour, and the inference is that many cases of neuroblastoma-*in-situ* are arrested and regress completely and spontaneously, possibly as the result of activation of the host's immune mechanisms (p. 541).

SPONTANEOUS REMISSION

It is a paradox that an established neuroblastoma, the most malignant and invasive of all paediatric tumours, can nevertheless undergo complete remission and spontaneous cure. For practical purposes it is the only malignant tumour of childhood which may follow this course even when it has become disseminated (Fig. 18.3).

Estimates of the incidence of spontaneous remission vary, but it appears that no more than 2–4% of actual tumours (excluding those '*in-situ*') undergo permanent clinical remission. This is more likely to occur in patients less than 12–15 months old and even more rarely in children who are more than two years of age at the time of diagnosis.

'GANGLIONEUROBLASTOMA'

The presence of fully differentiated ganglion cells in a neuroblastoma suggests that some neuroblasts actually mature into ganglion cells, either spontaneously or in response to treatment (Bill, 1968). Alternatively, in a remission neuroblasts may die and completely disappear, leaving the field to benign ganglion cells derived from another cell line. Against the latter is the capacity of neuroblasts in tissue culture to differentiate into mature ganglion cells. With treatment, partial remission occurs many times more frequently than complete spontaneous remission, but it has yet to be determined whether satisfactory response to treatment is the death and disappearance of neuroblasts or their maturation to ganglion cells, or both.

CATECHOLAMINE METABOLISM

There is an extensive literature concerning the complex metabolites of neural crest tumours, and four of the biologically active substances they secrete are adrenaline, nor-adrenaline, l-dopa and dopamine.

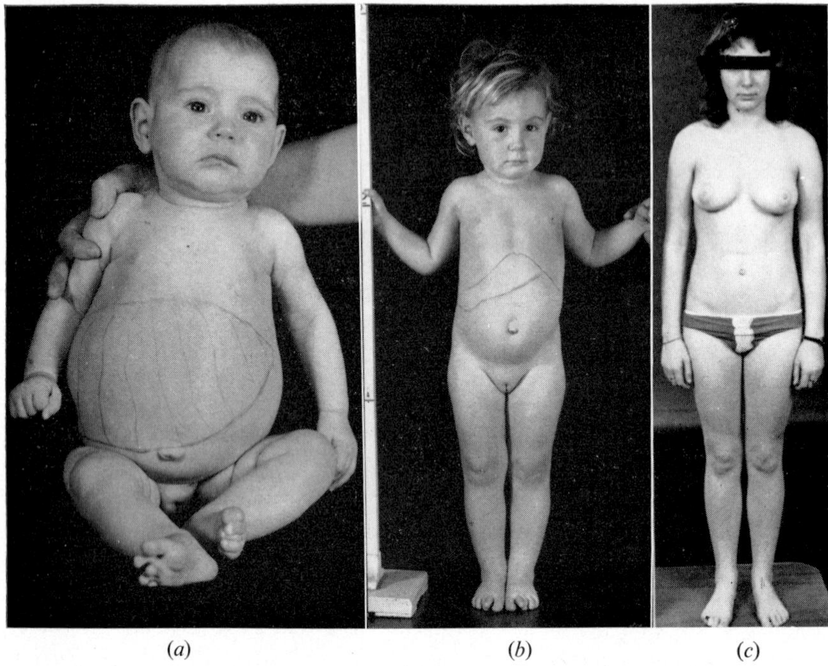

(*a*) (*b*) (*c*)

Figure 18.3. NEUROBLASTOMA; an example of spontaneous cure without treatment; (*a*) a girl aged 10 months presented with massive enlargement of the liver due to metastatic neuroblastoma proven by needle biopsy; (*b*) at 3½ years of age when laparotomy and open liver biopsy revealed whitish strands of mature ganglioneuroma throughout the still enlarged liver, and (*c*) normal growth, and no hepatomegaly, at 17 years of age.

Phaeochromocytomas (p. 565) typically produce the adrenaline (upper limit of normal excretion in urine: 70 μg/24 hrs) and nor-adrenaline responsible for the hypertension which is a distinctive feature of this tumour.

Ganglioneuromas (p. 552) are also actively secreting tumours, but their metabolites only rarely produce clinical symptoms, e.g. diarrhoea.

Neuroblastomas are not uniform or consistent in the types and amounts of metabolites they secrete, and several tests are customarily used to detect individual substances or to measure the total amount of catecholamines excreted in the urine. In general, neuroblastomas produce increased amounts of catecholamines, or their precursors, as evidenced by increased levels of metabolites in the urine, for example 3-methoxy 4-hydroxy mandelic acid (MHMA), a major metabolite of adrenaline and nor-adrenaline. Estimations of these substances in the urine form the basis of diagnostic tests, best performed on a 24-hour specimen of urine, and less reliably as a screening test on a random sample. As a rule, a rate of excretion in the urine three times the normal level is taken as the minimum required for a positive result.

IMMUNOLOGICAL ASPECTS

The biological behaviour of neuroblastoma has long been the subject of extensive studies (Hellstrom & Hellstrom, 1968, 1971; Hellstrom *et al.*, 1968) which have disclosed important interactions between the host and the tumour cells. A patient's leucocytes can be significantly cytotoxic for his own neuroblastoma cells, and there is also present, at times, a humoral agent capable of blocking the action of immunologically active leucocytes. This blocking antibody is present in patients dying of neuroblastoma, and greatly diminished or absent in those in whom the tumour has been controlled. The point has not yet been reached where these substances can be regularly applied in treatment, but these lines of research indicate the possibility of eradicating neoplastic cells, utilizing the high specificity of immunological processes.

They also point to a potential conflict in the effects of cytotoxic agents, all of which are to some extent immunosuppressants; although capable of adversely affecting tumour cells directly they may at the same time depress beneficial immune responses, thus depriving the host of defences which might otherwise be brought to bear on the cells of the tumour. The immunosuppressant effects of cytotoxic agents can be minimized by intermittent courses with intervals to allow for recovery.

Investigations of the inhibition of cell-mediated immune cytotoxic effects on the cells of rat hepatoma have indicated that the blocking factor is an antigen-antibody complex in which the antibody is chiefly of the IgG class (Baldwin *et al.*, 1974), while material from human neuroblastoma suggests that IgG_1, IgG_3 and IgG_4 may function as the antibody portion of specific blocking factor (Jose & Skvaril, 1974).

In addition, the ability of a malignant tumour to generate local or systemic excess of membrane-derived antigen may assist it to escape destruction by specific cellular immune processes (Jose & Seshadri, 1974).

AGE

Although migration of cells from the neural crest continues until about the age of ten years, neuroblastomas are essentially tumours of infancy and early childhood (Fig. 18.4). In the Index Series 83% were less than five years of age at the time of diagnosis, and 35% were less than two years of age.

There is a distinct though small heredito-familial incidence, with reports of several pairs of twins both affected (Wagget *et al.*, 1973) and in another family each of four siblings had a neuroblastoma (Chatten & Voorhees, 1967).

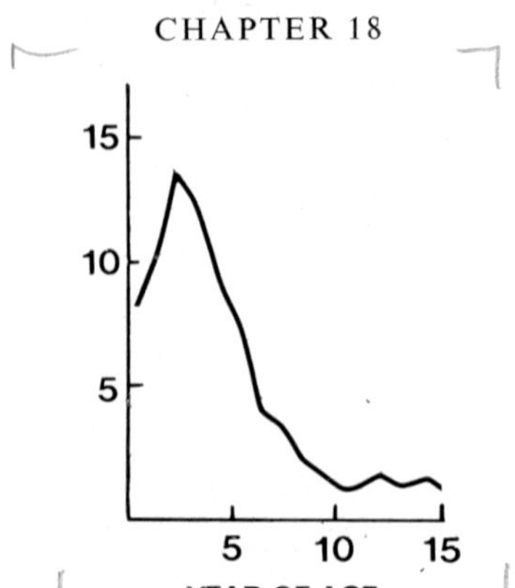

Figure 18.4. NEUROBLASTOMA; incidence according to age, showing the peak in the first quinquennium (for source of figures see Fig. 2.2, p. 48).

SITES

Extending from the posterior cranial fossa to the coccyx, the scatter of cells derived from the neural crest accounts for the extraordinary variety of sites in which this tumour may arise. In order of frequency, as shown in Table 18.1, there are as follows.

1. *The abdomen.* The adrenal medulla, or cells in the adjacent retroperitoneal tissues on the posterior abdominal wall, are the two commonest sites (50–80% of most reported series) and account for 5–7% of all solid malignant tumours of childhood. Because of their proximity and the large size of the tumour at the time of diagnosis, it is not always possible to determine exactly where the tumour arose.

2. *The thorax.* A thoracic neuroblastoma is usually paravertebral, i.e. in the posterior mediastinum (p. 460) and probably arises from cellular precursors of the autonomic ganglia (Clatworthy & Newton, 1970).

3. *The pelvis.* Here, too, neuroblastomas probably arise from autonomic derivatives of the neural crest, usually beneath the peritoneum covering the lateral or posterior wall (p. 709).

4. *The spine*, especially soft tissues in the extradural plane, is the site of a relatively uncommon but distinctive clinicopathological type of neuroblastoma which causes compression of the spinal cord (Lepintre, Schweisguth *et al.*, 1969), a mode of presentation also found in Ewing's tumour (p. 739) and Burkitt's lymphoma (p. 328).

Neuroblastomas arising in this site tend to cause spinal compression and paraplegia of rapid onset while the tumour is still small and undisseminated, and they consequently have a significantly better prognosis than those arising elsewhere, e.g. in the abdomen where they are latent, hence larger and often disseminated, before the diagnosis is made.

Table 18.1. Neuroblastoma; the sites of the primary tumour in 144 cases in the Index Series (RCH, 1950–1972)

Site			No.	
Abdominal	adrenal	71	103	(72%)
	retroperitoneal	?32		
Mediastinal			19	(13%)
Spinal			6	(4%)
Pelvic			3	(2%)
Cervical primary			1	
Intracranial			1	
Uncertain or unknown			11	
Total			144 patients	

Although some neuroblastomas arise in the epidural space, in most of the patients presenting with spinal cord symptoms compression is the result of extension in continuity of a paravertebral thoracic or abdominal neuroblastoma.

5. *In the cervical region* neuroblastomas are much less common (Table 18.1). They probably develop in the cervical sympathetic trunk or ganglia, giving rise to a swelling in the posterior or deep triangle of the neck.

6. *The posterior cranial fossa* (p. 258) and the olfactory bulb (p. 362) are, on rare occasions, the primary site of a neuroblastoma.

MACROSCOPIC APPEARANCES

The tumour is usually reddish, soft and friable and contains areas of necrosis which are yellow, irregular and often calcified, giving the tumour a gritty texture. There is radiographic evidence of calcification in approximately 50% of cases. The vessels of the tumour are extremely fragile, causing spontaneous haemorrhage or semifluid necrotic loculi prone to burst and spill during removal. The paucity and tenuous nature of the vessels may also account for difficulty in demonstrating the vascular pattern by angiography (p. 554). Some tumours, or areas within a tumour, are firmer, characteristically white, lobulated and rubbery, and contain a more fibrillary stroma.

The site of origin to some extent determines the macroscopic appearance of the primary tumour. In the adrenal gland it is usually large, encapsulated and mobile (Fig. 18.5a) but some are quite small and overshadowed by extensive deposits in adjoining para-aortic lymph nodes forming a nodular mass of matted retroperitoneal metastases. Retroperitoneal tumours tend to infiltrate deeply and are usually irremovably fixed to the posterior abdominal wall (Fig. 18.5b). In the thorax, the primary tumour is usually extensively fixed to the vertebral bodies, surrounds the aorta, and extends in nodular sheets beneath the mediastinal pleura in the paravertebral gutter (Fig. 16.9, p. 462).

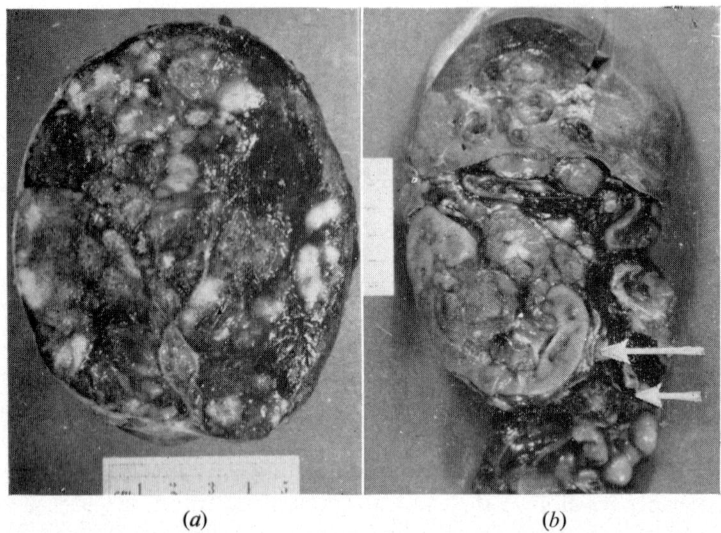

(*a*) (*b*)

Figure 18.5. NEUROBLASTOMA; macroscopic appearance of a primary tumour arising (*a*) in an adrenal gland, where it tends to remain encapsulated and relatively confined; most of the tumour is necrotic and only the white areas are viable; (*b*) in retroperitoneal tissues the tumour extends widely between and behind the vena cava (upper arrow) and the aorta (lower arrow), invading and displacing the kidney, and filling the sub-hepatic spaces.

MICROSCOPIC FINDINGS

The tumour is composed of masses of small cells with scanty cytoplasm, in lobular masses separated by delicate fibrovascular septa, the density of the cells varying from one part to another (Fig. 18.6a). Most tumours contain eosinophilic neurofibrillary tissue surrounding and separating individual cells or groups of cells. This is the characteristic pattern of a neuroblastoma (Fig. 18.6a) and with special stains, nerve processes can be demonstrated in the fibrillary areas. Rosettes are found in about a third of these tumours (Fig. 18.6c).

The neuroblast (Fig. 18.6a) is also characteristic, a small cell with an average diameter of 12 μ in paraffin sections, an irregular hyperchromatic nucleus containing closely packed, dense and clumped chromatin, a distinct nuclear membrane and usually one small nucleolus (Fig. 18.6a, b). The outline of the nucleus is irregular, and there is characteristically variation in the size of the nuclei from field to field.

Differentiation of variable degree, is found in most neuroblastomas. One form is maturation to a completely differentiated ganglion cell two or three times larger than a neuroblast, with a moderate amount of eosinophilic cytoplasm, a large round nucleus containing scattered chromatin and a single prominent nucleolus (Fig. 18.6d). All variations from a mature ganglion cell to an undifferentiated neuroblast can often be found in the one tumour. The commonest and simplest form of differentiation is a slight increase in the

(*a*)

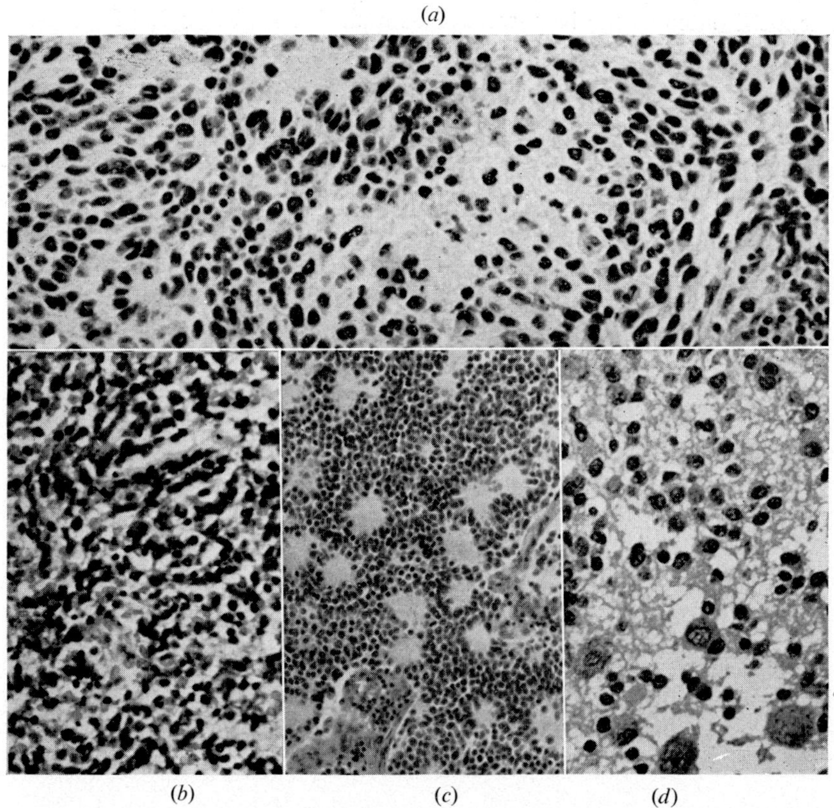

(*b*) (*c*) (*d*)

Figure 18.6. NEUROBLASTOMA; (*a*) typical 'scattered wheat' pattern with hyperchromatic neuroblasts separated by pale fibrillary neuroglial tissue (H & E. × 200); (*b*) undifferentiated type, composed of neuroblasts with little or no cytoplasm and no interspersed neurofibrillary tissue (H & E. × 200), impossible to identify histologically unless neurofibrillary differentiation can be found in other areas of the tumour; (*c*) the formation of rosettes (H & E. × 100); (*d*) neuronal differentiation with several large ganglion cells ('ganglioneuroblastoma') below (H & E. × 200).

amount of cytoplasm, rounding out of the nuclear outline, and clumping of the nuclear chromatin; another is the formation of the neuro-fibrillary material described above.

Rice (1965) classified a group of neuroblastomas incorporated in the Index Series into three groups: (i) undifferentiated tumours; (ii) those showing some differentiation (fibrillary tissue, etc.), and (iii) those with neuronal and ganglioneuromatous differentiation. There were significant differences in the behaviour of the three groups, but in an individual case a prognosis based entirely on histological differentiation can be misleading. One of the objects of a current prospective Australian National Trial is to determine to what extent the outcome can be correlated with particular histological features.

SPREAD (for clinical consequences see p. 552)

(i) **Local spread**

Except for those arising in the adrenal gland, some of which show a surprising tendency to remain encapsulated (Fig. 18.5a), local invasion and wide infiltration are highly characteristic. Large blood vessels are often surrounded and compressed (Fig. 18.5b), but very rarely invaded. Occasionally an adjacent vertebral body is infiltrated directly; more often vertebral involvement is metastatic.

(ii) **Lymph node metastases**

As in all embryonal tumours (except medulloblastomas) neuroblastomas have a special tendency to spread at an early stage to the lymph nodes of the para-aortic chain, and may then spread upwards to the retroclavicular nodes, particularly on the left side, to present as a mass of glands in the deep triangle of the neck.

Other nodes remote from the primary and the para-aortic chain may also be involved by blood borne metastasis.

(iii) **Haematogenous spread**

This is also a feature of neuroblastomas, although detectable pulmonary metastases occur extremely rarely, and only in the terminal stages of the disease. More commonly spread by the bloodstream is to:

1. *The bone marrow*

There is a special tendency for this tumour to spread to the bone marrow at an early stage, forming groups of cells larger and more irregular than those of the marrow; the nuclear chromatin of the neuroblasts is also more coarse and clumped (Fig. 18.7, see colour plates, following p. 140). Very occasionally the cells are so undifferentiated that the type of malignancy cannot be identified. Other tumours known to metastasize to the marrow in childhood are rhabdomyosarcoma, Wilms' tumour and hepatoblastoma, but in these tumours metastases in the marrow can usually be identified by their cellular morphology, and develop late in patients in whom the diagnosis has already been established.

2. *Bone*

Metastases develop as a single destructive lesion, e.g. in the orbital margin or as a diffuse infiltration of the growing ends of long bones (Fig. 22.14, p. 744) which resembles leukaemic infiltration radiographically.

3. *The liver*

Hepatic metastases occur more frequently in patients less than two years of age, and take one of two different forms;

(*a*) Spherical or irregular masses causing irregular, knobbly enlargement of the liver; or

(*b*) Diffuse infiltration, sometimes around individual cells or lobules, mostly in patients less than one year of age, and occasionally already present at birth.

A particular feature of some in the second group is that the infiltration may be so evenly distributed throughout the whole liver that although massively enlarged (Fig. 18.8a) it may yet retain its normal shape. Further, selective hepatic arteriography may show no distortion of the arterial pattern, and scanning (p. 77) may also be negative because of the diffuse distribution. If the primary tumour is latent (Fig. 18.8b) needle biopsy may be the only means of determining the cause when this type of hepatomegaly is the presenting feature and the results of other tests are equivocal or negative. One histological type of *hepatoblastoma* is composed of small cells not unlike neuroblasts (p. 606) and this is a potential source of diagnostic error.

Finally, it should be noted that massive hepatic metastases in neuroblastoma are not invariably fatal, and do not always have the poor prognosis as hepatic metastasis from other types of tumour (Fig. 18.3).

HISTOLOGICAL DIFFERENTIATION OF NEUROBLASTOMA FROM OTHER MALIGNANT TUMOURS

As with most paediatric tumours, sections of good quality are essential for diagnosis, especially in the difficult case in which the pattern is not characteristic and diagnosis rests upon the morphology of individual tumour cells.

Ewing's tumour, rhabdomyosarcoma and other embryonal or anaplastic tumours may resemble a neuroblastoma; in difficult cases the important points in making the correct histological diagnosis (see Table 5.1, p. 84) are as follows;

(*i*) *Imprints* of the cut surface of the fresh tumour are particularly helpful; Leishman's stain is the most suitable, for it reveals the smudged, coarse irregularity of the nuclear chromatin and the spider-web-like prolongations of cytoplasm characteristic of the neuroblast (Fig. 18.9, see colour plates, following p. 140).

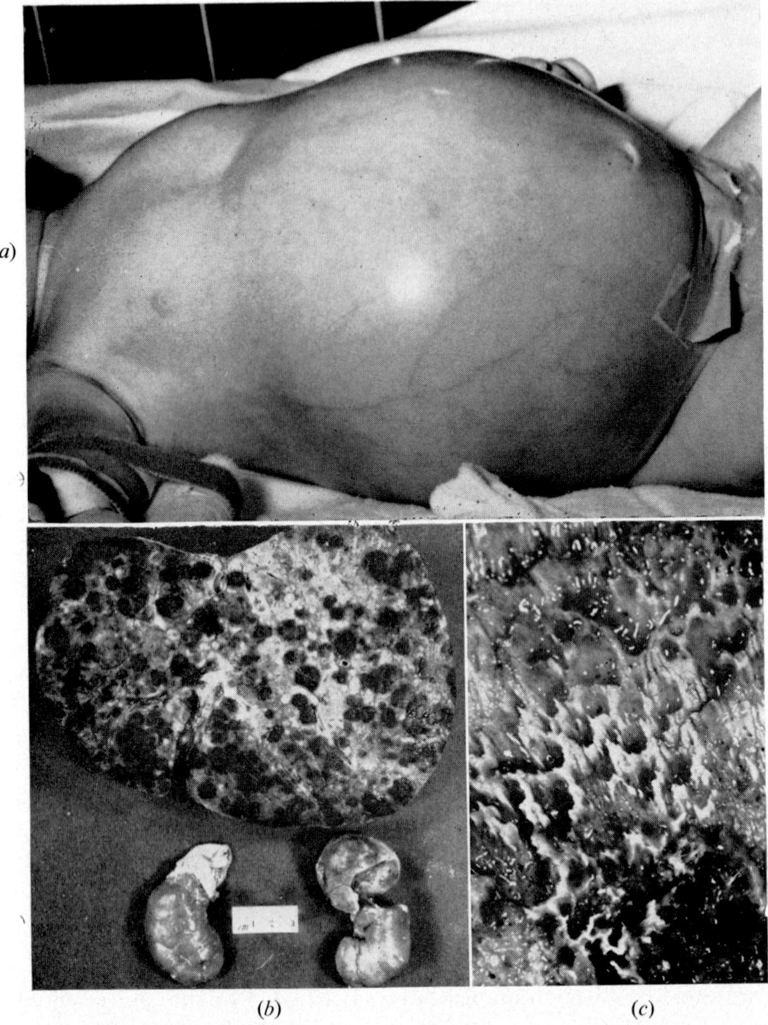

(*a*) (*b*) (*c*)

Figure 18.8. NEUROBLASTOMA; (*a*) massive (fatal) enlargement of the liver in an infant caused by diffuse hepatic metastasis; (*b*) another example with multiple areas of metastases in the liver; and (*c*) on the inner table of the calvarium causing circular spicules of new bone, from a latent, roughly spherical encapsulated primary tumour less than 4 cm in diameter arising in the left adrenal gland (*b*).

(*ii*) *PAS stains* will demonstrate PAS positive material in the cells of a rhabdomyosarcoma or a Ewing's tumour; material which is absent in neuroblasts (Fig. 18.9), although it may be present in differentiating cells and in ganglion cells.

(*iii*) *Fresh, frozen sections* stained for acid and alkaline phosphatase sometimes provide useful information, being strongly positive in differentiated neuroblasts, though usually negative when they are undifferentiated.
(*iv*) *Tissue cultures*, when available, are also helpful; neuroblasts grow readily in suitable media and the spider-web-like fibrillary processes can be clearly seen. Even cells from an undifferentiated neuroblastoma will differentiate in tissue culture (Burdman & Goldstein, 1964).

The histological features of *ganglioneuroma* are shown in Fig. 18.10, and silver stains demonstrate nerve processes intimately mixed with the connective tissue of this tumour. In some cases the stroma closely resembles that of a neurofibroma (p. 822) and contains scarcely any ganglion cells.

Bolande & Towler (1970) suggested that there may be a relationship between neuroblastoma and von Recklinghausen's disease.

'Ganglioneuroblastoma'

An otherwise characteristic ganglioneuroma is occasionally found to contain islands of neuroblasts which can be difficult to distinguish from lymphocytes. No matter how well-differentiated the ganglioneuroma element may be, the presence of neuroblasts within it removes it from this category; such a tumour should be described as a 'neuroblastoma with areas of ganglioneuroma' (Fig. 18.10) and not infrequently gives rise to fatal metastases. Although the term 'ganglioneuroblastoma' is undesirable because it may give an erroneous indication of benignancy to what is essentially a neuroblastoma, in any series of neuroblastomas those showing features of differentiation in the direction of ganglion cells behave more favourably than less well-differentiated tumours.

MODES OF PRESENTATION OF NEUROBLASTOMAS (Table 18.2)

It is said that if syphilis was the 'great imitator' of the past, neuroblastoma is a worthy successor in this century, at least in childhood. As well as the variety of sites in which it arises, each with a set of regional signs (Donahue, Garrett *et al.*, 1974), metastases almost anywhere can occur from a latent neuroblastoma; in addition, metabolites from such a tumour give rise to a complex of clinical effects which practically constitute a syndrome.

1. '*Malignant malaise*' is a convenient general term for this ill-defined but typical clinical picture which includes a few or most of the following:

Change in personality: irritability, fretfulness, loss of 'joie de vivre';
Lethargy, lassitude and tiredness;
Loss of energy, appetite and weight;
Irregular fever, episodes of sweating with or without fever;
Aches and twinges in the limbs, transient and recurrent;
Pallor, a variable degree of anaemia and an elevated ESR.

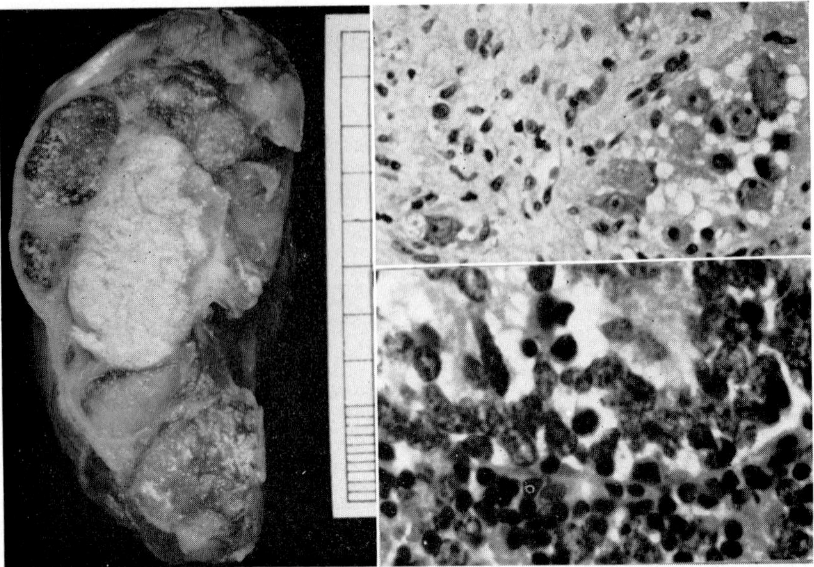

Figure 18.10. 'GANGLIONEUROBLASTOMA'; (*a*) a paravertebral mass with a central, yellow area of necrosis, tan, firm, fleshy areas, and loculi of dark, gritty tissue; (*b*) section of the fleshy area, containing ganglioneuroma with well differentiated ganglion cells (H & E. × 200); and (*c*) dark areas composed of neuroblasts with granular nuclear chromatin, surrounded by lymphocytes (H & E. × 520).

[(*a*) *Left*. (*b*) *Top right*. (*c*) *Bottom right*.]

All young children are, of course, prone to minor illnesses accompanied by some of the symptoms listed, and the commonest cause is repeated bacterial or viral infection. Nevertheless, 'malignant malaise' is such a recognizable clinical picture that a latent neuroblastoma should be considered in the differential diagnosis and confirmation should be sought, hopefully with some prospect of improving the current poor prognosis by earlier diagnosis.

Fever

The possibility of a latent malignant tumour in a child with unexplained fever as the presenting feature can be difficult to assess. Neuroblastoma, Wilms' tumour, Ewing's tumour, leukaemia and, to a lesser extent than previously considered, Hodgkin's disease, may all present with fever as the sole or chief complaint. That necrosis or infarction in the tumour is usually the cause of the fever in such cases has been challenged, and the disappearance of fever after removal of a tumour with neither complication suggests that

Table 18.2. Neuroblastoma; the modes of presentation in the 89 children in the Index Series (RCH. 1950–1972) with a primary neuroblastoma arising in the abdomen

	No.	
'Malignant malaise'	36	(41%)
Abdominal pain	12	
Abdominal mass	11	
Pain in bone (x-ray positive)	11	
Peripheral lymphadenopathy	5	
Diarrhoea	2	
Orbital metastases	2	
Lumps in the scalp	2	
Multiple subcutaneous nodules	1	
Intraperitoneal haemorrhage	1	
Agranulocytosis	1	
Myasthenia gravis	1	
Not certain	4	
Total	89 patients	

tumour metabolites themselves may be the cause of fever. As stated in an annotation in the *Brit. Med. J.* (1974):

> 'In every case where the cause of fever is in doubt, the patient and the nursing staff should be carefully questioned for clues; every accessible part of the body must be carefully examined for evidence of infection; . . . the opinion of a bacteriologist sought, . . . rather than indiscriminately bombarding the laboratory with swabs, sputum, urine and blood cultures'.

Screening tests

Excretion of catecholamine metabolites in the urine (Hinterberger & Bartholomew, 1969) is recognized as occurring in more than 90% of neuroblastomas (Gitlow *et al.*, 1970; Sharman, 1973). As a basis for screening children who may have a neuroblastoma, more than one substance in a 24-hour specimen of urine should be estimated; significantly elevated levels of MHMA or VMA will provide positive evidence in 70% of patients; elevated total catecholamine increase the figure to 80% (with some false positives if assessed on this figure alone), while the demonstration of high levels of dopamine increases the detection rate to more than 90%.

La Brosse (1968a,b) developed a widely used spot test for VMA in hospitals (Evans *et al.*, 1971), but as it involves mixing unstable reagents, and refrigeration, it is impractical outside a hospital.

An alternative method of screening children for neoplasms is based on elevated levels of carcinoembryonic antigen (CEA) in the plasma. This is estimated by detecting an ion-sensitive antigenic site in the CEA molecule, and can be employed as a diagnostic assay, or for monitoring patients during treatment and follow up. Reynoso, Chu *et al.* (1972), in a preliminary report, found elevated levels of plasma CEA in six patients with active neuroblastoma; in one patient with an apparent clinical cure the value was normal. Although not specific for neuroblastoma, elevated levels of CEA appear to be confined to a small group of tumours, thus reducing the possibilities to be investigated (Donohue, Garrett *et al.*, 1974).

In the absence of laboratory data the most useful initial investigations available in general practice are carefully centred and correctly exposed x-rays of the abdomen (Fig. 18.11) and the mediastinum, for evidence of speckled calcification or a mass which would indicate the presence of a neuroblastoma.

Other modes of presentation (Table 18.2) are as follows:

2. *Abdominal pain* may be the symptom which leads to examination of the abdomen and discovery of a mass. Occasionally the pain is sudden in onset and severe, but more often mild and intermittent.

3. *An abdominal mass* or abdominal distension discovered by one of the parents, is equally common as the mode of presentation. In some cases it is the primary tumour, but more often it is a matted mass of metastatic nodes, and in a few, mostly infants, it is an enlarged liver diffusely infiltrated with metastatic tumour (see p. 548) (Figs. 18.3, 18.8).

4. *Pain in a bone*, with radiographic changes, e.g. a metastasis causing local destruction, is occasionally the first evidence of a neuroblastoma. In the syndrome of 'malignant malaise', fleeting pains in the limbs without radiographic changes are not uncommon.

Positive radiological findings are an indication to search for a latent primary tumour, but if it cannot be demonstrated, the diagnosis can be made on the histological evidence of a drill biopsy of the affected bone.

5. *Metastases in peripheral lymph nodes*, commonly in the cervical region (see p. 225) may be the first sign of a latent neuroblastoma. Biopsy of the node(s) will indicate the cause.

6. *Multiple subcutaneous (or intramuscular) metastatic nodules* are another form of presentation, particularly in early infancy (see 'Stage IV–S', p. 558). The somewhat bluish nodules beneath the skin have led to the term 'blueberry muffin baby' (Shown & Durfee, 1970).

7. *Proptosis* due to metastatic deposits in the bones of the orbit, often accompanied by peri-orbital ecchymoses (Blake & Fitzpatrick, 1972), are more common in children than primary tumours of the orbit (see Fig. 15.6, p. 409).

8. *Diarrhoea*, caused by tumour metabolites acting on the alimentary musculature, is an unusual but well-documented phenomenon (Williams,

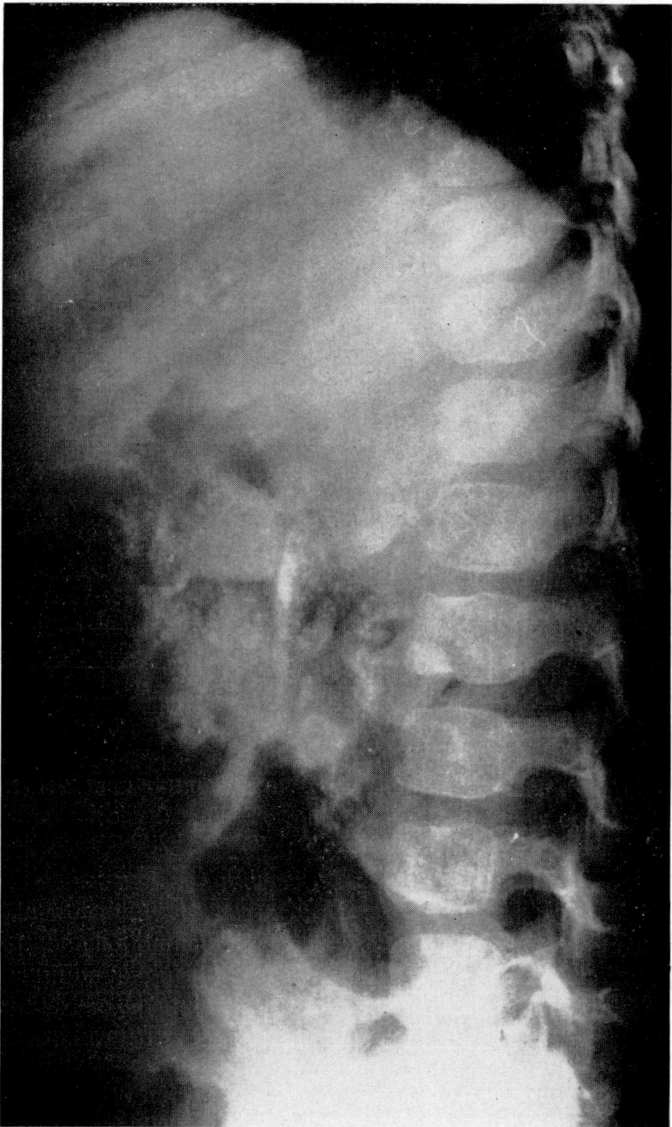

Figure 18.11. NEUROBLASTOMA; extensive calcification in a primary tumour (in the left adrenal) and in numerous retroperitoneal lymph node metastases, in an 18-month old girl on the day she presented with a para-orbital metastasis.

House *et al.*, 1972). It can also occur in ganglioneuroblastoma (Stickler & Hallenbeck, 1962), and in benign ganglioneuromas (Rosenstein & Engleman, 1963; Sindhu & Anderson, 1965) which secrete pharmacologically active substances (Käser *et al.*, 1973).

9. *Intraperitoneal haemorrhage* as the mode of presentation was seen once in the Index Series, in a neonate with massive and fatal bleeding from a large adrenal neuroblastoma which ruptured during birth.

10. *Agranulocytosis* due to extremely widespread metastases in the marrow is another rare form of presentation.

Other modes of presentation

In the literature there are reports of several bizarre presentations such as hypertension, opsoclonus (Soloman & Chutorian, 1968), cerebellar ataxia (Korobkin *et al.*, 1972), myasthenia gravis (Robinson & Howard, 1969), oculo-cerebellar myoclonus (Lemerle *et al.*, 1969), and myoclonic encephalopathy (Senelick, Bray *et al.*, 1973).

INVESTIGATIONS

The following investigations are required to establish the diagnosis and to assess the extent of dissemination.

1. Full blood examination, including ESR.
2. X-rays of the abdomen (Fig. 18.11), and a skeletal survey, to confirm or detect bone involvement.
3. Angiography (described on p. 69 and p. 507) to demonstrate the site and extent of the tumour (Fig. 18.12).
4. Marrow biopsy is positive in a large proportion of cases (60–70%) at the time of diagnosis, and the histological findings can be sufficient to make the diagnosis on this evidence alone (Fig. 18.7, see colour plates, following p. 140).
5. The levels of urinary catecholamines (see p. 551) in a 24-hour specimen, are significant when greater than three times the normal levels (Table 18.3).

DIAGNOSTIC CRITERIA

As a general rule, a histological diagnosis is mandatory before commencing treatment, and suitable material can often be obtained from a metastasis in a lymph node or a drill biopsy of a bony metastasis. However, when neither of these sources is available, (*a*) positive marrow smears, supported by the evidence of (*b*) aortography and selective arteriography (Fig. 18.12), and (*c*) significantly elevated levels of urinary catecholamines, are sufficiently reliable to establish the diagnosis of neuroblastoma and to commence definitive treatment without the need for further confirmation.

DIFFERENTIAL DIAGNOSIS OF ABDOMINAL NEUROBLASTOMA

The variety of the modes of presentation indicates the number of conditions to be excluded, and investigations in addition to those listed above are often required.

In 'malignant malaise', various causes of failure to thrive, such as malabsorption syndromes, immunological deficiencies (e.g. hypogammaglobulinaemia), and various causes of anaemia, etc. should be excluded.

Abdominal pain; excretory urography, a barium meal or a cholecystogram may be required.

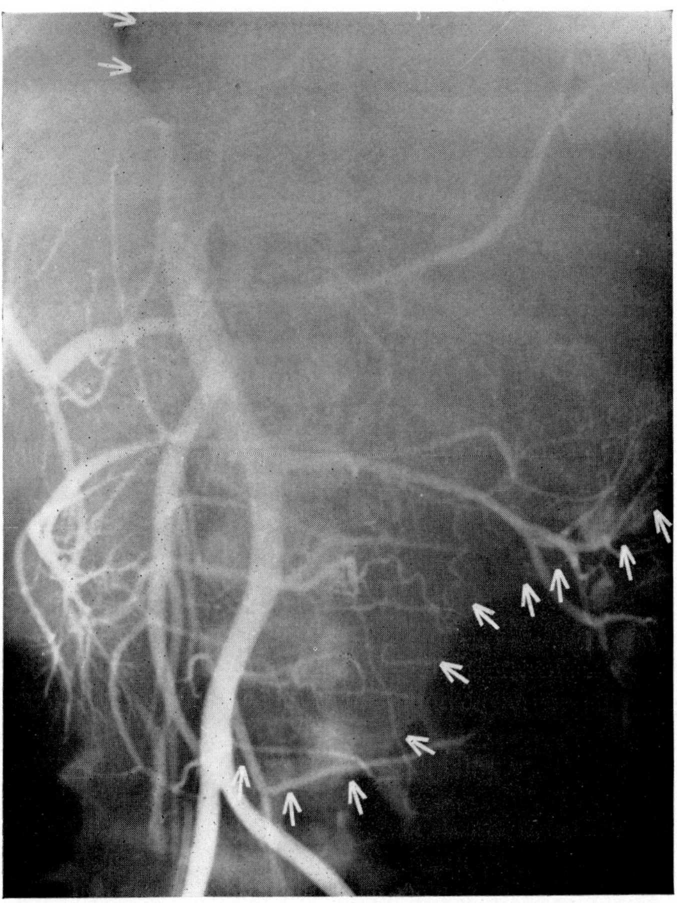

Figure 18.12. NEUROBLASTOMA; aortogram of a massive left adrenal primary, displacing the left kidney laterally and the aorta to the right.

Table 18.3. Catecholamines. Metabolites secreted by abdominal tumours including those derived from the neural crest, and other products such as renin

Tumour	Catecholamines etc.						Other
	Total Catecho- lamines	Dopa & dopa- mine	Nor adren- aline	Adren- aline	VMA	MHMA	
Neuroblastoma	+	+	+	0	+	++	
Ganglioneuroma	+				+	±	
Phaeochromocytoma	++ or +++	0	+	+	++	±	
Wilms' tumour	Normal	0	0	0	0	0	+Renin

Abdominal mass; Wilms' tumour (p. 516), hepatic tumours (p. 598) and other recognized causes (p. 492) should be considered, but angiography usually demonstrates clearly the viscus in which the tumour has arisen.

Bone lesions; primary tumours of bone other than Ewing's tumour are rare in the first five years of life, but as this age group is chiefly affected by both neuroblastoma and Ewing's tumour, confusion was not uncommon before the introduction of specific histological techniques (p. 84) to determine whether a lesion was a primary Ewing's tumour or a metastasis from a neuroblastoma.

Multiple subcutaneous metastatic nodules are recognized as one of the clinical patterns (Stage 'IV–S', see p. 558) and the diagnosis can be readily made by biopsy of one of the lesions.

SPINAL COMPRESSION

When deterioration of neuromuscular function in a child less than three years of age progresses so rapidly that the ability to walk is lost in the course of a week, or power and movement deteriorate in one or both arms, compression of the spinal cord by a neoplasm is the most likely cause (Fagan & Swischuk, 1974).

Benign causes of spinal compression are much less common, the onset of the disability is usually much slower, and the loss is less severe, e.g. when due to tethering of the cord in spina bifida occulta (see tumours of the spinal cord, p. 292).

Rare benign causes of spinal cord signs with a relatively rapid onset are:
(i) Infection in an intraspinal epidermoid cyst, most commonly in the lower lumbar or sacral region (p. 291);
(ii) Enterogenous intraspinal cyst, typically thoracic and accompanied by radiographic evidence of a vertebral anomaly, i.e. the split notochord syndrome (p. 450);
(iii) Extradural coccal abscess, presumably haematogenous in origin;
(iv) Tuberculosis; spinal caries with a gibbus and partial paraplegia is still common in some developing countries.

DIFFERENTIATION FROM OTHER MALIGNANT CAUSES OF SPINAL COMPRESSION

These include:
Ewing's tumour;
Metastatic medulloblastoma;
Malignant lymphomas;
Primary tumours of the spine (p. 288).

Ewing's tumour arising in a vertebra is usually accompanied by radiographic evidence of bone destruction in one of the pedicles or laminae, but the typical radiographic changes seen in long bones (p. 740) are usually lacking when a vertebra is involved.

Medulloblastomas (p. 248) typically present with signs and symptoms of a tumour in the posterior cranial fossa, but on rare occasions a latent medulloblastoma gives rise to metastases in the CSF, which lodge in the spinal theca and grow rapidly, leading to compression of the spinal cord. This occurs more often as a complication in a patient already known to have an intracranial medulloblastoma.

Hodgkin's lymphoma, other malignant lymphomas and leukaemia, may form deposits in the epidural fat, usually late in the course of the disease. Burkitt's lymphoma is a common cause of spinal compression and paraplegia in countries where it is endemic (p. 330).

CLINICAL STAGING OF NEUROBLASTOMA

Before the plan of treatment is formulated, the extent of dissemination is determined from the results of the investigations listed above. Patients with an abdominal primary are classified according to a scheme of staging based on the extent of dissemination at the time of diagnosis (Evans, D'Angio & Randolph, 1971).

Stage I. Tumour confined to the organ or tissue of origin.
Stage II. Tumour extending in continuity beyond the organ or tissue of

origin but not crossing the midline; ipsilateral regional nodes may be involved; tumours arising in midline structures can also be included in this group.
Stage III. Tumour extending across the midline, or metastases in regional lymph nodes on both sides.
Stage IV. Distant metastases, e.g. in bone, distant lymph nodes, marrow or in soft tissues, e.g. in the orbit (p. 408).
Stage IV–S. Those otherwise in Stage I or II but with metastases confined to one or more of the following: the liver, subcutaneous tissues, muscles or bone marrow, but without any metastasis in bone as determined by negative findings in a complete skeletal survey, and drill biopsy if necessary.

TREATMENT

One of the major difficulties in regard to treatment and prognosis is the high proportion of patients, variously reported as up to 70%, in whom dissemination, chiefly in the marrow, is present at the time of diagnosis (Rice, 1965; Koop & Johnson, 1971). In abdominal neuroblastoma, metastases in the marrow are found in up to 75% of cases (Koop & Schnaufer, 1975).

Three methods of treatment, surgical excision, radiotherapy and cytotoxic chemotherapy, are all used in most cases, but opinions concerning the optimum sequence and timing differ. Because of the extent of local infiltration and/or distant metastases, total surgical excision is rarely a feasible objective. Nevertheless, subtotal or even partial removal of the primary tumour may benefit the patient by facilitating the other two methods, as well as the patient's own immunological defences.

Because complete surgical removal of the primary tumour is unlikely, pre-operative radiation and chemotherapy may be followed by exploration after a suitable period for full therapeutic effect. Subtotal removal of the tumour may then be attempted, for the primary has almost always been considerably reduced in size.

The suggested protocol for coordinated treatment currently employed in an Australian National Trial can be summarized as follows.

STAGE I

When the clinical and radiographic evidence indicates that the tumour is likely to be removable, operation is undertaken about the third day after commencing chemotherapy, usually vincristine (VCR) and cyclophosphamide (CPA).
Chemotherapy (doses for patients more than 12 months old): Vincristine (1·8 mg/m^2 IV) weekly for 6 weeks, combined with cyclophosphamide (350 mg/m^2 IV) in weeks 1 and 2, and also in weeks 3 and 4 if no radiotherapy is given.

Surgical excision is undertaken 2–3 days after the first injections of VCR and CPA.

Radiotherapy is optional, but given in most cases, starting 3–4 weeks after operation; the total dose of a regime extending over 3–5 weeks varies according to factors such as the age of the patient (0–12 months of age, 1000–1500 rads; 1–4 years of age, 1500–4000 rads). During irradiation, cytotoxic agents other than vincristine are discontinued.

Maintenance chemotherapy is recommended after radiotherapy has concluded (i.e. at about 7 weeks), in the form of recurrent courses of cyclophosphamide (250 mg/m^2/day orally for 5 consecutive days) given every 3 weeks for 1–2 years.

In infants less than 12 months old the oral dose is reduced to 200 mg/m^2.

STAGE II

The sequence of treatment depends upon a decision to operate early (before radiotherapy), or later when it appears likely that much of the tumour cannot be removed.

Early surgery. Operation is performed within one week of diagnosis, preceded by the first doses of chemotherapy (as above); chemotherapy is continued for 12 weeks after operation (VCR weekly; CPA during weeks 1, 2, 8, 10 and 12). Radiotherapy (as above) is commenced in week 3, and extends over 3 weeks during which CPA is omitted. Maintenance chemotherapy (as above) is then continued for 1–2 years.

Later operation. Chemotherapy (as above) is given weekly for 12 weeks, with CPA in weeks 1, 2, 8, 10, 12, omitting one dose if it falls due 6 days before or after the date of operation. VCR (as above) is also given at weekly intervals.

Radiotherapy (as above) is commenced in week 3 and extends over 4 weeks.

Operation is performed during week 9, 10 or 11, after allowing time for full ‘tumour effect’, and after reassessment, including further aortography.

Maintenance chemotherapy (as above) is then given from week 13 onwards, for 2 years.

STAGE III

The plan of treatment, and the modifications determined by early or late operation, are the same as for Stage II, with the addition of a third cytotoxic agent, vinblastine (VBL) (2·5 mg/m^2 IV once a week) in weeks 7, 9 and 11.

Maintenance chemotherapy (as above) with the optional addition of a third cytotoxic agent, e.g. VBL or any one of adriamycin, daunorubicin, actinomycin D, methotrexate or procarbazine (see Appendix III for dosages etc.); the third agent chosen is given in the last 3 weeks of each 12 week cycle.

STAGE IV

Chemotherapy varies according to the timing of surgery and/or radiotherapy. The first course comprises three cytotoxic agents (e.g. VCR, VBL and CPA) given intravenously at intervals of one week; all three agents are given in weeks 1 and 2; VCR weekly throughout the 12 weeks, alternating the other two, i.e. VBL in weeks 3, 5, 7, 9 and 11 and CPA in weeks 4, 6, 8, 10 and 12.

Prednisolone (50 mg/m^2/day) is given orally, daily, on days 1 to 8.

Radiotherapy, when employed, can for example be commenced in week 3 if no major surgery is performed; only VCR is given during the 4 weeks of radiotherapy, alternating the other agents weekly thereafter up to 12 weeks.

Surgery, if it becomes feasible, may be performed in week 9 or 10, i.e. 3 weeks after radiotherapy has been concluded.

Maintenance chemotherapy. If the disease progresses in spite of treatment, a decision whether to continue treatment will have to be made. When the tumour response is favourable, maintenance chemotherapy is usually continued for 2 years, and may include CPA (orally for 5 days) at recurring 3 week intervals, accompanied by either daunorubicin (45 mg/m^2 IV), on two occasions 7–10 days apart, in weeks 9 and 11 of each 12 week cycle, or VCR at weekly intervals for 3 weeks, i.e. in weeks 10, 11 and 12.

STAGE IV–S

The optimum plan is somewhat uncertain because of the varying influence of age, rate of tumour growth, etc. on the prognosis, but 5-year tumour-free survivals occur in 60–80% of patients in Stage IV–S, and in infants, survival rates as high as 90% have been reported. The plan of chemotherapy is therefore less intensive than for Stage IV and closer to Stage II; some authorities favour none at all.

Modification of dosages

The following factors influence the dosage:

(i) The age of the patient; in those less than 12 months old, the dose of cytotoxic agents should be reduced by 15–20%; in Stage I and Stage IV–S, chemotherapy may be omitted altogether.

(ii) The development of leucopenia (below 1500 neutrophils/cmm) is an indication to reduce or omit chemotherapy until the count has improved.

(iii) Other symptoms or signs of toxicity (see Appendix III) may also indicate that cytotoxic agents should be reduced or temproarily discontinued.

(iv) Concurrent radiotherapy and chemotherapy should be avoided, except for vincristine which does not significantly affect leucopoiesis.

RESULTS

In the Index Series the results obtained are in general accord with reports of other larger series.

From 1948 to 1970, 101 children with a neuroblastoma were treated at the Royal Children's Hospital, with an overall 2 years + survival rate of 25%.

In the 72 patients treated between 1963, when cyclophosphamide and vincristine became available, and 1972 (to permit assessment of at least a 2-year survival rate), the results confirm the importance of the age at the time of diagnosis in determining the outcome, those less than 2 years having the best prognosis and those less than 1 year old even better.

0–11 months	(17 patients):	47% 2+ year survival
12–23 months	(14 patients):	35% 2+ year survival
2–3 years	(28 patients):	14% 2+ year survival
3 years +	(13 patients):	15% 2+ year survival

The overall survival rate in these 72 patients was 26%. The results also show the effect of the site of the primary tumour on the prognosis.

Abdominal primary (54 patients): (including abdominothoracic and abdominospinal tumours)	8% 2 year + survivors (median survival time: 5 months)
Thoracic primary (14 patients): (including thoracospinal (dumbbell) tumours)	70% 2 year + survivors (median survival time: more than 72 months)
Pelvic primary (3 patients):	100% 2 year + survivors (median survival time: more than 113 months)
Cerebellar primary (1 patient):	5 year + survival

PROGNOSIS

Inability to demonstrate any improvement in results since the introduction of chemotherapy has been reported by several authors, notably Sutow *et al.* (1970). However, in the Index Series the 4-year survival rate of 62 cases treated before 1963 was approximately 16%, and in the 39 cases treated since both cyclophosphamide and vincristine were employed (1963–1970) the 4-year survival rate was 41%, a statistically significant improvement, but not necessarily entirely due to the efficacy of chemotherapy.

Cohen (1969) pointed out that the prognosis appeared to depend more directly on the age of the patient, the site of the primary, and the degree of differentiation of the tumour cells than on the methods of treatment employed.

As borne out by the few cases in the Index Series, the prognosis of neuroblastoma arising in the pelvis appears to be even more favourable than in those arising in the mediastinum. Ghazali (1974) reviewed a series of seven children with a pelvic neuroblastoma, six of whom are very long term survivors (up to 20 years) and had apparently been cured by partial removal as virtually the only method of treatment employed. In the majority, the tumour underwent spontaneous remission, to ganglioneuroma or to complete disappearance. It is significant that six of these seven patients presented between the ages of 3 months and 15 months, the age group in which the prognosis appears to be the most favourable.

II. PHAEOCHROMOCYTOMA

This tumour also arises in cells derived from the neural crest (Fig. 18.2), specifically from chromaffin-positive cells, and in most cases the tumour is in the adrenal medulla. It is a rare neoplasm in childhood for less than 5% of all phaeochromocytomas occur before adolescence.

AGE : SEX

Examples have been reported in young children, but the overall range is from 7–70 years of age, with a peak in young adult life. Most children affected are between 10 and 15 years of age; before puberty boys are more often affected than girls, but after puberty there is no sex preponderance (Stackpole *et al.*, 1963). Girls with a phaeochromocytoma tend to present soon after the onset of puberty.

SITES

While most phaeochromocytomas occur in the adrenal gland (Robinson, Kent & Stocks, 1973), they may also arise in medullary rests in a variety of sites in the abdomen (Fig. 18.1): in the organ of Zuckerkandl, in retroperitoneal tissues, in cells related to the coeliac ganglion, and on rare occasions in the appendix, or in the thorax (p. 459). The proportion arising in extra-adrenal sites is greater in children than in adults (Glenn, Peterson & Mannix, 1968).

Multiple tumours, have been reported in 10%–40% of collected series, and bilateral tumours occur with sufficient frequency (20%) to require exploration of *both* adrenal glands, and reinvestigation 1–2 months after removal of a phaeochromocytoma, to determine whether a second tumour is present (see p. 568).

An association between neurofibromatosis and phaeochromocytoma has been reported in adults (Lopez 1958; Chapman *et al.*, 1959), and is occasionally seen in children. Other associations noted are renal artery stenosis and von Hippel-Lindau disease (p. 832).

SIPPLE'S SYNDROME

The association of phaeochromocytomas with a group of other conditions has been reported with increasing frequency (Kaiser, Beavan *et al.*, 1973) since Sipple (1961) first noted the combination of phaeochromocytoma and medullary carcinoma of the thyroid gland (p. 372). Multiple neurinomas of the mucous membrane of the tongue, mouth or larynx, were initially reported as a separate entity by Bazex & Dupré (1958), but this 'bumpy lip' syndrome has been observed in association with phaeochromocytoma, medullary carcinoma of the thyroid and hyperparathyroidism (Gorlin *et al.*, 1968; Kaiser *et al.*, 1973).

Steiner *et al.* (1968) proposed two groupings of endocrine adenomatosis, i.e. multiple endocrine tumours, typically occurring in adults:
Type 1: Tumours of the pituitary, parathyroids and pancreas, ('multiple endocrine neoplasia Type 1'); and
Type 2: Phaeochromocytoma, medullary thyroid carcinoma, and parathyroid tumours ('multiple endocrine neoplasia Type 2').

Levy, Habib & Lyon (1970), among others, have emphasized the characteristic facies in children with some of the components of Type 2, notably a long thin face, a scaphocephalic cranium, greatly thickened and everted lips, multiple submucosal neurinomas ('bumpy lip'), and 'amyloid' (medullary) carcinoma of the thyroid gland. Vance *et al.* (1972) suggested that the primary lesion in some of these cases may be a tumour of islet cells of the pancreas ('nesidioblastosis') and that the secretions of non-insulin producing tumours may be the cause of at least some of the endocrine disturbances which occur elsewhere.

MACROSCOPIC APPEARANCES

The tumour is usually encapsulated and rarely large, usually 2–3 cm in diameter, but ranging from 1–10 cm in large series. The cut surface is usually pale grey or pink (Fig. 18.13a), but in some cases dusky brown or variegated, with areas of necrosis and haemorrhage. When a specimen is fixed in formaldehyde, the tumour turns the solution brown within 24 hours, a very characteristic finding.

MICROSCOPIC FINDINGS

The tumour has an 'endocrine pattern', i.e. groups of cells divided into lobules by delicate septa of vascular connective tissue (Fig. 18.13b). The cells are oval or spindle shaped, and have a wispy vacuolated cytoplasm. About 10% of the cells show granules which stain brown after oxidation with chromium salts (Fig. 18.13c). The cells with granules often lie at the periphery of the lobules, but may be distributed irregularly.

The nuclei are round or oval, and vesicular, with relatively well dispersed chromatin and bear no resemblance to ganglion cells. However, single cells or groups of cells resembling ganglion cells are occasionally present. In some

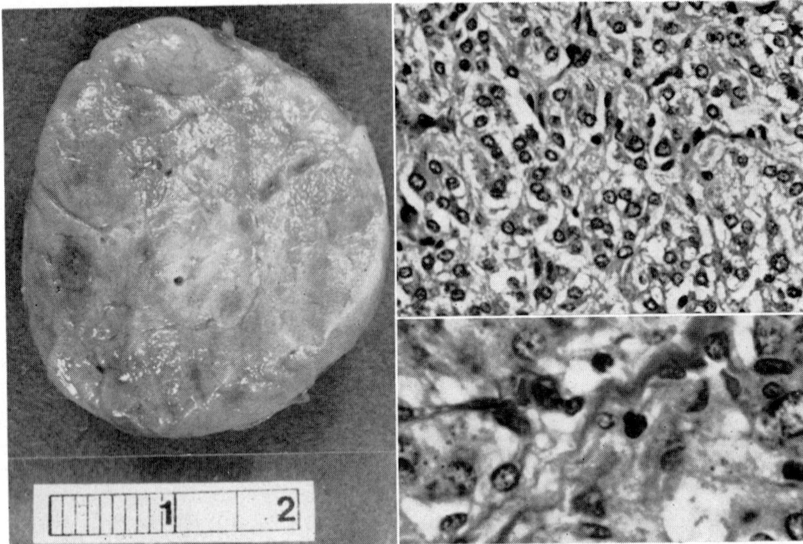

Figure 18.13. PHAEOCHROMOCYTOMA; (*a*) cut surface of a tumour of usual size (approx. 3 cm diameter) freshly removed from the left adrenal; the tumour is uniform, firm and slightly lobulated; (*b*) nests of cells resembling those in the adrenal medulla, with some nuclear polymorphism (H & E. × 200); (*c*) granules of chromaffin material in the cytoplasm of the tumour cells after fixation in dichromate solution (H & E. × 520).

[(*a*) *Left*. (*b*) *Top right*. (*c*) *Bottom right*.]

examples the cells are more pleomorphic, but pleomorphism cannot be correlated with the degree of malignancy. Indeed, some degree of pleomorphism has been reported to be a favourable finding for in most of the apparently malignant tumours the cells are uniform in type.

As in other endocrine tumours, e.g. adrenal cortical adenoma (p. 581), the cellular morphology of a phaeochromocytoma is unreliable as a guide to whether the tumour is benign or malignant; nuclear polymorphism is usual in benign lesions and may be less marked in some proven malignant examples. In adults 8–10% of phaeochromocytomas are unquestionably malignant, and in children the proportion is reported to be approximately the same. One of the five cases in the Index Series recurred locally and infiltrated paravertebral muscles, eventually invading the inferior vena cava.

Electron microscopy of phaeochromocytoma cells shows that some contain 'type 1 dense core vesicles', the type of vesicles found in neuroblasts, in the neurons of ganglioneuromas, and similar to those in normal cells in the adrenal medulla; however, the proportion of cells with vesicles in a phaeochromocytoma is less than in the normal adrenal medulla.

Biochemical and enzymic studies indicate that the rate of synthesis and turnover of catecholamines in the cells of a phaeochromocytoma is very rapid, five times the rate in neuroblastomas and ten times more rapid than ganglioneuromas; however, the ability of the granules to release their catecholamines seems to be much less in tumour cells than in normal adreno-medullary cells.

Histologically the differential diagnosis of a phaeochromocytoma is from adrenal cortical adenoma (p. 572) and carcinoma (p. 575), and from non-chromaffin paragangliomas (p. 586).

MODES OF PRESENTATION

The clinical features are not due to the size or pressure effects of the tumour, which is rarely palpable (in approximately 6% of cases in children; Cornell, 1972), but to the metabolites it secretes, which cause α- and β-adrenergic effects, especially hypertension.

Severe headaches, usually commencing suddenly, and accompanied by nausea, profuse sweating, palpitations, agitation, anxiety and pallor, are the typical effects and are characteristically episodic.

CLINICAL FINDINGS

Hypertension can usually be found during 'attacks', which are at first paroxysmal with symptomless intervals. Later, the paroxysms are super-imposed on a plateau of sustained hypertension.

Papilloedema is usually present; exudates and retinal haemorrhages appear later.

Loss of weight and increased basal metabolic rate are not unusual, and in some cases may resemble thyrotoxicosis, including an elevated BMR.

Thirst and polydypsia may be sufficiently severe to suggest diabetes insipidus, and may falsely suggest a lesion of the posterior lobe of the pituitary, especially when headaches and vomiting are also present.

Paroxysmal tachycardia occurs in less than 10% of phaeochromocytomas in children.

INVESTIGATIONS

As well as the usual examination and basic investigations (p. 506), there are two which are practically diagnostic in children with a phaeochromocytoma.

1. Catecholamines in the urine

The excretion of VMA (vanyllyl mandelic acid) measured in a 24-hour specimen of urine is greatly increased (Gitlow, Bertain *et al.*, 1972) and has replaced pharmacological tests based on alterations in the blood pressure following a test dose of phentolamine (see below).

Non-chromaffin tumours of sympathetic tissues, e.g. neuroblastoma, secrete increased amounts of dopa, dopamine and/or nor-adrenaline, but not adrenaline. The presence of large amounts of adrenaline in the urine thus virtually excludes a neuroblastoma (Table 18.3, p. 556) as the source of the excess catecholamines.

In unusual but well-documented cases of phaeochromocytoma, dopa and dopamine are produced in large quantities and as these substances may not produce any hypertension, the tumour may appear to be non-functioning, and there is consequent delay in diagnosis.

2. Aortography and selective arteriography

Phaeochromocytomas are highly vascular, and commonly arise in or near the adrenal gland or in the retroperitoneal tissues (Fig. 18.1). Angiography almost always demonstrates the site of the tumour by the presence of a vascular blush, and this can be detected when the tumour is as small as 2–3 cm in diameter (Fig. 18.14).

Other investigations which have been described are as follows.

3. Excretory pyelography as a means of demonstrating an adrenal phaeochromocytoma has been shown to be unreliable, giving rise to 4 false negative findings in 6 cases reported by Bloom and Fonkalsrud (1974).

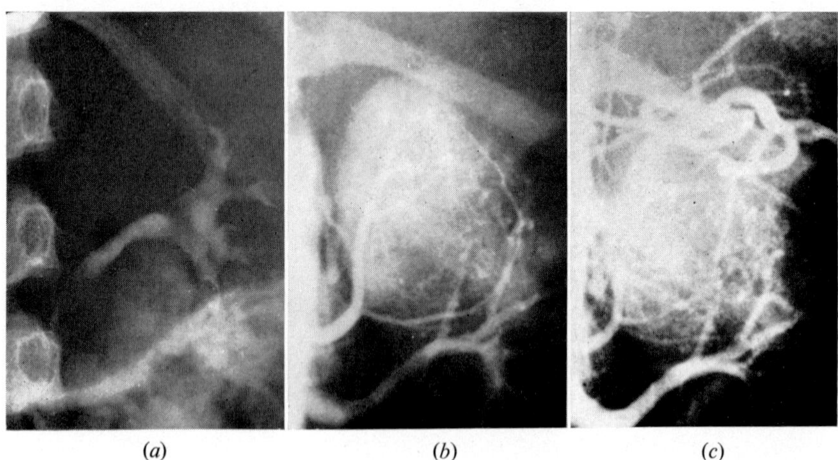

(*a*) (*b*) (*c*)

Figure 18.14. PHAEOCHROMOCYTOMA; (*a*) excretory pyelogram showing lateral displacement of the kidney and the upper calyces ('drooping lily' appearance); (*b*) aortogram demonstrating a small, highly vascular adrenal tumour supplied by an inferior adrenal artery as large as the renal artery; and (*c*) the late capillary phase with filling of tortuous venous channels.

4. Measurement of the tumour's secretions (e.g. assay of total adrenaline/nor-adrenaline) in serial samples of venous blood. This is useful in confirming the site of an adrenal phaechromocytoma, (see case report below), but is more valuable in locating one arising elsewhere, i.e. an extra-adrenal tumour, which can then, if required, be clearly demonstrated by retrograde venography.

5. Nephrotomography combined with pyelography is recommended by Remine *et al.* (1974) as a 'noninvasive' investigation, safer than arteriography, which was effective in localizing tumours 2·5 cm in diameter or larger, in a series of 138 cases at the Mayo Clinic. Regrograde venography was reserved for extra-adrenal tumours, and those not demonstrated by tomography. The surgical mortality in this series was 2·9% and the recurrence rate 9·8% at the time of review.

6. Radiocholesterol (^{131}I-19-iodocholesterol) combined with scintillography and image-enhancement has been employed by Sturman *et al.* (1974) to outline the adrenal cortex and hence demonstrate its distortion by a phaeochromocytoma as small as 2 cm in diameter.

DIFFERENTIAL DIAGNOSIS

The following conditions may produce similar presenting symptoms and are to be excluded by appropriate investigations:
Hypoglycaemia and hyperinsulinism (see p. 664);
Intracranial tumour;
Alternative causes of hypertension or elevated catecholamines;
Acute anxiety state and panic reactions;
Migraine (hemicranial and/or 'abdominal');
'Periodic' syndrome or 'cyclical vomiting';
Diabetes;
Hyperthyroidism;
Paroxysmal tachycardia.

An intracranial tumour may be suggested by headache, nausea and papilloedema, but the absence of separation of sutures, 'beaten silver' skull, or erosion of the clinoid processes is helpful.

It is particularly important to avoid an operative procedure such as ventriculography which can precipitate a fatal exacerbation of hypertension in a patient with a phaeochromocytoma. Hypertension is *not* a feature of intracranial tumours, and its presence should determine the appropriate choice of investigations.

Neuroblastoma and Wilms' tumour are, in some cases, accompanied by hypertension, in neuroblastoma due to the secretion of nor-adrenaline

(p. 556), and in Wilms' tumour by compression of the kidney or distortion of the renal artery causing renal ischaemia or, in some differentiated tumours, the production of excess renin (p. 505). Although these tumours may present with symptoms of hypertension, and both are usually located in the upper part of the abdomen, also the commonest site of phaeochromocytoma, each of the three conditions can be identified by angiography.

Other points which distinguish these three conditions are:

(i) Phaeochromocytomas are very rarely palpable;

(ii) Calyceal distortion on pyelography is usual in Wilms' tumour, and absent in the other two tumours;

(iii) Urinary catecholamines are not elevated in Wilms' tumour and neuroblastomas do not secrete adrenaline (Table 18.3).

TREATMENT OF PHAEOCHROMOCYTOMA

Management is complicated by two factors:

1. Phaeochromocytomas may be multiple (Bloom & Fonkalsrud, 1974);
2. 'Crises', i.e. episodes of extreme hypertension, arrythmia (and occasionally death) can occur at any time, but particularly during investigation and operation.

1. Multiple tumours

The incidence of multiple tumours in the one patient varies in different reported series from 10–40%. The possibility of more than one tumour presents several problems.

Two or more tumours may be present when the diagnosis is made; removal of one tumour may not relieve the symptoms or they may recur soon after operation.

A small second tumour may be difficult or impossible to demonstrate until the larger, 'dominant' tumour has been removed.

Alternatively a second tumour may not develop until many months or years after the first was removed (Harrisson *et al.*, 1974), and it may develop:

(*a*) *In the same adrenal gland*, sometimes at or very close to the site of the original tumour, a finding open to interpretation as 'local recurrence' of a tumour which may be malignant; or

(*b*) *In the contralateral adrenal.* According to Cornell (1972) the proportion of cases with more than one phaeochromcytoma is higher in children (30%) than in adults (4%) and the contralateral adrenal should always be examined at the time of operation.

(*c*) *In a variety of extra-adrenal sites*, e.g. in retroperitoneal tissues, the pelvis, thorax (Wilson *et al.*, 1974) or, least commonly in the cranial cavity. The proportion of extra-adrenal phaeochromocytomas is also greater in childhood (31% : 10%) than in adults (Bloom & Fonkalsrud, 1974).

In one series, a 'recurrence' or a second phaeochromocytoma occurred in 3 out of 7 patients less than 15 years of age at diagnosis (Harrison *et al.*, 1974); the shortest interval was 9 months and the longest 21 years, but in most reports of recurrence, symptoms reappeared within 5 years.

In the Index Series (Robinson *et al.*, 1956, 1973) one child had three operations for the removal of a total of six separate phaeochromocytomas.

2. 'Crises'

Exacerbations of hypertension and headache are due to α-adrenergic activity of catecholamines excreted by the tumour, while severe tachycardia, with or without arrhythmia, is due to β-adrenergic effects. Either can occur as the presenting signs and symptoms, and in addition they can appear, or become worse, at certain points in the management of a patient with a phaeochromocytoma.

(*a*) *During or following excretory pyelography*, particularly when abdominal compression is applied as part of the procedure.

(*b*) *During aortography or arteriography;* the injection of contrast material causes a sudden flush of blood through the tumour, liberating pressor substances into the bloodstream. For this reason, selective venography has been recommended as safer and because the venous catheter can be used to sample venous blood and hence determine the amount and the source of catecholamines.

(*c*) *In an anaesthetized patient*, especially when muscle relaxants have been used, transfer of the patient to the operating table and positioning for operation involves rotary movements of the trunk which 'massage' an adrenal or retroperitoneal tumour, thus liberating additional metabolites.

(*d*) *Squeezing the tumour* during dissection and removal has similar (potentially lethal) effects.

Control of the blood pressure and heart rate from the time of diagnostic suspicion is essential for the safe removal of the tumour, and mortality rates of up to 50% have been reported when attempts are made to remove a phaeochromocytoma discovered at laparotomy, without adequate pharmacological preparation.

BIOCHEMICAL INVESTIGATIONS

1. The amounts of individual and total catecholamines in a 24-hour specimen of urine are usually diagnostic, for they are almost always many times the normal level of MHMA (less than 8 μg/24 hours), 3-0-methyl-catecholamines (less than 1–5 μg/24 hours), or total catecholamines (less than 100 μg/24 hours).
2. Response to α-adrenergic blocking agents, as a diagnostic test, requires the injection of a small dose of phentolamine via an intravenous infusion. In

normal subjects there is a small and brief fall in blood pressure; in a patient with a phaeochromocytoma a fall exceeding 35 mm systolic and 25 mm diastolic should occur, and should persist for at least five minutes, typically returning to the pre-test pressure in 20–30 minutes.

3. Rarely, when a phaeochromocytoma is suspected but cannot be confirmed in any other way, a stimulation test may be justified, viz, provoking release of catecholamines by administering a very small dose of histamine acid phosphatase. In a patient with a phaeochromocytoma this typically produces a brief fall in blood pressure followed by a profound and sustained increase. The test is now outmoded for it is hazardous, and an antidote, e.g. phentolamine, must be available for immediate injection.

PHARMACOLOGICAL PREPARATION

The aims are to:

(i) Control the hypertension;

(ii) Correct the excessive vasoconstriction produced by the catecholamines secreted by the tumour; and

(iii) Prevent or treat tachycardia and arrhythmia (Katz *et al.*, 1968).

(i) Hypertension and vasoconstriction can be relieved by α-adrenergic blockers such as phenoxybenzamine (1 mg/kg), or the shorter acting phentolamine. Sodium nitroprusside, which acts directly on vascular smooth muscle, has a brief but rapid action and its administration as an infusion increases the flexibility of control. It is particularly effective in treating acute hypertensive episodes, and during operation.

(ii) Tachycardia and arrhythmia are due to excessive stimulation of the myocardium by β-adrenergic metabolites. Ideally a predominantly β-blocker such as practolol should be used.

The details of management vary considerably; many advocate pre-operative vasodilation with an α-blocker for 2–3 days, and gradual expansion of the blood volume with a plasma protein solution and/or blood; others prefer to augment the blood volume over 1–3 hours, i.e. during operation, using sodium nitroprusside as the vasodilator. The important point is that vasodilation and adequate augmentation of the blood volume should have been achieved before the tumour is actually removed. The necessary increase in blood volume can exceed 25% or even 30%.

If, despite this, hypotension develops after operation, more fluid, plasma or blood should be given, rather than vasoconstrictors which tend to recreate the effects of the tumour, and are rarely required if the blood volume has been adequately expanded.

It is noteworthy that arrhythmias associated with hypertension usually disappear when the blood pressure is reduced, and sodium nitroprusside is particularly useful in this regard because of its rapid action.

The choice of anaesthetic agent is determined by the method of preparation. If halothane (or a similar agent) which sensitizes the heart to catecholamines, is used, there is an increased incidence of arrhythmias, and these anaesthetic agents should be avoided.

It is most important that the anaesthetist knows how the patient has been prepared for operation, and is fully conversant with the pharmacological control of what may happen during operation. The blood pressure and pulse rate should be monitored throughout the operation, and ideally displayed continuously. A recent case illustrates these points.

A boy aged 6 years presented with a history of headache early in the morning for 3 weeks, epigastric pain, occasional vomiting, and recent loss of weight (2 kg in 3 months). Blood pressure by brachial cuff was 180/120, and total catecholamines in the urine were 2014 μg/24 hours. The response to a test dose of phentolamine (2 mg) was a fall in systolic pressure from 180 to 80 mmHg, and this persisted for 25 minutes.

Total adrenaline/nor-adrenaline (ng/ml) in samples of venous blood obtained via percutaneous needling of the femoral vein, gave the following results: confluence of iliac veins: 15·1, right renal vein: 15·3, left renal vein: 106, cava above renal veins: 22·3, hepatic vein: 5·5, superior cava at right atrium: 24·4 ng/ml, clearly indicating the source of secretion, in the left adrenal gland, and absence of a tumour in the right adrenal.

Phenoxybenzamine (1 mg/kg daily) was commenced, and 2 days later aortography and selective suprarenal arteriography showed a highly vascular tumour 4 cm in diameter in the left adrenal gland (Fig. 18.14). After preparation for a further 3 days the tumour (Fig. 18.13) was removed. The blood pressure and urinary catecholamines returned to normal within 7 days and have remained so for 18 months so far.

Although α-blockade had been instituted 2 days before aortography (and for 5 days before operation), there were sudden rises in blood pressure: (*a*) during aortography (to 210 mmHg systolic); (*b*) on positioning in preparation for operation (to 240 mmHg); and (*c*) during dissection of the tumour (from 110 to 180 mmHg). In each case the rise was quickly corrected, by phentolamine on the first occasion, and by sodium nitroprusside during operation.

Eight hours after operation, during which 300 ml of blood in excess of blood loss were given, the systolic blood pressure suddenly fell from 140 to 70 mmHg, and was quickly restored to 130 mmHg by rapidly infusing 300 ml of plasma. There were no further significant variations and all drugs were discontinued 2 days later.

During the following 12 months, the level of MHMA in a 24-hour specimen of urine was measured every 3 months, and ranged from 1·8 to 3·4 μg/1. This is to be repeated every 6 months in the second year, and then annually for 3 years.

III. NEUROFIBROMA

The adrenal medulla is one of the rarest sites in which a neurofibroma may arise. They may develop in medullary cell rests in the retroperitoneal tissues (Fig. 18.1) or in the posterior mediastinum (p. 465).

The histological features are described on p. 822, and the association with von Recklinghausen's disease in the section on the phakomatoses (p. 825).

The clinical features are those of a tumour of the posterior abdominal wall, similar to a retroperitoneal teratoma (p. 584) except for the tendency of a neurofibroma to extend into one of the intervertebral canals (Fig. 16.4, p. 448) to produce a dumb-bell tumour (p. 466), and to cause signs of compression of the spinal cord as the mode of presentation.

B. TUMOURS OF THE ADRENAL CORTEX

The adrenal cortex and medulla are in reality two distinct endocrine glands, the cells of the medulla being derived from the neural crest, and the cortex from splanchnic mesoderm. As in endocrine glands in general, excess secretion may be the result of hyperplasia, a benign adenoma or, when sufficiently differentiated, an adenocarcinoma. Disorders of the adrenal cortex include each of these possibilities, for many cortical adenocarcinomas are functional.

IV. ADENOMA OF THE ADRENAL CORTEX

Multiple minute nodules on or in the adrenal cortex are occasionally found incidentally at post mortem, and are not usually associated with any history or evidence of disturbance in endocrine secretion. The nodules sometimes appear to be separate from the gland, but more commonly they simply project from its surface and they are rarely more than a few millimetres in diameter. Microscopically the nodules consists of adrenal cortical cells, often resembling those in the zona reticularis.

Larger masses of cells compressing the adjacent parenchyma of the gland are true tumours and are properly described as adenomas.

Macroscopically an adenoma is 2–10 cm in diameter, tan to rich chocolate brown in colour, and usually oval or spherical (Fig. 18.15a), but some are lobulated. Areas of haemorrhage occur in the larger tumours, and there may be chalky areas of necrosis.

To the naked eye, an adenoma appears to be well encapsulated, but microscopically there may be infiltration of the capsule; however, this is not usually to be taken as an indication of malignancy, nor is the considerable nuclear pleomorphism so often present. The pattern of an adenoma closely resembles the adrenal cortex, and is composed of polygonal cells with eosinophilic cytoplasm containing fine droplets of neutral fat, a round nucleus slightly larger than in the normal adrenal cells, and may have a prominent nucleolus. The cells are arranged in columns or packets surrounded by thin-walled capillaries and fine strands of fibrous tissue, readily recognizable as an 'endocrine' pattern (Fig. 18.15b). Neuroblasts may be found in the intercellular septa in adenomas in young children.

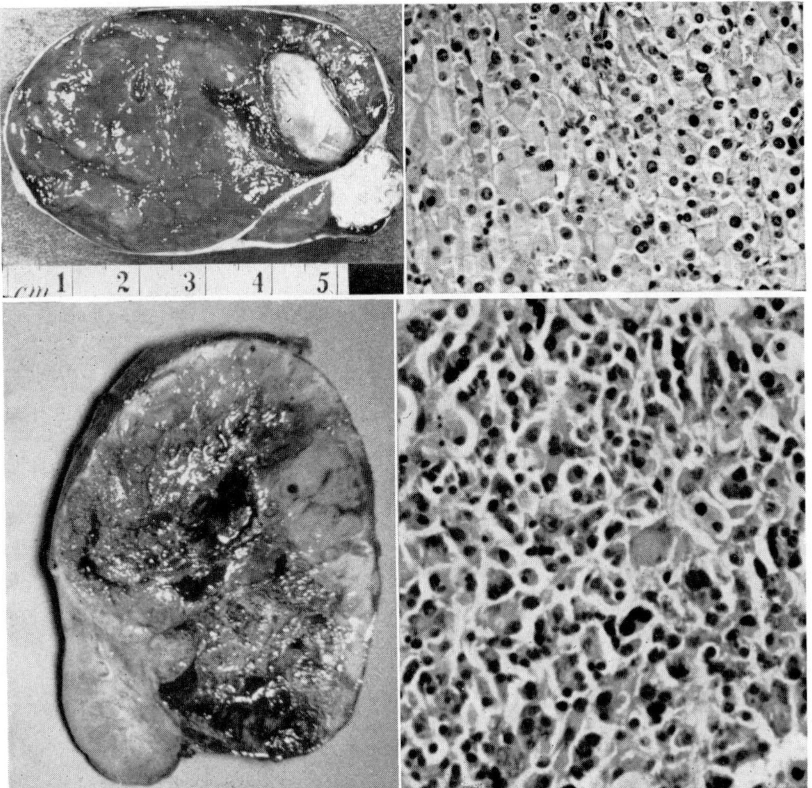

Figure 18.15. TUMOURS OF THE ADRENAL CORTEX; (*a*) CORTICAL ADENOMA, characteristically uniform, encapsulated, chocolate brown, and in some, as in this case, necrosis and the formation of microcysts; (*b*) the structure mimics adrenal cortex but the cells may show some nuclear irregularity (H & E. × 130); (*c*) CORTICAL CARCINOMA, a large tumour 19 × 12 × 10 cm which has invaded the left kidney and destroyed its upper pole; haemorrhage and necrosis are usual; as in adenoma (*d*) the cells mimic the structure of the adrenal cortex, but with some areas of small, uniform cells and others with bizarre hyperchromatic nuclei and marked pleomorphism (H & E. × 130).

[(*a*) *Top left.* (*b*) *Top right.* (*c*) *Bottom left.* (*d*) *Bottom right.*]

Adenomas are to be distinguished histologically from carcinoma of the adrenal cortex (q.v.) and in a large adenoma this may be difficult. In spite of some microscopic evidence of invasion and cellular pleomorphism, most adrenal tumours in childhood are benign.

In the Index Series there were five adenomas weighing from 45–145 g. In all but one the cut surface of the tumour was a uniform light brown; the other was pink. In contrast, the adrenal cortical carcinomas were much larger, the viable tissue was white or pale pink, and there were extensive areas of haemorrhage and necrosis.

The clinical features of cortical adenomas, including the elaboration of steroids and the differential diagnosis, are described in the following section on adenocarcinoma of the adrenal cortex.

V. CARCINOMA OF THE ADRENAL CORTEX

This very rare tumour almost always arises in the adrenal gland itself in childhood, and only a very small number occur in ectopic cortical tissue (Fig. 18.1) including ectopic cortical cells in the testis. A small nodule (2–3 mm in diameter) of adrenal cortical cells is a not uncommon incidental finding on the surface or the spermatic cord during operation for a hernia or an undescended testis (see p. 886).

The rarity of cortical carcinomas is indicated by the five in the Index Series (Dreher *et al.*, 1969) which covers a period of some 23 years. In order to provide a broader picture, Mr Douglas Cohen has generously supplied the data of six additional patients with a cortical carcinoma (hitherto unreported) treated at the Royal Alexandra Hospital for Children in Sydney; together with the cases in the Index Series, they will be referred to as the Combined Series, which contains 11 carcinomas and 10 adenomas arising in the paediatric age group.

AGE : SEX

No age is exempt, but most cortical carcinomas arise in adults more than 25 years old. In childhood they tend to affect the younger age groups, and six of the eleven carcinomas in the Combined Series occurred in children less than 2 years old. Females are said to be slightly more often affected in all age groups, but six of the eleven patients in the Combined Series were males.

MACROSCOPIC APPEARANCES

The tumour is usually large (Fig. 18.15c) white or pink, or occasionally yellowish in colour. Even when very large and subsequently shown to be malignant, the tumour may appear to be well encapsulated, although usually extremely necrotic and friable. Adenomas, on the other hand, tend to be firm, smaller, well encapsulated and characteristically brown or tan, or occasionally pink in colour (see above).

Tumours which announce their presence by the clinical effects of their endocrine secretion are said to be diagnosed relatively early, while the tumour is still small. In the literature there are reports of carcinomas as small as 2·5 cm in diameter identified and removed successfully. However, this was not the case in the Combined Series, in which most of the carcinomas weighed more than 150.

MICROSCOPIC FINDINGS

Cortical carcinomas consist of cells with an oval or pleomorphic nucleus (Fig. 18.15d) and a variable amount of cytoplasm often so scanty that they resemble the cells of a neuroblastoma. Mitoses are usually numerous and the nuclei are hyperchromatic. Characteristically the appearances vary from one part of the tumour to another, and in some areas there are cells with eosinophilic cytoplasm. The nuclei also differ; they are rounded, heavily outlined with chromatin and have a prominent nucleolus in adrenal carcinoma, whereas in neuroblastoma they are smaller, more oval and more variable in size.

SPREAD

Possibly because of the mesodermal origin of the adrenal cortex, cortical carcinomas tend to metastasize to the lungs without involvement of the regional lymph nodes (Burrington & Stephens, 1969). The pulmonary metastases, like the primary, usually show a considerable degree of differentiation and secretory activity.

ENDOCRINE SECRETION

The quantity and the types of substances secreted by cortical adenocarcinomas vary considerably from one tumour to another; they may secrete predominantly adrogens, glucocorticoids, a mixture of these or, extremely rarely, oestrogens or aldosterone.

Even more rare are 'non-hormonal' adrenocortical tumours, in which no endocrine function can be detected. Using strict criteria, Lewinsky *et al.* (1974) found 20 out of 178 tumours of the adrenal cortex; 2 of the 20 were in the paediatric age group, in males aged 2½ and 14 years respectively.

In general, the steroids secreted are not only increased in amount but also disordered in proportion, so that abnormal amounts of precursors and metabolites are produced. These may appear in increased amounts in the plasma or the urine, or in both. Estimation of these steroids to determine the nature of the causative pathological process is mentioned in the differential diagnosis of adrenal hypercorticism (p. 578) and summarized in Table 18.4.

MODES OF PRESENTATION OF CORTICAL CARCINOMAS

1. *An abdominal mass* is reported to be the commonest presenting feature in several series, and in the Combined Series a mass was palpable in the upper part of the abdomen in six of the eleven children with a carcinoma. However, in the series reported by Burrington & Stephens (1969) a tumour was palpable in only one of eight children with a carcinoma.
2. *An endocrine dyscrazia* is the other mode of presentation (Table 18.4) and this takes one of the following forms:
(*a*) Mixed syndromes, chiefly virilization with some Cushingoid features;
(*b*) Virilization;
(*c*) Cushing's syndrome, and very much less commonly
(*d*) Feminization or hyperaldosteronism.

In some children with a carcinoma (in three of the eleven cases in the Combined Series) there is no detectable abnormality in endocrine secretion.

INVESTIGATIONS

These are required to establish the diagnosis and assess the extent of the tumour before commencing treatment and these are as follows:
(i) X-rays of the abdomen and the lung fields;
(ii) The usual examination of the peripheral blood (WCC, Hb%, ESR);
(iii) Angiography (aortography and selective arteriography), and the subsequent pyelogram, to determine the presence or the site of an abdominal tumour;
(iv) Estimations of steroids in the serum and urine (see p. 581).

Table 18.4. Adrenal cortical hypersecretion. Endocrine effects observed in the Combined Series

		Clinical endocrinopathy				
Cause of hypersection	No. of patients	Virilization	Mixed syndrome	Cushing's syndrome	Feminization	None
Carcinoma	11	3	3	2	1	2
Adenoma	10	6	2	1	0	1
Hyperplasia	3	0	0	3	0	0
Totals	24	9	5	6	1	3

Previously reported:
Dreher, G.H., Williams, S.W., Howard, R.N., Campbell, P.E., Davies, H.E. & McCarthy, N. (1969). *Aust. Paediat. J.*, **5** : 62.
Cohen, D.H. *et al*. 1975 (personal communication).

DIFFERENTIATION OF OTHER ABDOMINAL MASSES

In children presenting with an abdominal mass no evidence of endocrine hypersecretion, Wilms' tumour (p. 495) or neuroblastoma (p. 538) are more likely than an adrenal tumour, and the findings on angiography and pyelography are usually diagnostic. Elevated urinary catecholamines would point to a neuroblastoma (p. 539) or to a phaeochromocytoma (p. 562), and their differentiation is described on p. 516.

A non-functioning adrenal carcinoma raises the possibility, suggested by Stowens (1959), that some non-secreting tumours of the adrenal cortex might in fact be paragangliomas (p. 586) which are very similar histologically, except for their negative chromaffin reaction. However, when the distinction turns on this reaction, it is important that the staining solution should be freshly prepared and suitably acidic, otherwise chromaffin positive cells may appear to be negative.

CLINICAL FEATURES OF HYPERADRENOCORTICISM

Hypersecretion of the adrenal cortex in children (Hayles, Hahn *et al.*, 1966) may be the result of a functioning carcinoma, or an adenoma or due to bilateral hyperplasia. The clinical syndrome produced by each of these conditions depends upon the predominant type(s) of hormone(s) secreted, i.e. androgens, cortisol, or, extremely rarely, oestrogens or aldosterone. As most adrenal cortical tumours, particularly carcinomas, may produce more than one hormone, mixed clinical syndromes are common (Table 18.4).

1. *Virilization* occurs when androgenic steroids are secreted in excess, producing isosexual precocity in males and masculinization in girls. In boys the clinical manifestations of virilization are enlargement of the penis, the appearance of pubic hair, excessive growth with an advanced bone age, acne and deepening of the voice. In girls, virilization commencing after birth causes acne, deepening of the voice, enlargement of the clitoris, and accelerated growth with an advanced bone age (Prévot, Mourot *et al.*, 1972).
2. *Cushing's syndrome* develops, in either sex, when the secretion is chiefly cortisol (McArthur *et al.*, 1972) and this is more likely to occur in a carcinoma than in an adenoma or cortical hyperplasia. Cushing's syndrome is a rarity in childhood, particularly before the age of ten years (Gilbert & Cleveland, 1970), and obesity, hypertension and stunted growth are the usual features.
3. *A mixed syndrome* of virilization with some Cushingoid features, due to hypersecretion of both androgens and cortisol, is one of the commonest consequences of a cortical carcinoma or adenoma.
4. *Feminization* in males, due to excess secretion of ostrogens is one of the rarest modes of presentation of an adrenal cortical tumour (Table 18.5). In the literature up to 1965 there were only 52 cases reported in males of all ages (Gabrilove, Sharma *et al.*, 1965), and in most cases the tumour appeared to

be malignant. A carcinoma was the cause in approximately 75% of the cases reviewed by Di George *et al.* (1959).

Feminizing adrenal tumours in girls are even more rare than in boys, but Snaith (1958) reported isosexual precocity in a 5½-year old girl with an anaplastic but encapsulated adrenocortical tumour.

From a review of the literature, Leditschke & Arden (1974) collected only five cases of a feminizing adrenal tumour in boys, and added a sixth of their own (Table 18.5) a boy who developed gynecomastia, accelerated growth and advanced bone age, at the age of five years. The tumour was successfully removed and thought to be an adenoma.

They noted that although most feminizing adrenal cortical tumours in adult males were malignant, those occurring in prepubertal boys appeared to be predominantly benign. Another example, also apparently benign, has been reported by Abodowsky and Maira (1972).

This was not the case in the only instance encountered in the Index Series, not previously reported.

A 12-year old boy presented with a large abdominal tumour, subsequently found to be a large, infiltrating carcinoma of the left adrenal. Gynecomastia was present, each breast being 7 cm in diameter but only 1·5 cm thick. At operation the tumour was removed (Fig. 18.15c), but myriads of 'millet seed' metastases in the left lung were seen through the abdominothoracic incision and confirmed by subsequent biopsy. Death occurred 3 months after operation.

An interesting and probably relevant point in the history suggests that the tumour may have been induced by radiation, for radium needles had been inserted into a superficial haemangioma of the chest wall, at the level of the fifth rib on the left side, when he was 2 years old, 10 years before he developed the carcinoma in the left adrenal gland.

5. *Primary hyperaldosteronism* is the rarest manifestation of adrenal hypercorticism in children, usually due to bilateral hyperplasia, and causes hypokalaemia, muscular weakness, polyuria, hypertension and cardiomegaly. This is to be distinguished from secondary aldosteronism, which is the more common, occurring in a variety of conditions such as the nephrotic syndrome, cirrhosis of the liver or cardiac failure.

OTHER CAUSES OF VIRILISM AND CUSHING'S SYNDROME

In the Combined Series of eleven carcinomas, the clinical picture was as follows: virilization with Cushingoid features (3), virilization (3), Cushing's syndrome (1), and feminization (1); in the remaining 3 patients with an abdominal mass due to an adrenal cortical tumour there was no clinical or biochemical evidence of abnormal or excessive secretion.

Adrenal cortical hyperplasia. Nearly all adrenal tumours develop after birth, but in a few cases a tumour has arisen before birth and produced congenital virilization indistinguishable clinically from virilization caused by

Table 18.5. Adrenal feminizing tumours

Case	Age	Bone age (yrs)	Height (cm)	Weight (kg)	17-Ketosteroids (normal: 0–4 mg)	17-Hydroxy corticoids (normal: 6–8 mg)	Oestrogens (normal: 8–23 μg)	Tumour Side	Size (cm)	Weight (g)	Pathological diagnosis	Result
Wilkins (1948)	4 yr 8 mo	10	112	—	4·1	—	Sl increase (5 rat units/ 24 hrs)	R	3×2	—	Adenoma	No recurrence 14 years post-op. Alive (1965)
Fontaine *et al.* (1954)	5 yr	12	142	29·5	5–10	—	Increased (5–6 mice units /24 hrs)	L	—	26·6	Carcinoma (with vascular spread)	No recurrence 10 year post-op. Alive (1963)
Mosier *et al.* (1961)	7 yr	—	123	24·6	9·1	5·0	4 μg	L	2	—	Adenoma	No recurrence 5 years post-op. Alive (1965)
Bacon & Lowrey (1965)	6 yr	12	132	26	53	2·4	Increased (20 rat units)	L	9×8×6	205	Adenoma (with neoplastic thrombus)	Recurrence $7\frac{1}{2}$ years post-op. Died
Castleman *et al.* (1972)	6 yr 8 mo	8	128	28	124	0·6	'Normal'	R	8	250	Carcinoma, pulmonary metastases	Died on operating table
Leditschke* & Arden (1974)	5 yr	8·5	120	22·68	21	24	140 μg	L	9·5 × 7·5×4·5	260	Adenoma	No recurrence 1 year post-op. Alive (1974)

* This table, after Leditschke & Arden (1974), is reproduced with permission of the authors and the *Australian Paediatric Journal*.

congenital adrenal hyperplasia. The latter develops *in utero* as the result of a deficiency in one or other of two enzymes, inherited as an autosomal recessive trait. The enzymic defects are in 21- or 11-hydroxylation, of which the former is by far the more common. Both lead to diminished secretion of cortisol, and hence to loss of the feed-back control on the pituitary which normally limits the secretion of ACTH. The consequent excess secretion of ACTH stimulates the adrenal cortex causing hyperplasia with excess production of androgenic steroids. When this occurs in a female *in utero*, masculinization with fusion of the labia and hypertrophy of the clitoris occurs; in affected males the genitalia are normal at birth. Approximately one-third of those so affected (of either sex) are also 'salt-losers', leading to life-threatening dehydration and electrolyte disturbances.

Secondary hypercorticism may occur, possibly as the result of a hypothalamic lesion, and cause excess secretion of ACTH by the pituitary. This results in bilateral adrenal hyperplasia, typically occurring after the age of ten years.

Cushing's syndrome has also been reported to occur with tumours arising in the lung, thymus, liver, pancreas and kidney, and in these cases it is thought that ACTH-like substances are secreted by the tumour cells. The same type of secretion probably accounts for the development of Cushing's syndrome in the syndrome of 'nesidioblastosis' (Vance *et al.*, 1972) which includes tumours of the islet cells of the pancreas, adrenocortical adenomas and other endocrine adenoma (p. 563). Cushing's syndrome is sometimes due to hyperplasia.

Tumours of the adrenal gland more commonly occur in the first decade of life, whereas hyperplasia typically occurs after this age.

DIFFERENTIATION OF CORTICAL ADENOMA, CARCINOMA AND HYPERPLASIA

The points on which these can be distinguished, summarized in Table 18.6 are as follows:

1. *A palpable adrenal tumour* narrows the possibilities by excluding hyperplasia, and the results of biochemical investigations may give some indication as to whether the tumour is benign or malignant. Because of the fallibility of histological differentiation, the final distinction may only be possible retrospectively when a long term follow up after operative removal of a tumour indicates that no recurrence or metastasis has occurred.
2. *Stimulation and suppression tests.* (*a*) ACTH given intravenously to normal children produces an increase in plasma and urinary corticoids, and this also occurs in cases of hyperplasia, but not in patients with an adenoma or a carcinoma. (*b*) In general, small doses of dexamethasone will suppress the secretion of corticosteroids in normal children, larger doses are required to

Table 18.6. Adrenal cortical tumours; Some features which may distinguish adenoma, adenocarcinoma and hyperplasia (figures in the Combined Series, Table 18.4)

Test/evidence	Carcinoma	Adenoma	Hyperplasia
Palpable abdominal mass	+	±	—
Calcification (adrenal area)	+	±	—
Abnormal angiogram	++	+	—
Cushing's syndrome ('pure')	—	—	+
Abnormal steroids in urine	+	—	—
Mixed syndromes	+	+	—
Feminization	+	+	—
Suppression test (dose of dexamethasone required)	+++	+++	+
ACTH stimulation test	—	—	+

suppress secretion in cases of bilateral adrenal hyperplasia, and even very large doses may fail to suppress secretion in adenomas and carcinomas.

3. *The age of the patient.* If the onset of the hypercorticism occurs in the first year of life, a carcinoma is more likely to be the cause than either an adenoma or hyperplasia.

4. *The more sudden the onset* of adrenal dyscrazia in a child, the more likely it is to be due to a carcinoma.

5. *Calcification* in x-rays of the adrenal area does not occur in hyperplasia, but is not uncommon in both adenoma and carcinoma.

6. *The nature of the endocrine dyscrazia.* Adrenal cortical hyperplasia tends to cause 'pure' Cushing's syndrome, while adenomas and carcinomas typically produce a mixed syndrome of virilism with Cushingoid features. Feminization, in either sex, occurs with adenomas but in some cases the tumour is a carcinoma (Table 18.5).

7. *The size of a tumour* is not always a reliable guide, but in general tumours weighing less than 150 g are usually benign. As noted in the literature, the only absolute criterion of malignancy is the presence (or later appearance) of recurrence or metastasis.

8. *The histology of the tumour.* It may be difficult to distinguish between cortical adenoma and carcinoma and in a few cases the only certain evidence of malignancy is the presence of metastasis, at the time of operation or after excision of the primary tumour. In the Combined Series, the following features were helpful in distinguishing adrenal adenomas and carcinomas.

(*a*) Adenomas are usually encapsulated and there is usually no capsular invasion; carcinomas show extensive invasion of adjacent structures and vessels.

(*b*) Adenomas preserve an organoid pattern resembling adrenal cortex structurally and cytologically; the cells form solid cords, occasionally acini, and are sometimes compartmented by delicate fibrous septa. Cytoplasm is usually abundant and eosinophilic, and lipofuchsin may be present.

Carcinomas show little structural organization, mitoses are numerous, nuclear hyperchromatism and pleomorphism are prominent, and there is widespread necrosis.

(*c*) Bizarre hyperchromatic nuclei are common in adenomas and are not necessarily indicative of malignancy; these large hyperchromatic nuclei, which are probably the result of degenerative changes, may contribute to the difficulty in diagnosis.

TREATMENT OF CORTICAL CARCINOMA

Surgical removal of the tumour is required. Supportive and post-operative substitution therapy are particularly important when excising an adrenal tumour causing Cushing's disease or Cushingoid features in a child (Raiti *et al.*, 1972). Cortisone is usually administered intravenously to prevent acute adrenal insufficiency during or following the removal of the tumour; treatment should be commenced 1–2 days before operation and continued after operation for at least 7–10 days, in diminishing doses, given orally as soon as possible.

Patients with hyperadrenocorticism appear to be more prone to infection, possibly related to the eosinopenia noted in a significant proportion of cases; a broad spectrum antibiotic 'cover' before and for 1–2 weeks after operation is also required.

Operation

Adrenal cortical carcinomas are usually large, and although some may appear to be encapsulated, the capsule and the substance of the tumour tend to be friable. Removal without rupture and spillage requires generous access, and an abdominothoracic incision is usually advisable to avoid excessive handling (Glenn, Peterson & Mannix, 1968) even when the size of the tumour does not make this mandatory.

When an adrenal carcinoma is adherent and frankly infiltrating, extensive resection of neighbouring organs and tissues may be feasible. In such cases the tumour bed, or any residual irremovable tumour, should be outline with metal clips to delineate the area to be irradiated subsequently.

Chemotherapy

The substance OP'-DDD is toxic to the cells of adrenal carcinomas and has been reported to be of benefit in some cases (Bergenstal *et al.*, 1960), but it is chiefly an antagonist to the secretion of the tumour, with toxic side effects, and has no demonstrable antineoplastic action.

Radiotherapy

It was initially thought that cortical carcinomas were resistant to radiotherapy, but with modern techniques useful regression can be effected, and uncertainty as to whether the tumour is benign or malignant has prompted the application of radiotherapy to the tumour bed in most cases. Irradiation is definitely indicated if there is any spillage of the tumour during removal, or when excision is incomplete and some of the tumour is left *in situ*.

RESULTS: PROGNOSIS

The outlook in frankly malignant carcinoma of the adrenal is poor, chiefly because of the high proportion of patients with metastases at the time of diagnosis.

In view of the acknowledged difficulties in distinguishing cortical adenoma from adenocarcinoma on histological grounds, the diagnosis of 'carcinoma' without corroborative evidence of local recurrence or metastasis is always open to some doubt. In some of the cases reported as long term survivals after removal of a 'carcinoma', the tumour may have been an adenoma.

In the Index Series, all five patients with a cortical carcinoma died of metastases; the longest survival after operation was 8 months, and two patients died within 5 months. However, three of the six patients in Cohen's series have survived; two of the three are free of disease, and the third is alive but has a local recurrence which developed one year after operation.

Able (1969) reported survival of all four children with a carcinoma in his series, and Stewart, Morris Jones & Jolleys (1974) four out of five cases surviving free of disease 1–12 years after operation.

C. TUMOURS OF RETROPERITONEAL TISSUES

The retroperitoneal tissues, particularly in the upper half of the abdomen, are a common site of tumours in childhood, and the factors which tend to delay the diagnosis are the same as in those arising in other tissues or viscera in this area.

Benign retroperitoneal swellings are probably less common than malignant tumours (Arnheim, 1950), although small hamartomas of connective tissues may occur more frequently than they are recognized. Neurofibroma (p. 822) arising below the level of the diaphragm may also present in this region.

Retroperitoneal lymphangiomas (p. 674) occasionally cause symptoms which lead to exploration and recognition.

Neuroblastoma (p. 543) *and 'ganglioneuroblastoma'* (p. 550) are by far the commonest tumours of the retroperitoneal tissues in childhood (De-

Lorimier, Bragg & Linden, 1969). In the Index Series, as in others reported, approximately 50% of abdominal neuroblastomas arose in autonomic cells derived from the neural crest (Fig. 18.1) located in the retroperitoneum.

Sarcomas of various types, e.g. rhabdomyosarcoma (p. 783) and embryonal fibrosarcoma (Fig. 21.12, p. 710), are also found in the retroperitoneum; either may reach a very large size before producing signs or symptoms. Occasionally, haemorrhage or rupture of the tumour into the peritoneal cavity presents with the clinical picture of an 'acute surgical abdomen'.

Tumours which have a particular tendency to arise in retroperitoneal tissues are as follows:

I. Teratoma;
II. Paraganglioma;
III. Phaeochromocytoma (see tumours of the adrenal medulla p. 562).

I. RETROPERITONEAL TERATOMA

Teratomas are less common in the retroperitoneal tissues than in the ovary (p. 716), testis (p. 882) and mediastinum (p. 456) and very much less common than sacrococcygeal teratomas (see teratomas, p. 45 and p. 711).

Most retroperitoneal teratomas present during the first two decades of life, and a high proportion cause symptoms during infancy.

AGE : SEX

In two extensive reviews of cases in children (Arnheim, 1950; Engel, Elkins & Fletcher, 1968) a total of 56 were diagnosed before the age of 15 years; the incidence in boys and girls was approximately equal. In the more recent series, 20 out of 30 patients were less than 15 years of age, and 43% were less than 10 years old.

SITE

The tumour is almost always situated just above the upper pole of one kidney and occurs with equal frequency on the right and left side.

PATHOLOGY

By definition, teratomas contain elements derived from more than one emybronic layer, and the tumours are moderately large, 10–15 cm in diameter. Those in which all the tissues are fully differentiated are classed as benign (see p. 45), and the term malignant is reserved for those with embryonic tissue lacking maturation. This distinction appears to be more reliable in retroperitoneal teratomas than in those arising in the mediastinum or the pelvis.

On histological criteria, 6–10% of retroperitoneal teratomas are classed as malignant, and the accuracy of this prediction was confirmed by subsequent metastasis and death in all three examples classified as malignant in the 30 cases reported by Engel *et al.* (1968).

MODES OF PRESENTATION

In spite of the close relationship with the kidney, urological symptoms and signs are rare.

1. *An abdominal mass* was the first indication of abnormality in most cases, particularly in the younger children.
2. *Gastrointestinal symptoms*, such as abdominal distension, nausea, vomiting and pain, were the main complaints leading to a diagnosis in the remainder.

INVESTIGATIONS

In those presenting with a palpable abdominal mass, the plan of investigation is the same as described in the section on Wilms' tumour (p. 506).

DIFFERENTIAL DIAGNOSIS

The presence of large plaques of dense calcification on plain x-rays is probably one of the most helpful findings, for they differ from the linear peripheral calcification seen in 5% of patients with a Wilms' tumour, and from the multiple, small, scattered flecks of calcification seen in 50% of neuroblastomas.

Arteriography and the subsequent pyelogram will exclude a renal tumour, in which distortion of the pelvicalyceal system occurs.

If the distinctive calcification of a teratoma is lacking, neuroblastoma would be the more likely diagnosis in a child less than five years of age, and absence of increased catecholamines in the urine (p. 551) could be helpful in distinguishing a teratoma. In some cases the diagnosis is only made at laparotomy, or on histological grounds.

TREATMENT

Complete excision

This is all that is required in most cases, and when large, this can be a formidable undertaking. If the mass is found to be infiltrating surrounding tissues, or when subsequent examination shows that it contains immature embryonic tissue, post-operative irradiation and chemotherapy should be considered.

Radiotherapy
Although embryonal carcinoma (see endodermal sinus tumour, p. 692) is generally classed as radio-resistant, radiotherapy in the dose range 1500–3000 rads (depending on the age of the patient) can be employed. The problems presented by irradiating marrow in the vertebral bodies are the same as in Wilms' tumour, and radiotherapy is usually deferred until the marrow has recovered from the effects of the primary course of chemotherapy.

Chemotherapy
On the assumption that the malignant element of a teratoma is often composed of 'endodermal sinus' tumour, the treatment recommended is a primary course of combination chemotherapy with actinomycin D, 5-fluorouracil and cyclophosphamide, or vincristine, actinomycin D and cyclophosphamide, or adriamycin, followed by repeated courses lasting 5–7 days, for a period of 1–2 years.

PROGNOSIS: RESULTS

The two reported series quoted, and an earlier review of retroperitoneal teratoma in all age groups (Palumbo, 1949), show a progressive decrease in operative mortality (54 %, 29 %, 14 %) between 1949 and 1968, a decline which reflects better operative technique and improved general management.

In those classed as malignant on histological grounds, the prognosis has been grave and almost uniformly fatal. However, few if any of the fatal cases reported in the past received the benefit of integrated surgery, radiotherapy and modern chemotherapy now available.

II. PARAGANGLIOMA
(syn. 'chemodectoma')

Paragangliomas arise in non-chromaffin cells derived from the neural crest, in the carotid and aortic bodies (p. 467), in chemoreceptor cells in the glomus jugulare (p. 366) and in the ear (p. 367). Similar but smaller groups of cells are scattered throughout the body, more widely in children than in adults. Stowens (1959) noted non-chromaffin cells in almost every part of the body in childhood, including the bone marrow, as encapsulated groups 1 mm in diameter, each related to a capillary, and without any demonstrable neural connections. Some of the cells in these groups contain chromaffin granules and are therefore potential sites of phaeochromocytoma (p. 562).

On rare occasions a chromaffin-negative cell in the adrenal gland gives rises to a paraganglioma, and Stowens also suggested that some of the 'non-functioning adenomas' and 'adenocarcinomas' of the adrenal cortex may be in reality paragangliomas.

AGE : SEX

The largest collected series of paraganglioma in childhood contained 36 cases (Helpap & Grouls, 1971); the peak incidence was between 10 and 15 years of age (in 16 of the 36), while in 7 cases the tumour appeared before the age of 10 years.

There were 20 girls and 14 boys, and in 2 cases the sex was not reported.

SITES

The sites varied widely; the carotid body was the commonest (13 cases), retroperitoneal tissue was second (6 cases) and then, equally common with 4 each, the mediastinum (p. 467), the glomus femorale and glomus jugulare (p. 366).

MACROSCOPIC APPEARANCES

The size of a paraganglioma tends to be related to its site; the largest are found in the abdomen and mediastinum, where they may reach 10–15 cm in diameter. The tumour is very vascular, encapsulated, and tan to red in colour, with yellowish areas of necrosis and darker haemorrhagic areas.

MICROSCOPIC FINDINGS

The typical appearance is an endocrine pattern with packets of cells, 'cell balls' (Zellballen), separated by delicate strands of connective tissue. Most of the cells contain abundant, slightly eosinophilic cytoplasm and a round or oval vesicular nucleus. Some cells are small and rounded with a hyperchromatic nucleus; others are rather pleomorphic with a large irregular nucleus, and some are multinucleated (Ackerman, 1955).

The cytoplasm may contain fine granules which are PAS positive. The chromaffin reaction is by definition negative, an important point on which the histological diagnosis depends. The reaction is apt to be misleading unless the tissue is fixed in a solution containing chromium salts; fixation in neutral formalin does not preserve the chromaffin material on which differentiation from a chromaffin-positive phaeochromocytoma depends.

Both malignant and benign paragangliomas have very similar histological findings, and nuclear pleomorphism alone is not a reliable indication of malignancy. In rare cases, as in phaeochromocytoma, only metastasis makes the distinction certain. Even 'metastases' in paraganglioma and phaeochromocytoma may be open to another interpretation in some cases, for multicentric primary tumours are known to occur.

SPREAD

Local infiltration is the most important aspect. Although metastases are sometimes found in lymph nodes, their rate of growth is usually slow, and infiltration of adjacent soft tissues precedes lymphatic metastases.

Blood-borne metastases to the lungs, marrow and liver occur in malignant examples, and in the series of 36 cases quoted, approximately 25% had local or distant metastases, a higher proportion than in adults with a chromaffin-negative paraganglioma.

ENDOCRINE SECRETION

Although chromaffin-negative and typically non-functioning, some paragangliomas in adults apparently produce metabolites similar to those associated with phaeochromocytomas, i.e. catecholamines capable of producing hypertension and a positive response to phentolamine (p. 569).

There appears to be only one case report of a functional paraganglioma in a child, a 12-year old boy reported by Glenner *et al.*, (1962); pressure on the tumour caused increases in pulse rate and blood pressure, and the tumour was demonstrated to secrete levarterenol.

MODES OF PRESENTATION

Of the 21 patients with a retroperitoneal paraganglioma collected by Olson and Abell (1970), six were between 5 and 19 years of age.

1. *An abdominal mass* was the mode of presentation in three of these six cases.
2. *Pain in the back*, severe and persistent in nature, was a notable complaint and led to x-rays which demonstrated a mass in the retroperitoneal tissues.

Paragangliomas arising in other sites produce signs or symptoms related to the region.

(*a*) In the mediastinum, some are so large as to present with mediastinal compression (p. 445), while others cause general systemic effects such as fever, malaise and weight loss without any localizing signs initially, in the case reported by Barrie (1961).

(*b*) Those arising in the region of the carotid body present as a firm swelling in the neck, less commonly with dysphagia, Horner's syndrome, syncope, headache, or cranial nerve palsies (Lederer, Skolnik *et al.*, 1958).

(*c*) Tumours of the glomus jugulare, or arising in adjacent subsidiary microganglia (p. 366), cause symptoms such as earache, tinnitus, deafness, bleeding from the ear, or an aural 'polyp' (p. 367).

INVESTIGATIONS

Those required in a child with an abdominal mass (p. 506) or a mediastinal tumour (p. 461) are described in the appropriate sections. In the abdomen, aortography and selective arteriography are the most informative, and usually demonstrate the site and size of the tumour.

Biochemical tests (e.g. catecholamines, 17-ketosteroids etc.) on 24-hour collection of urine provide a basis for diagnosis by excluding a neuroblastoma, phaeochromocytoma etc. (see Table 18.4).

DIFFERENTIAL DIAGNOSIS

When a paraganglioma arises in the retroperitoneal tissues, this includes neuroblastoma and Wilms' tumour, and the less common causes listed in Table 17.1 (p. 491).

1. *Wilms' tumour* (p. 495). The extrarenal site, and displacement without distortion of the pelvi-calyceal system, are usually sufficient to exclude this tumour.

2. *Neuroblastoma* can be difficult to exclude, because approximately 50% of those in the abdomen arise in the same retroperitoneal sites as paraganglioma, and calcification is not uncommon in both conditions.

The age of the patient is some guide; most neuroblastomas occur in children less than 5 years old, while abdominal paragangliomas are uncommon in this age group. In Helpap & Grouls' series, the youngest of the six children with an abdominal paraganglioma was $5\frac{1}{2}$ years old, and those typically affected are in the third quinquennium.

Absence of increased excretion of catecholamines in the urine is to be expected in truly 'non-functioning' paragangliomas (Table 18.4), but normal levels are insufficient grounds for excluding a neuroblastoma.

Neuroblastoma metastases in the marrow are so common (in 50–70% of cases) that the diagnosis can often be confirmed by a positive marrow smear see Fig. 18.7, colour plates, following p. 140).

Because of their rarity, the final diagnosis of a paraganglioma usually requires exploration and biopsy.

TREATMENT

Excision should be as complete as possible, but their vascularity and densely adherent margins can cause considerable technical difficulties.

Even when the primary appears to have been completely removed, the propensity for local recurrence, especially in childhood, would indicate the use of post-operative radiotherapy and chemotherapy.

Radiotherapy
Paragangliomas are relatively radiosensitive and in those arising in the abdomen or thorax, a total of 2500 rads, in fractions over 3–4 weeks, would be appropriate.

Chemotherapy
There has been insufficient experience with this rare tumour to make any useful recommendations concerning the place of cytotoxic agents.

PROGNOSIS

This depends largely on whether the tumour is inherently benign or malignant. Only two of the six retroperitoneal paragangliomas reported by Olsen and Abell (1970) were malignant; in Helpap and Grouls' series, 20% recurred locally, and a total of 26% were considered to be malignant.

Mediastinal and retroperitoneal paragangliomas have a higher incidence of malignancy than those arising in other sites. Considering all age groups, the proportion of malignant tumours appears to be 20–30%, possibly slightly higher in those less than 15 years of age.

Most authors have found cellular morphology alone of little value in prognosis, and pleomorphism does not appear to be associated with a lower survival rate.

The prognosis in patients without local invasion or metastases is reported to be uniformly good, and the four children without metastases in Olsen & Abell's series (1970) were all free of disease when last reviewed.

OTHER RETROPERITONEAL TUMOURS

A variety of benign and malignant tumours have been reported in retroperitoneal tissues (Ackerman, 1955). Retroperitoneal lymphangiomas and 'mesenteric' cysts are described in the section on omentum and mesenteries (p. 673).

Neuroblastoma arising in retroperitoneal tissues (see p. 544) are otherwise the same as those arising in the adrenal gland.

Retroperitoneal fibrosarcomas occasionally present as an abdominal mass in the early months of life, sometimes at birth, accompanied by signs and symptoms of intestinal obstruction.

REFERENCES

Neuroblastoma

BALDWIN, R.W., PRICE, M.R. & ROBINS, R.A. (1972). Blocking of lymphocyte mediated cytotoxicity for rat hepatoma cells by tumour specific antigen-antibody complexes. *Nature, New Biology*, **238** : 185.

BECKWITH, J.B. & PERRIN, E.V. (1963). In situ neuroblastomas: a contribution to the natural history of neural crest tumors. *Amer. J. Path.*, **43** : 1089.

BECKWITH, J.B. & MARTIN, R.F. (1968). Observations on the histopathology of neuroblastomas. *J. Pediat. Surg.*, **3** : 106.

BILL, A.H. (1968). The regression of neuroblastoma. *J. Pediat. Surg.*, **3** : 103.

BLAKE, J. & FITZPATRICK, C. (1972). Eye signs in neuroblastoma. *Trans. Ophthalmol. Soc. U.K.*, **92** : 825.

BOLANDE, R.P. & TOWLER, W.F. (1970). A possible relationship of neuroblastoma to von Recklinghausen's disease. *Cancer*, **26** : 162.

BRITISH MEDICAL JOURNAL (1974). Fever in malignant disease (leading article). *Brit. Med. J.*, **1** : 591.

BURDMAN, J.A. & GOLDSTEIN, M.N. (1964). Longterm tissue culture of neuroblastomas. 3. In vitro studies of nerve growth—stimulating factor in sera of children with neuroblastoma. *J. Natl. Cancer Inst.*, **33** : 123.

CHATTEN, J. & VOORHEES, M.L. (1967). Familial neuroblastoma. Report of a kindred with multiple disorders including neuroblastoma in four siblings. *New Engl. J. Med.*, **277** : 1230.

CLATWORTHY, H.W.Jr. & NEWTON, W.A. (1970). Mediastinal ganglion cell tumours in children. *Proc. Centenary Congress, Melbourne*, **1** : 185.

COHEN, D. (1969). Neuroblastoma: factors affecting survival. *Zeitschr. für Kinderchirurg.*, **6** : 389.

DELORIMIER, A.A., BRAGG, K.U. & LINDEN, G. (1969). Neuroblastoma in childhood. *Am. J. Dis. Child.*, **118** : 441.

DONOHUE, J.P., GARRETT, R.A. *et al.* (1974). The multiple manifestations of neuroblastoma. *J. Urol.*, **111** : 260.

EVANS, A.E., BLORE, J., HADLEY, R. & TANINDI, S. (1971). The LaBrosse spot test: a practical aid in diagnosis and management of children with neuroblastoma. *Pediatrics*, **47** : 913.

EVANS, A.E. (1972). Treatment of neuroblastoma. *Cancer*, **30** : 1595.

EVANS, A.E., D'ANGIO, G.J. & RANDOLPH, J. (1971). A proposed staging for children with neuroblastoma. *Cancer*, **27** : 374.

FAGAN, C.J. & SWISCHUK, L.E. (1974). Dumb-bell neuroblastoma or ganglioneuroma of the spinal canal. *Am. J. Roentgenol.*, **120** : 453.

GHAZALI, S. (1974). Pelvic neuroblastoma: a better prognosis. *Ann. Surg.*, **179** : 115.

GITLOW, S.E. *et al.* (1970). Diagnosis of neuroblastoma by qualitative and quantitative determination of catecholamines and metabolites in urine. *Cancer*, **15** : 1377.

HELLSTROM, I.E. & HELLSTROM, K.E. (1968). Regression of neuroblastoma. *J. Pediat. Surg.*, **3** : 103–106.

HELLSTROM, I.E., HELLSTROM, K.E., PIERCE, G.E. *et al.* (1968). Demonstration of cell-bound and humoral immunity against neuroblastoma cells. *Proc. Nat. Acad. Sci.*, **60** : 1231.

HELLSTROM, K.E. & HELLSTROM, I. (1971). Some aspects of the immune defense against cancer. *Cancer*, **28** : 1266–1271.

HINTERBERGER, H. & BARTHOLOMEW, R.J. (1969). Catecholamines and their acidic metabolites in urine and in tumour tissue in neuroblastoma, ganglioneuroma and phaeochromocytoma. *Clin. Chim. Acta*, **23** : 169.

JOSE, D.G. & SESHADRI, R. (1974). Circulating immune complexes in human neuroblastoma; direct assay and role in blocking specific cellular immunity. *Int. J. Cancer*, **13** : 824.

JOSE, D.G. & SKVARIL, F. (1974). Serum inhibitors of cellular immunity in human neuroblastoma: IgG subclass of blocking activity. *Int. J. Cancer*, **13** : 173.

JOUTE, P.A., WADMAN, S.K. & VAN PATTEN, W.J. (1970). Congenital neuroblastoma: symptoms in the mother during pregnancy. *Clin. Ped.*, **9** : 206.

KÄSER, H., SERRANO, G.L. *et al.* (1973). Ganglioneuroma in a girl with chronic diarrhoea and hypokalaemia. *Helv. Paediat. Acta*, **28** : 485.

KOOP, C.E. & JOHNSON, D.G. (1971). Neuroblastoma: An assessment of therapy in reference to staging. *J. Pediat. Surg.*, **6** : 595.

KOOP, C.E. & SCHNAUFER, L. (1975). The management of abdominal neuroblastoma. *Cancer*, **35** : 905.

KOROBKIN, M. & CLARK, R.E. & PALUBINSKAS, A.J. (1972). Occult neuroblastoma and acute cerebellar ataxia in childhood. *Radiology*, **102** : 151.

LA BROSSE, E.H. (1968a). Biochemical diagnosis of neuroblastoma: use of a urine spot test. *Proc. Amer. Ass. Cancer Res.*, **9** : 39.

LABROSSE, E.H. (1968b). 3-Methoxy-4-Hydroxyphenylglycol in neuroblastoma. *J. Pediat. Surg.*, **3** : 148.

LEMERLE, J. *et al.* (1969). Trois cas d'association à un neuroblastome d'un syndrome oculo-cerebello-myoclonique. *Arch. Franç. Péd.*, **26** : 547.

LEPINTRE, J., SCHWEISGUTH, O., LABRUNE, M. & LEMERLE, J. (1969). Hourglass neuroblastomas: a study of 22 cases. *Arch. Franç. Péd.*, **26** : 829.

REYNOSO, G., CHU, T.M. *et al.* (1972). Carcinoembryonic antigen in patients with different cancers. *J. Amer. Med. Assoc.*, **220** : 361.

RICE, M.S. (1966). Neuroblastoma in childhood: a review of 69 cases. *Aust. paediat. J.*, **2** : 1.

ROBINSON, M.J. & HOWARD, R.N. (1969). Neuroblastoma presenting as myasthenia gravis in a child aged 3 years. *Pediatrics*, **43** : 111.

ROSENSTEIN, B.J. & ENGELMAN, M.D. (1963). Diarrhoea in a child with a catecholamine-secreting ganglioneuroma. *J. Pediat.*, **63** : 217.

SENELICK, R.C., BRAY, P.F. *et al.* (1973). Neuroblastoma and myoclonic encephalopathy: 2 cases and a review of the literature. *J. Pediat. Surg.*, **8** : 623.

SHARMAN, D.F. (1973). Catabolism of catecholamines. *Brit. med. Bull.*, **29** : 110.

SHOWN, T.E. & DURFEE, M.F. (1970). 'Blueberry muffin' baby: neonatal neuroblastoma with subcutaneous metastases. *J. Urol.*, **104** : 193.

SINDHU, S. & ANDERSON, C.M. (1965). Ganglioneuroma as a cause of diarrhoea and failure to thrive. *Aust. paediat. J.*, **1** : 56.

SOLOMON, G.E. & CHUTORIAN, A.M. (1968). Opsoclonus and occult neuroblastoma. *New Engl. J. Med.*, **279** : 475.

STICKLER, G.B., HALLENBECK, G.A. *et al.* (1962). Catecholamines and diarrhoea in ganglioneuroblastoma. *Amer. J. Dis. Child.*, **104** : 598.

SUTOW, W.W., GEHAN, E.A. *et al.* (1970). Comparison of survival curves, 1956 verses 1962, in children with Wilms' tumour and neuroblastoma. *Pediatrics*, **45** : 800.

WAGGET, J. AHERNE, G. & AHERNE, W. (1973). Familial neuroblastoma: report of two sib. pairs. *Arch. Dis. Childh.*, **48** : 63.

WILLIAMS, T.H., HOUSE, R.F.Jr., BURGERT, E.O.Jr. & LYNN, H.B. (1972). Unusual manifestations of neuroblastoma: chronic diarrhoea, polymyoclonia—opsoclonus and erythrocyte abnormalities. *Cancer*, **29** : 475.

Phaeochromocytoma

BAZEX, A. & DUPRÉ, A. (1958). Mucosal myelin neuromas with mid-facial and laryngeal localization: neuromas of the lips, tongue, eyelids etc.; possibly new disease entity. *Ann. derm. syph. Paris.*, **85** : 613.

BLOOM, D.A. & FONKALSRUD, E.W. (1974). Surgical management of pheochromocytoma in children. *J. Pediat. Surg.*, **9** : 179.

CHAPMAN, R.C., KEMP, V.E. & TALIAFERRO, I. (1959). Pheochromocytoma associated with multiple neurofibromatosis and intracranial hemangioma. *Amer. J. Med.*, **26** : 883.

CORNELL, S.H. (1972). Pheochromocytoma of the lumbar sympathetic chain demonstrated by angiography. *Am. J. Roentgenol.*, **115** : 175.

GITLOW, S.E., MENDLOWITZ, M. & BERTANI, L.M. (1970). The biochemical techniques for detecting and establishing the presence of a pheochromocytoma. A review of 10 years experience. *Amer. J. Cardiol.*, **26** : 270.

GLENN, F., PETERSON, R.E. & MANNIX, H. (1968). *Surgery of the Adrenal Gland.* Macmillan, New York and London.

GORLIN, R.J., SEDANO, H.O., VICKERS, R.A. & CERVENKA, J. (1968). Multiple mucosal neuromas, pheochromocytomas and medullary carcinoma of the thyroid: a syndrome. *Cancer*, **22** : 293.

HARRISSON, T.S., FREIER, D.T. & COHEN, E.L. (1974). Recurrent pheochromocytoma, *Arch. Surg.*, **108** : 450.

HUME, D.W. (1960). Pheochromocytoma in the adult and child. *J. Surg.*, **99** : 458.

KAISER, H.R., BEAVAN, M.A. *et al.* (1973). Sipple's syndrome: medullary thyroid carcinoma, pheochromocytoma and parathyroid disease. *Ann. Intern. Med.*, **78** : 561.

KATZ, R.L. & WOLF, C.E. (1971). Pheochromocytoma. In *Highlights of Clinical Anesthesiology* (Mark, L.C. & Ngai, S.H., eds.). Harper & Rowe, New York.

LEVY, M., HABIB, R. LYON, G. *et al.* (1970). Neuromatose et epithélioma à stroma amyloide de la thyroide chez l'enfant. *Arch. Franç. Pédiat.*, **27** : 561.

LOPEZ, J.F. (1958). Pheochromocytoma of the adrenal gland with granuloma cell tumor and neurofibromatosis: report of a case with fatal outcome following abdominal aortography. *Ann. Intern. Med.*, **48** : 187.

REMINE, W.H., CHONG, G.C. *et al.* (1974). Current management of pheochromocytoma. *Ann. Surg.*, **179** : 740.

ROBINSON, M.J. & WILLIAMS, A.L. (1956). Clinical and pathological details of 2 cases of phaeochromocytoma in childhood. *Arch. Dis. Childh.*, **31** : 69.

ROBINSON, M.J., KENT, M. & STOCKS, J. (1973). Phaeochromocytoma in childhood. *Arch. Dis. Childh.*, **48** : 137.

SIPPLE, J.H. (1961). The association of pheochromocytoma with carcinoma of the thyroid gland. *Amer. J. Med.*, **31** : 163.

STACKPOLE, R.H., MELICOW, M.M. & USON, A.C. (1963). Pheochromocytoma in children. *J. Pediat.*, **63** : 315.

STEINER, A.L., GOODMAN, A.L., GOODMAN, A.D. & POWERS, S.R. (1958). Study of a kindred with pheochromocytoma, medullary thyroid carcinoma, hyperparathyroidism and Cushing's disease. *Medicine*, **17** : 371.

STURMAN, M.F., MOSES, D.C. *et al.* (1974). Radiocholesterol adrenal images for the localization of pheochromocytoma. *Surg. Gynec. & Obstet.*, **138** : 177.

VANCE, J.E., STOLL, R.W. *et al.* (1969). Nesidioblastosis in familial endocrine adenomatosis. *J. Amer. Med. Assoc.*, **207** : 1679.

WILSON, A.C., BENNETT, R.C. *et al.* (1974). An unusual case of intrathoracic phaeochromocytoma. *Aust. N.Z. J. Surg.*, **44** : 27.

Tumours of the Adrenal Cortex

ABLE, L.W. (1969). The adrenal glands. In *Pediatric Surgery* (Mustard, W.T. *et al.*, eds.). Year Book Medical Publishers Inc., Chicago.

ABODOWSKY, N. & MAIRA, J. (1972). Feminizing tumour of the adrenal. *Rev. Chil. Paediat.*, **43** : 25.

BACON, G.E. & LOWREY, G.H. (1965). Feminizing adrenal tumour in a 6 year old boy. *J. Clin. Endocrin.*, **25** : 1403.

BERGENSTAL, D.M., HERTZ, R., LIPSETT, M.B. & MOY, R.H. (1960). Chemotherapy of adrenocortical cancer with O, P'-DDD. *Ann. Intern. Med.*, **53** : 672.

BURRINGTON, J.D. & STEPHENS, C.A. (1969). Virilizing tumours of the adrenal gland in childhood: report of 8 cases. *J. Pediat. Surg.*, **4** : 291.

CASTLEMAN, B., SCULLY, R.F. & MCNEELY, B.U. (1972). Case records of the Massachusetts General Hospital. *New Engl. J. Med.*, **287** : 1033.

CUMMINS, G.E. & COHEN, D. (1974). Cushing's syndrome secondary to ACTH secreting Wilms' tumor. *J. Pediat. Surg.*, **9** : 535.

DI GEORGE, A.M. & PASCHKIS, K.E. (1959). Some aspects of tumors of the endocrine glands. *Ped. Clin. N. Amer.*, **6** : 583.

DREHER, G.H., WILLIAMS, S.W., HOWARD, R.N., CAMPBELL, P.E., DAVIES, H.E. & MCCARTHY, N. (1969). Cushing syndrome in a three month old girl. *Aust. pediat. J.*, **5** : 62.

FONTAINE, R., SACREZ, R., KLEIN, M. *et al.* (1954). Puberté precoce avec développement des seins chez un garçon porteur d'un tumeur de la surrénale. *Arch. Franç. Pediat.*, **11** : 417.

GABRILOVE, J.L., SHARMA, D.C. *et al.* (1965). Feminizing adrenocortical tumours in the male: a review of 52 cases including a case report. *Medicine*, **44** : 37.

GILBERT, M.G. & CLEVELAND, W.W. (1970). Cushing's syndrome in infancy. *Pediatrics*, **46** : 217.

GLENN, F., PETERSON, R.E. & MANNIX, H. (1968). *Surgery of the Adrenal Gland*. The Macmillan Company, New York.

HAYLES, A.B., HAHN, H.B., SPRAGUE, R.G., BAHN, R.C. & PRIESTLEY, J.I. (1966). Hormone secreting tumours of the adrenal cortex in children. *Pediatrics*, **37** : 19.

LEDITSCHKE, F.J. & ARDEN, F.M. (1974). Feminizing adrenal adenoma in a 5 year old boy. *Aust. Paediat. J.*, **10** : 217.

LEWINSKY, B.S., GRIGOR, K.M. & SYMINGTON, T. (1974). The clinical and pathological features of non-hormonal adrenocortical tumors. *Cancer*, **33** : 778.

MCARTHUR, R.G., CLOUTIER, M.D., HAYLES, A.B. & SPRAGUE, R.G. (1972). Cushing's disease in children: findings in 13 cases. *Mayo Clin. Proc.*, **47** : 318.

MOSIER, H.D. & GOODWIN, W.E. (1961). Feminizing adrenal adenoma in a 7 year old boy. *Pediatrics*, **27** : 1016.

PRÉVOT, J., MOUROT, M. *et al.* (1972). Two cases of masculinizing adrenal tumours in infants. *Ann Chir. Infant.*, **13** : 327.

RAITI, S., GRANT, D.B., WILLIAMS, D.I. & NEWNS, G.H. (1972). Cushing's syndrome in childhood: post-operative management. *Arch. Dis. Childh.*, **47** : 597.

SNAITH, A.H.A. (1958). A case of feminizing adrenal tumor in a girl. *J. Clin. Endocrinol. Metab.*, **18** : 318.

STEWART, D.R., JONES, P.M. & JOLLEYS, A. (1974). Carcinoma of the adrenal gland in children. *J. Pediat. Surg.*, **9** : 59.

STOWENS, D. (1959). *Pediatric Pathology*. Williams & Wilkins, Baltimore.

VANCE, J.E., & STOLL, R.W. *et al.* (1969). Nesidioblastosis in familial endocrine adenomatosis. *J. Amer. Med. Assoc.*, **207** : 1679.

WILKINS, L. (1948). A feminizing adrenal tumour causing gynaecomastia in a boy of 5 years contrasted with a virilizing tumour in a 5-year old girl. *J. Clin. Endocrin.*, **8** : 111.

Retroperitoneal Tumours

ACKERMAN, L.V. (1955). Tumors of the retroperitoneum, mesentery and omentum. *Atlas of Tumour Pathology*, Section VI, Fascicles 23–24. Armed Forces Institute of Pathology, Washington, D.C.

ARNHEIM, E.E. (1950). Retroperitoneal teratomas in infancy and childhood. *Pediatrics*, **8** : 309.

BARRIE, J.D. (1961). Intrathoracic tumours of carotid body type (chemodectoma). *Thorax*, **16** : 78.

DELORIMIER, A.A., BRAGG, K.U. & LINDEN, G. (1969). Neuroblastoma in childhood. *Amer. J. Dis. Child.*, **118** : 441.

ENGEL, R.M., ELKINS, R.C. & FLETCHER, B.D. (1968). Retroperitoneal teratoma: review of the literature and presentation of an unusual case. *Cancer*, **22** : 1068.

GLENNER, G.G., CROUT, J.R. & ROBERTS, W.C. (1962). A functional carotid-body like tumour secreting levarterenol. *Arch. Path.*, **73** : 230.

HELPAP, B. & GROULS, V. (1971). Nicht-chromaffine Paranganglioma im Kindersalter. *Zeit. für Kinderheilkunde*, **109** : 333.

LEDERER, F.L., SKOLNIK, E.M., SOBOROFF, B.J. & FORNATTO, E.J. (1958). Nonchromaffin paraganglioma of the head and neck. *Ann. Otol.*, **67** : 305.

OLSON, J.R. & ABELL, M.R. (1970). Nonfunctional nonchromaffin paragangliomas of the retroperitoneum. *Cancer*, **23** : 1358.

PALUMBO, L.T. (1949). Primary teratomas of the lateral retroperitoneal spaces. *Surgery*, **26** : **149**.

STOWENS, D. (1959). *Pediatric Pathology*. Williams & Wilkins, Baltimore.

Chapter 19. Tumours of the liver and bile ducts

Table 19.1. Tumours of the liver and bile ducts

Benign conditions	Malignant tumours
Liver	
Hepatomegaly	Hepatoblastoma
Infective	Hepatocarcinoma
Parasitic: e.g. hydatidosis	Hepatic metastases:
Toxic: e.g. post-irradiation and chemotherapy (p. 525)	e.g. neuroblastoma
	Wilms' tumour
	lymphomas
Storage diseases:	Histiocytosis-x (p. 206)
e.g. lysosomal, glycogen etc.	
Miscellaneous:	
cirrhosis, cystic fibrosis etc.	
Focal nodular hyperplasia	Lymph node metastases
(syn. benign 'adenoma')	(in porta hepatis):
	e.g. lymphosarcoma
	leukaemic deposits
Haemangioma	Displacement of liver forwards
(syn. haemangioendothelioma)	e.g. retrohepatic Wilms' tumour
Mesenchymal hamartoma	
(including 'Giant congenital' cyst)	Soft tissue sarcomas of liver
Lymphangioma	e.g. haemangiosarcoma
Teratoma	Other abdominal tumours (p. 491)
Bile ducts	
Choledochal cyst	Rhabdomyosarcoma
Enlarged gall bladder	
cholelithiasis	
mucocele	

In children primary malignant tumours of the liver are less common than hepatic metastases; benign tumours are rarer than either, an important consideration in the investigation and diagnosis of a child presenting with enlargement of the liver (Table 19.1).

The nomenclature of the malignant hepatic tumours is still the subject of debate; terms such as hepatoma, hepatic carcinoma, hepatoblastoma, mesenchymal tumour, mixed tumour, sarcoma etc., have all been applied to neoplasms containing areas with several different histological patterns, in keeping with the classification of similar mixed tumours as 'embryonal' (p. 38), for example Wilms' tumour.

Recent reviews have indicated that differences in histological pattern could be correlated with specific clinical behaviour. Ishak & Glunz (1967) classified malignant hepatic tumours in children into hepatoblastomas and hepatocarcinomas, further subdividing hepatoblastomas into those which are predominantly epithelial and those containing both epithelial and mesenchymal elements.

Kasai & Watanabe (1970) based their classification on the types of cell in the epithelial areas of the tumour, and divided these into four subtypes, ignoring the mesenchymal component as variable and less important. They found that children with an epithelial hepatoblastoma had a better prognosis, especially when it contained 'fetal' cells, i.e. cells closely resembling those in the fetal liver (Fig. 19.3), and a worse prognosis when the cells were more primitive and anaplastic.

Keeling (1971) suggested classification of tumours into three major types, the system adopted in reviewing the histology in the Index Series.

The three major types of liver tumours are:

Hepatoblastoma;

Rhabdomyoblastic hepatoma (syn. rhabdomyoblastoma); and

Hepatocarcinoma (syn. hepato-cellular carcinoma).

For practical purposes, the rare rhabdomyoblastic tumours have been grouped with the hepatoblastomas, to which they are closely related, and two types of tumours are described in this chapter:

I. Hepatoblastoma.

II. Hepatocarcinoma.

Because of the difficulty in relating our experience to reports in the literature based on other systems of classification and nomenclature, the findings in the Index Series provide the basis for the descriptions which follow.

Series of children with hepatic tumours have been reported recently by Exelby *et al.* (1971), Sinniah *et al.* (1974), Ein and Stephens (1974, a&b) and Clatworthy *et al.* (1974).

I. HEPATOBLASTOMA

There are 16 tumours in the Index Series classified as hepatoblastomas, to which have been added two cases of rhabdomyoblastic hepatoma.

AGE : SEX

The ages of the 16 patients ranged from 4 months to 10 years; 75% were less than 3 years of age. This is in accord with other series, in which this tumour is reported to arise most often in the first 3 years of life (Fig. 19.1) and to be uncommon after the age of 5 years (Keeling, 1971).

There were ten males and six females, a ratio of nearly 2 : 1, also noted in other series.

SITE

In most cases the tumour arises in the right lobe of the liver (11 out of 16) and this is believed to be due only to the greater size of the right lobe.

MACROSCOPIC APPEARANCES

These are very variable. Most are large, and displace or distort the lobe in which they arise (Fig. 19.2a). The tumour is usually 'encapsulated' and discrete, and arises as a single tumour in an otherwise normal liver; when more advanced, there are multiple nodular extensions into the adjacent liver parenchyma.

The surface is usually bossellated, and the colour of the cut surface varies

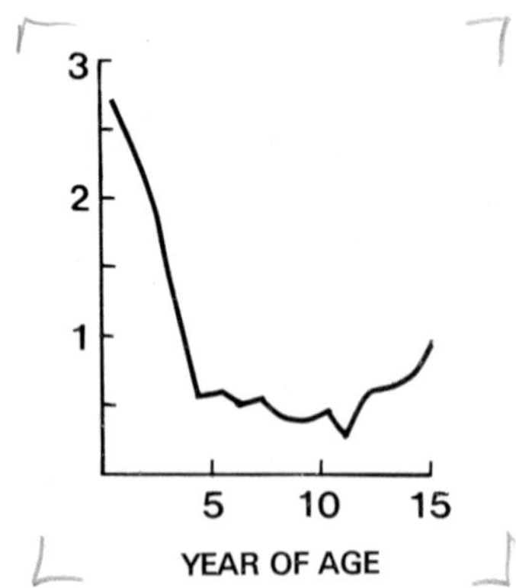

Figure 19.1. MALIGNANT TUMOURS OF THE LIVER; incidence according to age, showing the peak attributable to hepatoblastoma in the first quinquennium and an upward trend due to hepatocarcinoma commencing in the third (for source of figures see Fig. 2.2, p. 48).

according to the amount of bile or fat present; most are white with areas of haemorrhage and necrosis. The more differentiated tumours are green or yellow, more uniform in texture, and extremely vascular with very large aneurysmal vessels running in fibrous septa between lobules of tumour; they are also studded with dilated sinusoidal vessels giving the cut surface a sponge-like appearance (Fig. 19.2b).

MICROSCOPIC FINDINGS

In nearly all hepatoblastomas, epithelial cells resembling liver cells predominate, and in the more differentiated tumours the resemblance is striking. The cells are arranged in cords separated by sinusoids, often show fatty changes, and may secrete bile into acinar-like spaces.

Most tumours contain several kinds of cells, some with larger nuclei or areas more anaplastic in appearance, others with a tendency to form tubules and rosette-like structures. Cords of cells forming papillary festoons are also occasionally seen.

About half of these tumours also contain masses of tissue resembling fetal mesenchyme; this may blend into epithelial areas, but more commonly the stromal mesenchymal component is quite discrete. Ducts can be seen forming in this stroma; osteoid tissue, bone, occasionally cartilage and, rarely, strap cells with cross striations, are visible. Osteoid is common (Fig. 19.4b) and often intimately related to epithelial cells, suggesting that it is secreted by them.

The multiplicity of cell types is typical and the following varieties, using the nomenclature suggested by Kasai & Watanabe (1970), will be briefly described.

(*a*) *Fetal cells* closely resembling those normally seen in the fetal or infant liver (Fig. 19.3). They are granular or clear, arranged in columns and often form acini; this was the dominant cell type in 6 of the 16 cases in the Index Series.

(*b*) *Embryonal cells* are larger and less differentiated (Fig. 19.4a) with a tendency to form cords, prominent acini and rosettes. They may contain glycogen but do not secrete bile, and are commonly associated with a spindle celled stroma, merging with it to become a 'mixed' hepatoblastoma found in 14 of the 16 cases.

(*c*) *Anaplastic cells* are small, with scanty cytoplasm and a dark nucleus (Fig. 19.4c) morphologically resembling neuroblastoma, even to the extent of irregular giant cells. It is important to recognize this variant because of the frequency of metastatic neuroblastoma in the liver which is a potential source of diagnostic confusion (see p. 606).

(*d*) *Hepatocarcinoma* cells (see p. 614) were found in some portion in 2 of the 16 cases, and this emphasizes the difficulties in classification.

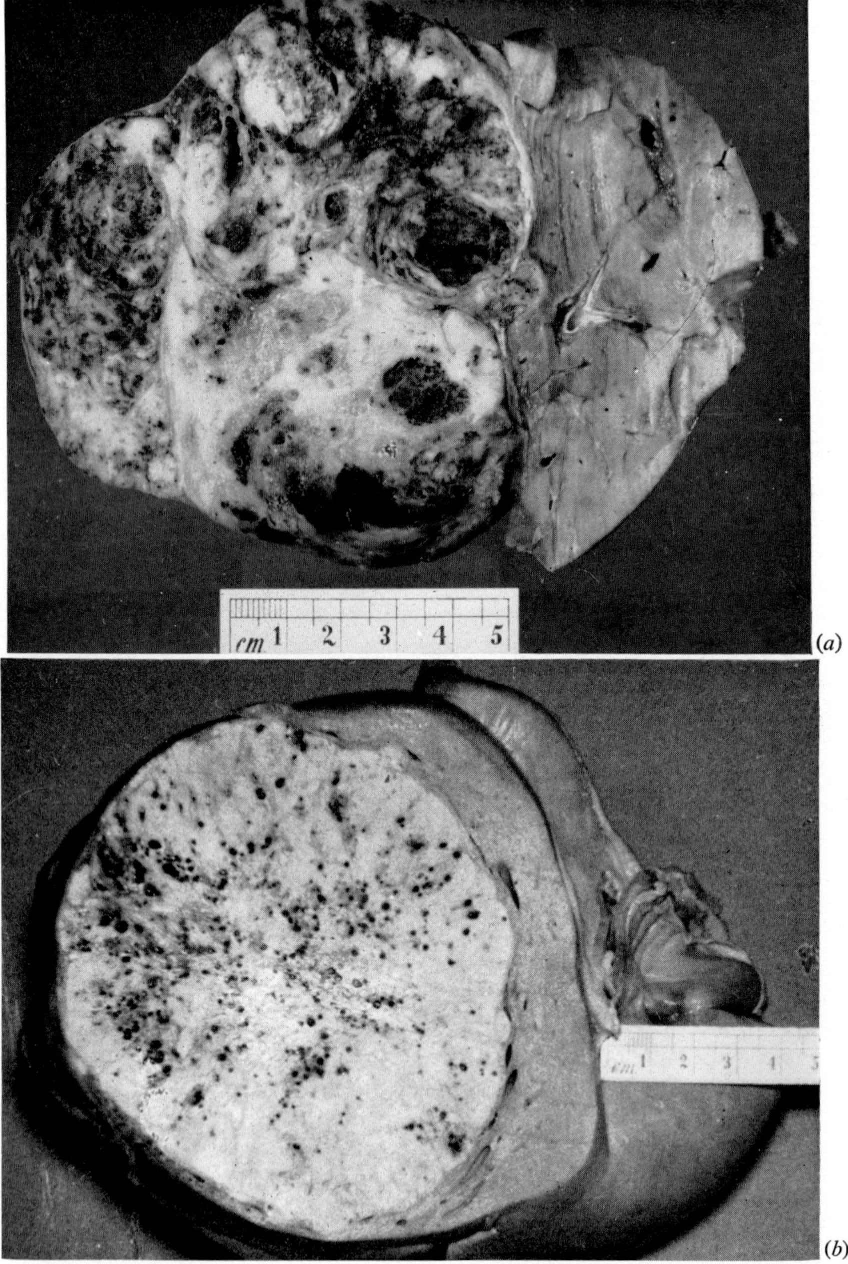

(a)

(b)

Figure 19.2. HEPATOBLASTOMA; (*a*) cut surface of a lobectomy specimen; a large, lobulated, undifferentiated tumour with areas of haemorrhage and necrosis; (*b*) a more differentiated example with a more uniform but sponge-like surface imparted by numerous dilated sinusoidal vessels. (Reproduced from 'Primary Hepatic Cancer in Infancy and Childhood' in *Progress in Pediatric Surgery*, Vol. 7. Urban and Schwarzenberg, 1974, with the permission of the publishers.)

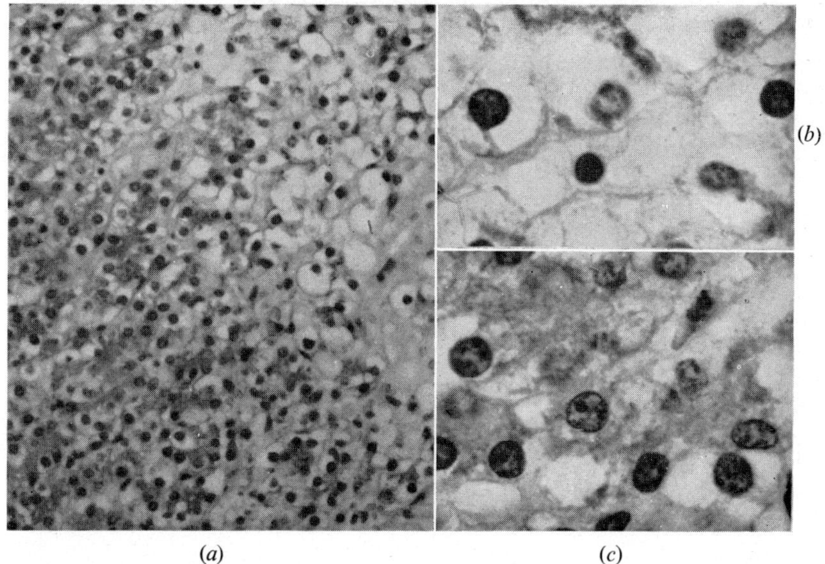

Figure 19.3. HEPATOBLASTOMA; (*a*) typical 'fetal' cells grading from granular cells (left) to clear cells (H & E. × 130); (*b*) clear cells; and (*c*) granular cells in greater detail showing rounded nuclei and distinct cell borders, closely resembling normal liver cells (H & E. × 430). (Reproduced from 'Primary Hepatic Cancer in Infancy and Childhood' in *Progress in Pediatric Surgery*, Vol. 7. Urban and Schwarzenberg, 1974, with the permission of the publishers.)

(*e*) **Rhabdomyoblastic type**

The two such tumours in the Index Series were in children aged 8 and 10 years, somewhat older than most of those with a hepatoblastoma. The predominant cell is spindle-shaped with abundant eosinophilic and strap-like cytoplasm containing glycogen and longitudinal myofibrils. No definite cross striations were seen, but the cells showed the nuclear polymorphism and gross irregularity typical of rhabdomyosarcoma (Fig. 19.4d).

SPREAD

As well as progressive infiltration spreading into the adjacent parenchyma, metastasis chiefly occurs *via* the hepatic veins to the lungs. There they form discrete rounded nodules, almost always with fatty changes in the cells of the metastases.

Spread beyond the lungs is unusual and occurred in only two patients in the Index Series, in each case to bone.

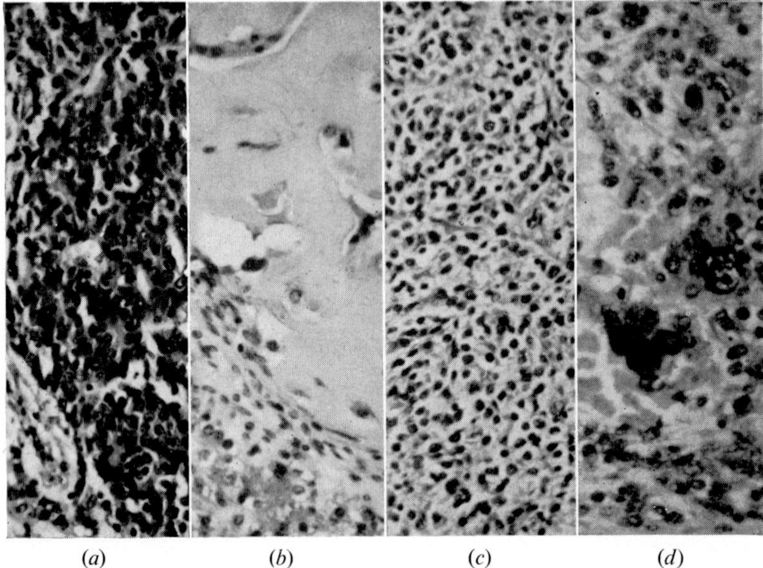

(*a*) (*b*) (*c*) (*d*)

Figure 19.4. HEPATOBLASTOMA; the varied appearances frequently found within one tumour; (*a*) embryonal cells as a dense mantle surrounding sinusoidal vessels; (*b*) osteoid tissue apparently secreted by epithelial cells (below); (*c*) small anaplastic cells with slightly irregular hyperchromatic nuclei and wispy cytoplasm, bearing a superficial resemblance to neuroblastoma; (*d*) rhabdomyoblastic type with elongated cytoplasmic extensions and pleomorphic nuclei, some of which are of giant size and multinucleated (all H & E. × 130).

MODES OF PRESENTATION

1. *Progressive enlargement of the abdomen*, and/or a mass in the upper abdomen, is by far the commonest presenting picture.
2. *A form of 'malignant malaise'* (see neuroblastoma, p. 549) is also commonly seen, i.e. anorexia, loss of weight and listlessness. These complaints lead parents to seek medical attention, and examination then reveals a painless abdominal mass.
3. *A pathological fracture* is a rare but recognized mode of presentation, e.g. a fracture of the femur, following trivial trauma. This has been shown to occur in an area of osteoporosis associated with liver disease (Teng *et al.*, 1961), including hepatic malignancies. The mechanism may be disturbance of the synthesis of proteins forming the ground substance of bone or hypercholesterolaemia directly affecting bone structure. Osteoporosis was noted particularly in 8 out of 9 cases of hepatoblastoma in the Index Series (see

p. 614). Alternatively a pathological fracture may very rarely be caused by a metastasis.

4. *Precocious puberty* is one of the rarest presentations with hepatoblastoma, and in five cases reported by Hung, Blizzard *et al.* (1963), circulating gonadotropins liberated by the tumour caused hyperplasia and hypersecretion of the interstitial (Leydig) cells in the testes.

Table 19.2. Hepatic tumours; signs and symptoms present at diagnosis in 16 children with a hepatoblastoma (Index Series)

Symptoms	No. of patients	Signs	No. of patients
Abdominal swelling	11	'Enlarged liver', or hepatic mass	15
Anorexia	10	Mobile abdominal mass*	1
Vomiting	5	Pallor	4
Loss of weight	5	Splenomegaly	4
Abdominal pain or colic	4	Collateral subcutaneous veins	2
Malaise, listlessness	4	Emaciation	1
Irritability	3	Jaundice	1
Fever	3	Spider naevi	1
Pallor	3	'Liver palms'	1
Loose stools	2	Haemangioma of eyelid	1

* An unusual pedunculated hepatoblastoma.

CLINICAL FEATURES

The symptoms and signs present at the time of diagnosis in the Index Series are shown in Table 19.2.

The typical findings can be summarized as a greatly enlarged liver causing distension of the upper abdomen, in a child less than five years of age who has been anorexic and irritable, with some pallor and recent loss of weight. In children, unlike adults, jaundice is exceptionally rare with an hepatic tumour.

It will be apparent that this picture resembles the usual mode of presentation of an abdominal neuroblastoma, or Wilms' tumour, and the same investigations described on p. 506 are required.

In summary, these are as follows:

(i) *Plain x-rays of the abdomen* and the chest, and a skeletal survey.

(ii) *Aortography and selective arteriography*, in this case coeliac or hepatic arteriography (Fig. 19.5).

(iii) *Inferior cavography* (p. 507).

(iv) *A liver scan* (p. 77, e.g. with ^{113m}Indium, ^{75}Selenium or ^{198}Aurium, (Andrews *et al.*, 1973).

(v) *Investigations in preparation for treatment*, such as a full blood examination, typing and matching of blood.

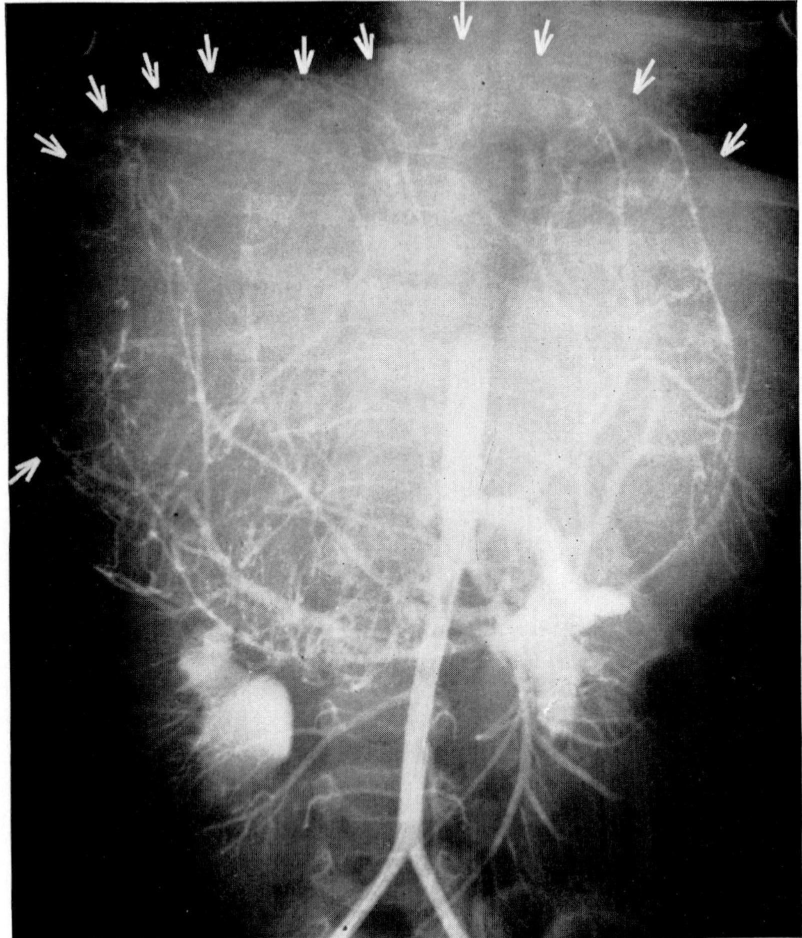

Figure 19.5. HEPATOBLASTOMA; aortogram of an inoperable tumour involving both lobes, supplied by irregular vessels arising from bowed branches of both right and left divisions of the hepatic artery.

Tests of liver function have not generally been found to be helpful (e.g. a mild increase in serum bilirubin (in three cases) and some elevation of SGOT in five out of nine cases).

Tests for α-fetoprotein may be helpful (Stillman & Zamcheck, 1970), and when standards have been fully established they may prove to be indispensible in monitoring patients during treatment. This protein is normally present in the human fetus after six weeks of gestation, and disappears from the circulation soon after birth. It can also be identified by immunofluorescence in the cells of hepatic tumours (Nishioka *et al.*, 1972). Complete removal of the tumour may be followed by disappearance of α-fetoprotein from the blood, and its return may be the first evidence of recurrence. The test may prove to be most useful (*a*) in screening populations with a high incidence of this tumour, (*b*) in detecting asymptomatic cases, (*c*) determining whether all of the tumour has been excised, and, (*d*) in monitoring patients during subsequent follow-up.

DIAGNOSIS

The results of the radiological investigations are usually diagnostic (Kreel, Jones & Tavil, 1968), particularly selective hepatic arteriography (Fig. 19.5) subsequently shown to be accurate in all of the cases in the Index Series in which it was performed (Andrews, Steven *et al.*, 1973).

DIFFERENTIAL DIAGNOSIS

With the accuracy of diagnosis obtained by angiography (Hiller, 1967; Novy, & Wallace *et al.*, 1974), this discussion becomes somewhat academic, but when specialized radiological investigations are not available, or before they are performed, alternative diagnoses which should be considered are those described fully in relation to Wilms' tumour (p. 516).

Only two clinical aspects will be mentioned here.

(*a*) A hepatic mass lies close to the costal margin and, typically, palpating fingers cannot get between the mass and the costal margin, as they usually can in a neuroblastoma, and usually but not always in a Wilms' tumour. Occasionally, a large Wilms' tumour in the right kidney extends upwards behind the liver, displacing it downwards, forwards and to the left. When this occurs the liver may appear to be greatly enlarged, and the true situation may only become apparent on angiography.

(*b*) Hepatic masses, as a rule, move with the liver during respiration, but a large and heavy tumour in a small patient does not always follow the rule.

DIFFERENTIATION FROM OTHER MALIGNANT TUMOURS OF THE LIVER

1. *Hepatocellular carcinoma.* This tumour can rarely be distinguished from hepatoblastoma with certainty before biopsy or operative material is examined histologically. Some indication can be gained from the age of the patient; in children more than eight years of age a hepatic tumour is more likely to be a hepatocellular carcinoma, but there is sufficient overlap of the age groups affected to make this unreliable (Fig. 19.1).

2. *Malignant mesenchymoma of the liver* (Andersen, 1951; Donovan &

Santulli, 1946) characteristically contains a variety of mesenchymal tissues; variations in their degree of differentiation present difficulties in distinguishing histologically between benign and malignant mesenchymoma on the one hand, and hepatic mesenchymal hamartoma and hepatoblastoma on the other. It is possible that a malignant mesenchymoma of the liver and a hepatoblastoma would be considered by some histopathologists to be the same entity, in the light of recent classifications of liver tumours.

3. *Rhabdomyosarcoma* of the bile ducts (p. 621) is a rarity which may present some of the features of a primary tumour of the liver.

METASTATIC TUMOURS OF THE LIVER

Neuroblastoma is the most common source of hepatic metastases; when the primary tumour is small and inconspicuous, gross hepatomegaly may be the presenting picture (Fig. 18.8a, p. 548). Sometimes the metastases are focal and confined to one or other lobe, more commonly the right, but in one form the neuroblastoma cells are infiltrated diffusely throughout the liver (p. 547).

The rare type of undifferentiated hepatoblastoma composed of small dark cells can also cause difficulties in distinguishing them from metastatic neuroblastoma (p. 602). However, the primary neuroblastoma can usually be demonstrated, and the Index Series contains no example of a hepatoblastoma metastasizing to the adrenal gland or retroperitoneal tissues.

Wilms' tumour, rhabdomyosarcoma arising in the pelvis, and the rare pancreatic carcinoma (p. 662) occasionally metastasize to the liver. This is not often a diagnostic problem because the primary tumour has usually been recognized before metastases in the liver become apparent.

Gastric and colonic carcinomas (p. 641) are extremely rare in childhood, and metastases in the liver are almost unknown.

Toxic hepatitis, possibly due to the combined effects of radiotherapy and the exacerbated cytotoxic effects of actinomycin D, can occur following treatment for Wilms' tumour (p. 525) or a malignant hepatic tumour. The findings of arteriography and scintillography may be misleading, but recurrence of the tumour or hepatic metastases can be excluded by needle biopsy (p. 526).

DIFFERENTIATION OF BENIGN HEPATIC MASSES

In most reported series, malignant tumours of the liver out-number benign masses, as in the Index Series, but difference in numbers was not large: 16 malignant tumours, and 12 benign masses (5 haemangiomas, 5 mesenchymal hamartomas and 2 liver cell adenomas, p. 611).

Haemangiomas, *lymphangiomas* and the rare *giant congenital cyst* (Saboo, Belsare *et al.*, 1974) have all been described, more commonly in the right than the left lobe. Some present as a large mass which may be difficult or impossible to distinguish from a malignant tumour before exploration.

In children the two important benign masses are:

1. Haemangioma, and
2. Mesenchymal hamartoma.

HAEMANGIOMA OF THE LIVER

In children, haemangiomas with signs suggestive of a malignant tumour usually present in the first 2 years of life as (a) *a mass* in the upper part of the abdomen, or (b) in early infancy with signs of *cardiac failure* due to multiple arteriovenous fistulae in the haemangioma, as occurred in 3 or the 5 in the Index Series.

Macroscopically the liver is greatly enlarged and looks 'haemorrhagic'.

Microscopically, cords of liver cells are widely separated by dilated vascular sinuses lined by plump endothelial cells. Small projections of endothelial cells may invaginate into the lumen of the vascular channels, and these may mimic a sarcomatous appearance. Mitotic figures may be present, but in children these tumours are almost invariably benign.

CLINICAL FEATURES

In an infant the presence of a mass in the upper part of the abdomen, comprising or attached to the right lobe of the liver, is the chief finding. Haemangiomas of the skin are often present, and provide a clue to the diagnosis. The presence of cardiovascular or haematological complications are also indications that the tumour may be a haemangioma.

A large haemangioma in the newborn or in early infancy is often life-threatening. High output cardiac failure due to large arteriovenous communications, or necrosis of the Glisson's capsule causing rupture and massive intraperitoneal haemorrhage, have been reported. A general haemorrhagic diathesis with thrombocytopenia, due to the trapping of platelets in the haemangioma, is also a possibility although uncommon, probably because of the brisk rate of blood flow through the lesion.

INVESTIGATIONS

Aortography followed by selective hepatic arteriography will confirm the diagnosis by demonstrating extreme hypervascularity, and rapid venous filling due to shunting. Angiography also demonstrates the extent of the lesion and whether one or both lobes are involved (Fig. 19.6).

A liver scan (p. 77), using reticulo-endothelial or blood-pool methods, (Andrews *et al.*, 1973) will provide confirmation and further delineation if required.

TREATMENT OF HAEMANGIOMA

Haemangiomas of the liver have the same tendency as cutaneous lesions to spontaneous resolution by sclerosis, and may with time become much smaller. However, this cannot be awaited in a young infant with serious

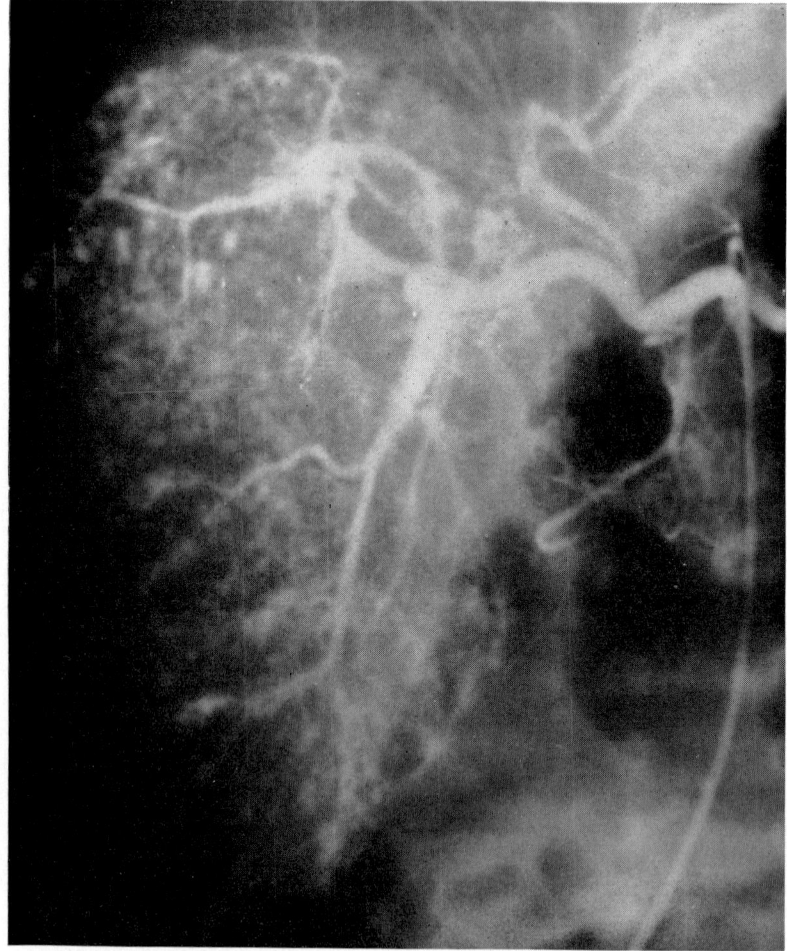

Figure 19.6. HAEMANGIOMA OF THE LIVER in an infant 3-days old; hepatic arteriogram showing saccular sinusoidal vascular spaces confined to the right lobe (note hypertrophy of the right branch of the artery).

cardiac embarrassment due to high output failure, and without treatment there is a high mortality. The distribution of the angioma, in one or both lobes, has a bearing on the choice of treatment.

DeLorimier *et al.* (1967) collected 25 reported cases and found a mortality of 88%, chiefly due to cardiac failure. Spontaneous resolution may occur with sufficient speed to produce remission of symptoms, but Matolo & Johnson (1973) found fewer than five cases in which this had occurred.

Radiotherapy has been employed successfully to hasten resolution (Lee, Newstedt & Siddall, 1956), but the well-known disadvantage of irradiation in children make it undesirable in non-malignant conditions.

Corticosteroids have been shown to assist resolution in haemangiomas (Goldberg & Fonkalsrud, 1969; Brown, Neerhout & Fonkalsrud, 1972), possibly by increasing the susceptibility of the terminal vascular bed to normally occurring vasoconstrictors. Response is somewhat unpredictable in superficial angiomas, and there may be no time for a 'failed trial' when other methods are available. Corticosteroids clearly have a role in treatment when involvement of both lobes rules out these alternatives.

Ligation of the branch of the hepatic artery supplying the lobe containing a haemangioma has been employed successfully (DeLorimier *et al.*, 1967), and Mattioli *et al.* (1974) reported ligation of the main hepatic artery, e.g. for bilobar haemangioma in the newborn, without detectable ischaemic damage to the liver, demonstrating that in this lesion and age group, portal flow can apparently provide sufficient oxygenation.

Considerable enlargement and tortuosity of the hepatic artery and its major branches occur in both uni- and bilobar haemangiomas, making it difficult to identify the vessel to be ligated, and the operative findings should be carefully correlated with the preoperative hepatic arteriogram.

Resection of the angioma, i.e. right or left hepatic lobectomy, has been performed successfully on several occasions (Shuller *et al.*, 1949; Matolo & Johnson, 1973; Sompii, Niemi *et al.*, 1974) and is probably the method of choice when a large haemangioma is confined to one lobe of the liver.

Braun, Ducharme *et al.* (1975) reviewed their series of 10 patients, 7 of whom had been successfully managed without operation, and recommended conservative management initially, i.e. steroids and aggressive treatment of cardiac failure and haematological complications, reserving operation for those in whom these measures fail.

MESENCHYMAL HAMARTOMA
(syn. cystadenoma, cystic hamartoma)

MACROSCOPIC APPEARANCES

Most mesenchymal hamartomas are multiloculated cystic lesions, with variable amounts of solid tissue in the septa. The cysts may contain clear fluid resembling lymph, haemorrhagic fluid, or mucus (Fig. 19.7b).

MICROSCOPIC FINDINGS

The walls of the loculi contain varying amounts of dense fibrous tissue and clusters of irregular dysplastic bile ducts or liver cells. Areas of myxoid degeneration in the stroma are common, and there is often loose, spindle-celled 'embryonal' connective tissue. Some of the cysts have an epithelial lining, commonly of bile duct type, but often no epithelium can be identified, and in some specimens the appearance of the spaces is consistent with a lymphatic origin, i.e. a lymphangiomatous component dominates the histological picture.

MODE OF PRESENTATION

In most cases a mesenchymal hamartoma is discovered as a mass in the upper part of the abdomen, often without symptoms other than epigastric fulness and anorexia. In others there are general symptoms of malaise and loss of weight.

INVESTIGATIONS

Angiography, e.g. selective hepatic arteriography (Fig. 19.7) is the most informative investigation; others required are the same as for tumours in the upper part of the abdomen (p. 506).

DIFFERENTIAL DIAGNOSIS

Differentiation from hepatoblastoma is discussed on p. 614. Other benign lesions of the liver are as follows.

1. *A choledochal cyst* (p. 492) should theoretically be included in this group but as a general rule the mass fluctuates in size, and is only palpable intermittently. The other two components of the triad, colicky pain and jaundice, are helpful when present, for pain and jaundice are very rare in children with a hepatic tumour.

2. *Lymphangioma* of the liver presents as a large, multilocular cystic mass usually confined to the right lobe. The cysts range from 1 cm to many centimetres in diameter; most contain straw-coloured fluid, but in some it may be turbid or haemorrhagic. Microscopically the cystic spaces are lined by flattened endothelial cells, and there are small focal or nodular aggregates of lymphoid tissue in the walls, which also contain smooth muscle fibres.

In some cases lymphangiomatosis of the liver is associated with similar malformations of the spleen and the skeleton (Asch *et al.*, 1974).

3. *Adenoma* of the liver. This is occasionally found at laparotomy or autopsy as a localized swelling resembling a cirrhotic nodule, and distinct from the surrounding normal parenchyma. In two cases in the Index Series, both in

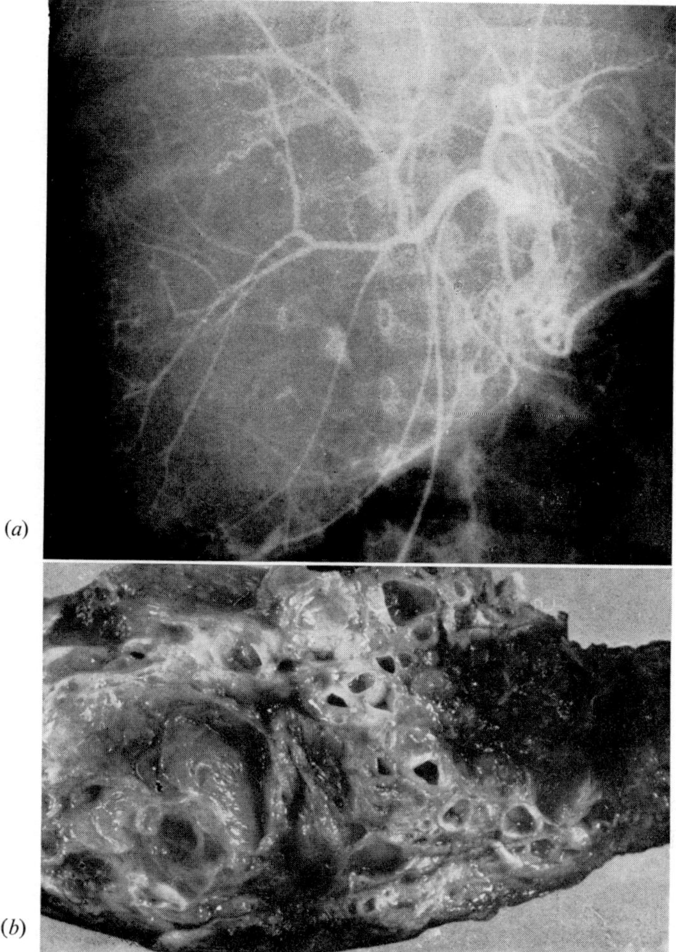

Figure 19.7. MESENCHYMAL HAMARTOMA OF THE LIVER; (*a*) hepatic arteriogram of disordered right lobe sparsely supplied by vessels individually indistinguishable from 'tumour' vessels, although benign (cf. Fig. 19.5 and 19.6); (*b*) cut surface of an example containing many small cysts.

older children, the adenoma was large enough to be identified as a lobulated palpable mass. In such cases exploration and biopsy are indicated, but removal of the nodule does not appear to be essential.

Microscopically an adenoma is composed of apparently normal liver cells, while the rest of the liver is also normal, except for mild cirrhosis in some cases. The cause and the nature of this lesion are uncertain and its malignant potential has yet to be determined.

4. *Other benign causes of massive hepatomegaly* in childhood include hydatid disease (p. 492) and amoebic abscess, in regions where these diseases occur. Generalized enlargement of the liver due to galactosaemia, familial lipoidoses and thalassaemia can usually be excluded by appropriate haemato-logical and biochemical tests, by angiography or, in selected cases, by needle biopsy.

TREATMENT

The treatment of hepatoblastoma is described on p. 614, following the section on hepatocarcinoma. It consists primarily of resection, combined with chemotherapy and radiotherapy unless excision has clearly been complete.

II. HEPATOCARCINOMA

AGE : SEX : SITE

The tumour is less common than hepatoblastoma and arises in an older age group, in children more than five years old and mostly in the third quin-quennium (Fig. 19.1).

The right lobe is again more often affected than the left.

MACROSCOPIC APPEARANCES

These differ from hepatoblastomas in that there is a high incidence of pre-existing liver disease, particularly cirrhosis. The tumour thus arises in an abnormal liver (Becker, 1974) and tends to be multicentric, varying in colour from nodule to nodule; some are white while others are bright green due to the formation of bile (Fig. 19.8). The tumour is more invasive than a hepatoblastoma and has a greater propensity for invading the branches of the portal vein and the tributaries of the hepatic veins. In one case in the Index Series the tumour grew down the portal vein, completely blocking it and causing portal hypertension.

MICROSCOPIC FINDINGS

The cells of the 'adult' type of hepatocellular carcinoma are more polygonal and more obviously epithelial (Fig. 19.8b) than those of embryonal tumours (Fig. 19.4). The cells vary considerably in size and shape and are arranged in trabeculae separated by sinusoidal spaces. Many of the cells are bizarre or irregular, and contain a hyperchromatic nucleus; mitoses are common. In

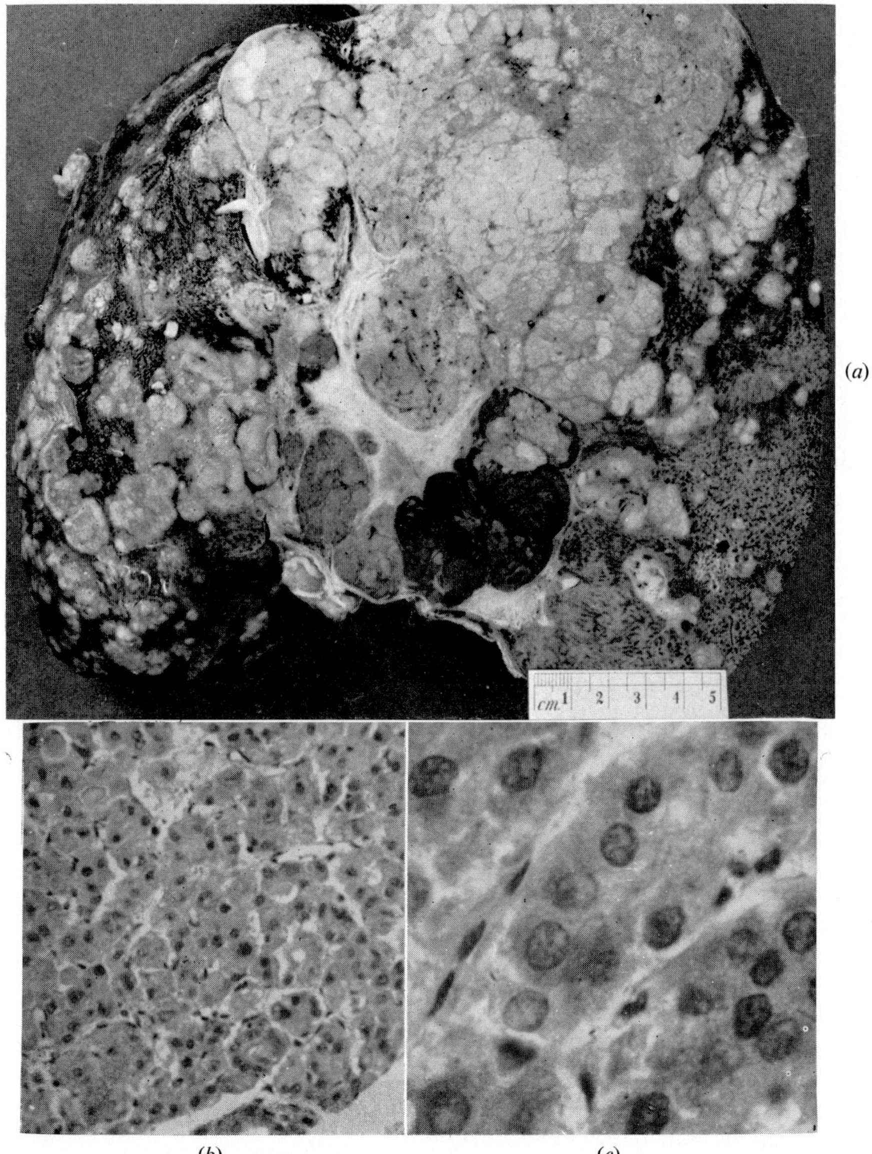

Figure 19.8. HEPATOCARCINOMA, of the adult type; (*a*) horizontal section of the liver at necropsy shows multiple, nodular, variegated masses, yellow, green or white in colour. The liver is fatty but not cirrhotic; (*b*) cords of epithelial cells separated by delicate sinusoids (H & E. ×130); (*c*) cellular detail of well-differentiated nuclei closely resembling normal liver parenchyma (H & E. ×430), in a vertebral marrow metastasis. (Reproduced from 'Primary Hepatic Cancer in Infancy and Childhood' in *Progress in Pediatric Surgery*, No. 7. Urban and Schwarzenberg, 1974, with the permission of the publishers.)

some areas the cells secrete a considerable amount of bile, but differentiation into recognizable ducts rarely if ever occurs.

SPREAD

The routes of spread are the same as described in hepatoblastomas (p. 601), except for the greater tendency of hepatic carcinoma to infiltrate blood vessels.

DIAGNOSIS

The clinical features are indistinguishable from hepatoblastomas, except that hepatocarcinoma tends to occur in an older group.

The investigations (p. 603) and the differential diagnosis (p. 605) are as described above.

MANAGEMENT OF HEPATIC TUMOURS

Although extrahepatic tumours can be excluded by arteriography and scintillography, these investigations cannot be relied upon to distinguish between hepatoblastoma, hepatocarcinoma and mesenchymal hamartoma (Ishida *et al.*, 1966; Sutton & Eller, 1968). In all three conditions the pattern of vessels depicted by selective hepatic artiography may be very similar; the supposed differences between 'malignant' and 'benign' vascular patterns (Goldstein, Nieman *et al.*, 1974) are in our experience unreliable (cf. Figs. 19.5, 19.7).

Generalized osteoporosis, however, has been a constant finding (most apparent in the long bones in the limbs) in 8 out of 9 of our patients with a hepatoblastoma; in one the mode of presentation was a pathological fracture of the shaft of the femur. Osteoporosis was not apparent in a retrospective review of cases of mesenchymal hamartoma, hepatocarcinoma or adenoma.

The age of the patient is some guide to the diagnosis, for hepatocarcinoma typically occurs in older children (5–15 years), while hamartomas and hepatoblastomas are usually found in children less than 4 years of age. In most reported series hepatoblastomas outnumber hamartomas; in the Index Series the proportion was 16 : 4.

Needle biopsy of hepatic tumours is somewhat controversial, but the danger of provoking a haemorrhage from a haemangioma can be averted by excluding this condition by angiography (Fig. 19.6). The risk of disseminating tumour cells is not sufficient to forgo the advantages of establishing the diagnosis before operative exploration, but this depends on an ability to obtain adequate and representative cores of tissue, and an experienced histopathologist prepared to make a diagnosis on relatively limited material.

Preparations for hepatic lobectomy include hypothermia which, without a pre-operative histological diagnosis, may prove to have been an unnecessary additional risk.

Mesenchymal hamartomas are benign lesions, and excision *in toto* is not essential, although lobectomy may be the best treatment in some cases. Their macroscopic structure varies from one case to another. Lobectomy may be necessary when a hamartoma is deeply embedded, mostly solid, or when the histological diagnosis (e.g. on frozen sections) uncertain. Some present on the surface of the liver as an encapsulated and predominantly cystic tumour which can be treated adequately by evacuating its contents, resecting septa, partially obliterating the cavity with mattress sutures, and temporary drainage of the remainder.

Hepatocarcinomas are theoretically curable by hepatic lobectomy, but they tend to be multicentric and invasive, and in our experience they are seldom completely resectable. In most reported series there are few survivors, and none in the 4 in the Index Series.

Hepatoblastoma is thus the chief indication for hepatic lobectomy in the paediatric age group, and the survival rate has improved with accumulated experience (Nixon, 1965; Martin & Woodman, 1969; Nickaldon *et al.*, 1907). The liver has remarkable powers of regeneration, and the portion remaining after excision of a tumour enlarges rapidly, so rapidly that tenderness and increase in size may suggest recurrence of the tumour. One of the long term survivors in the Index Series is well, with no evidence of disease and growing normally, 2 years after removal of all but half of the left lobe of the liver.

HEPATIC LOBECTOMY

The operation should be carefully planned following thorough investigation, including selective hepatic arteriography and vena cavography (Raffucci & Ramirez-Schon, 1970). Continuous monitoring of the central venous pressure throughout the operation is almost indispensible in following the effects of blood loss and in determining the rate of replacement transfusions. All intravenous lines should be inserted *via* vessels in the upper limbs, for measurements and infusions from below are interrupted by cross clamping the inferior cava.

Excessive blood loss, and hepatic insufficiency due to ischaemia during operation, can be avoided by the use of hypothermia, and by placing a non-crushing vascular clamp across the gastrohepatic ligament before commencing the resection. The clamp can be left in place for 50 minutes at a time when the body temperature, measured rectally, is between 20 and 25°C.

A transverse supra-umbilical incision is recommended, and can be readily converted into a thoraco-abdominal approach if necessary. Complete mobilization of the liver is obtained by dividing all its peritoneal attachments, and special care should be taken to avoid prolonged traction on or distortion of the inferior vena cava when the liver is brought out into the incision.

Vessels may tear, causing severe bleeding; air embolism into the hepatic veins can also occur. The complex metabolism in the remaining liver may be seriously disturbed by vascular stasis unless protected by hypothermia. The physiological aspects involved in major resections of the liver have been described by Stone *et al.* (1969).

Having ensured adequate exposure, the whole of the liver is inspected to determine the extent of the tumour and its operability. At this point frozen sections are required, not only to confirm the diagnosis but also to determine whether questionable areas are indeed involved.

A detailed knowledge of the surgical anatomy is essential, particularly the intrahepatic segmental structure (Fig. 19.9, 19.10) and the pattern of the vessels (Goldsmith & Woodburne, 1957; Wilson & Wolf, 1965). It should be especially noted that the hepatic veins (Fig. 19.10a), although fairly constant in position, do not drain the same areas as supplied by the analogous branches of the portal vein (Fig. 19.10b), hepatic artery and bile ducts, all three of which run a parallel course which does not correspond to the direction taken by the relevant tributary of the hepatic veins (Fig. 19.10c), a fact which complicates segmental excision. Attention should also be paid to variations in the pattern of the major hepatic arteries, for there is a real risk of ligating unnecessarily an artery essential to the survival of the remaining liver.

Other important points are the relationship of the middle hepatic vein (Fig. 19.11) to the tumour, and whether the tumour extends from one lobe across the interface into the other. This may be difficult to determine until

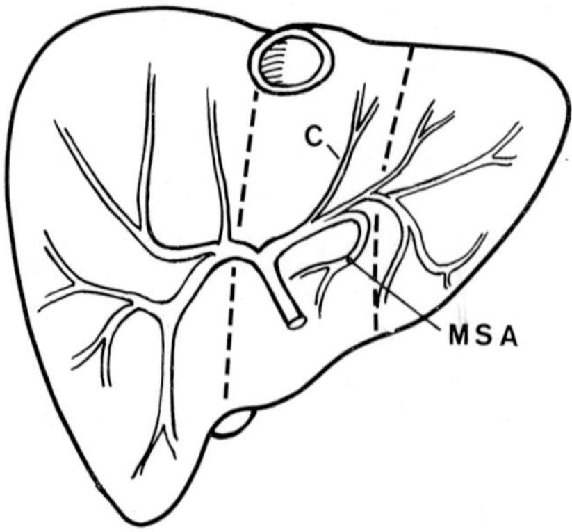

Figure 19.9. HEPATIC ANATOMY; the division into the right, left and 'middle' lobe, according to the distribution of the hepatic artery; the branches of the left hepatic artery to the caudate lobe (C) and the medial superficial artery (MSA) are indicated.

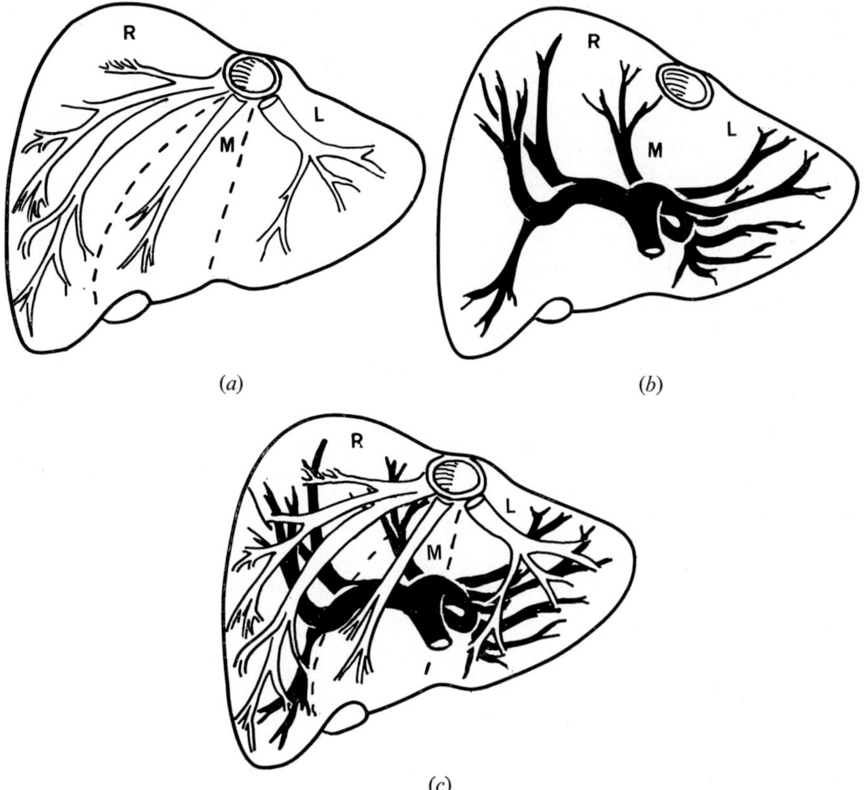

Figure 19.10. HEPATIC VASCULAR PATTERN; (*a*) the right, 'middle' and left hepatic veins joining the inferior cava; (*b*) the divisions of the portal vein; and (*c*) the portal and systemic vessels superimposed to illustrate lack of correspondence.

dissection is in progress, for the surface of the tumour may bulge into the opposite lobe without actually invading it.

Right hepatic lobectomy

When the right lobe is to be removed, the laparotomy incision can be extended upward into the eighth right costal interspace, and the diaphragm incised down to the vena cava, thus providing adequate exposure of the short and friable posterior hepatic veins (PV in Fig. 19.11).

The structures in the porta hepatis are separately identified, and those entering the affected lobe are ligated. It may take five minutes of vascular occlusion before a difference in the colour of the surface of the liver, demarcating the line between the lobes, becomes apparent.

The gall-bladder is freed from its bed (but not removed) and prepared for retrograde injection of dilute methylene blue into the biliary tree, so that bile ducts opening onto the cut surface can be picked up and closed.

One of the major objectives is to avoid leaving behind a large volume of liver devoid of adequate blood supply and lacking bile ducts, and yet to ensure the removal of an adequate margin of uninvolved liver tissue along with the tumour.

The line of resection in a right hepatic lobectomy passes from the left edge of the gall-bladder fossa to the vena cava, avoiding injury to the middle hepatic vein (M in Fig. 19.11). All the liver to the right of the main interlobar fissure can then be removed.

A little more of the liver can be excised, if necessary, by an 'extended right hepatic lobectomy' which includes right lobectomy plus removal of the medial segment of the left lobe, i.e. all of the liver to the right of the *left* segmental fissure.

When the lateral segment of the left lobe is to be removed, the line of section should be kept near the falciform ligament to avoid the branches of the middle hepatic vein which drain the anterior segment of the right lobe.

When completing resection of the right lobe, the right hepatic vein(s) and the multiple small veins on the anterior aspect of the vena cava (Fig. 19.11) are ligated close to the cava; a visible line of demarcation then develops, and the capsule of the liver is incised along this line, completing separation of the right lobe by blunt dissection, using the handle of a scalpel, or a finger, ligating and dividing vascular and biliary channels as they are encountered.

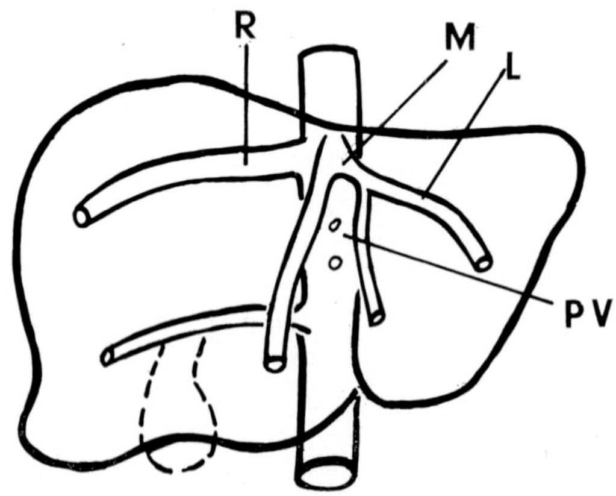

Figure 19.11. HEPATIC VEINS; the common pattern, in which the middle (M) and left (L) hepatic veins join before entering the cava; alternatively each may enter separately. The inferior right hepatic vein and the short posterior veins (PV) are also indicated (see text).

Left hepatic lobectomy

When the left lobe is to be removed, division and transfixation-ligation of the clamped left hepatic vein is performed after the parenchymal transection has been completed. The size of the left lobe in a normal liver varies with the age of the patient. The neonate has a disproportionately large left lobe, which becomes relatively smaller throughout childhood.

After lobectomy, the raw surface of the liver is covered with neighbouring tissue, such as the falciform ligament, the omentum, or any available flaps of peritoneum. Adequate drainage through a separate stab incision is mandatory, using a sump drain attached to low pressure suction (e.g. Redivac®) or a plastic bottle compressed before attachment to the drain tube. Blood loss during operation should be carefully measured and replaced continuously.

Intravenous glucose should be given generously after lobectomy to avoid hypoglycaemia which is likely to occur following loss of stored glycogen. Human serum albumin is also given intravenously until sources of protein can be taken orally, to furnish protein required during regeneration of the liver. Vitamin K is required to ensure adequate haemostasis.

Antibiotics (penicillin, streptomycin and wide spectrum antibiotics) are necessary, to reduce the risk of autogenous infection occurring in residual devitalized liver.

Unless surgical shock has developed (usually due to inadequate replacement of blood loss) the recovery of patients after major hepatic resections is remarkably rapid, and regeneration of the remaining liver may actually be alarming.

In two patients in the *Index Series*, progressive increase in the size of the remaining lobe and tenderness over it, in the months following operation, caused concern that the tumour had recurred.

In one case, the enlargement was subsequently shown to be due to rapid regeneration of the liver; the patient has thrived and is a long term survivor with no evidence of residual tumour.

In another case with similar findings, but accompanied by malaise and weight loss, a liver scan showed multiple, large 'cold' areas consistent with metastases. When further investigated by needle biopsy, the 'metastases' proved to be areas of focal 'hepatitis' thought to be due to toxic effects of radiotherapy and actinomycin D, which occurred in the liver after removal of a Wilms' tumour in the patient described on p. 525.

Regeneration of the liver can be monitored by serial liver scans (Samuels & Grosfeld, 1970), but these may falsely indicate recurrence or metastases unless interpreted in the light of other findings (see p. 526).

Chemotherapy and radiotherapy

Although primary tumours of the liver are relatively resistant to radiotherapy, and intensive chemotherapy has had only a limited trial, useful palliation may be obtained with these measures in hepatoblastoma and in some cases both may be essential for cure.

In the Index Series, a girl aged 2 years with a liver edge extending 8 cm below the costal margin, was proven by angiography and biopsy to have a huge inoperable hepatoblastoma. Irradiation with 3000 rads (in 3 weeks) followed by a 2-week course of mitomycin C produced some improvement, but the tumour was still inoperable. A further course of chemotherapy with vincristine, 5-fluoro-uracil and prednisolone for 10 weeks reduced the tumour to a size which made subtotal excision possible, and operation was followed by another 4 weeks of chemotherapy. The child is well with no evidence of disease 6 years later.

Mitomycin C, vincristine and other cycle-active cytotoxic agents (p. 102) are those most likely to aid regression of the tumour in the critical early stages of a hepatoblastoma, but no established regimen has evolved as yet.

A regime of chemotherapy using vincristine, 5-fluorouracil and cyclophosphamide has been employed by Holton *et al.* (1975) with success in hepatoblastoma, but, as in other reports, no improvement in the poor prognosis of hepatocarcinoma. Radiotherapy in the absence of chemotherapy has only a limited part to play.

Neither form of treatment appears to have much to offer children with a hepatocarcinoma, and as in other series, there were no survivors in children in the Index Series with this tumour.

PROGNOSIS

The outlook is very much better with a hepatoblastoma than a hepatocarcinoma; in children, as Foster (1970) has shown in adults, the prognosis depends primarily on whether the whole of the tumour can be removed, together with a safe margin of uninvolved liver if possible.

Reliance on total excision of the tumour, by whatever means, warrants an extended lobectomy and removal of part of the remaining lobe if this is feasible. The operative mortality may be as high as 25%, but this would still be acceptable if the other 75% have a 66% chance of surviving for 2–5 years, as this represents a considerable increase in salvage rate. The number of children treated by hepatic lobectomy is still small, but the results so far confirm the benefits of major resection.

Absence of a fall in α-fetoprotein after apparent total excision of a hepatic tumour, has been correctly interpreted as evidence of incomplete removal, and a second exploration to remove more of the liver (containing residual tumour) has been reported as successful in a few cases.

As well the histological type of tumour, the presence or absence of metastases before operation, the feasibility of complete excision, and the presence of pre-existing cirrhosis, appear to have a direct bearing on the outcome. An abnormally high ESR may reflect the presence of metastases, and the ESR before operation was normal in each of the long-term survivors in the Index Series.

Pre-existing cirrhosis is found more commonly in adults with a hepatocarcinoma than in children with this tumour. Multiple primary tumours appear to occur more frequently in cirrhotic livers, and the prognosis is correspondingly worse.

TUMOURS OF THE BILE DUCTS

Malignant tumours of the bile ducts in childhood are extremely rare, and by far the commonest is rhabdomyosarcoma. No benign neoplasm has been reported to have arisen primarily in the bile ducts in childhood.

RHABDOMYOSARCOMA OF THE BILE DUCTS

In a review of the literature Akers and Needham (1971) collected 24 cases in children, of which 17 were fully documented. The authors added one patient of their own, who was well without evidence of tumour $3\frac{1}{2}$ years after subtotal excision followed by radiotherapy and chemotherapy, and this appears to be the only survivor reported so far.

SITE : AGE : SEX

The common bile duct was the chief site (19 of the 24 cases); in three the tumour was thought to arise in ducts within the liver, while the common hepatic duct was the primary site in two instances.

Most of the children were between 2 and 6 years, with a peak at 4 years; the sex incidence was approximately equal.

MACROSCOPIC APPEARANCES

The tumour usually arises in the wall of the common bile duct as yellow, shiny, gelatinous, grape-like polypoidal projections growing from and along the thickened and enlarged duct, i.e. sarcoma botryoides (Davis, Kissane & Ishak, 1969). The polypoid masses are prone to haemorrhage and necrosis, and the affected duct may rupture, as occurred in the only case in the Index Series. The gallbladder is usually distended with 'white' bile.

SPREAD

Spread is primarily by progressive infiltration within the wall of the ducts, upwards towards the liver or towards the pancreas, or in both directions. Invasion of adjacent structures, especially the liver, is usual and produces cystic spaces into which project typical grape-like vesicles.

Distant metastases are not common, possibly because of the limited life span, but in a few cases metastases have been reported in long bones, the skull or the lungs (Kissane & Smith, 1967).

MICROSCOPIC FINDINGS

The usual pattern is an embryonal sarcoma, occasionally with cross striations, although these are not commonly found. Beneath the biliary epithelium, which may be intact or ulcerated, there is a denser zone of neoplastic cells, the so-called 'cambium' layer, also seen in sarcoma botryoides presenting at the vulva (see Fig. 21.7, p. 703).

The various types of rhabdomyosarcoma and their histology and prognostic significance are described on p. 784.

MODES OF PRESENTATION

The common presenting picture is a young child with fever, malaise, abdominal pain, jaundice and a palpable mass in the right upper quadrant of the abdomen. The initial diagnosis is usually hepatitis, but the obstructive nature of the jaundice and increase in the size of the mass soon indicate otherwise and lead to laparotomy.

INVESTIGATIONS

Liver function tests and liver biopsy are usually normal; a cholecystogram and/or intravenous cholangiogram are helpful in demonstrating biliary obstruction, and may delineate polypoidal filling defects. A barium meal often shows an indentation in the wall of the duodenum by an extraluminal tumour.

DIFFERENTIAL DIAGNOSIS

Jaundice, an early sign in this tumour, is uncommon apart from hepatitis in children 2–6 years of age. Other causes of jaundice in this age group are as follows.

1. *A choledochal cyst* typically causes intermittent jaundice, a mass in the right hypochondrium, and downward displacement of the duodenum, all of which may be found with a tumour of the bile ducts. However, the short-lived intermittent episodes of pain and jaundice, and the disappearance of the subcostal mass within 12–36 hours, are not typical of a tumour. The age

group of patients presenting with a choledochal cyst is also perhaps a little older, but the initial episode may be at 4–5 years of age or earlier.

2. *Cholelithiasis* is very uncommon in young children, particularly in boys, although hereditary spherocytosis producing pigment stones in the bile ducts can cause obstructive jaundice, and possibly an enlarged gall-bladder. Cholecystography usually demonstrates the calculi or a non-functioning gall bladder, while a family history and a positive red cell fragility test will effectively identify spherocytosis as the cause of pigment calculi.

3. *Hydatid cysts* in the liver in children less than five years of age occur in endemic areas, and enlargement of the liver by a cyst can present as a 'swelling' in the right hypochondrium. Rupture of a hydatid cyst into the biliary tree causing pain and obstructive jaundice is exceptionally rare in childhood.

The findings on selective hepatic arteriography and/or a liver scan (p. 77) are sufficiently reliable to make the diagnosis of hydatid disease with certainty.

DIFFERENTIATION OF OTHER MALIGNANT TUMOURS

1. *Primary tumours of the liver* (p. 598) are more common than rhabdomyosarcoma of the bile duct, but they rarely cause jaundice and they can be demonstrated by angiography (p. 604).

2. *Secondary deposits in lymph nodes* in the porta hepatis, e.g. from neuroblastoma, lymphosarcoma, Hodgkin's disease or leukaemia, may cause clinical findings very similar to a tumour of the bile ducts, and unless the primary tumour has already declared itself, the diagnosis is made only at exploration and biopsy.

Hamartomas, inflammatory polyps and lipomas obstructing the bile ducts have been recorded very occasionally.

Carcinoma of the bile ducts (Longmire, McArthur *et al.*, 1973) has yet to be reported in patients less than 20 years of age.

DIAGNOSIS

The diagnosis can only be made with certainty at laparotomy, and because of the rarity of rhabdomyosarcoma of the bile ducts, frozen sections, or an interim drainage procedure while paraffin sections are examined, are required.

TREATMENT

Total excision is desirable, but the tumour has usually progressed beyond the scope of even radical measures. Nevertheless, as much as possible of the tumour should be removed, and provision made for biliary drainage, for example by choledochojejunostomy (Roux-en-Y).

When the general condition is poor, temporary drainage proximal to the obstruction may provide some time to prepare the patient for a radical operation.

Chemotherapy and radiotherapy

Recent reports of the results in children with rhabdomyosarcoma (Donaldson *et al.* 1973; Kilman, Clatworthy *et al.*, 1973) have shown considerable improvement in the prognosis when aggressively treated with chemotherapy, augmented by radiotherapy.

A suggested regime for the treatment of rhabdomyosarcoma is described on p. 790.

PROGNOSIS

Results reported in the literature, before the development of current schema of treatment for rhabdomyoblastoma, are extremely poor. In the only long term survivor reported total excision was not possible, and residual tumour was apparently controlled by adjuvant therapy. In all the other patients, biliary obstruction was unrelieved or recurred quickly, and in most cases death occurred within six months (Davis *et al.*, 1969).

The Index Series contains one example which is typical of the cases described in the literature, in almost every detail.

A boy aged $2\frac{1}{2}$ years presented with a ten-day history of jaundice, abdominal pain, vomiting and diarrhoea, and pale faeces; the provisional diagnosis was viral hepatitis. The jaundice was obstructive in type and after decreasing over a few days, returned one week later, accompanied by signs of general peritonitis, a leucocytosis of 30, 500/cmm, and an opacity in the right hypochondrium in x-rays of the abdomen.

At laparotomy there was biliary peritonitis due to rupture of a dilated common hepatic duct proximal to a necrotic, haemorrhagic, fleshy tumour, 8 cm in diameter, which surrounded both the cystic and common bile ducts. The gall-bladder was distended and contained 'white' bile. Drainage of the ruptured duct was established, and biopsy of the tumour (paraffin sections) revealed rhabdomyosarcoma. The lymph nodes in the porta hepatis were free of tumour.

One week later radical pancreaticoduodenectomy was performed, one of the technical problems being the attachment of the tumour to the wall of the portal vein.

Actinomycin D and radiotherapy were commenced after operation, and the patient improved for three months, until the tumour recurred and led to death six months after the onset of symptoms.

REFERENCES

The Liver

ANDERSEN, D.H. (1951). Tumors of infancy and childhood. I. Survey of those seen in pathology laboratory of Babies Hospital during 1935–1950. *Cancer*, **4** : 890.

ANDREWS, J.T., STEVEN, L.W., ARKLES, L.B., SEPHTON, R.G. & MARTIN, J.J. (1973). Reticulo-endothelial and blood-pool scanning in the diagnosis and differentiation of space occupying lesions of the liver. *Aust. N.Z. J. Surg.*, **43** : 14.

ASCH, M.J., COHEN, A.H. & MOORE, T.C. (1974). Hepatic and splenic lymphangiomatosis with skeletal involvement: report of a case and review of the literature. *Surgery*, **76** : 334.

BECKER, F.F. (1974). Hepatoma: nature's model tumor. *Am. J. Path.*, **74** : 179.

BRAUN, P., DUCHARME, J.L. *et al.* (1975). Haemangiomatosis of the liver in infants. *J. Pediat. Surg.*, **10** : 121.

BROWN, S.H.Jr., NEERHOUT, R. & FONKALSRUD, E.W. (1972). Prednisone therapy in management of large hemangiomas in infants and children. *Surgery*, **71** : 168.

CLATWORTHY, H.W., SCHILLER, M. & GROSFELD, J.L. (1974). Primary liver tumours in infancy and childhood. *Arch. Surg.*, **109** : 143.

DELORIMIER, A.S., SIMPSON, E.B., BAUM, R.S. *et al.* (1967). Hepatic artery ligation for hepatic hemangiomatosis. *New Engl. J. Med.*, **277** : 333.

DONOVAN, E.J. & SANTULLI, T.V. (1946). Resection of left lobe of liver for mesenchymoma: Report of a case. *Ann. Surg.*, **124** : 90.

EIN, S.H. & STEPHENS, C.A. (1974a). Malignant liver tumors in children. *J. Pediat. Surg.*, **9** : 491.

EIN, S.H. & STEPHENS, C.A. (1974b). Benign liver tumors and cysts in childhood. *J. Pediat. Surg.*, **9** : 847.

EXELBY, P.R., EL-DOMERI, A., HUVOS, A.G. & BEATTIE, E.J.Jr. (1971). Primary malignant tumors of the liver in children. *J. Pediat. Surg.*, **6** : 272.

FORTNER, J.G., SHIU, M.H. *et al.* (1974). Major hepatic resection using vascular isolation and hypothermic perfusion. *Ann. Surg.*, **180** : 644.

FOSTER, J.H. (1970). Survival after liver resection for cancer. *Cancer*, **26** : 493.

GOLDBERG, S.J. & FONKALSRUD, E.W. (1969). Successful treatment of hepatic hemangioma with corticosteroids. *J. Amer. med. Assoc.*, **208** : 2473.

GOLDSMITH, N.A. & WOODBURNE, R.T. (1957). The surgical anatomy pertaining to liver resection. *Surg. Gynec. Obstet.*, **105** : 310.

GOLDSTEIN, H.M., NEIMAN, H.L. *et al.* (1974). Angiograph findings in benign liver cell tumours. *Radiol.*, **110** : 339.

HILLER, H.G. (1967). Paediatric hepatic arteriography. *Australasian Radiology*, **11** : 30.

HOLTON, C.P., BURRINGTON, J.D. & HATCH, E.I. (1975). A multiple chemotherapeutic approach to the management of hepatobiastroma. *Cancer*, **35** : 1083.

HUNG, W., BLIZZARD, R.M. *et al.* (1963). Precocious puberty in a boy with a hepatoma and circulating gonadotropin. *J. Pediat.*, **63** : 895.

ISHAK, K.G. & GLUNZ, P.R. (1967). Hepatoblastoma and hepatocarcinoma in infancy and childhood. *Cancer*, **20** : 396.

ISHIDA, R., TSUCHIDA, Y., SAITO, S. & SAWAGUCHI, S. (1966). Mesenchymal hamartoma of the liver: case report and literature review. *Ann. Surg.*, **164** : 175.

KASAI, M. & WATANABE, I. (1970). Histologic classification of liver cell carcinoma in infancy and childhood and its clinical evaluation. *Cancer*, **25** : 551.

KEELING, J.W. (1971). Liver tumors in infancy and childhood. *J. Path.*, **103** : 69.

KREEL, L., JONES, E.A. & TAVIL, A.S. (1968). A comparative study of arteriography and scintillation scanning in space occupying lesions of the liver. *Brit. J. Radiol.*, **41** : 401.

LEE, M.E., NEWSTEDT, J.R. & SIDDALL, S.H. (1956). Large abdominal tumors of children (other than Wilms' tumor or neuroblastoma). *Ann. Surg.*, **143** : 803.

MARTIN, L.W. & WOODMAN, K.S. (1969). Hepatic lobectomy for hepatoblastoma in infants and children. *Arch. Surg.*, **98** : 1.

MATOLO, N.M. & JOHNSON, D.G. (1973). Surgical treatment of hepato hemangioma in the newborn. *Arch. Surg.*, **106** : 725.

MATTIOLI, L., LEE, K.R. & HODER, T.M. (1974). Hepatic artery ligation for cardiac failure due to hepatic hemangioma in the new born. *J. Pediat. Surg.*, **9** : 859.

NIKAIDO, H., BOGGS, J. & SWENSON, O. (1970). Liver tumours in infants and children: clinical and pathological analysis of 22 patients. *Arch. Surg.*, **101** : 245.

NISHIOKA, T., IBATA, K., OKITA, T., HARADA, T. & FUJITA, T. (1972). Localization of α-fetoprotein in hepatoma tissues by immunofluorescence. *Cancer Res.*, **32** : 162.

NIXON, H.H. (1965). Hepatic tumours in childhood and their treatment by major hepatic resection. *Arch. Dis. Childh.*, **40** : 169.

NOVY, S. & WALLACE, S. *et al.* (1974). Angiographic evaluation of primary malignant hepatocellular tumors in children. *Am. J. Roetgenol.*, **120** : 353.

RAFFUCCI, F.L. & RAMIREZ-SCHON, G. (1970). Management of tumors of the liver. *Surg. Gynec. Obstet.*, **130** : 371.

SABOO, R.M. & BELSARE, R.K. *et al.* (1974). Giant congenital cyst of the liver. *J. Pediat. Surg.*, **9** : 561.

SAMUELS, L.D. & GROSFELD, J.L. (1970). Serial scans of liver regeneration after hemihepatectomy in childhood. *Surg. Gynec. Obstet.*, **131** : 453.

SHULLER, T., ROSENZWEIG, J.L. & AREY, J.B. (1949). Successful removal of hemangioma of the liver in an infant. *Pediatrics*, **3** : 328.

SINNIAH, D., CAMPBELL, P.E. & COLEBATCH, J.H. (1974). Primary hepatic cancer in infancy and childhood. *Progress in Pediatric Surgery*, **7** : 141.

SOMPII, E., NIEMI, K. *et al.* (1974). Cavernous hepatic hemangioma in the newborn infant: case report of a successful resection. *J. Pediat. Surg.*, **9** : 239.

STILLMAN, A. & ZAMCHECK, H. (1970). Recent advances in immunologic diagnosis of digestive tract cancer. *Am. J. Dig. Dis.*, **15** : 1003.

STONE, H.H. (1975). Major hepatic resections in children. *J. Pediat. Surg.*, **10** : 127.

STONE, H.H. *et al.* (1969) Physiological considerations in major hepatic resections. *Amer. J. Surg.*, **117** : 78.

SUTTON, C.A. & ELLER, J.L. (1968). Mesenchymal hamartoma of the liver. *Cancer*, **22** : 29.

TENG, C.T., DAESCHNER, C.W. *et al.* (1961). Liver disease and osteoporosis in children. *J. Pediat.*, **59** : 684.

WILSON, H. & WOLF, R.Y. (1965). Hepatic lobectomy : indications, technique and results. *Surgery*, **59** : 472.

The Bile Ducts

AKERS, D.R. & NEEDHAM, M.E. (1971). Sarcoma botryoides (rhabdomyosarcoma) of the bile ducts with survival. *J. Pediat. Surg.*, **6** : 474.

DAVIS, G.L., KISSANE, J.M. & ISHAK, K.G. (1969). Embryonal rhabdomyosarcoma (sarcoma botryoides) of the bilary tree. *Cancer*, **24** : 333.

DONALDSON, S.S., CASTRO, J.R., WILBUR, J.R. & JESSE, R.H. (1973). Rhabdomyosarcoma of the head and neck in children. *Cancer*, **31** : 26.

KILMAN, J.S., CLATWORTHY, H.W.Jr. *et al.* (1973). Reasonable surgery for rhabdomyosarcoma: a study of 67 cases. *Ann. Surg.*, **178** : 346.

KISSANE, J.M. & SMITH, M.G. (1967). *Pathology of Infancy and Childhood.* The C.V. Mosby Co., St. Louis.

LONGMIRE, W.P.Jr., MCARTHUR, M.S. *et al.* (1973). Carcinoma of the extrahepatic biliary tract. *Ann. Surg.*, **178** : 333.

Chapter 20. Tumours of the alimentary canal, spleen, pancreas, omentum and mesenteries

The three major differences between malignant tumours of the bowel in children and in adults are: (*a*) their great rarity in children; (*b*) the preponderance of sarcomas; and (*c*) their occurrence in the small bowel rather than the stomach or colon. Only 1% of all the malignant tumours in the Index Series arose in the alimentary canal. Although the gastro-intestinal tract may be subjected to many irritants during childhood, they are apparently not sufficient, in the course of the limited period of time, to cause the malignancies seen in adults.

The early symptoms of an alimentary malignancy in children are not distinctive, and resemble those due to more common childhood ailments. Delay in diagnosis is usual and understandable, for parents may not seek medical advice for mild symptoms in the early stages, and when they do, the clinician usually has a low index of suspicion of malignancy and may not be sufficiently concerned to arrange for a full scale investigation.

In this chapter tumours are described under the following headings:

TUMOURS OF THE OESOPHAGUS AND STOMACH

The oesophagus is among the rarest sites of tumours in childhood. Squamous carcinoma arising in the mucosa appears to be confined to one case in the literature (Moore, 1958).

Yannopoulos & Stout (1962) reviewed the world literature concerning leiomyoma and leiomyosarcoma in childhood, including an earlier series collected by Golden & Stout (1941), and added 20 personal cases. Of the total series of 34, only two arose in the oesophagus, in each case in a patient more than 13 years of age. The most recent case reported (Nahmad & Clatworthy, 1973) also occurred in the third quinquennium, in a 14-year old girl with a submucosal leiomyoma involving the whole length of the oesophagus; the oesophagus was excised and eventually replaced successfully with a segment of colon.

The symptoms caused by oesophageal tumours (dysphagia, vomiting) are often insidious until haematemesis occurs and leads to investigation. Barium swallow, oesophagoscopy and biopsy, should lead to the diagnosis before exploration.

No tumour of the oesophagus was seen in the period covered by the Index Series.

Tumours of the stomach although rare, are more common than in the oesophagus.

Carcinoma of the stomach was represented by fewer than 20 patients less than 15 years of age in a series of 501 cases of carcinoma 'in the young' collected by McNeer (1941). In some 75% of 19 cases in the paediatric age group a mass was palpable in the abdomen, accompanied by loss of weight, pain and vomiting. Surgical excision along the same lines as in adults would appear to be the most appropriate treatment, with a similar prognosis.

Leiomyosarcoma and leiomyoma of the stomach (Botting *et al.*, 1965) are possibly more common than carcinoma (of the stomach) in childhood. A recent review of the literature by Wurlitzer and colleagues (1973) yielded 32 cases, to which they added two from the records of the Children's Hospital of Los Angeles.

The most common mode of presentation was haematemesis which occurred in 51% of those judged to be sarcomas, and in 31% of the benign cases; melaena was also common, and anaemia a natural consequence.

Contrast studies showed a polypoid filling defect, with or without ulceration, but radiographic findings were of little or no assistance in distinguishing benign and malignant smooth muscle tumours. This is a difficulty not only in pre-operative clinical diagnosis, and in assessing macroscopic appearances at operation, but also in interpreting the microscopic findings. The histological diagnosis was frequently found to be incorrect in the light of the subsequent behaviour of the tumour. Unmistakable metastases or infiltration of adjacent structures were present in 10 of the 16 tumours described in sufficient detail to be classified as malignant.

Differential diagnosis before operation includes bezoars, foreign body granuloma, gastric duplications and lymphosarcoma of the stomach, all of which occurred in our patients in the period covered by the Index Series; there was no case of leiomyosarcoma of the stomach and one leiomyoma was seen.

A girl aged 14 months presented with anaemia and a palpable mass in the upper part of the abdomen. At laparotomy a gastric mass $8 \times 5 \times 4{\cdot}5$ cm was resected, together with the spleen. The gastric mucosa over the inner aspect of the tumour was ulcerated. The cut surface was pink, firm and whorled and there was a central necrotic area containing areas of calcification.

Microscopically the mass was composed of spindle cells with vesicular, cigar-shaped nuclei with blunt ends. The cytoplasm was plump and tapering, and some cells were vacuolated. Collagen formation was prominent in some areas, and there were scattered foci of calcification. In some respects the tumour resembled the 'bizarre leiomyoma' of Stout.

She is well with no evidence of disease 18 years later.

Prognosis

In the series reviewed by Wurlitzer *et al.* (1973), five of the eight patients with a leiomyosarcoma followed for five years after surgery were free of disease, chiefly those treated by subtotal gastrectomy or a more radical resection dictated by uncertainty as to whether the tumour was benign or malignant.

Teratoma of the stomach has also been described (Matias & Huang, 1973; Nandy & Sengupta, 1974) as a cause of haematemesis and a gastric filling defect, while regional enteritis though extremely rare in the stomach and duodenum in childhood may have radiological appearances which may suggest a tumour.

Laparotomy is required to make the diagnosis, and it may be difficult to determine the extent of resection of the stomach required. In young children the long-term effects on growth and development after radical or total gastrectomy as a general rule, are to be avoided if possible, but a leiomyosarcoma may be an exception, and in most of the cases reported a subtotal gastrectomy was performed.

TUMOURS OF THE SMALL INTESTINE

Abdominal pain

The factors which most often cloud the clinical assessment of children with these tumours is their rarity in childhood, and the common occurrence of recurrent, colicky abdominal pains, often psychosomatic in origin, or attributed to constipation or to 'chronic' appendicitis. Any unusual features in the admittedly wide range of minor abdominal symptoms, should remind the clinician of the possibility of malignancy, rare though it may be, and should suggest that appropriate investigations should be undertaken.

It is difficult to offer any dogmatic guidance as to which children presenting with abdominal pain should be selected for investigation, but points in the history which would indicate that full scale radiological investigation should be considered, are as follows:

(i) *Loss of weight*, particularly if recent, significant in amount (more than 2 kg), and when no alternative cause can be found.

(ii) *A significant degree of anaemia* without obvious cause.

(iii) *Episodes of pain* recurring at more or less regular intervals for more than an hour, and with intervals of freedom for more than 1–2 weeks.

(iv) *Periods of continuous pain*, even mild pain, if it lasts for more than 1 or 2 hours, especially when it is *not* periumbilical or central, and is accompanied by persistent vomiting or retching.
(v) *Suspicion of an indefinite mass* anywhere in abdomen, having excluded a full bladder and faeces in the colon.
(vi) *Abdominal distension.*

INVESTIGATIONS

A well-centred and properly exposed plain film of the abdomen is a simple and useful screening test; even when not completely conclusive the findings may indicate the need for more extensive investigations.

Contrast studies (Fig. 20.1) may be indicated by the pattern or the severity of the symptoms, or by indefinite but puzzling findings in plain films of the abdomen.

Palpation of the abdomen under anaesthesia should perhaps be employed more often, in selected cases, to confirm or exclude an impression that there is an ill-defined abdominal mass, especially in an uncooperative or fearful toddler, and when there is still uncertainty after repeated examination of the abdomen.

A reasonable index of suspicion, tempered by a realistic perspective and experience, should create the clinical approach most likely to detect a tumour of the gut as early as possible, when the symptoms are indefinite and the signs less than conclusive.

Primary tumours arising in the small intestine are as follows:

I. Lymphosarcoma (and reticulum cell sarcoma);
II. Carcinoid tumours (p. 809);
III. Leiomyosarcoma.

In childhood, sarcomas of the bowel are far more common than carcinomas, and a lymphosarcoma arising in lymphoid tissue is the commonest malignant tumour of the alimentary canal. Possibly because of the concentration of lymphoid tissue in Peyer's patches, the distal ileum is more often the site of the primary than any other part of the gut.

I. LYMPHOSARCOMA OF THE SMALL INTESTINE

Because of the preponderance of lymphosarcoma this tumour is described in detail; some closely related tumours have similar effects, e.g. reticulum cell sarcoma, and can only be distinguished on histological findings.

AGE : SEX

The age group maximally affected is 3–10 years, with a peak at about 5 years.

Boys are very much more often affected than girls (Mestel, 1959), in a ratio of approximately 10 : 1 in large reported series, and in the Index Series.

SITE

The terminal ileum is by far the commonest site (Marcuse & Stout, 1950; Pickett & Briggs, 1967; Bartram & Chrispin, 1973; Fu *et al.*, 1972).

Lymphosarcomas also arise elsewhere in the small bowel, in the colon, the appendix and, least commonly, in the stomach.

MACROSCOPIC APPEARANCES

There are two main types: the polypoid and the annular.

The polypoid type tends to grow into the lumen and is more likely to cause obstruction, especially in the form of an intussusception (Mestel, 1959) at a relatively early stage.

The annular type spreads both circumferentially and along the length of the bowel, causing it to become greatly thickened; it also permeates the muscular coats to appear beneath the serosa. Ulceration of the mucous membrane and erosion of the tumour and the muscle, leads to an aneurysmal extension of the lumen, and this is responsible for one of characteristics of this tumour: the size which it can attain without causing intestinal obstruction.

Ulceration or necrosis may lead to perforation and a local abscess or spreading peritonitis, or, more rarely, to an aneurysmal segment composed largely of tumour tissue (Norfray *et al.*, 1973).

The lymph nodes become involved and are often greatly enlarged.

The mesentery is invaded diffusely and greatly thickened. Infiltration may extend into the omentum, or as a sheet of cells spreading into retroperitoneal tissues.

A chylous type of ascites develops when there is extensive obstruction of lacteals, and an exudative reaction to peritoneal seeding may contribute to the intraperitoneal fluid.

In some cases the naked eye appearances at operation are potentially misleading; greatly enlarged lymph nodes and a markedly thickened mesentery, strongly suggesting extensive infiltration, may be largely or entirely due to lymphatic obstruction and widespread engorgement of lacteals with fatty material very similar to the creamy colour of lymphosarcomatous tissue.

This raises two possibilities: (*a*) a tumour judged to be inoperable may not be, and the patient may be denied the significant advantage of a radical resection; (*b*) in some of the patients with an unexpectedly satisfactory course after apparently only partial removal, most or all of the tumour may in fact have been completely removed.

STAGING

The stage of the disease at the time of presentation has an important bearing on survival, and the best results naturally occur in the early stages. The simplified system of staging used in the Index Series is as follows.

Stage I. The tumour is confined to the wall of the bowel.

Stage II. Involvement of the bowel and the local lymph nodes.

Stage III. Extensive spread to retroperitoneal nodes or tissue planes, or distant metastases, e.g. in the liver.

HISTOLOGICAL TYPES

Lymphosarcomas of the alimentary canal are either lymphocytic or lymphoblastic in type (see p. 171), and occasionally a reticulum cell sarcoma with very similar macroscopic appearances is found on microscopic examination.

There are thus three histological types of sarcomas of the small intestine:

Lymphocytic lymphosarcoma;

Lymphoblastic lymphosarcoma; and

Reticulum cell sarcoma.

Until recently, the first of these appeared to have the best prognosis, but differences in the outcome may not be as great since the introduction of intensive chemotherapy.

MICROSCOPIC FINDINGS

The two histological types of lymphosarcoma and their differentiation from reticulum cell sarcoma are described in the chapter on malignant lymphomas (p. 178).

SPREAD

Local contiguous infiltration in the most important route, at first in the submucosal plane, then through the wall of the bowel, into the adjacent mesentery and finally the retroperitoneal tissues.

Lymph nodes are involved early, particularly those at the mesenteric attachment, then, progressively, relays of nodes extending to the para-aortic groups around the coeliac axis, and eventually upwards to the deep supraclavicular nodes.

Transperitoneal seeding, and retrograde lymphatic embolism to the serosa of the bowel adjacent to the primary tumour also occur.

Blood-borne metastases to the lungs or the liver occur late in the course of the disease.

MODES OF PRESENTATION

The clinical patterns described below are usually found, in retrospect, to have been preceded, for a variable period of time, by loss of weight and intermittent, indefinite symptoms of abdominal pain, anorexia, constipation or diarrhoea.

In most of the 15 patients in the Index Series, the early features were chiefly anaemia, failure to thrive or loss of weight, all of mild or moderate degree.

Only two of 15 patients did not have a history of abdominal pain; the passage of blood per rectum occurred in four children and in three of these the tumour was the cause of an intussusception.

The modes of presentation in order of frequency are as follows:

1. *Intussusception or intestinal obstruction* occurred in five children, three of whom had recurrent pain for 2–4 months before culminating in an acute attack. The youngest of the five children in this group was 3 years of age; the age alone suggests the presence of an underlying cause, for the peak age of the 'idiopathic' type of intussusception is between 4 and 9 months.

In the two children who presented with subacute intestinal obstruction, radiological investigations were inconclusive (apart from confirming the presence of obstruction) and the real cause was only determined at laparatomy.

2. *A non-tender abdominal mass.* A mass was eventually palpable in all but one of the 15 children in the Index Series; when the mass is not an intussusception, it is an indication that the tumour has reached a relatively advanced stage. In some of these cases symptoms had been present for less than 2 weeks, but in others symptoms had been present intermittently for several months.

The commonest site of a palpable mass was the right iliac fossa; the suprapubic region was next, and the mass was in the epigastrium or hypochondrium in three children.

The tumour tends to be rounded and mobile when only the bowel and the adjacent local lymph nodes are involved, but in most cases the tumour has infiltrated the adjacent mesentery or loops of bowel, and the mass is then larger, ill-defined and fixed.

3. *Misdiagnosis as an appendical abscess* is an error which can readily occur in a child with mild or moderate abdominal symptoms and a tender mass in the right iliac fossa, the usual location of the distal ileum, and the commonest site of a lymphosarcoma. Here again the duration of the history, with abdominal pain for some weeks, should alert the clinician to the possibility that the cause is other than a recent acute appendicitis. However, even at operation the findings may initially be misleading; necrotic tumour may look like pus or fibrin, and a walled-off perforation in malignant tissue in the bowel may at first resemble an appendical abscess.

Hepatomegaly due to metastases was noted at the time of presentation in only two cases; in three others chylous ascites masked the presence of a tumour.

INVESTIGATIONS

A full blood examination may show only a secondary hypochromic anaemia, but a leukaemic picture occurs in a small proportion (5–10%) of cases of intestinal lymphosarcoma, and usually in a much greater proportion in the terminal stages. The bone marrow may contain metastatic cells.

Tests for occult blood in the faeces, when properly performed and positive, are especially significant in a child with vague abdominal symptoms, and should be regarded as an indication for a barium meal and 'follow-through'.

Peritoneal paracentesis is indicated in children with unexplained ascites, and can lead to the diagnosis by revealing malignant cells in material prepared for exfoliative cytology (p. 88).

Radiographs of the abdomen may show a 'ground glass' area displacing the gas shadow of the small bowel if the tumour is large enough, and contrast studies may show a persistent filling defect in the ileocaecal region (Fig. 20.1).

It should be noted that negative findings in contrast studies of the small bowel do not exclude the possibility of a tumour, and when a mass is suspected, aortography and selective arteriography of the coeliac axis may show the arterial supply of the mass stemming from the superior mesenteric artery (Fig. 20.2). The other more common abdominal neoplasms such as Wilms' tumour and neuroblastoma are usually excluded by the aortogram and subsequent pyelogram.

Cystography and venocavography may be required in some cases, and the level of catecholamines in the urine (p. 551) should be estimated when a neuroblastoma cannot be excluded.

A liver scan (p. 76) is indicated when the liver is enlarged, and hepatic metastases may be already large enough to be demonstrated at the time of presentation.

Laparotomy and biopsy are required to confirm the diagnosis in most cases, for barium studies are often inconclusive when the tumour arises in the ileum, and contrast studies are unnecessary or even illadvised when there is complete or nearly complete intestinal obstruction.

DIFFERENTIAL DIAGNOSIS

In the case of small lymphosarcomas presenting early with an intussusception or intestinal obstruction, the diagnosis is usually made on the findings at operation.

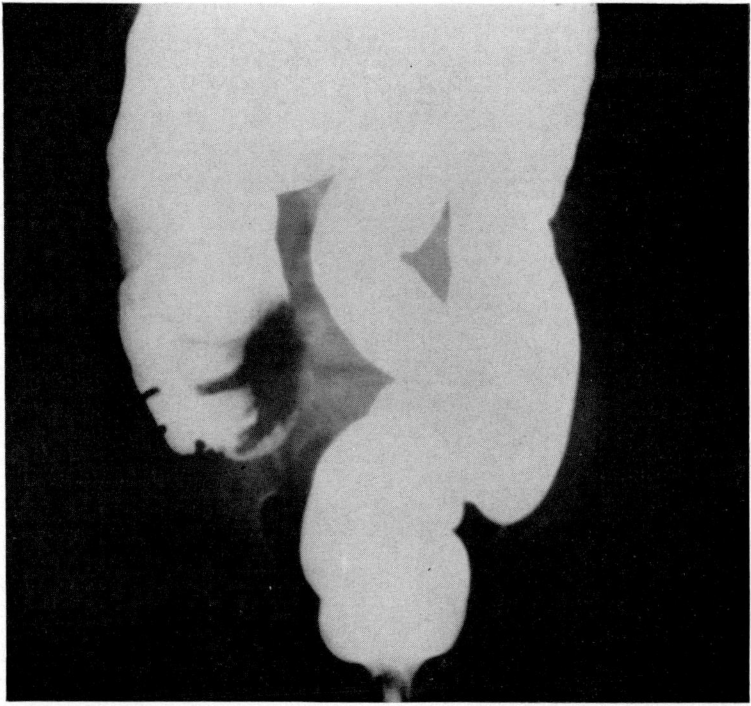

Figure 20.1. LYMPHOSARCOMA OF THE TERMINAL ILEUM; a contrast study with barium showing a persistent filling defect in the region of the caecum in a six-year old boy with a history of severe abdominal colic for three weeks.

A Meckel's diverticulum, benign polyp (p. 646), leiomyoma, haemangioma, eosinophilic granuloma, duplication cyst or a lymphangiomatous segment of the gut or mesentery (p. 673), may all produce somewhat similar clinical findings. In most cases these can be identified and excluded at operation, but in a few cases, for example massive enlargement of lymph nodes due to viral mesenteric adenitis, frozen sections may be required.

A large abdominal mass, particularly when in the upper half of the abdomen, raises a list of possibilities headed by Wilms' tumour and neuroblastoma (p. 491). The site of the tumour and hence the type can be determined with a high degree of accuracy before operation by aortography and angiography (p. 636).

An appendical abscess is statistically the most likely cause of a mass in the right iliac fossa, particularly when supported by a short history, fever and leucocytosis.

Lymphoid hyperplasia of the ileum with pseudopolyposis, caused by marked hyperplasia of follicles in the mucosa and submucosa (Danis, 1974; Schenken

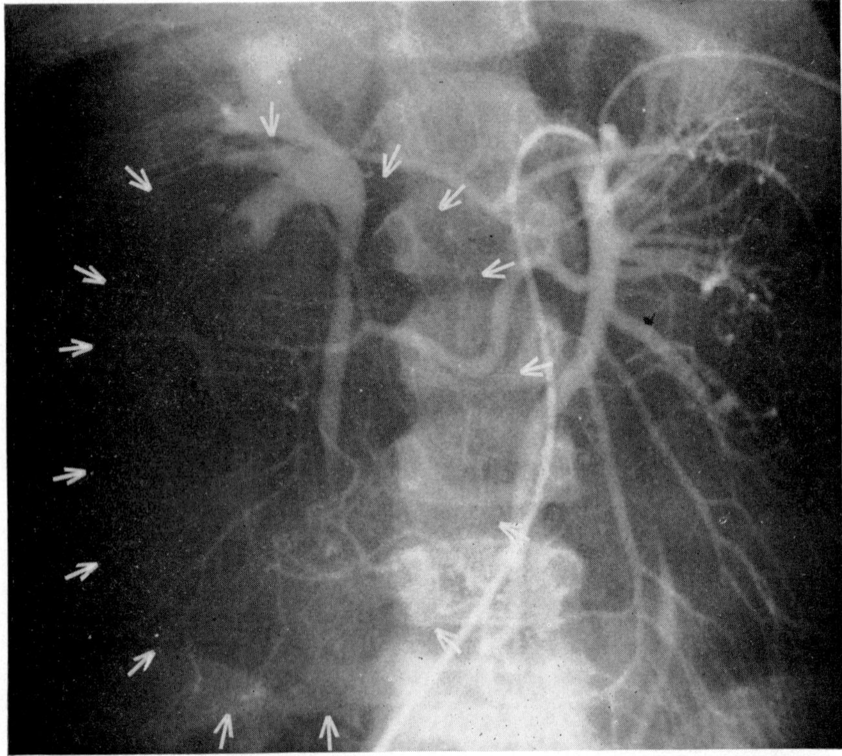

Figure 20.2. LYMPHOSARCOMA OF THE ILEUM; an aortogram showing loss of 'arcade pattern', and tumour circulation arising from the ilio-caecal branches of the superior mesenteric artery.

et al., 1975), is a rare condition which can resemble primary lymphosarcoma in causing an intussusception, recurrent abdominal pain or radiological evidence of a lesion partially obstructing the distal ileum.

Laparotomy is usually required to distinguish the two conditions. In lymphoid hyperplasia the serosal surface is normal in appearance, and the segment affected is sharply defined with a thickened wall and palpable polypoid projections into the lumen. The diagnosis may be made on frozen sections, but resection of the segment involved may be necessary because of intussusception or haemorrhage, or when neoplasia cannot be excluded.

Regional enteritis is another possible cause, often accompanied by chronic malaise, loss of weight and anaemia. A barium meal and careful follow-through is a useful investigation, but when inconclusive, or when the symptoms are acute, the diagnosis should be clarified by laparotomy without delay.

A chronic inflammatory ileo-caecal mass due to tuberculosis, or to *Pasteurella* (now Yersinia) *pseudotuberculosis rodentii*, may produce findings very similar to a lymphosarcoma of the gut. The correct diagnosis may be made at laparotomy, but is sometimes only made on the histological findings in the operative specimen.

Retroperitoneal lymphosarcomas are especially difficult to distinguish from those arising in the ileocaecal region, before laparotomy. There were five retroperitoneal lymphosarcomas in the Index Series; three were of the Burkitt type (p. 328), two of which presented as an upper abdominal mass; in one of these the diagnosis was made by biopsy of an enlarged supraclavicular lymph node.

Tuberculous peritonitis may closely resemble the chylous or ascitic form of lymphosarcoma. Here, too, laparotomy and biopsy may be required, although tuberculosis may be suspected when an active pulmonary focus can be demonstrated radiographically, for this is almost always present in children with tuberculous peritonitis.

TREATMENT OF LYMPHOSARCOMA

Surgery

The standard plan is radical surgical excision combined with chemotherapy and radiotherapy (Aur, Hustu *et al.*, 1971). However, good results can be obtained by surgery alone in Stage I, when the tumour is confined to the gut, with or without involvement of the epimural lymph nodes. Staging can usually be determined accurately at laparotomy, but the misleading macroscopic appearances described on p. 631 should be borne in mind and clarified before the situation is classed as non-resectable (Stage III). This conclusion should only be reached after careful examination of apparently affected tissues, and if necessary multiple frozen sections from doubtful areas.

When resection is possible, a generous segment of bowel should be resected, including at least 4–5 cm of bowel beyond the visible extent of the tumour, as well as the related portion of mesentery with its nodes and lymphatics, extending as far as the root of the mesentery, but preserving the main superior mesenteric vessels. Not infrequently this amounts to an extended right hemicolectomy which is well tolerated in children.

Chemotherapy can be commenced before laparotomy when the diagnosis has been made by exfoliative cytology of the ascitic fluid, but more often as soon as diagnosis is made at operation, and preferably before commencing the resection.

Radical curative surgery should be attempted if at all possible, because of the improved prospects of survival. In one of the long term survivors in the Index Series, the resection was extended to include partial pancreatectomy, right hemicolectomy and removal of the transverse colon.

Palliative surgery should be considered when the tumour is inoperable and there is intestinal obstruction, e.g. a bypass operation, followed by chemotherapy and radiotherapy, but there were no survivors in the Index Series when this plan was employed.

Chemotherapy

The regime recommended for lymphosarcoma is described on p. 175.

Radiotherapy

Following partial or complete removal of the primary tumour, the mesenteric and para-aortic lymph nodes from the diaphragm to the pelvis are usually irradiated to a dose of 2500 rads (over approximately 3 weeks), integrated with the regime of chemotherapy.

When exploration reveals advanced disease beyond the scope of operative excision, the results of all forms of treatment are extremely poor, but palliative radiotherapy (to 2000 rads) preceded or followed by cytotoxic agents, may be of some value.

RESULTS IN THE INDEX SERIES

Of the 17 sarcomas of the bowel, 15 were lymphosarcomas, one a leiomyosarcoma (Fig. 23.10, p. 810) and one a reticulum cell sarcoma. In ten of the 15 lymphosarcomas the tumour was resected; five of the ten had no additional treatment and are long-term survivors. Among the ten survivors (out of 17) five had a lymphocytic lymphosarcoma, three a lymphoblastic lymphosarcoma, one a leiomyosarcoma and one a reticulum cell sarcoma. The seven deaths (five in Stage III, two in Stage II) all occurred in children with a lymphoblastic tumour.

Reticulum cell sarcoma of the gut

Although only one of the tumours just described was a reticulum cell sarcoma, there are three other cases in the Index Series classified as 'abdominal' reticulum cell sarcoma because the primary site was not identified. The findings in all three children were remarkably similar.

Generalized symptoms of malaise, fever, abdominal pain and vomiting were the presenting picture, and on examination there was marked enlargement of the liver, spleen, deep external iliac and inguinal lymph nodes. In each case the diagnosis of disseminated reticulum cell sarcoma was made by biopsy, of inguinal nodes in two cases and a cervical node in the third. In one child the marrow also contained deposits of reticulum cell sarcoma.

Chemotherapy alone was the treatment used in each case; daunorubicin and prednisolone in one; combination courses of actinomycin D, daunorubicin and prednisolone in the second; actinomycin D and prednisolone followed by vincristine and cyclophosphamide in the third.

Complete remission and long term survival for more than five years with no evidence of disease was the outcome in each case. As none had a laparotomy the site of the primary is unknown, but all three appear to have been in 'Stage IIIB', i.e. malignant lymphoma with dissemination and general symptoms.

Lymphosarcoma

Of the 15 lymphosarcomas, eight are alive and free of disease, six of them for more than 5 years after operation; in two of these six, resection was thought to have been incomplete; three of the five who presented with an intussusception are alive and well, and in one of these the resection was extensive because the intussusception was irreducible.

All five children who presented with a large fixed palpable mass had a lymphoblastic type of lymphosarcoma in Stage III; all died quickly without responding to treatment.

PROGNOSIS

The following can be identified as favourable factors:

(i) *Those at the lower end of the age range*, i.e. between 3 and 5 years of age;

(ii) *Lymphocytic* rather than lymphoblastic lymphosarcoma;

(iii) *The polypoid type*, which tends to present early by causing an intussusception;

(iv) *Those in whom resection can be performed* (i.e. Stage I or II) and those in whom the tumour could be completely or almost completely removed;

(v) *Absence of distant metastases*, e.g. in cervical nodes, malignant ascites, or transperitoneal seedling.

II. CARCINOID TUMOURS
(syn. argentaffinoma)

The term 'carcinoid' (carcinoma-like) proposed by Oberndorfer in 1907 has been retained although only a small proportion are actually malignant. Argentaffinoma would be a better term.

SITE: AGE

Carcinoid tumours of the alimentary canal arise from Kulchitzky cells in the crypts of Lieberkuhn, and 90% occur in the appendix or ileocaecal area (Barclay & Robb, 1968). The rectosigmoid region is the second commonest site and the tumour may arise in any part of the bowel. Carcinoid tumours also occur as one form of bronchial adenoma (p. 473) or in the pancreas (p. 670).

The reported incidence in surgical specimens of the appendix is 0·05–0·69%, and in childhood the incidence lies closer to the lower figure. The true incidence is difficult to determine because many are never identified; the tumour is usually symptomless, in many cases the appendix is not examined adequately, and some tumours are only discovered incidentally at autopsy.

Stowens (1959) was unable to demonstrate argentaffin cells in the bowel of children before the age of 4 years, and the youngest case of carcinoid tumour ever reported was 5 years of age (Willox, 1964). In most of the cases in childhood the patient was more than 8 years old.

Females are affected much more often than males.

In the Index Series there are four cases and in each instance the tumour was found in the appendix; three of the four were girls, and all were between 8 and 14 years of age.

MACROSCOPIC APPEARANCES

This slowly growing but potentially malignant tumour is usually firm, yellowish, and less than 1 cm in diameter; 72% arise in the distal third of the appendix, and in most reported cases there is no evidence of inflammation. However, in the Index Series, three of the four cases had histologically proven inflammation in the appendix distal to the tumour.

Carcinoids are usually single, but may be multiple, and when recognized in the appendix during operation, the rest of the bowel, especially the ileum, should be carefully examined.

MICROSCOPIC FINDINGS

The tumour consists of solid clumps or strands of small, uniform polyhedral cells containing granules which stain deeply with silver stains in the same way as in the Kulchitzky cells from which they arise (Soga & Tazawa, 1971). Infiltration of the muscle of the bowel wall and lymphatic channels is almost universal, and invasion through to the peritoneal surface is common.

SPREAD

In spite of these common histological findings, spread from a carcinoid tumour of the appendix is extremely rare, and only 2 instances of metastases appearing after appendicectomy have been reported in the literature (D'Ingianni, 1946).

In tumours arising anywhere else than in the appendix, the prognosis is not as good. Metastases to local lymph nodes are reported in 30% of carcinoid tumours arising in the small intestine, and in a lesser proportion when the primary is in the colon.

Haematogenous spread to the liver has been described, but is extremely rare, and virtually unknown when the primary is less than 1 cm in diameter.

In children the tumour is usually discovered incidentally when examining the appendix after the operation has been concluded. The symptoms leading to operation are those of appendicitis; when the tumour obstructs the lumen of the appendix this may contribute to the development of acute inflammation, as occurred in three of the four cases in the Index Series.

MANAGEMENT

Because of the extreme rarity of metastasis from a carcinoid tumour of the appendix in children, removal of the appendix and a search of the bowel is all that is required when the tumour is recognized during appendicectomy.

No further operation or treatment is required if the tumour in the appendix is first recognized after the operation has been concluded. In the Index Series the four children affected are all well 5–18 years after appendicectomy.

However, when a carcinoid tumour is found in the ileum, usually in an adolescent or an adult, excision of a generous segment of the ileum is advised. When there are metastases in the epimural lymph nodes, a wider excision, including the mesentery and the area of lymphatic drainage, is necessary. An excision of this extent is also indicated when the primary tumour is more than 2 cm in diameter.

TUMOURS OF THE LARGE BOWEL

CARCINOMA OF THE COLON AND RECTUM

Carcinoma of the colon or rectum in childhood is rare (Hoerner, 1958), and in series containing all age groups, tumours arising in children usually account for less than 1% of the total. The actual proportion arising in children is probably even less (Johnson, Judd & Dahlin, 1959; Donaldson Taylor *et al.*, 1971). Phifer (1923) quoted a review by Weinlechner of 5,279 patients with carcinoma of the colon, of whom only 18 (0·34%) were less than 14 years of age.

The development of a carcinoma of the colon or rectum is recognized as a possible complication of two conditions commencing in childhood; ulcerative colitis and multiple polyposis, and these are discussed under separate headings.

Even so, carcinoma of the colon in children is reported to arise more commonly *de novo* than as a complication of either of these two conditions.

The risk of developing carcinoma of the colon or rectum in patients with Crohn's disease, although much less than in ulcerative colitis, is greater than in the general population. Weedon *et al.* (1973) found 12 instances of carcinoma (2·7%) in a study of 449 cases of Crohn's disease, and concluded that resection on the grounds of risk of malignancy alone was not indicated, but close long-term follow up was required.

AGE : SEX

Cain and Longino (1970) collected reports of 100 children with carcinoma of the colon and added three cases of their own. Most of the 'children' reported were between 10 and 18 years old, and only 12 cases have been described in children less than 10 years of age; 94% arose in children more than 9 years of age. The youngest patient was 9 months old, recorded by Kern & White (1958) who noted a sharp increase in the number of cases at the age of puberty, and thereafter a steady increase in incidence with age.

The incidence in boys is twice as high as in girls.

SITE

The distribution of carcinoma of the colon and rectum in children is probably the same as in adults, but figures for 'colon and rectum' are often reported as one group, and the age limit of children in some reported series is extended to 16 or 18 years. Carcinomas occur more commonly in the lower sigmoid and rectum than in the rest of the large bowel, in a ratio of approximately 2·5 : 1. Excluding those in the rectum, 27% of carcinomas arise in the sigmoid colon (the commonest single segment affected), but 43% occur in the length of the large bowel proximal to the splenic flexure (Cain & Longino, 1970).

PATHOLOGY

In most instances carcinoma of the colon and rectum arise *de novo*, i.e. unassociated with polyposis or ulcerative colitis. The relationship of carcinoma to adenomatous polyps (Table 20.1) is still uncertain (Kottmeier & Clatworthy, 1965); some authors have reported simple polyps and carcinoma in the one patient (Satyanand & Rana, 1969; Cain & Longino, 1970), but as pointed out by Dozois, Judd *et al.* (1969) in a similar context, an analysis in detail is required to determine whether carcinoma actually developed in a polyp or in an area free of polyps in a patient with polyposis.

From the pathological point of view, instability of the mucosa of the bowel may be expressed as the development of either polyps or as carcinoma. This becomes important in management only when it can be shown that: (*a*) most carcinomas arise in polyps; and (*b*) that most of the polyps are chiefly or solely in one segment of the alimentary canal; when these two statements are true, prophylactic resection of the segment at risk would be logical. In most cases this is not feasible and a plan of surveillance by repeated endoscopic or radiological examinations is an alternative.

MICROSCOPIC APPEARANCES

Of the various types of adenocarcinoma found in children (Kern & White, 1958), approximately 50% are the highly malignant mucin-producing adenocarcinoma, in contrast to only 5% of this type in adults (O'Brien, 1967). Mucinous carcinomas are highly invasive and metastasize early to regional lymph nodes and to the liver; transperitoneal seeding is also typical.

MODES OF PRESENTATION

These are generally similar to those seen in adults.

1. *Abdominal pain and change in the bowel habit* (constipation or diarrhoea) are the earliest symptoms. In children the duration of symptoms is usually less and progression more rapid than in adults. The passing of blood in the stools occurs in 20% of carcinomas of the colon, but is more common when the tumour arises in the rectum.
2. *Symptoms of obstruction* are common in children, and intussusception with the tumour as the leading point has been reported. Lethargy, anaemia and weight loss tend to occur late.
3. *An abdominal mass* is present in some 60% at the time of diagnosis, and abdominal distension in about 50%.

As in adults, carcinomas of the right half of the colon in children are usually large and polypoid and because of the fluid state of the faeces at this point, tumours of the proximal colon are less likely to produce obstruction and more likely to develop lymphatic or hepatic metastases before the diagnosis is made.

Tumours arising in the descending or sigmoid colon tend to encircle the bowel just as in adults, and cause obstruction relatively early.

DIAGNOSIS

The symptoms so often mimic other common disorders of childhood that early diagnosis is unfortunately the exception. When a mass is palpated in the pelvis or lower abdomen an appendical abscess is usually the initial diagnosis. The tumour can be missed at appendicectomy, and may remain undetected until persistent or more severe symptoms call for investigation, e.g. a barium enema.

Depending on the site of a palpable mass, an intravenous pyelogram or a cystogram is required to determine whether the urinary tract is involved.

Gross melaena, persistently positive tests for occult blood in the stools, or anaemia are indications for a diligent search for the cause.

DIFFERENTIAL DIAGNOSIS

A tumour arising in the pelvis (p. 683) or a lymphosarcoma of the small intestine (p. 630) should be considered in the differential diagnosis, and angiography usually indicates the presence of a tumour, although laparotomy is required to make the diagnosis.

A simple polyp, the commonest cause of frank bleeding per rectum in childhood, can usually be palpated, for most hamartomatous polyps are within reach of the examining finger.

A history of ulcerative colitis (p. 645) or familial polyposis (p. 650) obviously indicate the need for thorough investigation, e.g. double contrast colograms, endoscopy and biopsy.

TREATMENT

Radical excision is indicated, but in a high proportion of cases the tumour is found to be incurable because of extensive lymphatic or portal venous spread, and only palliative procedures such as palliative resection or proximal colostomy can be performed. Occasionally colostomy and active treatment of the patient's general condition may be required in a debilitated child before radical excision.

Chemotherapy

5-fluorouracil (p. 106) has been reported to be an effective cytotoxic agent in children with adenocarcinoma, but experience is limited because of the rarity of the tumour.

Radiotherapy

Radiotherapy may be useful for palliation.

PROGNOSIS

The prognosis is generally poor because of late diagnosis and the frequency of highly malignant mucinous carcinomas. The 5-year survival rate is less than 10%, although the outlook may be better in well-differentiated carcinomas.

The Index Series contains no case of carcinoma of the colon or rectum in the period 1950–1972, but there were three earlier examples.

1. A boy with severe epispadias and incontinence had bilateral ureterocolic anastomoses at the age of 4½ years; 3 years later this was replaced by an ileal conduit. At the age of 14 years he developed diarrhoea, melaena, lethargy and anorexia. Examination revealed a malignant mass in the upper rectum at the site of the previous anastomoses with the ureters. An invasive mucoid adenocarcinoma was resected, but lymphatic spread had already occurred and the child died 6 months later. The relationship to the previous ureteric anastomoses may be significant.

2. A 9-year old girl presented in 1933 with abdominal pain, bloody diarrhoea and a mass palpable over the sigmoid colon. Resection of an adenocarcinoma brought relief of symptoms for nearly 4 years, until she succumbed from a cerebral metastasis.

3. A boy aged 12 years in 1940 developed mucus diarrhoea followed by the passage of blood, tenesmus, poor appetite and lack of energy. A fixed, annular adenocarcinoma of the upper rectum was found and a colostomy was performed, as only partial resection was possible; the child died 4 months later with widespread metastases in the peritoneal cavity, the liver and the lungs.

CARCINOMA AND ULCERATIVE COLITIS

In children with ulcerative colitis, the incidence of carcinoma of the colon is probably less than 5%. Jackman *et al.* (1940) reported six cases of carcinoma in a series of 95 children with ulcerative colitis, and Wilcox and Beattie (1956) recorded seven children under 16 years of age who had colitis for 6–11 years before developing a carcinoma.

Devroede *et al.* (1971) made an actuarial analysis of a group of 396 children who developed ulcerative colitis before the age of 14 years and were followed for up to 43 years. A carcinoma developed in only 3% during the first 10 years after the onset, but in those with 10 years of symptoms, carcinoma of the colon or rectum developed in 20% of the cohort in each decade. At 35 years after the onset of symptoms, the incidence of carcinoma was estimated to be 43%, and the sexes were equally affected. For no known reason, those in whom the colitis began when they were between 5 and 9 years of age had a higher incidence of carcinoma than those younger or older.

They also found that the risk of carcinoma was greater when the colitis affected the entire colon, and the rate was higher in those in whom the disease was initially limited to the rectum than in those without rectal disease.

THE INDEX SERIES

No child with ulcerative colitis treated at the Royal Children's Hospital has developed a tumour before the age of 15 years, but in three cases a carcinoma appeared between 15 and 20 years of age, and in each case the disease had been active for more than 10 years.

A girl presented at 7 years of age with a history of frequent semi-fluid bowel actions (3–4 a day) since she first attended school 6 months before. Symptoms persisted more or less continuously for 4 years, with fluctuations in severity, up to 15 stools a day. X-rays showed that the entire colon, rectum, and distal ileum were involved. Some improvement at 10 years of age was followed by relapse at 12 years of age, and improvement again between 14 and 16 years of age.

At a routine review including a barium enema at 17 years of age, there was an irregular filling defect in the right half of the transverse colon. No metastases were present at laparotomy for removal of a scirrhous adenocarcinoma, by total proctocolectomy, almost exactly 10 years after symptoms first began.

One year after operation metastases in the liver appeared and death soon followed.

The probability of a carcinoma in only 3% of children with ulcerative colitis during the first 10 years, suggests that few if any in this age group should have a total proctocolectomy, or total colectomy with ileorectal anastomosis, solely on the grounds of this risk (Goligher, 1973). However, after 10 years of continuous symptoms or relapses totalling 10 years, the incidence of carcinoma is sufficiently high to become an indication for surgical intervention even when not indicated by the severity of the symptoms. However, generalizations are likely to be misleading, and surgical excision should only be performed after weighing all the factors, of which the probability of carcinoma is one.

Close supervision, by means of barium enema, sigmoidoscopy, colonoscopy and biopsy of suspicious areas to detect early malignant changes, is essential. Improved techniques in examining rectal biopsies, and in detecting 'carcino-embryoma antigen' in peripheral blood (p. 552) hold promise of more detailed surveillance.

Adequate arrangements for continuing supervision of adolescents when they have passed out of the paediatric age range are essential.

POLYPS, POLYPOSIS AND CARCINOMA

The term 'polyp' is often used without qualification, and with consequent confusion as to the exact nature of the lesion described. It is used here to describe a mass of tissue attached to the mucous membrane and protruding into the lumen of the bowel, and polyps are classified histologically as 'juvenile' (i.e. hamartomatous), inflammatory, lymphoid, adenomatous and carcinomatous (Fig. 20.3).

1. **Juvenile polyp** (syn. hamartomatous polyp)

The familial incidence, if any, of this type of polyp is still incompletely determined; the majority encountered in surgical practice appear to be sporadic (Toccalino & Guastavino *et al.*, 1973), but familial occurrence has also been reported (Veale, McColl *et al.*, 1966; Sachatello *et al.*, 1970; Gathright & Cofer, 1974).

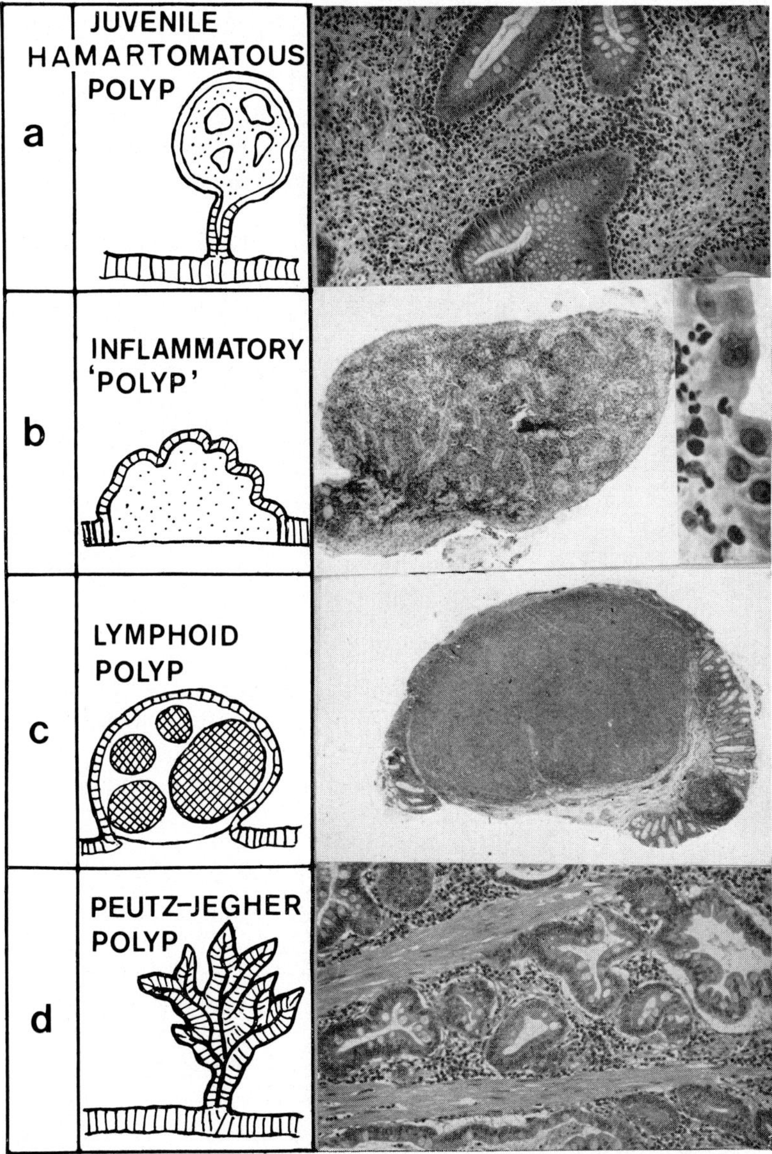

Figure 20.3. INTESTINAL POLYPS; the four commonest types, (*a*) the common juvenile (hamartomatous) polyp containing cystic spaces lined by colonic columar and goblet cells; (*b*) inflammatory polyp composed of highly vascular granulation tissue, partially covered by actively growing cuboidal cells infiltrated with polymorpho-nuclear leucocytes (inset); (*c*) lymphoid polyp almost entirely composed of lymphocytes and active follicles, with colonic mucosa covering the base on either side; (*d*) Peutz-Jeghers polyp (from the jejunum of a nine-year old girl); radiating cores of smooth muscle are clothed by cells appropriate to its site, in this case jejunal mucous membrane (see also Table 20.1, p. 651).

Rectal bleeding is the commonest presenting symptom, followed by mucous diarrhoea; pain is rare. Low polyps may prolapse through the anus, and are occasionally self-amputating by attrition of the pedicle outside the anus, or passed per rectum having separated from the point of attachment.

Macroscopically a juvenile polyp is a pedunculated, rounded lesion (Fig. 20.3a) and the cut surface is multicystic or solid, not papillary. The surface is usually slimy and often ulcerated.

Microscopically, it is composed of regular rectal or colonic glands, set in a fibroblastic stroma which rarely contains any smooth muscle. The glandular acini are rounded and discrete (Fig. 20.3a) and some are distended with mucus. Occasionally some of the mucus escapes into the stroma producing appearances which may suggest a carcinoma to a pathologist not accustomed to paediatric material. However, the cells of the mucous glands are regular, usually in a single layer and show no cytological features suggestive of malignancy.

Glands are usually scanty when compared with the amount of stroma. The stroma is often inflamed, and the surface is almost always ulcerated and covered by a layer of granulation tissue in which the blood vessels are occasionally so prominent as to suggest an angioma.

2. **Inflammatory polyp**

Sometimes a polypoid lesion macroscopically very similar to a juvenile polyp, but somewhat more sessile, is removed from a child with rectal bleeding. This type of lesion appears to be composed entirely of granulation tissue (Fig. 20.3b), contains no glands and is referred to as an 'inflammatory' polyp, although the etiology is unknown.

3. **Lymphoid polyp** (Fig. 20.3c)

These are much rarer than juvenile polyps, and the familial incidence is probably higher (Louw, 1968). Most present with rectal bleeding.

Macroscopically, the lesion differs from the classical juvenile polyp in that it is grey, dome-shaped and sessile; it may become ulcerated, and tends to be friable.

Microscopically, it is a sharply demarcated, submucosal, rounded mass of lymphoid tissue with the mucosa and muscularis mucosae stretched over it. The microscopic appearance of the lymphoid tissue may be alarming, and the lesion has been mistaken for a lymphoma. However, careful examination usually shows a follicular pattern which can be confirmed by reticulum stains. The cells of this lesion often appear to be large and active; bizarre forms are sometimes seen and mitoses may be numerous.

The Index Series. In the period covered by the Index Series there were 80 cases of non-familial polyps of the gut. Of these, 69 (86 %) arose in the rectum, three in the sigmoid, six in the remainder of the colon and two in the small intestine. Approximately 85% were single lesions in patients who presented with bleeding, pain, prolapse, and occasionally a history of self-amputation of the polyp. All but one were hamartomatous or inflammatory polyps.

4. **Adenomatous polyp**

This is found only very rarely in children, and some authorities doubt that they develop before the age of 10 years. Their relationship to potential carcinomatous changes is a source of concern and the subject of controversy. Most adenomatous polyps probably remain benign, but a proportion of them eventually undergo malignant metamorphosis. There are isolated case reports of adenomatous polyps discovered in other parts of the bowel in children with an adenocarcinoma of the colon (Louw, 1968), and also a history of previous removal of polyps in children later found to have a carcinoma (Cain & Longino, 1970). The single adenomatous polyp thus arouses suspicion that it may be the forerunner of polyposis and/or carcinoma (Table 20.1).

MANAGEMENT OF CHILDREN WITH POLYPS

In most children with a single polyp, it can be reached and identified by the examining finger and removed without difficulty. If subsequent histological examination shows it to be other than hamartomatous or inflammatory, a barium enema and sigmoidoscopy are required, to determine whether other polyps are present. If these investigations show that there are more polyps beyond the reach of sigmoidoscopic removal, laparotomy has usually been performed, after confirming the findings by repeating the double contrast enema to avoid an unnecessary operation.

The introduction of colonoscopy has modified management, for removal, at one sitting, of all polyps occurring in various parts of the large and small bowel is a significant advance made possible by laparotomy and multiple enterotomies when combined with endoscopic identification of individual polyps through a fiberoptic colonoscope (Folkman, 1973; Wolff & Shinya, 1973).

Simple removal or fulguration of accessible individual polyps is all that is required, unless they are numerous and clustered, or widely scattered.

When an adenomatous polyp is found, surveillance by double contrast enema and/or sigmoidoscopy or colonoscopy at intervals of 6–12 months, is necessary.

MULTIPLE POLYPOSIS

True multiple polyposis of the colon and/or rectum, although extremely rare, occasionally develops in late childhood or early adolescence (Abrahamson, 1967), and at least six clinico-pathological types have been described

I. Familial polyposis coli;
II. Juvenile polyposis (Tables 20.1, 20.2);
III. Peutz-Jeghers' syndrome;
IV. Gardner's syndrome;
V. Turcot's disease;
VI. Cronkhite-Canada syndrome.

I. FAMILIAL POLYPOSIS COLI

This involves the large bowel only; the polyps are adenomatous and have a high malignant potential. A positive family history is an important factor in diagnosis for the disease is transmitted by an autosomal dominant gene to approximately half the progeny. However, even when the family history is elicited carefully, it is positive in only about half of the cases identified.

SEX : AGE

Males and females are equally affected, and symptoms do not usually appear until 10–13 years of age. All children of known affected families should be observed carefully for early signs from the age of 10 years by repeated sigmoidoscopies. However, four children less than 2 years of age are recorded as developing multiple polyposis, and a carcinoma has been reported before the age of 13 years in 6% of children of affected families.

It has been suggested (and refuted) that both the polyposis and subsequent malignant change occur earlier in each succeeding generation, and that such a family should eventually be self-eliminating. The interval between finding polyposis and the development of carcinoma may be as short as one year. However, as a general rule, carcinomatous change in children with multiple polyposis does not occur before the age of 10 years. Regardless of age, the appearance of a single adenomatous polyp in a child with a positive family history must be viewed with concern as heralding generalized polyposis, and the polyps should be excised as they appear.

Every child of an affected family who develops multiple polyposis and is more than 10 years of age is a candidate for surgery. The polyps are true tumours (adenomas) and the same type of polyp is seen in familial polyposis, in Gardner's syndrome (*q.v.*) and in Turcot's disease (*q.v.*). They are usually pedunculated, often with a long, narrow, flat pedicle, and may be as large as 3 cm in diameter. Sessile examples are less common. The polyp is lobulated and the lobules are separated by deep clefts.

Microscopically, it is composed of closely packed, branching colonic glands lined by cells with dense hyperchromatic nuclei. Mitoses may be seen. In appearance and cellularity the glands are more obviously proliferative than in the hamartomatous juvenile polyp. Malignant change is heralded by invasion of the stroma by glandular formations, usually best seen at the base.

Table 20.1. Intestinal polyps; differential diagnosis, and prognosis of various types

Disease (mode of inheritance)	Type of polyp	Site(s)	Associated conditions	Incidence of malignant change
Familial polyposis (Autosomal dominant)	Adenomatous	Colon (and rectum)	Usually none	Very high (? 100% with time)
Peutz-Jeghers' syndrome (Autosomal dominant)	Specific, 'hamartomatous' (indigenous epithelium)	Small bowel jejunum, ileum (anywhere in bowel)	Mucosal pigmentation Ovarian cyst/tumour	Low (? 1–3%)
Gardner's syndrome (Autosomal dominant)	Adenomatous	Colon and rectum (stomach, small bowel)	Multiple osteomas. Multiple epidermal cysts. Desmoid tumours	Very high (? 100% with time)
Turcot's syndrome (? variant of Gardner's syndrome)	Adenomatous	Colon	Tumours of the CNS	? same as Gardner's syndrome
'Disseminated' polyposis (Sporadic)	Adenomatous	Anywhere in bowel	Nil	? some tendency
Cronkhite-Canada syndrome (Sporadic)	Adenomatous	Anywhere, generalized	Mucocutaneous pigmentation. Alopecia Onychodystrophia	?
Common Juvenile polyp (Sporadic)	Hamartomatous	Rectum (colon)	Nil	Nil

TREATMENT

Total proctocolectomy would be required to remove all of the area subject to carcinomatous change. However, total colectomy and ileoproctostomy is a feasible alternative, for there is some tendency for the adenomatous polyps to disappear or regress, and those remaining in the short rectal stump can usually be dealt with by fulguration and the area kept under surveillance. If the rectal stump is retained, it should be inspected at intervals of 6 months, indefinitely; if a carcinoma develops, and this is reported to occur in up to 25% of cases (Moertal *et al.*, 1970) the rectum is excised and an ileostomy fashioned.

The Soave technique, originally designed for Hirschsprung's disease and involving dissection and excision of the mucosa of the rectum, leaving a muscular tunnel, has been used in multiple polyposis to remove the mucosa of the rectum, in conjunction with total colectomy, bringing down the terminal ileum inside the rectal musculature and the sphincters (Safaie-Shirazi & Soper, 1973). This is a highly desirable alternative to excision of the rectum, and has the considerable advantages of preserving sphincteric and sexual function (in the male) while removing the potentially malignant rectal mucosa.

II. JUVENILE POLYPOSIS

Sachatello & Griffin (1975) noted that although 40–50 patients with 'multiple juvenile polyps' have now been reported, it is still not certain whether they represent a single syndrome with variable penetrance or several different syndromes. They classified those reported into the following groups (Table 20.2).

1. Juvenile polyposis coli.
2. Generalized juvenile gastrointestinal polyposis.
3. Juvenile polyposis of infancy.

1. Juvenile polyposis coli

Now recognized as an entity distinct from familial polyposis, (McColl *et al.*, 1964), this is the commonest type of juvenile polyposis, with a spectrum extending from the usual sporadic form with 1 or 2 rectal polyps, to those (few) with a colonic mucosa covered with 'hamartomatous' polyps. In some 50% of the group as a whole there is a family history of the same condition, and in a few, of true familial polyposis (Gathright & Cofer, 1974).

In most cases removal of the single or few rectal or colonic polyps is all that is required, followed by observation. A small minority may require colectomy, but conservative removal of polyps at colonoscopy or laparotomy should be attempted before proceeding to a major resection.

Table 20.2. Classification of juvenile polyposis (after Sachatello & Griffen, 1975)

Disease	1. Juvenile polyposis coli	2. Generalized juvenile polyposis	3. Juvenile polyposis of infancy	(Peutz-Jeghers' syndrome for comparison)
Histology of polyp(s)	Juvenile (hamartomatous) polyp (Fig. 20.3a)	Juvenile (hamartomatous) polyp (Fig. 20.3a)	Juvenile (hamartomatous) polyp (Fig. 20.3a)	Specific type of hamartoma (Fig. 20.3d)
Genetic Basis	Uncertain	Dominant	Recessive	Dominant, non-sex-linked
Sites of polyps (in order of frequency)	Rectum colon, (Rarely small bowel)	Stomach, large and small bowel	Stomach, large and small bowel	Jejunum, ileum, anywhere (p. 654)
Other specific manifestations	None known	None known	High incidence of congenital anomalies	Mucocutaneous melanin pigmentation. Ovarian cyst or tumour
Modes of presentation	Painless rectal bleeding; Prolapse of polyp	Haematemesis, anaemia; Diarrhoea, hypoprotein-aemia; Melaena	Intussusception; Diarrhoea-hypoprotein-aemia; Bleeding, anaemia; Prolapse of rectum	Intussusception. Melaena anaemia
Natural history	No increased risk of carcinoma	No increased risk of carcinoma	Not known (death before 2 years of age)	Slightly increased risk of malignancy (?1–5%)

2. **Generalized juvenile gastrointestinal polyposis**

A small number of patients have been reported with juvenile (hamartomatous) polyps in the stomach and small and large bowel. The gastric and colonic lesions have usually not become apparent at the same time (Sachatello, Pickren and Grace, 1971). The mode of presentation is chiefly recurrent bleeding from the gastric polyps, which may be so numerous or severe as to require gastrectomy. There appears to be no increased risk of carcinoma.

The distribution of the polyps in this group may be similar to the pattern in Peutz-Jeghers syndrome, and the differential diagnosis rests on correctly identifying the type of polyp (Fig. 20.3), and the absence of pigmentation.

3. Juvenile polyposis of infancy

Some 7 cases have been reported (Sachatello *et al.*, 1974). All have a similar clinical picture, presenting with diarrhoea containing either mucus or blood in the first few weeks of life. The diarrhoea causes anaemia, hypoproteinuria, failure to thrive, increased susceptibility to infection, and recurrent rectal prolapse (at 4 to 9 months) with ulceration of and bleeding from the prolapsed mucosa. Although biopsy of the polyps has been misinterpreted as adenomatous, they appear to be hamartomatous.

Treatment initially depends upon determining the extent and number of polyps, control of diarrhoea, correction of anaemia and hypoproteinuria, and parenteral alimentation when required.

Surgical treatment is directed to local removal of as many rectal polyps as feasible, possibly removal of segments of bowel heavily affected with polyps, and selective removal of individual larger polyps in the stomach and/or small bowel.

III. PEUTZ-JEGHERS' SYNDROME

In this syndrome, of which 327 cases had been reported up to 1969 (Dozois, Judd *et al.*, 1969), the criteria for diagnosis are: (*a*) abnormal mucosal pigmentation (Dormandy, 1957), typically at both oral and anal mucocutaneous junctions, the inside of the lip and buccal mucosa (and sometimes on the fingers and toes); and (*b*) polyposis of the alimentary canal (Jeghers, McKusick & Katz, 1949).

The condition is transmitted as an autosomal dominant trait, and in 45% of cases other members of the family are affected. The polyps in this syndrome have now been observed to occur in all parts of the alimentary canal, in order of frequency, jejunum, ileum, colon, rectum, stomach, appendix and oesophagus.

Ovarian cysts occur in some of the affected females, and may prove to be part of the syndrome.

Scully (1970) has described a distinctive and possibly unique type of sex cord tumour of the ovary, estimated to occur in approximately 5% of girls with Peutz-Jeghers' syndrome.

AGE: SEX

The sexes are affected with approximately equal frequency. Most cases are first diagnosed in adults; some present with symptoms in adolescence, and a few are found in children, almost always in those more than 10 years of age.

MACROSCOPIC APPEARANCES

To the naked eye, the polyps in this syndrome do not differ greatly from adenomatous polyps (p. 649). Rarely there is a solitary polyp, or only a few, but in most cases they are numerous, and sometimes there are myriads of minute nodules just visible to the naked eye. Polyps develop progressively, i.e. in groups or waves, throughout the life of the patient.

MICROSCOPIC APPEARANCES

Although now classed as a type of hamartoma, the polyps differ from the hamartomatous juvenile type. The Peutz-Jeghers polyp arises in the submucosa as an overgrowth of the cells indigenous to the region in which it develops.

The structure of the polyp (Fig. 20.3d, p. 647) is a stroma containing muscle fibres of the muscularis mucosae, forming a tree-like central core, with branches clothed by cells appropriate to the area, parietal cells in the stomach, Brunner's glands in the duodenum, goblet and Paneth cells in the small intestine, and tall columnar cells in the colon and rectum.

MODES OF PRESENTATION

1. *Recurrent attacks of colicky abdominal pain* occur when one of the polyps is large enough to become grasped in peristatic waves, and may culminate in an intussusception.
2. *An abdominal mass* is palpable in about a third of the patients, and is usually a 'chronic' or relapsing intussusception.
3. *Melaena or haematemesis* is the presenting feature in another third.

DIAGNOSIS

The presence of oral, labial or buccal pigmentation is diagnostic. The areas of pigmentation are not present at birth, but develop within the first five years and thereafter remain static.

Radiological confirmation of the polyps can usually be obtained when they are of any size. When very numerous and widespread in patients presenting with bleeding, the actual site of the haemorrhage can be difficult to determine.

DIFFERENTIAL DIAGNOSIS (See Table 20.1).

1. *Familial polyposis* is virtually confined to the colon; in the Peutz-Jeghers' syndrome, polyps are more frequent in the jejunum and ileum.
2. *In Gardner's syndrome* the polyps are also familial and multiple, but the polyps are adenomatous and scattered throughout the alimentary tract.

3. '*Disseminated*' *polyposis* appears to be non-familial; the polyps are few in number, adenomatous in type, and may affect any part of the alimentary canal.

MALIGNANT CHANGE

Estimates of the risk of malignancy arising in a Peutz-Jeghers' polyp have varied over the years. At one time thought to be as high as 20%, the incidence is now thought to be much lower, and from a recent critical analysis (Dozois, Judd *et al.*, 1969) evidence of a carcinoma was conclusive in only 11 of 327 cases, an incidence of some 3%. The authors also noted that even in these 11 cases the commonest sites of the carcinoma (the stomach and duodenum) were not those in which Peutz-Jeghers' polyps most frequently arose, indicating that the carcinoma may have arisen *de novo* and not in a polyp.

Of the 11 patients who developed a carcinoma, the three youngest were 13, 16 and 21 years of age.

TREATMENT

Because of the wide distribution of the polyps, and the natural history of more polyps developing in 'waves' or groups with the passage of time, 'prophylactic' resection of any one segment is not feasible.

When complications such as intussusception or haemorrhage occur, removal of the polyp(s) responsible, or of bowel secondarily involved, e.g. in an intussusception, may require resection of bowel, but whenever possible, enterotomy and polypectomy are preferable. Other polyps more than 2 cm in diameter should be removed individually, at a second operation if they are numerous or if the first operation is performed as an emergency.

Polyps in the stomach or colon are an indication for resection, because these are the sites in which carcinoma has most often occurred. However, the surgical procedure required varies from one patient to another.

Because operations are likely to become necessary at intervals throughout the patient's life, multiple enterotomies and polypectomies are in general the operation of choice, reserving resection of bowel for complications, for the unusual case in which a large number of polyps are clustered together in one segment, or for persisting haemorrhage not controlled by polypectomy.

IV. GARDNER'S SYNDROME

In this syndrome there are: (*a*) multiple adenomatous polyps in the bowel, chiefly in the colon, but also in the appendix, the small bowel, duodenum and the stomach (Wolf, Richards & Gardner, 1955; Gardner, 1962). The other criteria are: (*b*) connective tissue tumours, such as osteomas of the jaws (p. 331), and (*c*) multiple epidermoid cysts, mostly on the back.

Symptoms related to the alimentary canal are the chief mode of presentation, i.e. diarrhoea, the passage of mucus and blood per rectum or, less commonly, swellings in soft tissues unrelated to the alimentary symptoms.

V. TURCOT'S DISEASE

This extremely rare condition may prove to be a variant of Gardner's syndrome, and usually presents with tumours of the central nervous system.

VI. THE CRONKHITE-CANADA SYNDROME

This condition appears to be non-genetic and includes mucocutaneous melanin pigmentation, alopecia, atrophic changes in the finger nails, and generalized gastro-intestinal polyposis (Cronkhite & Canada, 1955).

OTHER 'POLYPS'

The Index Series. There may prove to be other rare or unusual types of polyposis, genetic or sporadic, for some of the cases in the Index Series cannot be fitted into any category yet established.

1. One child has multiple hamartomatous polyps of the small and large bowel, clubbed fingers and toes, and a negative family history for any of these features or for any of the familial entities described above. There is no mucocutaneous pigmentation. The symptoms and signs are frequent loose bowel actions, occasional bleeding and chronic anaemia.
2. Another child had two fibrous (?inflammatory) polyps in the jejunum, with no other associated signs or symptoms or relevant family history.

Neurofibromas occasionally present as a single or multiple submucosal mass or masses, usually in the small bowel, and may become somewhat pedunculated.

Benign tumours rarely develop in the bowel, but may be polypoid; these include lipoma, leiomyoma, fibroma, haemangioma (Abrahamson & Shandling, 1973) and ganglioneuroma.

HAEMANGIOMA OF THE ALIMENTARY CANAL

This unusual condition involves all layers of the bowel wall as well as the adjacent mesentery or omentum. Angiomatous 'polyps' projecting into the lumen are seldom confined to the mucosa or submucosa. Any segment of the bowel may be involved, and in about one third of cases there are also angiomas in the skin or mouth. Killingback *et al.* (1974) report 8 cases of which 5 were less than 15 years of age at the time of diagnosis. Rissier (1960) reviewed 114 patients of all ages with intestinal angiomas, of whom 35 had similar lesions in both skin and oral mucosa. The commonest alimentary sites were: small bowel (60), colon (53) and stomach (16); more than one segment was affected in approximately 10% of cases.

The presenting symptoms are bleeding, anaemia, pain, intussusception or malabsorption with diarrhoea; only very rarely is the lesion palpable as an abdominal mass.

The diagnosis may be suspected from the accompanying superficial angiomas, but contrast studies and aortography may not be conclusive, and not infrequently the diagnosis can only be made with certainty at laparotomy.

Treatment is, ideally, total resection of the affected segment and the adjacent angiomatous tissue, but this is not always feasible because of extensions into the parietes. Satisfactory relief of symptoms can be obtained by removing the intestinal component alone.

TUMOURS OF THE SPLEEN

Primary tumours of the spleen are extremely rare in childhood; malignant tumours are probably more common than benign neoplasms, but a variety of non-neoplastic conditions such as cysts and hamartomas are more common than either.

Among the few malignant tumours primarily or chiefly affecting the spleen, haemangio-endothelioma appears to be the commonest in children (Lazarus & Marks, 1946); reticulum cell sarcoma and lymphosarcoma have also been reported in the spleen (Das Gupta *et al.*, 1965) or involve the spleen when disseminated in the abdomen (see abdominal reticulum cell sarcoma, p. 638).

Deposits in the spleen in Hodgkin's disease (p. 190) and leukaemia (p. 151) are the commonest malignant conditions causing splenomegaly.

DIAGNOSIS

Consideration of the many causes of splenomegaly would be inappropriate here, and it is assumed that examination and investigations have excluded obvious sources of infection, storage histiocytoses and blood diseases, e.g. thalassaemia, leukaemia etc. (see Table 9.3, p. 146).

Causes of benign swellings in the upper part of the abdomen are described on p. 492, and malignant tumours in this region are listed on p. 491.

DIFFERENTIAL DIAGNOSIS

The following are mentioned because of the serious consequences of misdiagnosis, or because the condition affects the spleen primarily and may not be revealed by the usual investigations.

1. *Wilms' tumour* of the left kidney. In more than one case in the Index Series diagnosis of Wilms' tumour was delayed because the renal mass in the left hypochondrium was thought to be an enlarged spleen. When no cause can be found for a massively enlarged 'spleen', a pyelogram is required to clarify the diagnosis.

2. *Epidermoid cyst of the spleen* is a rare condition which may develop from embryonic ectodermal rests. Sirinek & Evans (1973) collected 54 cases from the literature; females outnumbered males 3 : 2. In 80% of the cyst was solitary and unilocular; 75% were situated at the lower pole and 65% were subcapsular. The diagnosis can be made before exploration by selective splenic arteriography (Bron & Hoffman, 1971).

3. *Hydatid cyst.* Even in areas where *Taenia echinococcus* is endemic, a hydatid cyst in the spleen is a great rarity, particularly in childhood. There were only two such cases in the series of 100 cases of hydatidosis treated at the Royal Children's Hospital between 1948 and 1966.

Involvement of the spleen is said to occur more commonly in areas where the endemic species is the infiltrative *Echinococcus alveolaris*.

4. *Ectopic pancreatic tissue*, and focal nodular hyperplasia (p. 458) are rare causes of splenomegaly.

TREATMENT

When uncertainty as to the diagnosis is resolved by laparotomy, the cause of splenomegaly can often be identified from the macroscopic appearances. If not, the alternatives are biopsy or splenectomy. Biopsy of the spleen presents difficulties primarily because the portion removed may not be representative, and hence misleading, but also because the structure and texture of the spleen are ill-suited to the excision of a wedge of tissue.

The adverse effects of splenectomy in diminishing immune defence mechanisms, leading to overwhelming and fatal infections, is more likely to occur following splenectomy in those less than four years of age (Horan & Colebatch, 1962) than in older children. The spleen should be preserved in this age group whenever feasible.

Fonkalsrud and Walford (1970) have demonstrated that a large epidermoid cyst can be excised without removing the spleen.

TUMOURS OF THE PANCREAS

Tumours of the pancreas are rarities in children and the clinical picture they present varies according to the type of cell from which they arise. Pancreatic adenomas and adenocarcinomas may arise in either the exocrine or endocrine (islet) cells, as shown in the classification in Fig. 20.4.

Hyperplasia or micro-adenomatosis is included in this section because the clinical signs and symptoms produced in children may be similar to or identical with those caused by functional adenoma or carcinoma.

The tumours are as follows:

Exocrine I. Adenoma;
II. Carcinoma.
Endocrine: III. Adenoma of β cells (syn. insulinoma);
IV. Adenoma of non-β cells and
Carcinoma of non-β cells.

I. ADENOMA OF THE EXOCRINE PANCREAS

Solid adenomas of the exocrine pancreas are possibly more common than clinical reports would indicate. Being small, circumscribed and unproductive of symptoms, they are mostly found at autopsy, or occasionally as an incidental observation during an abdominal operation (Willis, 1948).

Cystadenomas large enough to cause symptoms are uncommon (Becker, Wilson & Pratt, 1965), but have been reported in young children, e.g. a cystadenoma in a 16-month old child (Gunderson & Janis, 1969), in an 18-month old girl (Grosfeld *et al.*, 1970), and in a 2-year old (Gille, Barbier *et al.*, 1972).

The mode of presentation is distension of the upper part of the abdomen, with little or no symptoms; the swelling is non-tender and usually does not move on respiration. Occasionally symptoms occur from pressure on surrounding structures.

A post-traumatic pseudocyst of the pancreas is much more common than a cystadenoma, and the radiological findings in the two conditions may be very similar. However, the episode of trauma is usually sufficiently severe to be a feature of the clinical history.

Congenital cysts of the pancreas, either unilocular or multilocular (McPherson & Heersma, 1948; Miles, 1959), or related to von Hippel-Lindau disease (p. 832), have been reported.

Treatment

Excision of a cystadenoma in the body or tail of the pancreas is a relatively simple procedure. When it arises in the head of the gland, complete removal may require pancreaticoduodenectomy, and although a major undertaking this is quite feasible in children (Fonkalsrud *et al.*, 1966).

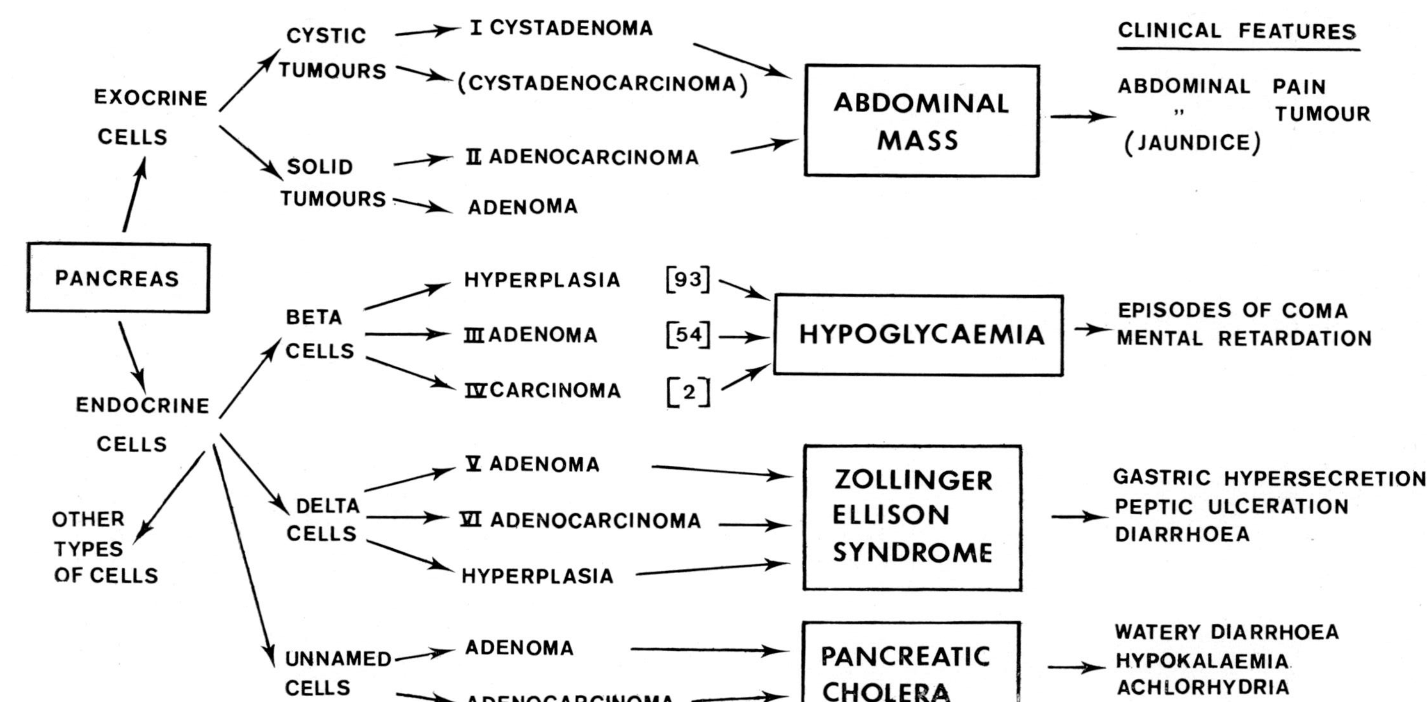

Figure 20.4. TUMOURS OF THE PANCREAS. Hyperplasia, cystadenoma, adenoma and adenocarcinoma, arising in exocrine and various endocrine cells, indicating the effects and clinical aspects of each type of abnormality. The numbers in brackets indicate the relative incidence reported by Welch (1969).

II. CARCINOMA OF THE EXOCRINE PANCREAS

This appears to be an extremely rare tumour; Welch (1969) collected from the world literature 14 cases of carcinoma arising from exocrine tissue in childhood. However, the tumour may not be as rare as this would indicate. More comprehensive autopsy studies of children dying of tumours, and more accurate identification of their histogenesis by electron microscopy, has yielded additional cases. Tsukimoto *et al.* (1973) reviewed 16 cases in the world literature and added 12 cases from autopsy data on Japanese children.

AGE : SEX

The ages of the 14 patients collected by Welch (1969) ranged from 3 months to 15 years; both sexes were equally represented. There appeared to be two age peaks; ten were less than 5 years of age, and four were between 10 and 15 years of age.

The histological types in the 14 tumours were described as adenocarcinoma (6), undifferentiated (3), cylindrical cell (2), ductal, carcinoma simplex, and medullary carcinoma.

Most of the tumours arose in the head of the pancreas.

The mode of presentation is chiefly abdominal pain and a palpable upper abdominal mass. Even when the tumour arises in the head of the pancreas jaundice is uncommon, and a palpable distended gall-bladder even less common. Anaemia, and melaena or haematemesis also occur; anorexia and weight loss are less common.

In many cases, exploration reveals that there are metastases in the para-aortic lymph nodes or further afield, and that the tumour is already beyond the scope of pancreaticoduodenectomy. In the 14 cases quoted excision was attempted (only partly) in only one case, and all 14 died of their disease within 10 months.

It is very probable that in early reports in the literature there was confusion between exocrine and islet-cell carcinomas. More recently Grosfeld *et al.* (1970) reported three children with an exocrine pancreatic tumour of which two, aged 10 and 12 years, were successfully treated by pancreaticoduodenectomy. They emphasized the value of intra-operative mesoportal venography in assessing operability, and of electron microscopy in determining the histogenesis of the tumour.

III. ADENOMA OF THE ISLET CELLS
(syn. insulinoma)

Identification of the various types of cells which make up the islets of

Langerhans is not yet complete, although the β (or B) cells have long been recognized as the site of insulin production and of benign insulinoma; less than 60 examples have been reported in childhood (Schwarz & Zwirew, 1971).

Hypersecretion producing hyperinsulinaemia and hypoglycaemia can occur as the result of hyperplasia, an adenoma, some adenocarcinomas of the B cells, and also in association with an ill-defined group of conditions causing idiopathic hypoglycaemia. The relative frequency of the causes of excess secretion of insulin, as collated from the literature by Welch (1969), was as follows:

hyperplasia (including micro-adenosis)	93 (62%)
benign insulinoma	54 (36%)
functional adenocarcinoma	2 (1%)

Whipple's triad of: (*a*) symptoms of hypoglycaemia on fasting; (*b*) a blood glucose less than 50 mg/dl during the period of symptoms; and (*c*) relief of symptoms by the intravenous administration of dextrose, is no longer accepted as an adequate set of criteria for the diagnosis of autonomous hyperinsulinism, for it can occur with other types oı hypoglycaemia.

Measurements of the levels of insulin in the plasma are now considered to be essential in proving the diagnosis, and the methods employed must be accurate at low concentrations to avoid misleading results (Annotation, *Lancet*, 1974).

AGE : SEX

Welch (1969) in a review of the literature collected 54 cases of functioning tumours of the B cells in children; 22 of them were less than 2 years old, while 32 were fairly evenly spread throughout the paediatric age group. There were 31 girls and 23 boys.

According to Rickham (1975), 14 insulinomas have presented in the newborn, and in one the tumour was as small as 2·5 mm in diameter.

SITE

In the 54 cases quoted, there was more than one adenoma in 14%. The tumour arose in the head of the pancreas in 25%, in the body or tail in 73%, and 2% were located outside the pancreas. Functional ectopic islet tissue has been reported in the duodenal wall, the hilum of the spleen, in retroperitoneal tissue, the wall of the stomach, in Meckel's diverticulum, and even in a mediastinal teratoma (Honicky & de Papp, 1973).

MODES OF PRESENTATION

Symptoms may appear in infancy (Mann, Rayner & Gourevitch, 1969), or even in the newborn (Todd, Rickham & Coulter, 1972), and when hyperinsulinism is due to hyperplasia (micro-adenomatosis), the onset is most commonly in the first two years of life.

To some extent the symptoms vary with the age of the patient, and although not invariably so, the presenting pattern may be: convulsions and coma in infants; sweating, pallor, irritability and restlessness (due to compensatory release of adrenaline) in toddlers; and sometimes macrophagia and obesity in older children.

There is a wide range of presenting symptoms and for practical purposes, two are sufficiently common in children to be considered important:

1. *'Epileptiform' seizures*

Convulsions in childhood are not uncommon and after investigation most cases appear to be idiopathic, non-recurring, and often associated with a high fever. A fasting blood sugar should be one of the tests performed before reaching this conclusion.

Recurrent seizures, even when mild, and particularly those not controlled by reasonable doses of anticonvulsants, should lead to suspicion that they are due to hypoglycaemia, especially when accompanied by any of the symptoms of the presenting patterns described above.

2. *Variations in the nature of the attacks*

In those due to hypoglycaemia the pattern may vary from one attack to another. Episodes resembling deep sleep, delirium or a temper tantrum may all be caused by hypoglycaemia at subconvulsive levels.

Disturbances of cerebral function of lesser degree lead to swings of mood, inconsistency of temperament, and loss of concentration with failure at school. It will be apparent that many of these symptoms could easily be attributed to a non-organic behavioural disorder.

DIAGNOSIS

The rarity of hypoglycaemia due to hyperinsulinism undoubtedly leads to delay in diagnosis which may extend over several years. Sooner or later the relationship of symptoms or 'attacks' to fasting, or the failure to control convulsions by usually effective doses of anticonvulsants, raises the possibility of hypoglycaemia and leads to estimation of the blood glucose. Blood should be obtained while symptoms are present or after an adequate period of fasting, for a single estimation may fail to detect pathological levels of hypoglycaemia, and should be repeated at least twice before accepting a negative result.

INVESTIGATIONS

1. *Glucose and insulin levels*

The crucial investigations (Schein *et al.*, 1973), ideally performed while symptoms are present, are those which demonstrate.

(a) A plasma glucose level significantly lower than 'low normal' values for the age of the patient, e.g. 45–55 mg/dl (2·5–3 m mol/l), as established for the particular laboratory and method (Table 20.3), at a time when there is

(b) an inappropriately high level of plasma insulin (normally inhibited by hypoglycaemia), thus reflecting 'autonomous' secretion and liberation of insulin.

Table 20.3. Plasma glucose levels in normal infants and children (R.C.H. laboratory figures)

	Plasma Glucose		
Age	S.I. Units m mol/l	'Old' Units mg/dl	Conversion factor
1 day	0·7–2·9	15–52	×18·02
2 days	0·9–3·2	17–57	
3 days	1·6–3·3	28–60	
4 days	2·1–3·4	38–62	
5–30 days	2·2–3·6	40–64	
1 month and over	3·6–5·4	64–98	

The most useful investigation is to estimate both plasma glucose and plasma insulin at levels of 1–2 hours throughout a 12-hour day, after an overnight fast (Pagliara *et al.*, 1973; Shatney & Grage, 1974), observing changes in the two parameters in relation to each other during the prolonged fast, and response to normal meals. As a general rule, hyperplasia of the B cells causes excessive release of insulin in response to appropriate stimuli; an insulinoma releases excess insulin more or less continuously and, typically, is not significantly affected by the usual stimuli (meals and fasts) which normally provoke or inhibit release of insulin.

Fasting can lead to a very low levels of plasma insulin in normal infants and children, e.g. below 5–10 μu/ml; hence plasma insulin levels of 5–10 μu/ml at a time when the blood glucose level is below 50 mg/dl, are to be considered as 'distinctly abnormal' (Pagliara *et al.*, 1973) and strongly suggestive of an insulin secreting tumour.

2. *Arteriography and scintillography*

Having established that there is excess (autonomous) secretion and liberation of insulin, demonstration of the source is of considerable assistance in preparation for exploration.

The introduction of selective coeliac arteriography (Alfidi, Dae *et al.*, 1971) combined with subtraction techniques (Boijsen & Sameulsson, 1970), has enabled the diagnosis of insulinoma before operation with an accuracy greater than 90% (Fulton *et al.*, 1975).

Scintillography with ^{75}Se-methionine (Davies, 1973) has shown that in an insulinoma the lower turnover of protein (methionine) compared with surrounding pancreas, causes a 'cold spot', but the resolving power of this method is less than that of arteriography.

Insulinomas in children, appear to be smaller than those found in adults, and a tumour less than 1·5 cm in diameter is the rule rather than the exception. This is at the lower limit of detection by arteriography, whereas the minimum lesion demonstrable by scintillography is rarely less than 2–2·5 cm in diameter.

DIFFERENTIAL DIAGNOSIS

Most conditions which cause or are associated with hypoglycaemia in childhood are transient rather than persistent or recurrent.

Ketotic hypoglycaemia is responsible for the majority of cases of hypoglycaemia in childhood. Those affected have a predisposition to hypoglycaemia, after a prolonged fast or precipitated by intercurrent infections and fever. The attacks are cyclic, and ketonuria is a marked feature. There is a rapid response to glucose, but no reaction to glucagon. Between attacks glucose and glucagon tolerance tests are normal and there is not, at any time, excess release of insulin.

'Tolerance tests'

These are useful between attacks in excluding some of the possible causes of hypoglycaemia.

1. *The leucine tolerance test* will identify those sensitive to this amino acid; when leucine is given orally or intravenously, there is a sharp decrease in plasma glucose and plasma insulin rises as plasma glucose falls.
2. *The fructose tolerance test* is primarily of use in detecting hereditary fructose intolerance; when fructose is given orally the blood fructose level rises but there is a marked fall in blood glucose.
3. *The tolbutamide test* is more useful in adults than in children; failure of the blood glucose to rise to normal levels 2–3 hours after administering tolbutamide is evidence of excessive release of insulin, but neither the leucine tolerance test nor the tolbutamide test will differentiate, absolutely, between various causes of hypoglycaemia, i.e. between islet hyperplasia, adenoma, or leucine sensitivity.

DIFFERENTIATION OF HYPERPLASIA, ADENOMA AND CARCINOMA

Hyperplasia occurs as an increased number of islets, or an increase in the population of B cells (micro-adenomatosis) in a pancreas with the normal number of islets. In both, hyperinsulinism is the result, usually in the form of excess insulin released in response to the usual stimuli, i.e. inappropriately large amounts but released at appropriate times.

Transient hyperplasia in the newborn occurs in infants born to diabetic and prediabetic mothers, in some cases of haemolytic disease of the newborn, in Beckwith's syndrome (exomphalos, macroglossia and visceromegaly), and in those with leucine sensitivity.

Hyperplasia is the commonest explanation of 'idiopathic' hypoglycaemia persisting beyond the age of two months, or appearing after that age, and in most cases can be controlled by administering glucocorticosteroids, partly on an empirical basis, but also because of their effect in increasing blood glucose. When the hypoglycaemia cannot be controlled by steroids or diazoxide and when hyper-insulinaemia is present, an adenoma of the B cells is the most likely cause, and exploration of the pancreas is warranted (Annotation, *Lancet*, 1974).

Endocrine adenocarcinoma

It was believed for many years that malignant tumours of the B cells were confined to adults, but examples of malignant insulinomas have been reported in children (Hurez *et al.*, 1961; Stokes *et al.*, 1966). The carcinoma may be secretory or non-secretory, and the ratio of one to the other is difficult to determine because exocrine carcinoma has only been distinguishable from malignant insulinoma since electron microscopy became available. In the past, 'functioning' endocrine carcinoma could be identified by their biochemical effects (causing hypoglycaemia) and by the general pathological features of malignancy, e.g. the occurrence of metastases; non-functioning carcinomas on the other hand, may have developed from either islet cells or exocrine cells.

Insulin-secreting carcinoma of the B cells is the rarest cause of hypoglycaemia in childhood, and one inadequately documented case, not previously reported, may be the only example in the Index Series.

A 9-year old boy presented with a swelling in the neck found on biopsy to be carcinomatous metastases in an enlarged cervical lymph node. For the preceding 10 months he had severe diarrhoea and loss of weight. The history also revealed that from the age of 6 months until they ceased spontaneously at the age of 7 years, he had almost daily convulsive attacks lasting a few seconds, followed by drowsiness for half an hour.

Barium meal revealed an identation in the wall of the stomach and at laparotomy there was an inoperable malignant tumour involving most of the pancreas, with metastases in adjacent lymph nodes. A biopsy was reported as 'scirrhus adenocarcinoma'. He was treated with radiotherapy, but died 2 years later with widespread metastases in lymph nodes, lungs and ribs.

It is tempting to postulate that this child had a functioning B cell adenoma from the age of 6 months to 7 years, that the adenoma then became malignant, lost its ability to secrete insulin, and 2 years later it made its presence known by metastases in the cervical lymph nodes.

A malignant nonsecretory 'nesidioblastoma', in a 13-year old girl has recently been reported by Babut, Le Calvé *et al.* (1974), and a functional carcinoma of B cells in childhood by Cubilla & Hadyn (1975).

TREATMENT OF ORGANIC HYPERINSULINISM

The current plan of management of children with symptomatic hypoglycaemia is a trial of diazoxide (15 mg/Kg/day), for up to 2 months. In most of these children the hypoglycaemia can be controlled, and they are assumed to be examples of hyperplasia of the B cells (Victorin & Thorell, 1974).

Surgical treatment

Failure to control hypoglycaemia with diazoxide, in the presence of hyperinsulinaemia, is an indication for surgical exploration (Harrison *et al.*, 1973), and experience has shown that most of those who fail to respond to cortisone are less than one year of age.

At operation they are found to have hyperplasia or an adenoma, and exploration of the pancreas often proves to be a long and difficult procedure.

When an adenoma is the cause, it is most likely to be in the body or the tail of the pancreas (73%). The adenoma is almost always less than 1·5 cm in diameter and only infrequently visible on the surface of the gland; even then it is only slightly more pink in colour than the rest of the pancreas.

Recognition of an adenoma may be facilitated by preoperative infusion of methylene blue (5 mg/Kg) as described by Gordon *et al.* (1974) who employed this method in locating an insulinoma 1·6 cm in diameter in the tail of the pancreas. The tumour was persistently stained a deep reddish blue, contrasting with the fading and paler tinge of the rest of the pancreas.

When an adenoma is discovered in the body or the tail of the pancreas and removed, it is still necessary to remove all the pancreas to the left of the superior mesenteric vessels (approximately 80% resection) because more than one adenoma is present in 14% of cases.

When no tumour can be found after a thorough search of the body or the tail, the head of the pancreas is explored, and this can only be done effectively by mobilizing the duodenum (by Kocher's manoeuvre) so that the posterior aspect of the head of the pancreas can be inspected, and palpated bimanually. When a tumour is found in the head of the pancreas (the site in 25% cases) it is removed and if confirmed by frozen sections, no further excision of the pancreas is required because an adenoma in this site is very likely to be the only adenoma present. The successful removal of a solitary adenoma can usually but not invariably be confirmed by an immediate, intra-operative rise in the blood sugar, which should be monitored continuously during exploration (Shatney & Grage, 1974).

When no adenoma can be found in the head of the pancreas, all the pancreas to the left of the superior mesenteric vessels should be excised (sometimes referred to as 'blind resection'), for this may include an undiscovered adenoma, as in one case in the Index Series.

Even when no adenoma can be identified in such an operative specimen, this removal, of approximately 80% of the pancreas, in cases of hyperplasia, may prove to be effective in reducing the amount of insulin secreted. If not, a subsequent operation is required to remove part of the head of the pancreas, leaving only the portion immediately adjacent to the common bile duct, the two excisions amounting to resection of some 90% of the whole gland.

It is not necessary to remove the spleen, even when 80–90% of the pancreas is resected, although its preservation requires a lengthy dissection of the splenic artery and vein along the upper border of the pancreas, dividing the numerous minute vessels which run between the splenic vessels and the pancreas.

Operative findings

In the series of 54 children with a functioning adenoma collected from the literature by Welch (1969), six had a benign adenoma diagnosed at autopsy, following death from uncontrolled hypoglycaemia. Of the remaining 48 cases, 34 had a single adenoma, eight had multiple adenomas, and one had an ectopic insulinoma in the liver.

In the period covered by the Index Series, one patient had a single adenoma in the head of the pancreas; the other, a 19-day old infant, had a minute adenoma (5 mm diameter) not discovered at operation, but found in the tip of the tail of the pancreas in the operative specimen following 'blind resection' (Robinson *et al.*, 1971).

RESULTS

Welch (1969) reviewed the results of operation in a collected series of 93 patients who had a 'graded' or 'subtotal' pancreatectomy for hypoglycaemia; 57 (61%) were normoglycaemic and required no further treatment; 23 (25%) were normoglycaemic but required some medication; and 11 were not improved by operation.

Of the 87 survivors, 14 (15%) were reported to have some impairment of neurological function. This figure is unexpectedly low and possibly an underestimate, for from our experience one of the tragedies of hypoglycaemia due to hyperplasia or adenoma, is that even when there has been only a few months delay in diagnosis, and when subtotal pancreatectomy has been successfully performed, the survivor is moderately or severely mentally retarded (Fonkalsrud, Trout *et al.*, 1974), presumably the result of the cerebral cortex being deprived of the glucose essential not only for current function but future development.

IV. ADENOMA AND CARCINOMA OF NON-B CELLS

'NESIDIOBLASTOSIS'

It has become apparent that there are several types of cell in the islets of Langerhans, that each elaborates a characteristic hormone (Vance *et al.*, 1969), and that adenomas and carcinomas of other than B cells occur (Verner, 1968).

The B cells account for 75% of the islet cells and elaborate insulin as described above. The α cells secrete glucagon, and both benign glucagonomas (Croughs *et al.*, 1972) and carcinomas (McGavran *et al.*, 1966) have been described.

Other islet cells, currently designated as 'delta' cells or 'G' cells, have been shown to secrete gastrin, and these or very similar cells also occur in the antrum of the stomach (Bhagavan *et al.*, 1974) in the duodenum and, in smaller numbers, scattered throughout the small bowel.

Considerable complexity is presented by the secretion of more than one type of biologically active substance by a variety of cells, in the pancreas and in various other sites. O'Neale, Kipnis *et al.* (1968) reported that 'ACTH secreting tumours' of islet cells have also been found to secrete gastrin, melanotropin, norepinephrine, serotonin, parathormone, vasopressin and glucagon.

THE ZOLLINGER-ELLISON SYNDROME

Hypergastrinaemia occurs when 'delta cells' are the site of either hyperplasia, an adenoma or a carcinoma; a carcinoma is the most common, and this is the basis of the Zollinger-Ellison syndrome (ZES) (Zollinger & Ellison, 1955; Zollinger & Coleman, 1974), i.e. a low grade functioning carcinoma (gastrinoma) of the non-β (delta or G) cells. 'Gastrinomas' cause hypergastrinaemia leading in turn to hypersecretion of gastric juices (including hyperchlorhydria) and to peptic ulceration, characteristically in the jejunum, but alternatively in the stomach or duodenum.

Diarrhoea (Rawson *et al.*, 1960) has been described as being the only symptom in the early stages of the ZES in some cases, and Welch (1969) suggested that this may explain the diarrhoea noted in 6 of 22 supposedly 'non-functioning' carcinomas of the pancreas in children. This possibility is complicated by the existence of another syndrome, 'pancreatic cholera', believed to be due to hypersecretion of yet another type of functioning islet cell tumour (benign or malignant) which elaborates a substance which may be 'gastric inhibitory polypeptide' (Elias, Pollak *et al.*, 1972). A malignant 'non β' cell tumour of the islet cells, which presented with pancreatic cholera has also been reported by Schafer (1964).

In patients with ZES, the gastrinoma causes hypergastrinaemia with serum gastrin as high as 1000 pg/ml (which is diagnostic), although in some cases as low as 150–650 pg/ml, and wide variations from day to day have been noted in individual patients. High levels of gastrin, wherever the source is located, and whether the gastrinoma is benign or malignant, cause a marked increase in the number of parietal cells, hence in the total volume and total acidity of the gastric secretions, which in turn produce severe peptic ulceration (Greider *et al.*, 1974; Zollinger, 1975a,b).

DIAGNOSIS

Peptic ulceration is a rare condition in children, and occurs most often as a complication of severe head injuries or extensive burns.

When peptic ulceration is not related to antecedent disease, and particularly when the ulcer is in the jejunum, a gastrinoma should be considered. The simplest screening test is a gastric test meal and very high levels of total acid, when associated with a large total volume, are suggestive of a gastrinoma. This can usually be confirmed by demonstrating hypergastrinaemia (Jaffe, Peskin & Kaplan, 1972), although estimations on several occasions may be necessary to demonstrate high levels of serum gastrin, because of variations from day to day.

Scanning with ^{75}Se-labelled methionine has recently been developed to the point where it can demonstrate the presence of a gastrinoma (Davies, 1973), and can also distinguish scintillographically between an insulinoma and a gastrinoma. As gastrin contains methionine, it is selectively taken up in a gastrinoma, and in favourable circumstances this may show as a 'hot spot' where there is a major collection of delta cells.

The distribution of nucleide-labelled methionine in the pancreas is highest at sites of high protein turnover, and is higher in exocrine tissue than in beta cells; hence an insulinoma will show as a 'cold spot', when large enough to reach the level of resolution.

TREATMENT

Most patients with ZES have more than one site of gastrin secretion, e.g. hyperplasia of gastrin secreting ('delta') cells, or multiple adenomas, or a carcinoma with functioning metastases. Further, the cells secreting gastrin may be in the pancreas, the duodenal wall or elsewhere, e.g. in the liver. Because of the difficulty in identifying and removing *all* gastrin secreting tissue, an alternative which has been adopted is to remove the 'target' cells, i.e. the parietal cells in the gastric mucosa, by total gastrectomy. Any lesser gastric resection has been followed by persistence or even exacerbation of gastric hypersecretion, and by complications which are often fatal (Wilson & Ellison, 1966).

Total pancreatectomy or pancreaticoduodenectomy should not be performed, because this does not always remove all gastrin producing tissue, e.g. in the liver, in latent metastases in lymph nodes, or a gastrinoma outside the scope of the resection.

In a series of 15 children with ZES (Wilson, Schulte *et al.*, 1971), seven were treated by total gastrectomy and all were well and free of symptoms; eight children had a less extensive gastric resection and six subsequently died.

In the only two survivors in this group, an apparently solitary gastrinoma situated in the wall of the duodenum was identified and removed successfully. This is the only exception to the rule that total gastrectomy is the operation of choice; in such patients gastric hypersecretion ceases as soon as the gastrinoma is removed, and this can be confirmed by monitoring gastric secretion throughout the operation (Isenberg *et al.*, 1973).

TUMOURS OF THE OMENTUM AND MESENTERIES

Many types of tumour have been reported to arise in the omentum or mesenteries on rare occasions (Stout *et al.*, 1963), including fibromatoses (p. 798), xanthogranuloma (p. 853), lipomatous tumours (p. 810), leiomyoma, neurofibroma (p. 822), mesenchymoma (p. 812), haemangioma (Rissier, 1960), lymphangioma (Singh *et al.*, 1971), omental or mesenteric cysts (Walker & Putnam, 1973), haemangioendothelioma (Hansen *et al.*, 1973), and chemodectoma (Carmichael, 1970).

Secondary involvement of peritoneal surfaces or the greater omentum by metastatic neuroblastoma (p. 546) or lymphosarcoma (p. 632), is more common than any of the primary tumours.

In the period covered by the Index Series, three types of benign intraperitoneal tumour-like masses have been seen: (*a*) duplication cysts of the alimentary canal, usually noncommunicating cystic lesions, attached to the small bowel; (*b*) fibrous histiocytoma of the mesentery (p. 676); and (*c*) a variety of unilocular or multilocular mesenteric 'cysts' (Hardin & Hardy, 1970; Caropreso, 1974), including lymphangiomas and lymphangiomatous hamartomas.

LYMPHANGIOMA OF THE MESENTERY OR OMENTUM

There were 13 patients with an intra-abdominal lymphangioma.

AGE : SEX

Their ages ranged from 1 month to 13 years, with a peak between 5 and 10 years; there were nine boys and four girls.

SITES

The location of the lymphangioma was as follows: in the mesentery of mid-small bowel (6), upper jejunum (2), mesocolon (2), lower ileum (1). In two cases the lymphangioma was chiefly in the greater omentum.

MACROSCOPIC APPEARANCES

The appearance of the mass is determined by its site, whether it is diffuse or pedunculated, and by the size of the cyst(s) it contains (Landing & Farber, 1956). Diffuse lesions, composed predominantly of small cysts, typically arise in the mesentery and some of them involve the wall of the alimentary canal.

The lesion consists of a collection of cysts filled with lymphatic or chylous fluid, arising in or from the mesentery; while most partially envelop the bowel (almost always the small bowel), in some cases the mass is pedunculated. Very occasionally the lesion involves the mucosa and the wall of the bowel as well as the mesentery.

MICROSCOPIC FINDINGS

Two features which identify the cysts as lymphatic in origin (see cystic hygroma p. 305) are the presence of (i) irregular bundles of smooth muscle in their wall, and (ii) islands of lymphoid tissue, sometimes organized in the form of follicles, in the fibrous tissue septa forming the walls of the cysts.

Pedunculated lesions may undergo torsion, and this occasionally produces confusing histological appearances. One case in the Index Series arose from the root of the mesentery as an irregular mass of mixed cystic and solid haemorrhagic tissue, 9 cm in diameter, containing fleshy areas composed of masses of smooth muscle cells, and fibroblasts with numerous mitotic figures. This quasi-neoplastic histological picture was somewhat alarming, but the subsequent course has been entirely benign.

CLASSIFICATION OF ABDOMINAL LYMPHANGIOMAS

Three clinicopathological types of intra-abdominal lymphangioma occur.

1. *Retroperitoneal lymphangiomas* (Wayne, Burrington *et al.*, 1973), similar in structure to cystic hygromas. Their mode of presentation is usually ill-defined abdominal pain, vomiting, general malaise, and fever, findings probably due to absorption of the altered blood frequently found in some of the cystic spaces at laparotomy (Ackerman, 1955).

The initial diagnosis is often acute appendicitis, or less specifically an 'acute surgical abdomen', and this clinical picture is also seen in the pedunculated type of lymphangioma.

2. *A protein-losing enteropathy* with diarrhoea causing low levels of serum proteins, peripheral oedema and failure of growth. This was seen in two patients, in whom lymphangiomatous tissue in the mesentery extended up to but not into the wall of the adjacent small bowel. The bulky lymphangioma caused kinking and intermittent obstruction of the lumen of the small bowel.

A similar protein-losing enteropathy occurs in 'lymphangiectasis', a condition which can be identified by the presence of large lymph spaces in a suction biopsy of the mucosa of the duodenum or the upper jejunum. Laparotomy was initially employed in some of our cases, but no lymphangiomatous tissue could be identified; although the lacteals were grossly distended with chyle suggesting lymphatic obstruction, this could not be identified or localized with certainty.

A distinction has been made (Werbeloff *et al.*, 1969) between *secondary lymphangiectasia*, (due to a variety of causes, e.g. obstruction of lymphatics by retroperitoneal and/or mesenteric lymph nodes affected with tuberculosis, the lymphomas or malignant metastases, etc.) and *primary lymphangiectasia*, a congenital disorder of mesenteric lymphatics (Waldemann, 1966) causing leakage of chyle into the lumen of the bowel and a protein-losing enteropathy. The latter is too diffuse to permit a cure by any feasible resection, whereas a relatively localized and resectable retroperitoneal lymphangiomatous mass may be the cause of secondary lymphangiectasia.

3. *A large multilocular lymphangioma* containing cysts of various sizes from 1–10 cm, lying free in the peritoneal cavity except for a pedicle, 3–4 cm in diameter, attached to the transverse mesocolon; two of the 13 cases in the Index Series were of this type. A similar but unilocular mass, also attached to the mesocolon, has been described by Ban, Hirose *et al.* (1972).

MODES OF PRESENTATION

Large lymphangiomatous masses can be completely asymptomatic, and usually draw attention to their presence only when a complication such as spontaneous haemorrhage into one or more loculi arises. When uncomplicated, signs are confined to some abdominal distention or dullness to percussion, both on which can be readily overlooked.

1. *An abdominal mass* was the mode of presentation in five of the 13 cases, and when confined to the mesentery, it was usually more discrete, and mobile in a transverse direction.
2. *Acute abdominal pain* was the main complaint in five children, and in most of these torsion of the cystic mass or of an adjacent loop of bowel was the cause.
3. *Subacute pain with a palpable mass and fever* were the findings in two patients, and acute appendicitis was the initial diagnosis. Altered blood and turbid chylous fluid, rather than infection, is the probable cause of general symptoms of 'toxaemia', and material from apparently infected loculi is usually found to be sterile. However, infection (with *E. coli*) was proven in one of our cases.

DIAGNOSIS

Excluding those presenting with chronic diarrhoea, or with torsion and necrosis of a loop of bowel, the initial diagnosis was usually acute appendicitis or an 'acute surgical abdomen', and this is also usual in lymphangiomas in retroperitoneal tissues (Wayne, Burrington *et al.*, 1973).

Pre-operative radiographs of the abdomen may show displacement of the gas shadows by an opaque mass, but the correct diagnosis and the exclusion of appendical inflammation is generally made at operation.

When a clearly defined mobile abdominal mass is palpable, it is more likely to be a tense duplication cyst than a lymphangioma.

TREATMENT

Excision of the lesion is required, and in some cases (in three of the series of 13) it is possible to confine the excision to lymphangiomatous tissue without removing a segment of the bowel.

In the other ten patients resection of a length of bowel of up to 30 cm, as well as the lymphangioma, was necessary because the vascular arcades were embedded in the abnormal tissue; in two of these ten specimens the lymphangiomatosis was subsequently found to extend into the wall of the bowel.

OTHER TUMOURS OF THE OMENTUM AND MESENTERIES

Leiomyoma

Tumours of smooth muscle are rare in childhood; most of them arise in the alimentary canal (p. 628) and less commonly in the urinary or the respiratory tract (p. 478). One of the few cases of leiomyoma in a child arose in the greater omentum (Love & Pemberton, 1973) and presented as a suprapubic pelvic mass in a 9-year old girl with a history of anorexia, loss of weight, lethargy and constipation; the tumour filled the pelvis but was confined to the omentum and readily removed.

Stout *et al.* (1963) collected 24 solid tumours of the omentum; of these only one, a neurofibroma, occurred in a child.

Haemangioendothelioma

This tumour has been reported in the mesentery, as a large, platelet-trapping lesion causing thrombocytopenia (Hansen *et al.*, 1973). Angiography was found to be helpful, both in delineating the lesion and in assessing response to treatment with corticosteroids. This lesion should be resected when feasible because of a low but definite malignant potential (Kauffman & Stout, 1961). When extensive and locally inoperable, corticosteroids and irradiation have been advocated.

Fibrous histiocytoma (syn. 'atypical' (? malignant) histiocytoma)

This unusual lesion has been described in a variety of sites, notably in the mediastinum (p. 459), and occasionally in the peritoneal cavity. The nature of the condition is uncertain for it combines some of the features of a neoplasm with those of a histiocytic proliferation (see p. 219).

The Index Series contained one example.

A boy aged 11 presented with a history of anorexia, listlessness and fever for 6 weeks. He complained of pain in the left hypochondrium, where a tender mass 5×8 *cm* was palpable.

Examination of the blood revealed slight anaemia (haemoglobin 8·7 g/dl), thrombocytosis (platelets 600,000/cmm) and hyperglobulinaemia (total serum protein 7·1 g/dl; albumen 2·5 g/dl, α-1 globulin 0·4 g/dl, α-2 globulin 1·9 g/dl, β-globulin 1·5 g/dl, γ-globulin 0·8 g/dl). Platelet counts on a number of occasions varied from 280,000/cmm to 1,300,000/cmm.

A barium enema showed an extrinsic mass indenting the colon at the splenic flexure, and at operation a fixed, infiltrating tumour in the transverse mesocolon was removed together with the spleen and a segment of the colon.

One month later fever and malaise recurred and the platelet count again rose to 840,000–880,000/cmm (haemoglobin 13 g/dl, leucocytes 9,600/cmm). At a further laparotomy two spherical masses, each 4 cm in diameter, were found; one in the greater omentum was completely excised; the other, lying between the rectum and the bladder, was enucleated and partially removed. No other treatment was given. He is well and free of all symptoms 14 months after the second excision, with platelet counts averaging 500,000/cmm.

The initial tumour was bossellated, $10 \times 9 \times 8{\cdot}5$ cm, and composed of two types of cells: fibroblasts, and histiocytic cells which appeared to be phagocytic, but many had a large single nucleolus suggesting active proliferation; no mitotic figures were seen. The second operation yielded tumours similar to the first except that they were more sclerotic and more extensively infiltrated with plasma cells and lymphocytes.

The diagnosis has been much discussed without reaching finality, for the lesions do not resemble any mesenteric tumour described in the literature. They have some of the features seen in a lymphoid hamartoma, a benign lesion associated with iron deficiency anaemia and hyperthrombocytaemia (p. 470), but their histology is not the same, and most closely resembles the atypical malignant fibrous histiocytoma described by Soule & Enriquez (1973).

REFERENCES

Oesophagus and Stomach

BOTTING, A.J., SOULE, E.H. & BROWN, A.L. (1965). Smooth muscle tumours in children. *Cancer*, **18** : 711.

GOLDEN, T. & STOUT, A.P. (1941). Smooth muscle tumours of the gastrointestinal tract and peritoneal tissues. *Surg. Gynec. & Obstet.*, **73** : 784.

MATIAS, I.E. & HUANG, V.C. (1973). Gastric teratoma in infancy. Report of a case and review of the world literature. *Ann. Surg.*, **178** : 631.

MCNEER, G. (1941). Cancer of the stomach in the young. *Amer. J. Roentgenol.*, **45** : 537.

MOORE, C. (1958). Visceral squamous cancer in childhood. *Pediatrics*, **21** : 573.

NAHMAD, M. & CLATWORTHY, H.W.Jr. (1973). Leiomyoma of the entire oesophagus. *J. Pediat. Surg.*, **8** : 829.

NANDY, A.K., SENGUPTA, P. *et al.* (1974). Teratoma of the stomach. *J. Pediat. Surg.*, **9** : 563.

WURLITZER, F.P., MARES, A.J., ISAACS, H., LANDING, B.H. & WOOLLEY, M.M. (1973). Smooth muscle tumours of the stomach in childhood and adolescence. *J. Pediat. Surg.*, **8** : 421.

YANNOPOULOS, K. & STOUT, A.P. (1962). Smooth muscle tumors in children. *Cancer*, **15** : 958.

Lymphosarcoma of the Bowel

AUR, R.J.A., HUSTU, H.O. & SIMONE, J.V. *et al.* (1971). Therapy of localized and regional lymphosarcoma of childhood. *Cancer*, **27** : 1328.

BARTRAM, C. & CHRISPIN, A.R. (1973). Primary lymphosarcoma of the ileum and caecum. *Pediat. Radiol.*, **1** : 28.

DANIS, R.K. (1974). Lymphoid hyperplasia of the illum—always a benign disease? *Am. J. Dis. Child.*, **127** : 656.

FU, YAO-SHI, & PERZIN, K.H. (1972). Lymphosarcoma of the small intestine: a clinicopathologic study. *Cancer*, **29** : 645.

KILLINGBACK, M., COOMBES, B., FRANCIS, P. (1974). Intestinal and cutaneous haemangiomatosis. *Med. J. Aust.*, **1** : 749.

MESTEL, A.L. (1959). Lymphosarcoma of the small intestine in infancy and childhood. *Ann. Surg.*, **149** : 87.

MARCUSE, P.M. & STOUT, A.P. (1950). Primary lymphocarcoma of the small intestine. *Cancer*, **3** : 459.

NORFRAY, J., CALENOFF, L. & ZANON, B. (1973). Aneurysmal lymphoma of the small intestine. *Am. J. Roentgenol.*, **119** : 335.

PICKETT, L.K. & BRIGGS, H.C. (1967). Cancer of the gastro-intestinal tract in childhood. *Ped. Clin. North Amer.*, **14** : 222.

SCHENKEN, J.R., KRUGER, R.L. and SCHULTZ, L. (1975). Papillary lymphoid hyperplasia of the terminal ileum: an unusual cause of intussusception and gastro-intestinal bleeding in childhood. *J. Pediat. Surg.*, **10** : 259.

Carcinoid Tumours

BARCLAY, G.P.T. & ROBB, W.A.T. (1968). A clinicopathological study of carcinoid tumours. *Surg. Gynec. Obstet.*, **126** : 483.

D'INGIANNI, V. (1946). Carcinoid of the appendix with metastases. *New Orleans Med. Surg. J.*, **99** : 158.

SOGA, J. & TAZAWA, K. (1971). Pathologic analysis of carcinoids: histological revaluation of 62 cases. *Cancer*, **28** : 990.

STOWENS, D. (1959). *Pediatric Pathology*. Williams & Wilkins, Baltimore.

WILLOX, S.W. (1964). Carcinoid tumours of the appendix in childhood. *Brit. J. Surg.*, **51** : 110.

Colon and Rectum

CAIN, A.S. & LONGINO, L.A. (1970). Carcinoma of the colon in children. *J. Pediat. Surg.*, **5** : 527.

DONALDSON, M.H., TAYLOR, P. *et al.* (1971). Colon carcinoma in childhood. *Pediatrics*, **48** : 307.

DOZOIS, R.R., JUDD, E.S., DAHLIN, D.C. & BARTHOLOMEW, L.G. (1969). The Peutz-Jeghers' Syndrome: Is there a predisposition to the development of intestinal malignancy? *Arch. Surg.*, **98** : 509.

HOERNER, M.T. (1958). Carcinoma of the colon and rectum in persons under 20 years of age. *Ann. J. Surg.*, **96** : 47.

JOHNSON, J.W., JUDD, E.S. & DAHLIN, D.C. (1959). Malignant neoplasm of the colon and rectum in young persons. *A.M.A. Arch. Surg.*, **79** : 365.

KERN, N.H. & WHITE, W.C. (1958). Adenocarcinoma of the colon in a nine month old infant. *Cancer*, **11** : 855.

KOTTMEIER, P.K. & CLATWORTHY, H.W.Jr. (1965). Intestinal polyposis and associated carcinoma in childhood. *Am. J. Surg.*, **110** : 709.

O'BRIEN, S.E. (1967). Carcinoma of the colon in childhood and adolescence. *Canad. Med. Assoc. J.*, **96** : 1217.

PHIFER, C.H. (1923). Cancer of the rectum and sigmoid in childhood and adolescence. *Ann. Surg.*, **77** : 711.

SATYANAND, L. & RANA, B.S. (1969). Primary carcinoma of rectum in children and young adults. *Ind. J. Cancer*, **8** : 38.

Ulcerative Colitis and Carcinoma

DEVROEDE, G.J., TAYLOR, W.F., SAUER, W.G., JACKMAN, R.J. & STICKLER, G.B. (1971). Cancer risk and life expectancy of children with ulcerative colitis. *New Engl. J. Med.*, **285** : 17.

GOLIGHER, J.C. (1973). Surgical aspects of ulcerative colitis in childhood. *Proc. Roy. Soc. Med.*, **66** : 1034.

JACKMAN, R.J., BARGEN, J.A. & HELMHOLZ, H.F. (1940). Life history of 95 children with chronic ulcerative colitis. *Am. J. Dis. Child.*, **59** : 459.

WEEDON, D.D., SHORTER, R.G. *et al.* (1973). Crohn's disease and cancer. *New Eng. J. Med.*, **289** : 1099.

WILCOX, H.R.Jr. & BEATTIE, J.L. (1956). Carcinoma complicating ulcerative colitis during childhood. *Am. J. Clin. Path.*, **26** : 778.

Polyps and Polyposis

ABRAHAMSON, J. & SHANDLING, B. (1973). Intestinal hemangioma in childhood and a syndrome for diagnosis: a collective review. *J. Pediat. Surg.*, **8** : 487.

ABRAHAMSON, J. (1967). Multiple polyposis in children. *Surgery*, **61** : 288.

BHASIN, R.P., MCALINDON, J.A. *et al.* (1974). Recurrent juvenile duodenal polyposis *J. Pediat. Surg.*, **9** : 553.

CRONKHITE, L.W. & CANADA, W.J. (1955). Generalized gastrointestinal polyposis: an unusual syndrome of polyposis, pigmentation, alopecia and onychotrophia. *New Engl. J. Med.*, **252** : 1011.

DORMANDY, T.L. (1957). Gastrointestinal polyposis with mucocutaneous pigmentation (Peutz-Jeghers' syndrome). *New Engl. J. Med.*, **256** : 1093, 1141, 1186.

DOZOIS, R.R., JUDD, E.S., DAHLIN, D.C. & BARTHOLOMEW, L.G. (1969). The Peutz-Jeghers' syndrome: Is there a predisposition to the development of intestinal malignancy? *Arch. Surg.*, **98** : 509.

FARMER, R.G., HAWKS, W.A. & TURNBULL, R.B. (1964). The spectrum of the Peutz-Jeghers' syndrome: report of 3 cases. *Am. J. Dig., Dis.*, **8** : 953.

FOLKMAN, M.J. in discussion of WOLFF, W.I. & SHINYA, M. (1973). A new approach to colonic polyps. *Ann. Surg.*, **178** : 367.

GARDNER, E.J. (1962). Follow-up study of a family group exhibiting dominant inheritance for a syndrome including intestinal polyps, osteomas, fibromas, and epidermal cysts. *Am. J. Hum. Genet.*, **14** : 376.

GATHRIGHT, J.B. & COFER, T.W. (1974). Familial incidence of juvenile polyposis coli. *Surg. Gynec. Obstet.*, **138** : 185.

JEGHERS, H., MCKUSICK, V.A. & KATZ, K.H. (1949). Generalized polyposis and melanin spots of the oral mucous membrane, lips and digits: syndrome of diagnostic significance. *New Engl. J. Med.*, **241** : 993.

LOUW, J.H. (1968). Polypoid lesions of the large bowel in children with particular reference to benign lymphoid polyposis. *J. Pediat. Surg.*, **3** : 195.

MCCOLL, I., BUSSEY, M.J.R., VEALE, A.M.O. & MORSON, B.C. (1964). Juvenile polyposis coli. *Proc. Roy. Soc. Med.*, **57** : 896.

MOERTEL, C.G., HILL, J.R. & ADSON, M.A. (1970). Surgical management of multiple polyposis: the problem of cancer in the retained bowel segment. *Arch. Surg.*, **100** : 521.

SACHATELLO, C.R., HAHN, I.S. & CARRINGTON, C.B. (1974). Juvenile gastrointestinal polyposis in a female infant: report of a case and review of the literature of a recently recognized syndrome. *Surgery*, **75** : 107.

SACHATELLO, C.R. & GRIFFEN, W.O. (1975). Hereditary polypoid diseases of the gastro-intestinal tract: a working classification. *Am. J. Surg.*, **129** : 198.

SACHATELLO, C.R., PICKREN, J.W. & GRACE, J.T. Jr. (1970). Generalized juvenile gastro-intestinal polyposis: a hereditary syndrome. *Gastroenterology*, **58** : 699.

SAFAIE-SHIRAZI, S. & SOPER, R.T. (1973). Endorectal pull-through procedure in the surgical treatment of familial polyposis coli. *J. Pediat. Surg.*, **8** : 711.

SCULLY, R.E. (1970). Sex cord tumor with annular tubules: a distinctive ovarian tumour of the Peutz-Jeghers syndrome. *Cancer*, **25** : 1107.

TOCCALINO, H., GUASTAVINO, E. *et al.* (1973). Juvenile polyps of the rectum and colon. *Acta Paediat. Scand.*, **62** : 337.

VEALE, A.M.O., MCCOLL, I., BUSSEY, H.J.R. & MORSON, B.G. (1966). Juvenile polyposis. *J. Med. Genet.*, **3** : 5.

WOOLF, C.M., RICHARDS, R.C. & GARDNER, E.J. (1955). Occasional discrete polyps of the colon and rectum showing inherited tendency in a kindred. *Cancer*, **8** : 403.

WOLFF, W.I. & SHINYA, H. (1973). A new approach to the management of colonic polyps. In *Advances in Surgery*, Vol 7 (Hardy, J.D., Zollinger, R.M. *et al.*, eds.). Year Book Medical Publishers Inc., Chicago.

The Spleen

AULDIST, A.W. & MYERS, N.A. (1974). Hydatid disease in children. *Aust. N.Z. J. Surg.*, **44** : 402.

BRON, K.M. & HOFFMAN, W.J. (1971). Preoperative diagnosis of splenic cysts. *Arch. Surg.*, **102** : 459.

DAS GUPTA, T., COOMBES, B. & BRASFIELD, R.D. (1965). Primary malignant neoplasms of the spleen. *Surg. Gynec. & Obstet.*, **120** : 947.

FONKALSRUD, E.W. & WALFORD, R.L. (1960). Transitional cell splenic cyst excised without splenectomy. *Arch. Surg.*, **81** : 634.

HORAN, M. & COLEBATCH, J.H. (1962). Relation between splenectomy and subsequent infection. *Arch. Dis. Childh.*, **37** : 398.

LAZARUS, J.A. & MARKS, M.S. (1946). Primary malignant tumours of the spleen. *Am. J. Surg.*, **71** : 479.

SIRINEK, K.R. & EVANS, W.E. (1973). Non-parasitic splenic cysts: case report of epidermoid cyst with review of the literature. *Amer. J. Surg.*, **126** : 8.

The Pancreas

ALFIDI, R.J., DAE, S.B., CRILE, G. & HAWK, W. (1971). Arteriography and hypoglycaemia. *Surg. Gynec. & Obstet.*, **133** : 447.

ANNOTATION (1974). Diagnosis of insulinoma. *Lancet*, **2** : 385.

BABUT, J.M., LE CALVÉ, J.L. *et al.* (1974). Tumeurs maligne du pancreas chez l'enfant: a propos d'un cas. *Ann. Chir. Infant.*, **15** : 59.

BECKER, W.F., WELSH, R.A. & PRATT, H.S. (1965). Cystadenoma and cystadenocarcinoma of the pancreas. *Ann. Surg.*, **161** : 845.

BHAGAVAN, B.S., HOFKIN, G.A., WOEL, G.M. & KOSS, L.G. (1974). Zollinger-Ellison syndrome: ultrastructure and histochemical observations in a child with endocrine tumorlets of gastric antrum. *Arch. Path.*, **98** : 217.

BOIJSEN, E. & SAMUELSSON, L. (1970). Angiographic diagnosis of tumors arising from the pancreatic islets. *Acta Radiol.*, **10** : 161.

CROUGHS, R.J.M., HULSMANS, H.A.M. & ISRAEL, D.E. (1972). Glucagonoma as part of polyglandular adenoma syndrome. *Amer. J. Med.*, **52** : 690.

CUBILLA, A.L. & HADJU, S.I. (1975). Islet cell carcinoma of the pancreas. *Arch. Path.*, **99** : 204.

DAVIES, E.R. (1973). The radiological and scintigraphic investigation of spontaneous hypoglycaemia. *Clin. Radiol.*, **24** : 177.

ELIAS, E., POLAK, J.M., BLOOM, S.R. *et al.* (1972). Pancreatic cholera due to production of gastric inhibitory polypeptide. *Lancet*, **2** : 791.

FONKALSRUD, E.W., TROUT, H.H. *et al.* (1974). Idiopathic hypoglycaemia in infancy: surgical management. *Arch. Surg.*, **108** : 801.

FONKALSRUD, E.W., WILKERSON, J.A. & LONGMIRE, W.P. (1966). Pancreaticoduodenectomy for islet cell tumours of the pancreas in infancy and childhood. *J. Amer. med. Assoc.*, **197** : 586.

FRIESEN, S.R. (1968). A gastric factor in the pathogenesis of the Zollinger-Ellison syndrome. *Ann. Surg.*, **168** : 483.

FULTON, R.E., SHEEDY, P.F. *et al.* (1975). Preoperative angiographic localization of insulin producing tumors of the pancreas. *Am. J. Roentgenol.*, **123** : 367.

GILLE, P., BARBIER, G., LECLERC, D. & BAUER, J. (1972). Cystadenome pancréatique chez un enfant de 2 ans. *Ann. Chirurg. Infant.*, **13** : 437.

GORDON, D.L., AIRAN, M.C. & SUNAVICH, S. (1974). Visual identification of an insulinoma using methylene blue. *Brit. J. Surg.*, **61** : 363.

GREIDER, M.H., ROSAI, H. & MCGUIGAN, J.E. (1974). The human pancreatic islet cells and their tumors. II Ulcerogenic and diarrhoeogenic tumors. *Cancer*, **33** : 1423.

GROSFELD, J.L., CLATWORTHY, H.W.Jr. & HAMOUDI, A.B. (1970). Pancreatic malignancy in childhood. *Arch. Surg.*, **101** : 370.

GUNDERSEN, A.E. & JANIS, J.F. (1969). Pancreatic cystadenoma in childhood: a report of a case. *J. pediat. Surg.*, **4** : 478.

HARRISON, T.S., CHILD, C.G., *et al.* (1973). Surgical management of functioning islet-cell tumors of the pancreas., *Ann. Surg.*, **178** : 485.

HONICKY, R.E. & DE PAPP, E.W. (1973). Mediastinal teratoma with endocrine function. *Am. J. Dis. Child.*, **126** : 650.

HORAN, M. & COLEBATCH, J.J. (1962). Relation between splenectomy and subsequent infection. *Arch. Dis. Childh.*, **37** : 398.

HUREZ, A., BEDOUELLE, *J.*, *et al.* (1961). Carcinoma of the islets of Langerhans with severe hypoglycaemic manifestations in a nine year old. *Arch. Franç. Pédiat.*, **18** : 625.

ISENBERG, J.I., WALSH, J.H. & GROSSMAN, M.I. (1973). Zollinger-Ellison syndrome. *Gastroenterol.*, **65** : 142.

JAFFE, B.M., PESKIN, G. & KAPLAN, E.L. (1972). Diagnosis of Zollinger-Ellison tumors by gastrinimmuno-assay. *Cancer*, **29** : 694.

MCGAVRAN, M.H., UNGER, R.H. *et al.* (1966). A glucagon secreting α-cell carcinoma of the pancreas. *New Engl. J. Med.*, **274** : 1408.

MCPHERSON, T.C. & HEERSMA, H.J. (1948). Diagnosis and treatment of pancreatic cysts in children. *J. Pediat.*, **33** : 213.

MANN, J.R., RAYNER, P.H.W. & GOUREVITCH, A. (1969). Insulinoma in childhood. *Arch. Dis. Childh.*, **44** : 435.

MILES, R.M. (1959). Pancreatic cyst in the newborn. *Ann. Surg.*, **149** : 576.

O'NEAL, L.W., KIPNIS, D.M. *et al.* (1968). Secretion of various endocrine substances by A.C.T.H. secreting tumours—gastrin, melanotropin, norepinephrine, serotonin, parathormone, vasopressin and glucagon. *Cancer*, **21** : 1219.

PAGLIARA, A.S. *et al.* (1973). Hypoglycemia in infancy and childhood. *J. pediat.*, **82** : 558.

RAWSON, A.B. *et al.* (1960). Zollinger-Ellison syndrome with diarrhoea and malabsorption: observations in a patient before and after removal of a pancreatic islet cell tumour without resort to gastric surgery. *Lancet*, **2** : 131.

RICKMAN, P.P. (1975). Islet cell tumors in childhood. *J. Pediat. Surg.*, **10** : 83.

ROBINSON, M.J., CLARKE, A.M. *et al.* (1971). Islet cell adenoma in the newborn. Report of two patients. *Pediatrics*, **48** : 232.

SCHAFER, W.H. (1964). Non-beta islet cell carcinoma of the pancreas presenting as diarrhoea. *Ann. Int. Med.*, **61** : 539.

SCHEIN, P.S. *et al.* (1973). Islet cell tumours: current concepts and management. *Ann. Int. Med.*, **79** : 239.

SCHWARTZ, J.F. & ZWIREN, G.T. (1971). Islet cell adenomatosis and adenoma in an infant. *J. Pediat.*, **79** : 232.

SHATNEY, C.H. & GRAGE, T.B. (1974). Diagnostic and surgical aspects of insulinoma: a review of 27 cases. *Am. J. Surg.*, **127** : 174.

STOKES, J.M., WOHLTMANN, H.J. & HARTMANN, A.F. (1966). Pancreatectomy for refractory hypoglycemia in children. *Arch. Surg.*, **93** : 40.

TODD, R.M., RICKHAM, P.P. & COULTER, J.B.S. (1972). Islet cell tumour of the newborn. *Helv. Paediat. Acta.*, **27** : 131.

TSUKIMOTO, I. *et al.* (1973). Pancreatic carcinoma in children in Japan. *Cancer*, **31** : 1203.

WELCH, K.J. (1969). Pancreatic neoplasms. In *Pediatric Surgery*, 2nd ed., p. 758. Year Book Medical Publishers Inc., Chicago.

WILLIS, R.A. (1967). *Pathology of Tumours*. C.V. Mosby Co., St. Louis.

WILSON, S.D. & ELLISON, E.H. (1966). Survival in patients with the Zollinger-Ellison syndrome treated by total gastrectomy. *Am. J. Surg.*, **111** : 787.

WILSON, S.D. & SCHULTE, W.J. *et al.* (1971). Longevity studies following gastrectomy in children with the Zollinger-Ellison syndrome. *Arch. Surg.*, **103** : 108.

VANCE, J.E., STORR, R.W. *et al.* (1969). Nesidioblastosis in familial endocrine adenomatosis. *J. Amer. Med. Assoc.*, **207** : 1679.

VERNER, J.V. (1968). Clinical syndromes associated with non-insulin producing tumours of the pancreatic islets. *International Symposium, Erlangen.* Georg Thieme Verlag, Stuttgart.

VICTORIN, L.H. & THORELL, J.I. (1974). Plasma insulin and blood glucose during longterm treatment with diazoxide for infant hypoglycaemia. *Acta Paediat. Scandinav.*, **63** : 302.

ZOLLINGER, R.M. (1975a). Ulcerogenic tumours of the pancreas. *Aust. N.Z. J. Surg.*, **45** : 1.

ZOLLINGER, R.M. (1975b). Islet cell tumors of the pancreas and the alimentary tract. *Am. J. Surg.*, **129** : 103.

ZOLLINGER, R.M. & COLEMAN, D.W. (1974). *The Influence of Pancreatic Tumors on the Stomach.* Charles C. Thomas, Springfield.

ZOLLINGER, R.M. & ELLISON, E.H. (1955). Primary peptic ulceration of the jejunum associated with islet cell tumours of the pancreas. *Ann. Surg.*, **142** : 709.

Omentum and Mesentery

ACKERMAN, L.V. (1955). Tumors of the retroperitoneum and mesentery. *Atlas of Tumor Pathology*, Section VI, Fascicles 23–24. Armed Forces Institute of Pathology, Washington D.C.

BAN, J.L., HIROSE, F.H., LACHMAN, R.S. & MOORE, T.C. (1972). Pedunculated cystic lymphangioma of the splenocolic ligament in a child. *Amer. J. Surg.*, **124** : 410.

CARMICHAEL, J.D. (1970). Mesenteric chemodectoma. *Arch. Surg.*, **101** : 630.

CAROPRESO, P.R. (1974). Mesenteric cysts: a review. *Arch. Surg.*, **108** : 242.

HANSEN, R.C., CASTELLINO, R.A. *et al.* (1973). Mesenteric hemangioendothelioma with thrombocytopenia: report of a case with arteriographic findings. *Cancer*, **32** : 136.

HARDIN, W.J. & HARDY, J.D. (1970). Mesenteric cysts. *Amer. J. Surg.*, **119** : 640.

KAUFFMAN, S.L. & STOUT, A.P. (1961). Malignant hemangioendothelioma in infancy and childhood. *Cancer*, **14** : 1186.

LANDING, B.H. & FARBER, S. (1956). Tumors of the cardiovascular system. *Atlas of Tumor Pathology*, Fascicle 7, p. 124. Armed Forces Institute of Pathology, Washington D.C.

LOVE, W.G. & PEMBERTON, L.B. (1973). Leiomyoma of omentum. *J. pediat. Surg.*, **8** : 329.

RISSIER, H.L. (1960). Haemangiomatosis of the intestine. Discussion, review of the literature and report of two cases. *Gastroenterologia* (*Basel*), **93** : 357.

SINGH, S., BABOO, M. & PATHAK, I.C. (1971). Cystic lymphangioma in children: report of 32 cases including lesions at rare sites. *Surgery*, **69** : 947.

SOULE, E.H. & ENRIQUEZ, P. (1973). Atypical fibrous histiocytoma, malignant fibrous histiocytoma, malignant histiocytoma and epitheloid sarcoma. *Cancer*, **30** : 128.

STOUT, A.P. *et al.* (1963). Primary solid tumors of the great omentum. *Cancer*, **16** : 231.

WALDMAN, T.A. (1966). Protein-losing enteropathy. *Gastroenterology*, **50** : 422.

WALKER, A.R. & PUTNAM, T.C. (1973). Omental, mesenteric and retroperitoneal cysts: a clinical study of 33 new cases. *Ann. Surg.*, **178** : 13.

WAYNE, E.R., BURRINGTON, J.D. *et al.* (1973). Retroperitoneal lymphangioma: an unusual cause of the acute surgical abdomen. *J. Pediat. Surg.*, **8** : 831.

WERBELOFF, L., BANKS, S. & MARKS, I.N. (1969). Radiological findings in protein-losing enteropathy. *Brit. J. Radiol.*, **42** : 605.

Chapter 21. Pelvic tumours

Table 21.1. Benign swellings and malignant tumours arising in the pelvis

Benign conditions	Malignant tumours
The ovary	
Benign teratoma	Malignant teratoma (syn. endodermal sinus tumour; yolk sac tumour)

Simple cyst
  follicular
  luteal
	Dysgerminoma (syn. germinoma)

Luteoma (syn. lipoid cell tumour)	Androblastoma (syn. arrhenoblastoma, Sertoli-Leydig cell tumour)
Granulosa-theca cell tumours	

Cystadenoma
  mucinous
  serous
	Cystadenocarcinoma
	  mucinous
	  serous

Parovarian cyst	Choriocarcinoma

Fibroma	Metastatic involvement
	  lymphosarcoma
	  Burkitt's lymphoma
	  leukaemic deposits

Haemangioma	Rhabdomyosarcoma
Rare 'germ cell' tumours	
The uterus and fallopian tubes	
Papilloma of the cervix	Rhabdomyosarcoma (botryoides)
Tubovarian abscess	Carcinoma: cervix, uterus
Hydrometra	Embryonal carcinoma
Haematometra	
Vagina	
Hymenal: epidermoid cyst, polyp	Rhabdomyosarcoma (botryoides)
Cyst of Gaertner's duct	Endodermal sinus tumour (syn. yolk sac tumour)
Hydrocolpos	Clear-cell carcinoma
Haematocolpos	Embryonal carcinoma
Neurofibromatosis	
Papillary adenoma	
Prostate	
Prostatic abscess	Rhabdomyosarcoma

Table 21.1. continued

Benign conditions	Malignant tumours
Bladder and urethra	
Full bladder	Rhabdomyosarcoma
Vesical polyp	Leiomyosarcoma
Leiomyoma	
Urachal abscess	
Ureterocele	
Bone tumours (see also p. 723)	
Aneurysmal bone cyst	Ewing's tumour
Eosinophilic granuloma	Chondrosarcoma
Other benign lesions (see p. 725)	Osteosarcoma
	Chordoma (see p. 289)
Retroperitoneal tissues (see also p. 709)	
Ganglioneuroma	Malignant teratoma
Teratomas (presacral)	Neuroblastoma
Fetus-in-fetu	Lymphosarcoma
Ectopic (pelvic) kidney	Liposarcoma
Lipoma	Fibrosarcoma
Anterior myelomeningocele	Other soft tissue sarcomas (p. 777)
Bowel	
Faecal masses	Lymphosarcoma (p. 630)
Appendical abscess	Other bowel tumours (p. 641)
Duplication cyst	

Malignant pelvic tumours are distinguished by their wide variety, especially those arising in the ovary (Ein, Darte & Stephens, 1970). They form only a small proportion of malignant tumours in childhood, and generally have a gloomy prognosis.

The most common tumour in the pelvis, however, is the benign ovarian teratoma, and differential diagnosis is therefore of some importance (Table 21.1).

MODES OF PRESENTATION

1. *A benign or a malignant tumour* in the pelvis may be discovered incidentally as the result of radiological examination which shows calcification in dentigerous tissues (Fig. 21.1).

Alternatively they present as one of the following clinical entities.

2. *A mass* discovered unexpectedly during routine palpation of the lower abdomen or, in some cases during an examination undertaken because of recurrent or acute abdominal pain.

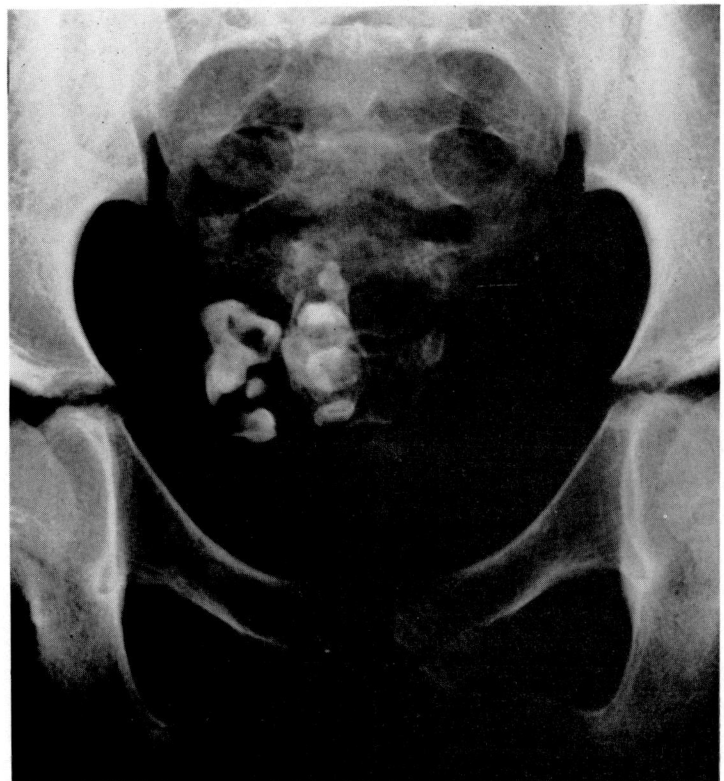

Figure 21.1. TERATOMA OF THE OVARY; x-ray of the pelvis showing 'organized' areas of calcification typical of dental derivatives of the ectodermal component of a teratoma.

3. *Urinary obstruction*, often as an acute retention, causing strangury, dribbling or haematuria.

Symptoms resulting from urinary obstruction are seldom obscure, but in the very young painless retention with overflow and incontinent dribbling can be overlooked or misinterpreted as frequency. When a palpable mass is separate from an overfilled bladder, and there is no radiological evidence of calcification, the most likely diagnosis is a malignant tumour.

4. *Vaginal bleeding* or a blood-stained watery discharge from the vulva.
5. *Virilization*, a very rare occurrence in childhood.

BENIGN SWELLINGS

Several benign swellings arise in the pelvis; many of them are not neoplasms

but they may resemble a malignant tumour in their mode of presentation, and these are, in approximately descending order of frequency:
—a distended bladder
—a mass of faeces in the rectum or colon
—an appendical abscess
—benign ovarian tumour or cyst
—mesenteric cyst
—ectopic pelvic kidney (with or without hydronephrosis)
—anterior sacral meningocele
—presacral teratoma
—cystic duplication of the alimentary canal.

CLINICAL INDICATIONS OF BENIGNITY

1. *Mobility* is a reliable clinical sign of a benign pelvic mass. The exceptions are fixed inflammatory masses such as an appendical or a urachal abscess, but these can usually be correctly identified by their site, the nature of peritoneal signs, and evidence of infection, e.g. rapid onset, fever and leucocytosis. All other benign masses are mobile, or relatively mobile when compared with the fixed immobility of a malignant mass.
2. *Benign masses tend to be frankly fluctuant* or soft in consistency, and vary in size from time to time; a malignant mass is hard and enlarges progressively.
3. *Acute onset with pain* and shock may indicate torsion. The underlying condition is generally benign but urgent operation is nevertheless required.

In the Index Series no malignant tumour in the pelvis presented with torsion, reflecting their fixity; three out of 23 benign ovarian tumours underwent torsion, and this also occurred in two other masses which were benign cystic developmental remnants.

4. *A symptomless mass* accompanied by radiographic evidence of areas of calcification is almost always diagnostic of a benign ovarian teratoma. However, diffuse calcification (in smaller areas and more diffuse) may occur in a neuroblastoma arising in the pelvis.

The co-existence of calcified dental derivatives and malignant tissue in one ovarian tumour in the Index Series shows that a predominantly 'benign' teratoma can also contain malignant elements; the presence of such areas of calcification is not an absolute guarantee that all of the lesion is benign.

CLINICAL INDICATIONS OF MALIGNANCY

Before discussing the presentation of individual tumours, some general observations on malignant lesions are in order.

1. *Age*. In the Index Series, the peak age of malignant tumours of the bladder, prostate, ovary, uterus, or retroperitoneal tissues was three years, whereas

the peak age for benign cysts or tumours of the ovary was eleven years. Except for those in the ovary, benign neoplasms of the pelvic viscera are almost unknown, and certainly less common than malignant tumours.

2. *The clinical signs* of a malignant tumour are usually distinctive; it is hard, immobile and steadily increases in size.

3. *Urinary obstruction* and a palpable mass in the lower abdomen or pelvis separate from the bladder almost always indicate a malignant tumour. In benign lesions causing obstruction (e.g. urethral valves, prolapsed ureterocele, urethral polyp, meatal ulcer) there is no other mass than the distended bladder itself.

4. *Bleeding* from the vagina, or a blood-stained watery discharge, in a young child is always ominous. In 25% of malignant tumours of the uterus or vagina this was the presenting symptom; three out of five non-teratomatous tumours of the ovary produced uterine bleeding, whereas no bleeding occurred in 23 benign ovarian teratomas.

5. *A polypoid grape-like mass* presenting through the vagina or vulva is usually so-called sarcoma botryoides, and is almost invariably malignant (Fig. 21.7a).

INVESTIGATION OF CHILDREN WITH A PELVIC MASS

Tests applicable to all children with a mass of unknown origin, both for diagnosis and to assess their extent, are as follows:

1. Full blood examination;
2. Bone marrow biopsy;
3. Excretion of catecholamines (MHMA; see p. 551) for neuroblastoma;
4. X-rays of the chest;
5. Skeletal survey;
6. X-rays of the abdomen and pelvis for dentigerous remnants and calcification;
7. Serum α-fetoprotein; this tends to be raised in hepatic tumours (p. 605) and in embryonal carcinomas of the ovary (or testis), but not with other pelvic neoplasms.

When there is suspicion of a malignant mass in the pelvis, most of the investigations listed below are required, but their selection and the order in which they are performed will vary according to the clinical findings, and these can be classified as follows:

(*a*) A palpable mass and no urinary symptoms

The most likely sites are the ovary, other genital structures or the retroperitoneal tissues. The investigations usually required are:

1. *A barium enema* to determine the position of the mass and hence its probable origin, and its extent;

2. *Micturition cysto-urethrogram* (MCU) to identify the site;
3. *Endocrine estimations* (see p. 575) if there are any signs of virilization;
4. *Aortography and selective arteriography* (and the consequent IVP) and inferior cavography, to determine the source of the tumour's blood supply, its extent, and whether there is any obstruction in the upper urinary tract (see p. 706);
5. *Laparotomy and biopsy*, or excision-biopsy, to obtain a histological diagnosis and to determine whether the tumour is resectable.

(*b*) **A palpable mass and urinary symptoms**

The most likely sites are the bladder or prostate and occasionally the retroperitoneal tissues. The same investigations as in (*a*) are required, and in addition:
1. *Retrograde urethrography* if a catheter cannot be passed, and an MCU is unobtainable, to show the extent of urethral involvement or prostatic obstruction;
2. *Endoscopy and cystoscopic biopsy* for bladder lesions, although it may not be possible to pass a cystoscope if there is marked urethral obstruction;
3. *A drill biopsy* through the perineum when the tumour mass primarily involves the prostate; cytotoxic drug cover (p. 109) should be considered.

A. TUMOURS OF THE OVARY

Apart from benign teratomas and simple follicular cysts, ovarian tumours in children are rarities (Norris & Jensen, 1972), but in tropical countries such as Africa and New Guinea, the higher incidence of lymphosarcoma of the ovary greatly increases the total number of primary ovarian tumours.

The classification of the ovarian tumours listed in Table 21.2 is based on that proposed by the W.H.O., as modified at the Royal Women's Hospital, Melbourne. Some of the tumours mentioned do not occur at all in childhood, while most of the others are seen only extremely rarely (Ein, 1970, 1973). Those more likely to be encountered in children marked with an asterisk (Table 21.2) are described in approximate order of frequency.

GERM CELL TUMOURS

HISTOGENESIS

The origin of extragonadal teratomas is thought to differ from that of teratomas arising in the ovary or the testis (p. 882). While ovarian teratomas are thought to arise from a single germ cell which has undergone the first

Table 21.2. Histological classification of ovarian tumours (Serov, S.F., Scully, R.E. & Sobin, L.M. (1973). *International Histological Classification*, No 9. W.H.O., Geneva), slightly modified for use in childhood

Benign[1]	Malignant
I. *'Epithelial' tumours*	
Serous tumours	
Serous papillary cystadenoma	Papillary adenocarcinoma
Superficial papillary tumours	
Serous adenofibromas	
Mucinous tumours	
*Mucinous cystadenoma	Mucinous adenocarcinoma
Mucinous adenofibroma	
Endometrial tumours	
Endometrial cystadenoma	Endometrial adenocarcinoma
adenofibroma	adeno-acanthoma
Mesonephroid (clear cell) tumour	
Brenner tumour	
Mixed epithelial tumours (i.e. containing multiple patterns)	
Undifferentiated	
	Carcinoma
Unclassified epithelial tumours	
II. *Sex cord stromal tumours*	
Granulosa-stromal cell tumours	
*Granulosa cell tumour[2]	
Thecoma-fibroma group of tumours[3]	
Androblastoma: Sertoli-Leydig cell tumour[3]	
Gynandroblastoma	
Unclassified	
III. **Lipid (lipoid) cell tumours*	
Luteoma	
IV. *Germ cell tumours*	
	*Dysgerminoma
	*Endodermal sinus tumour
	Embryonal carcinoma[4]
	Polyembryoma[5]
	Choriocarcinoma[5]
*Teratomas	*Malignant teratoma
Differentiated (benign)	Undifferentiated (immature or malignant)
Mixed forms	
Tumours containing multiple areas composed of the 6 tumours in this group.	
V. **Gonadoblastoma*	
A. Pure gonadoblastoma	
B. Mixed with dysgerminoma or other form of germ cell tumour	

Table 21.2. continued

Benign[1]	Malignant
VI. *Soft tissue tumours (not specific to the ovary)*	
Fibroma	Rhabdomyosarcoma
Haemangioma	Fibrosarcoma
Lymphangioma	Malignant lymphomas
VII. *Unclassified tumours*	
VIII. *Metastatic tumours*	
	Lymphosarcoma
	Leukaemic infiltration
	Neuroblastoma
	Wilms' tumour
IX. *Tumour-like conditions*	
Follicular cyst	
Endometrial cyst	
Inclusion cysts	
Parovarian cysts.	

1. Tumours of borderline malignancy also occur in childhood but are so infrequent that a separate column for them is not shown in the table
2. Most are benign
3. Most are benign but malignant forms occur
4. In practice almost impossible to distinguish from endodermal sinus tumour
5. Extremely rare, especially in children

meiotic division (Lindner *et al.*, 1975a), extragonadal teratomas are believed to arise from a somatic cell or displaced germ cell which failed to undergo meiosis and proceeded directly into mitosis (Lindner *et al.*, 1975b).

I. BENIGN TERATOMA OF THE OVARY (syn. 'Dermoid' cyst)

This is usually large by the time it presents, and the symptoms are the result of its size or of a complication such as torsion, infarction, haemorrhage or rupture (Forshall, 1960; Garfinkel & Rosenthal, 1962; Ahmed, 1971).

AGE

Benign teratomas tend to occur in the later part of childhood, from 5–15 years of age in most of the literature, and in the Index Series, have a peak incidence at about 11 years.

The ages of children in the Index Series with a malignant lesion were more widely spread, from 15 months to 11 years, with peak incidence at 3 years.

MODE OF PRESENTATION

Benign tumours most commonly present with pain, or the incidental discovery of a mobile mass; all cases of torsion in the Index Series occurred in benign lesions. Malignant masses are usually fixed to the walls of the pelvis, and produce pain, vaginal bleeding or virilization.

MACROSCOPIC APPEARANCES

Most benign teratomas of the ovary are unilocular cysts containing sebaceous material and hair (Fig. 21.2a), and an almost invariable squamous epithelial component that has given rise to the inaccurate term 'dermoid' cyst. As Willis pointed out (1962), a careful search of the wall of an ovarian teratoma almost invariably reveals a thickened area which contains tissues of other than ectodermal origin, and in some cases several types of epithelia, e.g. nervous tissue, bone, cartilage and even thyroid tissue (struma ovarii) can be seen (Fig. 21.2b).

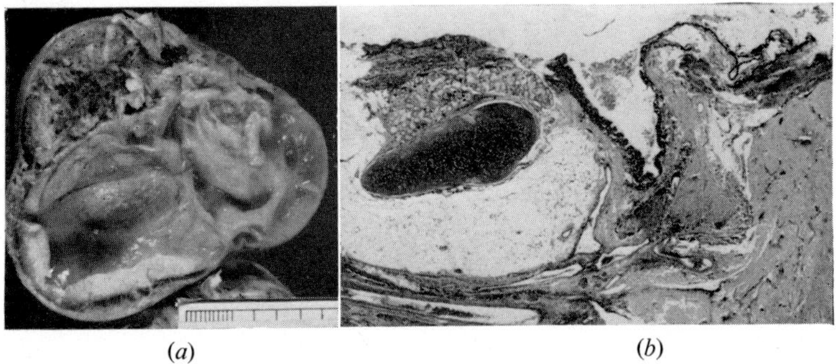

(*a*) (*b*)

Figure 21.2. BENIGN TERATOMA OF THE OVARY (cystic, differentiated); (*a*) cut surface of a large cystic cavity containing sebaceous material and hair (below), a solid mass of ectodermal tissues (above), and a soft greyish lobule (right) containing (*b*) a variety of epithelia, cartilage, fat, muscle, glandular tissue and neuroglia (right) (H & E. × 8).

II. MALIGNANT TERATOMAS

Ovarian teratomas rarely become malignant, but this occurs occasionally, and in the 25 patients in the Index Series there were two girls, aged 10 years and

12 years, in whom an ovarian tumour contained not only well-differentiated ectodermal tissue but also solid areas which were histologically malignant. In one the latter resembled a malignant granulosa-theca-cell tumour with other areas of primitive tissues; the other was an undifferentiated embryonal carcinoma with the papillary pattern seen in malignant sacrococcygeal teratomas, i.e. the pattern of an endodermal sinus tumour (Fig. 21.3). Malignant teratomas may be malignant *ab initio*. In general benign tumours becoming malignant are solid and cystic, whereas tumours which are malignant from the outset are commonly solid.

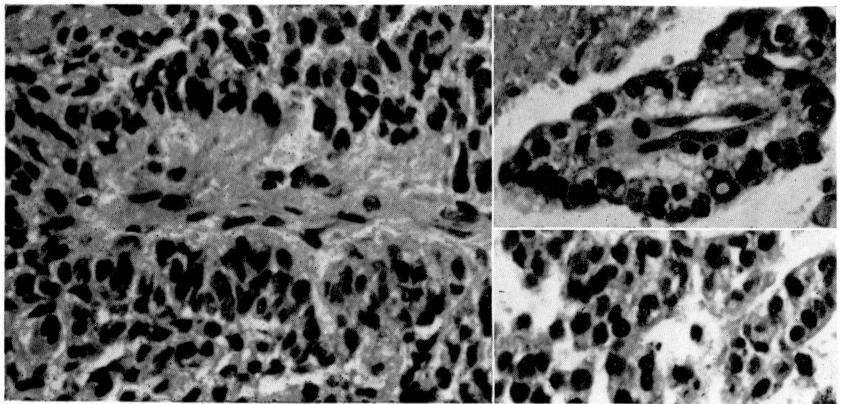

Figure 21.3. MALIGNANT OVARIAN TERATOMA (yolk sac, 'endodermal sinus' tumour, Teilum's tumour or embryonal carcinoma); (*a*) a mantle of cells around a blood vessel; in some areas the cells appear to be forming up to two layers. A pronounced tendency to papillary projections are typical of this tumour; (*b*) and (*c*) papillary structures resembling choroid plexus (H & E. × 130). The same pattern is seen in malignant sacrococcygeal and presacral teratomas.

[(*a*) *Left.* (*b*) *Top right.* (*c*) *Bottom right.*]

III. ENDODERMAL SINUS TUMOURS
(syn. embryonal (papillary) carcinoma, yolk sac tumour, Teilum's tumour)

These are highly malignant tumours, but in children they occasionally behave in a less malignant fashion. It is difficult to determine on histological evidence alone what their behaviour is likely to be (Huntington & Bullock, 1970).

In the Index Series there were three instances of undifferentiated embryonal carcinoma with the pattern of an endodermal sinus tumour and although they may have arisen in teratomas, no teratoid structures were found in multiple sections.

Macroscopically, they are usually large, soft, white and mucoid, with areas of haemorrhage. *Microscopically* they have a loose texture with small cavities, microcystic spaces and perivascular collections of cells forming a mantle 2–3 cells deep, separated from the wall of the vessel by loose connective tissue. The cells may be arranged in papillary projections on delicate vascular cores. The nuclei are round and vesicular and are surrounded by moderate amounts of pink cytoplasm, into which the nucleus commonly bulges. A more pronounced papillary pattern occurs in some examples of this tumour, and these have in the past been referred to as embryonal or papillary carcinomas.

It has been suggested that malignant sacrococcygeal tumours, orchioblastoma of the testis, the infantile carcinoma of the vagina, and this form of ovarian carcinoma, all have the same histogenesis and should be referred to as endodermal sinus tumours (Teilum, 1959).

IV. DYSGERMINOMA
(syn. germinoma)

This usually presents in young adults, only rarely in childhood, and then usually between 10 and 15 years of age. There was one case in the Index Series, an 11-year old girl who developed extensive metastases, but the degree of malignancy appears to vary considerably from case to case. This tumour may also be associated with ambiguous genitalia and intersex (see below).

MACROSCOPIC APPEARANCES

These are usually large tumours, white on section, with areas of haemorrhage and necrosis.

MICROSCOPIC FINDINGS

The pattern is typical and resembles germinomas arising elsewhere (p. 271), i.e. cords of large cells with a round, vesicular nucleus and a prominent nucleolus, interspersed with small dark cells resembling lymphocytes (Fig. 21.4); there may also be granulomatous areas.

Scully (1963) and Teter *et al.* (1964) have described atypical dysgerminomas containing various elements including germ cells, Sertoli cells and interstitial cells, referred to by Teter as a 'gonocytoma' and by Scully as a 'gonadoblastoma'. These tumours may or may not produce sex hormones, and are usually associated with intersex and sometimes ambiguous genitalia. They are believed to arise in dysgenetic gonads (p. 694).

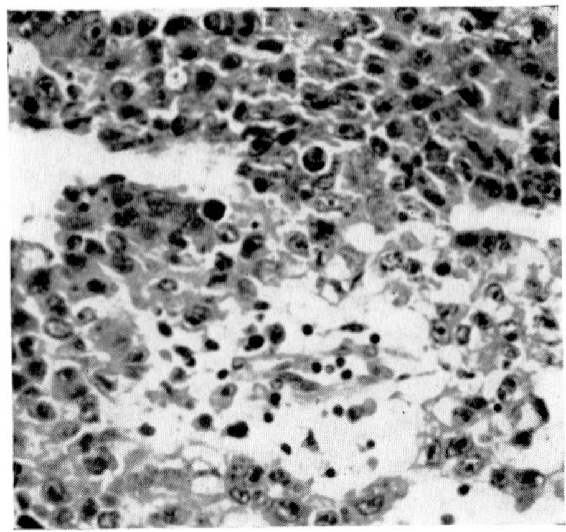

Figure 21.4. DYSGERMINOMA composed of large cells with abundant cytoplasm and a prominent nucleolus, and lymphocytes in the interlobular septa (H & E. × 300).

GONADOBLASTOMA

A gonadoblastoma is a rare tumour with a high potential for malignant transformation, composed of germ cells and also immature cells of the Sertoli and/or granulosa cell type; cells resembling Leydig and luteal cells are usually present as well (Scully, 1970).

In Scully's series, patients with this type of tumour were either (a) phenotypic females (80%), often with virilization, or (b) phenotypically abnormal males with 'cryptorchidism', hypospadias and female internal genitalia (20%). In 89% the sex chromatin was negative, and the commonest karyotypes were 46,X,Y and 45,X/46,X,Y, mosaics. The importance of the chromosomal constituents has recently been appreciated by Schellhas (1974) and elaborated by Mulvihill *et al.* (1975) who pointed out that the Y chromosome is a necessary prerequisite for the development of a malignancy; only in those cases of gonadoblastoma arising in a patient with a Y chromosome is a malignant tumour (estimated as approximately 25%) likely to arise. The type of malignancy is most commonly a germinoma (dysgerminoma, 'seminoma') but other types such as malignant teratoma, choriocarcinoma and embryonal carcinoma have been described.

MACROSCOPIC APPEARANCES

A gonadoblastoma arises in a dysgenetic gonad (ovary, 'streak-ovary' or testis) as a small firm tumour commonly calcified, but in approximately a third of Scully's series the tumour was only visible on microscopic examination. The tumour may also be overwhelmed by an associated malignant tumour and hence overlooked.

MICROSCOPIC FINDINGS

There are nests of germ cells with a large nucleus and fleshy cytoplasm, intimately mixed with smaller epithelial cells resembling immature Sertoli and granulosa cells. Leydig cells and stromal cells showing luteinization may also be present. Some of the germ cells may contain mitotic figures, and it is this type of cell in which a malignancy may arise.

A rare variant is composed of germ cells and sex cord stroma with a characteristic corded reticular pattern, as described by Talerman (1972).

V. LUTEOMA
(syn. lipoid cell tumour)

MODE OF PRESENTATION

These are usually palpable tumours in young girls who present with pseudo-precocious development (due to oestrogen), i.e. characteristically with menstruation (Scully, 1964).

In the Index Series there were two tumours which produced hormonal effects, e.g. an infant of 10 months who developed pubic hair, breasts and vaginal bleeding, and they are best described as luteomas (Campbell & Danks, 1963).

Macroscopically they are bright yellow, and histologically they are composed of festoons and sheets of large, clear cells resembling those of the corpus luteum (Fig. 21.5).

VI. GRANULOSA-THECA CELL TUMOUR

These may occur at any age from infancy to old age; the tumours are large and the cut surface shows prominent areas of cystic degeneration separated by soft, white to pinkish tumour tissue. Microscopically they are composed of islands of granulosa cells with theca cells surrounding and merging with them (Fig. 21.5c); Call-Exener bodies may be seen.

In spite of their large size most of these tumours behave in a benign fashion, although malignant forms have been reported. They are frequently associated with isosexual precocity, i.e. breast development, uterine bleeding and excess oestrogen excretion in the urine (Norris & Taylor, 1969; Fox *et al.*, 1975).

Both patients in the Index Series (aged 6 months and 4 years) presented with uterine bleeding.

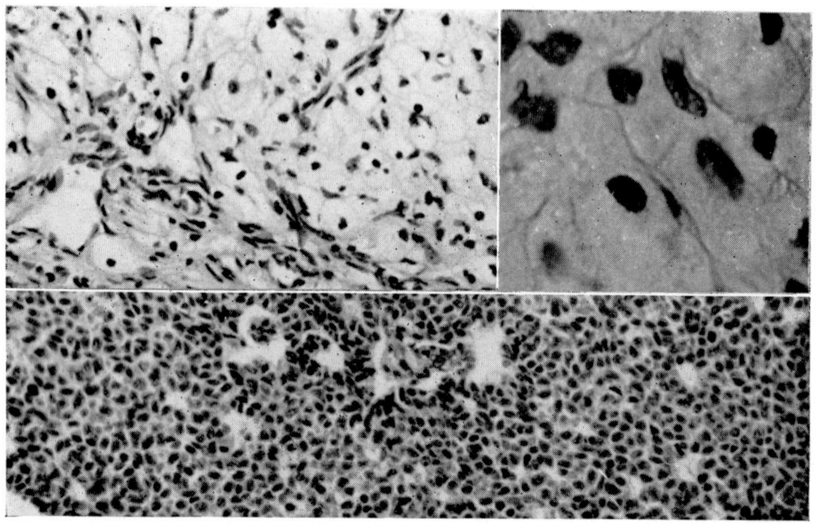

Figure 21.5. Luteoma (lipid-cell tumour), an example 4·5 × 3 × 2·5 cm causing precocious puberty in a 9-month old girl; (*a*) festoons of large lipid-filled cells (H & E. × 100); (*b*) clearly defined cystoplasmic borders and small dark nuclei (H & E. × 600); (*c*) Granulosa cell tumour containing regular, small dark cells tending to form rosettes around a small central space (H & E. × 100). [(*a*) *Top left.* (*b*) *Top right.* (*c*) *Bottom.*]

VII. ANDROBLASTOMA
(syn. arrhenoblastoma, Sertoli-Leydig cell tumour)

These are less common than granulosa-theca cell tumour and are thought to be derived from primitive gonadal mesenchyme which may differentiate to form cells resembling Sertoli cells or Leydig cells. Hormone effects are usual, and may be masculinizing (virilism and amenorrhoea) or feminizing. Some, however, are hormonally inert.

Macroscopically the tumours may be quite large, up to 20 cm in diameter, partly solid and partly cystic. *Microscopically* there are cords of cells resembling Sertoli cells and bearing a superficial resemblance to seminiferous tubules, (Fig. 21.6) usually embedded in undifferentiated mesenchyme containing groups of Leydig cells. They are so rare that it is very difficult to predict whether they will behave in a benign or malignant fashion; both courses have been reported in the literature, but most appear to be benign.

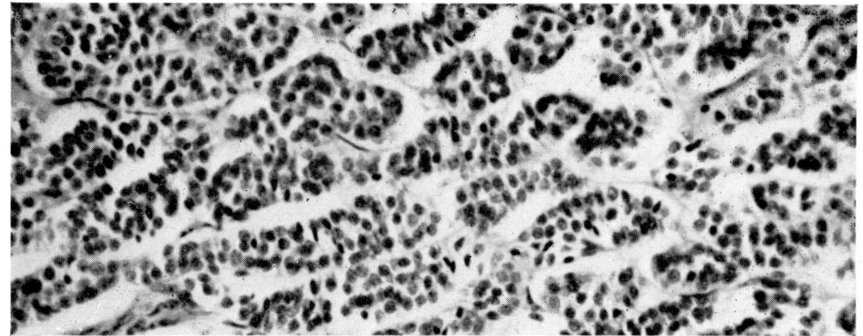

Figure 21.6. ANDROBLASTOMA; cords of dark cells with the suggestion of a central lumen and resembling the tubular cells of the neonatal testis or dysplastic undescended testis (H & E. × 200).

VIII. MUCINOUS CYSTADENOMA

Mucinous cystadenocarcinoma has rarely been reported before puberty. In the Index Series there are two examples, in girls aged 12 years at the time of diagnosis, and they are both well and apparently free of tumour several years after simple oophorectomy.

There were no cases of mucinous carcinoma, serous cystadenocarcinoma, gonadoblastoma or choriocarcinoma, in the Index Series.

SPREAD OF OVARIAN TUMOURS

This may occur:

(i) *Across peritoneal surfaces* to other parts of the pelvis (and possibly to the other ovary);

(ii) *By lymphatics* to the para-aortic nodes;

(iii) *By peri-uterine lymphatics* to the uterus, or to the contralateral ovary (see p. 698); or

(iv) *By the bloodstream* to the lungs and liver.

TREATMENT OF MALIGNANT OVARIAN TUMOURS

Surgical excision

The routes of spread indicate the range of metastases which can occur, and the need for radical excision. The decision to remove more than the affected ovary and the adjacent Fallopian tube should only be made at laparotomy and after biopsy and frozen sections, having assessed the extent of malignant fixation and infiltration. Alternatively, the histological diagnosis in frozen sections may be so uncertain that excision may have to be deferred to allow study of paraffin sections.

Harris and Boles (1974) noted that only a relatively small proportion of ovarian tumours in childhood prove to be malignant (e.g. 8–16%); some present at an early stage in which the tumour is confined to the ovary and readily removed by salpingo-oophorectomy, while others are found to be in an advanced stage with widespread dissemination usually beyond the scope of even radical excision. The authors recommended that where an ovarian tumour is found at the initial exploration, the contralateral ovary should be 'bivalved' to determine whether it contains a latent tumour.

One alternative is a second laparotomy, to perform hysterectomy and to excise the remaining ovary and tube if and when they become involved.

Because of the importance of an accurate histological diagnosis, it would be too radical to remove all the internal genitalia at the first excision, which is usually confined to removal of the tumour and the accompanying Fallopian tube.

Post-operative radiotherapy and chemotherapy

One of the special difficulties in the treatment of malignant ovarian tumours is that even when they have been completely removed, they have a tendency to recur in the pelvis, especially in the contralateral ovary or in the uterus. This may be due to regional metastatic permeation of lymphatics, which cannot be identifiable macroscopically at the time of original excision, or it may be the result of multicentric tumours arising in each ovary.

Such a 'recurrence' (or a second primary) is estimated to occur in 20% of malignant tumours of the ovary, and this naturally affects both the prognosis and decisions concerning post-operative irradiation. Because of the relatively high risk of a second lesion, the initial surgical excision is often followed by either irradiation or cytotoxic agents or both. Post-operative irradiation is usually delivered to the pelvis in a dosage which not only may destroy the function of the remaining ovary, but also cause atrophic changes in the uterus, including the endometrium, resulting in sterility.

Translocation of the remaining ovary out of the pelvis (p. 194), or protecting it in a suitable shield from the effects of irradiation, are of little avail in view of the significant risk of a tumour developing in the contralateral ovary, and in any case, a fertile ovary is practically useless if the uterus is too atrophic; successful implantation of a fertilized ovum is improbable.

Chemotherapy without radiotherapy (p. 568)

This offers an alternative method of management (Smith, Rutledge *et al.*, 1972, 1973) after the initial excision. It does not damage the uterus or the remaining ovary, and further surgery is reserved for those in whom there is a 'recurrence'. The floor of the pelvis is relatively accessible to palpation, and the best means of surveillance is probably repeated, careful bimanual palpation per rectum, under anaesthesia if necessary. In 80% of patients there is no recurrence, and no surgery is required; the other 20% can be identified by regular follow-up examinations.

The selection of the best course of management is difficult and should be decided after discussion with the parents, including the question of sterility and the significant risk of recurrence. The prognosis is as yet so poor with any combination of treatment that a compromise is reasonable, but the best chance of survival, at the cost of certain infertility, may be wide excision of all the internal genitalia.

RESULTS

In the Index Series, six out of seven patients with a malignant tumour of the ovary died within 2 years of diagnosis. Several combinations of treatment were employed, except complete and radical exenteration of the pelvis at the first operation. The sole exception, who is alive and well 10 years after diagnosis, had a simple oophorectomy without subsequent cytotoxic therapy or irradiation.

SOFT TISSUE TUMOURS OF THE OVARY

Malignant lymphomas and rhabdomyosarcomas may invade the ovary from adjacent sites, or arise there primarily. One primary rhabdomyosarcoma of the ovary was seen in a 3-year old girl who first presented with pulmonary metastases; only after thoracotomy and biopsy of the tumour was the primary site indicated and subsequently found.

B. TUMOURS OF THE UTERUS AND FALLOPIAN TUBE

These are exceedingly rare in childhood (Huffman, 1968). There are only 11 cases of adenocarcinoma of the body of the uterus reported in the world literature, and squamous carcinoma of the cervix is even more rare.

Adenocarcinomas are said to be more likely to arise in the cervix than the body of the uterus, and are believed to be derived from mesonephric structures (Fawcett *et al.*, 1966; Droegmuller *et al.*, 1970).

RHABDOMYOSARCOMA

Rhabdomyosarcomas of the uterus, cervix or broad ligament, particularly the embryonal type, are more common than any form of carcinoma; in children, sarcomas usually arise in girls less than 3 years of age, and the vagina is the more common site for this tumour (p. 701) in childhood.

MODES OF PRESENTATION

The most usual presenting features of uterine tumours are:
(*a*) *A palpable adbominal mass*, usually without dysuria; or
(*b*) *Vaginal bleeding*, or
(*c*) *A mass protruding into the vault of the vagina* (Fig. 21.7a).

DIAGNOSIS

This can only be made with certainty by biopsy. The usual investigations to exclude metastases are required, especially radiographs of the chest; involvement of the ureter or the bladder should be determined by micturating cysto-urethrography.

TREATMENT

There is usually extensive infiltration by the time the diagnosis is made. In general, radical excision supported by chemotherapy and followed by radiotherapy offers the best prospect of cure, but until recently the prognosis has been poor.

Surgical excision
In most cases partial exenteration of the pelvis is required, including radical hysterectomy, total cystectomy and fashioning an ileal conduit.

Chemotherapy and radiotherapy for rhabdomyosarcoma are on lines as described on p. 789, and the improved prognosis on p. 792.

In the Index Series there were 3 malignant tumours of the uterus. All were probably rhabdomyosarcomas, although cross striations were identified in only one.

C. TUMOURS OF THE VAGINA, BLADDER AND PROSTATE

These are rare, but rhabdomyosarcoma is again the commonest tumour, arising in derivatives of the urogenital sinus in childhood (Shachman, 1950; Batsakis, 1963).

The histological patterns are the same as in rhabdomyosarcomas arising elsewhere (p. 784), but the macroscopic appearances vary according to whether the primary arises beneath or close to a mucosal surface, or in deeper tissues. The classical sarcoma botryoides (see below) with its grape-like clusters of oedematous globules (Fig. 21.7a) is the usual form when the primary arises in the vagina or the bladder. In the prostate it usually forms a smooth, solid, whitish mass with an ill-defined margin where it is infiltrating surrounding tissues.

I. RHABDOMYOSARCOMA OF THE VAGINA

This is the classic site for sarcoma botryoides, which arises much more commonly in the vagina than the bladder or uterus in girls, whereas the bladder is the commonest site of this form of sarcoma in boys (Horn & Enterline, 1958).

AGE

Sarcoma of the vagina most often arises in girls less than 4 years of age, in some cases in infancy, and is occasionally present at birth.

SPREAD

The most important form is local infiltration of adjacent tissues and organs, and metastases to the lungs occur only rarely. Local invasion extends upwards into the wall or cavity of the uterus, forwards to involve the urethra and the bladder, but less commonly and less extensively backwards towards the rectum.

MODE OF PRESENTATION

A blood-stained discharge from the vulva occasionally draws attention to the area, and the lesion is found at endoscopy.

More commonly the sarcoma botryoides presents through the vulva as a watery, polypoid cluster of grape-like cysts (Fig. 21.7a).

DIAGNOSIS

The botryoid form of presentation is practically pathognomonic, for no benign lesion has this appearance except for the extremely rare mesonephric papillary adenoma (Janovski & Kasdon, 1963). Other tumours of the vagina such as carcinoma (Vawter, 1965), mesonephric adenocarcinoma (Droegmueller *et al.*, 1970) and squamous epithelioma (Pollack & Taylor, 1947) are infinitely less common and usually produce smooth, solid areas of induration.

Biopsy provides the confirmation of the diagnosis; the grape-like lesions often show very little cellularity (Fig. 21.7c), but such scattered cells as are present are pleomorphic, irregular and typically malignant (Fig. 21.7d).

TREATMENT

Radical excision usually involves cystectomy, hysterectomy, vulvectomy and a dissection of the inguinal nodes, but the rectum can usually be spared. An ileal conduit with bilateral implantation of the ureters is usually constructed at the definitive operation.

Chemotherapy alone (Ghavimi *et al.*, 1973) or combined with radiotherapy should be employed (see p. 789), but the prognosis has so far been poor. The remarkable improvement of the outlook in rhabdomyosarcoma in general (p. 792) may also apply to those arising in the vagina.

The one case in the Index Series, a girl aged 12 months at the time of diagnosis, died of pelvic recurrence eight months after operation.

OTHER TUMOURS OF THE VAGINA

The clear-cell adenocarcinoma of the cervix or vagina (Herbst *et al.*, 1971; Annotation, *Lancet*, 1974) related to maternal medication with high dosages of oestrogen during the first tremester of the pregnancy, is chiefly seen in late adolescence and young adults. The tumour appears to have a poor prognosis, and screening of those at risk is important so that the diagnosis can be made as early as possible (p. 5).

The pathology has been described in detail by Silverberg and De Giorgi (1972).

Embryonal carcinoma of the infant vagina. This rare but distinctive tumour usually arises in girls less than 2 years of age, and presents as a polypoid growth simulating the much more common rhabdomyosarcoma (sarcoma botryoides).

Microscopically it is composed of cells resembling those of embryonal adenocarcinoma of the testis (orchioblastoma, p. 871) or endodermal sinus tumour (Vawter, 1965; Norris, 1970), although Siegel *et al.* (1970) and Norris suggest an origin from mesonephric tissue. The histogenesis is at present uncertain, but the resemblance to embryonal carcinoma arising in the presacral region (p. 715) is striking.

A recent report (Siegel *et al.*, 1970) describes an apparent cure following radiotherapy alone.

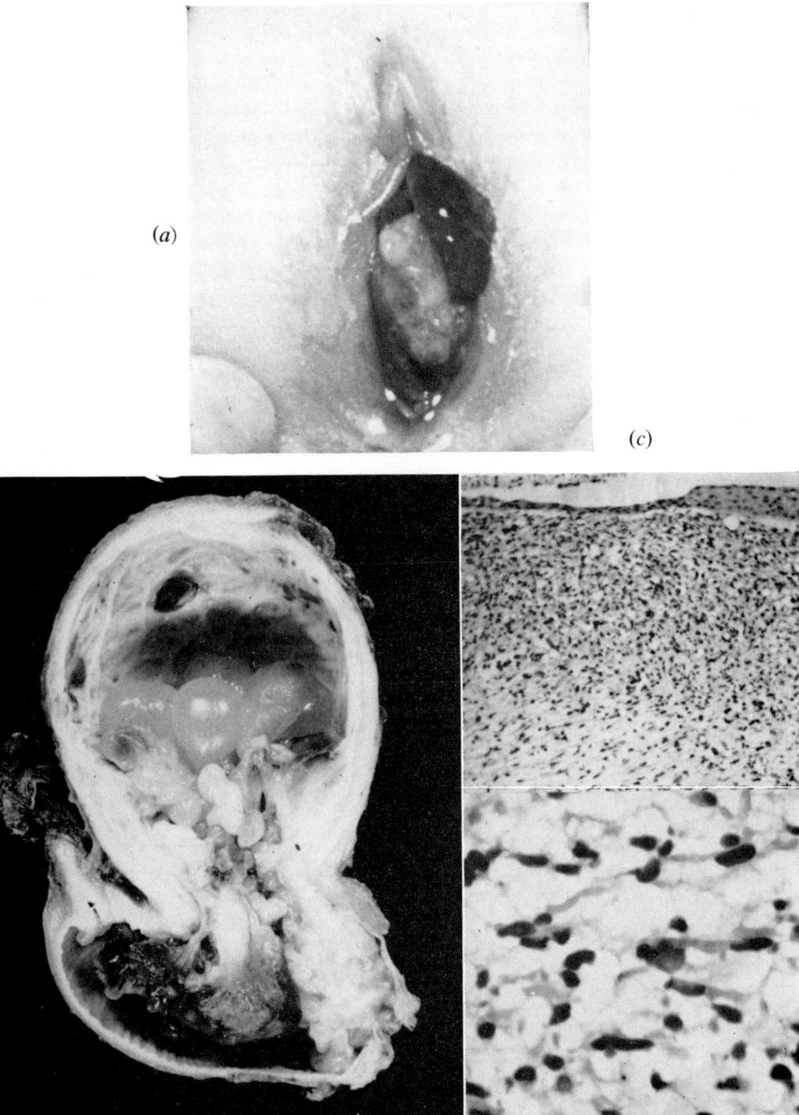

Figure 21.7. SARCOMA BOTRYOIDES; (*a*) small grape-like lesions presenting at the vulva, in this case due to a rhabdomyosarcoma of the bladder; (*b*) sagittal section of the bladder, vagina and uterus (posteriorly), showing a polypoid tumour of the base of the bladder projecting backwards into the vagina and forwards towards the introitus; (*c*) irregularly arranged rhabdomyoblasts, more closely packed near the surface, are covered by thinned but intact transitional bladder mucosa (top) (H & E. × 45); (*d*) cells with dark irregular nuclei and straps of cytoplasm, in a loose myxoid stroma (H & E. × 520).

II. RHABDOMYOSARCOMA OF THE BLADDER

AGE : SEX

This is more common in boys, and most are less than 4 years of age when symptoms arise (Jarman & Kenealy, 1970).

SITE

The trigone and posterior vesical wall are the commonest sites (Ghazali, 1973); occasionally the primary is situated in a urachal remnant at the apex of the bladder antero-superiorly.

SPREAD

Local invasion is the chief route, but hepatic and pulmonary metastases also occur, more commonly than with other sarcomas of the urogenital derivatives.

The tumour spreads locally in all directions, except posteriorly where it is usually confined at least for a time by Denonvillier's fascia, thus sparing the rectum.

MODE OF PRESENTATION

Dysuria due to intermittent obstruction of the internal opening of the urethra is the commonest presenting symptom. *Retention* of urine may also develop, suddenly or following a period of strangury and pain on voiding (Williams, 1964, 1968). An abdominal mass is more likely to be a distended bladder than the tumour itself, which usually causes vesical symptoms and signs before it is large enough to be palpable above the pubis.

INVESTIGATIONS AND DIAGNOSIS

Micturition cysto-urethrography will usually demonstrate one or more filling defects, and the radiographic appearance (Fig. 21.8) is diagnostic. Pyelography is required to determine whether the ureters are obstructed (Fig. 21.9), displaced or actually infiltrated. Endoscopy will exclude such benign conditions as a ureterocele, sacculations due to cystitis, a neurogenic bladder or the rare benign polyp. An accompanying biopsy will provide material for definitive histological diagnosis.

TREATMENT

Radical excision offers the best prospect of cure, combined with chemotherapy and irradiation, although the tumour is only moderately sensitive to irradiation.

En bloc dissection of the bladder and the urethra, including the prostate and posterior urethra in boys, the uterus and vagina in girls, is usually performed, after division of the pubic symphysis for adequate access. The excision is commenced distally, removing all the urethra, the vestibule in the female, and the urethra from the bulb upwards in males.

An ileal conduit is usually constructed at the same time, and a colostomy if the rectum is also involved, but this is unusual.

In females the ovaries can be preserved, retaining the arterial supply via the ovarian vessels in the lateral ligaments, and translocating the ovaries upwards (see p. 698) out of the field of post-operative irradiation.

Chemotherapy and radiotherapy are along the same lines as described on p. 791, and the prognosis has improved considerably in recent years (p. 792).

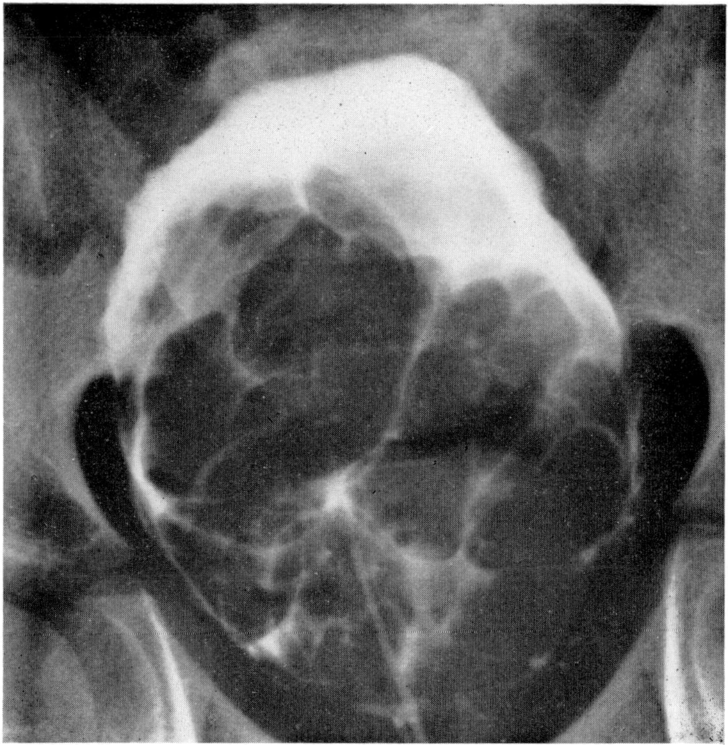

Figure 21.8. RHABDOMYOSARCOMA OF THE BLADDER; multiple globular filling defects caused by a polypoid tumour arising in the area of the trigone in a 4-year old boy.

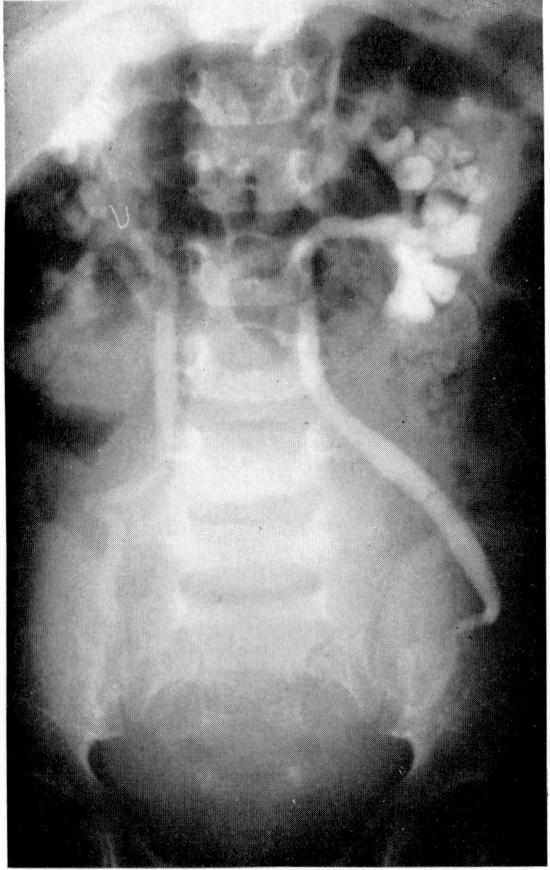

Figure 21.9. RHABDOMYOSARCOMA OF THE BLADDER; excretory pyelogram showing displacement and obstruction of the lower end of the ureters causing hydronephrosis and clubbing of the calyces.

EPITHELIAL TUMOURS OF THE BLADDER

Carcinomas of the bladder are extremely rare in childhood. The extremely well-differentiated papilloma sometimes seen in the bladder in childhood may not be the same as the similar type of lesion which occurs in adults, but rather a hamartoma analogous to epithelial polyps in the rectum (p. 647), the tongue (p. 317), and possibly, in the nasopharynx (p. 348).

The papillary tumour of the bladder in an 8-year old boy, described by Siegal and Pincus (1969) showed none of the histological features of invasiveness commonly seen in its counterpart in adults, and there was no sign of recurrence 7 years after simple transurethral resection and fulguration of the base.

OTHER MALIGNANT TUMOURS OF THE BLADDER

These are all extremely rare; transitional cell carcinoma and fibrosarcoma are occasionally reported. The bladder may also be invaded by neuroblastoma or involved in neurofibromatosis.

The Index Series contains nine patients ranging in age from 14 months to 8 years, with a peak at 3 years; five were males. All nine tumours were embryonal rhabdomyosarcomas.

Only four of the nine patients had a radical exenteration (with preservation of the rectum) and three of the four are alive and well at 18 months, 3 years and 5 years after operation. In the other five boys only biopsy or partial removal was performed and all have died, all but one within 3 months. None of these five received combination chemotherapy as currently employed (p. 790).

PROGNOSIS

From the Index Series and other reported series, aggressive surgical removal appears to produce better results than in rhabdomyosarcomas arising in some other sites (Nelson, 1968). The addition of chemotherapy and radiotherapy has considerably improved the outlook (Wilbur *et al.*, 1971), and recent reports (Kilman, Clatworthy *et al.*, 1973; Clatworthy, Braren & Smith, 1973) suggest that in Stage I cases there may be 75–80% of 2 year survivals, and a curability rate of better than 70%.

The improved outlook in rhabdomyosarcoma in response to recurring cycles of intensive combination chemotherapy (p. 792), and radiotherapy, notably in sites where excisional surgery is necessarily incomplete or confined to biopsy alone, may be grounds for a radical departure from the currently accepted treatment for rhabdomyosarcoma of the bladder, prostate or female genitalia.

As an alternative to radical excision, which leads to certain infertility and urinary diversion, probable impotence in the male, and sometimes a colostomy, surgery might be confined to biopsy to confirm the diagnosis, relying on chemotherapy and radiotherapy to destroy the tumour. This might involve some decrease in the survival rate, but this is not certain, and there would be unquestionably less disability (perhaps even approaching normality) in the survivors.

A decision against radical ablative surgery raises ethical considerations which would have to be weighed, and discussed with the parents when formulating a plan of treatment.

III. RHABDOMYOSARCOMA OF THE PROSTATE

SITE

The bladder is the more common site in boys, and the outlook is less hopeful when the tumour arises in the prostate.

PATHOLOGY: SPREAD

These are much the same as in tumours of the bladder (p. 704), and the ultrastructure has recently been studied by Sarkar *et al.* (1973).

MODES OF PRESENTATION

The symptoms are also much the same as those arising in the bladder; *retention of urine* may be sudden and acute, or slowly progressive resulting in chronic retention with overflow and little or no pain.

The tumour can be readily palpated per rectum as a smooth or slightly lobulated mass (Fig. 21.10).

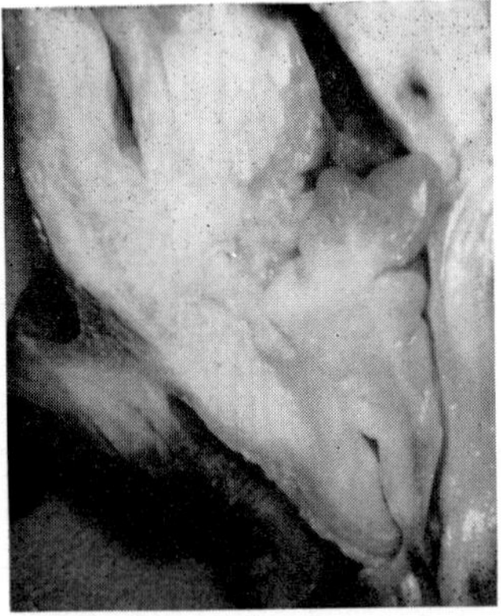

Figure 21.10. Rhabdomyosarcoma of the prostate; operation specimen of a dense whitish tumour with an ill-defined edge infiltrating the posterior urethra.

DIAGNOSIS

A prostatic abscess is the only benign lesion which might simulate these findings; it is extremely rare, and less common than a sarcoma.

The passage of a catheter may be very difficult or even impossible, but urethrography, retrograde or antegrade *via* a suprapubic needle, will demonstrate posterior displacement and elongation of the urethra, and upward displacement of the bladder (Fig. 21.11).

Biopsy. A needle or drill biopsy through the perineum, guided by a finger in the rectum, will provide material for histological diagnosis. Chemotherapy to cover the biopsy is usually employed (p. 109).

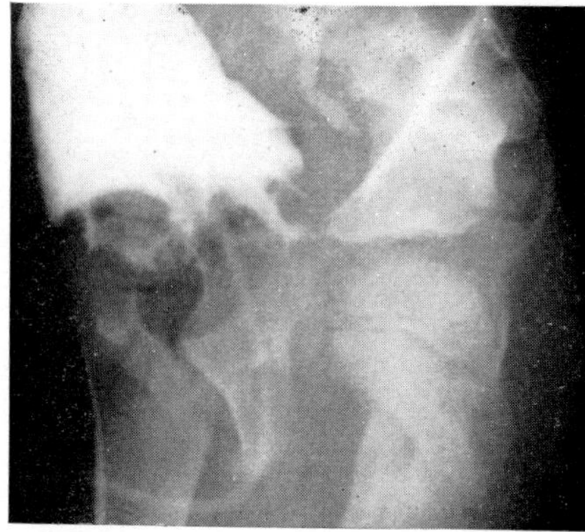

Figure 21.11. RHABDOMYOSARCOMA OF THE PROSTATE; elongation and upward displacement of the urethra, the typical radiographic appearance in a lateral view of a cystogram.

TREATMENT

Radical excision combined with chemotherapy and radiotherapy (p. 789) offers the best prospect of cure. The excision is the same as described for rhabdomyosarcoma of the bladder (p. 705) with the addition of complete removal of the entire urethra.

PROGNOSIS

In the past the outlook appears to have been worse when the tumour arose in the prostate, but the better survival rates now obtained (p. 792) offer a better outlook (Tefft & Jaffe, 1973).

In four of the eight patients in the Index Series, the treatment outlined above was employed, and all four are survivors, three of them for 3 years so far.

D. RETROPERITONEAL TUMOURS IN THE PELVIS

The most common tumours in this site, neuroblastomas (p. 538) and ganglioneuromas (p. 550) are described in Chapter 18.

PELVIC NEUROBLASTOMA

Neuroblastomas arising on the lateral wall of the pelvis or in the presacral region often contain areas of differentiation to ganglioneuroma; they rarely produce metastases, and have no tendency to extend into the neural canal.

The mode of presentation is usually urinary obstruction (with strangury and retention or urine), rectal symptoms (constipation, colic), or a mass in the iliac fossa, emerging from the pelvis and/or palpable on rectal examination.

The differential diagnosis includes rhabdomyosarcoma (of the prostate, bladder or other pelvic tissues) and intra-pelvic teratoma (p. 717) which may be benign or malignant. Each of these tumours can produce the same signs and symptoms as a pelvic neuroblastoma, and differentiation ultimately depends upon biopsy and histological evidence.

Surgical excision of a pelvic neuroblastoma is often incomplete and only indicated, in general, when there is urinary or rectal obstruction which demand relief. In the absence of significant obstruction, frequent reassessment of the size of the tumour, clinically and radiologically, may be all that is required.

Chemotherapy (p. 558) *and radiotherapy* (p. 559) are undesirable in infants, and may be omitted in Stage I and in Stage IV–S. In children who present

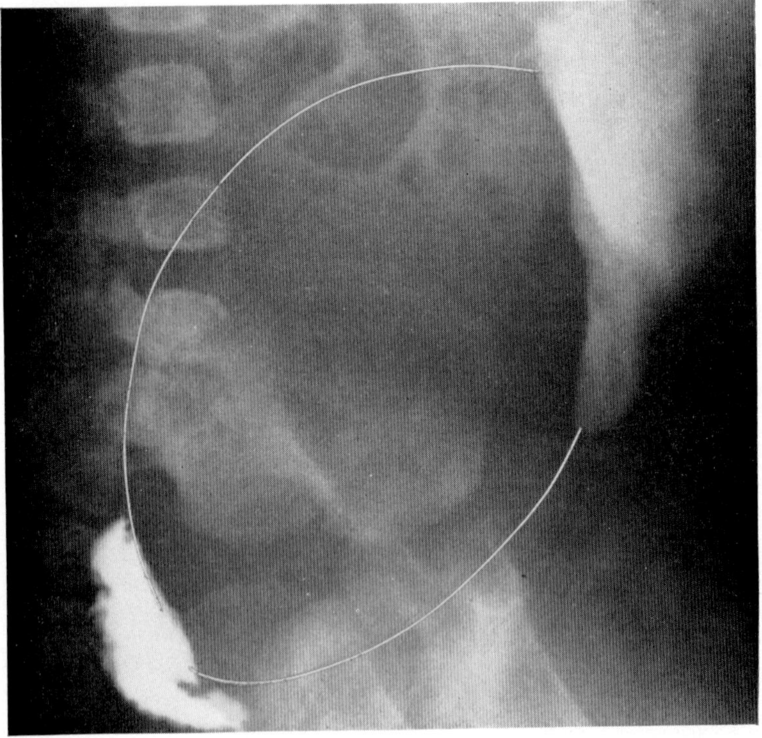

Figure 21.12. RETROPERITONEAL SARCOMA; an undifferentiated embryonic sarcoma; lateral view with the tumour outlined by simultaneous injections of contrast material into the bladder and rectum.

after the age of 2 years, adjuvant therapy is indicated before surgery and when there is extensive residual tumour after attempted excision.

The prognosis of pelvic neuroblastoma is unusually good (p. 561), chiefly due to the high proportion which undergo maturation or completely disappear (p. 539), as noted by Ghazali (1974) and supported by long-term (mean 113 months) survival in all 3 of the pelvic examples in the Index Series (p. 561) and in 3 of the 4 additional cases seen more recently.

There have been isolated case reports of other retroperitoneal tumours in the pelvis, e.g.

lymphosarcoma	leiomyosarcoma
liposarcoma	fibrosarcoma, and
malignant paraganglioma	undifferentiated retroperitoneal teratoma.

In the Index Series there were four such patients (undifferentiated sarcoma, fibrosarcoma, lymphosarcoma and leiomyosarcoma); all presented with lower abdominal pain and a palpable mass (Fig. 21.12), but without dysuria. All are dead, but in only one was radical excision attempted.

CHORDOMA

A chordoma is a malignant neoplasm arising from remnants of the notochord and is usually contiguous with the vertebrae or sacrum, causing erosion and destruction of bone (Fig. 13.22, p. 289).

This tumour can present anywhere along the spinal axis from the occiput to the coccyx. In children it is very rare and in the Index Series the few examples seen arose towards the upper end of the vertebral column; only one arose in the pelvis (Kamrin *et al.*, 1964).

E. SACROCOCCYGEAL TUMOURS

The great majority are benign, but a few are malignant, either *ab initio* or as the result of malignant transformation in a predominantly benign lesion (Lemire, Graham & Beckwith, 1971; Mahour *et al.*, 1975).

SITE

Most benign teratomas in this region are conspicuous or at least obvious at birth, usually as a massive tumour with its attachment lying between the coccyx and the anus (Fig. 21.13). The anus is often displaced forwards, and the surface of the mass is sometimes ulcerated.

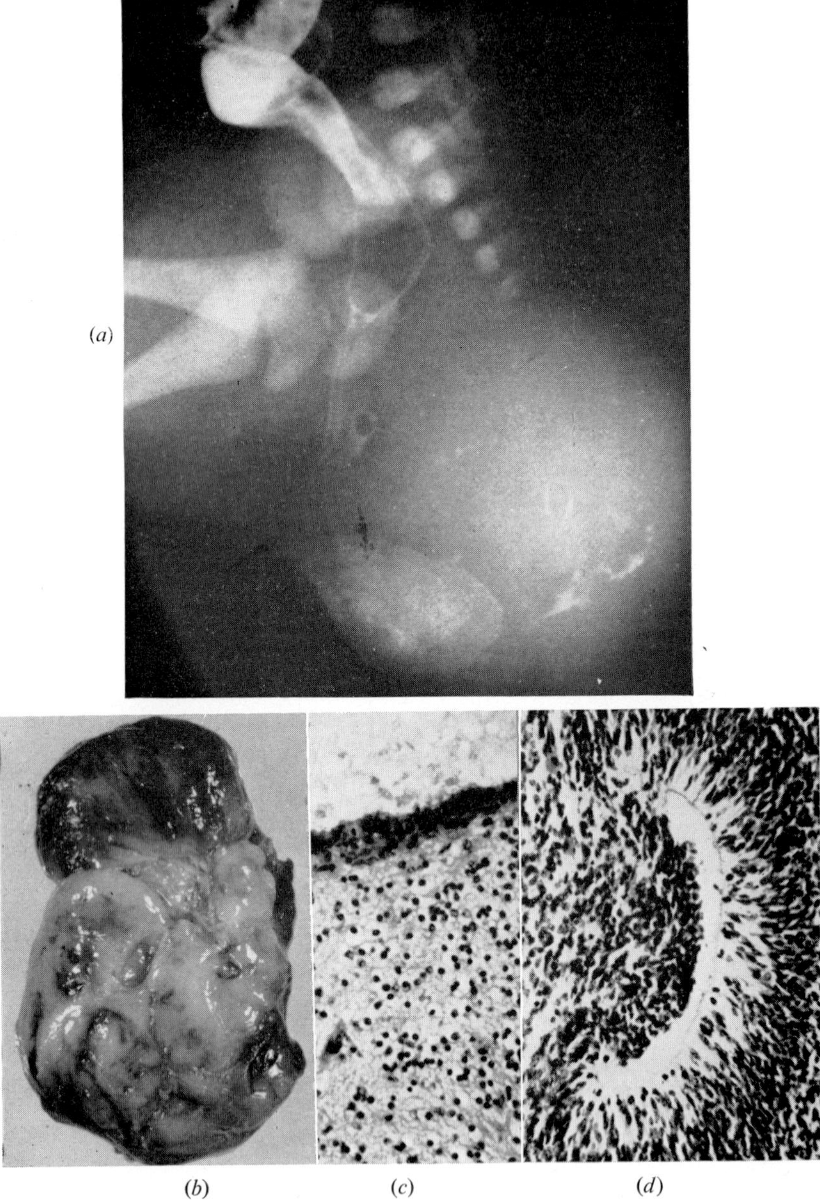

(a)

(b) (c) (d)

Figure 21.13. SACROCOCCYGEAL TERATOMA; (*a*) lateral x-rays of a large lesion containing flecks of calcification, showing a small intrapelvic extension outlined by contrast material in the rectum; (*b*) misleading sinister appearance of a solid teratoma composed of soft, grey diffluent tissue, composed of (*c*) immature but regular glial tissue beneath respiratory epithelium (H & E. × 130); (*d*) a primitive optic vesicle developing in a mass of neuroglial tissue (H & E. × 100). This tumour also contained many other differentiated epithelial and mesenchymal tissues, and proved to be completely benign.

SEX

Teratomas in the sacrococcygeal area (see teratomas, p. 45) are much more common in females, the usual ratio being 3 or 4 : 1.

AGE

There is a correlation between the age at the time of operation and the incidence of malignancy. Those removed before the age of one month are predominantly benign, while those removed later are variously reported to be malignant in from 25–66% of cases (Johnston, 1968; Izant, 1969; Chretien *et al.*, 1970).

Not the age of the patient but the size of the teratoma may be the determining factor; large masses, being obvious (and usually benign), are removed without delay, whereas small lesions not visible at birth may grow quite rapidly and first become clinically apparent at the age of one to four months. It is the latter group which may be malignant *ab initio*, and which also tend to arise on the *anterior* surface of the coccyx, where they may remain undetected until large enough to produce symptoms from pressure on the bladder, the rectum or less commonly the pelvic nerves.

HISTOGENESIS

The probable origin of extragonadal teratomas from a somatic or displaced germ cell which fails to undergo meiosis and proceeds directly to mitosis has been demonstrated by Lindner *et al.* (1975b). The different origin of gonadal teratomas is mentioned on p. 47.

I. BENIGN SACROCOCCYGEAL TERATOMAS

In most cases there is no intrapelvic extension and hence no interference with the function of bowel or bladder (Lemire *et al.* 1971), nor neurological signs. Occasionally there is a contiguous myelomeningocele; in some 10% of sacrococcygeal teratomas there is an associated but not necessarily significant sacral anomaly.

MACROSCOPIC APPEARANCES

They are usually large, up to 20 cm in diameter, and on section they contain masses of cysts separated by trabeculae which are usually soft, congested, rather mucoid in texture, and of variable thickness. Large masses of soft, grey diffluent tissue are often present, as well as sebaceous material, hair, dental derivatives and bone (Fig. 21.13).

MICROSCOPIC FINDINGS

The mass is composed of loose embryonal connective tissue in which are embedded epithelial structures in various stages of maturation, large areas of glial tissue, and usually cartilage and bone. An extraordinary degree of differentiation is sometimes found, for example intestinal structures complete with a smooth muscle coat and autonomic ganglion cells, or primitive retinal structures (Fig. 21.13d).

In most of the malignant examples no teratomatous elements are to be found even after a careful search. Their origin is still in dispute, but it now appears that the histology of the malignant areas is so similar to the endodermal sinus tumour (see p. 692), that this indicates their origin from germ cells, and this would favour the concept that the malignant tissues represent unilateral development of one of the elements of a teratoma (p. 717). This is also supported by the occasional instances in which derivatives of other than the ectodermal layer are found adjacent to malignant tissue.

INVESTIGATIONS

Plain radiographs of the mass show calcified structures in some 50% of cases, and when recognizable this will assist in diagnosis.

Micturating cysto-urethrograms, and occasionally intravenous pyelograms, are necessary to exclude intrapelvic extensions (Hendren & Henderson, 1970).

DIFFERENTIATION FROM OTHER SACRAL CONDITIONS

Although the clinical features of a teratoma are usually typical, several other conditions may need to be excluded.

1. *Meningocele and meningomyelocele.* Occasionally these coexist with, or as part of, a teratomatous mass; as the anus may appear to be flaccid and pouting in a simple benign teratoma, careful neurological examination of the limbs and the perineal skin reflex is required to exclude a neurological deficit due to a meningomyelocele. It has been suggested that pressure on the sac of a spina bifida cystica may produce a detectable bulge in the fontanelle, whereas it does not if the mass is a sacrococcygeal teratoma.
2. *Cystic lymphangiomas and haemangiomas*, although uncommon in this region, could produce similar findings. Radiographs showing calcification would probably exclude them, but if negative, an angiomatous mass can only be distinguished from a teratoma during excision.
3. *Cystic duplications of the colon*, if retrorectal, could also be difficult to exclude, except for the absence of calcification.
4. *Other tumours*, e.g. a neuroblastoma or ganglioneuroma, might also present very similar features, but usually arise higher in the pelvis. Chordomas

(see p. 711) are extremely rare in childhood particularly in infancy and are usually accompanied by radiological evidence of bone destruction.

TREATMENT

In most cases the mass is largely superficial and can be removed through a transverse perineal incision, excising the coccyx *in toto*, ligating the median sacral artery at an early stage in the dissection, as this may be the chief source of arterial supply to the teratoma.

If rectal and abdominal examination or radiographs indicate that there is an intra-pelvic extension of the mass, the first step should be laparotomy to identify and dissect free the intra-abdominal portion before commencing the perineal part of the operation (Hendren & Henderson, 1970).

The Index Series of 40 sacrococcygeal teratomas, 34 were benign histologically and two of these were associated with a sacral myelomeningocele. All were removed without special difficulty and all 34 patients are alive and well.

II. MALIGNANT SACROCOCCYGEAL TERATOMA

Almost all large series of sacroccygeal teratomas contain malignant examples (Vaez-Zadek *et al.*, 1972) which comprise some 10–30% of the whole group (Fig. 21.14).

CLINICAL FEATURES

In most cases of malignant teratoma, the tumour is first discovered when the patient is more than 2 months of age, but as mentioned on p. 713, this may be a reflection of the inherent nature of the tumour and not related to age *per se*. Gross *et al.* (1951) pointed out that there was a special category of teratoma which only became apparent later in infancy, and of those first discovered in infants 4–6 months of age, at least 50% are likely to be malignant. Izant (1969) reported that of those excised before the age of 1 month, the proportion which proved to be malignant was 18%, whereas in those excised *after* one month of age, the figure was 40%.

MICROSCOPIC FINDINGS

In malignant sacrococcygeal tumours the histological pattern in some ways resembles the choroid plexus of the cerebral ventricles (Chretien *et al.*, 1970) and these tumours may arise from choroid-like elements of neuroglial tissue. However, it is now believed that this tumour is of germ cell origin, i.e. a 'yolk-sac' or endodermal sinus tumour (Teilum, 1959), similar to those found

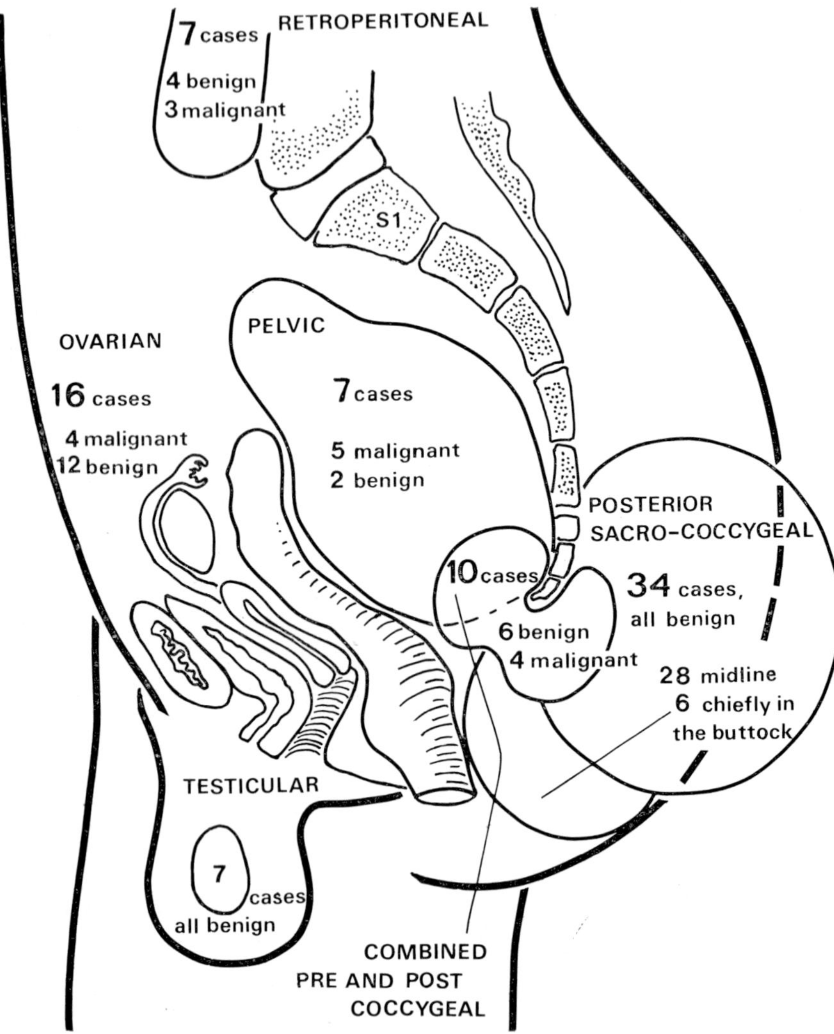

Figure 21.14. TERATOMAS; distribution of 81 subdiaphragmatic teratomas in a total of 107 cases reviewed at the Royal Alexandra Hospital for Children, Institute of Pathology, Sydney (1946 to October, 1974). All completely posterior examples were benign, while those combining pre- and post-coccygeal components, and those entirely intrapelvic, contain a progressively higher proportion of malignant teratomas (redrawn from 'Teratomas in Childhood', *Pathology* (1975) with the permission of the authors (Bale, P.M., Painter, D.M. & Cohen, D.H.) and the Editor of *Pathology*).

in the ovary, testes, mediastinum, brain and other sites (p. 45). They consist of masses of cells in a delicate fibrovascular stroma (Fig. 21.3) which project into spaces containing acid mucopolysaccharide and mucus. The tumour cells have vesicular nuclei, abundant cytoplasm, but despite their often benign appearance, mitotic figures are quite numerous and the outlook is uniformly bad. Usually, no element other than the embryonal carcinoma or yolk-sac pattern occurs in these neoplasms, and it is uncommon to find contiguous differentiated teratomatous elements (although they were present in one of the Index Series).

SPREAD

Extensive local infiltration tends to occur; more distant spread is *via* the bloodstream to the lungs, and to a variable extent *via* lymphatic channels to the para-aortic nodes.

PRESACRAL TERATOMAS

Most sacrococcygeal teratomas are visible at birth, but a proportion of them, as high as 15% in some series (Vaez-Zadeh *et al.*, 1972), arise internally on the anterior aspect of the sacrum, and present with symptoms of dysuria or a perineal swelling only later in infancy. Both presacral and the usual posterior teratomas are several times more common in females than in males; those first presenting after the age of 6 months are almost invariably malignant (Ghazali, 1973; Altman *et al.*, 1974; Mahour *et al.*, 1974).

From several reported series of pelvic teratomas (e.g. Fig. 20.14) there appears to be some correlation between the proportion of malignant examples and the site of origin. The proportion is least in those which are entirely retrococcygeal, and highest in the presacral group; all 9 of the presacral examples reported by Ghazali (1973) were malignant. However, a notable exception to this general tendency is the hereditary type of presacral teratoma. Ashcraft and Holder (1974) collected from 6 kindreds 17 such cases, of which only one was malignant.

DIAGNOSIS

In those without a teratoid mass visible at birth, there may still be a local abnormality (Scobie, 1971) indicative of a malformation, e.g. asymmetry of the buttocks, an overlong or curving natal cleft, or a deep paramedian retrococcygeal skin pit.

In such cases a rectal examination and careful palpation of the anterior aspect of the coccyx and sacrum may reveal a small swelling, and if present this should be explored. More often the diagnosis is only made when a visible swelling has gradually appeared or when symptoms arise from pressure on the bladder, the rectum, or the pelvic nerves (McDonald, 1973).

X-rays of the sacrum and coccyx may on occasions show destruction of bone which is always ominous, and only rarely is there any calcification in a malignant teratoma. Intrapelvic extensions should be identified or excluded by micturating cysto-urethrography, and may present considerable technical difficulties in their removal (Hendren & Henderson, 1970).

TREATMENT

Apart from the small initial size of the tumour, and the late presentation or late appearance of a swelling, there is little to distinguish malignant from benign teratomas (Donnellan & Swenson, 1968). When a malignant tumour is suspected, surgical exploration should probably be covered by cytotoxic drugs (p. 109), although the reported experience is not sufficiently extensive to prove their benefits.

A wide excision is necessary, if possible *en bloc* and clear of the abnormal tissue by as much margin as possible.

Post-operative chemotherapy and radiotherapy are also worth trying, but the prognosis is uniformly poor.

In the Index Series there were six examples of a malignant teratoma and four of the six were more than 12 months old when they presented. In the other two, the swelling had been present at birth but quite small; in one of these excision was not performed until the age of 6 months, by which time pulmonary metastases were present. Both the primary and the pulmonary metastasis contained well-differentiated ectodermal derivatives, but also areas of the papillary embryonic carcinoma now referred to as an endodermal sinus tumour (p. 692).

The outcome was uniformly bad; three of the six died within 6 months of diagnosis; one survived until 7 years of age, and the remaining two are alive but both have pulmonary metastases.

PROGNOSIS

As outlined above, adverse prognostic factors can be summarized as follows:

1. *Age*: Those more than one month old when the tumour is diagnosed.
2. *Size:* Small lesions, especially those not visible at birth, which grow rapidly.
3. *Site*: Those in which most or all of the mass in intrapelvic.
4. *Radiographic evidence or erosion* of the coccyx or sacrum.
5. *Absence of teratomatous elements*, as demonstrated histologically.
6. *The 'choroid plexus' pattern of embryonic carcinoma*, i.e. an endodermal sinus tumour.
7. *Recurrence* after initial excision.

REFERENCES

Ovarian Tumours

AHMED, S. (1971). Neonatal and childhood ovarian cysts. *J. Pediat. Surg.*, **6** : 702.

CAMPBELL, P.E. & DANKS, D.M. (1963). Pseudoprecocity in an infant due to a luteoma of the ovary. *Arch. Dis. Childh.*, **38** : 519.

EIN, S.H. (1973). Malignant ovarian tumours in children. *J. Pediat. Surg.*, **8** : 539.

EIN, S.H., DARTE, J.M.M. & STEPHENS, C.A. (1970). Cystic and solid ovarian tumours in children: a 44 year review. *J. Pediat. Surg.*, **5** : 148.

FORSHALL, I. (1960). Ovarian neoplasms in children. *Arch. Dis. Childh.*, **35** : 17.

FOX, H., AGRAWAL, K. & LANGLEY, F.A. (1975). A clinicopathologic study of 92 cases of granulosa-cell tumor of the ovary with special reference to the factors influencing prognosis. *Cancer*, **35** : 231.

GARFINKEL, B. & ROSENTHAL, A.H. (1962). Teratomas and follicular cysts of the ovary in children. *Am. J. Obst. & Gynec.*, **83** : 101.

HARRIS, B.H. & BOLES, E.T.Jr. (1974). Rational surgery for tumors of the ovary in children. *J. Pediat. Surg.*, **9** : 289.

HUNTINGTON, R.W. & BULLOCK, W.K. (1970). Yolk sac tumours of the ovary. *Cancer*, **25** : 1357.

LINDNER, D., MCCAW, B.K. & HECHT, F. (1975a). Parthenogenic origin of benign ovarian teratomas. *New Eng. J. Med.*, **292** : 63.

MULVIHILL, J.J., WADE, W.M. & MILLER, R.W. (1975). Gonadoblastoma in dysgenetic gonads with a Y chromosome. *Lancet*, **1** : 863.

NORRIS, H.J. & JENSEN, R.D. (1972). Relative frequency of ovarian neoplasms in children and adolescents. *Cancer*, **30** : 713.

NORRIS, H.J. & TAYLOR, H.B. (1969). Virilization associated with cystic granulosa tumours. *Obstet. & Gynec.*, **34** : 629.

SCHELLHAS, H.F. (1974). Malignant potential of the dysgenetic gonad. *Obstet. Gynce.*, **44** : 298, 455.

SCULLY, R.E. (1964). Stromal luteoma of the ovary. A distinctive type of lipoid-cell tumor. *Cancer*, **17** : 769.

SCULLY, R.E. (1970). Gonadoblastoma: a review of 74 cases. *Cancer*, **25** : 1340.

SMITH, J.P., RUTLEDGE, F. & WHARTON, J.T. (1972). Chemotherapy of ovarian cancer: New approaches to treatment. *Cancer*, **30** : 1565.

SMITH, J.P., RUTLEDGE, F. & SUTOW, W.W. (1973). Malignant gynecological tumors of children: current approaches to treatment. *Amer. J. Obstet. Gynec.*, **116** : 261.

TALERMAN, A. (1972). A distinctive gonadal neoplasm related to gonadoblastoma. *Cancer*, **30** : 1219.

TEILUM, G. (1959). Endodermal sinus tumor of the ovary and testis etc. *Cancer*, **12** : 1092.

TETER, J., PHILIP, J. & WECEWICZ, G. (1964). Mixed gonadal dysgenesis with gonadoblastoma *in situ*. *Amer. J. Obstet. Gynec.*, **90** : 929.

Tumours of Uterus and Fallopian Tube

FAWCETT, K.J., DOCKERTY, M.B. & HUNT, A.B. (1966). Mesonephric carcinoma and adenocarcinoma of the cervix in children. *J. Pediat.*, **69** : 104.

HUFFMAN, J.W. (1968). *The Gynecology of Childhood and Adolescence*. Saunders, Philadelphia.

WILLIS, R.A. (1962). *Pathology of Tumors in Childhood.* Thomas, Springfield.

Tumours of the Vagina

ANNOTATION (1974). Vaginal adenocarcinoma and maternal oestrogen ingestion. *Lancet*, **1** : 250.

Droegmueller, W., Makowski, E.L. & Taylor, E.S. (1970). Vaginal mesonephric adenocarcinoma in two prepuberal children. *Am. J. Dis. Child.*, **119** : 168.

Ghavimi, F., Exelby, P.R., D'Angio, G.J. *et al.* (1973). Combination chemotherapy of urogenital embryonal rhabdomyosarcoma in children. *Cancer*, **32** : 1178.

Herbst, A.L., Ulfelder, H. & Poskanzer, D.C. (1971). Adenocarcinoma of the vagina: association of maternal stilboestrol therapy with tumor appearance in young women. *New Engl. J. Med.*, **284** : 878.

Horn, R.C. & Enterline, N.T. (1958). Rhabdomyosarcoma: a clinicopathological study and classification of 39 cases. *Cancer*, **11** : 181.

Janovski, N.A. & Kasdon, E.J. (1963). Benign mesonephric papillary and polypoid tumours of the cervix in childhood. *J. Pediat.*, **63** : 211.

Norris, H.J., Bagley, G.P. & Taylor, H.B. (1970). Carcinoma of the infant vagina; a distinctive tumor. *Arch. Path.*, **90** : 473.

Pollack, R.S. & Taylor, H.C. (1947). Carcinoma of the cervix during the first two decades of life. *Am. J. Obstet. Gynec.*, **53** : 135.

Shachman, R. (1950). Sarcoma botryoides of the genital tract in female children. *Brit. J. Surg.*, **38** : 26.

Siegel, H.A., Sagerman, R. *et al.* (1970). Mesonephric adenocarcinoma of the vagina in a 7 month old infant simulating sarcoma botryoides. *J. Pediat. Surg.*, **5** : 468.

Silverberg, S.G. & DeGiorgi, L.S. (1972). Clear cell carcinoma of the vagina. *Cancer*, **29** : 1680.

Vawter, G.F. (1965). Carcinoma of the vagina in infancy. *Cancer*, **18** : 1479.

Tumours of the Bladder and Prostate

Batsakis, J.G. (1963). Urogenital rhabdomyosarcoma: histogenesis and classification *J. Urol.*, **90** : 180.

Clatworthy, H.W.Jr., Braren, V. & Smith, J.P. (1973). Surgery of bladder and prostatic neoplasms in children. *Cancer*, **32** : 1157.

Ghazali, S. (1973). Embryonic rhabdomyosarcoma of the urogenital tract. *Brit. J. Surg.*, **60** : 124.

Jarman, W.D. & Kenealy, J.C. (1970). Polypoid rhabdomyosarcoma of the bladder in children. *J. Urol.*, **103** : 227.

Kilman, J.W., Clatworthy, H.W.Jr. *et al.* (1973). Reasonable surgery for rhabdomyosarcoma: a study of 67 cases. *Ann. Surg.*, **178** : 346.

Nelson, A.J. (1968). Embryonal rhabdomyosarcoma: report of 24 cases and study of the effectiveness of radiation treatment upon primary tumor. *Cancer*, **22** : 64.

Sarkar, K., Tolnai, G. & McKay, D.E. (1973). Embryonal rhabdomyosarcoma of the prostate. *Cancer*, **31** : 442.

Siegel, W.H. & Pincus, M.B. (1969). Epithelial bladder tumours in children. *J. Urol.*, **101** : 55.

Tefft, M. & Jaffe, N. (1973). Sarcoma of the bladder and prostate in children, etc. *Cancer*, **32** : 1161.

Wilbur, J.R., Sutow, W.W., Sullivan, M.P., Castro, J.R. & Taylor, H.G. (1971). Successful treatment of rhabdomyosarcoma with combination chemotherapy and radiotherapy. *Amer. Soc. of Clin. Oncology*, Chicago, April 7.

Williams, D.I. (ed.) (1968). *Paediatric Urology*. Butterworth, London.

Williams, D.I. & Schistad, G. (1964). Lower urinary tract tumours in children. *Brit. J. Urol.*, **36** : 51.

Chordomas

Kamrin, R.P., Potanos, J.N. & Pool, J.L. (1964). An evaluation of the diagnosis and treatment of chordoma. *J. Neurol. Neurosurg. & Psychiatry*, **27** : 157.

Sacrococcygeal Tumours

ALTMAN, R.P., RANDOLPH, J.G. & LILLY, J.R. (1974). Sacrococcygeal teratoma: American Academy of Pediatrics Surgical Section Survey, 1973. *J. Pediat. Surg.*, **9** : 389.

ASHCRAFT, K.W. & HOLDER, T.M. (1974). Hereditary presacral teratoma. *J. Pediat. Surg.*, **9** : 691.

BALE, P.M., PAINTER, D.M. & COHEN, D.H. (1975). Teratomas in Childhood. *Pathology*, **7** : 209.

CHRETIEN, P.B., MILAM, J.D., FOOTE, F.W. & MILLER, T.R. (1970). Embryonal adenocarcinomas (a type of malignant teratoma) of the sacrococcygeal region. Clinical and pathologic aspects of 21 cases. *Cancer*, **26** : 522.

DONNELLAN, W.A. & SWENSON, O. (1968). Benign and malignant sacrococcygeal teratomas. *Surgery*, **64** : 834.

GHAZALI, S. (1973). Presacral teratomas in children. *J. Pediat. Surg.*, **8** : 915.

GROSS, R.E., CLATWORTHY, H.W.Jr. & MEEKER, J.A. (1951). Sacrococcygeal teratomas in infants and children. *Surg. Gynec. Obstet.*, **92** : 341.

HENDREN, W.H. & HENDERSON, B.M. (1970). The surgical management of sacrococcygeal teratomas with intrapelvic extension. *Ann. Surg.*, **171** : 77.

IZANT, R.I. (1969). Sacrococcygeal teratomas. In *Pediatric Surgery*, vol. 1, p. 849. Year Book Medical Publishers, Chicago.

JOHNSTON, J.H. (1968). In *Paediatric Urology* (Williams, D.I., ed.). Butterworth, London.

LEMIRE, R.J., GRAHAM, C.B. & BECKWITH, J.B. (1971). Skin covered sacrococcygeal masses in infants and children. *J. Pediat.*, **79** : 948.

LINDNER, D., HECHT, F., MCCAW, B.K. & CAMPBELL, J.R. (1975b). Origin of extragonadal teratomas and endodermal sinus tumours. *Nature*, **254** : 597.

MCDONALD, P. (1973). Malignant sacrococcygeal teratoma: report of four cases. *Am. J. Roentgenol.*, **118** : 444.

MAHOUR, G.H., WOOLLEY, M.W. *et al.* (1975). Sacrococcygeal teratoma: a 33 year study. *J. Pediat. Surg.*, **10** : 183.

MAHOUR, G.H., WOOLLEY, M.M., TRIVEDI, S.N. & LANDING, B.H. (1974). Teratoma in infancy and childhood: experience with 81 cases. *Surgery*, **76** : 309.

SCOBIE, W.G. (1971). Malignant sacrococcygeal teratoma: problem in diagnosis. *Arch. Dis. Childh.*, **46** : 216.

VAEZ-ZADEH, K., SIEBER, W.K., SHERMAN, F.E. & KIESEWETTER, W.B. (1972). Sacrococcygeal teratoma in children. *J. Pediat. Surg.*, **7** : 152.

Chapter 22. Bone tumours

Table 22.1. Benign lesions and malignant tumours of bone

Benign conditions	Malignant tumours
Simple bone cyst	Primary tumours
Osteomyelitis — coccal	Ewing's sarcoma
Osteomyelitis — tuberculous	Osteosarcoma
Cortical defect	Fibrosarcoma (of bone)
Aneurysmal bone cyst	Reticulum cell sarcoma (of bone)
Osteoid osteoma	Chondrosarcoma
Exuberant callus	Parosteal osteosarcoma
Incomplete (hairline) fracture	Haemangiosarcoma
Osteochondroma	Chordoma (p. 289)
Chondromyxoid fibroma	
Congenital fibromatosis	
Eosinophilic granuloma	Metastatic tumours
Calvarial lesions (p. 299)	Neuroblastoma
Osteoblastoma	Leukaemia
Chondroblastoma	Rhabdomyosarcoma
Haemangioma	Wilms' tumour
Melanotic progonoma (p. 334)	Malignant lymphomas
Fibro-osseous dysplasias (p. 331)	Carcinoma of thyroid
Intra-osseous lesions of the jaws (p. 323)	Retinoblastoma
Hyperparathyroidism (p. 383)	Histiocytosis X (p. 211)
Neurofibromatosis (p. 827)	Hand-Schüller-Christian syndrome
Hydatid disease of bone	Letterer-Siwe disease

Although the variety and sites of sarcomas of bone and soft tissues are many the range of presenting symptoms and signs is relatively small, i.e.:

1. Pain;
2. Swelling;
3. A pathological fracture;
4. A limp.

1. *Pain* is usually not always clearly localized, and is rarely severe in the early stages of a bone tumour; it is often intermittent and may have been recurring for some weeks when the patient first presents. Nocturnal pain has come to be particularly associated with bone lesions, while aches and pains

on commencing or after completing a period of vigorous activity suggest an origin in soft tissues.

2. *A swelling* is naturally the best guide to the site of a lesion, and may be obvious when the affected bone has little muscular investment; when the bone is more deeply situated it can be difficult to determine clinically whether the swelling has arisen in bone or in adjacent soft tissues.

3. *Fractures.* Incomplete ('hair-line') and greenstick fractures are not uncommon in childhood, and x-rays are essential not only for proper management, but also because the fracture may have occurred in an unsuspected area of pathological bone, a possibility which may also be suggested by the trivial nature of the injury.

On rare occasions a pathological fracture occurs as a result of a metabolic abnormality caused by a malignant tumour, without actual metastases at the site of the fracture. Both pancreatic carcinoma (p. 662) and hepatoblastoma (p. 602) have been reported as presenting in this way.

4. *A limp* unaccompanied by any complaint of pain or stiffness is not unusual in children. It is sometimes transient and of no significance, but may be the first sign of a variety of conditions including traumatic synovitis ('irritable hip' or 'observation hip'), Perthes disease and, sometimes, a bone tumour. A painless limp should always lead to a thorough general examination including careful palpation for oedema, induration, tenderness, or wasting of muscles, and to x-rays of the joint concerned to determine whether further investigations are indicated.

The symptoms discussed above, pain, swelling or a limp, lead to clinical examination and radiography including angiography, all of which play an important role in reaching the correct diagnosis. A check list of swellings affecting bone is shown in Table 22.1 and the Index Series of malignant bone tumours in Table 22.2.

Benign conditions are fortunately much more common; most of them share one or more of their presenting features with bone tumours, and although their benign nature is often apparent, their differentiation from malignant tumours is occasionally very difficult.

Table 22.2. Primary malignant bone tumours in the Index Series (RCH 1950–1972)

Ewing's tumour	24
Osteosarcoma	22
Fibrosarcoma	3
Reticulum cell sarcoma	2
Chordoma	4
Total	55

THE RADIOLOGY OF BONE LESIONS

This is the most informative initial investigation and may supply the definitive diagnosis, but even when the radiological findings strongly indicate a particular lesion, benign or malignant, they are not absolutely diagnostic, and a biopsy is almost always required.

High definition intensifying screens in the cassettes, or non-screen films, are desirable for they provide the greatest radiographic detail in bone. Varying the kilovoltage also allows more evidence to be obtained; by lowering it, more detail in the soft tissues appears, and by raising it, detail in dense bone can be seen more clearly.

Tomography may yield additional information when there are overlying loops of bowel or lung markings which interfere with interpretation.

Arteriography now plays an increasing role as a simple and safe means of obtaining additional information (see radiological findings, p. 741). Unfortunately, inflammatory lesions, especially osteomyelitis, because of their increased vascularity, often have arteriographic appearances similar to a neoplasm.

CLINICAL AND RADIOLOGICAL DIFFERENTIATION OF BENIGN LESIONS

The following benign conditions may need to be excluded in reaching the diagnosis of a malignant bone tumour.

1. Atypical osteomyelitis;
2. A 'sprain';
3. An incomplete ('hairline' or 'cortical') fracture of normal bone (e.g. the upper third of the tibia);
4. Simple bone cyst;
5. Osteoid osteoma;
6. Benign osteoblastoma;
7. Aneurysmal bone cyst;
8. Dysplasias of bone, e.g. cortical defect, fibrous dysplasia etc.;
9. Osteochondroma;
10. Tuberculous osteitis;
11. Hydatid disease of bone.

1. *Osteomyelitis.* The distinction can be made without difficulty when the findings are typical, i.e. with fever, leucocytosis, and especially the absence of any radiological changes in the affected bone for a week or more after the onset of symptoms. In bone tumours, abnormalities in x-rays are almost always already established when the patient first presents.

Difficulties in differentiation may arise in the following situations:

(*a*) *Atypical osteomyelitis*, subacute in onset with minimal constitutional symptoms and radiographic changes already established, or when the initial treatment with antibiotics has been tentative and inadequate in choice or dosage, the clinical signs and the radiological appearances may be confusing (Fig. 22.1). Rarefactive destruction or sclerotic changes, periosteal reaction and new bone formation due to infection, may closely resemble the changes seen in a malignant tumour such as Ewing's tumour or an osteosarcoma. However, the changes in osteomyelitis are generally rather circumscribed and the new bone is not of the 'sunray' type (p. 740).

(*b*) *In some cases of Ewing's tumour* there is fever, leucocytosis, extreme local tenderness and 'onion skin' layers of new bone formation. Even at exploration, material resembling pus may be released from the subperiosteal plane.

In both these situations serial x-rays may be helpful but can be equivocal, and a biopsy is more expeditious as the final court of appeal.

2. *A simple 'sprain'* is a rarity in children because their ligaments are usually stronger than the bones to which they are attached, and fractures are conse-

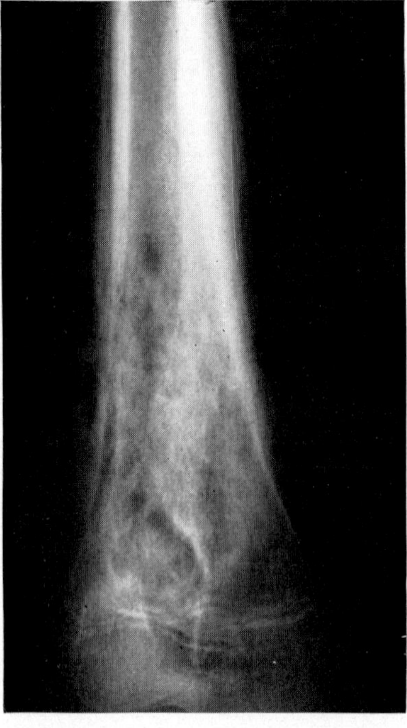

Figure 22.1. ATYPICAL OSTEOMYELITIS; lesion at the lower end of the femur, with rarefactive and destructive changes, and 'onion skin' layers of periosteal new bone. In such a lesion a tumour cannot be excluded on this evidence alone, and diagnosis rests on biopsy.

quently more likely to occur than sprains. Oedema and tenderness over a joint may be the first signs of a bone tumour, and when radiographic changes are minimal or absent, the real cause may only be suspected when resolution fails to occur after a period of rest, and further x-rays show that there has been progressive osteolysis.

3. *An incomplete (hairline) fracture* is often accompanied by pain, swelling, tenderness, and in some cases radiological evidence of periosteal new bone formation, all of which may indicate a tumour. The upper end of the tibia is a typical site for such a fracture (Fig. 22.2), and is also a common site for an osteosarcoma.

4. *A simple bone cyst*, typically in the diaphysis, often presents as a chronic ache, or with a shorter history of pain due to a pathological fracture. The radiographic findings are usually typical and diagnostic (Fig. 22.3), but if inconclusive, a biopsy yielding clear yellow fluid and a scanty lining containing a few osteoblasts and some multinucleated giant cells, is usually unmistakable (Neer, Francis *et al.*, 1966).

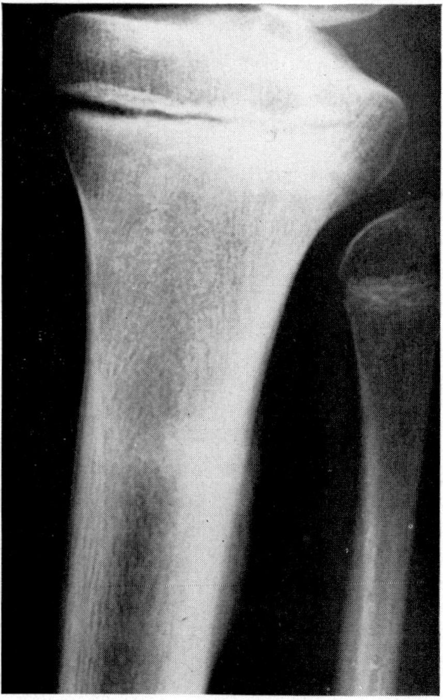

Figure 22.2. INCOMPLETE ('HAIRLINE' OR 'STRESS') FRACTURE in a typical site and level, in the upper end of the tibia; the 'fracture line' appears as an area of callus affecting one side of the bone, and an adjacent area of periosteal new bone.

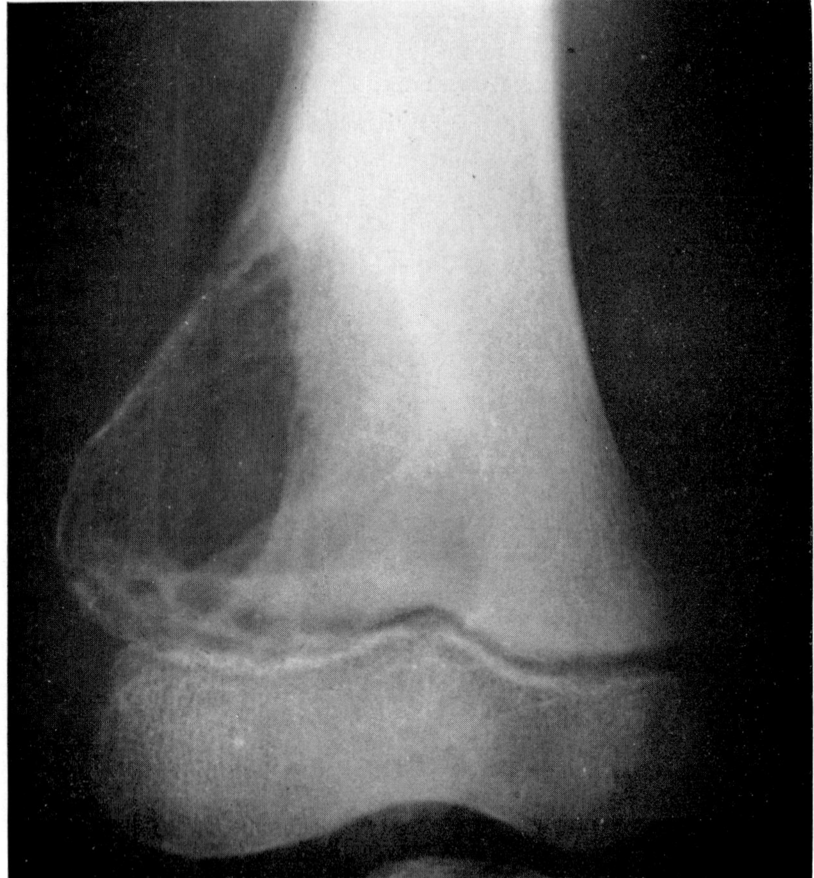

Figure 22.3. SIMPLE BONE CYST, typically in the metaphyseal region, with minimal expansion of the bone, and a trabecular texture.

5. *Osteoid osteoma.* The presenting feature is bone pain, usually intermittent, sometimes severe, and often wakens the patient at night. The extensive periosteal thickening may be palpable clinically, even in the deeply situated femur. The radiological findings (Fig. 22.4) are often diagnostic, i.e. dense new bone surrounding a centrally placed radiolucent nidus (Golding, 1954), but often difficult to interpret in unusual sites such as a vertebral body. In typical cases biopsy is not essential, but if there is any uncertainty, surgical excision, including the central nidus when possible, will provide material for biopsy as well as permanent and almost instant relief of pain (Dias & Frost, 1974).

6. *Benign osteoblastoma*, a rare lesion presenting chiefly in adolescents or in

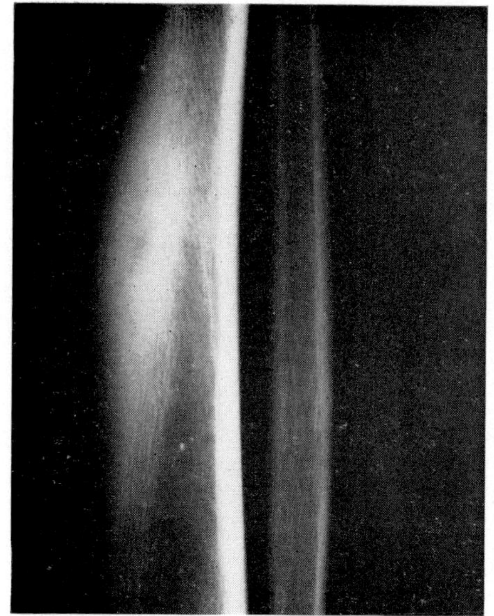
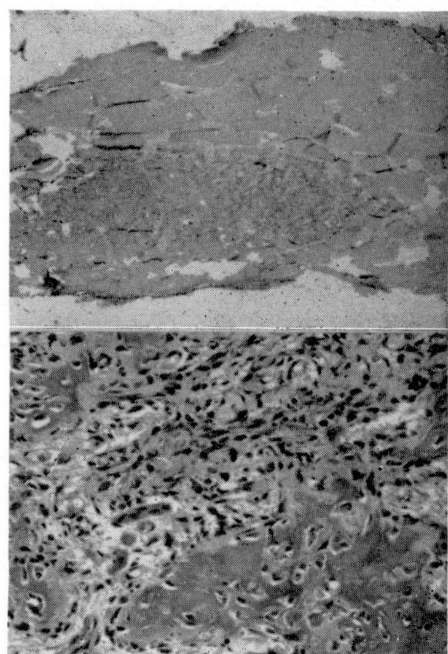

Figure 22.4. Osteoid osteoma; (*a*) dense, hypertrophic and sclerotic cortex with a small, central radiolucent nidus of decalcification; (*b*) low power view of the same nidus showing dense encircling cortical bone around an oval central mass of osteoid (H & E. × 30); (*c*) osteoid tissue in the nidus (H & E. × 530).

[(*a*) *Left*. (*b*) *Top right*. (*c*) *Bottom right*.

adults, has some of the features of osteoid osteoma, in that pain and a localized area of bone destruction with some new bone formation, are typical (Dahlin, 1967). More than half of the osteoblastomas of childhood arise in a vertebra, either in the body, or a transverse or spinous process (Marsh *et al.*, 1975).

X-rays show an area of destruction larger than the nidus of an osteoid osteoma, and within it a small area of bone formation (Fig. 22.5a). The histological findings are a highly vascular stroma containing large areas of osteoid tissue surrounded by numerous osteoblasts, some of which form giant cells (Fig. 22.5b).

The differential diagnosis includes osteoid osteoma (above), aneurysmal bone cyst (p. 730) and metastatic disease, but the site (when typical) and the radiological findings suggest the correct diagnosis, which should always be confirmed by biopsy.

Treatment is conservative in view of the benign nature of the condition, and even large examples can be cured by local excision when accessible, or by curettage. Depending on the site and extent of the lesion, a bone graft may also be required (e.g. in the cervical spine) to stabilize the weakened bone of origin.

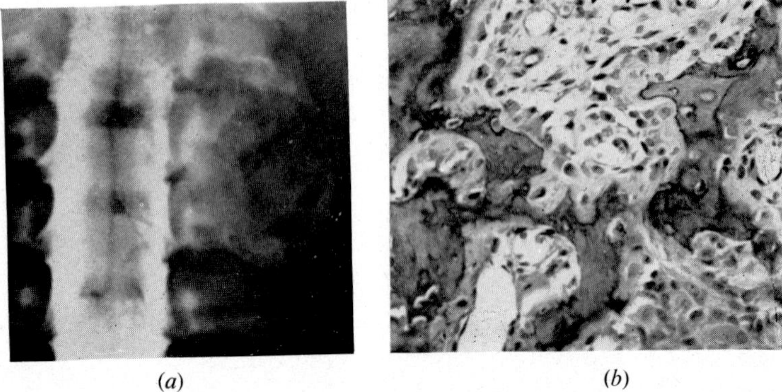

(a) (b)

Figure 22.5. BENIGN OSTEOBLASTOMA; (*a*) painful lesion arising in the transverse process of C3 and involving the adjacent processes; the myelogram shows no involvement of the theca; (*b*) biopsy showing masses of vascular osteoid tissue outlined by prominent osteoblasts, some forming giant cells, in a loose spindle-celled stroma (H & E. ×45).

7. *Aneurysmal bone cyst*. This also presents as a limp, pain or a pathological fracture (Godfrey & Gresham, 1959; Tillman, Dahlin *et al.*, 1968; Biesecker *et al.*, 1973). At an early stage it may resemble a simple bone cyst, and when aggressive and destructive, it can be indistinguishable on clinical grounds from a lytic type of osteosarcoma (Fig. 22.6). A trabeculated, cystic area expanding the bone is the main radiological feature. The high incidence of pathological fractures in the eggshell-thin bone, and the consequent periosteal new bone, may be confusing. However, the trabeculation is often typical and does not, in fact, occur in malignant bone tumours. Exploration reveals a very vascular 'sponge' with almost no solid elements, and a biopsy is found to be largely blood clot in which there are some thin-walled vessels and a few multinucleated osteoblasts (Lichtenstein, 1957).

8. *Dysplasias of bone*. Any of the several types can simulate a bone tumour (Harris *et al.*, 1962), (Fig. 22.8) and both radiological and histological data are often required to make the correct diagnosis, e.g. diffuse lesions affecting the jaws (p. 331).

A chondromyxoid fibroma (Ralph, 1962) can produce microscopic findings which may be difficult to interpret, but the radiographic appearances in no way suggest a tumour. The lesion is multicystic, eccentric, usually a short distance from the epiphyseal plate, and there is usually minimal or no expansion of the bone.

Cortical defects (Fig. 22.7a) and *congenital fibromatosis* (Fig. 22.7e) also have distinctive radiographic appearances (Selby, 1961).

9. *Osteochondroma*. This is one of the commonest benign bone lesions in children. Dominant inheritance with multiple lesions is described, but as a

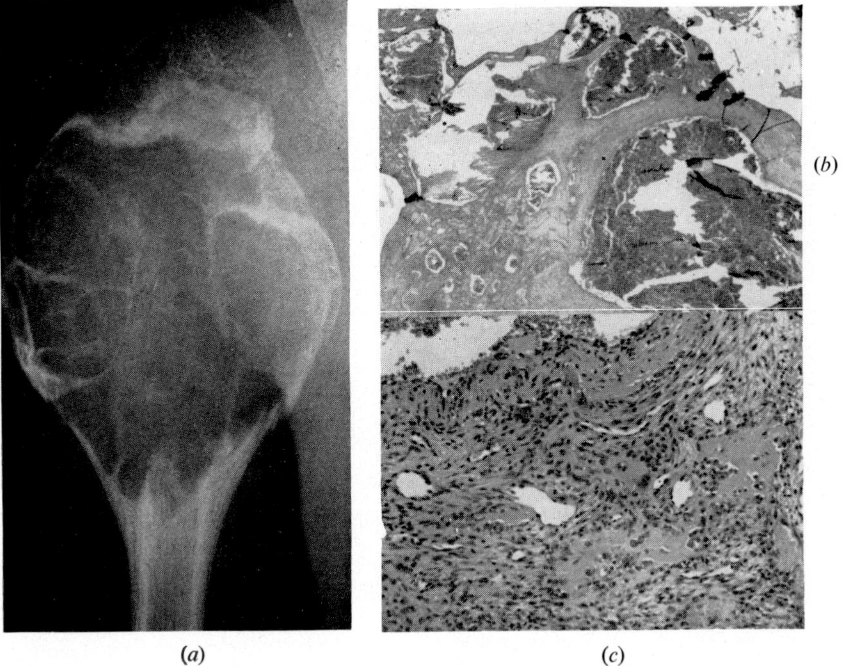

Figure 22.6. ANEURYSMAL BONE CYST; (*a*) a destructive multitrabecular lesion expanding the bone, thinning the cortex and causing a pathological fracture; (*b*) irregularly shaped vascular spaces, empty or filled with red cells; the walls are composed of sparsely cellular fibroblastic tissue (H & E. × 130); (*c*) detail showing fibroblastic stromal tissue forming the cyst walls. In this section some osteoid is being formed, a not infrequent finding (H & E. × 530).

rule the family history is negative and there is only one lesion, in the metaphysis, and most often at the upper end of the humerus or the lower end of the femur. Apparently sporadic cases may not all be examples of a new mutation, for an affected parent may have undetected small lesions only demonstrable by a complete radiological survey.

Symptoms may arise from pressure of soft tissues, nerves or vessels causing pain or limitation of movement, or simply the appearance of a swelling.

The lesion is composed of a base of cortical bone, with a cartilaginous cap which increases slowly in size until skeletal growth is complete. Very rarely the cartilage element undergoes chondrosarcomatous degeneration, and a sudden increase in growth rate and size may be the first evidence of this change.

X-rays show only the cortical base (Fig. 22.8a); the cartilaginous cap is radiolucent and may be considerably larger (Fig. 22.8b) with a smooth but

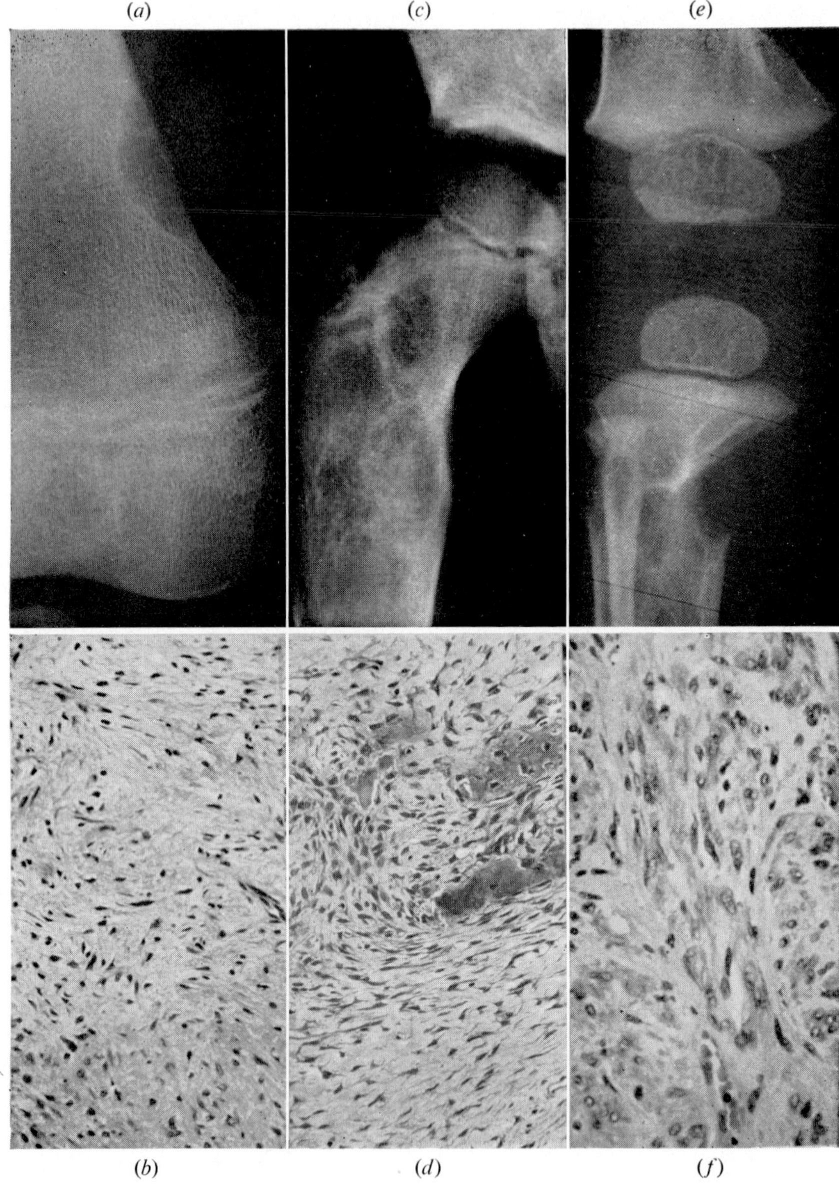

Figure 22.7. DYSPLASIAS; (*a*) FIBROUS CORTICAL DEFECT, usually single, in the commonest site: the posteromedial aspect of the lower end of the femur. The margin is well defined by minimal sclerosis, and there is no trabeculation; (*b*) bland, sparsely cellular fibroblastic tissue without any particular arrangement (H & E. × 70); (*c*) MONOSTOTIC FIBROUS DYSPLASIA, in the upper end of the femur. Scattered areas of irregular rarefaction, often expanding the bone, erode

the cortex from within; the epiphyseal plate is not involved. There are no radiological features which distinguish mono- from polyostotic dysplasia, nor the latter from the cystic osseous lesions of hyperparathyroidism; (*d*) more cellular tissue, in which irregular spicules of woven bone and osteoid are being formed (H & E. × 70); (*e*) CONGENITAL GENERALIZED (MULTIPLE) FIBROMATOSIS OF BONE; Typically this occurs in infants as multiple (often symmetrical) radiolucent areas in long bones (predominantly metaphyseal), enlargement of the bone ends but with loss of the overlying cortical bone weakening the bone, leading to deformity during weight-bearing. Lesions also occur in flat bones, in the calvarium (Fig. 14.4) and in soft tissues. If death from infection due to associated immune deficiency does not occur, the bone lesions can regress and may disappear; (*f*) more cellular than either of the other conditions and composed of plump fibroblasts arranged in ill-defined interlacing bundles (H & E. × 200).

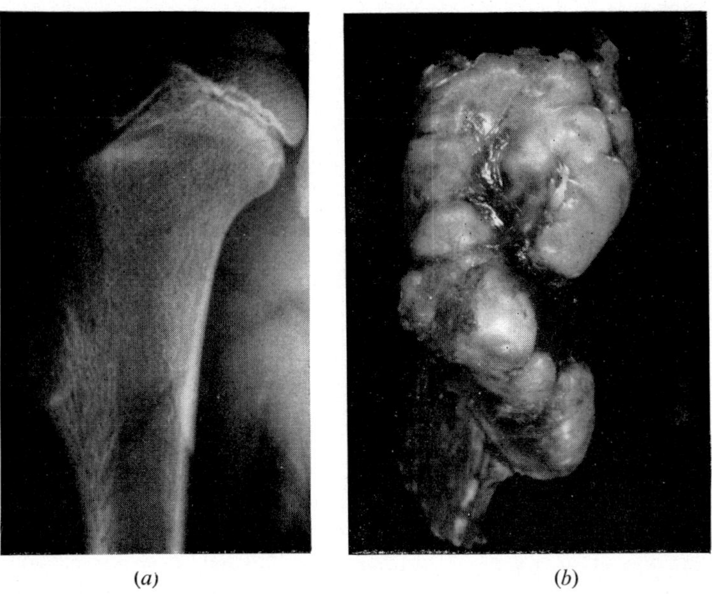

(*a*) (*b*)

Figure 22.8. OSTEOCHONDROMA; (*a*) the radiolucent caps of cartilage fails to appear in the x-ray, (*b*) but is palpable clinically and revealed at operation.

lobulated surface. Microscopically the chondrocytes show none of the characteristics of malignancy (p. 769).

Treatment is simple excision.

10. *Tuberculous osteitis* arises most commonly in the juxta-epiphyseal metaphysis. Constitutional symptoms, x-ray evidence of an active pulmonary lesion, and marked wasting of the muscles adjacent to the affected bone, out

of proportion to the duration and severity of the symptoms, are all typical of tuberculosis. The Mantoux test is usually helpful; in many cases the diagnosis can be made without a biopsy, but a synovial or lymph node biopsy may be necessary.

11. *Hydatid disease* in bone is extremely rare in children, even in communities where the disease is rife. It is only mentioned because in bone the lesions are quite unlike hydatid disease elsewhere; there is no discrete ectocyst and the resulting diffuse and destructive infiltration can resemble a malignant erosion (Fitzpatrick, 1965; Booz, 1972). Because the hydatid fluid is unconfined by a cyst wall, the Casoni and hydatid complement fixation tests are almost always positive. If unsuspected, or if the radiological picture is not recognized, the diagnosis can be made on biopsy.

PRIMARY MALIGNANT TUMOURS OF BONE

A complete list of bone tumours can be found in Table 22.1, and the tumours described here are as follows:

I. Ewing's tumour;
II. Osteosarcoma, p. 746;
III. Fibrosarcoma, p. 761;
IV. Reticulum cell sarcoma, p. 764;
V. Chondrosarcoma, p. 768;
VI. Histiocytosis X : Eosinophilic Granuloma, p. 206.

See also: chordoma, p. 288; and Tumours of the jaws, p. 326.

I. EWING'S TUMOUR
(syn. malignant endothelioma)

Ewing in 1921 described a round-celled non-osteogenic tumour and this was the most common bone tumour in the Index Series (Table 22.2).

Neuroblastomas are more common than Ewing's tumours in childhood, and because of their tendency to metastasize to bone, confusion between these two tumours can occur. However, neuroblastoma metastases in bone are a relatively uncommon presenting feature of this tumour (p. 551), and the age groups chiefly affected are also different, neuroblastoma being most common in children less than 5 years of age (p. 542).

AGE

Ewing's tumour (Fig. 22.9) usually arises in children between 5 and 15 years of age (Bhansali & Desai, 1963), only three of 24 patients in the Index Series were outside this age range (Table 22.3). Of 91 5-year survivors reviewed by

Falk & Alpert (1967), the youngest was 4 years old at diagnosis, and the average age was 18 years.

SITES

The diaphysis of a long bone is most commonly affected (Freeman, Sachatello *et al.*, 1972) chiefly the femur; less often a flat bone of the limb girdle (scapula, ilium), the vertebra (see p. 739) the ribs or small bones such as the os calcis or zygoma are affected.

The sites of the 24 Ewing's tumours in the Index Series are listed in Table 22.3.

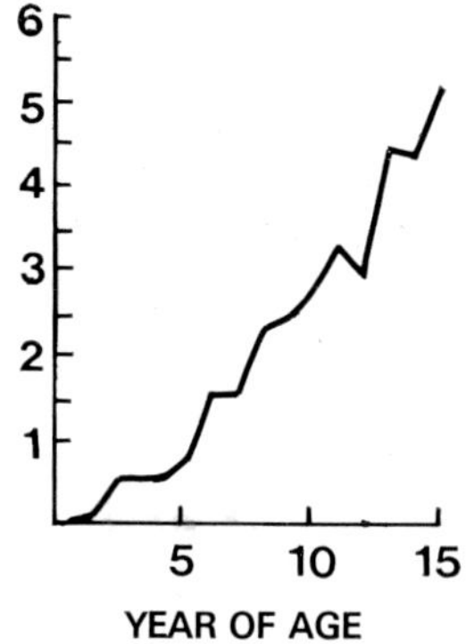

Figure 22.9. EWING'S TUMOUR; the incidence according to age. The tumour is rare before 5 years of age, but increases steadily throughout childhood and adolescence; the peak age incidence lies between 18 and 20 years of age (for source of figures, see Fig. 2.2, p. 48).

Table 22.3. Ewing's tumour, age at onset and site of 24 cases in the Index Series (RCH 1950–1972)

Age	No.	Sites	No.
0–5	3	Scapula	4
		Vertebrae	4
		Femur	4
5–10	9	Pelvis	3
		Orbit	2
		Humerus	2
10–15	12	Rib, tibia, os calcis Radius, ethmoid (1 each)	5
Total	24		24

MACROSCOPIC APPEARANCES

This tumour has a great tendency to infiltrate into adjacent soft tissues, and at biopsy the tumour is often found to have burst through the periosteum. The tumour is usually white, pale pink or grey, and soft, although quite tough where it is infiltrating fascia. Some are very haemorrhagic, producing purplish blood-stained fluid containing flocculent particles, in a cavity surrounding or adjoining the involved bone.

MICROSCOPIC FINDINGS

Paraffin sections reveal a very homogenous pattern of uniform, round or oval cells with delicate dust-like chromatin and a small or inconspicuous nucleolus. The cells may form diffuse sheets, but more characteristically lie in cords and strands in a fibrous connective tissue stroma, commonly in festoons around blood vessels (Fig. 22.10a). When these blood vessels are small, the cells around them may mimic the rosettes of a neuroblastoma, but the neurofibrillary material characteristic of neuroblastoma is absent. In several of the Ewing's tumours in the Index Series there were blood-filled lacunae with walls composed entirely of tumour cells so that the tumour appeared as a sheet of cells interspersed with vascular lakes of various sizes and shapes, and little stroma or supporting tissue (Fig. 22.10b).

New bone formation is very commonly found, but invariably beneath the periosteum, never in the soft tissue outside it. Subperiosteal new bone is soft, slightly gritty, and may erroneously suggest an osteosarcoma. New bone is never found in close relationship to tumour cells in Ewing's tumour.

The tumour cells have an affinity for PAS, but it is important to fix the tumour tissue soon after removal, because the glycogen which stains with PAS rapidly breaks down and is quite often negative in poorly prepared or post-mortem material.

The cells of Ewing's tumour are particularly delicate, easily distorted by manipulation, and require careful handling during biopsy (see p. 82) avoiding any crushing with forceps, ronguers, etc., which may make the material almost unrecognizable.

Touch preparations (Fig. 22.10d) of the surface of fresh material are of great value in many malignant neoplasms of childhood, and particularly valuable in Ewing's tumour (see Fig. 22.10, see colour plate following p. 170).

HISTOLOGICAL DIFFERENTIATION OF EWING'S TUMOUR

Certain features peculiar to the histology of bone tumours should be mentioned. The general appearances of a primary tumour are usually seen only by the operating surgeon; in most cases the pathologist receives a wedge of tissue or a drill biopsy. Although the limb may be subsequently amputated

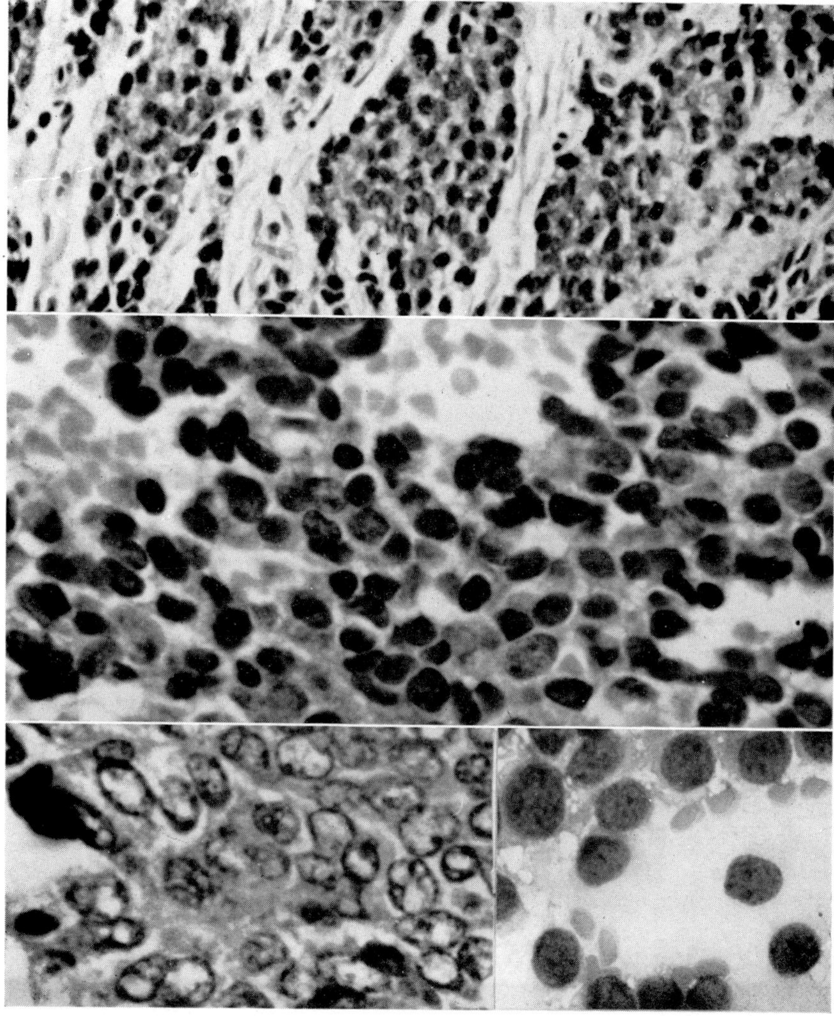

Figure 22.10. Ewing's Tumour; (*a*) infiltration outside the bone is very common, and here tumour cells are seen in cords infiltrating between strands of collagen (H & E. × 130); (*b*) the classical appearance, i.e. the nuclei are uniform and oval, and while some are dark, others have a delicate 'dusty' chromatin and one or two nucleoli. The cytoplasm is feathery, and vascular lakes (at top) appear to lack an endothelium (H & E. × 520); (*c*) a variant in which the nuclei are larger and appear to be vacuolated, probably the result of a fixation artefact (H & E. × 520); (*d*) imprint from cut surface showing nuclei with 'dusty' chromatin, each containing several very small nucleoli (H & E. × 520).

[(*a*) *Top.* (*b*) *Centre.* (*c*) *Bottom left.* (*d*) *Bottom right.*]

and submitted for examination, the tumour has usually been irradiated and the histological picture has considerably been altered by haemorrhage, necrosis or healing.

The diagnosis of a malignant bone tumour can almost always be made promptly if the soft part of the tumour, always present in an adequate biopsy, is carefully separated from the adjacent bone and processed without decalcification. The histological diagnosis can be confidently made within 24 hours, and it is rarely necessary to defer diagnosis until decalcified sections have been examined.

Imprint cytology (see p. 82)

This has proved to be particularly helpful in Ewing's tumour in which the delicate, spherical cells with abundant glycogen content (Fig. 22.11) are much more readily identified in this type of preparation.

Metastatic neuroblastoma and primary osteosarcoma are the two tumours most likely to be confused with Ewing's tumour in childhood. Neuroblastoma may be very difficult to exclude, especially if the material obtained or the histological preparations are inadequate. A careful search should be made for a latent primary neuroblastoma, and the level of MHMA excreted in the urine should always be determined in cases of Ewing's tumour.

An osteosarcoma is theoretically easy to identify, but the formation of reactive new bone in Ewing's tumour may be misinterpreted as indicating an osteosarcoma. Careful study shows that the cells of Ewing's tumour never grade into new bone, and that the new bone is quite obviously reactive, not neoplastic.

Reticulum cell sarcoma may be difficult to distinguish, except that in this tumour there is some variations in cell size, prominent nucleoli and the formation of reticulin.

Metastatic carcinoma is difficult to distinguish and causes confusion in adults, but not in children because of the extreme rarity of carcinomas.

SPREAD

This occurs quite rapidly in some cases, but late metastases are more characteristic of Ewing's tumour than other tumours of childhood.

Haematogenous spread to the lungs is most important, but there is a special tendency to metastasize to other bones. In one large series of 113 cases (Dahlin *et al.*, 1961), 20% developed fatal metastases more than 2 years after initial treatment.

MODE OF PRESENTATION

1. *A swelling* in or on a bone, with little or no pain, is the most common

mode; in some cases an incidental injury first draws attention to a pre-existing swelling.

2. *A history of stiffness and aching* after exercise, of some weeks duration, is common and often initially attributed to a strained muscle until a swelling is detected. Radiographic changes are usually well established when the patient presents; in long bones there is new bone formation, and penetration of the periosteum into the adjacent tissues is not uncommon.

3. *Progressive neural signs* culminating in paraplegia, occur in a small proportion of cases in which the tumour arises in a vertebra.

EWING'S TUMOUR OF THE SPINE

There is a distinctive type of Ewing's tumour which arises in the vertebrae, in a spinal or transverse process or a vertebral body, and invades the spinal canal producing compression of the spinal cord. The tumour is usually small and often almost entirely extradural, although it readily invades the dura itself. The attachment to, and origin in bone is often inconspicuous (see radiological features, p. 741). The tumour is white or pink, soft, lobulated and apparently encapsulated. Macroscopically it may be indistinguishable from a perispinal neuroblastoma (p. 556), but can be readily distinguished microscopically in sections stained with PAS; neuroblastoma cells are PAS negative while the cells of a Ewing's tumour are strongly positive (Fig. 22.11a, b, see colour plate, following p. 170).

INVESTIGATIONS

These are undertaken to confirm the diagnosis and to determine the extent of dissemination.

1. A full blood examination including the ESR.

2. Serum alkaline phosphatase; the level is a measure of active bone destruction or new bone formation. Serum electrophoresis has also been reported to show a characteristic prominence of IgM, β-lipoprotein and α_2-macroglobulin (Gupta, 1969) in Ewing's tumour.

3. Plain x-rays of the primary tumour provide excellent evidence of the diagnosis in as many as 90% cases.

Angiography, including selective arteriography, has been carefully assessed, and the findings reported in some detail (Yaghmai *et al.*, 1971), noting such features as neovasculature, hyperaemia, etc., which have been described as diagnostic in malignant bone tumours. However, many experienced radiologists have reluctantly come to the conclusion that while arteriography may be helpful in cases with atypical radiological findings, in general they have not added significantly to the information obtained from plain x-rays. Cases in which the radiological diagnosis proves to be the most difficult are those in which osteomyelitis is involved. The increased vascularity accompanying inflammatory lesions is very similar to the hyperaemia seen in vascular tumours, and may be difficult to distinguish by angiography.

4. X-rays of the lung fields, and a skeletal survey.

5. A spot test and a 24-hour specimen of urine for estimation of MHMA (p. 539) is also desirable because of possible confusion with metastatic neuroblastoma although tests for metabolites may be negative in 10–15% of cases of neuroblastoma (p. 551).

Radiological appearance of Ewing's tumour

In the shaft of a long bone the typical findings (Fig. 22.12a) are a combination of destruction and sclerosis surrounded by multiple laminae of periosteal new

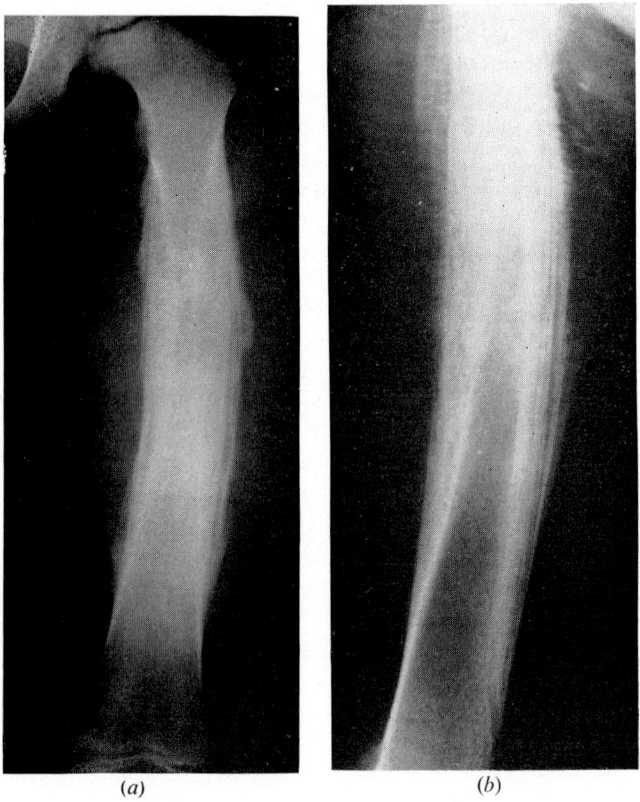

(*a*) (*b*)

Figure 22.12. Ewing's tumour; (*a*) gross thickening of the shaft of the femur, with 'onion-skin' layers of periosteal new bone predominating; (*b*) another example with both onion skin layers and 'sun ray' spiculations at right angles to the plane of the periosteum.

bone, i.e. 'onion skin' layers. When the tumour has broken through the periosteum, 'sunray' spiculation (Fig. 22.12b) is not infrequently seen.

When a Ewing's tumour arises in other sites, e.g. in bone forming the orbit, the scapula, ilium or zygoma, the radiological features are much less specific, and may be confined to erosion with minimal new bone formation. In some cases the tumour expands the bone and produces a 'soap bubble appearance, increased opacity throughout the affected area, and an increase in vascularity, as shown on angiography (Fig. 22.13).

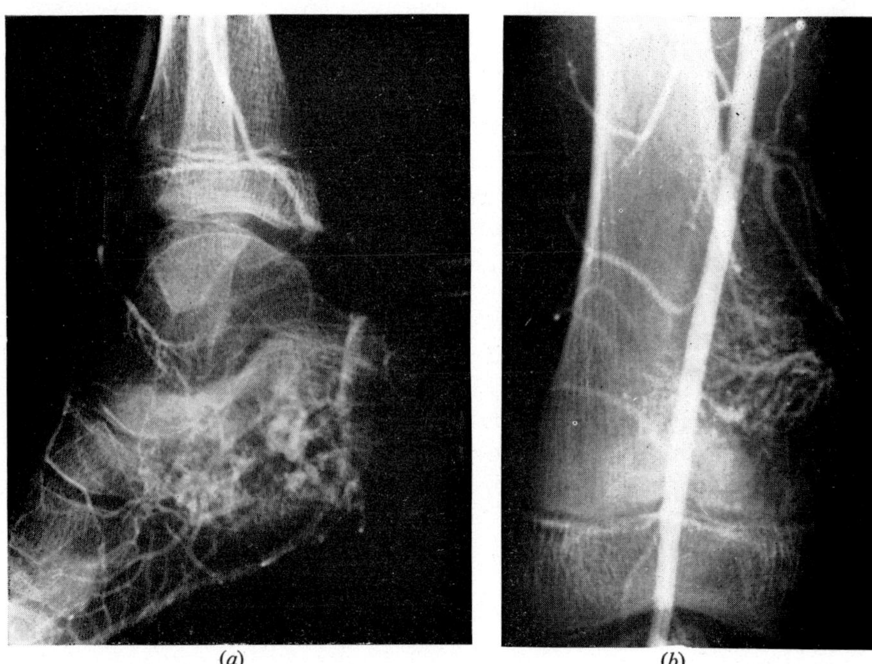

(*a*) (*b*)

Figure 22.13. ARTERIOGRAMS OF MALIGNANT BONE TUMOURS; (*a*) EWING'S TUMOUR arising in the os calcis, showing marked increase in vascularity, tumour vessels of irregular size, and vascular 'lakes', the typical features of a malignant bone tumour; (*b*) OSTEOSARCOMA of the lower end of the femur showing the same type of vascular features.

RADIOLOGICAL DIFFERENTIATION FROM OTHER MALIGNANT BONE TUMOURS

(*a*) **Primary bone tumours**

1. *Osteosarcoma*

The appearances vary greatly from one case to another, but destruction and new bone formation are always present, in varying proportions. There may be extensive or little or no reaction by the adjacent bone and periosteum. The periosteum is usually destroyed, with infiltration of adjacent soft tissues. Osteosarcomas usually arise in a somewhat older age group, close to the metaphysis of a long bone (Fig. 22.17), most frequently the upper end of the tibia and the lower end of the femur, at a period of rapid growth in height, and in patients above average height for their age.

2. *Fibrosarcoma*

The feature which distinguishes this tumour is the marked absence of any new bone formation (Fig. 22.20), either in the bone involved or in any extra-osseous component of the tumour. This lesion, too, is most common in the metaphysis.

3. *Reticulum cell sarcoma*

The radiological changes may stimulate Ewing's tumour; the degree of bone destruction is often more marked, but there is nothing diagnostic in the radiological findings (p. 766).

4. *Histiocytosis X*

The bone lesion in this disease is the eosinophilic granuloma (see p. 206), initially a single, well-circumscribed area of rarefaction, most frequently in the calvarium. In the uncommon more malignant form there are multiple erosions in many bones, also remarkable for the absence of bone reaction (Fig. 14.2b, p. 300).

(*b*) **Metastases in bone**

1. *Neuroblastoma*

This can present radiographically in the following ways:

(*a*) A solitary destructive secondary deposit in a bone, with much the same radiological characteristics as a fibrosarcoma (Fig. 22.14a) or a reticulum cell sarcoma, i.e. a rather non-specific osteolytic lesion.

(*b*) Multiple metastases. These are not uncommon in a neuroblastoma, and while rather non-specific in appearance, this tumour is suggested by the fact that it is by far the commonest cause of multiple metastases in bone in children. Rarely, multiple bone lesions occur in Histiocytosis X, or Wilms' tumour.

(*c*) Widespread infiltration of the more rapidly growing metaphyseal ends of long bones causing patchy bone destruction (Fig. 22.14c) is another form of metastasis from a neuroblastoma, and a very similar appearance can also be caused by leukaemic infiltration (see below).

2. *Leukaemia* (see p. 142)

Widespread infiltration of the marrow near the metaphyses of long bones is typical (Fig. 22.14b), but less destructive as a rule, and already present at the time of diagnosis in 20% of cases.

3. *Alveolar rhabdomyosarcoma and Wilms' tumour*
These may also give rise to metastases in bone; in most cases they are osteolytic in type, and occur relatively late, almost always after the diagnosis of the primary tumour has been clearly established. However, in two patients in the Index Series bone pain due to widespread metastases was the mode of presentation of an occult primary alveolar rhabdomyosarcoma.

Differentiation of non-malignant bone lesions
These are listed and described on p. 725. Subacute or chronic osteomyelitis with atypical clinical and radiological features may be so difficult to distinguish from Ewing's tumour that it is only possible on biopsy.

DIAGNOSIS OF EWING'S TUMOUR

The diagnosis must be established beyond doubt by biopsy before commencing treatment.

Biopsy of bone tumours. Some of the technical points have been set out by Suit (1975):

(i) The incision should be as short as consistent with adequate exposure, to avoid problems in wound healing caused by subsequent radiotherapy and chemotherapy.
(ii) The incision should be placed in an area of skin to be included in one of the portals used in subsequent radiotherapy.
(iii) The approach should be made, where possible, through an adequate 'soft tissue bed' of muscle and soft tissues, avoiding areas of subcutaneous bone, so that there is a layer of muscle between the skin incision and the site of the biopsy.
(iv) The biopsy should be confined to removal of extra-osseous extensions, where possible, to avoid weakening cortical bone which could predispose to a pathological fracture. When the tumour arises centrally and is confined to bone, removal of cortex should be limited to the minimum compatible with obtaining adequate material.

TREATMENT OF EWING'S TUMOUR

The objectives of treatment are: (i) to eradicate the cells of the primary tumour without destroying the bone in which it arises to the point where it is no longer useful; and (ii) to damage and if possible kill any cells which have already spread to form subclinical metastases which may remain latent for a long period.

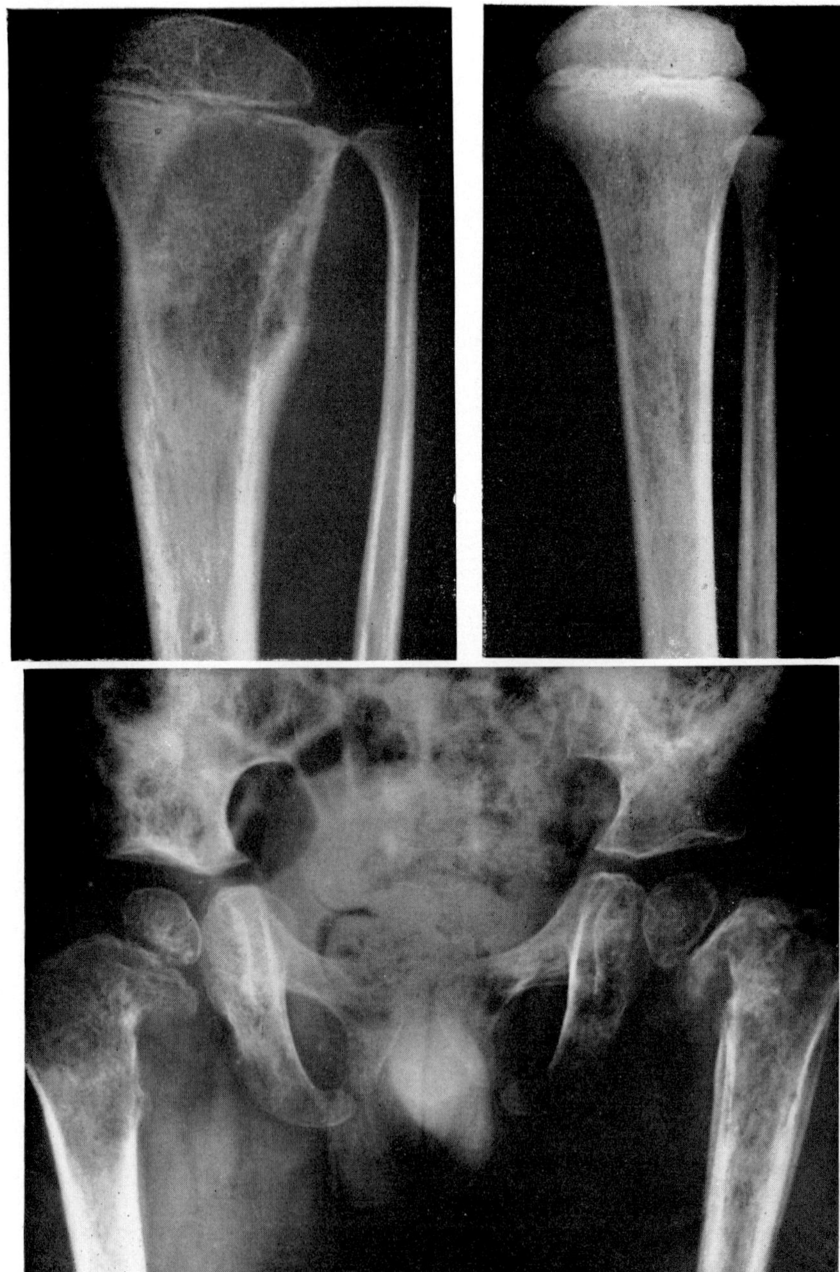

Figure 22.14. OTHER MALIGNANT BONE LESIONS; (*a*) localized metastasis (from a neuroblastoma) in the metaphysis extending to the epiphyseal plate, and producing periosteal new bone; (*b*) leukaemic infiltration of both tibia and fibula; (*c*) diffuse metastatic neuroblastoma in both femora and in the pelvis. Note onion-skin layers in the left femur.
[(*a*) *Top left*. (*b*) *Top right*. (*c*) *Bottom*.]

Surgery

Because of the common involvement of a significant length of the diaphysis and the early involvement of adjacent soft tissues, segmental or subtotal removal of the bone of origin is rarely feasible or successful. Depending on the site of the primary, ablative surgery may be possible, e.g. amputation in the case of a limb, but the response to irradiation and chemotherapy is so satisfactory, that local recurrence at the primary site following adequate treatment is uncommon. The feasibility of amputation should be reviewed after 6–18 months, because of the late appearance of metastases, as long as 2 years after apparent control of the primary tumour (Hustu, Pinkel & Pratt, 1972).

Radiotherapy

Ewing's tumour is classed as a relatively radiosensitive tumour, and treatment usually involves dosages of 4000–6000 rads given over a period of 4–6 weeks.

Chemotherapy

Ewing's tumour is far more sensitive to chemotherapy than either osteosarcoma or fibrosarcoma, a characteristic that may be expected from its ultrastructure and patterns in tissue culture, both of which resemble those of some of the reticulo-endothelial malignancies.

The range of antineoplastic drugs reported to have produced regression of the tumour and symptomatic relief includes cyclophosphamide, most of the cycle-active agents (actinomycin D, daunorubicin and adriamycin, mithramycin, vincristine and vinblastine), 5-fluoruracil and methotrexate.

Combinations of several of these agents can be expected to produce better responses than any one drug alone. Our current practice is to give, concurrently with the course of irradiation, vincristine (1·8–2·0 mg/m^2 IV) weekly and cyclophosphamide, also intravenously, to the limit of haematological tolerance. At the completion of radiotherapy, these two drugs plus actinomycin D are given intermittently, in alternating courses at increasing intervals for at least two and preferably three years. In Stage I cases with no late dissemination evident, modification of this regime may be justified.

SUMMARY OF TREATMENT

1. Local irradiation of the primary tumour, combined with chemotherapy.
2. Repeated courses of chemotherapy at increasing intervals of 1–4 months for at least 2 years, preferably using a combination of three drugs.
3. Review of the need for, or feasibility of, amputation at 6–18 months after the primary course of treatment.

PROGNOSIS

Falk & Alpert (1967) found, on reviewing reports of 987 cases up to the early 1960s, that 85% died within 2 years and only 8% survived for 5 years. Many of these had received inadequate treatment, even by former standards. More potent irradiation and more effective combinations of chemotherapeutic agents have become widely used during the past decade.

In the Index Series, several patients have shown prompt regression of their tumour with vincristine alone, and in one 14-year old, widespread nodular metastases in both lungs, arising 6 months after radiotherapy to the primary tumour, regressed completely for over 2 years following combination chemotherapy with vincristine, actinomycin D and daunorubicin.

The prognosis is better with tumours in the long bones or the jaw, and it is of course worse if the patient presents with metastases or is inadequately treated.

Improvements in results following initial intensive combination chemotherapy with a four drug regime (actinomycin D, vincristine, cyclophosphamide and adriamycin) and repeated course for up to 2 years, as well as radiotherapy (4000–6000 rads in 4–6 weeks), have been described from several centres, e.g. Rosen *et al.* (1974) who reported 12 consecutive patients surviving with no evidence of disease 10 to 37 months after commencing treatment.

II. OSTEOSARCOMA
(syn. osteogenic sarcoma)

This highly malignant tumour is fortunately a rarity in children, but in the Index Series it was the second commonest malignant bone tumour after Ewing's tumour. Little is known of the etiology, although minor trauma, possibly irrelevant, is a common feature in the clinical history. Virus infection (Moore *et al.* 1973) has also been suggested.

The supervention of an osteosarcoma as a complication of Paget's disease is seen in adults. Irradiation as an etiological factor is well documented (Marcove *et al.*, 1970). Arlen *et al.* (1971) collected 50 cases of osteosarcoma following therapeutic radiation in doses from 12,000–24,000 rads, with a mean latent interval of 9 years between exposure and neoplasia, and a slightly better prognosis (28% of 5-year survivals) than 'spontaneous' osteosarcomas.

In the Index Series of 22 cases of osteosarcoma, previous irradiation was implicated in four patients (20%), a much higher figure than in most series. These were an osteosarcoma of the occipital bone 8 years after radiotherapy for a cerebellar medulloblastoma, osteosarcoma of the jaw 6 years after radiation of an enlarged thymus, osteosarcoma of the scapula 6 years after radiation for pulmonary metastasis from a Wilms' tumour, and osteosarcoma of the upper end of the tibia 9 years after radiation for an aneurysmal bone cyst.

AGE : SEX : SITE

It is said to affect boys more frequently than girls (6 : 4), and mostly those between the age of 10 and 25 years (Fig. 22.15), at the peak of their bone growth rate. Osteosarcoma virtually never occurs in children less than 4 years of age; 90% arise in a long bone in a limb, and the lower end femur and the upper end of the tibia are the commonest sites (accounting for 50–65% of reported series), followed by the upper end of the humerus (Table 22.4).

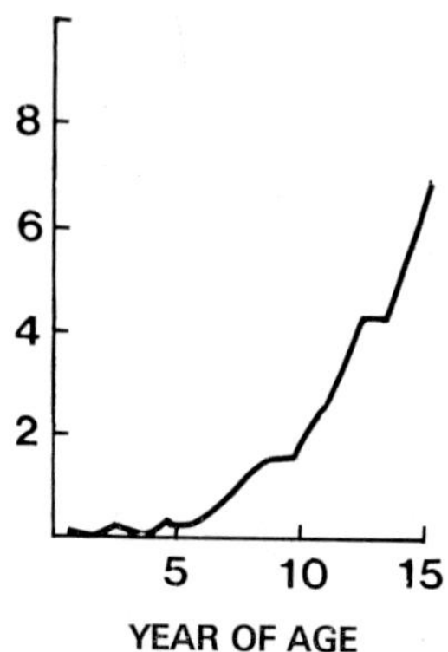

Figure 22.15. OSTEOSARCOMA; incidence according to age. The tumour is almost unknown in children less than 5 years of age, but there is a sharp increase in the third quinquennium (for the source of these figures, see Fig. 2.2, p. 48). The peak incidence occurs in young adults.

Table 22.4. Osteosarcoma age at onset and site of 22 cases in the Index Series (RCH 1950–1972)

Age	No.	Sites		No.
0–5	0	Femur		17
5–10	4	Tibia	1	2
		Humerus	1	
10–15	18	Mandible	1	3
		Rib	1	
		Occiput	1	
Total	22			22

MACROSCOPIC APPEARANCES

As in Ewing's tumour, there is rarely an opportunity to examine a complete, untreated specimen of osteosarcoma (p. 736). In children osteosarcoma tends to be predominantly osteolytic (see Fig. 22.17a) and osteogenesis may be minimal. The tumour is grey or yellowish, and characteristically gritty; extensive haemorrhage and necrosis, destruction of the cortex, and invasion of adjacent soft tissues are all common (Fig. 22.16a).

MICROSCOPIC FINDINGS

The diagnosis should not be made without the presence of '*malignant osteoid tissue*' i.e. abnormal osteoid formed by tumour cells and closely related to them, and this is a constant finding (Fig. 22.16c). The cells vary from large and irregular with polygonal cytoplasm and an almost epithelial appearance, to more spindle-shaped cells resembling fibroblasts.

Nuclear pleomorphism is a characteristic feature, and small irregular plates of osteoid tissue in direct contiguity with irregular, obviously neoplastic cells are typical (Fig. 22.16d).

Giant atypical mitotic figures are not infrequently seen, and multinucleated tumour giant cells are also common. Areas of cartilage or fibroblastic differentiation are quite usual.

One variant is an extremely vascular (telangiectatic) tumour which may be mistaken for an aneurysmal bone cyst, but careful microscopic study of the tissue between the vascular lakes reveals unmistakable features of malignant cells.

SPREAD

Extension up and/or down the shaft may occur, but is usually in continuity, and in general there is less invasion of the marrow cavity than in Ewing's tumour.

Metastases in the lung are very common, sometimes already present at the time of diagnosis, and may grow extremely rapidly.

Lymph nodes are almost never involved, but metastases have been described in the inguinal region on rare occasions.

MODE OF PRESENTATION

The most common clinical picture is pain (85%), followed by a swelling (Moore *et al.*, 1973). There is often a history of a minor injury of doubtful relevance. A pathological fracture is found in 3% of cases (Moore *et al.*, 1973).

Occasionally the onset is acute or subacute, accompanied by fever, and may resemble osteomyelitis (p. 725) or Ewing's tumour.

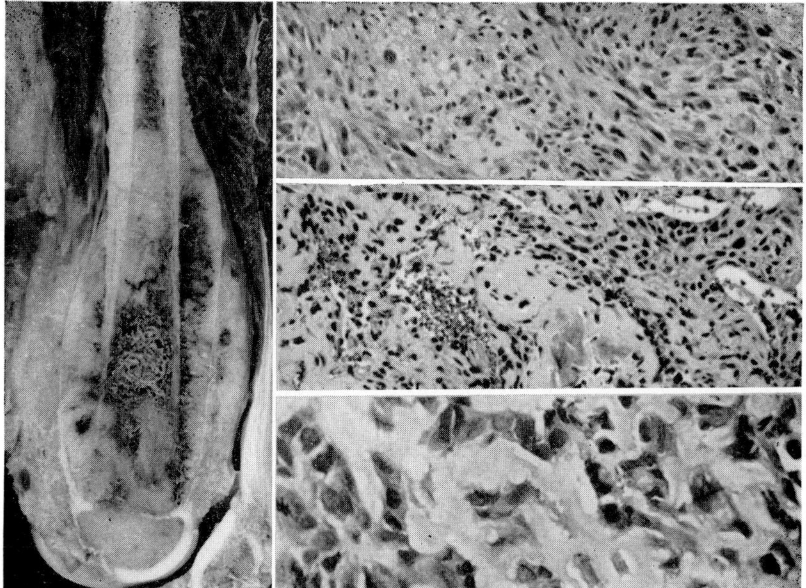

Figure 22.16. OSTEOSARCOMA; (*a*) arising in the metaphysis, invading the epiphysis, extending to produce a thin periosteal layer, and beyond into adjacent soft tissues. The medullary cavity is also involved and extends further than the extraosseous limits; (*b*), (*c*) and (*d*) variations in histology; (*b*) predominantly spindle cells, in an interlacing pattern resembling fibrosarcoma (H & E. × 130); (*c*) similar to (*b*) but with osteoid (centre), nuclear polymorphism and irregularity; several vascular lakes impart an angiomatous appearance ('telangiectatic' osteosarcoma) (H & E. × 100); (*d*) polygonal sarcoma cells with hyperchromatic nuclei and mitoses, forming delicate bands of osteoid tissue (H & E. × 520).
[(*a*) *Left.* (*b*) *Top right.* (*c*) *Centre right.* (*d*) *Bottom right.*]

INVESTIGATIONS

1. *X-rays.* The typical findings (Fig. 22.17) include the formation of new bone within the tumour, destruction of bone, areas of osteolytic and osteoblastic activity, a soft tissue mass extending from the surface of the affected bone, and reactive periosteal new bone (non-neoplastic bone) where the periosteum has been raised from the underlying cortex.
2. *Selective arteriography* indicates the extent of the lesion and its vascularity but interpretation has not yet been refined to the point where benign conditions can be completely excluded (Fig. 22.13, p. 741).

Yaghmai *et al.* (1971) examined the arteriographic features of bone tumours and described the points which indicate malignancy, namely:

(i) Hypervascularity and the formation of new 'pathological' vessels, of variable size and irregular shape ('neovasculature');

(ii) Areas of avascularity in the centre of the tumour, reflecting necrosis;
(iii) Arteriovenous fistulae, in most but not all types of bone tumours;
(iv) Rapid venous filling (in both benign and malignant lesions);
(v) Capillary 'staining' in extra-osseous extensions;
(vi) Tumour 'lakes', with delayed emptying of contrast material; and
(vii) Large abnormal veins in all malignant lesions, most obvious at the periphery of the tumour.

Benign tumours showed no 'pathological' vessels, no tumour 'stain', no venous lakes nor abnormal veins. Individually misleading findings were noted, such as a light 'tumour stain' in osteoid osteomas, and 'vacuoles' or 'cavity type' vessels in aneurysmal bone cysts, but these were not observed in malignant lesions. The authors reported that none of the arteriographic characteristics of malignant tumours was seen in acute or chronic osteomyelitis, in which there was only moderate hypervascularity.

3. *Bone scan* (p. 77). While helpful in determining the extent of a proven primary or recurrent tumour, this, too, is of limited value initially for it cannot distinguish between a neoplasm and inflammatory lesions.

4. *Serum alkaline phosphatase* is raised when there is a primary lesion, and

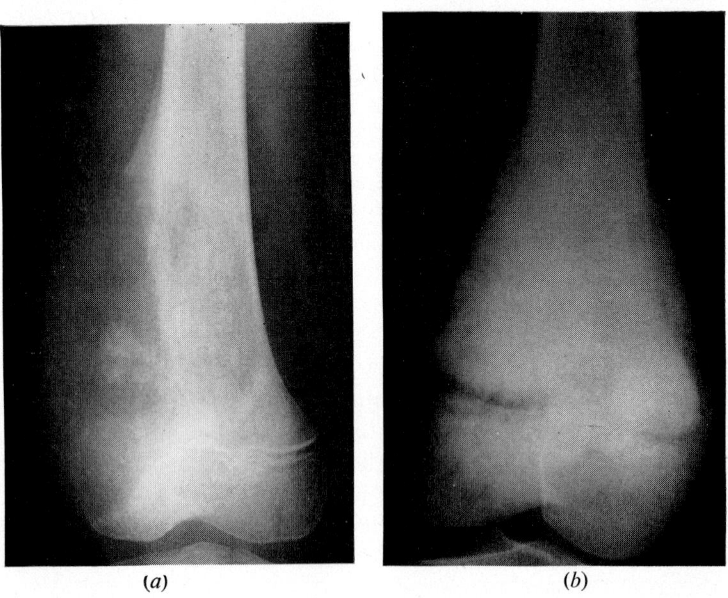

(*a*) (*b*)

Figure 22.17. OSTEOSARCOMA; (*a*) the osteolytic type; bone destruction predominates, and there is minimal new bone formation apart from 'Codman's triangle' at the upper limit; (*b*) an osteoblastic example with dense bone formation within the tumour, a less common type in childhood.

decreases following amputation. Its main usefulness is in detecting the presence of recurrences, but this can usually be demonstrated more clearly by radiography.

5. *X-rays of the lung fields* are necessary to determine whether there are pulmonary metastases.

DIAGNOSIS

It should be borne in mind that in childhood, Ewing's tumour is probably more common than osteosarcoma (see Table 22.2) at least in white children, and that in many parts of the world (see p. 12) osseous metastases from a neuroblastoma are more common than primary bone tumours.

Differentiation of an osteosarcoma from neuroblastoma is not often a clinical problem, for the presence of a mass in the abdomen (p. 553) or in the thorax (p. 460), can usually be demonstrated when the bony metastasis is first detected. Only rarely is an isolated metastasis in bone, without other clinical evidence of tumour, the mode of presentation of a latent neuroblastoma (p. 552)

DIFFERENTIAL DIAGNOSIS OF OSTEOSARCOMA

The groups of conditions which most closely simulate an osteosarcoma, and which should be considered in the differential diagnosis, are as follows:

(*a*) Other primary malignant bone tumours (described on p. 741);

(*b*) Metastatic tumours in bone (see p. 742);

(*c*) Benign lesions which may simulate a malignant bone tumour (see p. 725).

BIOPSY

Even when the clinical and radiological features are almost diagnostic, the grave outlook in osteosarcoma and the radical nature of the treatment required, demand confirmation by an adequate biopsy. The theoretical disadvantages of an open biopsy, e.g. the liberation of metastases and potential fungation at the site of biopsy, have not been borne out by experience (Dahlin & Coventry, 1967), and the necessity of an irrefutable diagnosis is paramount.

The technical points to be considered in biopsy of a suspected malignant bone tumour are mentioned on p. 743.

Parosteal fibrosarcoma (p. 761) may closely resemble osteosarcoma, but the better differentiated spindle cells, the typical cortical site of the primary, and the preponderance of tumour outside the bone, all constitute a distinct clinico-pathological entity, with a better prognosis, than osteosarcoma (p. 764).

In some cases the distinction between an osteosarcoma and Ewing's tumour, reticulum cell sarcoma of bone, osteomyelitis and metastatic neuroblastoma, can only be made after a searching histological examination of a biopsy, including special techniques described in Chapter 5, p. 83.

TREATMENT OF OSTEOSARCOMA

Until recently there had been no significant improvement in results for more than half a century (Sweetnam, 1971, 1973, 1974) chiefly because of the highly malignant nature of the tumour, the frequency of early haematogenous metastases, the resistance of the tumour to radiotherapy, and the ineffectiveness of single cytotoxic agents in conventional dosages.

Historically, various methods of treatment which have been employed are: amputation after open biopsy (Dahlin and Coventry, 1967); preoperative radiotherapy followed by delayed amputation in patients free of pulmonary metastases 6 months after diagnosis (Cade, 1967; O'Hara *et al.*, 1968); necrotizing preoperative radiotherapy followed by immediate amputation, and immunotherapy including transfer of specifically activated lymphocytes (Marsh, Flynn and Enneking, 1972, 1975). Results obtained varied to some extent, but the average overall 2-year survival rate rarely exceeded 25–30%, and in many series was as low as 5–6%, e.g. in a control series treated in earlier times, quoted by Sutow, Sullivan *et al.* (1974), and approximately 4% 2-year survival (only one out of 22 cases) in the Index Series.

In the last twelve months there have been reports of remarkably improved results with the use of chemotherapy, chiefly methotrexate, in extremely high dosage, as an adjunct to early amputation. The following plan of management is typical of those currently considered to be the most effective.

ADDITIONAL INVESTIGATIONS

When the clinical and radiological findings indicate a bone tumour, the following investigations are usually performed:

1. *Selective arteriography* to determine the extent of extra-osseous involvement of soft tissues.
2. *A bone scan*, e.g. with ^{99m}Tc (di- or polyphosphate) to assess the extent of intramedullary spread, in particular at the anticipated level of transection.
3. *Liver and renal function tests* (e.g. the creatinine clearance) and a full blood examination, as baselines for monitoring the toxic effects, detoxication and excretion of the cytotoxic agents employed.
4. *X-rays of the lung fields*, with tomography or a 'blood pool' scan (p. 77) when indicated, to determine whether there are pulmonary metastases, and if present their number, size and distribution.

Surgical treatment

Open biopsy and histological confirmation of the diagnosis of osteosarcoma is absolutely essential, not only to exclude benign lesions (p. 725), but also to identify other malignant tumours of bone, in particular Ewing's tumour, for which amputation is not usually required (p. 736).

Experience has demonstrated no disadvantages in open biopsy without a tourniquet, and a delay of 1 to 2 days to prepare and examine paraffin sections. Frozen sections may also be obtained, to confirm that the biopsy is adequate and representative, and for experience in comparing the histology in frozen and paraffin sections.

Amputation is performed as soon as the diagnosis has been established, possibly regardless of the presence of resectable pulmonary metastases. The extent of resection of the primary tumour depends on the bone of origin, whether it arises in the proximal or distal end, on the limits of extra-osseous extensions and, to some extent, on the structure of the subsequent prosthesis. In some cases a forequarter or hindquarter amputation may be required. In tumours of the lower limb an interim pylon prosthesis (p. 757) should be applied at the conclusion of amputation.

Chemotherapy

The rationale is to eradicate disseminated micrometastases, ideally at a time when the total cell number has been much reduced by amputation, and those remaining are likely to be susceptible to the action of cytotoxic agents. These are commenced after the result of the biopsy is known, or on the day after operation.

Vincristine (VCR), e.g. 1·75 mg/m^2 I.V. is given first, to arrest mitosis and facilitate the action of methotrexate.

Methotrexate (MTX), as an intravenous infusion containing 3000 mg/m^2, is commenced $\frac{1}{2}$ to 1 hour after the VCR, and completed in 6 hours.

Citrivorum factor (CF, i.e. folinic acid) the antagonist of MTX, is given in a dose of 5 to 15 mg depending on the size of the patient, commencing 2 hours after the infusion of MTX is completed. The dose of CF is given every 8 hours, intravenously for 24 hours and then orally for 24 hours. It is helpful but not essential to monitor the level of MTX in the blood in order to control the dose and duration of treatment with CF ('citrivorum rescue'), for without the antidote, the dose of MTX used would be as lethal to the patient as it is for the tumour cells.

Two weeks later a second course of VCR-MTX-CF is given, with the dose of MTX increased to 6000 mg/m^2; 4 weeks after the second course a third course is given, the dose of MTX being increased to 7500 mg/m^2 if possible, and the doses of CF accordingly.

Adriamycin (ADM) in a dose of 75 mg/m^2 is commenced one week after the third course, and is repeated one week after each subsequent course (i.e. VRC, MTX–CF, ADM) every 4 weeks until a maximum dose of 480 mg/m^2 of ADM has been given. Thereafter, the course of VCR, MTX–CF is repeated every 4 weeks for up to 2 years. The survival curves in one series suggests that it may be possible to discontinue chemotherapy after 18 months, but the optimum interval between courses and the duration of chemotherapy have yet to be determined.

PROGNOSIS

Interim reports indicate that with the regime described, or others using similar cytotoxic agents (Cortes *et al.*, 1974; Jaffe, Frei *et al.*, 1974; Rosen *et al.*, 1974; Sutow *et al.*, 1974), survival rates as high as 90% may be expected, i.e. more than three times higher than the best over-all results previously reported. Further clinical trials, substituting or adding other cytotoxic agents, may lead to even better results.

Undoubtedly there is a high cost to the patient: the loss of a limb; repeated malaise, nausea and vomiting (50%); recurrent alopecia (100%) and re-admission to hospital for 1–2 days every 4 weeks for up to 2 years; but with such a lethal tumour this is the price of life itself, and the best prospect of survival that can be offered at the present time. The mortality from complications of chemotherapy may be as high as 5%.

Factors adversely affecting the prognosis in the past, and which may still be unfavourable are:

1. *The age at diagnosis;* children in whom an osteosarcoma develops before the age of 10–12 years appear to fare even worse than adolescents or young adults.
2. *Tumours arising in the proximal segment* of an extremity, e.g. in the upper end of the humerus or femur, require a more extensive excision such as disarticulation through the shoulder or hip joint, or fore- or hindquarter amputation.
3. *The presence of pulmonary metastases.* Experience so far suggests that the regime of chemotherapy described above may produce partial remission, but relapse is common and surgical excision, e.g. segmental resection(s) or lobectomy, is usually confined to those with few metastases (2 or 3) and a favourable distribution, i.e. in one lobe, or confined to one lung, and not involving hilar or mediastinal structures.

Factors which do not appear to affect the outcome are the type of osteosarcoma, i.e. whether sclerotic or osteolytic (p. 750), the occurrence of a pathological fracture before diagnosis, and performance of open 'incision biopsy' of the tumour.

AMPUTATION FOR MALIGNANT BONE TUMOURS

An amputation is a mutilating operation dreaded by parents, and children old enough to understand; all the evidence should be thoroughly reviewed before the decision is made.

The histopathologist bears the greatest responsibility for this decision, and it is of the utmost importance that the best possible material is available for examination. Ideally, he should be present when biopsy is performed, to see the macroscopic appearances and to ensure that a representative specimen is obtained and properly processed.

When the decision to advise amputation has been reached, this should be conveyed to the parents, and their permission sought, with the same consideration required when they are initially informed of the diagnosis of a malignancy (p. 127); in osteosarcoma this may be at the first interview. In most cases the nature of the operation to be performed should be explained to the patient by the surgeon, except when the parents insist that they undertake this responsibility. The child should be told as much as is consistent with age and comprehension, and questions should be answered with complete (but considerate) frankness and honesty. The provision of a pylon or other prosthesis should also be explained, and the plan of treatment outlined.

Sites of election

Theoretically the entire bone of origin should be excised, e.g. amputation through the upper joint, or transection at the site of election proximal to the joint above the tumour. In practice this is seldom necessary, e.g. in osteosarcoma of the lower end of the femur amputation below the lesser trochanter is preferred because a better type of prosthesis can be fitted. Recurrence or secondary deposits in the stump are not common, e.g. in not more than 7% of cases reviewed by Moore *et al.* (1973). With the additional information provided by a bone scan (p. 77) and frozen sections of material taken from the proposed site at the time of operation (Lewis & Lotz, 1974), the incidence of recurrence in the stump is negligible (nil in the Index Series).

Amputations performed through the shaft of a long bone during childhood are complicated by subsequent growth of the remaining epiphysis, and this influences selection of the site of election, the operative technique, and subsequent management. With a malignant tumour such as osteosarcoma, it is generally better to sacrifice a growth centre than to run the risk of recurrence in the stump.

The humerus. Disarticulation at the shoulder joint is required for osteosarcoma of the upper end of the humerus. Trials of segmental excision of the upper humerus, and of fixation of a replacement internal prosthesis to the clavicle, are in progress. A forequarter amputation may be required when there is extension into soft tissues around the glenoid cavity or more proximally in the shoulder girdle. A prosthesis which restores the contour of the shoulder is available and a great deal can be done to conceal the extent of the operation.

The radius and ulna

With either an osteosarcoma or a Ewing's tumour of the forearm, the aim is to leave 50% of the shaft of the humerus, which produces a stump suitable for any of the several types of above-elbow prosthesis.

The tibia and fibula

A mid-thigh amputation is indicated, leaving a little more than half the shaft of the femur, for there is very little subsequent growth at the upper femoral epiphysis.

The femur

When there is an osteosarcoma of the lower end, a high femoral amputation can be performed (Jaffe, 1958; Hill, 1973), with the histological precautions mentioned above.

If tumour cells are found in material from the medulla at the site of transection, amputation at a more proximal level is required. Depending on the site, disarticulation through the hip joint may be necessary, but this is unusual.

In malignant bone tumours arising in the upper end of the femur, disarticulation at the hip is the minimum resection and, depending on the upper margin of extra-osseous extension, a hind quarter amputation may need to be considered.

In a Ewing's tumour at the upper end of the femur, the principles of management are the same as in the upper end of the humerus, and amputation is not usually indicated. On the rare occasions when a Ewing's tumour arises in the lower end of the femur, a high transection of the femur may be possible.

An above-knee suction-socket type of prosthesis can be fitted satisfactorily when there are 10 cm (4 inches) of femur, measured from the greater trochanter, but any lesser length will probably require a 'Canadian' type of artificial limb, i.e. a tilting table prosthesis (as used after disarticulation at the hip) which is much less desirable than a suction-socket prosthesis.

Operative technique

The incision. In amputations for a malignancy, a transverse scar is probably best, and there is no need for a long posterior flap. The scar should not lie antero-posteriorly in the forearm or lower leg, as it tends to be pulled upwards between the ends of the two bones.

Wherever possible, adhesions between the scar and the bone should be prevented by interposing muscle flaps, for an adherent scar is affected by the piston-like action of walking in a suction-socket, causing tension in the skin and pain.

The periosteum. Continuity should be restored by suturing the periosteum over the bone ends. In a below-knee amputation (very rarely required in cases of malignancy), the periosteum of the tibia and fibula should be closed as a single tube enveloping both bones so as to produce a synostosis.

The muscles should be sutured as thick flaps over the end of the bone, particularly in a high thigh amputation, but this is unnecessary more distally. The major vessels should be doubly ligated with non-absorbable sutures.

The nerves are pulled down, cut transversely and cleanly with a sharp scalpel, and allowed to retract well above the end of the stump.

The deep fascia should be carefully sutured to encourage the development of a firm cylindrical stump.

The skin is also carefully sutured, and suction drainage is desirable.

After care

Because of the advantages in maintaining or restoring morale, a prosthesis should be fitted as soon as possible.

Prostheses

In childhood, perhaps even more than in adults, the provision of a 'pylon' prosthesis which can be put on immediately after amputation, has particular advantages; the morale of the patient is aided by the presence of a 'leg and a foot' on waking from the anaesthetic; immediate ambulation is achieved; the patient can usually stand on the pylon the morning after amputation and walk unaided 50–100 yards within a week. An ischial-bearing ring is incorporated in the plaster above the pylon and prevents pressure on the suture line.

Close co-operation with the prosthetic technician in fitting a temporary limb is most important, particularly following amputations of the lower limb.

Physiotherapy

This is most important in amputations through the thigh, in which much of the adductor insertion is lost, and what remains should be strengthened. Furthermore, the extensors of the hip must also act as extensors of the knee and these, too, should be exercised to increase their efficiency.

Occupational therapy

After amputations of the upper limb, training in the use of a prosthesis is best carried out by an occupational therapist. In most cases an above-elbow type of prosthesis is required, and the patient often has difficulties in adjusting to the handicaps. The substitution of an cosmetic hand interchangeable with a functional split hook is an important point in helping the patient cope with the psychological problems involved.

Very few patients ever become confident in the use of the prosthesis required after a disarticulation at the shoulder joint, and most eventually prefer to have no prosthesis at all, or only a shoulder pad.

Psychological considerations
Even after thorough explanation and preparation, careful instruction in its use, and painstaking fitting and supervision of a prosthesis, there are still considerable anxieties for the patient. Much of the continuing technical supervision, and advice and assistance, can be supplied by the occupational therapist and the medical social worker, and their assessment of the problems which arise in the individual patient are a great help in guiding all who are involved in the integrated management of the child with an artificial limb, before, during and after amputation.

TREATMENT OF PULMONARY METASTASES

As pointed out by Morton, Joseph *et al.* (1973), and others, the presence of pulmonary metastases does not necessarily indicate that there is widespread dissemination of tumour throughout the body, on the contrary, metastases in the lungs are frequently the only foci of tumour found at autopsy, and this is particularly so in many cases of osteosarcoma.

While aggressive treatment with radiotherapy, chemotherapy and in selected cases excision, of pulmonary metastases in Wilms' tumour has yielded long term survivors in as many as 50% of cases (p. 523), the results in osteosarcoma have been less satisfactory.

Morton, Joseph *et al.* (1973) have described a means of selecting potentially operable cases in adults with a variety of tumours by estimating the '*tumour doubling time*' from the rate of growth of pulmonary metastases as seen in at least three serial x-rays of lung fields (Joseph, Morton & Adkins, 1971). When the doubling time was greater than 40 days, resection of metastases (usually by multiple wedge resections using a stapling device) produced a 5-year survival rate of 65%, compared with less than 2-year survival in comparable patients not submitted to operation.

The tumour doubling time and the survival rate were found to correlate with the extent of the patient's immune response as measured by the titre of tumour antibody indicating a more favourable biological state in these patients.

The authors recommended operation on the less affected lung first, when both were the site of metastases; approximately 90% of metastases were subpleural in location, and thorough exploration of the lung in both aerated and collapsed condition should precede any resection. Generally more metastases were found than indicated by pre-operative tomography.

An aggressive approach to pulmonary metastases using high dosage chemotherapy (p. 753) and, in selected cases, segmental or lobar resection(s) may prove worthwhile in children with osteosarcoma.

The Index Series, contains a sole survivor; the case is unusual in the atypical age of onset, misinterpretation of the initial radiographic findings, and in the fact of survival.

P.B., a girl aged 4 years 10 months, presented with pain and swelling in the upper third of the right tibia. Initial radiographs (Fig. 22.18a) suggested a hairline fracture, but 3 months later subsequent films showed progressive destruction of bone (Fig. 22.18b) which led to biopsy, a diagnosis of osteosarcoma and a mid-thigh amputation. She is alive with no evidence of metastasis 12 years later.

OTHER FORMS OF OSTEOSARCOMA

On rare occasions osteosarcoma has been reported as
(a) parosteal
(b) extra-osseous, or
(c) multiple primary tumours
(d) mixed histological types.

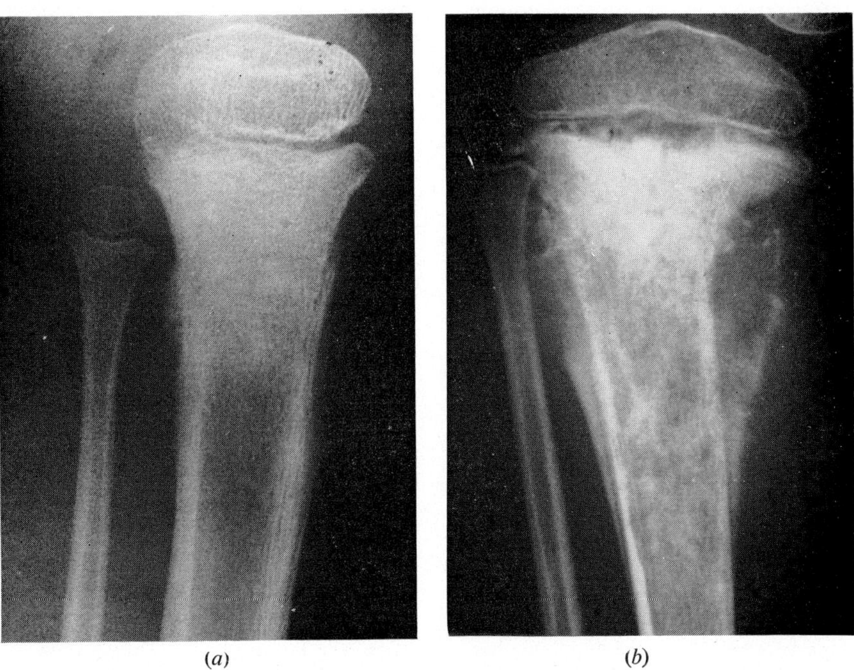

(*a*) (*b*)

Figure 22.18. OSTEOSARCOMA, an unusual example in a girl aged 4 years 10 months, who presented with a lesion of the upper end of the tibia (*a*) diagnosed as an incomplete fracture (cf. Fig. 22.2); (*b*) three months later x-rays showed typical features of an osteosarcoma, confirmed by biopsy and at amputation (see text). This patient is the only longterm survivor (12 years) in the Index Series.

(a) PAROSTEAL OSTEOSARCOMA (syn. juxta-cortical osteosarcoma)

The exact nature of this clinico-pathological entity is debatable. It is more typical of adults than children or adolescents, yet approximately 15–20% occur before the age of 20 years.

It is a slow growing tumour which arises in the periosteum and shows little or no tendency to invade the cortex. The metaphyseal region of the lower end of the femur, the humerus and the tibia appear to be the commonest sites. The histological features are essentially those of osteosarcoma yet there appears to be a reasonably good prognosis following amputation, with survival rates as high as 70–80% of cases (van der Heul & von Ronnen, 1967).

(b) EXTRA-OSSEOUS OSTEOSARCOMA

Although extremely rare, both osteosarcoma and chondrosarcoma have been reported to arise in soft tissues (Kauffman & Stout, 1963; Goldenberg *et al.*, 1967). The extra-skeletal origin may not be readily demonstrable radiologically, and is often proven only at operation. The few reports in children indicate that there is a slightly better outlook than when the tumour arises in bone.

(c) MULTIPLE OSTEOSARCOMAS

There are rare cases reported in which there are multiple skeletal foci of osteosarcoma in patients without detectable pulmonary metastasis (Singleton *et al.*, 1972; Davidson *et al.*, 1971), raising the possibility of multicentric origin.

In the Index Series there was one patient who might be in this category.

A nine-year old girl presented with anorexia and loss of weight, and on examination was found to have tumourous masses in the scalp, over the mandible and at the lower end of the right femur.

X-rays showed a sclerotic bony mass at each of these sites, also in practically all the long bones, and in the pelvic bones. She was given palliative treatment only and died 2 months later.

At autopsy nearly every bone contained areas of osteosarcoma with an atypical sclerotic appearance. There were also deposits in the soft tissues of the scalp, in skeletal muscle, and in a lymph node. There was no evidence of tumour in the lungs.

Microscopically the lesions in the scalp contained larger (15–20 μ) cells with irregular, hyperchromatic, pleomorphic nuclei containing 2–3 large prominent nucleoli. In some areas osteoid was being formed in the intercellular tissue. The findings in the bone lesions were similar, but showed no obvious deposition of bone.

Necropsy failed to resolve the question whether the lesions were multiple primaries or metastases from one of the bone lesions, none of which appeared to be larger or longer-standing than the others.

III. FIBROSARCOMA OF BONE

This is a relatively uncommon tumour of bone in children, both in the Index Series (Table 22.2) and in other much larger series in the literature (Eyre-Brook & Price, 1969). Table 22.5 shows the sites and the ages of the few in the Index Series.

Table 22.5. Fibrosarcoma of bone, age at onset and site of 3 cases in the Index Series (RCH 1950–1972)

Age	No.	Sites	No.
0–5	1	Tibia	2
5–10	0	Clavicle	1
10–15	2		
	—		—
Total	3		3

SITE

The tumour arises in the medullary cavity of long bones, but also in membrane bones such as the clavicle (Fig. 22.19), or from the periosteum as a parosteal fibrosarcoma.

AGE

The numbers are too small to indicate whether the tumour tends to occur in any particular period of childhood, but in general they are perhaps more common over the age of 5 years.

MACROSCOPIC APPEARANCES

A well-defined, firm, tumour is usual, and it may be possible to shell it out of its bony aspect, although some are poorly defined and adherent to adjacent soft tissues once the periosteum is breached. The cut surface is whitish and may show some whorling as seen in fibromas and soft tissue fibrosarcomas.

MICROSCOPIC FEATURES

The important feature is fibroblastic proliferation with a total absence of osteoid tissue. The cells are fairly uniform in any particular tumour, but

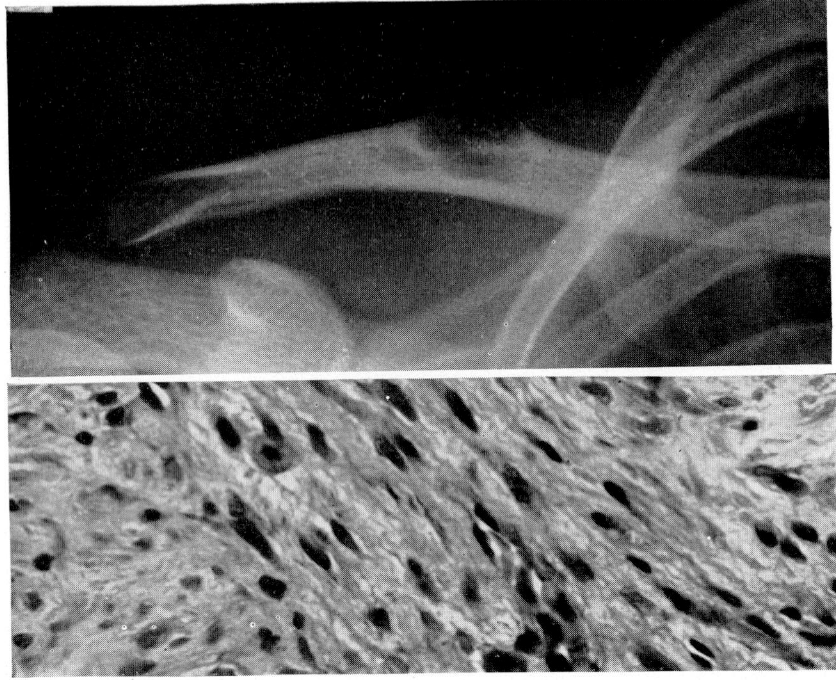

Figure 22.19. FIBROSARCOMA OF BONE; (*a*) arising in the clavicle causing a clear-cut defect without evidence of bone reaction; material from this lesion (*b*) shows mature looking fibroblasts interwoven in a herring-bone pattern (H & E. × 320). [(*a*) *Top*. (*b*) *Bottom*.]

individual examples show wide variations in the degree of differentiation, ranging from well-differentiated with formation of collagen but numerous mitotic figures, to an anaplastic pattern with pleomorphism and giant forms (Dahlin & Ivins, 1969).

SPREAD

Local infiltration, erosion of the adjacent bone and periosteum, and extension into contiguous soft tissues are common. Haematogenous metastasis to the lungs is the commonest type of dissemination, but often late.

RADIOGRAPHIC FINDINGS

The general picture is one of osteolysis with a notable lack of bone reaction (Fig. 22.20) in this respect resembling an eosinophilic granuloma (see Fig. 14.1, p. 299).

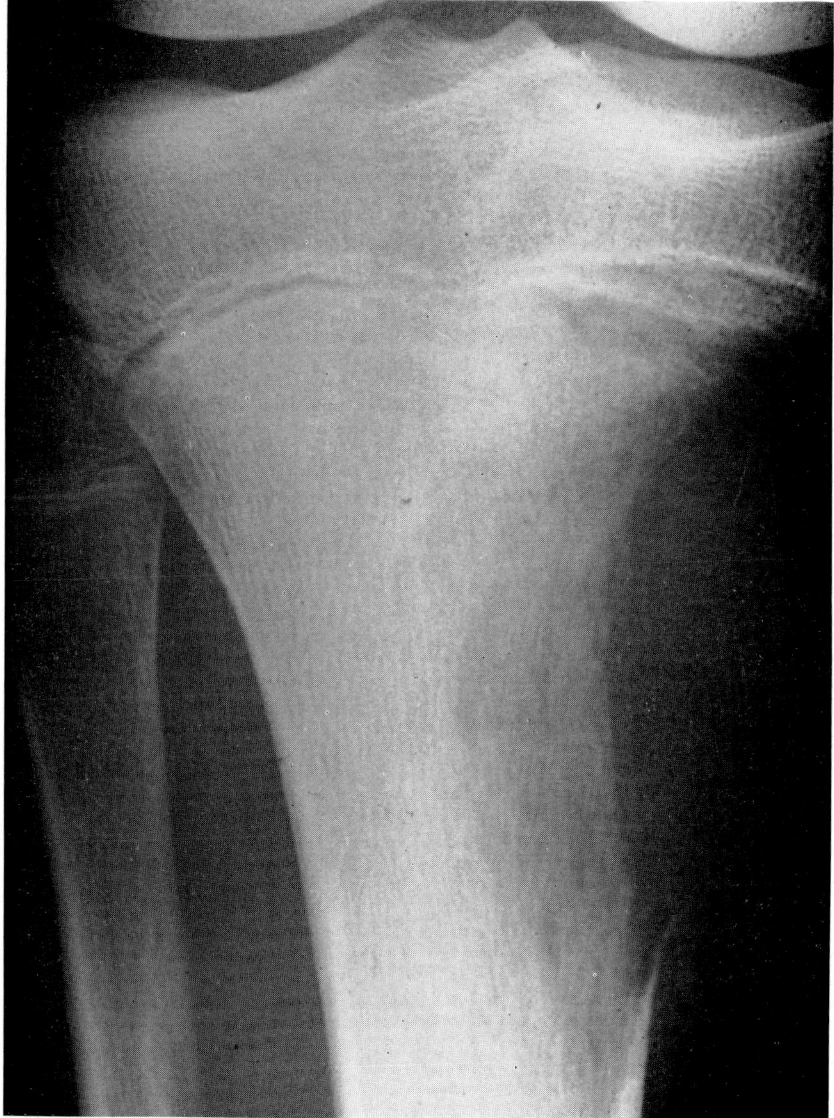

Figure 22.20. FIBROSARCOMA OF BONE; at the upper end of the tibia, with preservation of texture of the adjacent trabeculae and no radiological reactive changes.

DIAGNOSIS

Fibrosarcomas of bone are so uncommon that the diagnosis is almost always made on the histological findings in a biopsy. Technical points to be considered in performing a biopsy of what may be a malignant tumour are mentioned on p. 743.

TREATMENT

Treatment is influenced by the bone of origin, the location of the tumour (whether central or parosteal) and by the stage of the disease, including the extent of extra-osseous infiltration.

Wide local excision is recommended for localized parosteal tumours arising in a long bone in an extremity, and for central or parosteal fibrosarcoma in the head and neck.

Amputation is probably the safest method of treatment for the more aggressive intramedullary (central) tumour in an extremity.

Radiotherapy does not play a large part in treatment, because of the radioresistant nature of the tumour.

Chemotherapy may play a greater role in the future, and adriamycin shows promise of being effective in fibrosarcomas in general. Due to the rarity of the tumour, particularly in childhood, there are inadequate reports on which to base a plan of combination chemotherapy.

RESULTS: PROGNOSIS

In a series recently reported by Huvos & Higinbotham (1975) there were 11 children with a fibrosarcoma of bone; 3 with parosteal tumours treated by wide local excision alone, were long term survivors, while the survival rates in 8 children with a medullary (central) fibrosarcoma were 50% at 5 years and 38% at 10 years.

The overall results in reported series are approximately 35% 5-year survival in patients treated by wide local excision or amputation (with or without radiotherapy), and before the introduction of combination chemotherapy.

IV. RETICULUM CELL SARCOMA OF BONE
(syn. malignant lymphoma of bone)

This is one of the least common malignant tumour of bone in children; most cases occur in adults, and only some 10% occur before the age of 20 years (Francis *et al.*, 1954).

SITE

The diaphysis of a long bone is the most usual site, but a flat bone may occasionally be affected. The sites in approximate order of frequency are: the femur, humerus, pelvis, skull, tibia, ribs, scapula and vertebrae.

AGE : SEX

Although mostly affecting adults, 13 of the 47 patients reviewed by Shoji & Mieler (1971) were less than 20 years of age; two were less than 10 years old, and 11 were between 10 and 20 years.

Males are affected somewhat more frequently than females, in a ratio of 3 : 2, or 2 : 1.

MACROSCOPIC APPEARANCES

There are no characteristic macroscopic features that set apart reticulum cell sarcoma of bone from Ewing's tumour, which it closely resembles. The tumour tissue is usually pink or grey, fleshy, soft, with areas of haemorrhage and necrosis. Extension along marrow cavity is a prominent feature; often the tumour destroys the cortical bone and invades the adjacent soft tissue, and may, like Ewing's tumour, resemble pus.

MICROSCOPIC FINDINGS

The tumour is composed of sheets of cells with a vesicular, slightly indented nucleus and a prominent nucleolus. Cytoplasm is indistinct, often syncytial, and contains no significant amounts of glycogen. Festoons of cells around vascular lakes, so characteristic of Ewing's tumour, do not occur in reticulum cell sarcoma and this, together with a negative PAS reaction, helps to distinguish it from Ewing's tumour.

SPREAD

The tumour usually arises centrally, in *the medullary cavity*, and spreads along it in both directions. Infiltration and destruction of the cortical bone with penetration of the periosteum and extension into adjacent soft tissues, also occurs, but the rate of growth is often quite slow.

Lymphatic spread to regional nodes occurs in some cases, but possibly less often that some reported series would indicate; according to Shoji & Mieler (1971), regional nodes metastases were seen in only three of their 47 cases.

Dissemination to other bones, and also to viscera producing 'generalized reticulum cell sarcoma' of the spleen, liver, marrow and lungs, may occur late in the course of the disease.

MODES OF PRESENTATION

1. *Pain* at the site of the primary tumour is the predominant symptom, and

accompanied by local tenderness, was the chief feature in all 47 cases described by Shoji & Mieler (1971).

2. *A swelling* was less common as a presenting sign, but was present in 17 of the 47 cases.

INVESTIGATIONS

The usual investigations required when a bone tumour is suspected (p. 739) should be performed. Several types of radiographic changes typically commencing in the medullary region (Wilson & Pugh, 1955) have been described. These are:

(i) *Permeating decalcification* in irregular streaks, running parallel to the long axis of the diaphysis in a long bone;

(ii) '*Moth eaten*' *patchy decalcification;* and

(iii) *Frankly destructive changes*, with little or no new bone formation, often leading to a pathological fracture.

DIAGNOSIS

The radiological findings, although not distinctive in this tumour, will help to exclude benign lesions (p. 725) and other primary bone tumours (p. 741).

Biopsy to obtain histological confirmation is required in all cases.

TREATMENT

Surgery

When biopsy has been performed, and full investigations required in patients with a bone tumour have shown that the tumour is localized and without metastases, ablative surgery covered by chemotherapy (p. 181), may be considered. This applies to tumours arising in the distal portion of a limb, in which early amputation may be feasible, along the lines described on p. 754.

However, reticulum cell sarcoma is relatively radiosensitive and the plan of management favoured in most large series reported, especially when the tumour arises in other than long bones (Boston *et al.*, 1974) is radiotherapy.

Chemotherapy

Drug trials for reticulum cell sarcoma of bone have been too few to show whether the response differs much from the same tumour elsewhere. Most antineoplastic drugs have proved to be effective, especially actinomycin D, alkylating agents, the vinca alkaloids and corticosteroids.

A simple effective combination is actinomycin D and prednisolone, with either vincristine or cyclophosphamide; other regimens are described elsewhere (see p. 181).

To cover biopsy, vincristine (1·8–2·0 mg/m^{2}IV) is a suitable choice. When the diagnosis has been established, even with Stage I disease, a full course of the chosen combination is indicated, commencing before excision of the primary and/or regional nodes.

If dissemination has already occurred, a longer initial course of chemotherapy in the maximum dosage tolerated will be required. After completion of the primary treatment, when the patient is in full clinical remission, it is advisable (except possibly in cases in Stage I) to continue with recurrent courses of chemotherapy because of the highly malignant nature of the tumour.

In general, chemotherapy is repeated, at intervals of 2 months increasing to 4–6 months, for at least 2 years; in several patients in the Index Series chemotherapy has been continued for 3–4 years.

Radiotherapy

This is effective in reticulum cell sarcoma (Wang & Fleischli, 1968) although a minority are unpredictably more resistant and require a larger dosage for control of the primary tumour. The dose of radiotherapy depends upon the plan of treatment, which may be along the same lines as in osteosarcoma (p. 752), or in a lower dose and co-ordinated with chemotherapy to control the primary tumour as in Ewing's tumour (p. 745).

Doses of at least 4000–4500 rads are usually required, and radiotherapy as the sole form of treatment has been credited with 20–25% of 5-year cures. However, late local recurrence is recognized as a feature of this tumour and delayed amputation, 6–12 months after the primary tumour has been brought under control, should be considered when the site of origin makes amputation feasible.

SUMMARY OF TREATMENT

Stage I (primary only)

1. Chemotherapy to cover biopsy followed by completion of course, continuing repeated cycles for 2–3 years or more;
2. Combined with (*a*) early amputation if feasible, or alternatively (*b*) radiotherapy to the primary;
3. Consideration of late amputation if feasible.

Stage II (primary and regional nodes)

1. Radical excision of both primary and regional nodes if feasible;
2. Chemotherapy (and radiotherapy) as above, with a complete primary course of combination chemotherapy using three drugs, followed by maintenance chemotherapy as above.

Stage III (distant metastasis)

1. Primary course of actinomycin D and two or three other drugs in maximum dosage;
2. Repeated courses of maintenance chemotherapy as above;
3. Irradiation of any lesion causing pain or interference with function;
4. Consider excision or subtotal excision of the primary.

PROGNOSIS

Cases in which the tumour is confined to one bone naturally have a better prognosis and, in general, reticulum cell sarcoma arising in bone is said to have a somewhat better prognosis than in other sites. This has not been our experience in the Index Series in which those arising in the abdomen (p. 182) or in peripheral lymph nodes account for most of the long term survivors.

In a recent review of 43 cases, Shoji & Miller (1971) reported 5-year survival free of disease in 17 of 43 patients, and 10-year survival in 11 out of 30, approximately 30%; amputation had been performed in 11 of the 43 cases.

Generalized dissemination has a poor prognosis, but as some of our abdominal cases have shown (p. 638), the situation is by no means hopeless, and long term survivals, and possibly cures, can be obtained with intensive combination chemotherapy in repeated courses, reserving radiotherapy for localized resistant deposits.

V. CHONDROSARCOMA

AGE : SEX

This is a rare tumour in the paediatric group, except for a few cases in the third quinquennium which account for approximately 1–2% of all cases. The peak incidence is in mid-adult life. A slight male preponderance (3 : 2) is reported in large series.

SITES

In two of the largest series reported (Dahlin & Henderson, 1956; Marcove *et al.*, 1972) the sites, in order of frequency, were the ilium, ribs, upper end of femur, and scapula, which accounted for approximately 60% of cases in all age groups.

The tumour arises either centrally in the medullary cavity, or on the surface of a bone (juxtacortical type) and the point of origin may determine to some extent (a) the radiological findings, (b) the mode of presentation,

(c) the conditions to be excluded in differential diagnosis, and the extent of the excision required.

MACROSCOPIC APPEARANCES

The tumour is usually large, with a smooth but lobulated surface, and characteristically a mottled, bluish cut surface, interspersed with mucoid and cystic areas, and speckled calcification.

MICROSCOPIC FINDINGS

The diagnosis can be difficult, especially in well-differentiated tumours. The hallmark is said to be the presence of several binucleate and multinucleate cartilage cells with plump nuclei occurring in a single lacuna (Lichtenstein & Jaffe, 1943). Increased pleomorphism of the tumour cells, multinucleate giant cells, abnormal mitoses and fibroblastic or spindle-celled differentiation, all indicate a worse prognosis, whereas mucoid stromal degeneration and prominent lobulation point to a more benign potential.

SPREAD

Local infiltration of adjacent tissues, is a particular feature and the tumour is notorious for its slow growth and tendency to local recurrence, often on several occasions, despite wide excision, possibly because implantation during removal is a recognized phenomenon.

Metastasis to the lungs occurs infrequently, in about 10% of cases; regional lymph nodes are very rarely involved. Death is usually due to the general effects of massive and repeated local recurrences, and interference with the function of neighbouring structures.

MODES OF PRESENTATION

Several authors have remarked on the absence of pain or tenderness in chondrosarcomas, possibly due to the slow rate of growth. Latent tumours growing on the inner aspect of the ilium or ribs often reach a very large size before their presence is detected.

In superficial sites, the presenting feature is usually the tumour itself. Those arising centrally can cause pain, and occasionally a pathological fracture.

INVESTIGATIONS

The usual general investigations are required (p. 739), including x-rays of the lungs to exclude metastases.

The x-ray appearances of the tumour are partly determined by the point of origin; those arising centrally cause irregular lobulated radiolucent areas of destruction producing ballooning of the bone, whereas juxtacortical tumours produce only slight periosteal reaction and isolated, discontinuous streaks and patches of calcification, or mottled foci of calcification throughout the tumour.

DIFFERENTIAL DIAGNOSIS

The two most common benign conditions which may resemble a chondrosarcoma in its early stages are osteochondroma (p. 730) and enchondroma; only the former appears to have any potential for chondrosarcomatous degeneration.

The bone affected is also important in differentiation, for chondroid lesions located distally in the extremities are almost always benign.

The size of the lesion is significant; those less than 5 cm in maximum dimension are nearly all benign, while those 5–10 cm or larger should arouse suspicion of malignancy.

Other benign conditions to be excluded are as follows.

1. *Benign chondroblastoma* can be recognized by its site, in an epiphysis, and by the typical small angular cells with a round nucleus. Difficulty can arise when true cartilage is formed and dominates the histological picture. However, chondroblastomas are not invariably benign; some recur locally and metastases have been reported.
2. *Chondromyxoid fibroma* (p. 730). In this rare form of fibrous dysplasia chondroid and myxoid areas may be mistaken for chondrosarcoma when stellate, actively proliferating fibroblasts adjacent to myxoid areas are regarded as malignant. This is one of the situations where the radiological appearances are helpful in interpreting the histology; chondromyxoid fibromas have well-defined scalloped margins surrounding discrete areas of rarefaction.
3. *Synovial chondromatosis.* Although not strictly a bone tumour, dysplastic or metaplastic cartilage developing within synovial tissue should not be mistaken for a malignant tumour. The chondroid element is extremely well differentiated and shows none of the features of malignancy. The only peculiarity is the occasional development of this material within a joint space.
4. *Chondroid metaplasia in an area of fibrous dysplasia* caused difficulties in histological interpretation in one case in the Index Series.

A boy of 15 years of age with long-standing polyostotic fibrous dysplasia developed enlargement of a lesion in the fibula over a period of 12 months. The lesion was excised and found to be a lobulated mass of bluish chondroid tissue which expanded the fibula, breached the cortex at one point, and extended down the outer aspect of the shaft towards the ankle. Nine months after local but thorough excision, there is no evidence of recurrence.

Microscopic examination showed lobulation and mucoid change, but also numerous clusters of chondrocytes within a single lacuna. However, the cells showed no anaplasia, and the overall appearance was benign.

5. *Chondroblastic differentiation in osteosarcoma* is also a possible source of confusion, but polymorphic spindle cells are usually prominent, and 'malignant osteoid' (see p. 748) can be demonstrated. Aside from the upper end of the femur and tibia, the sites of osteosarcoma and chondrosarcoma are typically different.

The difficulty in distinguishing these two conditions is illustrated by another case in the Index Series.

A girl aged 9 years presented with an ache in the knee found to be due to a multilocular 'cystic' lesion at the upper end of the tibia. The initial diagnosis was an aneurysmal bone cyst (see p. 730) with an unusual amount of chondroid metaplasia. The lesion recurred after curettage, and was treated with radiotherapy (1000 rads in 2 weeks).

Six years later at 15 years of age the lesion reappeared and grew rapidly, and the limb was amputated through the femur. The histological diagnosis was osteosarcoma with marked chondrosarcomatous differentiation. The subsequent behaviour of the tumour was indolent and more typical of chondrosarcoma, with metastasis in the contralateral half of the pelvis, and subsequently in the femoral amputation stump. Death occurred at 16 years of age from complications of high dosage methrotrexate chemotherapy following disarticulation through the hip joint above the recurrence. The operative specimen contained tumour tissue regarded as an osteosarcoma, although much of the tumour showed chondrosarcoma-like areas.

TREATMENT OF CHONDROSARCOMA

Surgical excision. Because of the high incidence of local recurrence, osteochondromas have been traditionally treated by extremely radical, wide excision, and occasionally amputation as the initial operation, but perhaps more often as a secondary procedure to cope with persistent recurrences.

Disarticulation at the hip joint is usually required for chondrosarcoma of the upper end of the femur, while hindquarter amputation or hemipelvectomy may be required to remove a large tumour arising in the ilium.

Chondrosarcoma of the rib requires an extensive excision, including a long segment of the affected rib, the rib above and below it, as well as the full thickness of the intercostal tissues including the pleura (Marcove & Huvos, 1972), and the related extrathoracic musculature, repairing the defect with prosthetic material.

Radiotherapy has only a small role in the treatment of this radioresistant tumour, and high dosages are required.

Chemotherapy with single cytotoxic agents in standard dosages has proved to be of little use, but recently high-dose regimens as for osteosarcoma (p. 753) have been introduced. It will be some time before their effect can be evaluated, for as Marcove *et al.* (1972) and others have pointed out, 10-year survival rates are more informative than 2- or 5-year figures, in view of the slow growth and late recurrence typical of the tumour.

PROGNOSIS: RESULTS

There is no evidence that the age at diagnosis or length of history influence results. The grade of malignancy is some guide (Dahlin & Henderson, 1956), particularly the poor prognosis in highly malignant (Grade III) tumours.

There is ample evidence that survival rates in chondrosarcoma (2-year: 54%; 5-year: 37%) have been better than in osteosarcoma (2-year: 26%; 5-year: 18%), as reported by Marcove *et al.* (1972), who noted that longer survival could be correlated with more radical excision.

REFERENCES

ACKERMAN, L.V., SISSONS, H.A. & SHAJOWICZ, F. (1972). *Histological typing of Bone Tumours: International Histological Classification of Tumours.* No. 6, W.H.O., Geneva.

BHANSALI, S.K. & DESAI, P.B. (1963). Ewing's sarcoma. Observations on 107 cases. *J. Bone J. Surg.*, **45A** : 541.

BIESECKER, J.L., MARCOVE, R.C., HUVOS, A.G. & MIKE, V. (1970). Aneurysmal bone cysts. A clinicopathologic study of 66 cases. *Cancer*, **26** : 615.

BOSTON, H.C., DAHLIN, D.C., IVINS, J.C. & CUPPS, R.E. (1974). Malignant lymphoma (so called reticulum cell sarcoma) of bone. *Cancer*, **33** : 1131.

BOOZ, M.K. (1972). The management of hydatid disease of bone and joint. *J. Bone J. Surg.*, **54B** : 698.

BUNDENS, W.D.Jr. & BRIGHTON, C.T. (1965). Malignant haemangioendothelioma of bone. Report of two cases and review of the literature. *J. Bone J. Surg.*, **47A** : 762.

CABANELA, M.E., SIM, F.H. *et al.* (1974). Osteomyelitis appearing as neoplasms: a diagnostic problem. *Arch. Surg.*, **109** : 68.

CADE, S. (ed.) (1967). Symposium on limb ablation and limb replacement. *Ann. Roy. Coll. Surg. Eng.*, **40** : 203.

CORTES, E.P., HOLLAND, J.P. *et al.* (1974). Amputation and adriamycin in primary osteosarcoma. *New Eng. J. Med.*, **291** : 998.

DAHLIN, D.C., COVENTRY, M.B. & SCANLON, P.W. (1961). Ewing's sarcoma: a critical analysis of 165 cases. *J. Bone Jt. Surg.*, **43A** : 185.

DAHLIN, D.C. & COVENTRY, M.B. (1967). Osteogenic sarcoma, A study of 600 cases. *J. Bone J. Surg.*, **49A** : 101.

DAHLIN, D.C. & HENDERSON, E.D. (1956). Chondrosarcoma, a surgical and pathological problem. Review of 212 cases. *J. Bone Jt. Surg.*, **38A** : 1025.

DAHLIN, D.C. & IVINS, J.C. (1968). Fibrosarcoma of bone: a study of 114 cases. *Cancer*, **23** : 35.

DAVIDSON, J.W., CHACHA, P.B. & JAMES, W. (1971). Multiple osteosarcomata: report of a case. *J. Bone. Jt. Surg.*, **47B** : 537.

DIAS, L. DE S. & FROST, H.M. (1974). Osteoid osteoma—osteoblastoma. *Cancer*, **33** : 1075.

ENZINGER, F.M. (1970). Epithelioid sarcoma: a sarcoma simulating a granuloma or a carcinoma. *Cancer*, **26** : 1029.

EYRE-BROOK, A.L. & PRICE, C.H.G. (1969). Fibrosarcoma of bone. Review of 50 consecutive cases from the Bristol Bone Tumour Registry. *J. Bone J. Surg.*, **51B** : 20.

FALK, S. & ALPERT, M. (1967). Five year survival of patients with Ewing's sarcoma. *Surg. Gynec. Obstet.*, **124** : 319.

FINE, G. & STOUT, A.P. (1956). Osteogenic sarcoma of extraskeletal soft tissues. *Cancer*, **9** : 1027.

FITZPATRICK, S.C. (1965). Hydatid disease of the lumbar vertebrae. *J. Bone J. Surg.*, **47B** : 286.

FRANCIS, K.C., HIGINBOTHAM, N.L. & COLEY, B.L. (1954). Primary reticulum cell sarcoma of bone. Report of 44 cases. *Surg. Gynec. Obstet.*, **99** : 142.

FREEMAN, A.I., SACHATELLO, C., GAETA, J., SHAH, N.K., WANG, J.J. & SINKS, L.F. (1972). An analysis of Ewing's tumour in children at Roswell Park Memorial Institute. *Cancer*, **29** : 1563.

GELBERMAN, R.H. & OLSON, C.O. (1974). Benign osteoblastoma of the atlas. *J. Bone. Jt. Surg.*, **56A** : 808.

GODFREY, L.W. & GRESHAM, C.A. (1959). The natural history of aneurysmal bone cyst. *Proc. Roy. Soc. Med.*, **52** : 900.

GOLDENBERG, R.R., COHEN, P. & STEINLAUF, P. (1967). Chondrosarcoma of the extraskeletal soft tissues. *J. Bone. Jt. Surg.*, **49A** : 1487.

GOLDING, J.S.R. (1954). The natural history of osteoid osteoma: with a report of 20 cases. *J. Bone J. Surg.*, **36B** : 218.

GUPTA, R.M. (1969). Serum immunoelectrophoresis in patients with Ewing's sarcoma. *Lancet*, **2** : 1136.

HARRIS, W.H., DUDLEY, H.R.Jr. & BARRY, R.S. (1962). The natural history of fibrous dysplasia. An orthopedic, pathological and roentgenological study. *J. Bone J. Surg.*, **44A** : 207.

HENDERSON, E.D. & DAHLIN, D.C. (1963). Chondrosarcoma of bone: a study of 288 cases. *J. Bone J. Surg.*, **45A** : 1450.

HIGINBOTHAM, N.L., PHILLIPS, R.F., FARR, H.W. & HUSTU, H.O. (1967). Chordoma. Thirty-five year study at Memorial Hospital. *Cancer*, **20** : 1841.

HILL, P. (1973). Local recurrence in primary osteosarcoma of the femur. *Brit. J. Surg.*, **60** : 40.

HUSTU, H.O., PINKEL, D. & PRATT, C.B. (1972). Treatment of clinically localized Ewing's sarcoma with radiotherapy and combination chemotherapy. *Cancer*, **30** : 1522.

HUTTER, R.V.P., FOOTE, F.W. *et al.* (1966). Primitive multipotential primary sarcoma of bone. *Cancer*, **19** : 1.

HUVOS, A.G. & HIGINBOTHAM, N.L. (1975). Primary fibrosarcoma of bone. A clinicopathologic study of 130 patients. *Cancer*, **35** : 837.

JAFFE, H. I. (1959). *Tumors and Tumorous Conditions of the Bone and Joints.* Lea and Fibiger, Philadelphia.

JAFFE, N., FREI, E. *et al.* (1974). Adjuvant methotrexate and citrivorum factor treatment of osteogenic sarcoma. *New Eng. J. Med.*, **291** : 994.

JOSEPH, W.L., MORTON, D.L. & ADKINS, P.C. (1971). Prognostic significance of tumor doubling time in evaluating operability of pulmonary metastases. *J. Thorac. Cardiovasc. Surg.*, **61** : 23.

KAUFFMAN, S.L. & STOUT, A.P. (1963). Extraskeletal osteogenic sarcomas and chondrosarcomas in children. *Cancer*, **16** : 432.

LEWIS, R.J. & LOTZ, M.J. (1974). Medullary extension of osteosarcoma: implications for rational therapy. *Cancer*, **33** : 371.

LICHTENSTEIN, L. (1959). Aneurysmal bone cyst: observations on 50 cases. *J. Bone J. Surg.*, **39A** : 873.

MARCOVE, R.C., MIKE, V., HAJEK, J.V. *et al.* (1970). Osteogenic sarcoma under the age of 21: a review of 145 operative cases. *J. Bone J. Surg.*, **52A** : 411.

MARCOVE, R.C. & HUVOS, A.G. (1971). Cartilaginous tumours of the ribs. *Cancer*, **27** : 794.

MARCOVE, R.C., MIKE, V. *et al.* (1972). Chodrosarcoma of the pelvis and upper end of the femur: an analysis of factors influencing survival time in one hundred and thirteen cases. *J. Bone. Jt. Surg.*, **54A** : 561.

MARSH, B.W., BONFIGLIO, M. *et al.* (1975). Benign osteoblastoma: range of manifestations. *J. Bone. Jt. Surg.*, **57A** : 1.

MARSH, B., FLYNN, L. & ENNEKING, W. (1972). Immunologic aspects of osteosarcoma and their application to therapy; a preliminary report. *J. Bone. Jt. Surg.*, **54A** : 1367.

MOORE, G.E., GERNER, R.E. & BRUGAROLAS, A. (1973). Osteogenic sarcoma. *Surg. Gynec. & Obstet.*, **136** : 359.

MORTON, D.L., JOSEPH, W.L. *et al.* (1973). Surgical resection and adjunctive immunotherapy for selected patients with pulmonary metastases. *Ann. Surg.*, **178** : 360.

NESBIT, M.E.Jr. (1972/73). Bone tumors in infants and children. *Paediatrician*, **1** : 273.

O'HARA, J.M., HUTTER, R.V., FOOTE, F.W.Jr. *et al.* (1968). An analysis of 30 patients surviving longer than 10 years after treatment for osteogenic sarcoma. *J. Bone J. Surg.*, **50A** : 335.

NEER, C.S., FRANCIS, K.C. *et al.* (1966). Treatment of unicameral bone cyst. A follow up study of 175 cases. *J. Bone J. Surg.*, **48A** : 731.

PRICE, C.H.G. (1966). The prognosis of osteosarcoma: an analytic study. *Brit. J. Radiol.*, **39** : 181.

RAHIMI, A., BEABOUT, J.W. *et al.* (1972). Chondromyxoid fibroma: a clinico-pathologic study of 76 cases. *Cancer*, **30** : 726.

RALPH, L.L. (1962). Chondromyxoid fibroma of bone. *J. Bone J. Surg.*, **44B** : 7.

ROSEN, G., SUWANSIRIKNE, S. *et al.* (1974). High dose methotrexate with citrivorum factor rescue and adriamycin in childhood oesteogenic sarcoma. *Cancer*, **33** : 1151.

ROSEN, G., WOLLNER, N., TAN, C. *et al.* (1974). Disease free survival in children with Ewing's sarcoma treated with radiation therapy and adjuvant four-drug sequential chemotherapy. *Cancer*, **33** : 384.

SELBY, S. (1961). Metaphyseal cortical defects in the tubular bones of growing children. *J. Bone J. Surg.*, **43A** : 395.

SHOJI, H. & MILLER, T.R. (1971). Primary reticulum cell sarcoma of bone: significance of clinical features upon the prognosis. *Cancer*, **28** : 1234.

SINGLETON, E.B., ROSENBERG, H., DODD, G.D. & DOLAN, P.A. (1962). Sclerosing osteosarcomatosis. *Am. J. Roentgenol. Rad. Ther. Nucl. Med.*, **88** : 483.

SUIT, H.D. (1975). Role of therapeutic radiology in cancer of bone. *Cancer*, **35** : 930.

SUTOW, W.W., SULLIVAN, P. & FERNBACH, D.J. (1974). Adjuvant chemotherapy in primary treatment of osteogenic sarcoma. *Proc. Am. Assoc. Cancer Res.*, No. **77** : 20.

SWEETNAM, R. (1973). Amputation in osteosarcoma: disarticulation at the hip or high thigh amputation for lower femoral growths. *J. Bone J. Surg.*, **55B** : 189.

SWEETNAM, R., KNOWELDEN, J. & SEDDON, H. (1971). Bone sarcoma: treatment by irradiation, amputation or a combination of the two. *Brit Med. J.*, **2** : 363.

SWEETNAM, R. (1974). Tumours of bone and their management. *Ann. Roy. Coll. Surg. Eng.*, **54** : 63.

TILLMAN, B.P., DAHLIN, D.C., LIPSCOMB, P.R. & STEWART, J.R. (1968). Aneurysmal bone cyst: an analysis of 95 cases. *Mayo Clin. Proc.*, **43** : 478.

VAN DER HEUL, R.O. & VON RONNEN, J.R. (1967). Juxtacortical osteosarcoma: diagnosis, treatment and analysis of 80 cases. *J. Bone J. Surg.*, **49A** : 415.

WANG, C.C. & FLEISCHLI, D.J. (1968). Primary reticulum cell sarcoma of bone: with emphasis on radiation therapy. *Cancer*, **22** : 994.

WILSON, T.W. & PUGH, D. (1955). Primary reticulum cell sarcoma of bone with emphasis on roentgen aspects. *Radiol.*, **65** : 343.

YAGHMAI, I. *et al.* (1971). Value of arteriography in the diagnosis of benign and malignant bone lesions. *Cancer*, **27** : 1134.

Chapter 23. Sarcomas of soft tissues

Table 23.1. Benign swellings and malignant tumours of soft tissues

Benign swellings	Malignant tumours
Rhabdomyoma	Rhabdomyosarcoma
Fibroma	Fibrosarcoma
Synovioma (synovial harmartoma)	Synovial sarcoma
Giant cell tumour (fibroxanthoma of tendon sheath)	
Fibrous hamartoma	
Tumoural calcinosis	
Keloid	
Nodular (pseudosarcomatous) fasciitis	
Juvenile cervical fibromatosis	
Juvenile plantar and palmar fibromatosis	
Juvenile aponeurotic fibroma	
Juvenile angiofibroma of nasopharynx	
Juvenile (aggressive) fibromatosis	
Recurring digital fibroma (of Reye)	
Congenital generalized fibromatosis	
Neurofibroma	Neurofibrosarcoma
Leiomyoma	Leiomyosarcoma
Lipoma Diffuse lipomatosis Lipoblastomatosis	Liposarcoma
Angiomyolipoma	
Hibernoma	
Mesenchymoma (benign)	Mesenchymoma (malignant)
Vascular leiomyoma	Haemangio-endotheliosarcoma
Glomus tumour (chemodectoma)	Haemangiopericytoma (malignant)
Histiocytic tumours (juvenile xanthogranuloma)	Histiocytosis X (p. 206)
Myxoma	Myxosarcoma
	'Embryonic' sarcoma
Granular cell 'myoblastoma'	Alveolar 'soft part' sarcoma
	Extraskeletal osteosarcoma (p. 760) Extraskeletal chondrosarcoma
	Kaposi's sarcoma (p. 864)
	Epithelioid sarcoma
	Clear-cell sarcoma

As a group, sarcomas of the soft tissues are important because they comprise approximately 6% of all malignant tumours in childhood, although with one or two exceptions, each type is individually uncommon. There are also a number of soft tissue lesions which may resemble a sarcoma clinically (Table 23.1).

The histology of sarcomas presents some difficulties.

1. They may resemble a benign homologue or one of its variants, e.g. a fibrosarcoma may be difficult to distinguish from an aggressive and highly cellular but benign fibromatosis.
2. Variations in biological behaviour and hence the prognosis, in different sites, despite almost identical histological features.
3. Anaplasia and pleomorphism may make it difficult or impossible to determine the actual cell, or the site of origin. Multiple paraffin sections and/or special stains may be necessary to reach a histological diagnosis.

Management, too, may be difficult.

1. Misleading macroscopic appearances. At exploration or open biopsy, a false capsule of compressed malignant tissue may enable the tumour to be shelled out, thus predisposing to local recurrence. On the other hand, extensive fixation due to infiltration of adjacent tissues can occur in benign lesions, such as the fibromatoses.
2. Relative resistance to radiotherapy and chemotherapy is not uncommon, and somewhat unpredictable. These forms of treatment appear to have little or no effect on some soft tissue sarcomas, while in other examples of the same tumour, long term survival and cures can be obtained, even when surgical excision has been incomplete.
3. Sarcomas arising in inaccessible sites or in close proximity to vital structures seriously limit the possibility of surgical excision.

GENERAL CLINICAL FEATURES

Some guidance as to the type of sarcoma can be gained from the age of the patient and the site of origin, but the diagnosis always rests on the histological findings. It is not uncommon for a sarcoma to be initially mistaken for a benign lesion, e.g. a semimembranosus bursa, subacute lymphadenitis, a 'ganglion' of the wrist, a haematoma or an infection.

Familiarity with the typical clinical features of benign swellings commonly found in children is some assistance in determining when the clinical features are sufficiently atypical to require urgent exploration. However, as most sarcomas present simply as a swelling, with little or no pain nor tenderness, the general rule (see Farber's dictum) is that excision biopsy (p. 24) should be carried out in practically all cases and without delay.

Two benign conditions which may prove to be particularly difficult to exclude are:

1. *An intramuscular haematoma.* A history of injury is helpful, but may be lacking in a young child, and a deeply situated haematoma may not show any discolouration of the overlying skin. On the other hand, minor trauma can cause a haemorrhage into an as yet undiagnosed tumour which may then present as a 'haematoma' which fails to resolve, or with fever and tenderness suggestive of an infection.
2. *An intramuscular abscess de novo* in a healthy child is uncommon, except as idiopathic suppurative myositis in children in the tropics (Wong, 1973).

From the previous paragraphs it will be clear that infection in a haematoma can resemble a sarcoma and vice versa. If no pus is obtained, and particularly when encephaloid material escapes when a supposed abscess is incised, a biopsy of some of the material extruded should be carefully examined microscopically.

INVESTIGATIONS

Plain radiographs of the swelling are often unrewarding and show no more than some increase in tissue density (Fig. 23.1a), and usually no abnormality in the adjacent bone. Angiography may show only the increased vascularity, which also occurs in inflammatory lesions, but the demonstration of abnormal 'tumour' vessels (see Fig. 23.16) may be the first definite indication that a swelling is a sarcoma (Martel & Abell, 1973).

DIAGNOSIS

The chief difficulty in the early diagnosis of sarcomas, particularly those arising in the superficial tissues of the limbs or the trunk, is that there *are* no distinctive clinical features. Because of the rarity of sarcomas, benign conditions are much more common, resulting in a low index of suspicion of malignancy. A review of case histories of children with a sarcoma shows that a swelling had been present for weeks or even months before the diagnosis was first suspected.

In general, *signs which immediately arouse suspicion*, such as *hypervascularity*, *rapid increase in size*, *pain or oedema* of the overlying tissues, are seen only occasionally; in most cases the initial presentation of a sarcoma is much less dramatic.

The types of sarcoma, their origins and probable benign counterparts are listed in Table 23.2.

BIOPSY

Exploration and biopsy require judgement and experience in choosing the method most appropriate to the site and size of the lesion. The procedures

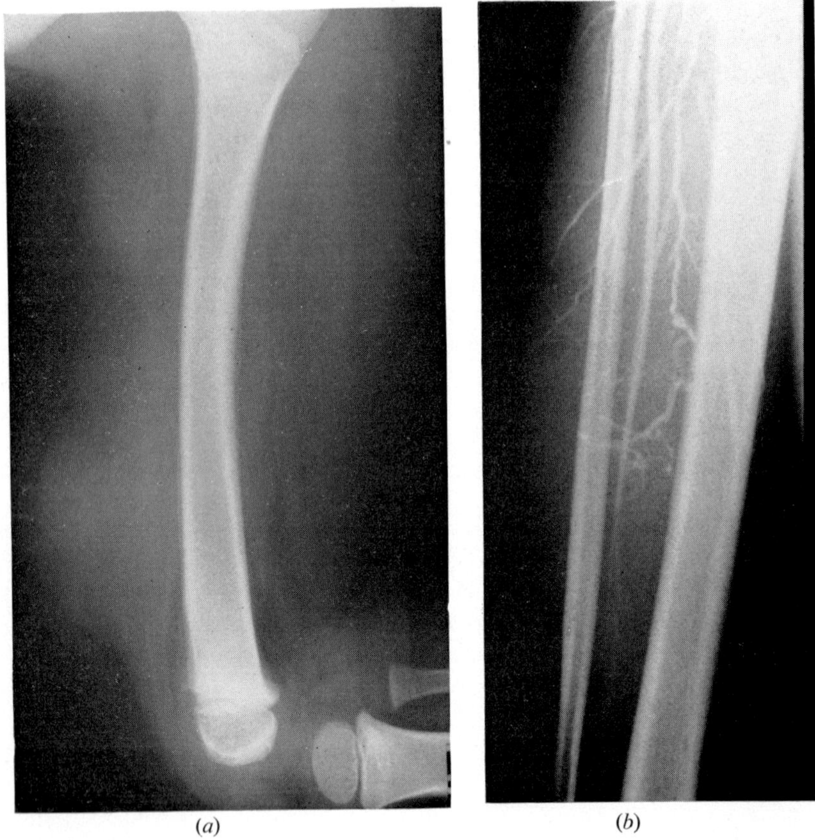

Figure 23.1. SOFT TISSUE SARCOMA; (*a*) rhabdomyosarcoma of the thigh outlined by a 'soft tissue' film; (*b*) femoral arteriogram of a child with a reticulum cell sarcoma of the calf showing vascularity, tumour vessels, and one distinct 'lake'.

available are drill biopsy, 'incision' biopsy (partial removal), 'excision' biopsy (i.e. apparent total removal) or, least commonly, an extensive or radical excision based on the evidence of frozen sections.

These various methods are described on p. 82.

Preoperative chemotherapy to minimize the risk of dissemination (p. 109) should be considered when a sarcoma is a possibility, and the potential disadvantages of cytotoxic agents interfering with the histological interpretation are mentioned on p. 25.

The correct histological diagnosis can be difficult even when adequate material is submitted, and even more difficult when only a small or non-representative specimen is obtained. In general, excision biopsy followed by thorough examination of paraffin sections of the tissue obtained is the preferred method, but in some situations a drill biopsy is better, e.g. a prostatic tumour (p. 708), or a swelling on the face.

DEFINITION

In this chapter, Willis' definition of a tumour has been followed, and 'soft tissues' include all connective tissues, except the skeleton (Chapter 22) the reticulo-endothelial system (Chapter 11), the glia (Chapter 13) and the supporting stroma of parenchymal organs. In the interest of clarity, neuroblastomas are also excluded from this chapter and described on p. 538.

CLASSIFICATION

The classification of soft tissue tumours proposed by the World Health Organization has been adopted, with some modifications, as the basis of the histological types described in this chapter (Table 23.2). Although most of the

Table 23.2. Classification of soft tissue tumours

Presumed origin	Benign	Malignant
Striated muscle	(? Rhabdomyoma)	Rhabdomyosarcoma (p. 783)
Fibrous tissue	Fibromatoses, etc.	Fibrosarcoma (p. 794)
Synovial tissue	Synovioma	Synovial sarcoma (p. 802)
Peripheral nerves	Schwannoma	Malignant Schwannoma (p. 825)
	Neurofibroma	Neurofibrosarcoma (p. 825)
Paraganglia	Phaeochromocytoma	Malignant phaeochromocytoma (p. 564)
	Chemodectoma	? Haemangiopericytoma (p. 821)
	Paraganglioma (unclassified)	Malignant paraganglioma (p. 586)
Smooth muscle	Leiomyoma	Leiomyosarcoma (p. 809)
Tendon, aponeurosis	Xanthoma	Clear-cell sarcoma (p. 806)
	Lipoma	Epithelioid sarcoma (p. 814)
Adipose tissue	Lipoblastomatosis	Liposarcoma (p. 810)
Mesenchyme	Mesenchymoma	Malignant mesenchymoma (p. 812)
Blood vessels	Haemangioma	Haemangio-endothelioma (p. 817) Haemangiopericytoma (p. 554)
Lymph vessels	Lymphangioma	Lymphangio-endothelioma (p. 817)
Tumours of uncertain origin		
Granular cell tumour (p. 857)		'Alveolar soft part' sarcoma (p. 816)
Melanotic progonoma (p. 334)		Kaposi's sarcoma (p. 864)

sarcomas listed occur in children, many of them are extremely rare and these are mentioned only briefly.

Both the absolute and the relative incidence of the different types of sarcomas and their sites vary considerably from one reported series to another, mainly due to the criteria adopted by the authors or to inadvertent bias in the samples. There are, however, genuine variations in incidence in different parts of the world, and this has become more apparent from data of surveys conducted by the UICC (Doll *et al.*, 1972).

HISTOLOGICAL DIAGNOSIS

As described in Chapter 5, the standard histological methods can be supplemented by special techniques such as imprint cytology (p. 82), histochemistry (p. 84), cell culture (p. 86), and electron microscopy (p. 85), all of which have been employed in examining material in the Index Series. The first two techniques have proved to be of considerable help in identifying cell morphology in difficult cases.

The clinical and operative findings are also of considerable importance, and with the close co-operation of the surgeon, and the techniques listed, the number of unclassifiable tumours in the Index Series has been reduced to less than 5%.

The Index Series soft tissue sarcomas seen between 1950 and 1972 number 142, i.e. 12% of the total number of solid tumours (i.e. excluding leukaemias). Soft tissue sarcomas are therefore fifth in order of frequency and slightly less common than lymphomas.

A number of benign tumours of connective tissue were found to be difficult to distinguish from sarcomas, and these have been excluded, but if their numbers were added to those which proved to be sarcomas, the total would further emphasize the importance of these two groups of conditions in clinical paediatric practice.

The sarcomas of soft tissues to be described are as follows:

I. Rhabdomyosarcoma;
II. Fibrosarcoma;
III. Synovial sarcoma;
IV. 'Clear-cell' sarcoma;
V. Leiomyosarcoma;
VI. Liposarcoma;
VII. Malignant mesenchymoma;
VIII. Epithelioid sarcoma;
IX. Alveolar soft part sarcoma;
X. Haemangio-endotheliosarcoma.

I. RHABDOMYOSARCOMA

This malignant tumour, arising from a rhabdomyoblast, is the commonest of all soft tissue sarcomas in childhood (Mahour *et al.*, 1967), variously estimated to comprise from 12–56% of all solid malignant tumours in the paediatric age group. The higher incidence of this tumour in recently reported series reflects the greater confidence with which the diagnosis can now be made (Santamaria, Colebatch & Campbell, 1970; Bale & Reye, 1975).

AGE

It can occur at any age in childhood, but more especially in younger patients (Figure 23.2); in the Index Series the great majority were less than 4 years of age, the youngest being 3 months old.

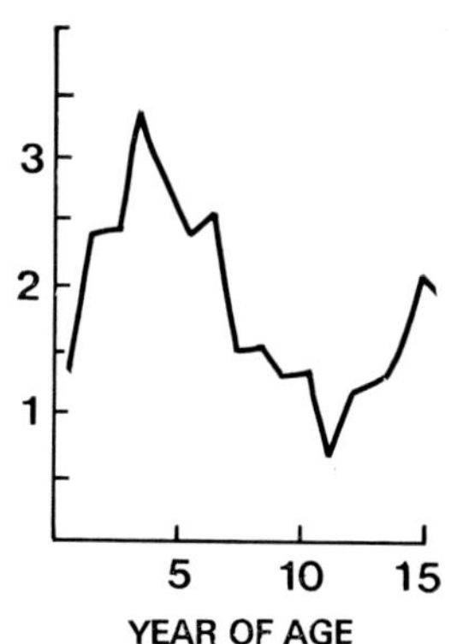

Figure 23.2. RHABDOMYOSARCOMA; incidence according to age showing a peak between 3 and 5 years, a fall in the third quinquennium, and commencement of a rise to a second peak between 15 and 18 years (for source of figures, see Fig. 2.2, p. 48).

SITES

Rhabdomyosarcomas are most frequently found in a relatively small number of typical sites (Albores-Saavedra *et al.*, 1965):
(*a*) *The head and neck*, particularly the orbit (p. 402), the nasopharynx (p. 358), less commonly the oropharynx (p. 345) and the inner ear (p. 364);
(*b*) *The pelvis*, especially the prostate or bladder (p. 704), the uterus and vagina (p. 701) and the spermatic cord (p. 891);
(*c*) *Less commonly in the extremities* (p. 789); and very rarely
(*d*) *On the trunk.*

In the Index Series the number arising in the extremities was unusually high, and the relative incidence is shown in Table 23.3.

MICROSCOPIC FEATURES

Rhabdomyosarcomas are highly malignant tumours composed of cells characterized by pleomorphism. Authorities differ as to whether it is essential to demonstrate cross striations to establish the diagnosis, and it is not our practice to insist on this as a diagnostic criterion (Fig. 23.3).

Three histological varieties (Horn & Enterline, 1958) occur in childhood:

(i) Embryonal,
(ii) Alveolar; and the
(iii) Pleomorphic type.

The first two types account for more than 90% of rhabdomyosarcomas. Recent studies suggest that it is a considerably underdiagnosed tumour in children, and the Index Series confirm this; 27 cases were initially diagnosed, but following a review of the entire series of tumours seen between 1950 and 1972, a further 20 cases were added by reclassifying those previously 'unclassified' (15), or diagnosed as neuroblastomas (2), synovial sarcoma (1) or as lymphomas (2). The alveolar histological pattern, the presence of glycogen in the cytoplasm, and in some instances the clinical course and the pattern in the metastases, were the grounds for reclassification. The small-celled alveolar type appeared to be the most likely to cause diagnostic difficulties.

Table 23.3. Rhabdomyosarcoma; types and sites of 64 cases in the Index Series (RCH 1950–1972)

Site	No.
Genito-urinary	27
Head and neck	15
Limbs and trunk	15
Other sites, axilla, etc.	7
Total	64
Histological type	**No.**
Embryonal	42
Alveolar	18
Pleomorphic	4
Total	64

Although three 'types' of rhabdomyosarcoma are described, a mixed histological pattern is common, particularly in the embryonal group, in which there are often wide variations within one tumour.

This view is supported by Bale and Reye (1975) who described variations in appearances from one block to another in many primary tumours, and also from primary to recurrent tumours.

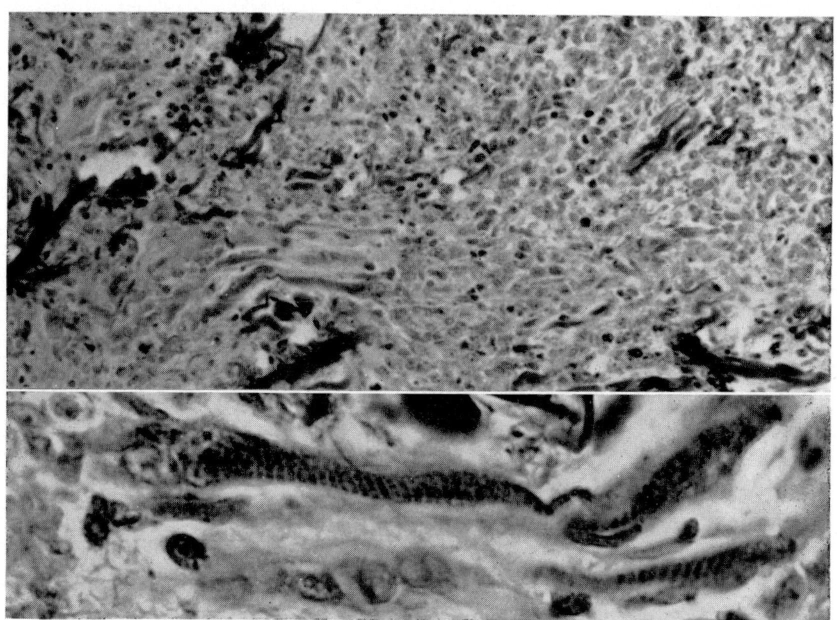

Figure 23.3. RHABDOMYOSARCOMA of the lip; (*a*) a cellular pleomorphic tumour, largely undifferentiated, but with a group of strap cells near the centre (PTAH × 130); (*b*) cross striations in several tumour cells. The large cell in the centre has several nuclei clustered at its expanded end (PTAH × 520).

[(*a*) *Top*. (*b*) *Bottom*.]

(i) Embryonal rhabdomyosarcoma (Fig. 23.3)

This is the least differentiated and can cause the greatest difficulty in diagnosis. While often very cellular, the botryoid type (*sarcoma botryoides*) common in the urogenital tract, may be sparsely cellular, often misleadingly so (Fig. 23.4a), the cells being widely separated by loose myxomatous matrix. The cells are arranged very irregularly, with rarely any parallelism of fibres or cell cytoplasm, and a completely chaotic pattern is characteristic. The nuclei are hyperchromatic, varying in size and shape, but giant and bizarre forms are infrequent, and mitoses are often scanty.

The diagnostic feature is the presence of longitudinal or transverse striations in the eosinophilic cytoplasm (Fig. 23.3), and this is prominent in a few of the tumour cells. Electron microscopy is helpful in demonstrating the striations, but the pattern of the tissue is more important than this single aspect in establishing the diagnosis.

Two variants of the embryonal type should be noted.

(*a*) *Tumours arising in the bile ducts* or gall-bladder (see p. 621); these rare tumours may have interlacing bundles of cells arranged like smooth muscle and can resemble a leiomyosarcoma. However, there are also myxoid areas characteristic of rhabdomyosarcoma, and these are helpful in making the diagnosis.

(*b*) *Polygonal, almost epithelial, cells* are seen in an equally rare variant arising in the uterus or the ovary. The cells are large and angular, but a few containing cross striations are found, in the primary tumour or in metastases, and the striations enable the correct diagnosis to be made.

(ii) Alveolar rhabdomyosarcoma

This appears to arise most commonly in the limbs or, less often, on the trunk. The characteristic feature is the tendency of the cells to be arranged in groups separated by delicate fibrovascular septa (Fig. 23.4b). The 'alveolar' appearance is the result of a single layer of cells lining each side of two closely placed but separate fibrovascular septa, mimicking in a somewhat fanciful way the alveoli of the fetal lung. This pattern often occurs amid sheets of otherwise undifferentiated cells. The tumour cells in the alveolar type are often quite uniform, with spherical or oval nuclei, a delicate nucleolus, and very scanty cytoplasm. Invariably, however, strap-like cytoplasmic processes can be identified by a careful search, and cross-striations can usually be demonstrated in these processes.

Alveolar rhabdomyosarcomas are occasionally mistaken for reticulum cell sarcoma or lymphosarcoma because of the relatively small size of the cells and their compact hyperchromatic nuclei (Fig. 23.4b). Some alveolar rhabdomyosarcomas may show pleomorphism with prominent cytoplasm, and the alveolar pattern may be rather inconspicuous.

(iii) Pleomorphic rhabdomyosarcoma

These are rare in children (e.g. only 4 of 64 rhabdomyosarcomas in the Index Series) and almost all arise in skeletal muscle. Their characteristic feature is extreme pleomorphism of the nuclei and abundant cytoplasm (Fig. 23.4c), often with prominent cross striations. The cells are usually arranged irregularly, but in some cases they are aligned in parallel groups; no alveolar pattern occurs.

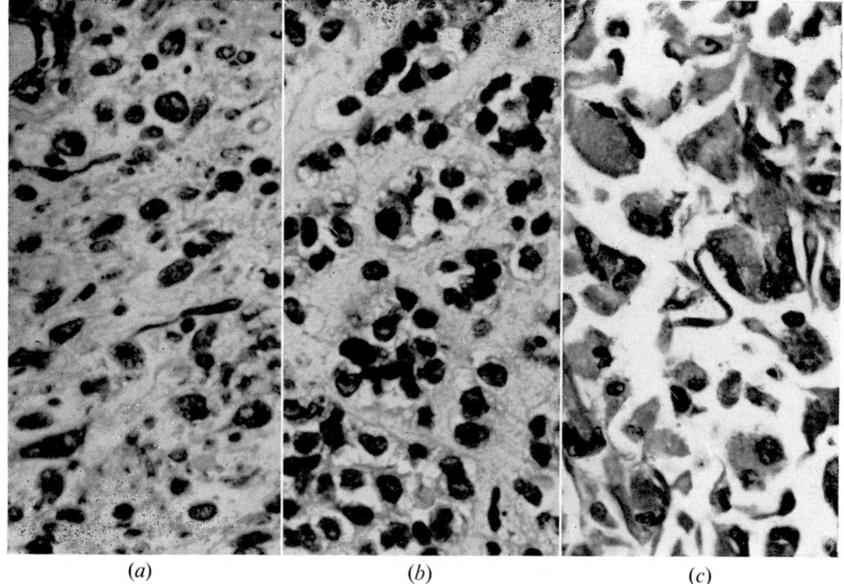

(*a*) (*b*) (*c*)

Figure 23.4. RHABDOMYOSARCOMA; the three histologic types; (*a*) the embryonal (botryoid) type with loose, myxoid stroma and small but very pleomorphic cells in totally disordered arrangement. Several 'tadpole' cells are present (H & E. × 520); (*b*) the alveolar pattern, of small dark layers on each side of two separate fibrovascular septa, and cells arranged in 'alveoli' (H & E. × 520); (*c*) pleomorphic pattern; the cells are irregular, but many have abundant eosinophilic cytoplasm, and the S-shaped cell (in the centre) has cross striations (H & E. × 520).

GROWTH AND SPREAD

All rhabdomyosarcomas grow rapidly and tend to metastasize early and widely. Exceptions are seen in the embryonal type, some of which have a greater tendency to infiltrate and to recur locally. This is particularly true of some of the botryoid embryonal tumours arising in the urogenital organs (see p. 703) or in the nasopharynx (p. 358).

Although most rhabdomyosarcomas grow rapidly, there is a small group in which progression is surprisingly slow and the prognosis correspondingly better.

Metastasis in regional lymph nodes is common, and in some sites, e.g. the nasopharynx, constitutes one of the modes of presentation (p. 356).

Rhabdomyosarcoma is also one of the few malignant neoplasms in children which may produce *bone-marrow metastases*, and in some cases this leads to the first manifestation of the disease (cf. neuroblastoma p. 552).

MODES OF PRESENTATION

As mentioned above, there are no distinctive clinical features by which one can readily identify a superficial swelling as a sarcoma (p. 779). When they arise in deeper tissues, in internal organs or on surfaces which communicate with the exterior, the signs or symptoms may arouse suspicion immediately. The following modes are characteristic of rhabdomyosarcoma.

(*a*) *A watery, blood-stained vaginal discharge* (p. 701);

(*b*) *A persistent, purulent, malodorous or blood-stained discharge* (or epistaxis) from the nose or ear (p. 364);

(*c*) *Retention of urine*, dysuria or strangury, in a boy less than 5 years of age, when the tumour arises in the prostate or bladder (p. 704);

(*d*) *A rapidly increase in the soft tissues of the orbit*, causing strabismus or proptosis (p. 403);

(*e*) *A tender swelling in the scrotum* close to but separate from the testis (p. 892).

(*f*) *Compression of the spinal cord*, causing paraplegia (p. 556) is a rare presentation (Watanabe *et al.*, 1974) but a rhabdomyosarcoma is one of the causes of a dumb-bell tumour (p. 460).

General non-specific symptoms such as irritability, loss of weight and appetite, are fairly common, but not as prominent as in the 'malignant malaise' occurring in children with a neuroblastoma (p. 549).

DIAGNOSIS

This can only be established by biopsy, and investigations are then required to determine what other effects the tumour has produced, and whether there are any detectable metastases.

INVESTIGATIONS

Radiographs of the primary tumour, including angiography, may be helpful in determining the site of origin and the extent of the tumour, and in excluding other conditions.

X-rays of the chest and a skeletal survey are necessary to detect metastases which would alter the management and the prognosis.

Haematological tests; a raised E.S.R. may be the first evidence of a latent malignancy, while anaemia or leucopenia suggest metastases in the marrow, and the need for a marrow biopsy. A full blood examination is required for pre-operative assessment and also for monitoring the effects of radiotherapy or cytotoxic agents during treatment.

Biopsy of the bone marrow occasionally provides the first firm evidence of a rhabdomyosarcoma. Negative findings at one site do not completely exclude the presence of metastases elsewhere. A marrow biopsy is not regarded as essential in all patients with a sarcoma, and is usually reserved for those with evidence of dissemination, when there are symptoms and radiographic changes suggesting bone metastases, or when peripheral blood counts are unaccountably low.

Management depends on a thorough assessment to:

(i) Identify the site and type of the primary tumour;

(ii) Determine as far as possible, the extent of local involvement; and

(iii) Whether there are distant metastases.

As well as radiography (e.g. of the lung fields), biopsy (or the primary, suspicious regional nodes, and the bone marrow), *other investigations appropriate to the site of the primary* are required, e.g. endoscopy in nasopharyngeal tumours (p. 355), or cysto-urethrography and pyelography in prostatic or vesical tumours (p. 704).

Treatment almost always includes surgery, chemotherapy and radiotherapy. Until relatively recently the possibility of cure was thought to depend to a large extent on extensive and radical removal of the primary. This belief has been modified recently by accumulating evidence that with integrated programmes of radiotherapy and chemotherapy, subtotal removal or in some cases only minimal resection in the form of a biopsy, is not inconsistent with cure (p. 793).

In the following section the treatment of rhabdomyosarcomas of the extremities is described, including the radiotherapy and chemotherapy which, with some minor modifications, can also be applied in rhabdomyosarcomas arising in other sites, i.e. in the orbit (p. 407), the nasopharynx (p. 358), the urogenital tract (p. 707), and the spermatic cord (p. 895).

TREATMENT OF RHABDOMYOSARCOMA

When the diagnosis has been made by drill biopsy or incision biopsy, a more radical excision may be indicated and there may be advantages in 'covering' this operation, as well as the original biopsy, with chemotherapy (p. 109); vincristine, with or without actinomycin D, is the usual choice.

Surgery

In the extremities, the scope of the excision depends on the accessibility of the site and the extent of local infiltration and involvement of important adjacent structures.

1. *The overlying skin* should be widely excised if the tumour is superficial and involves the dermis or subcutaneous tissues; the resulting defect can be closed by local mobilization, rotation flaps and/or full thickness skin grafts.
2. Total *removal of the muscle* in which the tumour arises, from origin to insertion, is desirable, as is the total excision of any continguous muscles which have been infiltrated (Suit *et al.*, 1973).

3. If a major *neurovascular bundle* has become involved, it may be desirable to remove the affected segment, but this might necessitate removing some of the muscles supplied by that bundle.

Depending on the disability resulting from such a removal, amputation (p. 754) might be preferable, but in general amputation for a soft tissue sarcoma is not often performed, and its abandonment does not seem to have been disadvantageous in patients treated with radiotherapy and chemotherapy (Kilman, Clatworthy *et al.*, 1973).

4. In some situations, e.g. in the nasopharynx, oropharynx and ear, mutilating operations are not warranted or unacceptable, and greater reliance is placed on chemotherapy and radiotherapy.

5. 'Prophylactic' excision of the related regional lymph nodes is not indicated, even when they are accessible. Where possible the nodes can be included in the field of radiotherapy given to the primary site; alternatively the nodes should be kept under close surveillance for evidence of metastases.

6. When lymph node metastases are present (Stage II), the choice between excision and radiotherapy is determined by the individual circumstances.

CHEMOTHERAPY OF SOFT TISSUE SARCOMAS

In the early years of cancer chemotherapy, sarcomas other than those of the reticulo-endothelial system appeared to be resistant to the drugs then available. Alkylating agents, however, have been shown for more than a decade to cause tumour regression in some cases, and vincristine and vinblastine likewise for nearly as long. In the past five years an increasing range of drugs has been used, with objective responses, better in some circumstances than will result from cyclophosphamide and other alkylating agents. The more rapidly growing and the more embryonic the tumour is, the more it is likely to respond to drugs acting on the cell-cycle (Fig. 6.2), such as vincristine, vinblastine, daunorubicin, adriamycin, mitomycin C, actinomycin D and methotrexate, given in adequate dosage. In many cases the best results have been obtained by the use of cyclophosphamide or dimethyl-triazeno-imidiazole-carboxamide or DTIC (a more recently introduced drug with some similar actions) in combination with one or more of the cycle-active agents. For example, in a mixed group of sarcomas in a somewhat older age group, the rate of objective response with adriamycin alone was reported as 22%, with DTIC alone it was 17%, but when both drugs were given in combination it was 41% (Gottlieb *et al.*, 1972).

The three drugs most commonly used in combination in the treatment of soft tissue sarcomas have been vincristine, actinomycin D and cyclophosphamide. If chemotherapy can be started before excisional surgery, one dose of at least two of these drugs may be given, up to 4 hours before operation, or preferably 48 hours before operation if the histopathological diagnosis has already been established (p. 25). Where residual or disseminated tumour is suspected or known, intensive therapy with all three drugs may begin as soon as the required period for wound healing has passed. Usually vincristine can be continued once weekly during this period and during any course of radiotherapy.

Intensive chemotherapy and irradiation cannot safely be given concurrently, and circumstances will determine their relative priorities. If there is evidence or a real risk of dissemination having occurred, intensive chemotherapy should be given first; if the risk of dissemination seems negligible but there is a risk of local recurrence, irradiation should be given priority.

Recently, a number of trials have been conducted with other combinations. Adriamycin or daunorubicin or mitomycin C as an alternative to actinomycin D, DTIC in place of cyclophosphamide, and methotrexate in addition to three other drugs—these and other variations have been producing responses in patients with tumours previously thought to be drug-resistant. Their safe and effective administration calls for a degree of expertise and special facilities (including monitoring the effects of cytotoxic agents, p. 116) which are normally available only in centres with experience in treating a large number of patients with tumours. The chemotherapy programme needs to be flexible to the extent that some drugs are better than others for certain tumours, and that the child's age, the size of the tumour and the site, etc., may call for individual variations.

Rhabdomyosarcoma

A common practice in this hospital has been to start chemotherapy (preferably before operation) with vincristine 1·8–2·0 mg/m^2/week IV, for 4–8 weeks (a current national protocol in U.S.A. gives it for 12 weeks), and during that period actinomycin D is also given, four doses each of 0·5 mg/m^2, over 7–10 days; the latter comes early in the plan of treatment if radiotherapy is deferred, otherwise it follows radiotherapy. Cyclophosphamide is begun about the sixth or seventh week and continued for 2 years (about 200 mg/m^2/day for 5 days orally) every 3–4 weeks. When there is a probability of dissemination, the cyclophosphamide is better given in high intermittent dosage, (e.g. 750–900 mg/m^2 IV every 3–4 weeks) interrupted every 3–4 months by another 8-day course of actinomycin D, plus two doses of vincristine. This sort of regimen, combined with surgery and radiotherapy, has already produced disease-free remissions for 3–4 years in several 'poor risk' patients.

The possibility that adriamycin and DTIC are a more effective combination is being investigated, and others have used mitomycin C and methotrexate with apparent success.

Other soft tissue sarcomas (listed on p. 782)

These are so uncommon that no adequate testing and comparison of the more recent drugs has yet been possible. Dramatic responses have been the exception, but tumour regression has followed chemotherapy, often without irradiation, in leiomyosarcoma, liposarcoma, haemangiosarcoma, haemangiopericytoma and possibly synovial sarcoma. The drugs used have included actinomycin D, daunorubicin, vincristine, alkylating agents and streptozoticin, usually in combinations of two or three agents.

In the Index Series a 9-year old girl with a large haemangiosarcoma in the buttock was treated with radiotherapy and with prolonged combination chemotherapy (vincristine, actinomycin D, methotrexate and later chlorambucil) and is free from overt tumour 3 years later.

RADIOTHERAPY

The aim is to destroy residual tumour cells in the primary site and/or in the regional nodes, and the dose is determined by the age and size of the patient, the site of the primary, the scope of the previous excision, and especially the proximity of tissues particularly vulnerable to irradiation (p. 124), e.g. an epiphysis, the gonads, or the eye. In general, the field irradiated should include the relevant regional lymph nodes draining the site of the primary tumour, unless these nodes were removed as part of the definitive operation. Megavoltage therapy in a dose of 2500–4000 rads over 3–4 weeks is usually employed.

PROGNOSIS IN RHABDOMYOSARCOMA

The median survival time of patients in the Index Series with a rhabdomyosarcoma was 19·2 months, indicating the poor overall prognosis before the introduction of integrated programmes of combined therapy. Factors which appear to influence the outcome are as follows:

1. *The age of the child;* those less than 10 years old at the time of diagnosis fare better than older children;
2. *The site;* the most favourable is the orbit (despite the relatively undifferentiated nature of these tumours) and the worst are those in the abdomen, where diagnosis is often made at a later stage;
3. *The histological pattern* (p. 785); in general, the embryonal type (especially the botryoid variety) is said to have a more favourable outcome, while the alveolar type is associated with the worst prognosis; however, Bale and Reye (1975) were unable to show any correlation between the histological types and survival rates, and our recent experience confirms this impression;
4. *The presence of metastases* (Stages II and III) in part reflect such factors as the degree of differentiation, the rate of growth, or delay in diagnosis, all of which are unfavourable, and the outcome is consequently worse;
5. *The completeness of the surgical excision.* Total removal of the primary

together with an adequate margin of adjacent tissue, while desirable, is not essential and less important than previously. 'Reasonable' excision (Kilman, Clatworthy *et al.*, 1973) rather than radical ablative surgery, when combined with radiotherapy and combination chemotherapy, is followed by higher survival rates than radical surgery alone.

In Stage I cases, survival rates of 65–80% are now being reported, (Sutow, Sullivan *et al.*, 1970; Erhlich *et al.*, 1971; Pratt, Hustu, Fleming & Pinkel, 1972; Donaldson *et al.*, 1973; Kilman, Clatworthy *et al.*, 1973; Jaffe, Filler *et al.*, 1973; Ragab, 1972/73).

In summary, the treatment of rhabdomyosarcoma varies to some extent according to its site of origin, but the general principles are as follows:

Surgical excision of the primary tumour where feasible. This should be as complete as possible but not radical or mutilating.

Radiotherapy to the site of the primary tumour, including the regional nodes in the same field if possible, and shielding adjacent vulnerable tissues.

Chemotherapy, usually in combinations of two, three or four cytotoxic agents as a primary course, with secondary courses at intervals of 1 to 3 months continuing for up to 2 years.

An Intergroup Study in progress since 1972 has been established to obtain answers to questions posed by results already obtained. The grouping of patients in this study is shown in Table 23.4 (after Heyn, 1975). The information expected from this controlled study can be summarized as follows.

Table 23.4. Clinical grouping for the Intergroup Study of rhabdomyosarcoma

Group I	Localized tumour completely resected (regional lymph nodes not involved).
Group II	
A.	Tumour grossly resected, with microscopic residual disease (lymph modes negative).
B.	Regional disease, completely resected; regional nodes involved and/or extension of tumour into an adjacent organ.
C.	Regional disease with regional nodes involved, tumour grossly resected, but with evidence of microscopic residual tumour.
Group III	
	Incomplete resection of tumour, or biopsy only, with gross residual disease.
Group IV	
	Distant metastatic disease present at diagnosis.

(a) The need for radiotherapy when the primary tumour has been completely excised. In addition to surgery and combination chemotherapy, a randomized subgroup of patients in Group I will be treated with radiotherapy, while the other half will not.

(b) The relative effectiveness of two regimes of multidrug chemotherapy: actinomycin D-vincristine for one year, and vincristine-actinomycin D-cyclophosphamide for 2 years. Patients in Group II are divided into two randomized subgroups for this purpose.

(c) The effect of adding adriamycin to the standard three drug regime. Patients in Groups III and IV are treated initially with combination chemotherapy, followed by radiotherapy, and surgery if feasible. The patients will then be randomly divided into two subgroups, one of which receives adriamycin in addition to the recurrent courses of vincristine-actinomycin D-cyclophosphamide which both subgroups receive.

II. FIBROSARCOMA

Tumours arising from fibrous tissue constitute a special problem in children, for it can be extremely difficult to determine whether they are benign or malignant. The many kinds of fibromatoses (p. 798) also contribute to these difficulties (Enzinger, 1965b).

SITES

In the Index Series most of the fibrosarcomas arose in the subcutaneous tissues of the limbs; three arose in bone and are described in the appropriate chapter (p. 761).

Rarely a fibrosarcoma arises in the supporting stroma of a viscus, and occasionally from the connective tissue sheath of a nerve (p. 825), as a neurofibrosarcoma (Soule *et al.*, 1968).

Very rarely a fibrosarcoma may develop in the retroperitoneal tissues (p. 584), or in a bronchus (p. 478) in which case the differential diagnosis from 'pseudosarcoma' (p. 470) is particularly important.

AGE

They occur throughout the paediatric age group, (Exelby *et al.*, 1973), with a slight peak between 1 and 5 years of age and a second between 10 and 15 years. A very occasional tumour appears to be congenital.

MACROSCOPIC APPEARANCES

Fibrosarcomas are not truly encapsulated, although frequently surrounded by a pseudocapsule of flattened cells. The tumour is usually white and firm, the degree of firmness depending on the amount of collagen produced by the tumour cells. Well-differentiated tumours are firm and rather rubbery; less differentiated tumours are soft and whitish, and may show areas of haemorrhage.

SPREAD

Most fibrosarcomas grow slowly (Stout, 1962), and although they are locally aggressive and tend to recur following excision, metastasis may occur rather late. Some are extremely indolent, which is unusual in childhood neoplasms.

In the Index Series two cases illustrate the propensity of fibrosarcomas to recur locally and spread slowly.

1. A boy aged 6 received a blow on the thigh and a subsequent depression at the site of injury was considered to be due to fat necrosis and atrophy. Some months later a lump slowly appeared at the edge of the depression. At 10 years of age the swelling was excised and considered to be a fibroma, although it was cellular and contained occasional mitoses; 3 years later (at 13 years of age), it recurred and was again excised; 4 years later a further recurrence 2 cm in diameter was excised and the histological diagnosis was a well-differentiated fibrosarcoma.

2. A boy aged 8 years presented with a swelling posterior to the right parotid, and biopsy showed a well-differentiated fibrosarcoma. Total excision was attempted but was incomplete. Radiotherapy was given, but the mass recurred, and after two further attempts at excision he died 2½ years later with pulmonary metastases which were so well differentiated that they could have been taken for fibromas (Fig. 23.5b).

MICROSCOPIC FEATURES

The classic feature is the 'herringbone' or 'fir tree' pattern, i.e. cells arranged in interlacing bundles intersecting in a 'V' formation (Fig. 23.5a). The nuclei may be rounded and plump, or slender and rather pointed. The tumour cells produce collagen, and abundant reticulum formation can be demonstrated by special stains. The cellularity and mitotic index give some indication of the tumour's malignant potential, but they do not always correlate well with the outcome which in many instances seems to depend more on the site of the tumour than on its histological structure.

The tumour cells are PAS negative (p. 85) and show marked acid phosphatase activity. Histological differentiation from a leiomyosarcoma or a synovial sarcoma may be difficult (p. 803) and may depend on electron microscopy; the pleomorphic type can usually be distinguished by its cytological characteristics (p. 40).

Congenital (juvenile) fibrosarcoma. Differentiation of this condition from fibrosarcoma is by no means easy, and rests chiefly on the presence of the tumour at birth or its appearance and rapid growth in the neonatal period. The incidence is equal in boys and girls, and the commonest sites are the extremities (eight of the eleven reported in the literature; Balsaver, Butler & Martin, 1967).

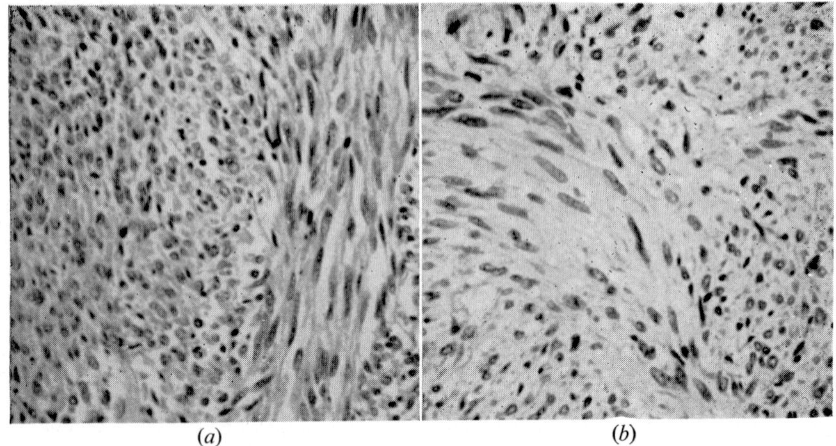

(*a*) (*b*)

Figure 23.5. FIBROSARCOMA; (*a*) a slightly unusual primary tumour (on the face); interlacing swathes ('herring bone' pattern) of plump tumour cells (H & E. × 200); (*b*) pulmonary metastases from this tumour grew extremely slowly, being less cellular and highly differentiated (H & E. × 200).

The clinical features are a large, rapidly growing, solid tumour with a violaceous colour suggestive of a vascular lesion. At operation the mass is firm, rubbery, poorly defined and partially or wholly unencapsulated. The cut surface is usually fleshy, lobulated, greyish white to tan, and occasionally contains friable areas of necrosis.

Microscopically the findings are typical of fibrosarcoma, i.e. spindle cells in a 'herring bone' or 'fir-tree' pattern, with little or no pleomorphism, moderate nuclear hyperchromatism and scattered mitotic figures.

Differentiation from true fibrosarcoma is usually based on the age of the patient and the presence of the tumour at birth. Its distinction from the aggressive forms of 'fibromatosis' (including 'juvenile progressive fibromatosis') is more difficult, and again rests on its presence at birth.

Excision is usually followed by local recurrence, often on more than one occasion, but the tumour can usually be controlled without amputation, and metastasis is extremely rare.

HISTOLOGICAL DIFFERENTIATION FROM BENIGN FIBROUS LESIONS

1. Fibromas

(*a*) *True, localized fibromas*, composed of fibroblasts and fibrocytes are uncommon in childhood, but hamartomas containing fibrous tissue are relatively common (Enzinger, 1965a). The classical subdivision of fibromas in adults, into '*fibroma durum*' and '*fibroma molle*', is somewhat artificial in childhood, although a fibroma of one or other kind sometimes arises in skin or the mucous membrane in a child. Fibromas are more common in younger children (Enzinger, 1965b), quite probably hamartomas rather than true tumours, and occasionally multiple.

(*b*) '*Dermatofibromas*' occasionally occur in older children, and their features are almost identical to those more commonly seen in adults. In current terminology they are fibrous histiocytomas, now recognized as occurring in a variety of sites, chiefly but not exclusively in subcutaneous soft tissues. The parent cell is thought to be a histiocytic type of cell which undergoes metaplasia to form fibroblasts and collagen. In children they are to be distinguished from fibrosarcomas and from histiocytoses (p. 219), depending on which type of cell dominates the histological picture.

(*c*) *The recurring digital fibroma* of Reye (Reye, 1956) is a rare and interesting conditions of the fingers or toes in infants and young children (Bloem *et al.*, 1974). It is often multiple (Fig. 23.6), shows a great tendency to recur following local excision, and is composed of plump, spindle-shaped fibroblasts containing spherical eosinophilic inclusions in the cytoplasm or in the nucleus, and occasionally free in the intercellular connective tissue. It is suggested that these inclusions represent a virus infection, but no virus has yet been isolated and the etiology is still unknown. They are only important because their cellularity and tendency to recur locally may be interpreted as evidence of

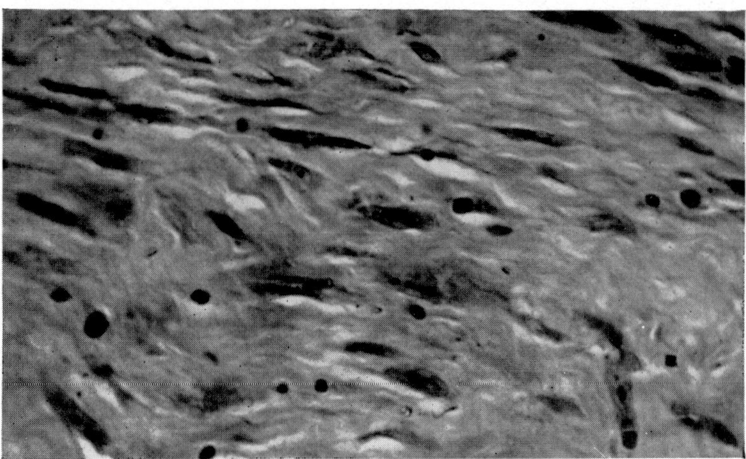

Figure 23.6. RECURRING DIGITAL FIBROMA OF REYE; this cellular fibroma differs from others occurring elsewhere in that it contains spherical, eosinophilic, intracytoplasmic inclusion bodies which stain brick red with Masson's stain, and appear here as sharply defined, round black blobs (Masson × 520).

malignancy, and this may lead to an excision which is more radical than justified. However, in one of the six patients reported by Reye, amputation of a digit became necessary because of repeated recurrences and infiltration of bone and tendon.

2. **The Fibromatoses**

This is a diverse and potentially misleading group of conditions (Stout, 1954), some of which are congenital while others appear in early infancy, later in childhood, or in adult life. The lesions may be localized or generalized (Plaschkes, 1974), and the more or less distinct entities seen in the paediatric age group are as follows.

(*a*) *A keloid* is a smooth, superficial, reddish-purple lesion arising in a laceration, healed pustule or surgical scar in predisposed individuals, or certain vulnerable areas (e.g. the front of the chest). It is composed of coarse, interlacing, homogenous bundles of collagen, often associated with thinning of the overlying epidermis. The lesion tends to recur following excision; it is not a tumour but the result of localized hyperplasia of fibroblasts with excessive formation of collagen.

An unusual but recognized type presents as a small papule following a trivial pustule in the skin of the front of the chest, and slowly spreads to form a firm, sessile, roughly spherical mass which recurs rapidly following excision, and extends by progressively involving normal skin around the site of attachment. This 'creeping keloid' is particularly difficult to treat. Clinically, its differentiation from sarcoma may be a problem, but histologically there is little or nothing to suggest malignancy.

(*b*) '*Nodular* (*pseudosarcomatous*) *fasciitis*' (Stout, 1961; Price, Silliphant & Shuman, 1961) is uncommon but not unknown in children. The features are the same as in adults: a swelling in a muscle or in subcutaneous tissue, growing at an alarming rate.

Histologically it is cellular and consists of plump, often irregular fibroblasts set in a mucoid stroma, with apparent destruction and infiltration of adjacent tissues. Mitoses may be seen, but they are always regular. This lesion is important because it can be readily mistaken for a fibrosarcoma (Butler, 1965); the mucoid stroma, the rather irregular disposition of the proliferating cells and the regular mitoses are distinctive features of this condition.

(*c*) *Fibromatosis colli* is a benign, poorly-localized overgrowth of fibrous tissue, e.g. perhaps in the sternomastoid muscle or more typically in various planes in the neck (Connolly, 1961) in infants and young children. In the early stages the lesion is often very cellular and consists of proliferating fibroblasts infiltrating between degenerating skeletal muscle which may contain multinucleated 'muscle giant cells' or bizarre nuclei. The etiology is still controversial, and although formerly attributed to perinatal trauma, a sternomastoid 'tumour' is currently believed to be an 'embryopathy' or a fibromatosis, i.e. a benign proliferation of fibroblasts.

Differentiation from a fibrosarcoma may theoretically pose a problem if the pathologist is not aware of the histology, especially when the 'tumour' has a fairly cellular picture and steadily increases in size for some weeks or months. Fortunately, it seems that a proven sarcoma of the sternomastoid muscle has never been reported (Gruhn & Hurwitt, 1951; Jones, 1968).

(*d*) *Palmar fibromatosis* is extremely rare in children, but similar to the more common *plantar fibromatosis*. The latter presents as a nodule in the plantar fascia and the histology in the early stages is often strikingly cellular, even to the production of mitotic figures, and confusion with fibrosarcoma is possible. Clinical experience suggests that when left alone these lesions tend to regress spontaneously in children. However, some believe that the lesion should be widely and completely excised to prevent local recurrence.

(*e*) *Juvenile aponeurotic fibroma* (syn. calcifying fibroma) is also a rare lesion, chiefly affecting the muscles and subcutaneous fat of the hands, and occasionally the foot and ankle (Booher & McPeak, 1959). It may also arise from the ligamentum flavum in the cervical region and present as a mass on the back of the neck.

Histologically it consists of infiltrating fibroblasts showing a peculiar focal degeneration and chondroid metaplasia in the stroma (Allen & Enzinger, 1970). They have a tendency to recur locally following inadequate excision, and calcification is not uncommon (Keaseby, 1953).

(*f*) *Nasopharyngeal 'fibroma'* (syn. juvenile angiofibroma) is very rare and appear to be almost confined to adolescent males, the youngest patient reported being 10 years of age (p. 352). They are locally invasive and composed of a fairly mature fibroblastic stroma intimately associated with thin-walled blood vessels. The lesion arises in the wall of the nasopharynx and frequently undergoes spontaneous regression. However, they are also known to invade the nasopharyngeal wall with destruction of bone; their position and their vascularity make them particularly difficult to eradicate (see p. 354).

(*g*) *Aggressive* (*juvenile*) *fibromatosis* (Fig. 23.7). This is most commonly found in children 1–2 years old; it can occur anywhere, but most frequently in the subcutaneous tissues of the thorax or the limbs. Clinically it appears as a swelling with some cicatrization in the overlying skin and subcutaneous tissue. The swelling is hard, diffuse and ill-defined, and adherent to the skin.

Histologically it consists of extremely cellular masses of fibroblasts producing delicate collagen fibres in a loose mucoid stroma. The collagen is often laid down in a wavy pattern simulating nerve bundles. In the subcutaneous fat the lesion infiltrates widely, tethering the epidermis to the deep fascia. Finger-like projections of loose cellular fibroblastic tissue extending into normal adipose tissue are very characteristic of this lesion. Rarely the stroma of the lesion contains giant cells and lipid.

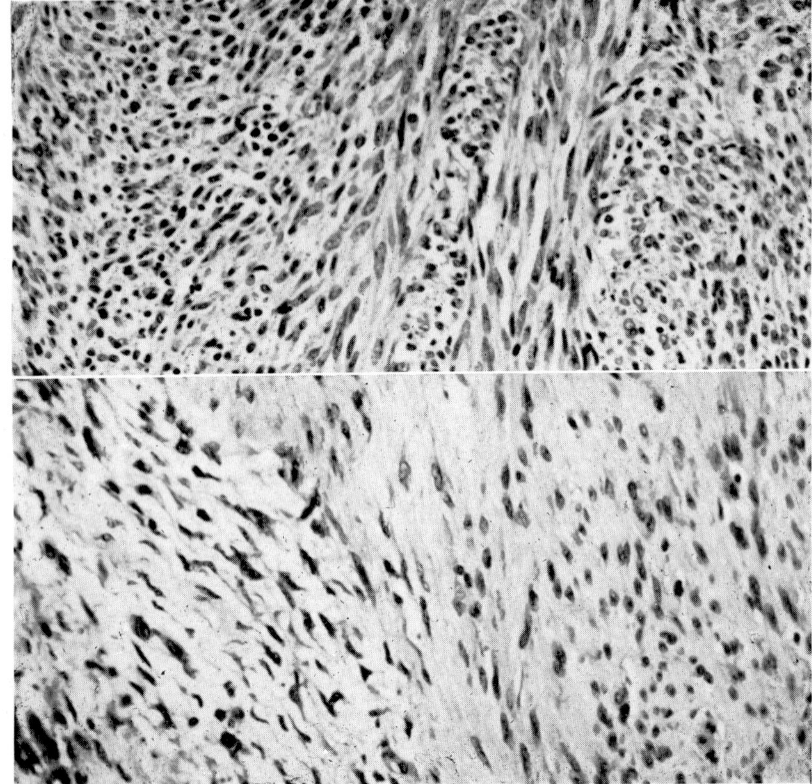

Figure 23.7. (*a*) FIBROSARCOMA composed of plump, closely packed cells with a 'herring bone' pattern (H & E. × 200), for comparison with (*b*) JUVENILE FIBROMATOSIS, an aggressive example from subcutaneous tissue; with a poorly defined interlacing pattern of spindle shaped plump fibroblasts. Note the band of wavy fibroblasts (lower left) suggestive of neurofibroma (Fig. 23.14b, p. 824).

[(*a*) *Top.* (*b*) *Bottom.*]

The natural history is one of spontaneous regression and even when there are considerable amounts of fibroblastic tissue, almost complete resolution ultimately occurs. Because of uncertainty as to the diagnosis and their rapid clinical progress, surgical excision is not infrequently performed, and local recurrence is extremely common. When the correct diagnosis is made, the lesion is simply observed, and spontaneous arrest and resolution usually follow.

(*h*) *Congenital generalized fibromatosis.* In this syndrome there are multiple, poorly localized masses of cellular fibroblastic tissue. Lesions in bone (p. 732), in soft tissue and viscera, including the intestine, are common; although most of the lesions ultimately heal, death from overwhelming infection in the first few weeks of life is a recognized hazard. The relationship of this particular condition to other forms of fibromatosis in children, and to localized areas of fibrous tissue in bone (i.e. various types of fibrous dysplasia), is uncertain.

(*i*) *Dermatofibrosarcoma protuberans* (Taylor & Helwig, 1962; Burkhandt *et al.*, 1966) is considered by some to be indistinguishable from a dermatofibroma (p. 797); it is a relatively benign neoplasm which, apart from a tendency to local recurrence, has none of the hallmarks of a truly malignant neoplasm (Burckhardt *et al.*, 1966).

CORRELATION OF HISTOLOGY AND BEHAVIOUR

In all the above conditions the problem of differentiating benign from malignant lesions arises. The chief difficulty is that whereas the clinician is presented with patients in a wide range of age groups, with fibrous lesions arising in various sites and having different clinical characteristics and rates of growth, e.g. lesions which may cease to grow, regress spontaneously or recur repeatedly (with or without distant metastasis), the histopathologist is presented with fibroblastic lesions showing a much smaller range of variations in pattern, cellularity, nuclear morphology and ability to form collagen.

In general, both histological and clinical data are required to reach a diagnosis. When the site of the lesion, the clinical history and the microscopic findings are all taken into consideration, it is usually possible to distinguish true fibrosarcomas from the fibromatoses.

The difficulties are well exemplified in a report by Stout (1962) of 23 cases of fibrosarcoma, and a review of 31 possible cases in the literature. In the total group of 54, metastases were found in only 4 patients, and metastasis could not be correlated with the mitotic index of the tumour.

This typifies the difficulty in assigning a degree of malignancy to any particular fibroblastic proliferation. In general, however, a high degree of *cellularity*, the presence of *mitoses*, particularly *bizarre mitotic figures*, a *reduced amount of reticulin and collagen* formation, and a *herringbone* or *'fir tree' pattern*, are indicative of fibrosarcoma, and these points serve to distinguish it from benign fibrous proliferations.

TREATMENT

Because of the relative radioresistance of fibrosarcoma, and the possible but unproven value of chemotherapy, surgical excision of the tumour assumes greater importance than in rhabdomyosarcoma (Hays *et al.*, 1970).

Surgery. Whenever possible the tumour and a generous margin of surrounding normal tissue should be excised. In the limbs the muscle of origin should be removed from origin to insertion, together with any adjacent muscle which has become infiltrated, following the same general principles as in rhabdomyosarcoma in an extremity (p. 789), except that amputation is rarely indicated.

Chemotherapy Drugs have been tested less extensively because of its low incidence. Tumour regression has occurred in some cases following a single drug, e.g. cyclophosphamide, methotrexate, daunorubicin or DTIC. The total reported experience to date however favours combination therapy for the best results: cyclophosphamide and methotrexate with actinomycin D, mitomycin C or vincristine; or adriamycin with DTIC; or bleomycin perhaps combined with a cycle-active agent.

In the Index Series one boy aged 10 years with a fibrosarcoma in the thigh had an apparently total excision of the tumour followed by methotrexate 20 mg/m^2 twice weekly for 4 months, and is well and free of disease 5 years later.

Radiotherapy, in doses up to 4500 rads, should be considered, but may be reserved for recurrences. When employed, careful shielding or a somewhat reduced total dosage may be required when there is an epiphysis or other vulnerable structure close to the area to be irradiated.

Recurrences are treated by further wide but not necessarily destructive excision, and chemotherapy.

PROGNOSIS

Generally the prognosis is good, with metastases occurring in only 5–10% of fibrosarcomas in childhood. Even when local recurrences appear they are often spread over many years and 10-year rather than 2 or 5-year survival rates are more relevant.

III. SYNOVIAL SARCOMA

(syn. synoviosarcoma, synovio-endothelioma, malignant synovioma, sarcomesothelioma)

This tumour accounts for approximately 7% of soft tissue sarcomas in those less than 16 years of age, and some 10% of sarcomas in all age groups (Cadman, Soule & Kelly, 1965). The figures quoted below are taken from their review of 134 cases at the Mayo Clinic.

AGE : SEX

Synovial sarcoma is not typically a tumour of young children; the peak incidence lies between 15 and 40 years of age. Only some 5% occur in children less than 10 years of age, and a slightly greater proportion between 10 and 15 years (Mackenzie, 1966).

There is no great preponderance in either sex, but the male : female ratio in two large series was reported to be 3 : 2 and 1·9 : 1.

SITES

In large series the commonest sites are the extremities, especially in the thigh or around the knee joint. Although the tumour may arise from the synovium of a joint, tendon sheath or a bursa, most synovial sarcomas appear to arise *de novo* where no synovium normally exists, presumably from an undifferentiated mesenchymal cell.

This tumour can appear in unexpected sites. Roth *et al.* (1975) reported cases of synovial sarcoma arising in cervical prevertebral tissues, from the base of the skull to the deep triangle of the neck; 7 of the 23 were between 10 and 15 years of age, and 13 of the 24 were less than 20 years of age.

MACROSCOPIC APPEARANCES

The typical tumour is greyish yellow, roughly rounded or ovoid, lobulated, and often appears to be encapsulated; haemorrhage and necrosis are unusual. In some examples the cut surface has a slightly mucoid appearance, and cystic spaces up to 1 cm in diameter are occasionally seen.

MICROSCOPIC FINDINGS

The distinctive feature is the biphasic cellular pattern (Fig. 23.8) composed of:
(*a*) *Plump endothelium-like cells* lining clefts or acinar structures, often with a mucoid substance; and
(*b*) *Spindle cells forming collagen*, in a background stroma with which the pseudo-epithelial areas mingle. The stroma may show foci of calcification and hyalinization. In typical 'differentiated' examples, diagnosis is a relatively simple matter, but when the 'epithelial' areas are absent, inconspicuous or poorly differentiated, and the spindle cells are preponderant, differentiation from a fibrosarcoma may be extremely difficult. The clefts should always be sought, for the certain diagnosis of a synovial sarcoma depends upon their presence.

'Benign' synoviomas occur, chiefly in the fingers, wrist and toes; their clinical and even their histological features can closely resemble their malignant counterpart (Wright, 1952). Benign synoviomas are composed of sparsely cellular fibroblastic tissue containing clefts and spaces, and the ground substance may be mucoid. The problem in distinguishing them from malignant synovioma is accentuated when the cells are well-differentiated.

In the Index Series two malignant synoviomas were well-differentiated tumours related to the elbow joint and the femur respectively. They were initially considered to be probably benign, but both recurred after local excision, and one has metastasized and led to the death of the patient.

SPREAD

The tumour tends to infiltrate locally along fascial and muscle planes; it may also spread along lymphatics as well as via the bloodstream, and it is recognized as one of the sarcomas likely to metastasize to regional nodes (p. 42). It has a marked tendency to recur locally, largely because of the development of a pseudocapsule of compressed malignant cells from which the mass can be 'shelled out', in the mistaken belief that it is benign.

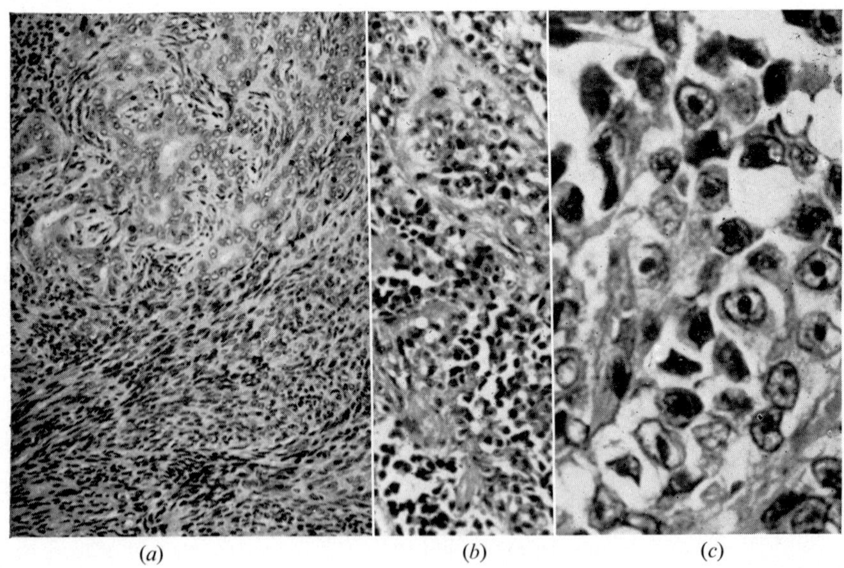

Figure 23.8. SYNOVIAL SARCOMA; (*a*) the classical 'biphasic' pattern of whorled spindle cell stroma (below) and cells arranged in a 'glandular' pattern resembling an epithelial tumour (above) (H & E. × 90); (*b*) another pattern in which synovial cells line clefts in the stroma, an appearance easily confused with alveolar acinar-like carcinoma, or the mucoid ground substance of rhabdomyosarcoma (H & E. × 180); (*c*) high power of (*b*) showing prominent nucleoli (H & E. × 468).

MODES OF PRESENTATION

A palpable mass or swelling, as described on p. 779 is a common and relatively non-specific mode of most sarcomas, and this is the presentation in more than 95 % of cases of synovial sarcoma.

Pain or tenderness is also fairly common (approximately 60 %) and any prolonged unexplained pain in the thigh or related to a joint is grounds for suspicion (Mackenzie, 1966).

Less commonly *general systemic symptoms* such as loss of weight are the first complaint, and occasionally pulmonary metastases give rise to the first evidence of the tumour, e.g. by causing haemoptysis.

INVESTIGATIONS

The radiological findings are not always positive, but faint irregular plaques of calcification have been reported in 30 % of cases, and infiltration or pressure erosion or adjacent bone occurs in 5–10 %.

Radiographs of the lungs are necessary to determine the extent of metastases.

Biopsy is required if there are any significantly enlarged regional nodes, e.g. in the inguinal region, and lymphangiography, is indicated to investigate the possibility of metastases in deep inguinal and para-aortic lymph nodes.

DIAGNOSIS

Although synovial sarcoma is occasionally suggested by the clinical and radiological findings, certainty depends upon histological findings.

In view of the relatively common occurrence of synovial sarcomas in the region of the thigh and the knee joint, swellings in these areas, including the popliteal fossa (p. 228), should be viewed with suspicion and explored without delay.

TREATMENT

As with sarcomas of the extremities in general, amputation perhaps offers the greatest prospect of cure when there is no evidence of metastasis. Because of the frequent occurrence of synovial sarcoma in the proximal part of the leg, and their marked tendency to recur (even after many years) a high amputation is theoretically indicated, but the advantages of disarticulation at the hip joint, compared with less radical surgery, may be marginal (e.g. 48 % mortality v 50 % recurrence).

In their review of 134 cases, Cadman *et al.* drew some conclusions from various methods of treatment which had been employed. They noted that in synovial sarcomas one should be wary of 5-year or even 10-year 'cures', for in six of their patients the tumour reappeared 6–11 years after apparently successful treatment.

When local excision alone was performed, the recurrence rate was 91%, and this was reduced to 50% when radiotherapy was given following local excision.

Amputation within one month of diagnosis was carried out in 23 patients, of whom 11 (48%) died of their tumour, but at least three of the remainder survived without evidence of tumour for more than 5–9 years. Radiotherapy, particularly hyperbaric irradiation, has produced better results recently, using mega voltage radiation to a dose of 6000–8000 rads in twenty fractions over 8 weeks.

Chemotherapy was not involved in the results quoted above, and adriamycin and cyclophosphamide both offer some prospects of improved results.

PROGNOSIS

The mean duration from onset of symptoms to death in 78 cases was 6·5 years, longer than most other comparably lethal sarcomas (Cadman *et al.*, 1965). The biological behaviour of some synovial sarcomas is unusual and a slow growth rate would explain the unexpected long-term survival (or 'cure') seen in some patients in whom the initial diagnosis was mistaken and in whom recurrences had occurred. In 6 of their 13 patients who may have been cured, the interval between onset of symptoms and definitive treatment was 6·2 years, three times as long as the average of those known to have died of their tumour. Mackenzie (1966) reported two patients alive and free of disease following excision of five and six recurrences.

Cade (1962) has emphasized the advantages of an integrated plan of treatment combining adequate surgery, radiotherapy and chemotherapy.

Two recent reviews (Cameron & Kostuik, 1974; Gerner & Moore, 1975) have emphasized the long natural history of this tumour and the tendency to late recurrence. Gerner and Moore reported a 5-year survival rate of 36% in their 34 patients, and inferred that results might be improved by resisting the temptation to persist with conservative measures for apparently 'encapsulated' recurrences of a tumour which nevertheless has a high malignant potential.

IV. 'CLEAR-CELL' SARCOMA

This connective tissue sarcoma, first described as a distinct entity by Enzinger (1965c), arises from tendons or aponeuroses in the extremities.

SITES

In the 21 cases collected by Enzinger, the commonest site was the region of the foot (tendo Achilles, plantar fascia and ankle), the knee, and less commonly the upper limb.

AGE: SEX

Most of the reported cases have been in young adults, with a median age of 24 years; five patients were between 13 and 16 years of age at the time of diagnosis; none was younger, and it appears that when the tumour arises in the paediatric age group it is exclusively in the third quinquennium. Males appear to be affected slightly more often than females.

MACROSCOPIC APPEARANCES

The tumour is usually small (average diameter 4 cm), roughly spherical, firm and smooth, or nodular and sometimes lobulated. Most are well defined swellings surrounded by dense fibrous tissue (8 of 21 were described as 'encapsulated'), and not fixed to the overlying skin. The cut surface is usually grey to white in colour, and sometimes mottled.

MICROSCOPIC FINDINGS

The typical pattern is of compact aggregates of cells separated by delicate septa of fibrous tissue; vascular structures are not prominent. The cells are epithelioid in appearance; the pale-staining amphophilic cytoplasm has indistinct borders; and the appearance of the 'clear' cells is enhanced by the presence of minute vacuoles. The nucleus is prominent (Fig. 23.9) and multinucleated giant cells were seen in 14 of the 21 cases described.

SPREAD

Infiltration of adjacent structures is indicated by the high recurrence rate after local excision (16 of 19 cases). Metastases in regional lymph nodes are common, and the most usual form of spread. The second commonest is metastasis to the lungs, although this may be long delayed.

The natural history is of one of slow but relentless growth and local recurrences, even after radical excision; eventually metastasis to the lungs occurs, less commonly to the heart, liver and brain. The behaviour of the tumour has some similarities to synovial sarcoma; the general plan of treatment (p. 805) and the results are also similar.

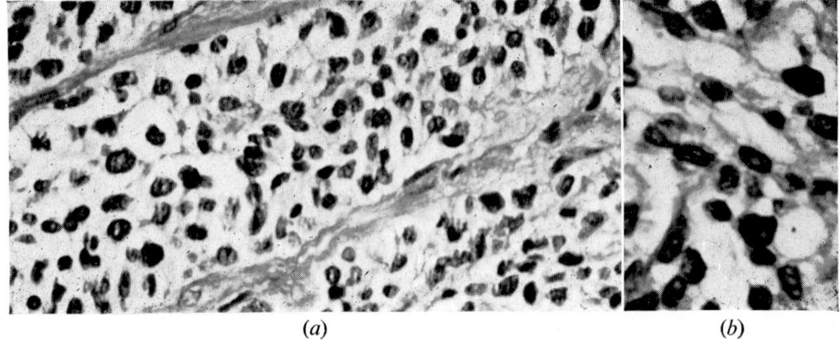

(a) (b)

Figure 23.9. CLEAR CELL SARCOMA; (*a*) cells arranged in a pattern resembling alveolar rhabdomyosarcoma, but with a more uniform nuclei and clear 'watery' cytoplasm (H & E. × 200); (*b*) shown in more detail at higher magnification (H & E. × 520).

MODE OF PRESENTATION

A small painless swelling was the chief clinical feature in all cases in the reported series; about half were associated with some mild pain or tenderness.

INVESTIGATION: DIAGNOSIS

Radiological findings were confined to non-specific soft tissue shadows, and films of the lung fields are required to exclude pulmonary metastases. Biopsy of the regional nodes is indicated when there is any significant enlargement.

Diagnosis rests upon excision biopsy and histological examination.

TREATMENT

Following establishment of the diagnosis by biopsy, a more extensive resection is required if the tumour was encapsulated and 'shelled out'. The extent of radical excision depends upon the site of the primary, but on general principles amputation would be justified by the high recurrence rate after even extensive local resection. When amputation is declined or contra-indicated, irradiation of the primary site, including the regional nodes is probably indicated.

The role of chemotherapy has not been established because of the rarity of the tumour, but on general principles the programmes recommended for rhabdomyosarcoma (p. 789) or synovial sarcoma (p. 805) would seem to be the most appropriate.

RESULTS

In the only series reported (Enzinger, 1965a) only 5 of the 19 patients reviewed were alive and free of disease, and the number of long term survivors may eventually be even less because of delayed appearance of pulmonary metastases, in one case as long as 8 years after the first definitive operation.

In the Index Series there was one clear-cell sarcoma, in a 12-year old boy who presented with aching knees (probably unrelated) and a semi-membranosus bursal cyst on one side. Palpation of this swelling led to the discovery of a small contiguous, firmer lesion (also probably unrelated) which was found at biopsy to be a solid tumour attached to the aponeurosis of gastrocnemius (Fig. 23.9). Extensive local excision of the calf muscles and tissues at the back of the knee was, uncharacteristically, followed within 2 months by widespread metastases in both femora, in the epidural fat causing spinal paresis, and in extrapleural tissues in the chest wall.

V. LEIOMYOSARCOMA

This is an exceptional rarity in children. In soft tissues it usually behaves in a relatively benign fashion, but when it arises in a viscus (p. 628) its malignant potentialities are said to be greater, and the incidence of pulmonary metastases as high as 50%.

SITES

It can arise in any tissue or organ which contains smooth muscle (Botting *et al.*, 1965) e.g. the skin, the wall of a blood vessel, or a hollow viscus, and occasionally in the small bowel (p. 638).

A leiomyosarcoma occasionally arises in the wall of a large blood vessel, more often a vein (Kevorkian & Cento, 1973) and mostly in adults. The few reported in children (Nesbit & Rob, 1975) were chiefly in the saphenous or femoral vein and produced signs resembling thrombosis with distal oedema and a filling defect on venography.

Radical excision of the vein, preserving the related artery, and radical removal of the regional nodes when feasible, has been followed by long term survival in a few cases. The tumour has had a high recurrence rate and mortality, but no case treated by modern methods has been reported.

The mode of presentation is a palpable swelling, in either superficial or deep structures (Yannopoulos & Stout, 1962). However, it occasionally presents with symptoms due to interference with the function of the viscus in which it arises, e.g. intestinal obstruction.

Radiological investigations of leiomyosarcomas of the alimentary canal usually demonstrate a mass, or its effects (p. 634), but the precise diagnosis can only be made by biopsy. As with fibrosarcoma, it may be extremely difficult to decide on histological grounds whether a given tumour is benign or malignant (Fig. 23.10).

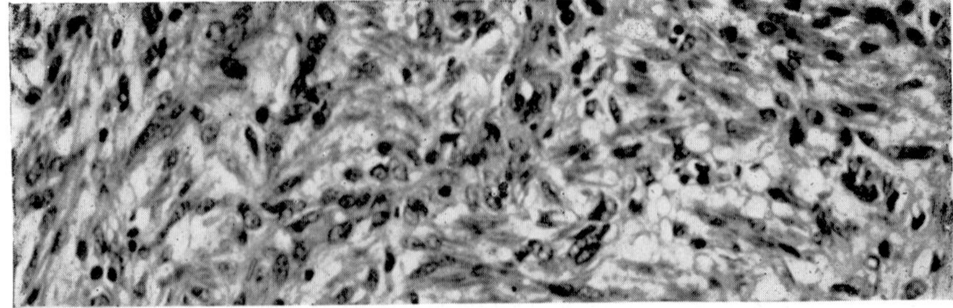

Figure 23.10. LEIOMYOSARCOMA, in this case from the small bowel (p. 638); the tumour cells are rather irregularly arranged, with only the suggestion of an interlacing pattern, and the nuclei are moderately pleomorphic (H & E. × 200).

Successful management requires adequate removal of the primary, and perhaps the proximal group of lymph nodes. In the limbs, amputation should be considered, either initially, or when local recurrences have appeared.

VI. LIPOSARCOMA

This is an extremely rare type of sarcoma in childhood, and occurs more often in adults. None was seen in the Index Series. Kauffman & Stout (1959) collected 15 cases from the literature and added 13 cases of their own, a series of only 28 cases in children up to that date.

AGE : SEX

Although typically an adult tumour, liposarcoma is occasionally seen in infancy or in adolescence. Kauffman & Stout in their series of 28 cases found that boys were affected approximately twice as often as girls (19 : 9) and 17 of the 28 occurred in children less than 5 years of age.

SITES

The thigh is the commonest site, followed in descending order of frequency by the cervical region, the thorax, the foot and the retroperitoneum (Enterline & Culberson, 1960; Enzinger & Winslow, 1962). Most liposarcomas develop in sites of naturally occurring adipose tissue, but some have been described as arising within muscle masses.

MACROSCOPIC APPEARANCES

The tumour is generally lobulated and resembles a lipoma, but has a grey rather than yellow cut surface, and is often myxoid in texture. It may appear to infiltrate local structures, although this is not always noticeable macroscopically.

MICROSCOPIC FINDINGS

Most liposarcomas are well differentiated and closely resemble the lesion lipoblastomatosis. According to Kauffman & Stout, these two lesions can be distinguished by the fact that liposarcomas infiltrate local tissues whereas in lipoblastomatosis (Fig. 23.11a, b, c) the lesions are nodular and non-infiltrative (Vellios *et al.*, 1958; Chung & Enzinger, 1973; Tabrisky *et al.*, 1974). Liposarcomas also tend to be diffuse with prominent myxoid change in the stroma, and are often vascular.

The diagnosis rests on the presence of lipoblasts, cells with oval or stellate cytoplasm, containing finely divided droplets of neutral fat. The nuclei may be round and regular, or show varying degrees of irregularity and hyperchromatism, occasionally with giant forms.

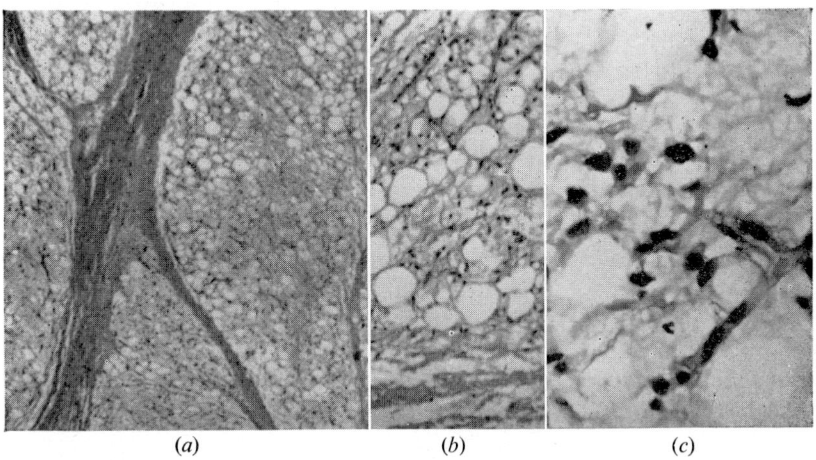

(*a*) (*b*) (*c*)

Figure 23.11. LIPOBLASTOMATOSIS; (*a*) the lobulated nature of the lesion (H & E. × 35); (*b*) mature fat cells differentiating from immature embryonal fatty tissue (H & E. × 130); (*c*) greater magnification of (*b*) to show the rich capillary plexus in the stroma (H & E. × 520).

TREATMENT

Surgical excision, removing a wide margin of macroscopically normal tissue is the treatment of choice. Radiotherapy or chemotherapy are not required, at least initially, since most liposarcomas though locally aggressive, almost never metastasize.

PROGNOSIS

The prognosis is good. None of the tumours in the 13 personal cases of liposarcomas reported by Kauffman & Stout gave rise to metastases, and this has been reported in only one case in the literature. In two cases local recurrence following excision was treated by further excision, and neither had a further recurrence at the time of the report.

VII. MALIGNANT MESENCHYMOMA

The term mesenchymoma was proposed by Stout (1948), who also suggested the term malignant mesenchymoma for tumours containing two or more types of malignant (sarcomatous) tissue, excluding 'fibrosarcoma' commonly found in many malignant tumours of soft tissue. Nash and Stout (1961) reported on 460 cases which met the criteria; 335 were malignant and 125 benign. Of these, 86 arose in children (50 malignant, 36 benign) and in the same period there were 621 sarcomas of soft tissue in children; thus the 50 malignant mesenchymomas represented 8% of the total (621), and in that particular series they were second only to rhabdomyosarcoma as the largest group of soft tissue sarcomas of childhood.

A diagnosis of malignant mesenchymoma was not made in the Index Series, nor since. The type of tumour described by Stout (1948) is accepted as an entity, but many of the cases described by Nash and Stout may well have been rhabdomyosarcomas. In this difficult diagnostic area the pathologist's interpretation obviously affects the classification.

AGE : SEX

Dividing the paediatric age group into three quinquennia, most of the tumours arose in the first (24 cases) and the third (12 cases); nine of the tumours were present at birth, and three were noticed before the age of 3 months.

Boys were affected more than twice as frequently as girls (29 : 13).

SITES

Most malignant mesenchymomas in the series quoted arose in superficial soft tissues of the limbs and trunk; others arose in deep soft tissues, and a few in viscera, notably in the liver.

MACROSCOPIC APPEARANCES

Nash & Stout could find no features common to all mesenchymomas which would help in recognizing them. Most appeared to be partially or completely encapsulated, but all were shown to be invading adjacent tissues microscopically. The colour of the tumour varies, and larger examples contain multiple areas of necrosis, and sometimes cystic areas.

MICROSCOPIC FINDINGS

In all cases the tumour was infiltrating and invasive. According to definition, each contained two or more sarcomatous elements, not counting fibrosarcoma, but including 'undifferentiated sarcoma'. Rhabdomyosarcoma was the type most often present, followed by malignant vascular tissue (angiosarcoma, lymphangiosarcoma and malignant haemangiopericytoma). In others there were, in various combinations, leiomyosarcoma, liposarcoma, chondrosarcoma, osteosarcoma and synovial sarcoma.

SPREAD

While local infiltration was common to all, the potentiality of an individual tumour to metastasize proved to be highly unpredictable, and information in the series quoted was incomplete. Metastases in regional lymph nodes were known to have developed in a few cases, and pulmonary metastases in others.

CLINICAL FEATURES

Neither the macroscopic appearances nor the clinical findings are distinctive, and as noted in most sarcomas in childhood, a swelling is the only finding on examination (p. 779); pain or tenderness are not common and present only in those growing fairly rapidly.

DIAGNOSIS

As malignant mesenchymomas have no special characteristics by which they may be recognized, diagnosis depends on histological findings, preferably on an excision biopsy (p. 950), covered by a cytotoxic agent given at an appropriate time before operation (p. 109).

TREATMENT

Once the diagnosis has been established, a more extensive excision of the region of the primary tumour may be indicated (p. 789), and amputation may need to be considered (p. 790). On the other hand, the variable and unpredictable degree of malignancy may not warrant radical ablative surgery, considering that rhabdomyosarcomatous tissue is the commonest component in malignant mesenchymomas, and that recent reports of co-ordinated surgery, chemotherapy and radiotherapy for rhabdomyosarcoma show significantly improved results (p. 792) with less reliance upon radical surgery (Kilman, Clatworthy *et al.*, 1973).

In a review of 21 infants with a malignant mesenchyma, 10 of them on the trunk or in an extremity, Holdsworth Mayer *et al.* (1974) reported 2 personal cases with no evidence of disease 44 and 62 months after surgical excision followed by combination chemotherapy using vincristine, actinomycin D and cyclophosphamide.

PROGNOSIS

The outcome of the patients in the series reviewed by Nash & Stout (1961) proved to be unexpectedly favourable, although the follow-up was not as detailed or for as long as they would have wished; of those less than 5 years of age at the time of treatment, 75% appear to have survived, as did 28% of those between 5 and 10 years of age, and 48% of children between 10 and 15 years. The numbers of cases in the subgroups were small, but the survival rates were higher than expected.

Factors reported as likely to be favourable were:

(*a*) Those less than 5 years of age at the time of diagnosis; with
(*b*) A tumour 5 cm or less in maximum dimension; and
(*c*) Mesenchymomas containing other than rhabdomyosarcoma.

VIII. EPITHELIOID SARCOMA

AGE : SEX

This rare type of sarcoma occurs mostly in young adults (median age 23 years), but in a review of 62 cases by Enzinger (1970), three were less than 10 years old, and 16 were between 10 and 19 at the time of diagnosis.

Males were affected four times as frequently as females.

SITES

In all but two of 62 cases the tumour arose in deep subcutaneous tissues of the extremities (Bryan, Soule *et al.*, 1974).

MACROSCOPIC APPEARANCES

The lesion is usually small, less than 2 cm in diameter, and firm, with a glistening greyish white cut surface showing yellow or brown flecks.

MICROSCOPIC FINDINGS

The typical appearance is of nodular granulomatous lesions each with a central area of degenerating cells and necrosis. Most of the cells are plump and spindle shaped, while some are large and polygonal with a strongly acidophilic cytoplasm.

SPREAD

The lesion has a marked tendency to infiltrate and grow along densely fibrous structures such as tendons and fascial sheets. The deceptively benign appearance is belied by a high rate of recurrence after local excision, and the development of pulmonary metastases in 30% of the series quoted.

Metastases in lymph nodes is by contrast rare, and occurred in approximately 10%.

CLINICAL FEATURES

Although superficial, the initial nodule is not usually subcutaneous, and presents as a slowly growing painless firm nodule without any distinctive features.

DIAGNOSIS

Epithelioid sarcoma is an unusual tumour and the diagnosis is usually made on histological examination of an excision biopsy of a nodule which has some similarities to small superficial lesions such as a glomus tumour, pilomatrixoma and others mentioned on p. 850.

TREATMENT

The high recurrence rate (85%) after local excision, and the incidence of pulmonary metastasis, are ample justification for radical local excision. The history frequently found in case reports is repeated recurrences at long intervals over several years, and in Enzinger's series some form of amputation (e.g. a finger or hand) was performed in 74% of cases with two or more recurrences.

X. ALVEOLAR SOFT PART SARCOMA
(syn. malignant granular cell tumour)

This highly malignant neoplasm, also known as malignant granular cell tumour (organoid type) and malignant granular cell myoblastoma, is particularly rare in childhood and usually confined to the third quinquennium. The name 'alveolar soft part' sarcoma derives from the histological structure in which nests of large cells with prominent and granular eosinophilic cytoplasm (Fig. 23.12) present a pseudoglandular pattern (Welsh & Bray, 1972). The characteristic features are the architecture of the cell masses, and granules in the cytoplasm which are PAS positive, diastase resistant, and sometimes appear crystalline with the light microscope and with electron microscopy (Shipkey *et al.*, 1964).

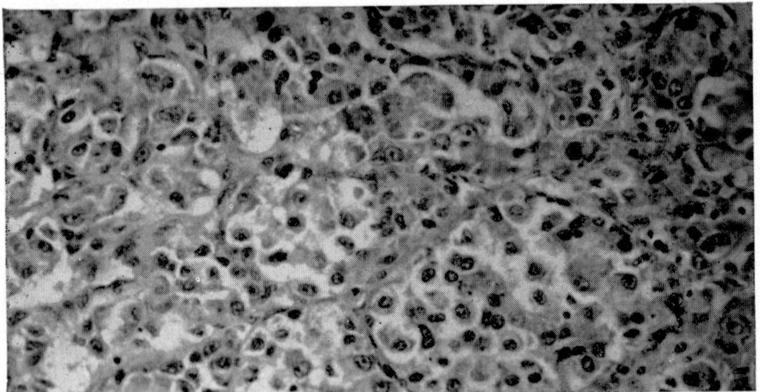

Figure 23.12. 'ALVEOLAR SOFT PART SARCOMA'; nests of large plump cells with a round nucleus, a prominent nucleolus and abundant eosinophilic cytoplasm, arranged in a characteristically alveolar pattern (H & E. $\times$ 200).

Fisher and Reidbord (1971) suggested that this tumour is derived from myogenous cells and represents a unique form of rhabdomyosarcoma. On the other hand Welsh and Bray (1972) suggest that there are similarities in the ultrastructure of alveolar soft part sarcomas and para-gangliomas of the carotid body type, which seems to be less likely than the former suggestion; certainly their behaviour is that of a highly malignant neoplasm.

SITES

The tumours are found most commonly in muscle masses in the limbs and trunk, and have a special proclivity for early metastasis via the bloodstream.

The Index Series. A 14-year old girl presented with bone pain; x-rays revealed multiple lytic lesions in several long bones, and multiple pulmonary metastasis. Biopsy of one of the lesions showed alveolar soft part sarcoma, and death soon followed. The primary was thought to have arisen in the muscles of the posterior abdominal wall.

TUMOURS OF BLOOD VESSELS AND LYMPHATICS

Malignant tumours of blood vessels are very rare indeed (e.g. only two in the 23 years represented in the Index Series). Because of difficulties in identifying the cell of origin, the terms 'angiosarcoma' and 'lymphangiosarcoma' have been widely used, but Kauffman & Stout (1961) have suggested the following more precise classification:

1. *Haemangio-endothelioma* (syn. endotheliosarcoma), for malignant tumours arising from the endothelial lining of blood vessels;
2. *Haemangiopericytoma*, arising from the adventitial cells or pericytes surrounding capillaries (Backwinkel & Diddams, 1970).
3. *Leiomyosarcoma*, when the tumour is clearly derived from smooth muscle in the vessel wall;
4. *Malignant lymphangio-endothelioma* when the origin is in the endothelial lining of lymphatics; this tumour is found only in adults, particularly in an oedematous arm resulting from radical mastectomy for carcinoma of the breast.

X. HAEMANGIO-ENDOTHELIOSARCOMA

MACROSCOPIC APPEARANCE

The tumour is white and extremely soft, but only moderately vascular.

MICROSCOPIC FEATURES

The typical cell is a spindle cells with a rounded nucleus, and plump cytoplasm containing glycogen. The cells form vascular spaces varying from capillary to venule in size, and there are numerous mitotic figures.

In the Index Series one of the two cases metastasized to the brain and to the skin, and led to the death of the patient. The other arose in the buttock and recurred after primary excision, but the patient is alive with no evidence of tumour 2 years after excision of the local recurrence.

Two other tumours in the Index Series were considered to be haemangiopericytomas, (Fig. 23.13) of questionable malignancy, one in the palm and the other in the axilla. In both cases local excision proved to be adequate, although the axillary lesion recurred once; the question of malignancy was raised solely because of moderate mitotic activity in the tumour cells.

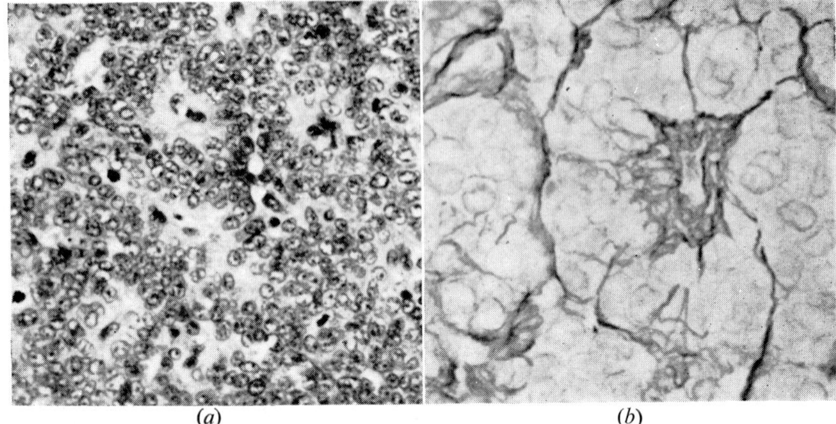

(*a*) (*b*)

Figure 23.13. HAEMANGIOPERICYTOMA; (*a*) the cells have a round, vesicular nucleus, and a capillary at the centre of each cell nest (H & E. × 200); (b) reticulin stain demonstrates that the reticulin frame work of each capillary surrounds its endothelial cells, and each is invested by surrounding pericytes outside the reticulin of the endothelial cells (Reticulin stain (Foots) × 520).

SPREAD

Because of their vascular origin haematogenous spread is the commonest route, but extensive local infiltration along contiguous tissue planes can also occur (Kauffman & Stout, 1961).

DIFFERENTIATION OF BENIGN TUMOUR-LIKE LESIONS OF BLOOD VESSELS

1. Haemangiomas

These are ubiquitous in infancy and childhood and, together with naevi and lymphangiomas, are the commonest benign 'tumours' in this age group. In view of their non-progressive nature, most of them are regarded as malformations or hamartomas rather than true neoplasms. They are composed of blood vessels of various sizes and, according to the predominant type of blood vessel, the following sub-types are recognized:

(*a*) *Benign haemangio-endothelioma*, typically composed of plump endothelial cells;

(*b*) *Capillary haemangioma*, with delicate thin-walled capillaries;

(*c*) *Cavernous haemangioma* composed of larger, rather dilated sinusoidal and venous channels.

In the most cases, however, all three types of vessels or cells are found, particularly in the larger lesions.

Their natural history is one of spontaneous resolution, by sclerosis or 'maturation', during which the pattern changes from a predominantly haemangioma-endothelial or capillary picture to a 'cavernous' pattern. There is also considerable fibrosis in the intervening stroma, and ultimately almost complete obliteration of the abnormal vascular bed.

2. **Venous haemangiomas**

These are small to medium in size, and thick-walled blood vessels usually predominate. Sometimes fibrous tissue, smooth muscle and fat are intimately associated with the vascular spaces.

3. **Racemose (cirsoid) haemangiomas**

These are actually multiple arteriovenous communications, in children most commonly found in the brain and meninges. The vessels are large, thick-walled and tortuous, with numerous sinusoidal out-pouchings and aneurysms. The latter tend to undergo spontaneous thrombosis, but those in the brain occasionally rupture.

4. **Haemangiomas in skeletal muscle and connective tissues**

These occur as part of a giant haemangioma (see below) or as isolated lesions. They are composed of thin-walled endothelial-lined capillaries, usually poorly defined, and 'infiltrate' widely. Displacement, degeneration and atrophy of skeletal muscle are common accompaniments. The important differential diagnosis is from malignant vascular tumours, and the aggressive clinical and histological appearance of benign but infiltrating haemangiomas in young infants can be particularly alarming.

5. **Giant haemangioma of infancy**

This occurs only in young infants and is a very large and extensive variant of the capillary haemangioma described above. Some are present at birth, but many appear within a few days or at most weeks after birth and may grow with almost incredible speed, encroaching on adjacent skin at the rate of up to 1 cm a day. In giant lesions, thrombocytopenia occurs (Shim, 1968), presumably due to trapping of platelets in the sinusoidal channels. In another type there are also features suggestive of a lymphangioma, and this variant may involve a whole limb, developing rapidly after birth, and increasing in size so quickly that it is mistaken for a malignant neoplasm.

6. **Haemangiomatosis**

This is either generalized (e.g. in von Hippel-Lindau (p. 832) or Sturge-Weber disease, (p. 832), or localized, and often associated with arteriovenous fistulae. The localized type often occurs in the neighborhood of a joint and may be accompanied by an overgrowth of fat and nervous tissue; they tend to recur after surgical excision. Histologically, a haemangiomatosis contains numerous capillaries and thicker walled vessels, separated by fat and loose myxoid connective tissue, together with many medullated and non-medullated nerve fibres.

7. **Benign haemangiopericytoma**

This is a rare tumour in childhood, appears to be composed of pericytes (O'Brien & Brasfield, 1965) and may be difficult to identify. Characteristically the cells are round, oval or spindle-shaped, fairly uniform in size, and arranged around vascular spaces lined by a single endothelial layer. Reticulin stains may demonstrate endothelial cells in a reticulum framework, with pericytes outside the reticulin.

8. **Glomus tumour** (syn. glomangioma, chemodectoma)

This is a rare localized tumour of specialized pericytes which occurs in subcutaneous tissue, chiefly in the fingers and toes, and typically beneath a fingernail or toenail (see p. 855). Morphologically there are two patterns, a compact and a cavernous form. The characteristic cell is small, with a round, dark nucleus, very scanty cytoplasm, and arranged in concentric rings around thin-walled blood vessels (Fig. 24.7, p. 856).

9. **Angioleiomyomas**

These are presumed to arise from smooth muscle fibres in the wall of a blood vessel, usually a vein. Some are extraordinarily sensitive to touch, and may be deep in the muscles of the leg or arm. Histologically they contain interlacing bundles of uniform leiomyocytes, and some have a rich nerve supply. Two such lesions have been seen in the Index Series.

10. **Pyogenic granuloma** (syn. granuloma pyogenicum, haemangioma of granulation tissue)

This common lesion in childhood occurs mostly on the face or trunk, and presents clinically as a small but rapidly growing crusted, sessile nodule which bleeds profusely and very easily. Histologically it is composed of an irregular open meshwork of capillaries, with a pattern suggesting granulation tissue, in a loose mucoid stroma. The surface is usually ulcerated, infiltrated with polymorphs and partially covered with blood clot; simple excision followed by a pressure dressing is usually effective.

The lesion is probably a distinctive form of infection affecting the blood vessels in the superficial dermis. It is sometimes confused clinically with spindle cell/epithelial naevi (juvenile melanoma, p. 846) but they can be readily distinguished histologically.

11. Benign lymphangioma

These are second in frequency to haemangiomas in childhood, and can occur in practically any part in the body, with a predilection for the neck (p. 389), the mediastinum (p. 448), the parotid (p. 305), the subcutaneous tissues of the trunk and limbs, the bowel wall and the mesentery (p. 673). Their histological pattern is similar wherever they arise: characteristic cystic spaces lined by a single layer of flattened endothelial cells. The larger spaces often have smooth muscle cells in their wall, and there are invariably clusters of lymphocytes forming either projections into the spaces or nodules in the connective tissue septa between them.

Occasionally a lymphangioma in the mediastinum or neck contains bizarre endothelial cells forming multinucleated cells, and when associated with overgrowth of fibroblastic tissue, they may cause difficulties in diagnosis.

Secondary changes such as haemorrhage, infection and fibrous obliteration, are very common, particularly in those in the neck and mediastinum. Malignant lymphangiosarcoma is an extreme rarity in childhood, but a few examples have been reported (Finlay-Jones, 1970).

TREATMENT

Haemangio-endotheliosarcomas and malignant haemangiopericytoma are infiltrating tumours with a variable malignant potential. As they tend to recur locally, radical local excision is indicated when the site of the tumour permits, and in the absence of pulmonary metastasis.

Radiotherapy alone may be curative (Dube & Paulson, 1974).

Chemotherapy has been shown to be an important aspect of treatment, e.g. in combinations of 2 to 4 drugs, integrated with radiotherapy, using vincristine, actinomycin D, cyclophosphamide and methotrexate (Ortega *et al.*, 1971).

TUMOURS OF PERIPHERAL NERVES

Malignant neoplasms arising in peripheral nerves are generally quite uncommon, and in children particularly so. Benign tumours such as neurofibromas and Schwannomas occur with sufficient frequency in childhood to be considered in the differential diagnosis of sarcomas and many benign soft tissue masses.

BENIGN TUMOURS

All benign tumours of peripheral nerves are believed to arise in either a

Schwann cell or a fibroblast. The two tumours in this category are the Schwannoma and the neurofibroma.

I. SCHWANNOMA (syn. neurilemmoma, 'acoustic' neuroma, neurinoma)

A Schwannoma is usually solitary, grows slowly and arises within a nerve, initially displacing it and later compressing it without destroying it. It may occur in a peripheral nerve, in autonomic nerves or in one of the cranial nerves, and is not necessarily associated with neurofibromatosis, although patients with von Recklinghausen's disease (p. 827) usually develop multiple Schwannomas during the course of the disease.

The tumour arises from the Schwann cells of the nerve sheath, and on electron microscopy they are characterized by the presence of a basement membrane.

Macroscopically they are usually encapsulated, and the cut surface is tan or grey, with areas of yellowish discolouration and occasionally cyst formation. They are intimately attached to the nerve of origin.

Microscopically it is composed of spindle shaped cells arranged characteristically in one of two different patterns, so-called Antoni 'type A' and Antoni 'type B'.

In Antoni type A, the cells tend to lie with their long axes parallel and aligned, in the form of a pallisade. When two groups of pallisaded nuclei are separated by an area of hyalinized collagen, the resultant structure is known as a 'Verocay body'. These tumours also contain abundant collagen believed to be produced by the Schwann cells.

Antoni type B tissue is much less cellular; the cells are again spindle-shaped and elongated, and separated by a poorly-staining myxomatous matrix which can be shown by appropriate stains to contain reticulum fibres and collagen. The individual tumour cells are sparse and the cell boundaries, more clearly visible than in Antoni type A tissue, are often twisted and irregular.

Most Schwannomas contain both types of tissue, mixed in various proportions, and the transition from one type to the other is often abrupt. Antoni type B is very similar to the tissue comprising neurofibromas (see below).

A moderate degree of nuclear irregularity is seen in some Schwannomas, but this is not considered to indicate malignant change. Some tumours contain areas infiltrated with lymphocyte-like cells. A Schwannoma occurring in the eighth cranial nerve is known as an acoustic neuroma.

II. NEUROFIBROMA

In children, neurofibromas are commonly an expression of the phakomatosis of von Recklinghausen's disease (p. 827), but an isolated tumour can also occur in patients with no stigmata of the generalized disease (generalized neurofibromatosis, multiple neurilemmal fibromatosis). Because the full expression of von Recklinghausen's disease may not develop until adult life, it can be difficult to decide in a particular patient whether a single tumour is the first manifestation of a generalized disease. A diagnosis of neurofibromatosis is not justified unless there are other stigmata, especially multiple *café-au-lait* patches, multiple neurofibromas (in particular the plexiform type), or a positive family history. A child with thoracic neurofibroma (p. 465) usually has other evidence of von Recklinghausen's disease; but in some cases the thoracic lesion is the first evidence of the disease, and further stigmata may not appear for a number of years (p. 831). In the Index Series neurofibromas developed in the brachial plexus in the neck (p. 465) on the median nerve in the forearm, and in the bowel.

Macroscopically a neurofibroma is characteristically soft, greyish, fleshy, and sometimes slightly mucoid or slimy on cross section; occasional tumours may be so pale as to be almost translucent. Lesions in the skin lie in the dermis and produce an elevated nodule with compression of the superficial dermis and stretching of the overlying skin; the deep aspect has an ill-defined edge which merges with the subcutaneous tissue.

Neurofibromas of peripheral nerves, or within the thorax (p. 465) are characteristically the plexiform type, composed of a cluster of rounded nodules externally resembling a bunch of small grapes (Fig. 23.14), the term 'a bag of worms' is commonly used to describe the feel of these tumours *in situ*.

Plexiform neurofibromas (Raffensperger & Cohen, 1972) differ from solitary neurofibromas more in gross architectural pattern than in cellular detail. In the plexiform type each neurofibromatous nodule is a greatly enlarged nerve twig, and each is surrounded by a delicate fibrous capsule. Surviving axons and occasionally even myelin sheaths may be found in the smaller lesions, although they are generally overwhelmed by mucoid intercellular matrix in larger lesions.

Microscopically a neurofibroma is composed of a loose stroma of Schwann cells, separated by a mucinous matrix containing collagen. The cytoplasmic processes of the Schwann cells are characteristically tortuous and often greatly elongated. Harken and Reed (1969) noted that the matrix of neurofibromas commonly stains positively with alcian blue for acid mucopolysaccharide, in contrast to the negative reaction of the similar matrix seen in Schwannomas.

Many benign tumours of the nerve sheath show features of both Schwannomas and neurofibromas, and this is not suprising since both are derived from Schwann cells. In children, areas of nuclear pallisading are common in otherwise typical neurofibromas, and in this age group the

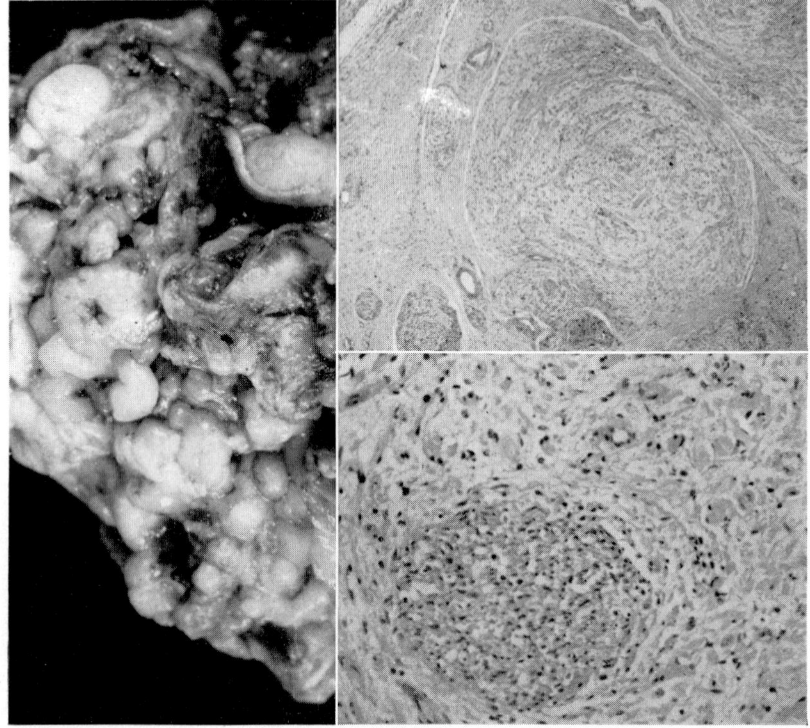

Figure 23.14. PLEXIFORM NEUROFIBROMA; (*a*) grape-like clusters of pale, glistening nodules of neurofibroma; (*b*) rounded lobules of abnormal nerve bundles distorted and greatly expanded by interfibrillary ground substance (H & E. × 30); (*c*) a nerve twig surrounded by mucoid neurofibrillary tissue (H & E. × 320).

[(*a*) *Left*. (*b*) *Top right*. (*c*) *Bottom right*.]

distinction between the two entities appears to be even more difficult than it is, occasionally, in adults.

MODES OF PRESENTATION

Neurofibromas are found in two main sites in children:

1. In the skin and subcutaneous tissue, e.g. of the trunk;
2. In relation to the spinal nerves, in the posterior mediastinum (p. 466), the thoracic inlet (p. 465) or the intervertebral foramina, where they may give rise to a mass lying partly within the thoracic cavity and partly in the spinal canal, i.e. a dumb-bell tumour, producing compression of the spinal cord (p. 448).

MALIGNANT TUMOURS OF PERIPHERAL NERVES

These occur most commonly as complications of neurofibromatous lesions and are largely confined to adult life. However, the occasional cases seen in childhood appear to fall into two groups: (*a*) those which are predominantly fibroblastic and resemble fibrosarcoma; and (*b*) those with neuroepithelial differentiation.

Malignant Schwannomas have been reported by Ghosh, Ghosh *et al.* (1973) as solitary tumours arising *de novo* (74%) or in patients with von Recklinghausen's disease (26%); only 9 of their series of 115 patients were less than 10 years old at diagnosis. Radical local excision yielded 79% of 5-year survivors in the group as a whole.

The Index Series contains one Schwann-cell tumour considered to show some features of malignancy. The tumour arose in the brachial plexus and produced multiple, separate masses, some of which appeared to be poorly encapsulated and infiltrating. The nuclei were hyperchromatic and contained mitotic figures. Other areas showed the typical Antoni type A tissue (p. 822) Verocay bodies (p. 822), and nuclear pallisading. Surgical excision was successful and there has been no evidence of recurrence.

No lesion considered to be a fibrosarcoma of nerve sheath origin was encountered. Two tumours were difficult to classify but could be primitive neuroectodermal tumours. One arose in the popliteal fossa and the other in the neck. The lesion in the popliteal fossa was localized and has not recurred following excision. The tumour in the neck was more diffuse and led to the death of the child. Both tumours were composed of cords of hyperchromatic cells with oval nuclei and a prominent nucleolus, set in a rather loose myxoid stroma, and they resembled to some degree the illustrations of the tumour described by Willis (1962) as a medullo-epithelioma of the cerebellum. Their origin from nerve tissue has not been proven by cell culture or electron microscopy, but they bear some resemblance to epithelioid Schwannomas.

THE PHAKOMATOSES

As a group, the four conditions customarily referred to as phakomatoses can produce a remarkable variety of clinical presentations. Although the majority are genetically determined and non-neoplastic, they are frequently involved in the differential diagnosis of a number of tumours in childhood. Each of the conditions is described in the following section, rather than separately in several chapters in which they are relevant, to avoid repetition.

The phakomatoses are as follows:

I. Tuberous sclerosis;
II. Neurofibromatosis (von Recklinghausen's disease);
III. Encephalotrigeminal angiomatosis (Sturge-Weber syndrome);
IV. von Hippel-Lindau disease.

von Recklinghausen was the first to describe the features of tuberous sclerosis, in the autopsy findings of a neonate with focal cerebral sclerosis and multiple cardiac tumours. Bourneville (1880) gave the condition its name, based on tubercles of sclerosis found in the cerebral cortex, associated with epilepsy and mental deficiency.

Van der Hoeve (1932) described as 'phakomas' the tumours of the optic disc and retina also found in this condition, and proposed the term phakomatosis. Co-existence of tuberous sclerosis and neurofibromatosis in the same patient or in the same kindred has been reported and also refuted, but this is the basis for referring to both conditions as 'phakomatoses'. It is now thought that there is a genetic basis for tuberous sclerosis, as there undoubtedly is for von Recklinghausen's disease.

I. TUBEROUS SCLEROSIS

Of several general reviews of this condition, one of the more recent, by Lagos & Gomez (1967) reviewed 71 cases seen at the Mayo Clinic between 1953 and 1964. They concluded that mental retardation may have been over-reported in earlier reviews, possibly due to bias in the samples which were drawn from institutions for the retarded and epileptic. The authors therefore divided their patients into two groups, group A: 26 patients (38 %) with normal intelligence, and group B: 43 patients (62 %) with mental retardation (Paulson & Lyle, 1966).

The various conditions which may occur in this syndrome are listed in Table 23.5. Some are present at birth while other lesions develop later (Fig. 23.15). One of the commonest stigmata are facial angiofibromas, formerly referred to as 'adenoma sebaceum' (of Pringle), chiefly found in the 'butterfly' area of the face. This was found in 83 % of the patients reviewed, and two thirds of those so affected had at least one other cutaneous abnormality, including *café-au-lait* patches. In most affected children, adenoma sebaceum is not present at birth but develops between 2 and 5 years of age, and rarely after 5 years of age.

The average age at diagnosis in the series of 71 cases quoted was 8½ years in those with mental retardation, and 17 years in those of average or normal intelligence.

RHABDOMYOMA

Rhabdomyomas of the myocardium (p. 481) not infrequently give rise to symptoms during early infancy as one of the modes of presentation of the disease.

Although almost confined to the cardiac muscle and to tuberous sclerosis, a series of nine extracardiac hamartomatous 'fetal' rhabdomyomas has been described (Dehner *et al.*, 1972). Most of the lesions were apparent before the

Table 23.5. Tuberous sclerosis; manifestations in various sites (after Lagos & Gomez, 1967)

Sex incidence		Equal
Epilepsy		93%
'Adenoma sebaceum'		83%
Other skin conditions:		
Leather ('shagreen') patches	66%	
Peri- and sub-ungual fibromas	17%	
Vitiligenous (achromatic) patches	15%	
Hyperpigmented areas	10%	
Café-au-lait patches	7%	
Abnormal electro-encephalogram		87%
Intracranial calcification		51%
Phakomas of the retina		53%
Osseous lesions:		
Osteoporosis, osseous 'islands'		
Cystic changes in phalanges		
Tumours:		
Haemangiomas and mixed tumours of liver, spleen, kidney		
Angioleiomyomas of kidney		
Rhabdomyomas of the myocardium (p. 481)		
Subependymal neurogliomas		
Sarcomatous tumours of the kidney		
Multiple mixed pulmonary tumours		
Gliomas and cysts of the retina (p. 428)		
Astrocytomas		
Meningioma		
Telangiectasia (oculo-cutaneous).		

age of 3 years, chiefly in the neck, particularly in the post-auricular region, and all appeared to be benign.

II. NEUROFIBROMATOSIS
(syn. von Recklinghausen's disease)

von Recklinghausen first described this condition in 1882, having initially observed it in a wild carp caught on a fishing expedition, and subsequently found in man. Its exact nature has remained the subject of debate for it is not certain whether it arises primarily in cells derived from the neural crest, in the mesenchymal stroma which supports them, or in both.

The resulting hamartomatous lesions are remarkable for the range of tissues, organs and systems in which they may arise, and for the variety of forms which they may take. The importance of the disease in relation to tumours in childhood lies in the differentiation of one form or another from

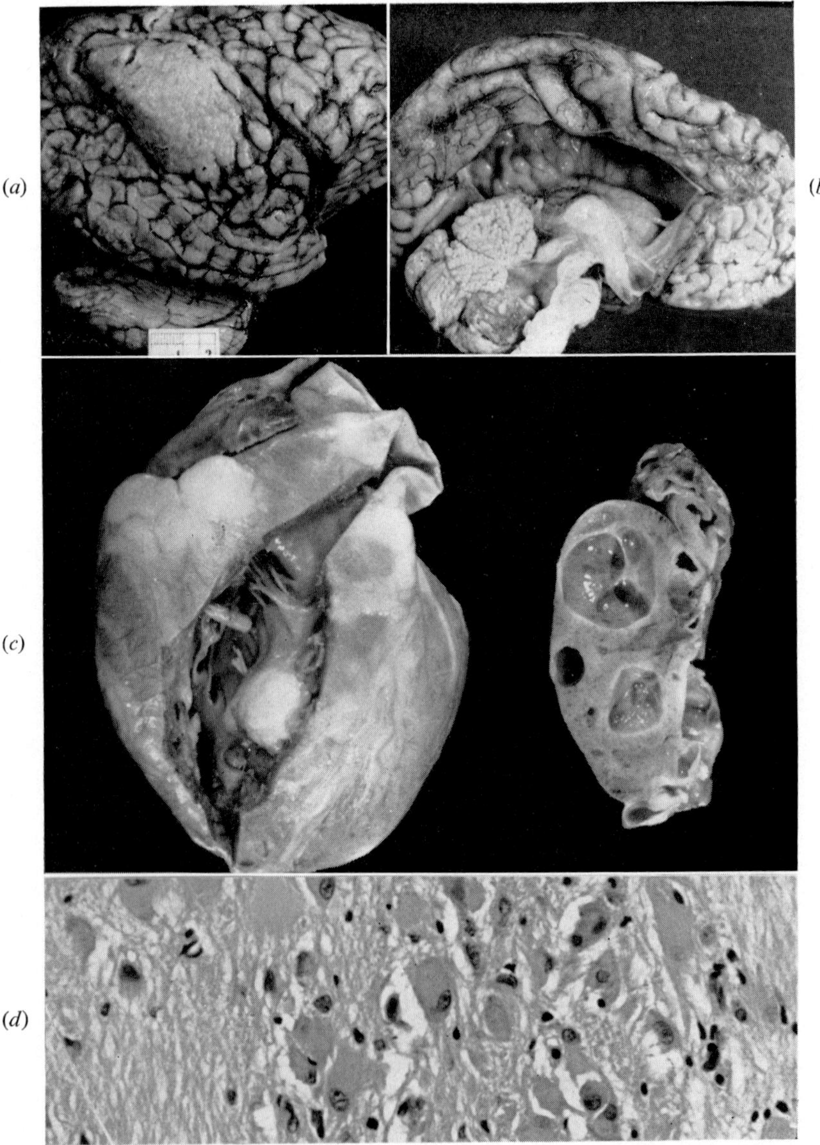

Figure 23.15. TUBEROUS SCLEROSIS; a composite of typical multiple lesions including; (*a*) a 'tuber' of unusually large size in the cerebral cortex; (*b*) 'candle guttering' on the interior of the lateral ventricle; (*c*) multiple 'rhabdomyomas' (hamartomas) in the heart, and in the kidney which is also cystic; (*d*) 'tuber' cells, swollen astrocytes with dense eosinophilic cytoplasm and large round nuclei (H & E. × 200).

truly benign neoplasms of soft tissues, from other kinds of hamartoma, and from malignant neoplasms. These distinctions are not always clear; even when histologically benign, a neurofibroma may be so inaccessible, so incorrigible or so destructive that it amounts to a malignant lesion. The small but definite incidence of truly malignant change (to a neurofibrosarcoma) in some of the lesions is also a source of clinical or pathological confusion.

The following summary is based on extensive reviews in the literature, and deals primarily with the manifestations apparent during childhood. Table 23.6 contains most of the entities which have been reported in childhood and adolescence.

Table 23.6. Neurofibromatosis: manifestations in various sites

Manifestation	Page
Tumours of the peripheral nerves	
* Neurofibroma (single, multiple; sessile, pedunculated)	
* Schwannoma (neurilemmoma, neurinoma)	
* Plexiform neurofibroma (localised, diffuse, regional)	
* Hemihypertrophy, regional giantism	
* Multiple neurilemmal fibromatosis	
* Interstitial hypertrophic polyneuritis	
(Any of the above types may affect the spinal cord, nerve roots, cauda equina, plexus or nerve trunks)	
Central nervous system	
Focal cerebral gliosis (mental retardation $\pm$ epilepsy)	
* Glioma of optic nerve, chiasma, anterior fossa	(p. 411)
* Astrocytoma of cerebellum (solid, cystic)	(p. 240)
* Acoustic neuroma (cerebello-pontine angle tumour)	(p. 822)
* Meningioma (spherical, en plaque)	(p. 281)
* Leptomeningeal melanosis	(p. 285)
Stenosis of the aqueduct of Sylvius-hydrocephalus	
Syringomyelia	
* Arachnoid cysts	
Bone lesions	
* Fibrous dysplasia (monostotic or polyostotic)	(p. 730)
* Metaphyseal fibrous dysplasia (bone 'cyst')	(p. 727)
Pseudarthrosis of the tibia	
Congenital shortening of lower limbs	
Hypertrophy or overgrowth of long bones	
* Vertebral lesions: scoliosis, vertebral collapse, herniations of intervertebral foraminae	(p. 448)
Regional 'tumours'	
* Spheno-orbital bone defects: pulsating exophthalmos	
* Thoracic neurofibroma	(p. 465)
* 'Parsnips' tumour of thoracic inlet	(p. 465)
* Dumbbell tumour (thoracospinal)	(p. 466)
* Neurofibroma or neurinoma of the alimentary canal	
* Pelvic neurofibromatosis	

Table 23.6. continued

Skin lesions	
Café-au-lait patches	(p. 830)
* Multiple subcutaneous neurofibromas	(p. 831)
Neurocutaneous melanosis	(p. 860)
Giant pigmented naevi	(p. 842)
* Malignant melanoma	(p. 841)
* Neurofibrosarcoma	(p. 832)
Associated (?related) tumours	
Ganglioneuroma	(p. 540)
Phaeochromocytoma } ?	(p. 562)
Chromaffin-negative paraganglioma } ?	(p. 562)
Adrenal cortical tumours } ?	(p. 562)
Neuroblastoma	(p. 538)
(Ganglioneuroblastoma)	(p. 549)

* Tumefactive lesions.

HEREDITY

The disease is inherited as an autosomal dominant trait with variable penetrance. A high rate of mutation has also been implied; some patients born to apparently normal parents may be examples of mutation, but it is very difficult to exclude the possibility that one or other parent possessed the gene yet had too few overt manifestations to allow diagnosis. Before regarding a patient as a new mutant, both parents should be thoroughly examined for minor expressions of the disease. The decision that a child is or is not a new mutant is of great importance in genetic counselling; if the disease is the result of mutation, the chance of subsequent siblings being similarly affected is negligible; when not due to mutation, the chance is approximately 50%.

INCIDENCE

This has been estimated as 1 per 2500–3300 births in 'western' communities (Crowe *et al.*, 1956).

CHILDHOOD

The commonest clinical findings in children is the *café-au-lait* patch. A few are present at birth, but most arrive later and are added to progressively during the first decade. Although the patch is a distinct clinical entity, it is not a unique lesion confined to neurofibromatosis, nor a *sine qua non* of neurofibromatosis (Feinman & Yakovac, 1970).

The pigment is melanin situated in the deeper layers of the epidermis. Yet this type of lesion is not prone to any of the changes found in 'pigmented naevi' (p. 844), and is only diagnostically significant: (*a*) when at least 0·5 cm in diameter; and (*b*) when there are five or more patches of this size; these are grounds for a presumptive diagnosis of von Recklinghausen's disease.

Physical signs are recognizable at birth in about 40% of patients, in 65% by the age of one year, and in a progressively greater proportion with increasing age. Patches are not essential for the diagnosis, and possibly 10% of cases have no abnormal pigmentation, but this figure probably decreases as a cohort of cases is followed into later years.

Multiple neurofibromas in subcutaneous tissues are distinctly unusual in young children, but develop as small sessile lesions in older children and progress to larger pedunculated tumours in adolescents and adults.

PATHOLOGY

Classification of histological appearances into distinct sub-categories and setting limits to the spectrum of the histological appearances in various lesions, pose particular difficulties.

Macroscopically the lesion may be one of the following:

1. *A discrete, more or less spherical lesion*, of almost any size, solid and compact, with a cut surface showing whorls resembling a fibroma.
2. *A focal plexiform lesion* composed of greatly enlarged individual nerve fibres which are also enormously elongated, and at the same time convoluted into masses, which appear to be but are not, knotted, compressed into as small a space as possible.
3. *Regional giantism* or hemihypertrophy, in which large areas or even whole regions of the body are increased in bulk by masses of the plexiform tissue described above, for example apparently confined initially to a single digit or, on a large scale, the whole of one buttock, the adjoining half of the perineum and extending into the related half of the pelvis as an ill-defined mass filling the iliac fossa. Partial excision of such a swelling, for symptomatic relief, produced masses of plexiform nerve fibres, but no clinical evidence of any neural deficit.

Microscopically the spectrum extends from neurofibromas through neurilemmomas and Schwannomas by persuasive degrees to a borderland in which lie gliomas, astrocytomas, meningiomas, fibrous dysplasia (monostotic or polyostotic) of bones (Hunt & Pugh, 1961) and, indirectly, to vascular lesions (Mena *et al.*, 1973).

The natural history and behaviour of the different types of lesions varies considerably too, for example: (*a*) focal cerebral gliosis (the probable cause of mental retardation and epilepsy) appears to be static from the outset and possibly congenital; (*b*) other lesions in the skin or subcutaneous nerves gradually appear as the patient grows older, and they progress (if at all) at an almost undetectable rate; (*c*) yet others, such as optic gliomas, extend more rapidly, but still relatively slowly, for months or a few years, before coming to a halt, although some continue to advance inexorably and invade the cerebral hemispheres; (*d*) lastly, another form suddenly springs to life in an almost static lesion in adults, to become a highly malignant neurofibrosarcoma.

The sites in which these various macroscopic, microscopic and clinical behavioural types arise, is virtually unlimited; every organ or tissue in the body may be affected by one type or another, each of which shows some predilection for a particular site (Vinken & Bruyn, 1972).

III. ENCEPHALO-TRIGEMINAL ANGIOMATOSIS (syn. Sturge-Weber syndrome)

In contrast to the previous group, the genetic background of this and the following condition is uncertain. The most obvious component of this syndrome is an extensive, bright-reddish 'port wine' stain, often confined to the facial skin supplied by the trigeminal nerve, in particular the ophthalmic division.

Calcification in the cerebral cortex, typically as parallel serpiginous lines, is attributed to stasis, thrombosis and calcification in cortical vessels, usually commencing in the occipital lobe and developing during the first year of life. These changes are associated with *petit mal* seizures and later mental retardation.

Congenital glaucoma and buphthalmos (p. 400) is due to naevi or angiomas of the choroid. Telangiectasia, and sometimes giantism, occur, especially in the arm.

The calvarium is thicker on the affected side and the capacity of the hemicranium less. Crossed hemiparesis and hemianopsia may also occur from extensive involvement of one cerebral hemisphere. When seizures are frequent, severe and difficult to control, hemispherectomy in selected cases has been followed by improvement in the general clinical condition, or at least easier and better pharmacological control of the seizures.

IV. VON HIPPEL-LINDAU DISEASE

In this condition the pattern of inheritance is uncertain, and the commonest pathological manifestations are caused by haemangiomas or vascular hamartomas (Grossman & Melmon, 1972).

Haemangiomas or angiomatous cysts may occur in a variety of sites; in the central nervous system they may be found as haemangiomatous cysts in the cerebellum and the spinal cord; lesions may also develop in the kidney, liver, testes and the pancreas. In the eye, they cause detachment of the retina and blindness (p. 427).

REFERENCES

ALBORES-SAAVEDRA, J., BUTLER, J.J. & MARTIN, R.G. (1965). Rhabdomyosarcoma: clinicopathologic considerations and report of 85 cases. In *Tumors of Bone and Soft Tissues.* Year Book Medical Publishing Company, Chicago.

ALLEN, P.W. & ENZINGER, F.M. (1970). Juvenile aponeurotic fibroma. *Cancer,* **26** : 857.

BACKWINKEL, D.K. & DIDDAMS, J.A. (1970). Hemangiopericytoma: case report and comprehensive review of the literature. *Cancer,* **25** : 896.

BALE, P.M. & REYE, R.D.K. (1975). Rhabdomyosarcoma in childhood. *Pathology,* **7** : 101.

BALSAVER, A.M., BUTLER, J.J. & MARTIN, R.G. (1967). Congenital fibrosarcoma. *Cancer,* **20** : 1607.

BLOEM, J.J., VUZEVSKI, V.D. & HUFFSTADT, A.J.C. (1974). Recurring digital fibroma of infancy. *J. Bone Jt. Surg.,* **56B** : 746.

BOOHER, R.J. & MCPEAK, C.J. (1959). Juvenile aponeurotic fibromas. *Surgery,* **46** : 924.

BOTTING, A.J., SOULE, E.H. & BROWN, A.L. (1965). Smooth muscle tumours in children. *Cancer,* **18** : 711.

BRYAN, R.S., SOULE, E.H. *et al.* (1974). Primary epithelioid sarcoma of the hand and forearm: a review of 13 cases. *J. Bone Jt. Surg.,* **56A** : 458.

BURKHARDT, B.R. & SOULE, E.H. *et al.* (1966). Dermatofibrosarcoma protruberans: study of 56 cases. *Am. J. Surg.,* **111** : 638.

BUTLER, J.J. (1965). Fibrous tissue tumours: nodular fasciitis, dermatofibrosarcoma protruberans, and fibrosarcoma, grade I, desmoid type. In *Tumors of Bone and Soft Tissue.* Year Book Medical Publishers, Chicago.

CADE, S. (1962). Synovial sarcoma. *J. Roy. Coll. Surg. Edinb.,* **8** : 1.

CADMAN, N.L., SOULE, E.H. & KELLY, P.J. (1965). Synovial sarcoma: an analysis of 134 tumors. *Cancer,* **18** : 613.

CAMERON, H.V. & KOSTUIK, J.P. (1974). A long-term follow up of synovial sarcoma. *J. Bone Jt. Surg.,* **56**B : 613.

CHUNG, E.B. & ENZINGER, F.M. (1973). Benign lipoblastomatosis: an analysis of 35 cases. *Cancer,* **32** : 482.

CONNOLLY, N.K. (1961). Juvenile fibromatosis: a case report showing invasion of bone. *Arch. Dis. Childh.,* **36** : 171.

DOLL, R., MUIR, C. and WATERHOUSE, J. (*Eds.*) (1972). Cancer Incidence in Five Continents. Vol. II. (U.I.C.C.)—Springer Verlag. Berlin, Heidelberg, New York.

DONALDSON, S.S., CASTRO, J.R., WILBUR, J.R. & JESSE, R.H. (1973). Rhabdomyosarcoma of the head and neck in children. *Cancer,* **31** : 26.

DUBE, V.E. & PAULSON, J.F. (1974). Metastatic hemangiopericytoma cured by radiotherapy: a case report. *J. Bone Jt. Surg.,* **56B** : 833.

EHRLICH, F.E., HAAS, J.E. & KIESEWETTER, W.B. (1971). Rhabdomyosarcoma in infants and children: factors affecting survival. *J. Pediat. Surg.,* **6** : 571.

ENTERLINE, H.T. & CULBERSON, J.D. *et al.* (1970). Liposarcoma. *Cancer,* **13** : 932.

ENZINGER, F.M. & WINSLOW, D.J. (1962). Liposarcoma: study of 103 cases. *Virchow's Arch. Path. Anat.,* **335** : 367.

ENZINGER, F.M. (1965a). Fibrous hamartoma of infancy. *Cancer,* **18** : 241.

ENZINGER, F.M. (1965b). Fibrous tumours of infancy. In *Sarcomas of Bone and Soft Tissues.* Year Book Medical Publishing Company, Chicago.

ENZINGER, F.M. (1965c). Clear-cell sarcoma of tendons and aponeuroses: an analysis of 21 cases. *Cancer,* **18** : 1163.

ENZINGER, F.M. (1970). Epithelioid sarcoma: a sarcoma simulating a granuloma or a carcinoma. *Cancer,* **26** : 1029.

Enzinger, F.M., Lattes, R. & Torloni, H. (1969). Histological Typing of Soft Tissue Tumours. W.H.O., Geneva.

Exelby, P.R., Knapper, W.H., Huvos, A.G. & Beattie, E.J. (1973). Soft tissue fibrosarcoma in children. *J. pediat. Surg.*, **8** : 415.

Fisher, E.R. & Reidbord, H. (1971). Electron microscopic evidence suggesting the myogenous derivation of so called alveolar soft part sarcoma. *Cancer*, **27** : 150.

Finlay-Jones, L.R. (1970). Lymphangiosarcoma of the thigh: case report. *Cancer*, **26** : 722.

Gerner, R. & Moore, G.E. (1975). Synovial sarcoma. *Ann. Surg.*, **181** : 22.

Ghosh, B., Ghosh, L. *et al.* (1973). Malignant schwannoma: a clinicopathologic study. *Cancer*, **31** : 184.

Gottlieb, J.A., Baker, L.H., Quagliana, J.M. *et al.* (1972). Chemotherapy of sarcomas with a combination of adriamycin and dimethyl-triazeno-imadazole carbosamide (D.T.I.C.). *Cancer*, **30** : 1632.

Grossman, M. & Melmon, K. (1972). Von Hippe-Lindau disease. In the Phakomatoses (Vinken, P.J. & Bruyn, G.W.—*Eds*). Handbook of Clinical Neurology, Vol. 14. American Elsevier Publishing Co. Inc., New York.

Gruhn, J. & Hurwitt, E.S. (1951). Fibrous sternomastoid tumor of infancy. *Pediatrics*, **8** : 522.

Harken, J.C. & Reed, R.J. (1969). Tumors of the peripheral nervous system. Atlas of Tumor Pathology. 2nd series. Fascicle 3. Armed Forces Institute of Pathology. Washington, D.C.

Hays, D.M., Mirabel, V.Q. *et al.* (1970). Fibrosarcomas in infants and children. *J. Pediat. Surg.*, **5** : 176.

Heyn, R.M. (1975). The role of chemotherapy in the management of soft tissue sarcomas. *Cancer*, **35** : 921.

Holdsworth Mayer, C.M., Favara, B.E. *et al.* (1974). Malignant mesenchymoma in infants. *Am. J. Dis. Child.*, **128** : 847.

Horn, R.C. & Enterline, H.T. (1958). Rhabdomyosarcoma: a clinicopathologic study and classification of 39 cases. *Cancer*, **11** : 181.

Jaffe, N., Filler, R., Farber, S. & Murray, J.E. (1973). Rhabdomyosarcoma in children: improved outlook with a multidisciplinary approach. *Amer. J. Surg.*, **125** : 482.

Jones, P.G. (1968). *Torticollis in Infancy and Childhood.* Charles C. Thomas, Springfield.

Kauffman, S.L. & Stout, A.P. (1959). Lipoblastic tumors of children. *Cancer*, **12** : 912.

Kauffman, S.L. & Stout, A.P. (1961). Malignant haemangio-endothelioma in infants and children. *Cancer*, **14** : 1186.

Kauffman, S.L. & Stout, A.P. (1965). Congenital mesenchymal tumours. *Cancer*, **18** : 460.

Keasbey, L.E. (1953). Juvenile aponeurotic fibroma (calcifying fibroma). *Cancer*, **6** : 338.

Kevorkian, J. & Cento, D.P. (1973). Leiomyosarcoma of large arteries and veins. *Surgery*, **73** : 390.

Kilman, J.S., Clatworthy, H.W.Jr. *et al.* (1973). Reasonable surgery for rhabdomyosarcoma: a study of 67 cases. *Ann. Surg.*, **178** : 346.

Mackenzie, D.H. (1966). Synovial sarcoma: a review of 58 cases. *Cancer*, **19** : 169.

Mahour, G.H., Soule, E.H., Mills, S.D. & Lynn, H.B. (1967). Rhabdomyosarcomas in infants and children: a clinicopathologic study of 75 cases. *J. Pediat. Surg.*, **2** : 402.

Martel, W. & Abell, M.R. (1973). Radiology of soft tissue tumours: a retrospective study. *Cancer*, **32** : 352.

Mena, E., Bookstein, J.J. *et al.* (1973). Neurofibromatosis and renovascular hypertension in children. *Am. J. Roentgenol. Rad. Ther. Nucl. Med.*, **118** : 39.

Nash, A. & Stout, A.P. (1961). Malignant mesenchymoma in children. *Cancer*, **14** : 524.

Nesbit, R.R. & Rob, C. (1975). Leiomyosarcoma of a vein: survival for six years. *Arch. Surg.*, **110** : 118.

O'Brien, P. & Brasfield, R.D. (1965). Haemangiopericytoma. *Cancer*, **18** : 249.

Ortega, J.A., Finkelstein, J.Z. *et al.* (1971). Chemotherapy of malignant haemangiopericytoma of childhood. *Cancer*, **27** : 730.

Pellerin, D. & Bertin, P. (1974). Abdominal, pelvic and perineal embryonic sarcomas in childhood: an analysis of 37 cases. *Progress in Pediatric Surgery*, **7** : 83.

Pinkel, D. & Pickren, J. (1961). Rhabdomyosarcoma in children. *J. Amer. Med. Assoc.*, **175** : 293.

Plaschkes, J. (1974). Congenital fibromatosis: localized and generalized forms. *J. Pediat. Surg.*, **9** : 95.

Pratt, C.B., Hustu, H.O., Fleming, I.D. & Pinkel, D. (1972). Coordinated treatment of childhood rhabdomyosarcoma with surgery, radiotherapy and combination chemotherapy. *Cancer Res.*, **32** : 606.

Price, E.B.Jr., Silliphant, W.M. & Shuman, R. (1961). Nodular fasciitis: a clinicopathological analysis of 65 cases. *Am. J. Clin. Path.*, **35** : 122.

Ragab, A.H. (1972/73). Childhood rhabdomyosarcoma. *Paediatrician*, **1** : 288.

Reye, R.D.K. (1956). Considerations of certain subdermal fibromatous tumours of infancy. *J. Path. Bact.*, **72** : 149.

Roth, J.A., Enzinger, F.M. & Tannenbaum, M. (1975). Synovial sarcoma of the neck: a follow up study of 24 cases. *Cancer*, **35** : 1243.

Santamaria, J.N., Colebatch, J.H. & Campbell, P.E. (1970). Rhabdomyosarcoma: a study of 27 cases. *Australas. Radiol.*, **14** : 438.

Shim, W.K. (1968). Hemangiomas of infancy complicated by thrombocytopenia. *Am. J. Surg.*, **116** : 896.

Shipkey, F.H., Lieberman, P.H., Foote, F.W.Jr. & Stewart, F.W. (1964). Ultrastructure of alveolar soft part sarcoma. *Cancer*, **17** : 821.

Soule, E.H., Mahour, G.H. & Mills, S.D. *et al.* (1968). Soft Tissue sarcomas of infants and children: a clinicopathologic study of 135 cases. *Mayo Clin. Proc.*, **43** : 313.

Stout, A.P. (1958). Juvenile fibromatosis. *Cancer*, **7** : 953.

Stout, A.P. (1948). Mesenchymoma, mixed tumor of mesenchymal derivatives. *Ann. Surg.*, **127** : 278.

Stout, A.P. (1961). Pseudosarcomatous fasciitis in children. *Cancer*, **14** : 1216.

Stout, A.P. (1962). Fibrosarcoma of infants and children. *Cancer*, **15** : 1028.

Suit, H.D., Russell, W.O. & Martin, R.G. (1973). Management of patients with sarcoma of soft tissues in an extremity. *Cancer*, **31** : 1247.

Sutow, W.W., Sullivan, M.P. *et al.* (1970). Prognosis in childhood rhabdomyosarcoma. *Cancer*, **25** : 1384.

Tabrisky, J., Rowe, J.H. *et al.* (1974). Benign mediastinal lipoblastomatosis. *J. Pediat. Surg.*, **9** : 399.

Taylor, H.B. & Helwig, E.B. (1962). Dermatofibrosarcoma protruberans: a study of 115 cases. *Cancer*, **15** : 717.

U.I.C.C. (1973). *Clinical Oncology*. Springer-Verlag, Berlin, Heidelberg, New York.

Vellios, F., Baez, J. & Shumacker, H.B. (1958). Lipoblastomatosis: a tumor of fetal fat different from hibernoma. *Am. J. Path.*, **34** : 1149.

Watanabe, I., Ohtomo, S. & Kimura, N. (1974). Dumbbell type rhabdomyosarcoma in an infant. *J. Pediat. Surg.*, **9** : 407.

Welsh, R.A., Bray, D.M. *et al.* (1972). Histogenesis of alveolar soft part sarcoma. *Cancer*, **29** : 191.

Willis, R.A. (1962). *Pathology of Tumours in Childhood.* Charles C. Thomas, Springfield.

WONG, H.B. (1973). Abdominal wall abscess. *Proc. Roy. Aust. Coll. Surg.*, Singapore, p. 393.

WRIGHT, C.J.E. (1952). Malignant synovioma. *J. Path. Bact.*, **64** : 585.

YANNOPOULOS, K. & STOUT, A.P. (1962). Smooth muscle tumours in children. *Cancer*, **15** : 958.

Phakomatoses

Neurofibromatosis

CROWE, F.W., SCHULL, W.J. & NEEL, J.V. (1956). *Multiple Neurofibromatosis*. Charles C. Thomas, Springfield.

FIENMAN, N.L. & YAKOVAC, W.C. (1970). Neurofibromatosis in childhood. *J. Pediat.*, **76** : 339.

FONT, R.L. & FERRY, A.P. (1972). The phakomatoses. *Internatal. Ophthal. Clin.*, **12** : 1.

HUNT, J.C. & PUCH, D.G. (1961). Skeletal lesions in neurofibromatosis. *Radiology*, **76** : 1.

MENA, E., BOOKSTEIN, J.J. *et al.* (1973). Neurofibromatosis and renovascular hypertension in children. *Am. J. Roentgenol. Rad. Ther. Nucl. Med.*, **118** : 39.

RAFFENSPERGER, J. & COHEN, R. (1972). Plexiform neurofibromas in childhood. *J. Pediat. Surg.*, **7** : 144.

VAN DE HOEVE, J. (1932). The Doyne Memorial Lecture: Eye symptoms in phakomatoses. *Trans. Ophthal. Soc., U.K.*, **52** : 380.

VINKEN, P.J. & BRUYN, G.W. (*Eds.*) (1972). The phakomatoses. In *Handbooks of Clinical Neurology*, vol. 14. Elsevier, New York.

Tuberous Sclerosis

DEHNER, L.P., ENZINGER, F.M. & FONT, R.L. (1972). Fetal rhabdomyoma. An analysis of nine cases. *Cancer*, **30** : 160.

LAGOS, J.C. & GOMEZ, M.R. (1967). Tuberous sclerosis: reappraisal of a clinical entity. *Mayo Clin. Proc.*, **42** : 26.

PAULSON, G.W. & LYLE, C.B. (1966). Tuberous sclerosis. *J. Dev. Med. Child. Neurol.*, **8** : 571.

Chapter 24. Tumours of the skin

Table 24.1. Benign swellings and malignant tumours of the skin

Benign conditions	Malignant tumours
Haemangioma: capillary	Primary tumours
Haemangioma: cavernous	Squamous cell carcinoma
Naevus: pigmented	Basal cell carcinoma
Naevus: junctional	Reticulum cell sarcoma
Naevus: activated	Malignant melanoma
Naevus: intradermal	Kaposi's sarcoma
Naevus: compound	Malignant Schwannoma
Naevus: 'giant hairy'	Secondary deposits
Naevus: spindle/epithelioid cell	(including subcutaneous metastases)
Blue naevus	Neuroblastoma ('blueberry-muffin' baby)
Sebaceous naevus	
Epidermoid cyst	Letterer-Siwe disease
Pilomatrixoma	Leukaemic deposits
Tricho-epithelirioma (syn. Brooke's tumour)	Lymphoma deposits
Adenoma sebaceum	
Pyogenic granuloma	
Granuloma annulare	
Syringoma	
Cylindroma	
Juvenile xanthogranuloma	
Dermatofibrosarcoma protruberans	
Dermatofibroma (syn. fibrous histiocytoma)	
Glomus tumour (syn. glomangioma)	
Reticulohistiocytoma	
Cutaneous leiomyoma	
Hidradenoma ('clear cell' tumour)	
Subcutaneous tissues	
Fibromatoses (see p. 798)	Haemangiopericytoma (malignant)
Glomus tumour	Haemangioendothelioma (malignant)
Granular cell 'myoblastoma'	Mesenchymoma (malignant)
Other benign tumours of soft tissues (see p. 796)	Other soft tissue sarcomas (see p. 781)

The skin is the site of a considerable variety of hamartomas and other benign conditions, both pigmented and unpigmented, arising during childhood. Some 'birth marks' are actually congenital, but many are misnomers and appear during the neonatal period—such as intracutaneous capillary haemangiomas, or progressively throughout childhood and adolescence, e.g. pigmented naevi (Table 24.1).

The relationship of the latter to malignant melanoma has been partly clarified by the identification of the so-called 'juvenile melanoma', now referred to as the spindle/epithelioid cell naevus (Spitz, 1948; Allen & Spitz, 1953), which can be excluded from consideration as a malignant condition.

Malignant tumours of the skin almost never arise in completely normal unblemished skin, and are found closely related to two abnormalities predisposed to the development of malignancy:

(*a*) The rare familial condition xeroderma pigmentosum; and

(*b*) The 'giant hairy' naevus, always present at birth and usually involving large areas of the skin.

However, the most prevalent causes of practically groundless anxiety, to both parents and medical profession, are the infinitely more common, in fact universal, pigmented naevi, most of which are not present at birth but develop progressively throughout childhood and adolescence (Nicholls, 1973).

Finally, malignant melanoma may arise in childhood from melanocytes in the meninges, cells which are occasionally present in large numbers as leptomeningeal melanocytosis (p. 285) a condition sometimes associated with a giant hairy naevus of the scalp.

NON-EPITHELIAL MALIGNANT TUMOURS OF THE SKIN

The rarity of carcinoma and malignant melanoma is matched by another group of tumours in childhood: a primary or metastatic malignant tumour of soft tissues in the upper layers of the dermis, presenting as a subepithelial lesion. These are as follows:

1. Malignant lymphomas
2. Rhabdomyosarcoma
3. Metastatic lesions.

1. *Malignant lymphomas.* Both lymphosarcoma and reticulum cell sarcoma may develop as a very superficial primary tumour in the skin (p. 179).

The clinical appearances vary, but in several examples in the Index Series the lesion was a firm, sharply demarcated, sessile, reddish plaque, up to 1 cm high, 1 to 4 cm in diameter, nontender and movable to some extent on subdermal areolar planes. The overlying epithelium was intact, stretched and shiny in some, slightly oedematous with early peau d'orange in others.

Biopsy is required for diagnosis, and excision biopsy, removing the lesion completely, is preferable when the site and size permit. Occasionally there is significant enlargement of a related regional node and this offers an alternative or additional source of biopsy material.

Treatment depends upon the extent of the tumour as revealed by the appropriate investigations (p. 174), and combination chemotherapy is the mainstay of treatment (see lymphosarcoma p. 175, reticulum cell sarcoma, p. 181).

2. *Rhabdomyosarcoma*, on rare occasions, presents as a superficial swelling in the skin, without any particular distinguishing features. Diagnosis rests on excision biopsy and histological examination. Treatment of rhabdomyosarcoma is described on p. 789.

3. *Metastatic cutaneous lesions* also occur, usually in the terminal stages, and in the Index Series these were seen in a variety of tumours notably hepatocarcinoma and synovial sarcoma.

Nodular subcutaneous swellings form part of the 'blueberry muffin' syndrome seen in neuroblastoma Stage IV S. (p. 552) and similar lesions may also develop in congenital leukaemia (p. 166). Less discrete plaques of metastatic infiltration very occasionally occur in acute monocytic leukaemia or in Hodgkin's disease.

Malignant tumours of the skin in childhood are:

I. Epidermal carcinoma and basal cell epithelioma;
II. Malignant melanoma;
III. Kaposi's sarcoma

I. EPIDERMAL CARCINOMA
(syn. squamous cell carcinoma, squamous epithelioma, epidermoid carcinoma)

These tumours never arise in normal skin in childhood; while some may develop in chronic scars caused by burns or irradiation, the majority develop in patients with xeroderma pigmentosum.

Xeroderma pigmentosum is inherited as an autosomal recessive trait (Lynch, 1967) which is expressed as a deficiency of the enzyme endonuclease (Cleaver, 1968, 1973) essential to the excision and patching of new bases in DNA molecules damaged by ultraviolet radiation; the manner in which this deficiency is related to carcinogenesis is unknown. There appears to be a milder form of the disease, inherited as a dominant autosomal trait (Anderson & Begg, 1960).

The skin of children with xeroderma is dry and inelastic from the outset, and has a marked sensitivity to ultraviolet light. Lesions subsequently develop in those areas most exposed to sunlight, the face, hands, knees and forearms. Neoplasms develop in the third stage of the disease (Siegelman & Sutow, 1965), the first stage being atrophic changes and the second, hyperkeratosis and hyperpigmentation of the epidermis.

A variety of premalignant and malignant lesions subsequently develop, and characteristically at the one time in one patient there are solar keratoses, kerato-acanthomas, basal cell carcinomas and squamous cell carcinomas. In addition, malignant melanomas and, least commonly, subcutaneous fibrosarcomas may also develop in this condition.

Once the diagnosis has been established, and this is possible at a very early age, on the basis of the family history and the intense 'freckling' on exposed surfaces (Fig. 24.1), the child should be kept under close and continuing surveillance so that neoplastic lesions can be detected and removed as early as possible in their evolution.

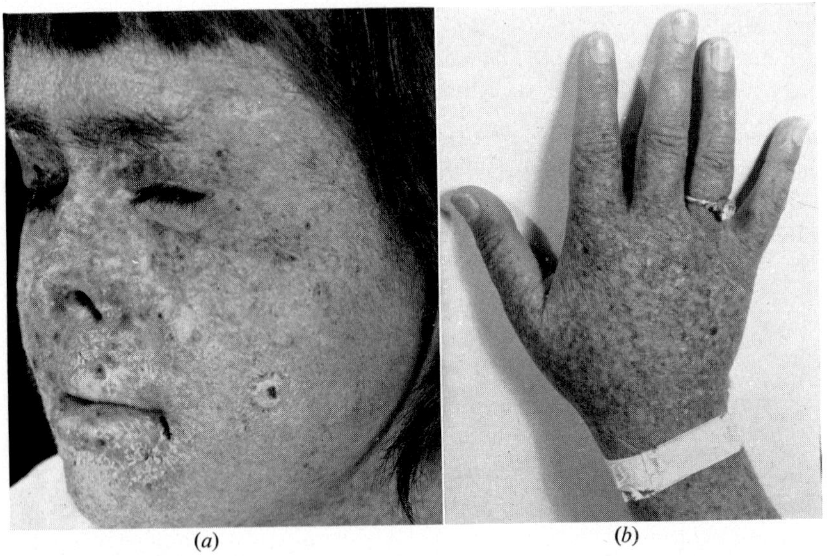

(*a*) (*b*)

Figure 24.1. XERODERMA PIGMENTOSUM; typical appearance of (*a*) the face, and (*b*) dorsum of the hand, of 15-year old girl with a positive family history; more than 25 malignant skin tumours of all kinds (except malignant melanoma) have already been excised from this patient.

Squamous cell carcinomas in this condition are usually well differentiated, and some of the tumours are intermediate between basal cell and squamous cell carcinoma (see also basal cell naevus syndrome, p. 848).

TREATMENT

Covering forearms and knees with suitable clothing, and protective skin creams for the face and hands from a very early age are required. Frequent re-examination, at intervals of 2–3 months, and early surgical excision of each neoplasm as it arises, form the basis of management.

Prophylactic chemotherapy, e.g. with bleomycin, is under trial, but the need for longterm management and the undesirable side effects of even mildly toxic chemotherapeutic drugs pose difficulties in selecting the most appropriate cytotoxic agent to be used over a long period of time.

Preservation of the facial appearance for as long as possible requires minimal but adequate excision and careful closure of each defect, by direct suture, re-arrangement of local flaps or skin grafts. In time, multiple scars and the inelasticity of the atrophic skin may indicate a need for more extensive reconstructive procedures, but skin from elsewhere on an affected individual will inevitably suffer the same histological changes when transferred to an area exposed to sunlight.

PROGNOSIS

In spite of close supervision and the most expert care, facial disfigurement eventually occurs and life is rarely prolonged beyond early adulthood.

Genetic counselling is made relatively easy by the strong motivation of parents to avoid having children once they have observed the course of the disease in a member of the family. The risk of subsequent affected children is 1 in 4, and another 25% will be asymptomatic carriers of the gene.

II. MALIGNANT MELANOMA
(syn. melanotic sarcoma)

This tumour is an exceptional rarity in childhood, but not entirely unknown in the paediatric age group; Lerman *et al.* (1970) collected 73 proven cases reported in the literature up to that date.

The clinical and histological features of malignant melanoma in children are sufficiently unusual to suggest that they may differ significantly from their adult counterpart, at least in Australia where there is, in adults, convincing evidence that the relatively higher incidence in Australia, compared with other parts of the world, is due to the cumulative carcinogenetic effects of solar radiation. The types of melanoma which arise in Hutchinson's freckle or in premalignant melanosis in adults do not occur in children.

In adults there is a significantly increased incidence of malignant melanoma in the inland (western) part of Queensland in which there is the highest incidence of pathological solar damage (including squamous and basal cell carcinomas) in Australia, and possibly the highest in any white population in the world. However, the area with the greatest incidence of malignant melanoma is the coastal region of Queensland. Further, in the coastal regions the areas of skin in which there is the highest incidence of malignant melanoma, are not the same as the sites of squamous and basal cell carcinoma in inland Queensland. One explanation may be that there is greater exposure to solar damage of different (and larger) areas of the body in the coastal region, where sunbathing is common; in contrast, the farming population of the inland (where ambient temperatures are higher, relative humidity much less and sea breezes absent) dress so as to prevent the effects of sunlight on all areas except those inescapably exposed, i.e. the face and neck, and the dorsum of the hands (Davis, 1971).

Black and Douglas (1973) have shown in animal experiments that one of the carcinogenetic effects of ultraviolet light is the oxidation of cholesterol to cholesterol α-oxide which enters the blood stream to reach unexposed skin, where it is capable of provoking the development of squamous carcinoma. It is conceivable that a similar mechanism may be responsible for the development, in those exposed to sunlight, of malignant melanoma in unexposed areas of skin (Lee, 1972; Annotation, *M.J.A.* 1974).

The importance of racial and/or hereditary pigmentary factors is illustrated by the fact that no case of malignant melanoma in an Australian aboriginal in Queensland has been reported in the last 20 years (Davis, 1971).

In the period 1963–1969, 1514 patients with malignant melanoma were reported in the Queensland Melanoma Project (Beardmore, 1972). Of these, 36 (approximately 2%) were between 10 and 20 years of age; apparently there was no case in a child less than 10 years of age. In males (of all ages) the trunk was the commonest site for a malignant melanoma, whereas in females the lower leg was the area with the highest incidence.

It is particularly noteworthy that in no less than 45% of this series of 1514 patients, a malignant melanoma arose in skin not known to have been the site of a pre-existing pigmented lesion.

Malignant melanoma most commonly develops in a pigmented naevus and the two types of lesion in which it may arise are:

(*a*) A giant hairy naevus;

(*b*) A junctional naevus.

(*a*) GIANT HAIRY NAEVUS

Reed, Becker & Becker (1965) reported six cases of congenital or neonatal malignant melanoma arising in a giant pigmented naevus, and Feins (1973) recently described the total excision, at the age of 4 weeks, of an extensive lesion of this kind involving most of the scalp. The association of the so-called 'giant hairy naevus' (Fig. 24.2) and malignant melanoma has been reported to be significant, but is difficult to assess. In a review of 41 malignant melanomas arising in childhood, Skov-Jensen *et al.* (1966) found that in 10 of the 41 cases a malignant melanoma had developed in a giant hairy naevus. The incidence of malignancy has been estimated variously (Reed, Becker & Becker, 1965; Lerman *et al.*, 1970; Penman & Stringer, 1971) to be as high as 30%, but the population at risk may be very much greater than has been estimated, and the incidence may thus be much less.

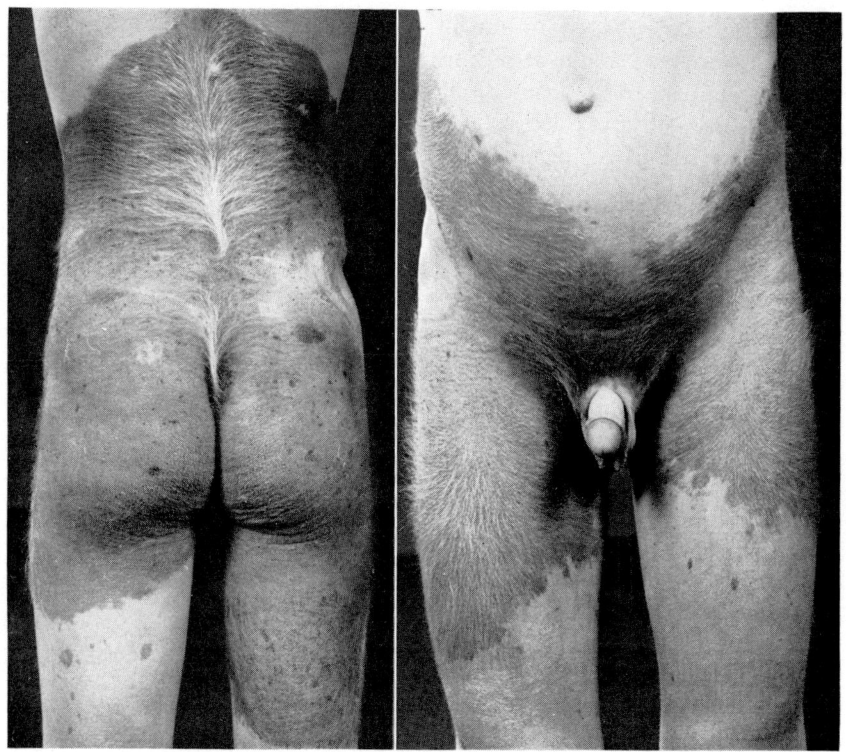

Figure 24.2. GIANT 'HAIRY' NAEVUS; an extensive lesion of the 'bathing trunk' type and distribution. The site of removal of an amelanotic malignant melanoma four years previously, can be seen near the right anterior superior iliac spine (see patient 2, p. 863).

One difficulty is to establish widely accepted criteria for the diagnosis of a 'giant' hairy naevus; most of the extensive congenital naevi seen at the Royal Children's Hospital have not been 'hairy'; none has been completely excised prophylactically, and over many years observation (admittedly not far into adult life) only one has undergone a malignant change (p. 863).

Another difficulty concerns interpretation of the microscopic findings; the only incontrovertible proof of malignancy in a melanoma is the development of metastases. Pathologists of great experience have seen metastases from lesions thought to be benign on microscopic evidence, and conversely, lesions with highly malignant histological appearances without any dissemination.

A final difficulty presented by patients with very extensive pigmented naevi, occupying more than 10% of the body surface, is that even if total prophylactic excision were considered desirable, it would present formidable technical problems, more so if all subcutaneous tissues beneath the pigmented are were to be excised, because this tissue, too, has also been reported to be on rare occasions a source of malignancy (Lund & Kraus, 1962).

Depending on the area involved, partial removal of such lesions may be warranted for other reasons than the risk of malignancy, e.g. on cosmetic grounds for lesions on the forehead or neck, or to improve hygiene and comfort when the perineum is the site of a bulky, fissured lesion.

(*b*) JUNCTIONAL NAEVI

The progressive development of ever greater numbers of this type of naevus throughout childhood and adolescence is well known, and has been documented in a sample of 1518 white children in Sydney, Australia by Nicholls (1973) who reported that males reach their peak number of such lesions at the age of 15 years, whereas females reach their maximum number at 20–29 years. Most adolescents have at least 10–12 such lesions, and many have a much greater number. The chief difficulty in management stems from the fact that it is impossible to determine which (if any) lesion on one individual might become malignant, and the statistical chance of this occurring is one in many millions. Although there is a somewhat higher statistical probability of malignancy in a naevus on the eyelids, the lower extremity, the genitalia or beneath a finger nail or toe nail, it is nevertheless unwarranted (as well as impossible) to attempt to remove every pigmented naevus in these areas from every child.

Supervision and re-examination at regular intervals is the alternative, and the signs of potential or impending neoplasia are as follows:

(i) *Increase in the thickness* of the dermis;

(ii) *Increase in the area* affected or in the depth of pigmentation in the lesion;

(iii) *Alteration in the surface layers*, with increase in coarseness and roughness, and the appearance of cracks or bleeding.

It should be noted that some of these changes commonly occur during puberty and adolescence without portending malignancy. Increase in the depth of pigmentation is not a reliable indication of neoplasia, as shown by the development of an amelanotic melanoma (at lease macroscopically) in two of the four malignant melanomas of the skin encountered in the Index

Series; in each case a melanoma was not even suspected until the lesion was examined microscopically. For this reason, non-pigmented benign skin lesions have been included in the discussion of the differential diagnosis.

DIFFERENTIATION OF MALIGNANT MELANOMA FROM OTHER SKIN LESIONS

These benign conditions can be classified in three groups:
(*a*) Pigmented lesions containing melanin (i.e. naevi);
(*b*) Non-pigmented lesions, a large group composed of hamartomas and benign tumours of the skin; and
(*c*) A small group of benign lesions containing pigment other than melanin.

(*a*) **Pigmented naevus**

The word 'naevus', derived from the Latin *nascor* (to be born), was initially applied to any 'mark or flaw present at birth'; by extension it came to be applied to any blemish (at one stage even to a flaw in character), and until the late 19th century, it was applied solely to vascular birthmarks. The subdivision of 'birthmarks' into vascular and pigmented naevi has left us saddled with a term which has too many different connotations, and as the great majority of melanin-containing lesions are not present at birth, the term 'naevus' is hardly appropriate for those which are gradually acquired in increasing numbers throughout childhood and adolescence.

Pigmented naevi are classified according to which layer of the skin is chiefly affected. These are, in order of frequency:

1. *The junctional naevus*, in which the naevus cells are in the epidermis, at its junction with the dermis. Pigmentation is usually light and uniform, producing a light brown discolouration of a small area of skin, which is flat, without a palpable edge, and the overlying epidermis is normal.
2. *An activated junctional naevus* is one which contains areas with variations in the depth of pigmentation at various points, with palpable thickening of its margin, and some hyperkeratosis of the overlying epidermis.
3. *An intradermal* (*or dermal*) *naevus* develops when cells from a junctional naevus bud off into the underlying dermis. In older children the lesion matures so that the 'junctional' component disappears, leaving inactive cells confined to the dermis.
4. *A compound naevus* is one in which the naevus cells are present not only in the epidermis in the junctional layers, but also in the dermis beneath. *A composite naevus* is the term used when most or all of the elements of the skin are involved and abnormally active, e.g. the prickle cells, squames, hair follicles and sebaceous cells; this represents a regional disturbance of development which could qualify as a hamartoma. Eventually nodularity and deep fissures develop in the skin of the affected area.

The café-au-lait patch in the skin in von Recklinghausen's disease is a pale brown, flat, oval area, usually on the trunk or limbs. Microscopically there is an increase in pigmentation in the cells of the basal layer of the epidermis. Frozen sections stained for dopamine reveal some increase in the number of melanocytes, and some increase in their activity. The dermis is usually normal and does not contain more melanocytes than normal skin.

Blue naevus (syn. benign dermal melanocytoma; blue naevus of Jadassohn-Tièche)
This lesion is typically in the dermis and presents clinically a dark blue, slate-blue or black, smooth, slightly raised area of skin, usually on the trunk, the limbs or the face. From our experience they are less common than spindle/epithelioid naevi (15 : 40 in the period covered by the Index Series).

Macroscopically they are clinically well defined areas of intense pigmentation deep in the dermis, often extending into subcutaneous fat. The whitish epidermis overlying the dark brown pigment is responsible for the clinical 'blue-black' or 'slate-blue-grey' appearance.

Microscopically they are composed of interlacing bundles of elongated, spindle-shaped cells, often so heavily pigmented that the outline of the nucleus is completely obscured. The melanin can be removed by treating the section with peroxide, and the nucleus is then revealed as round or oval, with a thick nuclear membrane and a prominent nucleolus. Fibrous tissue and nerve-like tissue are often present in the lesion. Junctional activity is not seen, but occasionally some epidermal naevus cells are present. Although they are moderately cellular lesions, especially in young children, they behave in a benign fashion.

In the Index Series, a 3-year old girl had a blue naevus excised from her forearm; 3 months later a similar lesion appeared in the cubital fossa some 4 cm proximal to the first, and this, too, was excised. Both were cellular blue naevi, and nothing further has appeared in the following 1½ years.

Spindle/epithelioid cell naevus (syn. juvenile melanoma)
This is a most important type of benign naevus because of the diagnostic problems it presents. It is composed of cells with a vesicular nucleus and a prominent nucleolus, features which suggest active growth and hence occasionally lead to confusion with malignant melanoma (Fig. 24.3). The term 'juvenile melanoma' is open to criticism as the lesion is not confined to children, and is not a melanoma if that term is considered to be synonymous with malignant melanoma. Although somewhat clumsy, the term 'spindle/epithelioid naevus' has been widely adopted because it is accurate and descriptive, and sets the lesion apart from both the junctional naevus, and from malignant melanoma.

Spindle/epithelioid cell naevi are not rare; there are 40 cases (20 boys and 20 girls) in the period covered by the Index Series, and approximately three new cases are seen each year. This is probably a low estimate of the incidence of a lesion not always subjected to excision.

Macroscopically the average size is 1 cm in diameter; the lesion is pink, raised, and may be ulcerated; some are pigmented but characteristically most are not.

Microscopically the typical lesion has an intact but often attenuated epidermal covering, and there is some oedema of the subpapillary dermal connective tissue. There is no junctional activity. Groups of cells with a prominent, round nucleus and a large single nucleolus lie in clusters in the dermis; they may extend below the level of the hair follicles and sweat glands, but rarely as deep as the subcutaneous fat. The cells have prominent, fleshy, pink-staining cytoplasm with sharp margins; they are often binucleated and occasionally multinucleated. Although the nucleolus is prominent the nuclear chromatin is regular and sparse, and mitoses are rare (Fig. 24.3).

Cells with an identical nucleus but a more spindle-shaped cytoplasm are also present as a rule; in some lesions all the cells are of this type, but both

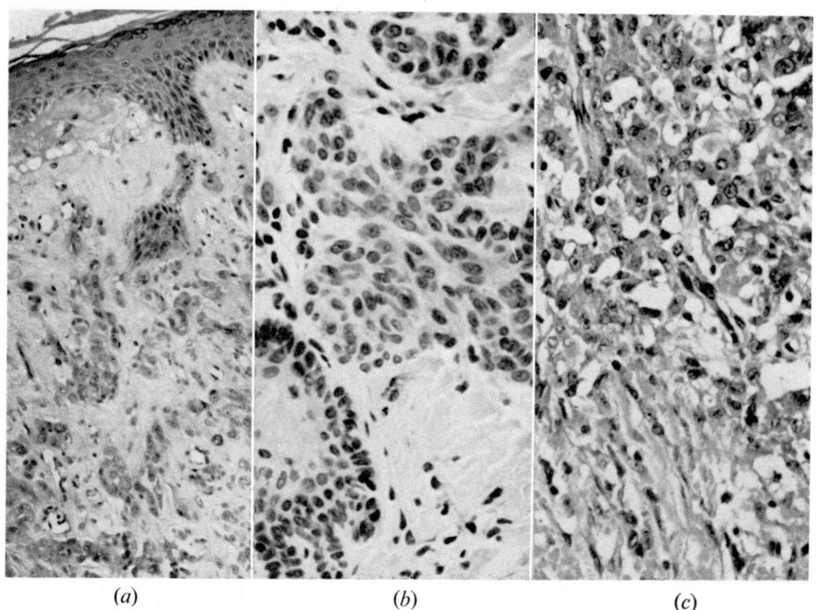

(*a*) (*b*) (*c*)

Figure 24.3. SPINDLE/EPITHELIOID CELL NAEVUS; (*a*) the most active area lies in the junctional region, (H & E. × 130) while the deepest (*b*) is composed of benign, well-differentiated naevus cells (H & E. × 200), in contrast to (*c*) malignant melanoma in which irregular, pleomorphic active cells are most apparent in the deepest part of the dermis (H & E. × 320).

types of cell are usually present, the plump fleshy cells lying closer to the surface and the spindle cells situated more deeply. The presence of both types of cell suggested the term spindle/epithelioid cell naevus (Graham, Johnson & Helwig, 1972).

Differentiation from malignant melanoma

This is an important distinction to make and is usually not difficult. In a spindle/epithelioid cell naevus, the naevus cells never invade the epidermis, do not form pseudo-acini, rarely form pigment, and show no nuclear anaplasia. The more deeply placed cells are always less active in appearance than those near the surface; the contrary is found in a malignant melanoma, the deeper cells being more invasive and showing greater anaplasia.

The multiple basal cell naevi syndrome

More than 50 examples have been reported (Gorlin *et al.*, 1965) of a rare syndrome inherited as an autosomal dominant (non-x-linked) condition. The expressivity is variable, for no one component is present in every case. The lesions which give the syndrome its name appear in childhood, at about puberty, or in young adults, as numerous nodules with various depths of pigment ranging from skin coloured to dark brown, chiefly on the face, neck, shoulders and the upper trunk (Howell *et al.*, 1966).

Associated features are multiple cysts in both jaws (keratocysts (p. 337) or odontogenic cysts), skeletal malformations (e.g. bifid ribs) and, less commonly, medulloblastoma, hyporesponsiveness to parathormone, and a wide variety of abnormalities.

Some of the children affected have a distinctive facies combining frontal and temporoparietal bossing and ocular hypertelorism.

The nature of the skin lesions varies from benign 'trichoepithelioma' (p. 851) to a typically aggressive and ulcerated basal cell carcinoma. None was seen in the Index Series.

Subnaeval folliculitis

Walton (1971) noted that rupture of the base of the hair follicles found in some benign naevi can cause an inflammatory reaction leading to hyperaemia, rapid increase in size and induration, which may suggest the development of a malignant melanoma. The correct diagnosis can be made on excision-biopsy.

(*b*) NON-PIGMENTED BENIGN LESIONS

A lesion presenting clinically as a discrete mass in the skin arises either in the epidermis, in its appendages (Fig. 24.4) or in the immediately subjacent dermis and grows upwards to elevate or possibly infiltrate the epidermis. The overwhelming majority are benign and can be recognized by their clinical features.

In most of these conditions the differential diagnosis turns on the age of the patient, and the site, size, rate of growth, colour and clinical characteristics of the lesion. In some cases the diagnosis is uncertain and, according to the general rule (p. 24), any swelling of uncertain nature should be excised without delay and examined histologically.

For descriptive purposes this group of conditions is subdivided into epithelial and fibrous lesions.

EPITHELIAL LESIONS

Four groups of benign epithelial lesions arise in the skin and they are classified according to the direction in which they differentiate, i.e. towards hair, sebaceous, apocrine or eccrine epithelium. In general, benign skin lesions develop chiefly in older children and adolescents, and they are morphologically identical with the same lesions seen in adults. Lever (1975) regards all of them as hamartomas, and the four lesions most likely to be encountered in children are as follows:

1. **Pilomatrixoma** (syn. benign calcifying epithelioma of Malherbe; trichomatrioma) (Fig. 24.5)

Macroscopically this is hard, encapsulated, elliptical or button-shaped, usually small, ranging from a few mm up to 2–3 cm in diameter, lying in fibro-fatty tissue at the junction of dermis and subcutaneous fat. They usually appear to be partially tethered to the skin clinically, although histologically they are separate from the epidermis and its appendages. They have a crisply defined edge and a fine granularity can be seen or felt when the overlying skin is further stretched taut (Jones & Campbell, 1971).

The lesion shells out fairly easily and is then seen as slightly lobulated, yellowish, firm to very hard, with a delicate, glistening transparent capsule. The cut surface is usually chalky, interspersed with wavy strata of pink or grey fleshy tissue. Many are calcified and feel gritty or even bony hard.

Microscopically there are two types of cells: small, dark spheroidal cells resembling those of the hair matrix, and pale eosinophilic 'shadow' cells. The mass of 'mummified' shadow cells provokes an intense foreign body reaction in the surrounding stroma, producing alternating triple laminae of viable cells, mummified shadow cells and granulation tissue containing large numbers of foreign body giant cells. In older lesions bone is laid down in the stroma.

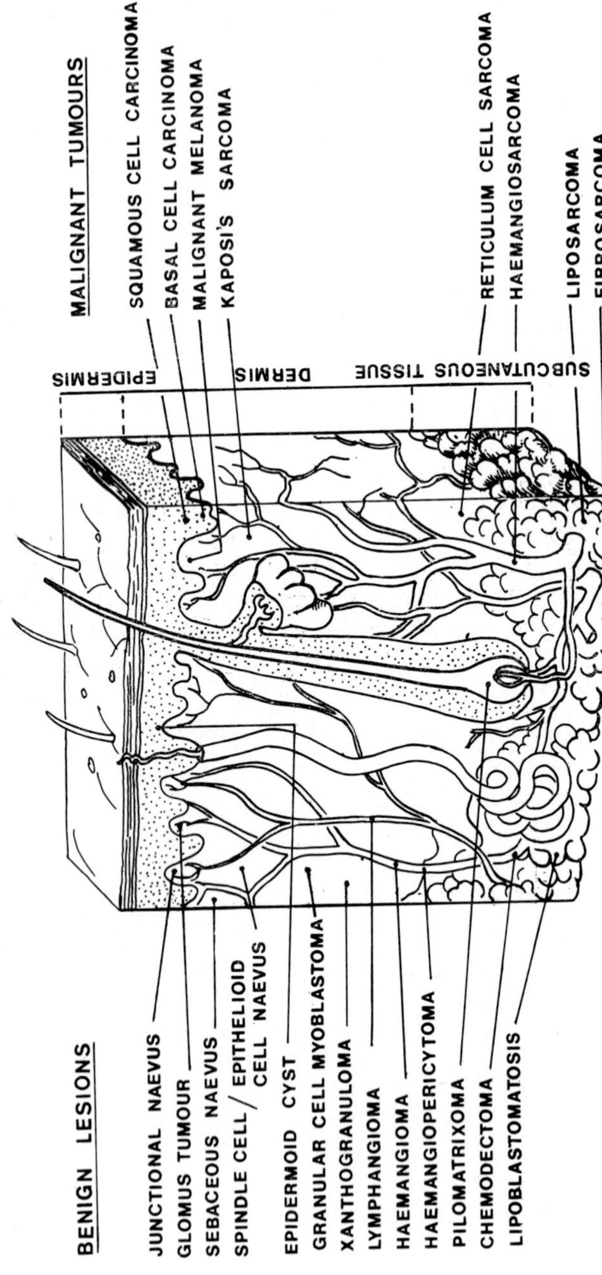

Figure 24.4. THE SKIN; a diagram showing sites of various benign conditions (listed on the left) and malignant tumours (on the right).

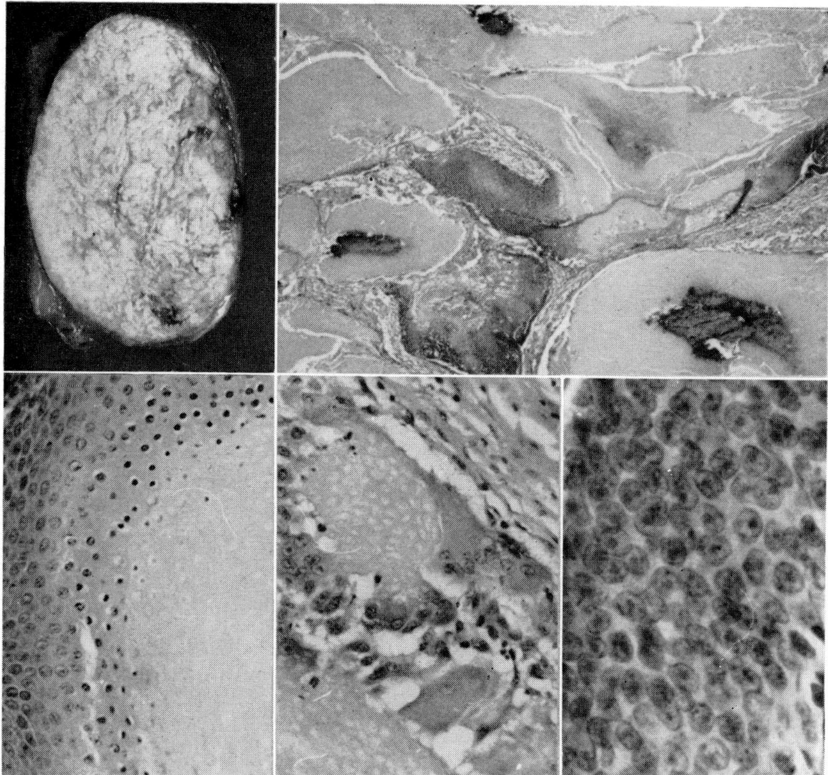

Figure 24.5. PILOMATRIXOMA; (*a*) the cut surface of a typical lesion (usually less than 3 cm in maximum dimension) is chalky and flaking; (*b*) the folded pattern of the viable epithelium and mummified tissue in which foci of calcification develop (H & E. × 30); (*c*) viable epithelium (left) grading through a 'pyknotic' area to mummified, keratinized 'ghost' cells (H & E. × 200); (*d*) eosinophilic ghost cells (centre) surrounded by foreign-body giant-cell reaction (H & E. × 200); (*e*) the growing cells in the viable epithelium ('matrix' cells) resemble basal cells of skin epithelium, hence the earlier term 'calcifying epithelioma' (of Malherbe) (H & E. × 520).

[(*a*) *Top left.* (*b*) *Top right.* (*c*) *Bottom left.* (*d*) *Bottom centre.* (*e*) *Bottom right.*]

The practical importance of pilomatrixomas is that they should not be confused with basal cell carcinomas, or other more malignant neoplasms composed of small cells, developing in the skin, e.g. metastatic neuroblastoma (p. 839), or a primary reticulum cell sarcoma of superficial tissues (p. 838).

2. **Trichoepithelioma** (syn. Brookes' tumour)

These may be single or multiple; multiple tricho-epitheliomas are thought to be inherited as a dominant trait, whereas single lesions are not; the lesions are otherwise identical. They are important because they usually first appear in older children or adolescents, and may be mistaken for a squamous carcinoma.

Macroscopically the lesion is firm, pink and rounded, up to 10 mm in diameter, and mainly confined to the skin of the face and neck.

Microscopically the margins are moderately well defined and the lesion is composed of rounded masses of squamous cells surrounding a keratin plug, rather like a poorly-formed hair shaft. These are the 'horn cysts' characteristic of a trichoepithelioma. Areas of less well differentiated epithelium may also be present and the whole lesion is often associated with a moderate inflammatory infiltrate. The differential diagnosis from squamous cell carcinoma can usually be made on the abrupt keratinization within the horn cysts.

3. **Sebaceous naevus**

This is usually located on the scalp, forehead or face, is present at birth, but only assumes its characteristic clinical features near puberty. In infants and young children it is smooth, slightly raised, hairless, and pink or faintly yellow; at puberty it becomes larger, more prominent, more nodular and a deeper yellow.

Microscopically this is a true hamartoma composed of immature sebaceous structures in the dermis, often associated with groups of naevus cells, hypertrophied hair follicles and a xanthoid papilliform epidermal layer. At puberty the lesion enlarges, and the sebaceous glands hypertrophy and dominate the histological picture.

4. **Epidermal cyst** (syn. 'sebaceous' cyst)

In children most of these lesions are not 'sebaceous' cysts but developmental in origin; only a few are acquired as a result of traumatic implantation. There are certain sites of predilection, e.g. the outer canthus of the eye (external angular dermoid), the scalp (see subgaleal dermoids, p. 301), the subcutaneous tissues of the neck (p. 376), and the upper trunk. Clinically they present as a rounded swelling rarely more than 2–3 cm in diameter, usually in the superficial subcutaneous tissues, and scarcely likely to be confused with a melanoma.

Macroscopically they are grey or yellow in colour, separate from the skin and shell out relatively easily. On section the cavity contains soft buttery material containing fine hairs, and the colour of the contents depends on the amount of sebaceous material present.

Microscopically the wall of the cyst is a layer of stratified squamous epithelium with granular cells and prickle cells, and in most cases adnexal structures embedded in the cyst wall.

5. **Eccrine and apocrine lesions** such as clear-cell hidradenomas, apocrine

mixed tumours and eccrine spiradenomas are very occasionally seen in childhood, but they are so rare that they can be excluded from practical consideration.

FIBROUS LESIONS

Tumours derived from fibrous tissue in the dermis are described in the section on tumours of soft tissues (p. 796); those commonly arising superficially in the skin in childhood are as follows:

1. **Juvenile xanthogranuloma** (syn. naevo-xantho-endothelioma)
This is a dermal rather than epidermal lesion, but may produce elevation of the skin to form a pink, reddish or pale yellow papule. They are often multiple, commoner in infants and young children, and appear to undergo spontaneous resolution with time.

Microscopically it is composed of histiocytic cells crowded together in the immediate subpapillary layer of the dermis, and the overlying epidermis is often thinned. The cells can be shown to contain neutral fat in abundance and scattered 'Touton giant cells' in the superficial parts of the lesion; older lesions may show an intermingled population of fibroblasts. These lesions are closely related to so-called dermatofibromas or histiocytomas of the skin. The histogenesis of juvenile xanthogranuloma is still in dispute; some believe that it represents an abortive form of a histiocytosis X (see p. 219). Xanthogranulomas are also somewhat similar in appearance to skin lesions associated with hyperlipaemia or hypercholesterolaemia, but the latter can be distinguished clinically by their more linear distribution, sometimes localized to the flexures, and by co-existing hyperlipaemia or hypercholesterolaemia.

2. **Dermatofibroma** (syn. histiocytoma, 'sclerosing' haemangioma)
This lesion is less common in children than in adults, but occasionally presents as a small, pink to red, raised lesion in the skin, often on the extensor surface of the knees or wrists, and with some scaling of the overlying epidermis.

Microscopically it contains fibroblasts arranged in an intricate, whorled pattern around vessels, and lipid can usually be demonstrated in the cytoplasm. The presence of clefts resembling capillary spaces in early lesions has led some to suggest that they are 'sclerosing haemangiomas.' The typical lesion contains large numbers of histiocytes resembling a juvenile xanthogranuloma, and provides a link between the more fibrous dermatofibromas and the more histiocytic xanthogranulomas. The histogenesis is unknown. Some are slightly to moderately pigmented and are mentioned again below.

3. **Dermatofibrosarcoma**
This slowly growing tumour originates in the dermis, beginning as an elevated

plaque from which individual nodules arise. The lesion may ulcerate, and local infiltration is the rule, and recurrence is not unusual, but metastasis is extremely rare. They appear to be very uncommon in childhood and extremely difficult to distinguish from a subcutaneous fibrosarcoma, to which they seem to be very closely related. The diagnosis depends upon part of the lesion containing areas typical of dermatofibroma while other areas in the same lesion appear to be more anaplastic and sarcomatous.

4. Reticulohistiocytoma

This is a rarity in childhood and presents as a raised papule in the skin, most commonly on the fingers and hands, and may ulcerate. Most authors consider them to be a bizarre type of granuloma, consisting of large multinucleated giant cells with a pale, glassy cytoplasm set in a loose fibrous stroma; in some examples there is an infiltrate of chronic inflammatory cells. The etiology is unknown.

5. Pyogenic granuloma

This common condition in children is only important because it may be confused with a malignant lesion, in particular malignant melanoma or squamous cell carcinoma. Clinically the lesion usually arises on the face, trunk or arm, often beginning as a small papule which rapidly enlarges, ulcerates, and bleeds copiously at the slightest trauma.

Microscopically it is composed of irregular capillary blood vessels set in an inflamed oedematous stroma infiltrated with polymorphs, and with an ulcerated surface. Some believe they are due to infection arising in a tiny haemangioma, while we and others suggest an extremely vascular granulation tissue in response to an unknown inflammatory agent. If left alone they eventually regress spontaneously, but they are usually treated by surgical excision because of their rapid growth, alarming clinical appearance, and troublesome bleeding.

6. Haemangiopericytoma

This is a rare tumour of low grade malignancy, usually arising in the subcutaneous tissues, commonly solitary, firm and non-tender; the lesion can usually be shelled out readily, but occasionally the tumour infiltrates adjacent structures. Recurrence after excision is common (30%), but metastases very rarely occur (Backwinkel and Diddams, 1970).

Microscopically the lesion is composed of endothelial-lined capillary vessels, each surrounded by a mantle of closely packed spindle-shaped cells resembling capillary endothelial cells but with less cytoplasm; some resemble smooth muscle cells, and a helpful point in diagnosis is that the tumour cells are extra-capillary, as can be demonstrated by reticulum stains which identify the reticulum in the wall of the vessel (Fig. 23.13, p. 818).

7. **Glomus tumour** (syn. glomangioma, chemodectoma)

AGE : SEX : SITES

This sometimes puzzling tumour occurs in older children; in a comprehensive review, Kohout & Stout (1961) collected 57 cases, of which 30 were between the ages of 11 and 15 years.

The sex incidence in the group as a whole was equal, but those arising in the classical situation, beneath a finger nail (Carrol & Berman, 1972), are much more common in girls at or about puberty. When this group is excluded, glomus tumours in all other sites (Table 24.2) are more common in boys.

Table 24.2. Glomus tumour; sites of glomus tumours in childhood (after Kohout and Stout, 1961)

Single lesions			
Upper limb:	Subungual	13	27
	Finger	7	
	Forearm	3	
	Hand	1	
	Arm	1	
	Elbow	1	
Lower limb:	Thigh	3	10
	Knee	3	
	Leg	3	
	Foot	1	
Elsewhere:	Penis	2	5
	Auricle	1	
	Forehead	1	
	Chest	1	
Multiple sites			15
Total			57

A glomus unit (Fig. 24.6) consists of an arteriole and a venule joined by an anastomotic vessel lined by endothelium and surrounded by smooth muscle cells and cuboidal glomus cells (pericytes), which have been shown by electron microscopy to be a type of smooth muscle cell. Although composed of the same types of pericytes, glomus tumours are to be distinguished from paragangliomas (p. 586), e.g. those arising from the glomus jugulare (p. 366),

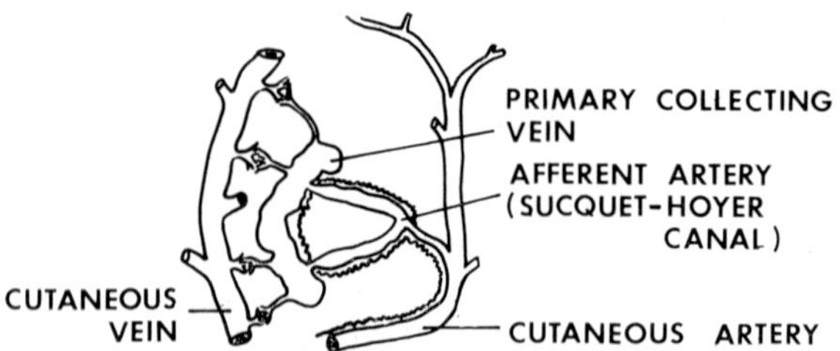

Figure 24.6. GLOMUS UNIT; a diagram of the components of the normal glomus, interposed between a small cutaneous arteriole and venule; the distribution of the 'glomus' cells (pericytes) is indicated by the wavey line (after Carroll, 1973).

or from chemoreceptor and baroreceptor cells associated with the great vessels in the thorax (p. 467).

Macroscopically a glomus tumour is usually small, up to 1 cm in diameter, but most are 4–5 mm, well defined and reddish blue in colour. Occasionally they are multiple, more commonly in children (26%) than in adults (2%), and sometimes related to a hereditary influence.

Microscopically the typical lesion is encapsulated and composed of numerous small blood vessels surrounded by several layers of small, dark-staining cells of uniform size with a rather vesicular nucleus and scanty cytoplasm. Each cell is surrounded by a fine reticulin fibre and set in a myxoid stroma. The typical cells are arranged very regularly around the vessels, and may mimic multilayered epithelium. Occasionally nerve fibres can be demonstrated connecting with the glomus cells.

In the Index Series some of the glomus tumours contained vascular spaces which were large and aneurysmal, while the glomus cells were only one or two layers thick, and hence much less conspicuous than usual (Fig. 24.7a).

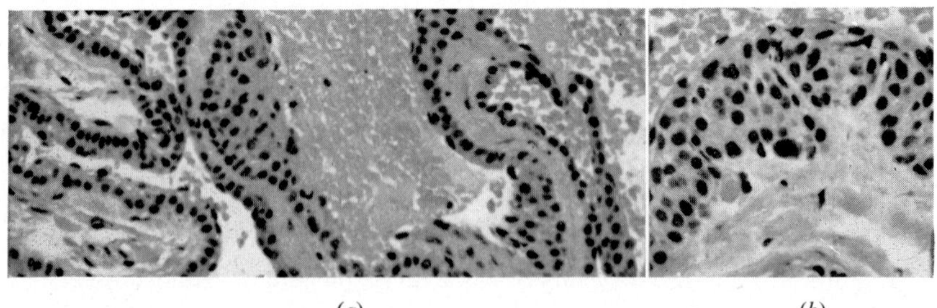

(*a*) (*b*)

Figure 24.7. GLOMUS TUMOUR; (*a*) glomus tumours have an obviously angiomatous pattern, in this case composed of 'aneurysmal' vessels with hyaline thickening in their walls, lined by glomus cells with small dark nuclei and 'cuboidal' cytoplasm (H & E. × 30); (*b*) in some areas there are multiple layers of glomus cells surrounding the vascular spaces (H & E. × 200).

MODES OF PRESENTATION

The most common is simply a visible and palpable dark grey nodule beneath the skin or, less easily visible, beneath a finger nail.

Pain is very seldom the chief complaint contrary to traditional accounts, and usually develops only after the nodule has been present for several years. However, in a few cases pain is extremely severe, paroxysmal and unpredictable, sometimes with hyperaesthesia or vascular colour changes in the overlying skin.

DIFFERENTIAL DIAGNOSIS

This includes other unpigmented lesions mentioned above, but also lesions accompanied by exaggerated tenderness, including schwannoma (p. 822) and, very rarely, an angioleiomyoma (Duhig & Ayer, 1959; Goodman & Briggs, 1965). None of these lesions is characteristically small, superficial or subungual. A tender neuroma is another possibility, but usually larger, and suggested by a history of trauma.

Microscopically the principal lesion to be distinguished is a haemangiopericytoma (p. 818), and as both lesions are derived from pericytes, this distinction can be difficult.

Treatment of a glomus tumour is 'excision biopsy' (p. 950), and those palpable as a superficial nodule present no particular difficulties, except that subungual lesions recur unless the nail is completely removed before removing the lesion beneath it.

On rare occasions a glomus tumour is so small that aside from subjective symptoms, which may be severe, a 'trigger point' is the only objective finding. Excision of a very small block of tissue (e.g. 2–3 mm a side) may be successful, when subsequently found to contain the glomus tumour (Sibulkin & Healey, 1974).

8. **Granular cell tumour** (syn. granular cell Schwannoma, myoblastoma, Abrikossoff's tumour, congenital epulis)

AGE : SITES

This benign tumour may develop in a variety of sites, most of them superficial and often immediately beneath a surface epithelium. One of the classic forms is the congenital epulis on the alveolar ridge in the region of the central incisors in the new born (p. 324).

In children the tumour occasionally arises in subcutaneous tissue as a firm swelling seldom more than 2–5 cm in diameter, and without any distinctive clinical features. Rarely it is found in the tongue or the bowel.

HISTOGENESIS

The current theory, based on the evidence of ultra-structure (Sobel *et al.*, 1971; Kay *et al.*, 1971) is that the tumour develops from Schwann cells, and the observations of light microscopy would support this since there is a close relationship with nerve twigs (Fig. 24.8b).

A 'malignant granular cell tumour' is described in older texts, but the present view is that these may have been 'alveolar soft part' sarcomas (p. 816) or malignant non-chromaffin paragangliomas (p. 586). Although these tumours have some resemblance to granular cell tumours, they are not thought to be related.

MICROSCOPIC FINDINGS

The cells are triangular or polygonal in shape. In cutaneous examples the cells are elongated or crescentic and arranged concentrically in layers around a small nerve fibre. The cells have abundant granular eosinophilic cytoplasm (usually PAS positive) with a small rounded nucleus containing chromatin in an open pattern (Fig. 24.8a).

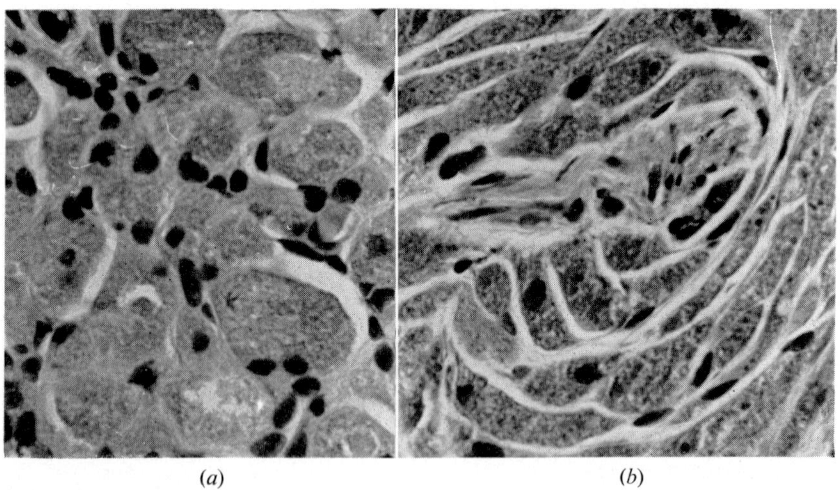

(*a*) (*b*)

Figure 24.8. GRANULAR CELL MYOBLASTOMA; a benign tumour, in this case from the thenar eminence of a 9-year old girl; (*a*) the cells have a small dark nucleus, and abundant granular cytoplasm which stains brick red with H & E. (× 650); (*b*) subcutaneous examples are often related to nerve twigs, shown here as a medullated nerve fibre surrounded by concentric rings of granular cells (H & E. × 520).

DIAGNOSIS

As the lesion has no particular clinical features, diagnosis rests on histological diagnosis, ideally following (total) excision-biopsy (p. 945).

DIFFERENTIAL DIAGNOSIS

The histological findings are on occasions difficult to distinguish from those of histiocytic tumours, in particular fibrous histiocytoma (p. 219) or xanthoma, for the granules of a granular cell tumour may occasionally resemble the vacuoles of histiocytic cells (Stout & Lattes, 1967).

TREATMENT

Surgical excision is required for diagnosis as a rule, and when completely removed no further treatment is necessary.

In the congenital alveolar form ('epulis') there appears to be a tendency to spontaneous remission (Cussen & MacMahon, 1975) and in this site complete excision, determined by histological findings, is neither necessary nor desirable (p. 325).

(*c*) BENIGN LESIONS WITH PIGMENT OTHER THAN MELANIN

In this small group of conditions the pigment is usually light in colour, and it is unlikely that they could be mistaken for pigmented naevi. However, the possibility of an amelanotic malignant melanoma in childhood means that colour alone is of little value in clinical differential diagnosis.

1. **Dermatofibroma** (syn. 'sclerosing' angioma, p. 853)
This is seen in older children as a honey coloured swelling; microscopically the lesion itself is devoid of pigment and the overlying epidermis, which imparts the colour, is merely thickened and somewhat irregular.

2. **Xanthogranuloma** (p. 853)
This contains lipofuchsin which gives it a yellow or even orange colour, in no way resembling melanin.

Haemosiderin can occur as a persisting end-product in any benign lesion in which blood is involved, e.g. in a thrombosed subepithelial angioma, or following a small haemorrhage into any of the benign lesions listed in Section (*b*). In one instance a small haemorrhage into an epidermoid cyst, led to presentation as a hard, black-purple swelling with a history of recent and sudden increase in size. Haemorrhage as the cause of sudden or rapid increase in the size of a lesion is always a possibility in both benign and malignant conditions.

CLASSIFICATION OF PREPUBERTAL MALIGNANT MELANOMA

In a thorough critical review of all reported cases by Trozak, Rowland & Hu (1975), 68 cases with proven local, regional or distant metastases were accepted, and other cases which may or not have been malignant were excluded. The 68 cases were then classified (with some modifications) according to the system proposed by Skov-Jensen *et al.* (1966), as follows.

Type I Congenital acquired transplacental malignant melanoma
3 cases (approx 4%).

Type II Metastatic malignant melanoma, with onset before puberty
44 cases (approx 65%).

Type III Metastatic malignant melanoma, with onset before puberty, arising in a naevus pigmentosus giganticus (syn. giant 'hairy' naevus)
21 cases (approx 31%).

Trozak *et al.* also recognized but excluded from further consideration 8 cases of malignant melanoma arising in leptomeningeal melanosis (Morris & Danta, 1968), a condition associated in some cases with giant pigmented naevus. The Index Series contained 2 examples of primary malignant meningeal melanoma (p. 285).

Type I

In each of the 3 cases (all fatal) the mother had demonstrable metastases before conception. In 2 of the 3 infants the metastic tumour did not become apparent clinically until 7½ and 8 months of age, possibly indicating initial but temporary immunological resistance. The contrary may have been exhibited in the third infant whose tumour was clinically apparent at 11 days of age, and his failure to reject a therapeutic skin graft from his maternal grandmother (Brodsky *et al.*, 1965) may also be explained by deficient immune response.

Type II

In this group of 44 children one had xeroderma pigmentosum and 2 others had a pre-existent extensive pigmented naevus resembling a giant naevus. In 9 of the 44 children the naevus in which the tumour developed had been present since birth. From 35 cases with adequate data, the 5-year survival rate was 34%, similar to adult cases with the same tumour in an equivalent stage. There were no 5-year survivors in types I and III.

Type III

Estimates of the incidence of malignant melanoma developing in a 'giant' naevus, collected by Trozak *et al.*, ranged from 1·8% to 10·7% in various series, some of which included adult patients. All 21 cases listed by the reviewers were dead by the age of 2 years. Factors which they considered might be responsible for the high mortality rate were: the irregular surface of giant naevi (causing delay in detecting a 'new' nodular lesion), involvement of skin extending across the midline (conducive to more widespread metastasis), development of the malignant focus in the deeper part of the lesion, contributing to delay in diagnosis and also placing the tumour closer to deep lymphatics and vessels.

MANAGEMENT OF PIGMENTED NAEVI IN CHILDREN

In view of their prevalence and multiplicity in childhood, there is no place for the wholesale removal of naevi, and when there are no unusual features they are best left alone and observed, without arousing parental anxiety.

The development of any change suggestive of malignancy is extremely rare, one in many millions, but nevertheless an indication for excision and microscopic examination, which frequently demonstrates that the lesion is benign.

Changes reported to be of particular concern (Trozak *et al.*, 1975) are haemorrhage, ulceration, cracks, crusting, rapid increase in size, satellite (outrider) lesions, and focal hyper-or hypopigmentation.

Surgical treatment

Excision-biopsy. The suspected lesion should be excised completely, including a margin of 0·5 to 1 cm of normal surrounding skin. Because of potential difficulties in histological interpretation, the biopsy should be carefully handled and properly processed without delay (p. 82). Closure of the defect can in most cases be performed by direct suture, and the resulting scar is usually no less desirable cosmetically than the original lesion.

Radical excision. If the histological diagnosis of malignant melanoma is firmly established, radical re-excision of the area (or excision of the rest of the lesion after incision-biopsy) is required, removing a surrounding area of normal skin and subcutaneous tissues. The depth of tissue to be removed is the subject of controversy, and currently recommended practice is to excise a block of tissue down to but not including the fascia covering muscle etc., for removal of fascia might open a deeper lymphatic field not hitherto accessible for metastasis.

Prophylactic removal of clinically uninvolved regional nodes (Clinical Stage I) is not recommended in general, although also the subject of debate and prospective trials.

Removal of clinically involved regional nodes is required, and when reasonably close to the primary lesion, it may be feasible to combine this with the radical excision of the primary tumour. Skin grafts may be required for the site of the primary tumour or the regional nodes, or both.

Chemotherapy

Various cytotoxic agents have been used in the treatment of malignant melanoma, and the most effective so far appears to be dimethyl triazeno-imidazole carboxamide (DTIC), as reported by Luce (1972). This may also be the choice to 'cover' excision biopsy (p. 109), completing the course if the diagnosis is subsequently proven histologically.

The role of regional perfusion (e.g. of a limb) with cytotoxic agents is still debatable. Early reports indicated that the primary tumour could be controlled or even destroyed by this means, but without detectable improvement in survival rates. In a more recent study of a larger series (Krementz & Ryan, 1972) regional perfusion was reported to have added 15% to the 5-year survival rate of adult patients in Stage I, and to have doubled the survival rate of patients in Stage II (with involvement of regional lymph nodes). Endolymphatic perfusion with radionucleides, following wide excision, is also under trial, and the early results appear to be promising, e.g. 85% of 3–5 year survivals in Stage I.

Immunotherapy

This has been employed (Lewis *et al.*, 1973; McCarthy *et al.*, 1973) e.g. by inducing a local delayed sensitivity reaction to an unrelated antigen (Hersh *et al.*, 1973). Delayed reaction to a chemical has been induced by sensitizing the patient topically to 2–4 dinitrochlorobenzene, and then treating the surface of the tumour 2–3 weeks later with the same substance. In favourable cases the reaction has been followed by disappearance of not only of the tumour so treated, but also other loci of tumour not treated directly.

General nonspecific stimulation of immunodefense mechanisms to augment host resistance (e.g. with BCG) has also been reported to be effective (Gutterman, McBride *et al.*, 1973).

In the present state of knowledge, immunotherapy is still largely experimental and should be approached with caution for there are instances reported in which a spreading effect or stimulation of blocking antibody have actually enhanced tumour growth in a small number of patients.

Radiotherapy

This plays a little or no part in the treatment of malignant melanoma because of the relative radioresistance of this tumour.

In summary, there is no place for 'incisional-biopsy' in malignant melanoma, with the possible exception of excising portion of a 'giant hairy' naevus. In all other instances adequate excision-biopsy, with a clear margin of normal tissue around the lesion, is the procedure of choice for any suspected area; this should include all connective tissue down to but not including the deep fascia, closing the defect by local flaps or a graft when necessary.

In the Index Series our experience is limited to six cases of malignant melanoma, none of which has previously been reported; four of the six arose in the skin; the other two arose in melanocytes in the meninges, and these are described on p. 285. The others are as follows:

1. A child was born with an indeterminate but non-pigmented atrophic-looking abnormality of the skin beneath the chin. At the age of 9 months a sessile nodule approximately 1 cm in diameter developed in this anomaly, and was excised. Macroscopically the lesion was at first thought to be a pyogenic granuloma, but microscopically it was composed of polygonal cells with a round nucleus and a prominent nucleolus, assuming the alveolar pattern seen in some examples of malignant melanoma in adults. No pigment could be demonstrated in the primary tumour, nor in the lesions found at autopsy when the child died of multiple metastatic deposits in the neck and mediastinum, at the age of 2 years.

2. A child born with very extensive 'giant hairy naevus' of the 'bathing trunk 'distribution developed a firm nodule beneath the skin of the pigmented area, at the age of 4 years. Excision-biopsy yielded a non-pigmented nodule just beneath the dermis but separate from it.

Macroscopically the tumour was an encapsulated mass of soft, white tissue containing irregular grey areas; to the naked eye it was not pigmented. Microscopically the cells closely resembled those of a malignant melanoma, but they were somewhat more regular, with a uniform round nucleus and a prominent nucleolus. Some of the cells were producing brown pigment, but the majority were non-pigmented. In some fields the tumour cells were arranged in cords, in a pattern reminiscent of a neuroepithelioma. Imprints of the tumour surface showed cells with abundant neutral fat and some glycogen in the cytoplasm. The brown pigment had the staining characteristics of melanin. Sections of the overlying hairy pigmented naevus showed intradermal naevus only, and no junctional activity. The microscopic findings also confirmed the absence of any attachment between the tumour and the epidermis.

A second wider excision was undertaken, closing the defect with a skin graft; the regional nodes were also removed at the second operation, and microscopic examination showed no evidence of metastatic tumour. Although the histological diagnosis is malignant melanoma, the ultimate proof of metastasis is lacking. The child is well with no evidence of tumour 3 years after operation (Fig. 24.2).

3. A diabetic boy 16 years of age developed a pigmented lesion *de novo* in the skin of the back, uniquely in apparently unblemished skin. Excision biopsy revealed a lesion histologically typical of malignant melanoma; there were no metastases. He is well and free of tumour 5 years later.

4. A girl aged 15 years, also a diabetic, presented with pigmented metastatic deposits of malignant melanoma in the inguinal lymph nodes, some months after destruction by diathermy of a 'mole' on the thigh on the same side. The presumed primary tumour was never examined histologically. She subsequently died of disseminated melanoma.

Both the diabetic adolescents would be outside the paediatric age group, if strictly defined, and have therefore not been listed in the Index Series of tumours.

An association between diabetes and malignant melanoma does not appear to have been noted in the literature, but is suggested by additional evidence from a third diabetic patient; a boy aged 14 years, who is attending the Diabetic Clinic at the Royal Children's Hospital, recently developed a pigmental lesion on the back which was excised elsewhere, diagnosed as a malignant melanoma and treated with radiotherapy.

Since 1971, the parent of three diabetic patients (one father, two mothers) has been reported to have died from a malignant melanoma. In one of these instances the non-diabetic mother who died had two diabetic sons both of whom have an identical (and unusual) 'adult' type of 'diabetic' curve in response to glucose tolerance tests, suggestive in these cases of a genetically determined type of diabetes in each of the siblings.

It is probably true that a diabetic clinic is one of the areas in a children's hospital where patients tend to continue to attend well into adolescence, and where there is a close *rapport* between the clinician in charge, the patients, and their parents. Both these factors would favour the collection of data concerning changes in pigmented lesions and malignant melanomas. It would be useful to determine whether others have observed an association between diabetes and malignant melanoma.

PROGNOSIS

Until Spitz (1948) described the 'juvenile melanoma' as a benign entity, it was widely believed that the prognosis of 'malignant' melanoma in children was almost uniformly good, and this can be attributed to the inclusion of the spindle/epithelioid cell naevus which is not a malignant melanoma at all.

Recent studies suggest that true malignant melanomas in children follow much the same course and have the same outlook as those arising in adults, with an overall figure of 33% of 5-year survivals (Lerman *et al.*, 1971). Lane *et al.* (1960) reported a survival rate in adults in Stage I of 71%, but noted that 41% of lymph nodes removed 'prophylactically' were found to contain microscopic metastases. McNeer *et al.* (1964) reported a 52% 5-year survival rate when the regional nodes were involved microscopically, but a survival rate of only 19% when the regional nodes removed were *clinically* enlarged as well as microscopically involved (Stage II).

III. KAPOSI'S SARCOMA

First described by Kaposi in 1872, this peculiar tumour is extremely rare except in Africa especially in the Congo, where it accounts for some 10% of all malignant tumours in all age groups (Cook, 1969; Templeton, 1972).

AGE : SEX

In Africa it is almost confined to males, occurs most commonly in young adults and occasionally in children.

MODES OF PRESENTATION

1. *Cervical lymphadenopathy*, involving multiple nodes in more than one

group, is the typical presentation in childhood. In many cases the tumour appears to be multicentric.

2. *Skin lesions* tend to occur in an older age group and present as firm, tender, painful nodules 5 mm in diameter, in descending order of frequency in feet, legs, hand or arm. Small lesions may show the sign of emptying on pressure and larger confluent lesions may be visibly pulsatile.

3. In other sites, include the eyelids and the salivary glands (including the lachrymal gland) the tumour may present as Mickulicz' syndrome (p. 310).

Microscopically the typical pattern is a spindle-cell tumour containing vascular spaces which appear to be formed by the tumour cells themselves. This may resemble granulation tissue, but the presence of mitoses, the irregular nuclear polymorphism, and the plump, swollen endothelial cells are typical of the Kaposi's sarcoma.

Course of the disease

For a highly vascular tumour, the natural history is curiously diluted by time, and without treatment the life span may be up to eight years. Spontaneous regression and disappearance of some of the lesion is not unusual, but rarely complete and permanent.

TREATMENT

Surgical excision is rarely feasible, whereas radiotherapy is highly effective, and the cure rate in cases diagnosed early is reported to be as high as 60%; even in Africa where late diagnosis is the rule, approximately 35% of those treated by radiation appear to be cured.

Chemotherapy has been employed where facilities for irradiation are not available. Nitrogen mustard (0.4 mg/Kg) has been used with success, but Vogel *et al.* (1973) have reported better results in rate and duration of response using combination chemotherapy with actinomycin D and vincristine.

REFERENCES

Xeroderma Pigmentosum

ANDERSON, T.E. & BEGG, M. (1950). Xeroderma pigmentosum of mild type. *Brit. J. Derm.*, **62** : 402.

ANNOTATION, Xeroderma pigmentosum (1974). *Lancet*, **1** : 792.

CLEAVER, J.E. (1968). Defective repair and replication of DNA in xeroderma pigmentosum. *Nature*, **218** : 652.

CLEAVER, J.E. (1973). Xeroderma pigmentosum, DNA repair and carcinogenesis. In *Current Research in Oncology*. Academic Press, New York, London.

GRAHAM, J.H., JOHNSON, W.C. & HELWIG, E.B. (1972). *Dermal Pathology*. Harper & Row, New York.

LYNCH, H.T., ANDERSON, D.E. *et al.* (1967). Cancer, heredity and genetic counselling in xeroderma pigmentosum. *Cancer*, **20** : 1796.

SIEGELMAN, M.H. & SUTOW, W.W. (1965). Xeroderma pigmentosum. *J. Pediat.*, **67** : 625.

Malignant Melanoma

ALLEN, A.C. & SPITZ, A. (1953). Malignant melanoma; a clinicopathological analysis of criteria for diagnosis and prognosis. *Cancer*, **6** : 1.

ANNOTATION (1974). Aetiology of melanoma. *Med. J. Aust.*, **1** : 779.

BACKWINKEL, K.D. & DIDDAMS, J.A. (1970). Hemangiopericytoma: case report and comprehensive review of the literature. *Cancer*, **25** : 896.

BEARDMORE, G.L. (1972). The epidemiology of malignant melanoma in Australia. In *Melanoma and Skin Cancer*. Government Printer, New South Wales.

BLACK, H.S. & DOUGLAS, D.R. (1973). Formation of a carcinogen of natural origin in the etiology of ultraviolet light-induced carcinogenesis. *Cancer Res.*, **33** : 2094.

BRODSKY, I., BAREN, M. *et al.* (1965). Metastatic malignant melanoma from mother to fetus. *Cancer*, **18** : 1048.

CUSSEN, L.J. & MACMAHON, R.A. (1975). Congenital granular-cell myoblastoma. *J. Pediat. Surg.*, **10** : 249.

DAVIS, N.C. (1971). Aetiological factors in melanoma (1971). In *Proc. Fifth World Congress of Plastic & Reconstructive Surgery*. Butterworth, London.

FEINS, N.R. (1973). Excision of giant hairy nevus in newborn. *J. Pediat. Surg.*, **8** : 825.

GORLIN, R.J., VICKERS, R.A. *et al.* (1965). The multiple basal cell nevi syndrome. *Cancer*, **18** : 89.

GRAHAM, J.H., JOHNSON, W.C. & HELWIG, E.B. (1972). Dermal Pathology. Harper & Row, New York.

GUTTERMAN, J.J. *et al.* (1973). Active immunotherapy with BCG for recurrent malignant melanoma. *Lancet*, **1** : 1208.

HERSH, E.M., GUTTERMAN, J.U. & MAVLIGIT, G. (1973). *Immunotherapy of Cancer in Man: Scientific Basis and Current Status*. Charles Thomas, Springfield, Illinois.

HOWELL, J.B., ANDERSON, D.E. & MqCLENDON, J.L. (1966). Multiple cutaneous cancers in children: the nevoid basal-cell carcinoma syndrome. *J. Pediat.*, **69** : 97.

JONES, P.G. & CAMPBELL, P.E. (1969). Pilomatrixoma: a not uncommon hamartoma of infancy and childhood. *Aust. paediat. J.*, **5** : 162.

KAY, S., ELZAY, R.P. & WILLSON, M.A. (1971). Ultrastructure observations on a gingival granular cell tumor (congenital epulis). *Cancer*, **27** : 674.

KREMENTZ, E.T. & RYAN, R.F. (1972). Chemotherapy of melanoma of the extremities: fourteen years clinical experience. *Ann. Surg.*, **175** : 900.

LANE, N., LATTES, R. & MALIN, J. (1960). Clinicopathological corelations in a series of 117 malignant melanomas of skin of adults. *Cancer*, **13** : 612.

LEE, J.A.H. (1972). Melanoma and skin cancer. In *Proc. Int. Cancer Conf.*, Sydney.

LERMAN, R.I., MURRAY, D., O'HARA, J.M., BOOHER, R.J. & FOOTE, F.W. (1970). Malignant melanoma of childhood. *Cancer*, **25** : 436.

LEVER, W.F. (1975). *Histopathology of the Skin*, 5th ed. J.B. Lippincott, Philadelphia.

LEWIS, M.G., MCLOY, E. & BLAKE, S. (1973). The significance of humoral antibodies in the localization of human malignant melanoma. *Brit. J. Surg.*, **60** : 443.

LUCE, J.K. (1972). Chemotherapy of malignant melanoma. *Cancer*, **30** : 1604.

LUND, H.Z. & KRAUS, J.M. (1962). *Melanotic Tumours of the Skin* (A.F.I.P. Section 1. Fascicle 3.) Armed Forces Institute of Pathology, Washington, D.C., p. 102.

MCCARTHY, W.H. (Ed.) (1972). Melanoma and Skin Cancer: Proceedings of the International Conference. Government Printer, Sydney.

McCarthy, W.H., Cotton, G. *et al.* (1973). Immunotherapy of malignant melanoma. *Cancer*, **32** : 97.

McNeer, G.E. & Das Gupta, T. (1964). Prognosis in malignant melanoma. *Surgery*, **56** : 512.

Morris, L.L. & Danta, G. (1968). Malignant cerebral melanoma complicating giant pigmented nevus: a case report. *J. Neurol. Neurosurg. Psych.*, **31** : 628.

Nicholls, E.M. (1973). Development and elimination of pigmented moles and the anatomical distribution of primary malignant melanoma. *Cancer*, **32** : 191.

Penman, H.G. & Stringer, H.C.W. (1971). Malignant transformation in giant congenital pigmented nevus. *Arch. Dermatol.*, **103** : 428.

Reed, W.B., Becker, S.W.Sr. & Becker, S.W.Jr. *et al.* (1965). Giant pigmented nevi, melanoma and leptomeningeal melanocytosis. *Arch. Dermatol.*, **91** : 100.

Sibulkin, D. & Healey, W.V. (1974). Invisible glomus tumor. *Arch. Surg.*, **109** : 111.

Sobel, H.J., Marquet, E. *et al.* (1971). Granular cell myoblastoma. An electron microscopic and cytochemical study illustrating the genesis of granules and ageing of myoblastoma cells. *Am. J. Pathol.*, **65** : 59.

Skov-Jensen, T., Hastrup, J. & Lambrethsen, E. (1966). Malignant melanoma in children. *Cancer*, **19** : 620.

Spitz, S. (1948). Melanomas of childhood. *Amer. J. Path.*, **24** : 591.

Stout, A.P. & Lattes, R. (1967). Tumors of the soft tissues. Armed Forces Institute of Pathology, Fascicle 1, Second Series. Washington, D.C.

Trozak, D.J., Rowland, W.D. & Hu, F. (1975). Metastatic malignant melanoma in prepubertal children. *Pediatrics*, **55** : 191.

Walton, R. (1971). Pigmented nevi. *Pediat. Clin. North Amer.*, **18** : 897.

Glomus Tumours

Carroll, R.E. & Berman, A.T. (1972). Glomus tumours of the hand. *J. Bone & Jt. Surg.*, **54A** : 691.

Kohout, E. & Stout, A.P. (1961). The glomus tumour in children. *Cancer*, **44** : 555.

Angioleiomyoma

Duhig, J.T. & Ayer, J.P. (1959). Vascular leiomyoma: a study of 61 cases. *Arch. Path.*, **68** : 424.

Goodman, A.H. & Briggs, R.C. (1965). Deep leiomyoma of an extremity. *J. Bone. Jt. Surg.*, **47A** : 529.

Kaposi's Sarcoma

Cook, J. (1968). Kaposi's sarcoma. In *Companion to Surgery in Africa* (Davey, W.W. ed.). Livingstone, Edinburgh, London.

Templeton, A.C. (1972). Studies in Kaposi's sarcoma. *Cancer*, **30** : 854.

Vogel, C.L., Primack, A. *et al.* (1973). Treatment of Kaposi's sarcoma with a combination of actinomycin D and vincristine: results of a randomized clinical trial. *Cancer*, **31** : 1382.

Chapter 25. Tumours of the testis and breast

A. TUMOURS OF THE TESTIS AND ADNEXAE

Both benign and malignant neoplasms of the testis and epididymis (Table 25.1) or their investing soft tissues are less common in children than in adults. In the Index Series of 1689 malignant conditions of all types, there were 8 tumours of the testis, epididymis or spermatic cord (Table 25.3) an incidence of 0.5%.

Hauser *et al.* (1965) estimated that only 2–5% of testicular tumours occur in childhood, and that whereas 90% were of 'germinal' origin in adults, only 60% of tumours of the testis in children were derived from germinal cells.

Mostofi (1973) noted that tumours of the testis are predominantly limited to three age groups: (a) infancy, (b) late adolescence and young adult life (15–35 years), and (c) men over 50 years of age. The paediatric age range encompasses only the first of these categories, but also includes a scattering of tumours typically developing in the second age group.

Table 25.1. Benign swellings and malignant tumours of the testis and adnexae

Benign swellings	Malignant tumours
Spermatic cord	
Encysted hydrocele	Paratesticular rhabdomyosarcoma
Lipoma	Metastatic deposits:
Inguinal hernia	leukaemia
Funiculitis	lymphomas, etc.
Epidermoid cyst	
Adrenal cortical rest	
Splenotesticular cord	
Henoch-Schönlein vasculitis	
Other benign tumours of connective tissue, e.g. haemangioma, etc.	Other sarcomas of soft tissue (p. 781)
Testis	
In infants	
Hydrocele	Orchioblastoma (syn. embryonal carcinoma)
Meconium peritonitis (tunica)	
Extratunical torsion	
Idiopathic infarction	

Table 25.1. continued

Benign swellings	Malignant tumours
Older boys	
Hydrocele	Rhabdomyosarcoma
Haematocele	
Orchitis	
Torsion of the testis	
Torsion of a hydatid of Morgagni	
Epidermoid cyst	
Teratoma	
Sertoli-cell tumour	Sertoli-cell tumour*
(syn. androblastoma,	Seminoma
gynandroblastoma,	
sertolioma)	
Interstitial cell tumour	Metastatic deposits;
(syn. interstitioma, Leydig-cell adenoma)	leukaemia
Splenogonadal fusion	lymphomas, etc.
Epididymis	
Epididymitis	
Epidermoid cyst	
Mesothelioma (syn. adenomatoid tumour)	
Retinal anlage tumour	
(syn. melanotic progonoma, neuroectodermal tumour)	
Scrotum and investments	
Haematoma	Rhabdomyosarcoma
Fat necrosis	
Other benign tumours of connective tissue,	Other sarcomas of soft tissue (p. 781)
e.g. lymphangioma, haemangioma etc.	
Skin (see p. 837)	

One case reported (see text)

CLASSIFICATION

The pathological classification employed in this chapter (Table 25.2) is based on that of Mostofi (1973), omitting some of the categories chiefly or solely applicable in adults, and with minor modifications related to paediatric practice.

The tumours to be described in this section are as follows:

I. Embryonal adenocarcinoma of infancy (syn. orchioblastoma, etc.);
II. Teratoma;
III. Seminoma;
IV. Interstitial cell tumour (syn. Leydig cell adenoma; interstitioma);

V. Sertoli-cell tumour (syn. androblastoma; gonadoblastoma; gynandroblastoma; sertolioma, etc.);
VI. Paratesticular rhabdomyosarcoma (of the spermatic cord);
VII. Retinal anlage tumour (syn. melanotic progonoma; neuro-ectodermal tumour of infancy, etc.);
VIII. Metastatic tumours of the testis.

Table 25.2. Classification of tumours of the testis (after Mostofi, 1974).

1. *Germ cell tumours*
(a) Tumours composed of a single cell type
  (i) Seminoma
  (ii) Embryonal carcinoma
  (iii) Choriocarcinoma
  (iv) Teratoma
(b) Others
  (v) Epidermal cyst
  (vi) Retinal anlage tumour

2. *Tumours of gonadal stroma*
  (i) Leydig-cell tumour (interstitioma, interstitial cell tumour)
  (ii) Sertoli cell tumour
  (iii) Tumours of primitive gonadal stroma

3. *Tumours with germ cell and gonadal stromal components*
  Gonadoblastoma

4. *Tumours of the adnexae*
(a) Benign
  (i) adenomatoid tumour
  (ii) adenoma
  (iii) soft tissue tumours
(b) Malignant
  (i) carcinoma
  (ii) sarcomas (paratesticular rhabdomyosarcoma)

5. *Metastatic tumours*
  (i) Malignant lymphomas
  (ii) Leukaemias
  (iii) Neuroblastoma
  (iv) Other

I. EMBRYONAL ADENOCARCINOMA OF INFANCY
(syn. orchioblastoma, endodermal sinus tumour, yolk sac tumour, Teilum's tumour, infantile embryonal carcinoma, etc.)

This neoplasm has been referred to by a variety of names, most of which indicate its adenocarcinomatous appearance. Teoh, Steward and Willis

(1960) suggested the term orchioblastoma, on the grounds that it was peculiar to the testis, derived from embryonic undifferentiated tubules of the immature testis, and that it was not teratomatous. This view was challenged by Young *et al.* (1969) who described 2 tumours (in a series of 18 from Memorial Hospital, New York) which contained teratomatous elements as well as embryonic adenocarcinomatous cells. This, and other evidence that morphologically identical tumours can arise elsewhere, led the latter authors to suggest that they were germinal tumours similar to or identical in histogenesis with the 'yolk sac' tumour of Teilum (1959), also referred to as an 'endodermal sinus' tumour and known to occur in the ovary (p. 692), vagina, sacrococcygeal region (p. 715), retroperitoneal tissues, and other extragonadal sites.

The current concept of the histogenesis of orchioblastoma is that it arises from germ cells, and that while the 'embryonal' carcinoma of the testis in adults probably has the same origin, it differs in histological pattern, has a higher degree of malignancy and a worse prognosis than the characteristic 'orchioblastoma' of infancy and early childhood.

AGE

The chief incidence is in infancy (Klugo *et al.*, 1972); almost all present in the first 4 years of life with a peak at 1–2 years, and only occasionally in older children up to 5 or 6 years of age. The tumour is invariably unilateral (Ravitch, Lernan *et al.*, 1966).

In the Index Series the oldest of the 6 patients was 15 months of age (Table 25.3).

MACROSCOPIC APPEARANCES

The testis is usually uniformly enlarged; the tumour is 2–4 cm in its

Table 25.3. Tumours of the testis in the Index Series (RCH. 1950–1972)

Type of tumour	Age at diagnosis	Survival
Orchioblastoma	4 months	9 years+
Orchioblastoma	5 months	10 years+
Orchioblastoma	9 months	22 years+
Orchioblastoma	12 months	7 years+
Orchioblastoma	14 months	6 years+
Orchioblastoma	15 months	4 years+
Teratoma	8 years	6 years+
Rhabdomyosarcoma of spermatic cord	6 years	16 years+

largest dimension, the cut surface is homogeneous, pink, occasionally slightly mucoid and, rarely, minute cystic spaces are seen. When examined at exploration it is often difficult to distinguish the tumour from normal testicular tissue (Fig. 25.1a) unless the compressed remainder of the testis can be identified. Macroscopic spread along the spermatic cord does not occur.

MICROSCOPIC FINDINGS

A glandular pattern dominates the picture and, characteristically, appearances vary from one area of the tumour to another. The glandular structures are typically irregular and lined by either short or tall cells (Fig. 25.1b), many of which have a clear cytoplasm (Fig. 25.1c). There is usually no basement membrane, and the deep aspects of the 'glands' merge with loose, interglandular, mucoid 'embryonal' stroma, often rich in acid mucopolysaccharide which stains positively with Alcian blue.

There are papillary projections and infoldings of epithelium into the lumen, a pattern identical with the 'endodermal sinus' pattern of extra-

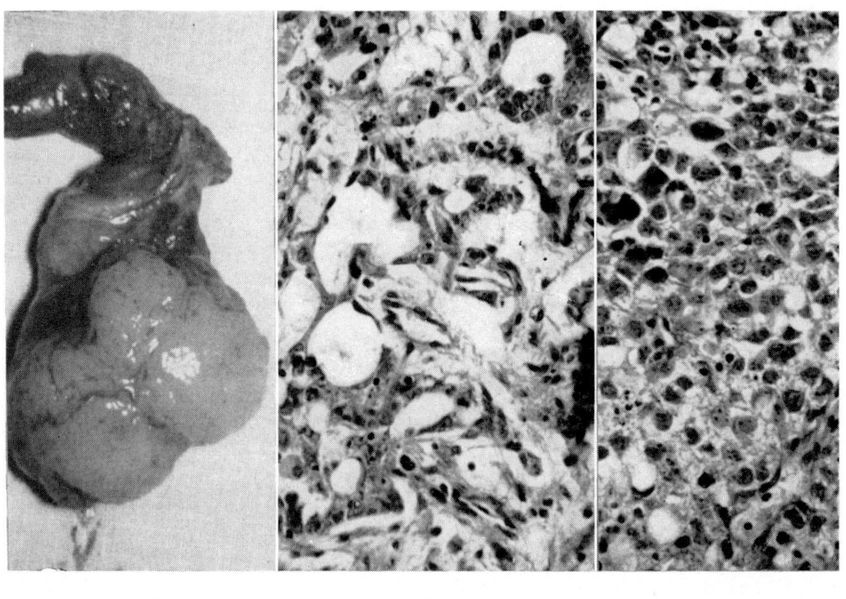

(*a*) (*b*) (*c*)

Figure 25.1. ORCHIOBLASTOMA (embryonal carcinoma); (*a*) the cut surface of the tumour bulges, and has replaced most of the testis. The tumour is soft, pale tan in colour and 'mucoid'; (*b*) glandular pattern; and (*c*) solid sheets of cells, both fields in the same tumour from a 1-year old boy (H & E. × 300).

gonadal 'yolk sac' tumours or Teilum's tumour (1959). At times this lacy, irregular pattern gives way to more compact sheets of darker cells forming more regular tubules. In other areas there are solid sheets of vacuolated embryonal clear cells with both carcinomatous and sarcomatous features.

Acid phosphatase activity in frozen sections is negative or weakly positive in the glands but strongly positive in the stromal tissue; stains for alkaline phosphatase, on the other hand, are usually strongly positive in the glands and weak or negative in the stroma. This distribution is similar to staining reactions in yolk sac (endodermal sinus) tumours and would support the concept that they are the same entity or very closely related.

SPREAD

Metastasis has been described in a small proportion of cases, usually to the para-aortic nodes at the level of the renal hilum (see p. 880). Because of uncertainty in distinguishing orchioblastoma from embryonal carcinoma of the adult type, the incidence of metastasis in some series containing all age groups is difficult to interpret.

STAGING

The simple system widely used for all tumours of the testis is as follows:

Stage I: Tumour confined to the testis, epididymis and/or spermatic cord.
Stage II: Metastases involving only para-aortic (renal hilar) lymph nodes and/or inguinal nodes in rhabdomyosarcoma of the cord (p. 891).
Stage III: Distant metastases, in the lungs or elsewhere.

The TNM notation, which may eventually replace this system appears in Appendix III (p. 947).

MODES OF PRESENTATION

The following applies to all tumours of the testes, for aside from differences in age (Table 25.4), there are few clinical features which distinguish one type from another. Paratesticular tumours such as rhabdomyosarcoma (p. 891), may be clearly separate from the testis, or merge with it.

Although tumours of the testicle are traditionally described as 'heavy', in infants and young children this can be difficult to assess and largely subjective.

1. *A painless swelling* of the testis, discovered by a parent, occasionally by the patient, and only rarely during a routine examination, is the commonest presenting picture. When the swelling is present at birth, its initial discovery

Table 25.4. Tumours of the testis in childhood*

Type of tumour	Age group typically or maximally affected	Benign (B) or malignant (M)	Approx. % of tumours of the testis in childhood	
Infantile (juvenile) embryonal carcinoma (syn. orchioblastoma)	4 to 40 months	M	55%	
Teratoma	0 to 5 years	B	35%	
Seminoma	10 years and over	M	<5%	
Leydig cell tumour (syn. interstitial-cell tumour)	2 to 6 years	B	<1%	
Sertoli cell tumour (syn. gonadal stromal tumour)	0 to 10 years	B	<1%	
Epidermoid cyst	0 to 5 years	B	<0·5%	} <5%
Retinal anlage tumour (syn. melanotic progonoma)	0 to 5 months	B	<0·25%	

* Based mainly on data from Mostofi & Price (1973) Tumors of the Male Genital System, Second Series, No. 8.

may be expressed as 'testicles of different sizes', with uncertainty as to which is abnormal.

2. *A dragging sensation or ache* in the groin occasionally draws attention to a testicular swelling in an older boy.

Endocrine abnormalities such as isosexual precocity are the first evidence of a functioning gonadal adenoma, e.g. an adenoma of the interstitial cells of Leydig (p. 886).

Virilization and macrogenitosomia occur with tumours or hyperplasia of the adrenal cortex (p. 577) and these enter the differential diagnosis.

Feminization is the rarest form of endocrine dyscrazia (p. 578) but is seen in phenotypic females with dysgenetic testes ('testicular feminization syndrome'), and the rare atypical interstitial cell tumour (p. 888).

DIFFERENTIATION OF BENIGN SWELLINGS

There are many benign swellings of the testis or spermatic cord and most can be identified on clinical grounds, e.g. a hydrocele of the tunica vaginalis, or an encysted hydrocele of the cord. However, Gross (1953) noted that *delay in diagnosis of a tumour of the testis is most often the result of an incorrect diagnosis of 'hydrocele'*, an error which might appear to be easily avoided, but a secondary hydrocele due to a tumour is common and may completely mask the underlying cause.

Non-neoplastic swellings to be included in the differential diagnosis are as follows.

In infants:
1. Neonatal hydrocele;
2. Meconium peritonitis (of the tunica vaginalis);
3. Neonatal infarction of the testis;
4. Neonatal torsion of the testis.

In older children:
5. Hydrocele or haematocele;
6. Torsion of the testis or one of its appendages;
7. Orchitis or epididymitis;
8. Ectopic splenic tissue ('spleno-gonadal fusion');
9. Epidermoid cyst;
10. Mesothelial hyperplasia, in a hernial or hydrocele sac.

1. Neonatal hydrocele

A lax hydrocele 2–5 cm in diameter is common in the first 3 months of life, and because the clinical findings are classical, symptoms are absent, and spontaneous cure is almost invariable, no investigation or treatment is required. In most cases a testis of normal size can be palpated within the hydrocele, or demonstrated as a shadow by transillumination. On the rare occasions when there are any unusual aspects, it might be reasonable to aspirate the fluid to demonstrate that the testis within is normal, and no larger than the other.

2. Meconium peritonitis

Escape of meconium into the peritoneal cavity *in utero* when the processus vaginalis is patent, can lead to a distinctive doughy or hard scrotal swelling with purplish discolouration of the overlying skin. The diagnosis is not difficult when accompanied by signs of neonatal intestinal obstruction, or plaques of calcification in the abdomen and/or the scrotum. However, these are not invariably present and when the testis cannot be palpated as separate from the tunical mass, its differentiation from a tumour may not be possible without exploration.

3. Infarction of the testis

Rarely an enlarged hard testis is found at exploration to be due to thrombosis of the spermatic vessels of unknown etiology. As the testis is almost always necrotic, orchiectomy is usually required and the diagnosis clarified by microscopic examination.

4. **Neonatal torsion of the testis**

This type of torsion is almost confined to the first few weeks of life, and occurs in an areolar plane outside the tunica. There is a tense haemorrhagic secondary hydrocele with some of the features of solid mass. As exploration, and usually orchiectomy are required, the diagnosis is not delayed.

5. **Haematoceles and hydroceles**

A hydrocele first appearing in a boy approaching puberty is sufficiently unusual to arouse suspicion. When the findings suggest a haematocele but without a history of significant trauma, a tumour should be suspected; some patients with a tumour have been observed for weeks, or months, until progressive enlargement of the swelling leads to exploration, and delayed diagnosis of a tumour.

6. **Torsion of the testis or its appendages**

Torsion is not always sudden in onset and the symptoms are not invariably acute. The exact diagnosis can seldom be made with certainty on clinical signs, and exploration should be undertaken without delay. When no torsion is found, the testis should be carefully palpated, compared with its fellow as to size and shape, and if necessary formally explored for a tumour (p. 879).

7. **Orchitis and epididymitis**

In the absence of mumps or chronic pyobacilluria, inflammation of the testis and/or epididymis is not common in childhood. Exploration is usually necessary, and occasionally an unexpected tumour is found.

8. **Ectopic splenic tissue**

Splenogonadal fusion (Watson, 1968; Hill, 1969) is almost confined to the left side and takes one of two forms.

(i) *a narrow cord of splenic tissue* ('splenotesticular' cord) parallel to the spermatic cord and attached to the region of the upper pole of the testis, and

(ii) *an irregular sequestrated piece of splenic tissue* contiguous with or between the epididymis and testis (Fig. 25.2). No other condition more closely resembles a tumour, but awareness of the condition and recognition of the typical brownish red colour of splenic tissue may lead to biopsy and diagnosis on frozen sections, and preservation of the testis, with or without attempting to dissect out the splenic tissue.

9. Epidermoid cyst

This rare cause of a testicular swelling (Price, 1969; Price & Mostofi, 1970) is only identifiable at exploration. Even then it may be confused with a teratoma of the testis (p. 882). In the period covered by the Index Series one epidermoid cyst was found at exploration, and as it was clearly cystic and shelled out readily, the testis was left intact. The ultimate distinction from a teratoma requires careful microscopic examination for other than epidermal derivatives.

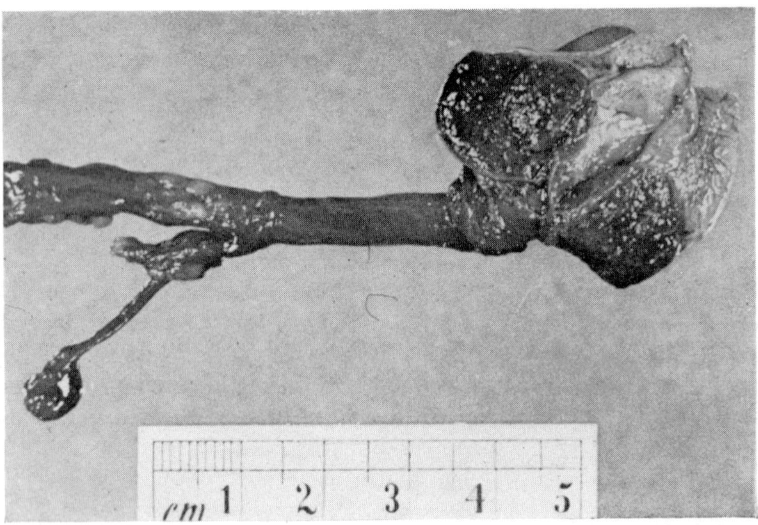

Figure 25.2. SPLENOGONADAL FUSION; the cut surface of the nodule of splenic tissue (2 cm in diameter) blending with the upper pole of the testis at its junction with the cord.

10. Mesothelial hyperplasia

Sometimes at operation on an inguinal hernial sac, but more often when the sac is examined microscopically, the presence of small, grey or brownish nodules of tissue have been reported to suggest a neoplastic process. Rosai and Dehner (1975) reviewed 13 examples, 9 of them in material from children, and noted cytological features which may resemble a primary or metastatic tumour.

In our experience mesothelial lesions in hernial sacs are fairly common, but seldom cause concern because their benign nature is clearly indicated by the presence of foreign-body giant cells, and appropriate stains show that the lesion contains lipid material.

INVESTIGATIONS

1. The usual investigations such as full blood examination are required, and x-rays of the chest to exclude pulmonary metastasis.
2. *Lymphangiography*, although desirable to demonstrate the para-aortic nodes, has a high failure rate in infancy, at least in our hands, and has not been employed in the Index Series.
3. *Excretory pyelography* is performed as one means of detecting lymph node metastases, which if present may extend to the level of the renal hilum and cause lateral displacement of the calyces or ureters.
4. *A gallium scan* (^{67}Ga, gallium citrate) may prove to be an important method of investigation (Winchell *et al.*, 1970), for tumours of the testis have an affinity for this radionucleide, and para-aortic lymph node metastases in embryonal carcinoma (Bailey *et al.*, 1973) can be detected with a high degree of accuracy. Precise staging by this or similar methods could make both lymphangiography and 'prophylactic' lymphadenectomy unnecessary.

EXPLORATION OF A SUSPECTED TUMOUR OF THE TESTIS

Opinions may differ as to the advantages of a median scrotal incision versus an inguinal approach for non-neoplastic conditions of the testis and epididymis, but when a malignant tumour is a possibility the inguinal route is essential because high transection of the cord may be required, and the incision can, if necessary, be included in the field of subsequent radiotherapy without irradiating the scrotum or the contralateral testis. The following technique is suggested.

Through an inguinal incision the inguinal canal is opened and the spermatic cord cleared at the level of the internal ring, ligating the cremasteric vessels which form the major collateral vessels supplying the testis. Two non-crushing vascular or rubber-shod clamps are then placed across the spermatic cord at the internal ring. The testis within its areolar fascial investments is dislocated from the scrotum and delivered into the inguinal incision.

The testis can then be brought through a small hole in an adhesive plastic drape which is then sealed around the spermatic cord, and smoothed down to adhere to the area of skin around the incision. The tunica vaginalis is opened and the testis inspected and palpated.

Biopsy in situ

Because of the very small proportion of testicular swellings in childhood which prove to be a malignant tumour, the general rule in adult practice, that orchiectomy represents the 'minimum biopsy' (to avoid local recurrence following biopsy of a tumour *in situ*, reported to occur in 20–25% of adults), should not be applied to children. The use of an adhesive drape may seem unnecessary, but is designed to make 'biopsy *in situ*' in childhood as safe as possible, and a satisfactory alternative to orchiectomy without preliminary biopsy.

With the spermatic cord clamped, the swelling can be dissected, incised and biopsies taken for frozen sections. If orchiectomy is decided upon, the upper and lower edges of the plastic drape are freed and brought together, enclosing the testis and cord in a plastic envelope. Gloves, gowns and instruments used during the biopsy are discarded.

The spermatic cord is divided between the two clamps already in place, securing the proximal end with a transfixion ligature (i.e. 'radical' orchiectomy), and the testis removed, still wrapped in its envelope to minimize spilling any tumour cells exposed during exploration.

Chemotherapy (p. 882) may be commenced as soon as the result of biopsy is obtained, or after examination of paraffin sections of the testis and tumour.

The administration of a single dose of a cytotoxic agent (e.g. vincristine) before operation to 'cover' biopsy or excision of a tumour, with the object of discouraging metastasis by cells liberated during operative interference, is controversial, but common practice at the Royal Children's Hospital. The rationale is discussed on p. 109 and the potential disadvantages, such as alterations in the histological findings, on p. 25.

RETROPERITONEAL LYMPHADENECTOMY

Lymphatic channels draining the testis and cord run parallel to the spermatic vessels to the first relay, the para-aortic nodes in the renal hilum (Ray *et al.*, 1974). The lymphatics interconnect freely so that bilateral metastases can occur, in nodes extending from the brim of the pelvis to above the renal vessels, and when lymphadenectomy is to be performed, bilateral clearance is required (Staubitz *et al.*, 1974). An undesirable aspect of the procedure is the incidence of autonomic complications such as loss of ejaculation, reported by Leiter & Brendler (1967) and by others more recently (e.g. Staubitz *et al.*, 1974). Removal of the first lumbar ganglia on both sides has been found to cause permanent loss of ejaculation, e.g. in as high as 54% of adults treated by sympathectomy for hypertension.

Since the introduction of retroperitoneal lymphadenectomy for testicular tumours in the 1950s there have been differences of opinion as to which tumours warrant treatment by this procedure.

Culp *et al.* (1973) reported in their periodic reviews of testicular tumours in adults that in all types of tumour, except germinoma, survival rates were improved by lymphadenectomy. In embryonal carcinoma, predominantly in adults, they found retroperitoneal lymph nodal or other metastases in all but 17 of 93 cases.

The question is whether treatment based on experience with embryonal carcinoma in adults should be applied in infants and young children with an orchioblastoma, a tumour with a similar histogenesis but distinctively different histological pattern and less propensity to metastasize.

Tefft, Vawter *et al.* (1967) employed bilateral retroperitoneal lymphadenectomy in the treatment of 6 cases of embryonal carcinoma in boys less than 2 years of age (in addition to radical orchiectomy and abdominal radiotherapy of 1755 to 2600 rads); all 6 were alive without evidence of disease 1½ to 5 years later. Histological examination of the material removed showed that *none* of the nodes excised contained metastasis.

In the Index Series, 6 patients aged 3 to 15 months, with an orchioblastoma were treated by 'radical' orchiectomy alone, and all are long term survivors (7 to 22 years) without evidence of disease.

There were no regional lymphatic metastases in 6 additional case reports reviewed by Ghangai (1968), who nevertheless recommended 'prophylactic' lymphadenectomy for this tumour regardless of the patient's age.

On the other hand one out of the 4 examples mentioned by Willis (1967), and 5 of the 15 cases of orchioblastoma described in the original report by Teoh *et al.* (1960) developed metastases and died of their tumour. Exelby (1975) reported a survival rate of 75% in a series from Memorial Hospital. We have also had the opportunity to examine specimens supplied by Professor James Gibson, from a 2-year old Chinese boy in Hong Kong. Radical orchiectomy for an orchioblastoma was followed by para-aortic lymph node and bilateral pulmonary metastases, with death in less than a year. McCullough *et al.* (1971) collected from the literature 8 cases of orchioblastoma with death due to metastases.

Even after allowing for possible confusion of orchioblastoma with the embryonal carcinoma of the adult type, and for the good results in many cases of orchioblastoma treated by orchiectomy alone (as in the Index Series), there are sufficient reports of fatal metastasis (Sabio *et al.*, 1974) to conclude that treatment should include something more than radical orchiectomy.

Additional treatment should be designed for those (perhaps as many as 25%) who already have 'micrometasasis', almost always subclinical, at the time of diagnosis. In the future, a gallium scan or similar tests may prove to be a reliable method of identifying these patients; for the present, the choice lies between radiotherapy and chemotherapy, or combinations of the two. Selection of the mode of treatment should be influenced by the fact that in the majority of patients no additional treatment is necessary, and if it is to be applied in all cases, the long term sequelae should be minimal. Chemotherapy would appear to be the most acceptable adjuvant treatment (Sabio *et al.*, 1974; Karamehmedovic *et al.*, 1975).

Prophylactic radiotherapy

Matsumoto *et al.* (1970) used radiotherapy (2000 to 3000 rads in 4 to 7 weeks) in 19 children with an orchioblastoma and all were free of evidence of disease at least one year after orchiectomy and radiotherapy, in contrast to 4 deaths, all within 15 months of diagnosis, in 9 patients treated by orchiectomy alone. However, in children less than 3 years of age, radiotherapy of the para-aortic area inevitably affects a considerable portion of the vertebrae and the marrow it contains, causing marrow suppression initially and disturbances of growth in later years. Radiation nephritis is also a potential sequel.

Chemotherapy

Although in adults with primary tumours of adenocarcinomatous type, tumour regression has often been demonstrated with several drugs used alone, e.g. mithramycin, actinomycin D, vinblastine, methotrexate, in children insufficient cases have been studied to justify firm recommendations. Three cytotoxic antibiotic drugs have given the most encouraging results: adriamycin, mithramycin and actinomycin D; vinblastine, vincristine and methotrexate are others which merit consideration. As a general guide, it would appear advisable to use a combination of *one* of the three antibiotic drugs plus a vinca alkaloid or methotrexate, repeated in courses at interval of 2 to 3 months for at least a year. In the first year of life, with its better prognosis and greater drug toxicity, chemotherapy should be more limited, except when residual tumour is suspected.

If there is any elevation of the plasma level of α-feto-protein or gonadotropins, serial estimations of them are an aid in monitoring and modifying treatment.

II. TERATOMA

Hauser *et al.* (1965) estimated that 60% of testicular tumours in children are germinal in origin, and some 30% of germ cell tumours are teratomas. As in other testicular tumours, the behaviour and the prognosis of basically similar types differ greatly in adults and in children. In adults a teratoma is one of the most malignant of testicular tumours; in childhood teratomas are almost entirely benign, perhaps without exception.

Phelan *et al.* (1957) collected the cases of teratoma in boys reported up to 1956, and reported one which appeared to be malignant histologically; the 61 additional cases reported between 1956 and 1973 were reviewed by Carney *et al.* (1973) who thought that while 7 were likely to have been malignant, there was only one in which metastases may have occurred, in the total series of 109 cases. Brosman and Gondos (1974) also reviewed the data available and concluded that there was no proven case of malignant teratoma of the testis in a child.

AGE

The tumour appears in the first five years of life as a rule, and some are present at birth.

MACROSCOPIC APPEARANCES

The testis is enlarged by the tumour, which largely replaces it. The cut surface varies from mainly solid but containing small cystic spaces, to a multicystic appearance with the cysts separated by thin septa. Least commonly the teratoma is composed of a single cystic loculus.

MICROSCOPIC FINDINGS

The usual pattern is a wide variety of tissues derived from all three germ layers. Glial tissue is often predominant and neural derivatives such as retinal tissue are not uncommon. Mesodermal structures include muscle, cartilage, bone and fibrous tissue. Immature tissue with numerous mitoses may be found, but in young children areas resembling embryonal carcinoma are very rarely present.

The modes of presentation, investigations, differential diagnosis and exploration, are the same as for orchioblastoma, described on p. 879.

A point of doubtful value in differentiation is that, in general, a teratoma grows much less rapidly than orchioblastoma.

TREATMENT

As teratomas in early childhood are invariably benign, 'radical' orchiectomy (p. 880) is all that is required.

There is a theoretical reservation in that if teratomas in childhood are always benign, and those presenting in late adolescence or adult life are nearly all malignant, at what age lies the breakaway point? In practice this presents little or no difficulty, for there is a gap of up to 5 to 10 years (e.g. from 8 to 16 years of age) in which teratomas seldom appear. Another safeguard is a thorough examination of serial sections of the operation specimen; if only mature elements are present, no further treatment is required; if questionably malignant tissue is found *in situ* in a teratoma from a boy past puberty, additional treatment such as lymphadenectomy, radiotherapy and/or chemotherapy should be considered.

III. SEMINOMA

AGE

Seminoma is one of the rarest tumours of the testis in childhood; less than 10 have been reported (Hauser *et al.*, 1965), mostly in pubescent boys or adolescents 12 to 16 years of age. The rarity of this tumour in the testis in children is in contrast to the occurrence in this age group of an almost identical tumour ('germinoma' or 'dysgerminoma') in other sites such as the cranium (p. 271).

RELATIONSHIP TO UNDESCENDED AND DYSGENETIC TESTES

Since reports by Gilbert (1941) and Campbell (1942) of a relationship between lack of descent and malignant tumours of the testis, this has been widely discussed in the literature. Most but not all tumours arising in undescended testes are seminomas. Dow *et al.* (1967) reviewed 2,100 cases of testicular tumour, of which 73 (approximately 3%) were associated with lack of descent. In 14 of these 73 cases the affected testis had been brought down by operation 1 to 26 years before the tumour appeared, and all 14 patients were more than 6 years old at the time of operation.

Gehring *et al.* (1974) reviewed a series of 529 men with malignant tumours of the testis, of which 37 (7%) were associated with lack of descent. In 29 of the 37 the tumour arose in a testis which was or had been undescended, but in the other 7 (24%) the tumour arose in the *contralateral* (normally descended) testis; one patient had bilateral tumours in intraabdominal testes. These figures (7% and 24%) are similar to those reported by Johnson (1968) who, like Sohval (1956), suggested that dysgenetic tissue in an undescended testis or in an apparently normally descended contralateral testis, may account for the propensity for malignant degeneration. In the 37 cases reported by Gehring *et al.* the average age at orchiopexy was 13·4 years and at diagnosis of the tumour 31·7 years, after an average interval of 18·3 years.

It is recognized that bringing down an undescended testis by operation does not decrease the chance that a malignant tumour will develop in it, but at least the testis is more accessible to observation and palpation, with a better prospect of detecting a tumour at an early stage.

In the period reviewed by Dow *et al.* (1967) the age of election for orchiopexy was generally held to be 7 to 9 years of age; it is now 4–5 years, before the commencement of adverse histological changes which appear at 5 to 6 years of age (MacNab, 1955) and are thereafter progressive.

It is possible that lack of descent and the development of a tumour are both expressions of a dysgenetic testis (Sohval, 1956) and not directly related to each other. Alternatively, deterioration in the structure of an undescended testis after the age of 5–6 years may contribute in some way to neoplasia.

SEMINOMA IN DYSGENETIC GONADS

Scully (1970) showed that gonadoblastoma arising in a dysgenetic gonad, e.g. a 'streak' ovary, or the 'testis' found in phenotypic females with the 'testicular feminization syndrome', are potentially malignant and that when a malignant tumour develops it is a germinoma ('dysgerminoma'), the female counterpart of the male seminoma. However, it has recently been found that a Y chromosome is a prerequisite for the development of a malignancy in a dysgenetic gonad. In 60% of patients with gonadal dysgenesis, the karyotype is 45, X, and it is the remaining 40% with a Y chromosome who are at risk, and in whom the dysgenetic gonad should be excised (Mulvihill *et al.*, 1975).

The findings of Dow *et al.* and Gehring *et al.* do not exclude the possibility that operation at 4 to 5 years of age may yet be followed by an incidence of tumour no less than in those operated on at a later age. However, the data collected by Altman and Malament (1967) indicate a relationship between age at the time of orchiopexy and incidence of a tumour, i.e. the older the child the greater the likelihood that a tumour will develop in the testis concerned.

The general conclusion is that although there is an increased likelihood of a tumour developing in an undescended testis, the risk is still too small to warrant routine orchiectomy for all such testes. Orchiopexy is justifiable, and the data presented by Dow *et al.* can be taken, at least for the time being, as grounds for operation at the currently accepted age of election, at 4 to 5 years of age.

MACROSCOPIC APPEARANCES

The contour of the testis is usually preserved and the cut surface of a seminoma reveals a soft, uniformly greyish pink tumour which rarely shows any areas of necrosis or haemorrhage unless very large.

MICROSCOPIC FINDINGS

The tumour cells are large and uniform with a round nucleus, prominent nucleolus and a well-defined nuclear membrane. The cytoplasm is relatively abundant, usually eosinophilic with a high content of glycogen, and the cells are arranged in columns and cords separated by a fibroblastic stroma that contains numerous lymphocytes. There may also be foreign-body granulomas.

SPREAD

Early lymphatic spread to the para-aortic lymph nodes (p. 880) is typical, and in seminoma there is progressive involvement of the abdominal and thoracic para-aortic nodes, extending to the supraclavicular group.

The modes of presentation, investigations and differential diagnosis are not distinctively different from other testicular tumours, as described on p. 874.

TREATMENT

Seminomas are so rare in childhood that there is insufficient information to determine the best method of treatment in this age group and whether their behaviour differs materially from those in adults. If data from adults can be taken as a guide, there are early lymphatic metastases to and beyond the para-aortic nodes as far cranially as the mediastinum. Culp *et al.* (1973) found that retroperitoneal lymphadenectomy did not increase the survival rate in adults with a seminoma, chiefly because metastases had already extended beyond the scope of the excision.

Radiotherapy

Both the primary tumour and its metastases are very radiosensitive, and following 'radical' orchiectomy (p. 880), radiotherapy in a dose of 3500 to 4000 rads in 3 to 4 weeks to median field extending from the inguinal ligaments to clavicles is usually administered (Castro, 1969; Culp *et al.*, 1973).

The combination of orchiectomy and radiotherapy in adults yields a 5-year survival rate of 95% in Stage I, but only 26% in Stage II, and 16% in Stage III (Culp *et al.*, 1973).

Chemotherapy with 'triple therapy', i.e. chlorambucil, actinomycin D and methotrexate has been employed, but does not appear to produce improvement in results (Culp *et al.*, 1973).

IV. INTERSTITIAL CELL TUMOUR
(syn. interstitioma, Leydig-cell adenoma)

This is reported to be the most common of the 'non-germinal' tumours of the testis, constituting approximately 30% of this group. Some 170 cases have been reported (Hopkins, 1970), but fewer than 50 in children.

In an earlier review of 22 Leydig-cell tumours in children, Savard *et al.* (1960) found that all had appeared between 3 and 6 years, only 3 developed gynecomastia, and that there were no criteria which could be relied upon to distinguish with certainty a Leydig-cell tumour from an ectopic adrenal cortical adenoma arising in an intratesticular cell rest.

AGE

In children, the tumour almost always develops in boys between 2 and 6 years of age, although in the normal testis, Leydig cells cannot as a rule be demonstrated until the age of about 11 years.

MACROSCOPIC APPEARANCES

The tumour is usually 1–2 cm in diameter and unilateral. The affected testis may be enlarged by the tumour, but also by local diffusion of the androgens it secretes. The cut surface of the tumour is golden to light tan or brownish in colour, and clearly encapsulated.

MICROSCOPIC FINDINGS

The pattern is typically 'endocrine', with sheets of cells divided into lobules by delicate connective tissue septa. There may be some nuclear pleomorphism or irregularity, but as in adrenal cortical adenoma (p. 573) this is not to be taken as indicative of malignancy. Metastasis has never been documented from an interstitial cell tumour arising before puberty, although at least 16 malignant examples have been reported in adults.

Occasionally areas of other types of non-germinal 'stromal' cells are found in an interstitial cell tumour.

MODES OF PRESENTATION

Precocious puberty developing in a boy between 2 and 6 years of age, associated with only slight enlargement of one testis is strongly suggestive of an interstitial cell tumour. Muscular development, macrogenitosomia, acne, deepening of the voice, a coarse growth of pubic hair and advanced bone age and growth, commonly develop before any enlargement of the testis can be detected (Allibone *et al.*, 1969). Significant enlargement of both testes is not typical of a Leydig cell tumour.

Gynecomastia may occur in a small proportion of cases (Johnstone, 1967).

Secretion in adenomas of endocrine tissues is not infrequently disordered as well as excessive (p. 577), and experiments with murine Leydig cell tumours suggest that they may elaborate not only androgens, but also oestrogens, and sometimes progesterone and corticosteroids. The ability of some tumours to secrete oestrogens would explain the occasional development, in man, of gynecomastia as well as virilization due to androgens (Mostofi & Price, 1973).

Gynecomastia has also been reported in some patients with a Sertoli-cell tumour (p. 890).

Feminizing interstitial cell tumour

In a recent review of this tumour, Gabrilove *et al.* (1975) found that like other interstitial cell tumours of the testis, the age incidence was bimodal, with peaks at 5–10 years and at 25–30 years of age. Interstitial cell tumours arising in the younger age group are almost all virilizing in their effects, while there are no endocrine manifestations in most of the adults with this tumour, some of which are malignant. However, feminization occurs with 20–25% of Leydig cell tumours in adults, and occasionally in prepubertal boys.

The authors collected from the literature 5 feminizing interstitial cell tumours in boys aged 3¾, 6, 6, 6, and 7 years respectively. All the tumours were unilateral and benign, and most were 2–3 cm in diameter.

Gynecomastia (without macrogenitosomia) and slight to moderate enlargement of one testis were the clinical manifestations. Confirmation by demonstrating increased levels of oestrogens in plasma and urine is necessary, for gynecomastia may occur in boys with (a) a virilizing Leydig-cell adenoma (see above), and also occasionally with (b) a Sertoli-cell tumour (p. 890). The rare feminizing adenoma of the adrenal cortex (p. 578) should also be included in the differential diagnosis.

Enlargement of one testis indicates the site of the tumour in most cases, but in one case (in an adult) neither testis was detectably enlarged and both were explored or biopsied on more than one occasion without finding a tumour. Radio-immuno-assay of the oestrogen levels in samples of blood from each spermatic vein, obtained by catheterization via the cava, showed that the source was in the right testis which was removed and sectioned, revealing a tumour 7 mm in diameter.

DIAGNOSIS

Recognition of precocious puberty is not difficult, and can be confirmed by an advanced bone age, and slightly or moderately increased levels of 17-ketosteroids in the urine.

DIFFERENTIAL DIAGNOSIS

Omenn (1971) noted that hyperplasia of the cells of Leydig leading to 'secondary' precocity can occur in response to hormones secreted in a variety of conditions such as a hepatoblastoma (Hung, Blizzard *et al.*, 1963), choriocarcinoma, or a teratoma containing adrenal cortical cells.

Adrenal cortical hyperplasia, *adenoma* or *adenocarcinoma* may all produce virilization and precocious puberty in males, but usually with some Cushingoid features (p. 576). A discrepancy between advanced development of pubic hair and relatively little enlargement of the testis is suggestive of a Leydig cell tumour rather than adrenal hypersecretion. Other differences have been summarized by Allibone *et al.* (1969) and are reproduced as Table 25.5.

Table 25.5. Differential diagnosis of Leydig cell tumour from virilizing adrenal hypersecretion (after Allibone *et al.*, 1969)

	Interstitial cell tumour of testis	Adrenal hyperplasia
Family history	Negative	May be positive
Nocturnal emissions	Frequent	Rare
Precocious sexual behaviour	Frequent	Infrequent
Urinary salt excretion	Normal	Often raised
Effect of cortisone on excretion of 17-ketosteroids	None	Reduction
Effect of ACTH on 17-ketosteroid excretion	Increased	Increased
Effect of ACTH on 17-hydroxysteroid excretion	Increased	No increase
Abnormal metabolites in urine (pregnanetriol, tetrahydro-s)	Absent	Present
Testicular enlargement	Usually unilateral	May be bilateral
Effect of steroid therapy on size of tumour	None	May be reduced

TREATMENT

When the results of investigations point to a Leydig-cell tumour but neither testis appears to be larger than the other, or only marginally, delivery of both testes through a median scrotal incision for close inspection and comparison may clarify the situation, as reported by Gittes *et al.* (1970). High ligation of the cord is not necessary for a benign adenoma of this type and the inguinal approach (p. 879) is, in this case, the less appropriate route.

Removal of the adenoma is theoretically all that is required, once other causes of precocious virilization have been excluded. However, the tumour usually occupies the centre of the testis which is reduced to a compressed peripheral layer around it, and simple orchiectomy may be required.

A recent case, since the Index Series closed, illustrated the point that orchiectomy is not invariably necessary.

A boy aged 6 years 11 months presented with a 6 week history of a sudden spurt in growth, frequent erections, the development of sparse but long pubic hair, and enlargement of one testis. The bone age from X-rays of the wrist was 12 years; and swelling approximately 1·5 cm in diameter was palpable at the upper pole of the left testis, and as well as other extensive investigations, tests showed considerable increase in the secretion of androgens.

At exploration (as described on p. 879) a vertical incision in the tunica albuginea at the upper pole revealed a spherical lesion embedded in the superficial part of the testis, and an encapsulated tan-coloured tumour 1 cm in diameter was readily shelled out from the surrounding tissues. The tunica was sutured and the testis returned to the scrotum. Histological examination showed a typical Leydig-cell adenoma without unusual microscopic features.

V. SERTOLI-CELL TUMOUR

(syn. gonocytoma, gonadoblastoma, androblastoma, granulosa-theca cell tumour, gonadal 'stromal' tumour)

This tumour is one of the rarest tumours of the testis in adults. Pugh and Cameron (1964) found only 6 (0·6%) in 995 testicular tumours in all age groups, but it is perhaps relatively more common in children, for Holtz and Abell (1963) found 4 Sertoli-cell tumours (12%) in 33 tumours of the testis in children.

There appears to be no doubt of its origin from the stromal (supporting) tissues of the testis (Rosvoll and Woodard, 1968). Mixed tumours containing Leydig cells, granulosa cells, Sertoli cells and cells resembling fibroblasts have been described, as well as tumours containing combinations of only one or two of these cell types (Scully, 1970).

Stromal tumours of the Sertoli type (i.e. gonadoblastomas) are the commonest type of neoplasm of the gonad in patients with the 'testicular feminization syndrome', i.e. phenotypic females with dysgenetic 'testes', who present (i) in childhood with an inguinal hernia, or (ii) after puberty with primary amenorrhoea ('delayed menarche'). In these patients the testes are sometimes situated in the inguinal canals, but more commonly one or both are in the abdomen.

MODES OF PRESENTATION

1. *A painless testicular swelling* is the commonest presentation and the tumour has no particular clinical features (see p. 874).
2. *Gynecomastia* occurs in a small proportion of cases, generally only after the tumour has been present for some time. Mostofi *et al.* (1959) collected reports of 7 Sertoli-cell tumours associated with gynecomastia, and 2 of these were in children.

DIAGNOSIS

The investigation, modes of presentation and differential diagnosis of tumours of the testis are described on p. 874.

The testicular swelling is almost invariably the only clinical finding, and diagnosis rests on exploration (described on p. 879) and biopsy findings.

TREATMENT

There is only one report in the literature of metastasis from a Sertoli-cell tumour in a child (Rosvoll & Woodard, 1968), an 8-year old Negro boy who had a tumour of the testis for 3 years before treatment. A pyelogram showed displacement of the left ureter by retroperitoneal lymph node metastases, and these were removed after orchiectomy. Radiotherapy and vincristine were given, and there was no evidence of disease 2 years after diagnosis.

As this case appears to be exceptional, if not unique, 'radical' orchiectomy is all that is required for Sertoli-cell tumours in children.

VI. PARATESTICULAR RHABDOMYOSARCOMA

The spermatic cord is one of the less common sites of rhabdomyosarcoma but approximately 150 cases have been reported, most of them in the last 20 years (Banowsky & Schultz, 1970; Malek *et al.*, 1972).

Various estimates of their incidence relative to tumours of the testis suggest that it may be difficult in some cases to distinguish this tumour from a predominantly sarcomatous element arising in a malignant teratoma.

Tanimura *et al.* (1968) collected 125 case reports of 'intrascrotal' rhabdomyosarcoma from the literature, of which only 25 arose in the spermatic cord; the remainder appeared to develop in the testis, the epididymis or in the soft tissues of the inguinoscrotal region. In a review of 387 swellings of the spermatic cord Badawi and Al-Ghorab (1956) reported that 222 were benign, 125 were malignant, and 40 were 'unclassified'.

A rhabdomyosarcoma is undoubtedly the commonest primary malignant tumour of the spermatic cord (Williams & Bannergee, 1969).

AGE

Paratesticular rhabdomysarcomas occur more frequently in children and adolescents (80%) than in adults (20%); Gowing and Morgan (1964) noted that in 10 out of 11 cases the patient was less than 20 years of age. Most arise between 10 and 18 years of age, with a peak at 14 to 15 years (Hayes *et al.*, 1969).

SITE

The tumour usually arises above the upper pole of the testis and is intra-scrotal, but in a few cases it is higher, more superficial, and may involve the deeper layers of the skin in the region of the pubic crest.

Rhabdomyosarcomas have been reported (a) in the spermatic cord, (b) in the testis itself, or (c) in adjacent connective tissues outside but close to the testis. The tumour grows quickly and when the diagnosis is made at a relatively late stage it may be difficult if not impossible to determine clinically or macroscopically the exact origin of the tumour. In those who present earlier, the clinical findings should indicate more clearly where the tumour arose and the differential diagnosis includes:

(a) swellings of the spermatic cord (below)

(b) tumours of the testis (p. 875), or

(c) benign scrotal conditions, such as fat necrosis (Ong & Solomon, 1974), a haematoma in scrotal connective tissues (*de novo* or in pre-existing lymphangiomatous tissue), or a haematocele (p. 877).

MACROSCOPIC APPEARANCES

The tumour is often large, firm, unencapsulated, infiltrating investing tissues, and may compress the testis or invade it. It is tan to reddish brown in colour (cf. splenotesticular fusion, p. 877) and the cut surface often shows areas of haemorrhage and necrosis.

MICROSCOPIC FINDINGS

The classification of this tumour into histological types is described on p. 784. Multinucleated giant cells are described as common in those arising in the spermatic cord.

SPREAD

1. *Local infiltration* is usually confined to adjacent fascial layers, but some tumours grow extremely rapidly and if diagnosis is delayed they may invade the skin of the scrotum or inguinal region, in which case the superficial inguinal nodes may be the site of metastasis.
2. *Lymphatic spread* is one of the features of rhabdomyosarcoma and the lymphatics of the testis and cord follow the spermatic vessels to para-aortic nodes at the level of the renal vessels (p. 880).
3. *Haematogenous* spread to the lungs is typical of all sarcomas, and pulmonary metastases may be present at the time of diagnosis, as noted in a third of patients in the series reported by Williams and Bannergee (1969).

MODES OF PRESENTATION

The tumour grows rapidly and is usually noticed and reported by the patient. The clinical history is usually measured in weeks when the tumour is a rhabdomyosarcoma, whereas with a fibrosarcoma or leiomyosarcoma the history tends to be much longer, and when the cause is a benign condition the swelling has often been present for years (Donaldson *et al.*, 1973).

CLINICAL FEATURES

The tumour is large, mobile, firm to hard, slightly nodular or lobulated, and can usually be identified as separate from the testis and epididymis. Even in cases presenting late with a large tumour, the skin is rarely involved, although the fascial investments of the cord may be infiltrated, and a secondary hydrocele is commonly present.

INVESTIGATIONS

When a tumour of the spermatic cord is suspected, the investigations required are similar to those for a tumour of the testis.

1. *X-ray of the chest* to detect pulmonary metastases, and a skeletal survey.
2. *An intravenous pyelogram* for evidence of para-aortic lymph node metastases e.g. displacement of the renal calyces or ureters, and also to locate the kidneys for the purposes of subsequent radiotherapy.
3. *Bone marrow biopsy* for metastatic rhabdomyosarcoma which occurs in advanced cases (Stage IV).
4. *Lymphangiography* is usually feasible in adolescents, the age at which a rhabdomyosarcoma arises, and may furnish firm evidence of lymphatic metastases.
5. *A gallium scan* (p. 881) may also prove to be an important means of identifying para-aortic metastases.

DIFFERENTIAL DIAGNOSIS

Of the many benign conditions presenting as a swelling in the inguinoscrotal region the following may cause some of the signs or symptoms of a rhabdomyosarcoma; their differentiation on clinical grounds is usually but not always possible.

1. A strangulated inguinal hernia

This was the initial diagnosis in a number of cases in the literature, but as the treatment is operative, there is no delay in establishing the correct diagnosis.

2. **An irreducible inguinal hernia**

A hernia containing adherent omentum, sometimes with a distal hydrocele loculus, is more commonly seen in older children and adolescents 10 to 15 years of age than in younger children. The diagnosis is clarified by exploration.

3. **Obliterating encysted hydrocele of the cord**

This is an unusual but minor complication of a previously small and perhaps unnoticed hydrocele of the cord, producing signs of mild inflammation, increase in the size and some tenderness, and may suggest a tumour, but the operative findings in no way suggest a neoplasm.

4. **Funiculitis**

A non-suppurative cellulitis of unknown etiology is occasionally found in the spermatic cord, and produces an oedematous swelling usually developing over several days. There may be a small central abscess, but culture is usually negative. This condition, too, can only be identified with certainty at exploration.

5. **Teratoma of the spermatic cord**

Rarely a teratoma (p. 882) arises in the cord, and apart from its slow growth may not be distinguishable from an early rhabdomyosarcoma before exploration.

6. **'Adenomatoid' tumour of the epididymis**

Broth *et al.* (1960) and McKay *et al.* (1971) described this condition as extremely rare in childhood. The histogenesis is debatable and an origin from mesothelium, mullerian or mesonephric remnants has been suggested.

Macroscopically it is usually small, discrete, white and hard, and the cut surface may appear whorled.

Microscopically, there is a dense fibrous stroma intersected with clefts lined by flattened or cuboidal epithelium. The tumour is benign, grows slowly, and is not likely to be mistaken for a rapidly growing rhabdomyosarcoma.

7. **Epidermoid cyst of the testis or epididymis**

This rare slowly growing lesion is more likely to be mistaken for a teratoma than a rhabdomyosarcoma. Its origin in this site is uncertain, but Price and Mostofi (1970) concluded that they are teratomatous.

8. **Ectopic splenic tissue**

This developmental oddity (p. 877) may be difficult to distinguish from a rhabdomyosarcoma. In the one case in the period covered by the Index

Series, ectopic splenic tissue 4 × 3 × 2 cm was firmly embedded in the region of the globus major of the epididymis (Fig. 25.2). Orchiectomy was performed and the splenic tissue was only identified on subsequent microscopic examination.

9. **Retinal anlage tumour** (syn. melanotic progonoma, etc.)
The epididymis is one of the sites of this extremely rare and probably hamartomatous condition (see below), typically found in the jaw (p. 334). The blackish or gun-metal grey colour of the tissue is a clue to the diagnosis at exploration.

10. **Wilms' tumour**
Two cases of ectopic Wilms' tumour arising as a primary in the inguinal canal in children, one of them in a boy aged 3 years, have been reported (Thompson *et al.*, 1973). The age group in which a Wilms' tumour typically arises (1–5 years) differs from that of rhabdomyosarcoma of the cord (10–15 years), but the diagnosis could only be made by exploration and biopsy.

TREATMENT OF RHABDOMYOSARCOMA OF THE CORD

Surgery

Inguinal exploration of the spermatic cord, as for a tumour of the testis (p. 879) is required, and the diagnosis can be confirmed by frozen sections.

Transection of the cord as high as possible, at or above the internal ring, i.e. 'radical' orchiectomy, is performed, and infiltrated investing fascia around the cord is removed.

Excision of the overlying skin may be necessary in the rare advanced case, and when the skin is involved the superficial inguinal lymph nodes should be explored and biopsied whether or not they are enlarged clinically.

A skin graft may be required for closure if the area excised is extensive.

Retroperitoneal lymphadenectomy
The frequency of lymphatic metastases in rhabdomyosarcoma suggests that bilateral lymphadenectomy should be performed, and this has been recommended by most authorities, e.g. Culp *et al.* 1973; Skeel *et al.*, 1975). However, Tanimura and Furuta (1968) were unable to show that lymphadenectomy produced any improvement in results, possibly because pulmonary metastases (already present at diagnosis in some of their cases) were more important in determining the outcome in the patients they reviewed.

With the recent considerable improvement in results in rhabdomyosarcoma, chiefly due to more intensive combination chemotherapy (e.g. Donaldson Castro *et al.*, 1973; Ghavimi *et al.*, 1975), there is a trend towards less radical ablative surgery and greater reliance on integrated programmes of chemotherapy and radiotherapy (Kilman, Clatworthy *et al.*, 1973).

In keeping with this trend, possible intra-abdominal lymph node metastases from paratesticular rhabdomyosarcoma should probably now be managed by laparotomy and biopsy of retroperitoneal tissues and nodes (Johnson, 1975), in particular the remnant of the spermatic cord proximal to the internal ring, the iliac nodes, and para-aortic nodes as high as the renal vessels, sampling each group, removing significantly enlarged nodes and marking their sites with metal clips. This will allow accurate staging, and determine whether radiotherapy is required, without the formal clearance of the lymphatic field implied in the term 'retroperitoneal lymphadenectomy'.

Radiotherapy

A typical course is a total dose of 3500 to 4000 rads in 4 to 6 weeks, delivered to an area which includes the inguinal incision, the superficial inguinal lymph nodes if investing fascia was involved, and a field extending from the level of the pubic crest to the diaphragm, shielding the kidneys as far as possible, and protecting the contralateral testis completely, by translocating it temporarily to the thigh if necessary.

Chemotherapy

The chemotherapy of rhabdomyosarcoma is described on p. 791.

PROGNOSIS

In the past, the outlook in rhabdomyosarcoma of the testis or cord has been better than in most other sites except the orbit, probably because a swelling in the scrotum (or the orbit) is likely to be detected and the tumour diagnosed at an early stage.

As yet, there have been few reports of cases arising in the spermatic cord or testis and treated by current methods of chemotherapy. In one of the more recent series, there were 4 long term survivors in a series of 6 (Burrington, 1969).

In the Index Series, the only example encountered, in an unusually young patient, had a satisfactory outcome following radical orchiectomy alone.

A boy of 6 years presented with a swelling situated just above the testis, involving both the cord and the epididymis, with a second lobule of tumour caudal to the testis and attached to the tunica. The tumour was white, with yellow areas of necrosis, and while most of the tumour was composed of undifferentiated spindle cell embryonal sarcoma, some areas contained cells with eosinophilic cytoplasm and clearly identifiable cross-striations.

The patient is well with no evidence of disease 16 years after excision of the testis and the cord at the level of the internal ring.

Factors which various authors have considered to be favourable (and some are obvious) are as follows.

(i) the histological type of rhabdomyosarcoma (p. 785),
(ii) a small tumour, and a short history.
(iii) patients younger than the usual age group affected.
(iv) absence of involvement of scrotal or inguinal skin.
(v) absence of palpable para-aortic lymph node metastases.
(vi) absence of pulmonary metastases at the time of diagnosis.

VII. RETINAL ANLAGE TUMOUR

(syn. melanotic adamantinoma; melanotic progonoma, neuro-ectodermal tumour of infancy)

The epididymis is a rare but recognized site for this tumour (Eaton & Ferguson, 1956; Zone, 1974). The histological findings are similar to those found in typical sites such as the jaw (p. 334) and the tumour is believed to develop from the neuroectodermal cells of the neural crest (Borello & Gorlin, 1966).

The diagnosis is usually first suggested by the deep pigmentation of the lesion, which is gun-metal grey to black in colour. Because of their tendency to recur locally unless completely excised, simple orchiectomy is probably the treatment of choice.

VIII. METASTATIC AND OTHER TUMOURS OF THE TESTES

Testicular enlargement, unilateral or bilateral, is one of the modes of presentation of *Burkitt's lymphoma* (p. 328). Rarely the testis is the site of metastases from a *lymphosarcoma*, or deposits of tumour cells in *Hodgkin's disease* or in *leukaemia* (p. 152) and the latter is said to be the commonest cause of bilateral metastatic malignant enlargement of the testes. *Primary lymphosarcoma* of the testis occurs more frequently in tropical than in temperate countries.

Testicular metastases are occasionally seen in neuroblastoma, usually in the late stages, in a patient in whom the diagnosis has already been established.

B. TUMOURS OF THE BREAST

Both benign and malignant tumours of the breast are very rare before the age of puberty. Fibro-adenoma (p. 901) is the benign tumour most often reported.

Malignant tumours are predominantly adenocarcinoma; papillary carcinoma of the mammary ducts occurs much less commonly.

Table 25.6. Benign swellings and malignant tumours of the breast

Benign swellings	Malignant tumours
Breast tissue	
Hyperplasia of the breast bud	Adenocarcinoma
Pubertal 'fibro-adenosis'	
Papilloma } of duct epithelium	papillary
Papillomatosis } of duct epithelium	non-papillary
Fibro-adenoma { 'juvenile'	ductal
Fibro-adenoma { 'adult'	scirrhus
Virginal hypertrophy	
Post-pubertal hyperplasia (in males)	
Stromal tissues	
Haemangioma	Metastatic deposits
Lympholipoma	leukaemia
Lymphangioma	lymphomas, etc.
Haematoma	
Cystadenoma phyllodes	
Fat necrosis	
Other benign swellings of connective tissues (p. 772)	Sarcomas of connective tissues (p. 781)

CARCINOMA OF THE BREAST

AGE : SEX

de Cholonoky (1943) reported that less than 0·1% of all carcinomas of the breast occurred in patients less than 20 years of age. Herrmann (1960) from collected reports, listed 14 primary carcinomas of the breast in patients aged 14 years or less; 12 of them were less than 12 years of age. Of the affected girls, most were 10–12 years old, and Fenstenstein (1960) reported that the incidence in boys and girls, in the age group 10–15, was approximately equal. However, McDivitt & Stewart (1966) reported that boys were much less often affected. Only three additional cases of carcinoma under the age of 15 years have been reported (Byrne, Fahey & Gooselaw, 1973) since Herrmann's review (1960).

PAPILLARY CARCINOMA

A carcinoma similar in appearance to the ductal carcinoma commonly seen in adult women is very occasionally found in girls; the youngest patient reported was 3 years old, but the majority occur in girls at or near puberty. Benign papilloma of the duct system (see below) is more common.

NON-PAPILLARY CARCINOMA

Macroscopically a non-papillary carcinoma is small, infiltrating, ill-defined, greyish-white, firm and occasionally scirrhus. *Microscopically* it is an infiltrating tumour with irregular duct formation. The cells of the tumour may be vacuolated, and droplets of secretion in the ducts may be prominent. The type described by Oberman & Stephens (1972) is more obviously glandular but irregular and slightly papillary, and it produces abundant PAS-positive mucinous secretion.

Carcinomas arising in young adult women are usually highly malignant, but many of the cases reported in pubertal girls appeared to behave in a rather benign fashion, and have been cured by simple mastectomy or even local excision. This applies more to carcinomas showing a glandular 'secretory' pattern than to the infiltrating scirrhus type which occasionally metastasizes to regional lymph nodes and bones, in the same way as in adults, although in pubertal girls even the metastases appear to be less aggressive than in adults (McDivitt & Stewart, 1966).

Nichini *et al.* (1972) described a 12-year old girl with well-developed breasts who presented with a swelling and oedema in one breast. Microscopy showed an infiltrating carcinoma composed of small, anaplastic, polygonal cells which blocked the lymphatics and caused an 'inflammatory' clinical picture. This tumour metastasized widely and was rapidly fatal.

SPREAD

The propensity to metastasize appears to be appreciably less, or at least to occur at a later stage, in pubertal girls than in adults. The axillary lymph nodes, and possibly the anterior intercostal nodes, may eventually be involved, followed in a few cases by distant metastases in the lungs and bones.

DIFFERENTIAL DIAGNOSIS

Although carcinoma of the breast is well known to be rare in childhood, the reaction to the discovery of a swelling in the breast is so conditioned by its implications in adult practice that the question of a malignancy inevitably arises.

Benign swellings in the breast are very much numerous and, in approximate order of frequency, they are as follows:

1. Hyperplasia of the breast bud;
2. Lympholipoma;
3. Fat necrosis;
4. Fibroadenoma;

5. Duct papilloma;
6. Cystosarcoma phyllodes.

1. *Hyperplasia of the breast bud.* The commonest swelling in the breast in childhood and adolescence is 'hyperplasia' or early development of the tissue which grows to become the normal breast. This may commence in girls as early as 2 years of age, but is more common between 7 and 9 years. The swelling is concentric with and develops immediately underneath the nipple as a firm, discrete, circular (discoid) lesion 2–3 cm in diameter and 1–2 cm in thickness. No problems arise when this type of development occurs in both sides at the same time, but anxiety and a potential diagnostic difficulty arise when it occurs on only one side and at an age when breast development is not generally expected to occur.

This is not 'premature' or 'precocious' puberty, for no other signs of puberty such as pubic hair or menarche appear. Having reached the dimensions described, development usually ceases and the swelling remains static for several years. In unilateral cases, the same type of development in the opposite breast usually appears within the year following recognition of the first swelling; both 'lesions' then mark time until the menarche, which occurs at the normal age.

The most important aspect of the condition is that if the general rule governing the need for biopsy in all swellings in the breast (in adults) is followed in children, the 'biopsy' may be, in effect, a total mastectomy. The swelling described represents the *whole* of the breast at the age of 5–10 years, and no breast tissue is left to develop if the swelling is removed. 'Tenderness' is often an accompanying complaint, but usually mild, possibly iatrogenic, and likely to be aggravated by frequent palpation (by patient or parents), amplified by their anxiety.

The correct diagnosis can be made from its size, shape, symmetrical position, mobility on deep structures, and the absence of any significant increase in size once it has been discovered; the diagnosis requires no histological confirmation.

Precisely the same lesion as described above is fairly common in the male breast after puberty (August *et al.*, 1972). Both breasts are affected as a rule, and the swelling eventually regresses spontaneously after being present for 1–2 years. Very rarely this limited form of hyperplasia progresses to gynecomastia, of which there are many causes, but the commonest is simply idiopathic.

It should perhaps be borne in mind that although exceptionally rare, carcinoma of the breast has been reported in at least two boys, one aged 6 years (Hartman & Magrish, 1955) and the other aged 13 years (Simmons, 1917).

2. *Lympholipomas* are simple hamartomatous malformations of the sub-

cutaneous tissues, not infrequently found on the trunk or limbs in early childhood. They have the clinical features of a lipoma except for the absence of distinct margins, and they have no potential for growth beyond the natural increase in the size of the child.

Following mild trauma, a small haematoma up to 5 cm in diameter may form in one of the minute cystic spaces within them, and the nature of the complication may not be recognized until it is explored or excised. Biopsy in this situation is simple and safe unless the lesion or the haematoma is located directly beneath the nipple; it would probably only cause anxiety if the lympholipoma occurred in the general area of the pectoral muscle.

3. *Fat necrosis* due to trauma, as seen in adults, probably occurs more commonly in the scrotum (p. 892) than in the breast in childhood, but is not unknown in children and adolescents and any uncertainty as to the diagnosis should be resolved by biopsy.

4. *Fibro-adenoma* occurs mostly in girls whose breasts are already well developed, and this is by far the commonest true tumour of the breast in late childhood and adolescence. While most resemble the typical lesion seen in adults, some fibro-adenomas in children grow so rapidly, and the histology may show such striking cellularity in the stroma and in ductular proliferation, that they constitute a clinicopathological entity, the 'juvenile fibro-aednoma'. In 181 girls between 10 and 19 years with a fibro-adenoma reported by Ashikari, Farrow & O'Hara (1971) only 12 fibro-adenomas were of the 'juvenile type', while 169 were the adult type.

The 'adult' type presents as a firm, mobile, rounded swelling unattached to skin or to deep structures. It is painless and asymptomatic; the lesions may be multiple and bilateral, and the clinical pictures merge into the spectrum of changes seen in pubertal fibro-adenosis.

Macroscopically the 'adult' fibro-adenoma is seldom larger than 2 cm in diameter, round, encapsulated, and firm or rubbery with a whorled cut surface. Microscopically it contains proliferated ducts in a fibrous stroma, and the ratio and arrangement of the stroma determine whether the pattern is a 'pericanalicular' or 'intracanalicular' (Fig. 25.3).

The 'juvenile type' presents with rapid painless enlargement of one breast, usually over a period of 10 months, without any discharge from the nipple. Examination reveals a large breast and when the enclosed lesion exceeds 10–15 cm in diameter, diluted veins are usually visible beneath the overlying tissues. However, even when the lesion is very large, it is still discrete and mobile. Some are soft, while others are firm but not hard. The nipple and areola may be eccentric due to asymmetric enlargement of the breast, a feature which distinguishes the lesion from a unilateral case of so-called 'virginal hypertrophy' (Lewis & Geschickter, 1943).

Macroscopically a juvenile fibroadenoma is grey to tan in colour, en-

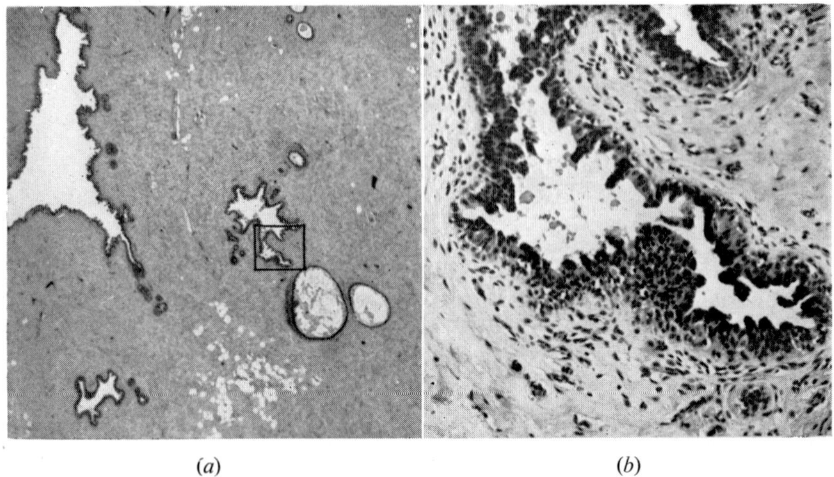

(*a*) (*b*)

Figure 25.3. Fibroadenoma of the breast, unusually arising in an otherwise normal 4-year old boy, as a unilateral swelling; (*a*) irregular ducts with some spherical cysts in a moderately dense fibroblastic stroma (H & E. × 13); (*b*) active proliferation of the cells lining the duct outlined in (*a*); note collagen in the stroma (right) (H & E. × 130).

capsulated and often lobulated. Microscopically ducts and stroma blend in a pattern basically similar to the 'adult' fibroadenoma, but the stroma is more cellular and the epithelium of the ducts may have 2–3 layers of cells. Occasionally the stromal cells show some pleomorphism, but the stroma itself is loose and slightly oedematous, a feature which distinguishes it from cystosarcoma phyllodes (see below).

Treatment. Fibroadenomas are benign, and mastectomy is unwarranted; local excision is curative. Some of the patients reported have been noted to be large and overweight, and a temporary hormonal imbalance may be implicated in the etiology.

The Index Series. A boy aged 4 years presented with a history of a swelling near the right nipple since the age of 2 months. The swelling had increased slowly in the previous 12 months. On examination there was a nontender, irregularly lobulated, soft swelling 4 cm in diameter, with a granular texture, in the subareolar region deep to the lower margin of the left nipple. The tumour was excised and found to be a fibro-adenoma containing multiple, minute cystic spaces. Microscopy showed a dense fibrous stroma with scattered glandular spaces lined by hyperplastic columnar epithelium folded in a papillary pattern. Some of the glandular spaces were cystic and filled with mucus.

5. *Duct papilloma.* This is rarely found in girls less than 15 years of age, although an occasional case arising in the age group 10–15 years has been reported (Diethrich, Hammond & Holtz, 1966). The lesion presents with

either a discharge from the nipple, sometimes blood-stained, or a nodule in the breast. In the former, the lesion may be so small that it is impalpable, and its localization may be difficult.

The Index Series. The only example of a duct papilloma (Fig. 25.4) was a girl of 13 years 9 months, who presented with a discharge from the nipple, beneath which a small mass was palpable.

Microscopically a miniature cauliflower-like lesion filled one of the subareolar ducts; microscopically it was papillary, predominantly fibrous, with the papillae covered by cuboidal epithelium. In some of the case reports in the literature the lesion was more diffuse and involved several ducts ('papillomatosis') with a more cellular structure composed of proliferating glands and ducts, in a delicate stroma.

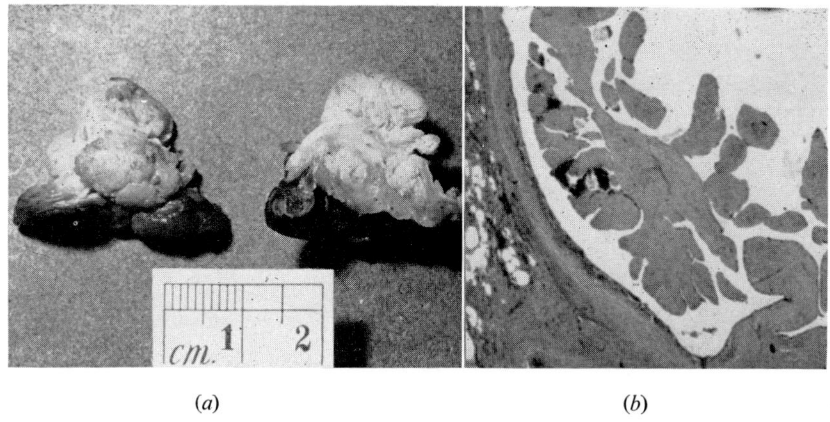

(*a*) (*b*)

Figure 25.4. DUCT PAPILLOMA; (*a*) small cauliflower-like mass projecting into the lumen of a subareolar duct; (*b*) scanning view of a simple papillomatous projection covered by a single layer of duct cells (H & E. × 13).

Treatment. Simple excision is adequate, removing a rim of surrounding tissue through a radial or preferably a partial circum-areolar incision, taking care not to damage other ducts beneath the nipple.

In those difficult to localize and presenting with a discharge, close inspection of the ducts under strong magnification and probing each duct orifice with the eye of a needle, followed by dilation with the finest lachrymal probe may help to identify the quadrant in which the source of the discharge lies.

6. *Cystosarcoma phyllodes* (syn. Brodie's serocystic disease). Some authorities have held that this lesion does not occur in children, but Simpson, van Dervoort & Lynn (1969) collected eight cases in children less than 13 years of age. Amerson (1970) described five girls, all black, who presented with enlargement of one breast, associated with pain in some cases. The

duration of symptoms was generally short, but ranged from 1 month to 1 year. All five had a mass which was soft, lobulated, discrete, and involved one breast asymmetrically. The diagnosis of cystosarcoma phyllodes was made on the histological findings of marked hyperplasia of epithelial ducts associated with cellularity of the stroma; the stromal areas tended to predominate. Whether these lesions are true cystosarcoma phyllodes as occurs in adults (Oberman, 1965), or a form of cellular juvenile fibro-adenoma, is difficult to decide on the basis of the descriptions and illustrations. In either case the results of simple excision (local or segmental) were uniformly good, and there was no instance of recurrence.

The Index Series contains no lesion of this type, no case of carcinoma, only one fibro-adenoma (which was 'adult' in type) and one intraductal papilloma, described above.

In the same period of time (1950–1972), some 250–300 girls between 5 and 11 years of age presented with the 'premature' development of one breast bud described on p. 900; in none of these was a 'biopsy' performed.

TREATMENT OF CARCINOMA OF THE BREAST

The degree of malignancy of carcinoma of the breast in prepubertal girls seems to be remarkably low, and a good proportion of the few cases reported in the literature appear to have been permanently cured by what would generally be regarded as inadequate excision in an adult.

Two clinical types of carcinoma in the 10–15 year age group can be identified:

(*a*) *Prepubertal or intrapubertal girls* 10–12 years of age in whom the tumour arises in a small breast; it is this group which appears to have the lowest degree of malignancy. When carcinoma is confirmed by frozen sections or preferably paraffin sections, and when there is no clinical evidence of enlargement of the axillary nodes, simple mastectomy appears to be all that is required.

(*b*) *Postpubertal girls* with a moderate or 'adult' degree of breast development at 13–15 years of age. While some authorities would advise the same operative treatment as would be employed for carcinoma in adult women (whatever that may be in their opinion), others would advise simple mastectomy, with or without dissection of the related axillary nodes.

However, Byrne, Fahey & Gooselaw (1973) have reported metastases in the axillary nodes in an 8½-year old girl with a carcinoma of the breast successfully treated by radical mastectomy; Hartman & Margrish (1955) also found metastases in the axillary lymph nodes in a carcinoma of the breast in a 6-year old boy, after conventional radical mastectomy.

The traditional Halsted type of radical mastectomy is a mutilating operation at any age, and even less desirable in adolescents. This attitude, coupled with the allegedly lesser degree of malignancy of carcinoma of the breast in girls in the age group 10–15 years, would warrant examination of alternative procedures.

A logical step in the continuing evolution of the treatment of carcinoma of the breast has been a controlled randomized trial (the 'Cardiff Breast Trial') of simple (total) mastectomy accompanied by biopsy of the medial pectoral group of axillary nodes, with postoperation irradiation of the axilla of those patients with positive findings of metastases in the sampled nodes. In an interim report (Roberts, Forest *et al.*, 1973) the early results of this plan of treatment have been, so far, not inferior to those of radical mastectomy. The procedure used in the trial, and which might be considered appropriate for a young adolescent with carcinoma of the breast is as follows.

Simple total mastectomy is performed through a transverse incision which diverges to include on an ellipse of skin containing the nipple. Dissection commences at the medial border of the breast, which is cleared from the surface of pectoralis major until the axillary tail is reached. At the upper border of the tail, the pectoral nodes are specifically sought if they are not immediately palpable, and they are removed for separate biopsy. A portion of the skin overlying the nodes is also removed for biopsy. After freeing and removing the axillary tail, the apex of the axilla is palpated; any nodes which are significantly enlarged are also removed for histological examination, and the incision is then closed.

Radiotherapy

If examination of paraffin sections of the biopsied nodes reveals metastases, the axilla (alone) is irradiated to a total dose of 3500 rads given in 30 fractions in the course of 3 weeks.

Chemotherapy

In adults with cancer of the breast it has become common practice to use a multi-drug combination such as vincristine, methotrexate, cyclophosphamide and 5FU, sometimes with prednisolone. On occasions, similar therapy may be indicated in a child with breast cancer.

OTHER MALIGNANT CONDITIONS OF THE BREAST

Patients with leukaemia occasionally present with enlargement of the breast due to infiltration of the breast tissue or to retromammary leukaemic deposits. More commonly the enlargement occurs during a relapse in a patient in whom the diagnosis of leukaemia has already been made.

Primary lymphosarcomas (p. 170) or 'reticulosarcomas' of the breast are extremely rare, and some reticulum cell sarcomas (p. 178) would be difficult to differentiate from anaplastic carcinoma except for the extreme rarity of the latter in childhood.

In areas where Burkitt's tumour is endemic, unilateral or bilateral enlargement of the breast is a recognized mode of presentation of this tumour.

Other types of sarcoma of the connective tissues of the breast have been reported as isolated cases.

REFERENCES

The Testis

ALLIBONE, E.C., ANDERSON, C.K. & ARTHURTON, M.W. (1969). Macrogenitosomia praecox due to an interstitial cell tumour of the testis. *Arch. Dis. Childh.*, **44** : 84.

ALTMAN, B.L. & MALAMENT, M. (1967). Carcinoma of the testis following orchiopexy. *J. Urol.*, **97** : 498.

ANSFIELD, F.J., KORBITZ, B.C., DAVIS, H.L. & RAMIREZ, G. (1969). Triple drug therapy in testicular tumours. *Cancer*, **24** : 442.

BAILEY, T.B., PINSKY, S.M. *et al.* (1973). A new adjuvant in testis tumor staging; Gallium —67 citrate. *J. Urol.*, **110** : 307.

BANOWSKY, L.H. & SCHULTZ, G.N. (1970). Sarcoma of the spermatic cord and tunica: review of the literature, case report and discussion of role of retroperitoneal lymph node dissection. *J. Urol.*, **103** : 628.

BORELLO, E.D. & GORLIN, R.J. (1966). Melanotic neuroectodermal tumor of infancy: A neoplasm of neural crest origin. *Cancer*, **19** : 196.

BROSMAN, S. & GONDOS, B. (1974). Testicular tumors in children in *Reviews in Paediatric Urology*. (Johnston, J.H. & Goodwin, W.E.—eds) American Elsevier, New York. p. 131.

BROTH, G., BULLOCK, W.K. & MORROW, J. (1960) Epididymal tumors: 1. Report of 15 new cases including review of the literature. 2. Histochemical study of the so-called adenomatoid tumor. *J. Urol.*, **100** : 530.

BURRINGTON, J.D. (1969). Rhabdomyosarcoma of the paratesticular tissues in children: report of 8 cases. *J. Pediat. Surg.*, **4** : 503.

CAMPBELL, M.F. (1942). Incidence of malignant growths of the undescended testis: a critical and statistical study. *Arch. Surg.*, **44** : 353.

CARNEY, J.A., KELALIS, P.P. & LYNN, H.B. (1973). Bilateral teratoma of the testis in an infant. *J. Pediat. Surg.*, **8** : 49.

CASTRO, J.R. (1969). Lymphadenectomy and radiation therapy in malignant tumours of the testes other than pure seminoma. *Cancer*, **24** : 87.

CULP, D.A., BOATMAN, D.L. & WILSON, J.B. (1973). Testicular tumours: 40 years experience. *J. Urol.*, **110** : 548.

DONALDSON, M.H., DUCKETT, J.W. & MULHOLLAND, S.G. (1973). Malignant genitourinary tumors. In *Clinical Pediatric Oncology* (Soutow, W.W., Vietti, T.J. & Fernbach, D.J. eds.). Mosby, St. Louis.

DONALDSON, S.S., CASTRO, J.R., WILBUR, S.R. & JESSE, R.H. (1973). Rhabdomyosarcoma of head and neck in children: combination treatment by surgery, irradiation and chemotherapy. *Cancer*, **31** : 26.

DOW, J.A., OTEEN, N.C. & MOSTOFI, F.K. (1967). Testicular tumors following orchiopexy. *South. Med. J.*, **60** : 193.

EATON, W.L. & FERGUSON, J.P. (1956). Retinoblastic teratoma of epididymis: case report. *Cancer*, **9** : 718.

El-Badawi, A.A. & Al-Ghorab, M.M. (1965). Tumors of the spermatic cord: a review of the literature and a report of a case of lymphangioma. *J. Urol.*, **94** : 445.

Exelby, P.R. (1975). Other abdominal tumors. *Cancer*, **35** : 910.

Gabrilove, J.L., Nicolis, G.L., *et al.*, (1975). Feminizing interstitial cell tumor of the testis: personal observations and a review of the literature. *Cancer*, **35** : 1184.

Gangai, M.P. (1968). Testicular neoplasms in an infant. *Cancer*, **22** : 658.

Gehring, G.G., Rodriguez, F.R. & Woodhead, D.M. (1974). Malignant degeneration of cryptorchid testes following orchiopexy. *J. Urol.*, **112** : 354.

Ghavimi, F., Exelby, P.R., D'Angio, G.J. *et al.* (1975). Multidisciplinary treatment of embryonal rhabdomyosarcoma in children. *Cancer*, **35** : 677.

Gilbert, J.B. (1941). Studies in malignant tumours. V. Tumors developing after orchidopexy. *J. Urol.*, **46** : 740.

Gittes, R. F., Smith, G. *et al.* (1970). Local androgenic effect of interstitial cell tumour of the testis. *J. Urol.*, **104** : 774.

Gowing, N.F.C. & Morgan, A.D. (1964). Paratesticular tumors of the connective tissue and muscle. *Brit. J. Urol.*, **36** : 78.

Gross, R.E. (1953). The *Surgery of Infancy and Childhood.* Saunders, Philadelphia, London.

Hays, D.M., Mirabal, V.Q. *et al.* (1969). Rhabdomyosarcoma of the spermatic cord. *Surgery*, **65** : 845.

Hill, M.Q. (1969). Ectopic splenic tissue in the gonad. *Canad. J. Surg.*, **12** : 457.

Holtz, F. & Abell, M.R. (1963). Testicular neoplasms in infants and children. *Cancer*, **16** : 982.

Hopkins, B.G. (1970). Interstitial cell tumor of the testis: case report and review of the literature. *J. Urol.*, **103** : 449.

Houser, R., Izant, R.J. & Persky, L. (1965). Testicular tumors in children. *Am. J. Surg.*, **110** : 876.

Hung, W., Blizzard, R.M. *et al.* (1963). Precocious puberty in a boy with a hepatoma and circulating gonadotropin. *J. Pediat.*, **63** : 895.

Johnson, D.E., Kuhn, C.R. & Guinn, G.A. (1970). Testicular tumors in children. *J. Urol.*, **104** : 90.

Johnson, D.G. (1975). Trends in surgery for childhood rhabdomyosarcoma. *Cancer*, **35** : 916.

Johnstone, G. (1967). Prepubertal gynaecomastia in association with an interstitial cell tumour of the testis. *Brit. J. Urol.*, **39** : 211.

Karamehmedovic, O., Woodtli, W. & Plüss, H.J. (1975). Testicular tumors in childhood. *J. Pediat. Surg.*, **10** : 109.

Kennedy, B.J. (1970). Mithramycin therapy in advanced testicular neoplasms. *Cancer*, **26** : 755.

Kilman, J.W., Clatworthy, H.W.Jr. *et al.* (1973). Reasonable surgery for rhabdomyosarcoma: a study of 67 cases. *Ann. Surg.*, **178** : 346.

Klugo, R.C., Fisher, J.H. & Retik, A.B. (1972). Endodermal sinus tumor of the testis in infants and children. *J. Urol.*, **108** : 359.

Leiter, E. & Brendler, H. (1967). Loss of ejaculation following bilateral retroperitoneal lymphadenectomy. *J. Urol.*, **98** : 375.

McCullough, D.L., Carlton, C.E. & Seybold, H.M. (1971). Testicular tumors in infants and children. Report of 5 cases and evaluation of different modes of treatment. *J. Urol.*, **105** : 140.

Macnab, G.H. (1955). Maldescent of the testicle. *J. Roy. Coll. Surg. Edinb.*, **1** 126.

McKay, B., Bennington, J.L. & Skoglund, R.W. (1971). The adenomatoid tumor: fine ultrastructure evidence for a mesothelial origin. *Cancer*, **27** : 109.

MALEK, R.S., UTZ, D.C. & FARROW, G.M. (1972). Malignant tumors of the spermatic cord. *Cancer*, **29** : 1108.

MATSUMOTO, K., NAKAUCHI, K. & FUJITA, K. (1970). Radiation therapy for the embryonal carcinoma of testis in childhood. *J. Urol.*, **104** : 778.

MOSTOFI, F.K. (1973a). Infantile testicular tumors. *Bull. N.Y. Acad. Med.*, **28** : 684.

MOSTOFI, F.K. (1973b). Testicular tumors: epidemiologic, etiologic and pathologic features. *Cancer*, **32** : 1186.

MOSTOFI, F.K., (1974). International histological classification of tumors. A report by the Executive Committee of the International Council of Societies of Pathology. *Cancer*, **33** : 1480.

MOSTOFI, F.K. & PRICE, E.B. JR. (1973), *Atlas of Tumour Pathology*, Second series, Fascicle 8. Tumors of the Male Genital System, Armed Forces Institute of Pathology, Washington D.C.

MOSTOFI, F.K., THEISS, E.A. & ASHLEY, D.J.B. (1959). Tumors of specialised gonadal stroma in human male patients. Androblastoma, Sertoli cell tumor, granulosa cell tumor of the testis and gonadal stromal tumor. *Cancer*, **12** : 944.

MULVIHILL, J.J., WADE, W.M. & MILLER, R.M. (1975). Gonadoblastoma in dysgenetic gonads with a Y chromosome. *Lancet*, **1** : 863.

OMENN, G.S. (1971). Ectopic hormone syndrome associated with tumors in childhood. *Pediatrics*, **47** : 613.

ONG, T.H. & SOLOMON, J.R. (1973). Fat necrosis of the scrotum. *J. Pediat. Surg.*, **8** : 919.

PHELAN, J.T., WOOLNER, L.B. & HAYLES, A.B. (1957). Testicular tumors in infants and children. *Surg. Gynec. & Obstet.*, **105** : 569.

PRICE, E.B. (1969). Epidermoid cysts of the testis. *J. Urol.*, **102** : 708.

PRICE, E.B. & MOSTOFI, F.K. (1970). Epidermoid cysts of the testis in children: a report of 4 cases. *J. Pediat.*, **77** : 676.

PUGH, R.C.B. & CAMERON, K.M. (1964). Relative malignancy of testicular tumours. *Brit. J. Urol.*, **36** (Suppl.) : 107.

PUGH, R.C.B. & SMITH, J.P. (1964). Teratoma of the testis. *Brit. J. Urol.*, **36** (Suppl. 2) : 28.

RAVICH, L., LERMAN, P.H. *et al.* (1966). Embryonal carcinoma of the testicle in childhood: review of literature and presentation of 2 cases. *J. Urol.*, **96** : 501.

RAY, B., HAJDU, S.I. & WHITMORE, W.F. (1974). Distribution of retroperitoneal lymph node metastases in testicular germinal tumors. *Cancer*, **33** : 340.

ROSAI, J. & DEHNER, L.P. (1975). Nodular mesothelial hyperplasia in hernial sacs : a benign reactive condition simulating a neoplastic process. *Cancer*, **35** : 165.

ROSVOLL, R.V. & WOODARD, J.R. (1968). Malignant Sertoli cell tumours of the testis. *Cancer*, **22** : 8.

SABIO, H., BURGERT, E.O. Jr. *et al.* (1974). Embryonal carcinoma of the testis in childhood. *Cancer*, **34** : 2118.

SAVARD, K., DORFMAN, R.I. *et al.* (1960). Clinical, morphologic and biochemical studies of a virilizing tumor of the testis. *J. Clin. Invest.*, **39** : 534.

SCULLY, R.E. (1970). Gonadoblastoma: a review of 74 cases. *Cancer*, **25** : 1340.

SKEEL, D.A., DRINKER, H.R. & WITHERINGTON, R. (1975). Rhabdomyosarcoma of the spermatic cord : report of 3 cases with review of the literature. *J. Urol.*, **113** : 279.

SOHVAL, A.R. (1956). Testicular dysgenesis in relation to neoplasm of the testicle. *J. Urol.*, **75** : 285.

STAUBITZ, W.J., EARLY, K.S., MAGOSS, I.V. & MURPHY, G.P. (1974). Surgical management of testis tumor. *J. Urol.*, **111** : 205.

TANIMURA, H. & FURUTA, M. (1968). Rhabdomyosarcoma of the spermatic cord. *Cancer*, **22** : 1215.

TEFFT, M., VAWTER, G.F. & MITUS, A. (1967). Radiotherapeutic management of testicular neoplasms in children. *Radiol.*, **88** : 457.

TEOH, T.B., STEWARD, J.K. & WILLIS, R.A. (1960). The distinctive adenocarcinoma of the infant's testis: an account of 15 cases. *J. Path. Bact.*, **80** : 147.

TEILUM, G. (1959). Endodermal sinus tumor of the ovary and testes: comparative morphogenesis of the so-called mesonephroma ovarii (Schiller) extraembryonic (yolk sac-allantoic) structures of the rat's placenta. *Cancer*, **12** : 1092.

THOMPSON, M.R., EMMANUEL, I.G., CAMPBELL, M.S. & ZACHARY, R.B. (1973). Extrarenal Wilms' tumor. *J. Pediat. Surg.*, **8** : 37.

WATSON, R.J. (1968). Splenogonadal fusion. *Surgery*, **63** : 853.

WILLIAMS, G. & BANNERGEE, R. (1969). Paratesticular tumours. *Brit. J. Urol.*, **41** : 332.

WILLIS, R.A. (1967). *Pathology of Tumours of Childhood.* Oliver & Boyd, London.

WINCHELL, H.S., SANCHEZ, P.D. *et al.* (1970). Visualization of tumors in humans using ^{67}Ga-citrate and the Anger whole body scanner, scintillation camera and tomographic scanner. *J. Nucl. Med.*, **11** : 459.

YOUNG, P.G., MOUNT, B.M., FOOTE, F.W. & WHITMORE, W.F. (1970). Embryonal adenocarcinoma in the prepuberal testis. *Cancer*, **26** : 1065.

ZONE, R.M. (1970). Retinal anlage tumor of the epididymis : a case report. *J. Urol.*, **103** : 106.

The Breast

AMERSON, J.R. (1970). Cystosarcoma phyllodes in adolescent females. *Ann. Surg.*, **171** : 849.

ASHIKARI, R., FARROW, J.H. & O'HARA, J. (1971). Fibroadenomas in the breast of juveniles. *Surg. Gynec. & Obstet.*, **132** : 259.

AUGUST, G.P. *et al.* (1972). Prepubertal male gynecomastia, *J. Pediat.*, **80** : 259.

BYRNE, M.P., FAHEY, M.M. & GOOSELAW, J.G. (1973). Breast cancer with axillary metastasis in an 8½ year old girl. *Cancer*, **31** : 726.

DE CHOLONOKY, T. (1943). Mammary cancer in youth. *Surg. Gynec. & Obstet.*, **77** : 55.

DIETHRICH, E.G., HAMMOND, W.W.Jr. & HOLTZ, F. (1966). Intraductal papillomatosis of the breast: report of a case in a 10 year old girl. *Amer. J. Surg.*, **112** : 80.

FENSTENSTEIN, M. (1960). Adenocarcinoma of the breast in a South African Bantu boy aged 14 years. *S. African. med. J.*, **34** : 517.

HARTMAN, A.W. & MARGRISH, P. (1955). Carcinoma of the breast in children: case report of 6 year old boy with adenocarcinoma. *Ann. Surg.*, **141** : 792.

HERRMANN, J. (1960). In *Cancer and Allied Diseases in Infancy and Childhood.* (Ariel, I.M. & Pack, G.T. eds.). Little Brown, Boston.

LEWIS, D. & GESCHICKTER, C.F. (1934). Gynecomastia, virginal hypertrophy and fibroadenosis of breast. *Ann. Surg.*, **100** : 779.

MCDIVITT, R.W. & STEWART, F.W. (1966). Breast carcinoma in children. *J. Amer. Med. Assoc.*, **195** : 388.

NICHINI, F.M., GOLDMAN, L. & LAPAYOWKER, M.S. *et al.* (1972). Inflammatory carcinoma of the breast in a 12 year old girl. *Arch. Surg.*, **105** : 505.

OBERMAN, H.A. (1965). Cystosarcoma phyllodes: a clinicopathologic study of hypercellular periductal stromal neoplasms of the breast. *Cancer*, **18** : 697.

OBERMAN, H.A. & STEPHENS, P.J. (1972). Carcinoma of the breast in childhood. *Cancer*, **30** : 470.

ROBERTS, M.M., FORREST, A.P.M. *et al.* (1973). Simple versus radical mastectomy: Preliminary report of the Cardiff Breast Trial. *Lancet*, **1** : 1073.

SIMMONS, R.R. (1917). Adenocarcinoma of the breast occurring in a boy of 13. *J. Amer. Med. Assoc.*, **68** : 1899.

SIMPSON, T.E., VAN DERVOORT, R.L.Jr. & LYNN, H.B. (1969). Giant fibroadenoma (benign cystosarcoma phyllodes): report of case in 13 year old girl. *Surgery*, **65** : 341.

Appendix I. The Index Series

MALIGNANT DISEASE IN CHILDHOOD

ROYAL CHILDREN'S HOSPITAL, MELBOURNE

(1689 tumours in 23 years, 1950–1972)

Neoplasm	No. of Cases	Percentage	Group Totals
1. Leukaemias	615	36	615 (36%)
2. Intracranial tumours	329	19	329 (19%)
Eye (Retinoblastoma : 9)	25	2	Other solid tumours 745 (45%)
3. Neuroblastoma	144	9	
4. Sarcomas (Soft tissue and bone, all sites)	142	8	
5. Malignant Lymphomas	120	7	
6. Wilms' tumour (Nephroblastoma)	112	7	
7. Teratoma (all types)	79	5	
8. Histiocytoses (Reticuloses, excl. leukaemia and other lymphomas)	58	3	
9. Miscellaneous	65	4	
	1689	100%	100%

1. LEUKAEMIA

Year	Lymphocytic	Granulocytic	Other	Total
1950	14	4	1	19
1951	22	2	1	25
1952	12	1	1	14
1953	12	5	1	18
1954	16	3	–	19
1955	6	5	–	11
1956	13	8	3	24
1957	9	3	1	13
1958	25	6	–	31
1959	10	9	2	21
1960	27	12	2	41
1961	15	6	2	23
1962	14	7	8	29
1963	23	2	6	31
1964	16	5	6	27
1965	15	5	9	29
1966	21	5	7	33
1967	17	4	8	29
1968	33	3	4	40
1969	22	4	2	28
1970	20	8	–	28
1971	29	4	–	33
1972	44	5	–	49
23 Year: Totals	435	116	64	615

2. CEREBRAL AND OCULAR TUMOURS

Medulloblastoma	95
Astrocytoma (well differentiated)	80
Astrocytoma (with anaplasia)	51
Ependymoma (incl. choroid plexus papillomas)	38
Meninges and other	25
Glioblastoma multiforme	16
Optic glioma	16
Craniopharyngioma	14
Retinoblastoma	9
Germinoma	8
Total	352

3. NEUROBLASTOMA

Adrenal	71
Abdominal	32
Thorax	19
Spinal cord	6
Sacrum	3
Cervical sympathetic	1
Cerebellum	1
Unknown	11
	144

4. NEOPLASMS OF SOFT TISSUE AND BONE

Rhabdomyosarcoma	64	
Soft tissue sarcomas	14	85
Synovial sarcomas	7	
Bone—Ewing's tumour	25	
—osteosarcoma	22	57
—other bone tumours	10	
		142

4a. RHABDOMYOSARCOMA

Site	Type			
	Alveolar	Embryonal	Pleomorphic	
Limbs and trunk	13	1	1	15
Head and neck	2	12	1	15
Genitourinary	1	26	0	27
Other	2	3	2	7
Total	18	42	4	64

5. MALIGNANT LYMPHOMAS

Neoplasm	Sites					
	L.N.	Mediastinal	Bowel	'Burkitt's'	Other	
Hodgkin's disease	33	0	0	0	0	33
Lymphosarcoma	29	16	13	3	7	68
Reticulum cell sarcoma	9	2	1	0	5	17
G.F. Lymphoma	2	0	0	0	0	2
					Total	120

5a. HODGKIN'S DISEASE

Mixed cell type	15
Lymphocyte dominant	10
Lymphocyte depleted	4
Nodular sclerosing	4
Total	33

6. WILMS' TUMOUR

Total 112

7. TERATOMA

Sacrococcygeal		
benign	26	
malignant	7	33
Ovarian		
benign	27	
malignant	2	29
Other sites		
benign	14	
malignant	3	17
		79

8. HISTIOCYTOSES

Eosinophilic granuloma	25	
Letterer-Siwe disease	11	
Unclassified malignant reticulosis	10	
Hand-Schüller-Christian disease	5	
Haemophagic reticulosis	4	(2 siblings)
Sinus histiocytosis	3	
Total	58	

9. MISCELLANEOUS TUMOURS

Hepatoblastoma	16
Testicular (malignant)	7
Salivary tumour	6
Phaeochromocytoma	5
Malignant hepatoma	4
Adrenal carcinoma	4
Basal cell carcinoma	4
Argentaffinoma	4
Ovarian, malignant	4
Thyroid carcinoma	3
Islet cell carcinoma	1
Renal carcinoma	1
Unclassified tumours	6
Total	65

Appendix II. Biochemical and haematological normal paediatric values

The following reference ranges have been derived from a review of the literature, from a detailed analysis of results of tests performed on patients treated at the Royal Children's Hospital, and in some cases from studies in our laboratory on healthy children. Results within these ranges can be considered to be 'within normal limits'.

The values are stated in traditional units and also in S.I. units*, with a conversion factor.

ABBREVIATIONS (as recommended by the International Federation of Clinical Chemistry*)

B	Blood	m	milli- (10^{-3})
d	day	mol	Mole
dl	100 ml	n	nano- (10^{-9})
eq	equivalent	Osm	Osmole
f	fasting	P	Plasma
fl	femto- (10^{-15})	p	pica- (10^{-12})
g	gramme	Pa	Pascal
h	hour	S	Serum
I	International	U	Unit
k	Kilo- (10^{3})	μ	micro- (10^{-6})
Lkc	Leukocyte	w	week
M	Month	y	year

**SI Units.* The International Federation of Clinical Chemistry has recommended that all laboratories use a common terminology when expressing results. The units of this system (Le Système International d'Unités) i.e. S.I. Units, express results in molecular terms (e.g. moles/litre) rather than in mass (e.g. mg/100 ml). It is the form required for publication in many journals and is being progressively introduced throughout the world.

HAEMATOLOGICAL NORMAL VALUES

Bleeding time (Ivy's method)	Up to 11 min
Coagulation time (Lee and White)	5–11 min
Prothrombin time (Quick)	10–14 seconds
Partial thromboplastin time (activated)	30–40 seconds
Plasma fibrinogen	150–400 mg/dl
Fibrin split products (TRCHI method)	Positive greater than 1/16
Serum iron	50–150 μg/dl (9–27 μmol/l)
Iron binding capacity	250–400 μg/dl (45–72 μmol/l)
Percentage saturation	16–33%
Fetal haemoglobin—at birth	60–90%
at 3 months	10–25%
at 6 months	<2%
Hb A_2	1·0 to 4·0%
Serum B_{12}	200–800 pg/ml
Serum folate	5–21 ng/ml
Red cell folate	160–640 ng/ml
Whole blood folate	50–300 ng/ml (with normal PCV)
Plasma haemoglobin	1–4 mg/dl (0·6–2·5 μmol/l)
Serum haptoglobin	30–200 mg Hb-binding per dl (8–124 μmol Hb-binding per l)
Cold agglutinin titre (4°C)	<1/64
Sedimentation rate (micro Westergren)	0–7 mm in one hour
Osmotic Fragility	Increased if haemolysis occurs over 0·5% NaCl. 50% haemolysis occurs between 0·40 and 0·45% NaCl. Complete haemolysis by 0·25–0·30% NaCl. After incubation at 37°C for 24 hours the range increases and is interpreted relative to a normal control.
Autohaemolysis	After incubation at 37°C for 48 h without added glucose 0·2–2·0% with added glucose 0–0·9%
Neutrophil alkaline phosphatase score (NAP)	16–100

BIOCHEMICAL NORMAL VALUES

BLOOD, PLASMA OR SERUM

Tests	Age	Reference Range Traditional Units	Reference Range S.I. Units	Conversion Factor SI→Trad. Mult. by	Comments
Acid/Base (P)					Arterial or capillary blood.
pH	1d	7·25–7·43			
	2d–1M	7·32–7·43			
	>1M	7·34–7·43			
$P\text{co}_2$		mm Hg	kPa	7·592	
		32–45	4·2–5·9		
Base Excess		meq/l	mmol/l	1·000	Based on paediatric hospital population.
		−4 to +3	−4 to +3		
Actual Bicarbonate		meq/1	mmol/l	1·000	
		18–25	18–25		
Acid Phosphatase (S, P)		Int. Units			Higher values seen in infants.
		0–2			
Albumin					See Proteins.
Alkaline Phosphatase (S, P)		KA Units	U/l		
	0–2y	10–32	250–800	0·041	
	2–10y	10–28	250–700		
	10–16y	10–32	250–800		
Ammonia (P)		μg/100 ml	μmol/l	1·703	Values up to 120 μg/dl (70 μmol/1) often seen in infants.
	0–2w	90–150	55–90		
	>1M	40–90	20–55		
Amylase (S, P)		Somogyi	U/l	0·546	
		40–160	75–300		

BLOOD, PLASMA OR SERUM (Continued)

Tests	Age	Reference Range Traditional Units	Reference Range S.I. Units	Conversion Factor SI→Trad. Mult. by	Comments
Aryl Sulphatase (B) Lkc		Units 45–290			
Aspartate Amino-transferase					See Transaminase, (SGOT).
Base Excess					See Acid/Base.
Bicarbonate					See Acid/Base.
Bilirubin (Total) (S,P)		mg/100 ml	μmol/l	0·0585	Higher values in newborn due to increase in unconjugated (indirect) fraction.
	Full-term				
	0–24h	< 5	< 85		
	24–48h	< 9	< 150		*Note* 20 mg/100 ml = 340 μmol/l.
	3–5d	< 12	< 200		
	> 1M	< 1	< 15		
	Premature				
	0–24h	< 8	< 135		
	24–48h	< 12	< 205		
	3–5d	< 24	< 410		
Calcium (Total) (S,P)		mg/100 ml	mmol/l	4·008	*Note* Lower limit of normal range in neonates not well defined.
	0–2w	7·5–11·0	1·9–2·8		
	3M–1y	9·0–11·0	2·3–2·8		
	> 1y	8·8–10·7	2·2–2·7		
Caeruloplasmin					See Copper Oxidase.
Carotenoids (S,P)		Units/100 ml			
	Birth	20 (Average)			
	18M	100 ,,			
	> 2y	30–200			

Chloride (S,P)		meq/l	mmol/l	1·000	
		98–107	98–107		
Cholestrol (Total)		mg/100 ml	mmol/l	38·66	
(S,P)	< 1y	110–220	2·8–5·7		
	1–16y	120–250	3·1–6·5		
Copper (S,P)		μg/100 ml	μmol/l	6·354	
	0–6M	< 70	< 11		
	2y	95–185	15–29		
	6y	85–175	13–127		
	> 10y	70–155	11–124		
Copper Oxidase		O.D. Units			
(S,P)		0·25–0·49			
Cortisol (S,P)		μg/100 ml	nmol/l	0·0362	Random levels of little value. Best measured as part of appropriate stimulation or suppression test. Higher values in morning. Average value 0900 hrs approximates 25 μg/100 ml (690 nmol/1)
		(see comments)			
Creatine Kinase (CPK)		U/l	U/l		
(S,P)		<40	< 85	0·48	
Creatinine (S,P)		mg/100 ml	μmol/l	0·0113	
	< 4y	0·1–0·7	10–60		
	4–10y	0·2–0·9	20–90		
	10–16y	0·3–0·1	30–100		
Dibucaine No.					See Pseudocholinesterase.
Dilantin (S,P)		μg/ml	μmol/l	0·2523	
(Therapeutic level)					
		10–20	40–80		
Free Fatty Acids f		μg/l	μmol/l	1·000	
(P)	1–6M	550–750	550–750		
	1–8y	450–1150	450–1150		
	> 8y	450–850	450–850		

BLOOD, PLASMA OR SERUM (Continued)

Tests	Age	Reference Range Traditional Units	Reference Range S.I. Units	Conversion Factor SI→Trad. Mult. by	Comments
FSH (S)	Adult	mIU/ml			
		1·1–4·0			
Galactose-I-PO. Uridyl Transferase (B) Ery		U/gHb			Galactosaemia < 3U/gHb
		15–47			Heterozygotes 5–12 U/gHb
Globulins					See Proteins
Glucose f (S,P)		mg/100 ml	mmol/l	18·02	
	1d	12–52	0·7–2·9		
	2d	17–57	0·9–3·2		
	3d	28–60	1·6–3·3		
	4d	38–62	2·1–3·4		
	5d	40–64	2·2–3·6		
	> 1M	64–98	3·6–5·4		
Glycerol f (P)		μg/100 ml	μmol/l	9·209	
		280–900	30–100		
Growth Hormone (S,P)		μU/ml (See comments)			Single levels of limited value. Best measured as part of appropriate stimulation test.
Haptoglobin (S,P)	Newborn	Undetectable			
	> 4M	Saturated by 50–150 mg/100 ml Haemoglobin			
17α-Hydroxyprogesterone (P)		μg/100 ml	nmol/l	0·033	Higher values in cord blood and first few days of life.
	< 4d	< 1·5	< 45		
	> 4d	< 0·5	< 15		

Insulin (P)		μU/ml			Random levels of little value.
		(See comments)			
Iron		μg/100 ml	μmol/l		
		50–150	9–27	5·586	
Iron Binding Capacity		250–400	45–72	5·586	
Lactate f (B)		mg/100 ml	mmol/l	8·904	
		9–16	1·0–1·8		
Lactate Dehydrogenase (S,P)		U/1			Higher values in infants, especially newborn.
	> 1y	70–140			
Lead (B)		μg/100 ml	μmol/l	20·72	
		< 40	1.9		
Luteinizing Hormone (S,P)		mIU/ml			
	Adult	0·5–2·0			
Magnesium (S,P)		mg/100 ml	mmol/l	2·432	
		1·7–2·5	0·7–1·0		
Methaemoglobin (B) Ery		% of Total Hb			
		0–2			
Methaemoglobin Reductase-NADH Dependent (B) Ery		Units			
		2–4			
Osmolality (S,P)		mOsm/kg H_2O	mmol/kg		
		270–295	270–295		
P_{CO_2}					See Acid/Base
pH					See Acid/Base
Phenylalanine (S,P)		mg/100 ml	mmol/l	16·39	
		1–3	0·06–0·18		
Phosphorus Inorganic (S,P)		mg/100 ml	mmol/l	3·098	
	< 2W	5·0–9·0	1·7–3·0		
	< 1y	4·0–7·0	1·3–2·3		
	2–16y	3·6–5·6	1·1–1·8		
	Adult	2·5–4·5	0·8–1·5		

BLOOD, PLASMA OR SERUM (Continued)

Tests	Age	Reference Range Traditional Units	Reference Range S.I. Units	Conversion Factor SI→Trad. Mult. by	Comments
Po_2 (P)		mm Hg	kPa	7·592	Arterial blood only.
		85–100	11·2–13·2		
Potassium (S,P)		meq/l	mmol/l	1·000	Ranges quoted on capillary blood specimens. Venous specimens average 0·2 mmol/l lower.
	2d–2w	4·0–6·4	4·0–6·4		
	2w–3M	4·0–6·2	4·0–6·2		
	3M–1y	3·7–5·6	3·7–5·6		
	1–16y	3·7–5·3	3·7–5·3		
Proteins (S)		g/100 ml	g/l	0·100	
Total Protein	1d–1M	5·0–7·0	50–70	0·100	
	1M–1y	5·5–7·5	55–75		
	1–4y	5·8–7·8	58–78		
	4–16y	6·0–8·0	60–80		
Albumin	1d–1M	2·5–4·0	25–40	0·100	
	1M–16y	3·2–4·8	32–48		
Globulins (Total)	1d–1M	1·5–3·5	15–35	0·100	
	1M–1y	1·9–3·5	19–35		
	1–4y	2·1–3·8	21–38		
	4–16y	2·4–4·0	24–40		
α_1	1d–16y	0·1–0·4	1–4	0·100	
α_2	1d–1M	0·3–1·0	3–10	0·100	
	1M–16y	0·5–1·1	5–11		
β	1d–1M	0·4–1·1	4–11	0·100	
	1M–16y	0·5–1·1	5–11		
γ	1d–1M	0·4–1·3	4–13	0·100	
	1–6M	0·2–0·8	2–8		

	6M–1y	0·3–1·0	3–10	
	1–4y	0·4–1·3	4–13	
	4–16y	0·6–1·6	6–16	
Protoporphyrin		μg/100 ml	μmol/l	56·2
(B) Ery		RBC's	erys	
		16–50	0·3–1·0	
Pseudocholinesterase		Units		
(S,P)		0·74–1·52		
Dibucaine No.		80% inhibition		
Pyruvate f (B)		mg/100 ml	mmol/l	8·702
		0·35–0·6	0·04–0·07	
Sodium (S,P)		meq/l	mmol/l	1·000
		133–143	133–143	
Testosterone (S,P)		ng/100 ml	nmol/l	28·84
	Prepubertal	0–220	0–8	
	Adult Male	300–950	10–33	
	,, Female	30–95	1·0–3·3	
Thyroid Function (S)				
P.B.I. (S)		μg/100 ml	μmol/l	12·69
	1–3d	6·6–13·7	0·520–1·08	
	1–2w	6·3–10·9	0·50–0·86	
	2–4w	5·3–10·9	0·42–0·86	
	1–4M	4·6–9·8	0·36–0·77	
	4M–1y	3·6–8·8	0·28–0·70	
	>1y	3·0–7·6	0·24–0·60	
Thyroxine		μg/100 ml	nmol/l	0.0777
(Total) (S)	1–3d	10·1–20·9	130–270	
	1–2w	9·8–16·6	125–215	
	2–4w	8·2–16·6	105–215	
	1–4M	7·1–15·0	90–190	
	4M–1y	5·5–13·5	70–175	
	>1y	5–12	65–155	

BLOOD, PLASMA OR SERUM (Continued)

Tests	Age	Reference Range Traditional Units	Reference Range S.I. Units	Conversion Factor SI→Trad. Mult. by	Comments
T_3 Resin Uptake		%			
(S)	1d–1M	85–120			
	1–6M	75–110			
	>6M	80–110			
Electrophoretic		%			
Index (S)	Children	65–80			
	Adults	61–75			
Free Thyroxine Index (S)	>6M	2·3–8·2			
Thyroxine Binding Globulin		μgT_4/100ml	nmolT_4/l	0·0777	
(Capacity) (S)	Infants	>40	>520		
	Children	30–40	390–520		
	Adults	30–40	390–520		
Diagnostic Thyroxine Ratio (S)		0·75–1·35			Limits in infancy uncertain.
Thyroid Stim.		μU/ml			Levels up to 6μU/ml seen in infants and children.
Hormone (S)	Adult	0–5			
Transaminase		U/l (Boehringer)	U/l	0·46	Highest values in newborn
(SGOT) (S,P)	<1y	9–50	20–110		Upper limit in infants not well defined.
	1–3y	6–30	13–65		
	3–16y	5–25	7–50		
Triglycerides		mg/100 ml	mmol/l	88·0	
f (S,P)	>1y	<120	<1·36		
Tyrosine (S,P)		mg/100 ml	mmol/l	18·1	Higher values in newborn especially low birth weight.
		0·8–1·3	0·045–0·072		
Urea (S,P)		mg/100 ml	mmol/l	6·006	Related to protein intake.
		15–40	2·5–6·7		Lower in breast fed infants.

Uric Acid		mg/100 ml 2–6	mmol/l 0·12–0·36	16·81	
Zinc		μg/100 ml 75–140	μmol/l 12–20	6 538	

URINARY VALUES

δ-Aminolaevulinic		mg/l < 5	μmol/l < 40	0·13	Fresh random sample. Wrap in foil to keep dark.
Amylase		Somogyi Units/100 ml 70–750			
Calcium		mg/kg/24 hr < 6	mmol/kg/d < 0·15	40·08	
Catecholamines (Total)		μg/mg creatinine < 1·5	mmol/mol creatinine < 1·0	1·5	
Copper		μg/24 h < 20	μmol/d < 0·3	63·5	
Coproporphyrin		μg/l < 300	μmol/l < 0·46	654	Fresh random sample. Wrap in foil to keep dark.
Creatinine Clearance		ml/min/ 1·73m² 85–145	ml/sec/ 1·73m² 1·4–2·4	60·0	
Cystine	Adult	mg/24 hr 30–100	mmol/d 0·13–0·42	240	
11-Deoxy : 11-Oxy					See 17 Ketogenic steroids.
Gonadotrophins		Mouse Uterine Units			
	Pre-pubertal	< 4			
	Adult	4–40			

URINARY VALUES (Continued)

Test	Age	Reference Range Traditional Units	S.I. Units	Conversion Factor SI→Trad. Mult. by	Comments
5-Hydroxyindole-Acetic Acid		mg/24 h	μmol/d	0·19	
		2–10	10–50		
17-Keto(=oxo) genic steroids		mg/24 h	μmol/d	0·288	
	0–2y	0·2–1·3	0·7–5		
	2–6y	1·5–6·0	5–20		
	6–8y	1·5–7·0	5–24		
	8–10y	1·5–8·0	5–28		
	12–13y	2·7–8·5	9–30		
	> 13y	5–13	17–45		
11-Deoxy : 11-Oxy Ratio (17 kegs)		< 0·8			
17-Keto(=oxo) steroids		mg/24 hr	μmol/d	0·288	
	0–14d	1·5–2·5	5–9		
	0–2y	0–0·2	0–0·7		
	2–6y	0–2·0	0–7		
	6–8y	0·2–2·1	0·7–7		
	8–10y	0·7–3·0	2–10		
	10–12y	1·0–7·5	4–26		
	12–13y	1·6–13	6–45		
	> 13 Male	2·5–13·0	9–45		
	> 13 Female	2·5–11·0	9–38		
Lead		μg/24 h	μmol/d	207	
		< 50	< 0·24		
3-Methoxy 4-Hydroxymandelic Acid (MHMA) (VMA)		mg/24 h	μmol/d	0·20	Values > 1·5 times upper limit of normal suggest neural crest tumour.
	0–1y	< 1·8	< 9		

	1–4y	< 3·0	< 15		
	4–10y	< 4·4	< 22		
	> 10y	< 7·2	< 36		
Oestrogens		μg/24 hr	μmol/d	280	
	Prepubertal	< 1	< 5	0·29	
	Adult male	8–23	28–80		
	Post menstrual	7–23	24–80		
	Pre-ov. peak	45–93	155–325		
	Luteal max	22–104	76–360		
Osmolality		mOsm/ kgH_2O 50–1400			Random specimens of little value. Consult laboratory.
Oxalate		mg/24 h	mmol/d	90	
	1–10w	< 15	< 0·2		
	1–10y	< 60	< 0·7		
	> 10y	< 100	< 1·1		
Porphyrobilinogen		mg/l	μmol/l	0·23	Fresh random sample.
		< 2	< 9		Wrap in foil to keep dark.
Pregnanetriol		mg/24 h	μmol/d	0·34	
	0–6y	0–0·2	0–0·6		
	7–16y	0·3–1·1	0·9–3·3		
	> 16y	0·2–3·5	0·6–10		
Protein		mg/24 h	mg/d		
	Adult	< 70	< 70	1·000	
Urobilinogen		Ehrlich Units/100ml 0–0·1			
Uroporphyrin		μg/l	μmol/l	830	
		0–40	0–0·05		

CSF VALUES

Tests	Age	Reference Range Traditional Units	S.I. Units	Conversion Factor SI→Trad. Mult. by	Comments
CSF					
Pressure	Newborn	30–80 mmH_2O			
	Children	50–100 mmH_2O			
	Adults	70–200 (Av. 125)			
Cells	1y	up to 10/mm^3			Only lymphocytes normally present.
	1–4y	up to 8/mm^3			
	4y	0–5/mm^3			
Specific Gravity		1·005–1·009			
Chloride		mEq/l	mmol/l		
		120–128	120–128	1·000	
Colloidal Gold		Negative			
Glucose		mg/100 ml	mmol/l		
		40–50	2·2–2·8 g/l	18·02	
Protein		15–40	0·15–0·4	0·100	Albumin – 80%
					Globulin – 20%
FAECES		μg/g dry wt.	μmol/g dry wt.		
Protoporphyrin		0–100	0–0·18	562	
Coproporphyrin		0–40	0–0·06	654	
Sweat		mEq/l	mmol/ l		
Sodium		< 60	< 60	1·000	
Chloride		< 60	< 60		
Tissues		% wet wt.			
Glycogen (Liver)		< 5			
Glycogen (Muscle)		< 1			

MEASUREMENTS

Head and Thorax (circumference in cm)

Age	Head	Thorax
Birth	34·8	34·8
2 months	40·1	38·9
4 months	42·7	42·4
6 months	44·2	43·7
1 year	46·7	46·5
2 years	48·8	49·3
3 years	49·8	51·6
4 years	50·8	53·3
5 years	51·6	55·1

Haematological normal values (cellular)

REFERENCE RANGES

The conversion of haematology values to S.I. units is in a transitional state. The date for the complete change has not been set, but for completeness both values will be given where applicable.

HAEMOGLOBIN

Age	Mean g/dl	Mean mmol/l	Range g/dl	Range mmol/l	Conversion Factor SI→Trad. Mult. by
Birth	18·0	11·2	14·0–22·0	8·7–13·7	1·61
2 weeks	15·0	9·3	12·0–18·0	7·5–11·2	
3 months	11·0	6·8	9·5–13·0	5·9– 8·1	
12 months	11·5	7·1	10·5–13·0	6·5– 8·1	
6 years	12·0	7·5	11·0–13·5	6·8– 8·4	
10 years	12·5	7·8	11·5–14·0	7·1– 8·7	
Puberty (males)	14·0	8·7	12·5–16·0	7·8– 9·9	
Puberty (females)	13·0	8·1	11·5–15·0	7·1– 9·3	

Age	P.C.V. %	P.C.V. S.I. Units	M.C.V. fl*	R.B.C. 10^{12}/l	Reticulocytes %
Birth	54±10	0·54±0·10	106	4·7–7·0	2·0–6·0
2 weeks	42± 7	0·42±0·07	96	4·3–6·0	0·3–1·5
3 months	37± 3	0·37±0·03	78	3·8–5·3	0·5–1·5
12 months	35± 3	0·35±0·03	77	4·0–5·5	0·5–1·5
6 years	38± 3	0·38±0·03	80	3·8–5·4	0·5–1·5
10 years	39± 3	0·39±0·03	80	3·8–5·4	0·5–1·5
Puberty (males)	43± 7	0·43±0·07	87	4·6–6·2	0·5–1·5
Puberty (females)	39± 5	0·39±0·05	87	4·2–5·4	0·5–1·5

* Femto litre (1×10^{-15})

LEUCOCYTES $\times 10^9$/l

Age	Mean	Range	Neutrophils	Lymph.	Monocytes	Eosinophils	Basophils
Birth	18·0	9·0–30·0	6·0–26·0	2·0–11·0	0·4 –3·1	0·02–0·85	0–0·64
1 week	12·2	5·0–21·0	1·5–10·0	2·0–17·0	0·3 –2·7	0·07–1·10	0–0·25
2 weeks	11·4	5·0–20·0	1·0– 9·0	2·0–17·0	0·2 –2·4	0·07–1·00	0–0·23
3 months	11·0	6·0–18·0	1·0– 9·0	3·0–16·0	0·1 –1·5	0·07–0·85	0–0·20
12 months	11·4	6·0–18·0	1·5– 8·5	4·0–10·5	0·05–1·1	0·05–0·70	0–0·20
2 years	10·6	6·0–17·0	1·5– 8·5	3·0– 9·5	0·05–1·0	0·04–0·65	0–0·20
6 years	8·5	5·0–14·5	1·5– 8·0	1·5– 7·0	0 –0·8	0 –0·65	0–0·20
10 years	8·1	4·5–13·5	1·8– 8·0	1·5– 6·5	0 –0·8	0 –0·60	0–0·20
Puberty	7·9	4·5–13·0	1·8– 8·0	1·2– 5·8	0 –0·8	0 –0·50	0–0·20

PLATELETS

Birth	100–400 × 10^9/l
1 week to Puberty	150–400 × 10^9/l

BONE MARROW

The published values for bone marrow percentages vary considerably. Ranges given below should be considered approximate only.

	New Born	Infancy	Childhood	Adult
Granulopoiesis				
Myeloblasts	0·2–3·5%	0·2–5·0%	0·2–3·5%	0·1–3·5%
Promyelocytes	0·2–5·0%	0·5–7·5%	0·5–10·0%	0·5–5·0%
Myelocytes	2·0–20·0%	5·0–15·0%	5·0–20·0%	5·0–20·0%
Metamyelocytes	5·0–25·0%	5·0–15·0%	5·0–20·0%	5·0–20·0%
Band Forms	5·0–30·0%	5·0–15·0%	5·0–20·0%	5·0–20·0%
Neutrophils	10·0–30·0%	5·0–15·0%	5·0–15·0%	7·0–25·0%
Eosinophils	0–3·0%	0–3·0%	0–3·0%	0·2–3·0%
Basophils	0–0·5%	0–0·5%	0–0·5%	0–0·5%
Erythropoiesis				
Pronormoblasts	0·5–1·0%	0–0·5%	0·5–5·0%	0·5–5·0%
Basophilic	0·5–10·0%	0–3·0%	0·2–5·0%	0·5–7·5%
Polychromatic	7·0–20·0%	0–5·0%	5·0–10·0%	2·0–15·0%
Pyknotic	7·0–20·0%	2·0–5·0%	5·0–10·0%	2·0–10·0%
Lymphocytes	5·0–10·0%	5·0–40·0%	5·0–35·0%	5·0–20·0%
Monocytes	0–0·2%	0–0·2%	0–0·2%	0–0·2%
Plasma Cells	0–1·0%	0–2·0%	0–2·5%	0·1–3·5%
Reticulum Cells	0–1·0%	0–2·0%	0·1–2·0%	0·1–2·0%
Megakaryocytes	0·1–0·5%	0·1–0·5%	0·1–0·5%	0·1–0·5%

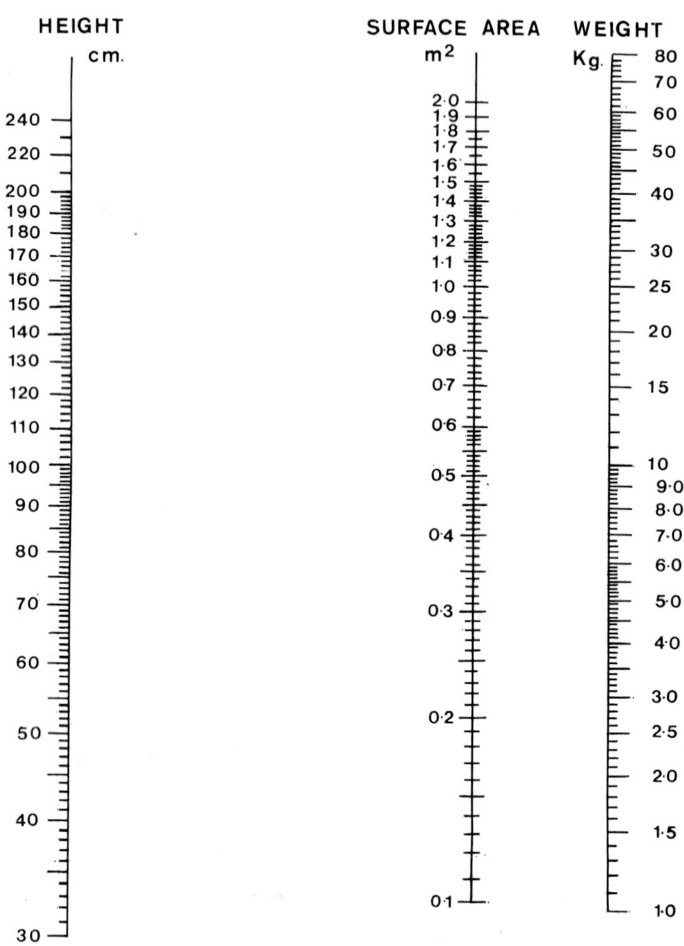

Nomogram for determining surface area from height and weight.

Appendix III. Antineoplastic drugs

ANTIMETABOLITES
- Methotrexate
- 6-Mercaptopurine
- Cytosine arabinoside
- 5-Fluorouracil
- Thioguanine

ALKYLATING AGENTS
- Cyclophosphamide
- Chlorambucil
- Busulfan

ALKALOIDS
- Vincristine
- Vinblastine
- Demecolcine

ANTIBIOTICS
- Dactinomycin
- Daunorubicin
- Adriamycin
- Mitomycin-C

MISCELLANEOUS
- L-Asparaginase
- Procarbazine
- DTIC

THERAPEUTIC INFORMATION ABOUT DRUGS (in alphabetical order)

IMPORTANT NOTE: The doses cited for the following drugs are those usual for children aged 12 months to 12 years. For those aged 13+ years and infants under 12 months, it is generally advisable to use lower doses, 10–25% below those quoted here.

Adriamycin
(doxorubicin hydrochloride)
Abbreviation: ADM. Trade name: Adriablastina.

Preparation Vial 10 mg of freeze-dried powder to be dissolved in 5 ml of sterile water or normal saline. Solution may be stored at 4°C for up to 24 hours.

Route of administration Intravenous; scalp tourniquet may be used.

Usual dose 40–60 mg/m^2 every 10–21 days,
OR 15 mg/m^2/day for 3–5 days, then rest 4–10 days, then repeat.

Mechanism of action Inhibits mitosis and synthesis of DNA and RNA.

Toxic effects
1. Epilation (severe)
2. Mouth ulcers; nausea, vomiting, diarrhoea
3. BM depression, neutropenia, thrombocytopenia
4. T wave and S-T changes in ECG; heart failure if total dosage exceeds 500 mg/m^2. OR with lower dosage if heart included in radiotherapy.

Uses 1. ALL 2. AML 3. Malignant lymphomas
4. Solid tumours—neuroblastoma, Wilms' tumour, rhabdomyo-

sarcoma, Ewing's sarcoma, soft tissue sarcomas, osteosarcoma, adenocarcinoma, primary liver cancer.

L-Asparaginase

Abbreviation: APG Trade names: Crasnitin; Colaspase.

Preparation Vial (10,000 international units) of powder to be dissolved in 5 ml normal saline or sterile water for I.V. use,
OR in 1–2 ml of sterile water for I.M. use.

Route of administration
1. Intravenous
2. Intramuscular

Usual dose 30,000 I.U./m^2 twice weekly,
OR 5,000–6,000 I.U./m^2/day for 2 weeks, or for 4 days in repeated courses.

Mechanism of action Enzyme that catalyses hydrolysis of 1-asparagine, thereby decreasing the supply of extracellular asparagine on which certain tumour cells are dependent. Action may be partly due also to associated glutaminase.

Toxic effects
1. Nausea, vomiting and anorexia,
2. Fever,
3. Hypersensitivity reactions ranging from urticaria to anaphylactic shock; adrenalin, hydrocortisone and oxygen should always be available when administering APG. Risk may be reduced by antihistamine, e.g. promethazine 25 mg, before each dose.
4. Depression of protein synthesis—albumin, fibrinogen, factor V, lipoproteins, etc.
5. Liver dysfunction.

Uses 1. ALL 2. Lymphosarcoma 3. ?AML 4. Malignant islet cell tumours of the pancreas.

Busulfan

Abbreviation: BSF. Trade name: Myleran.

Preparation Tablets 0·5 mg and 2·0 mg.

Usual dose 1·6 mg/m^2/day orally.

Mechanism of action An alkylating agent which damages cells by reaction with nucleoproteins.

Toxic effects
1. Nausea and vomiting,
2. Bone marrow depression, neutropenia, thrombocytopenia,
3. Lymphopenia,
4. Gonadal effects if given at or after puberty,
5. Interstitial pulmonary fibrosis (occasionally).

Uses 1. CML (adult and juvenile). 2. Subacute myeloid leukaemia.

Chlorambucil

Abbreviation: CAB. Trade name: Leukeran.

Preparation Tablets 2 mg and 5 mg.

Usual dosage 2·5–7·5 mg/m^2/day orally.

Mechanism of action An alkylating agent (a derivative of nitrogen mustard) which probably damages cells by reaction with nucleoproteins.

Toxic effects

1. Nausea and vomiting,
2. BM depression, neutropenia, thrombocytopenia,
3. Lymphopenia,
4. ?Gonadal effects.

Uses 1. Hodgkin's disease, 2. Other lymphomas, 3. Mixed tumours—?teratoma, 4. Histiocytosis-X.

Cyclophosphamide

Abbreviation: CPA. Trade names: Endoxan, Cytoxan.

Preparation Tablet 50 mg.

Vials 100 mg, 200 mg and 500 mg. Dissolve in 5, 10 or 25 ml (respectively) of sterile water or normal saline. Solution must be used within 3 hours.

Routes of administration

1. Oral
2. Intravenous

Usual dose

Intravenous intermittent: 25–35 mg/m^2 8-hourly for 4 days each month,
OR 450 mg/m^2 every 7–10 days,
OR 900–1200 mg/m^2 every 3–4 weeks
(Scalp tourniquet may be advisable)
Oral intermittent: 200 mg/m^2/day for 5 days each month.
Oral daily: 75 mg/m^2 every day.

Mechanism of action Activated *in vivo* to form an alkylating agent which probably damages cells by reaction with nucleoproteins.

Toxic effects

1. Lymphopenia,
2. Bone marrow depression, neutropenia, thrombocytopenia,
3. Haemorrhagic cystitis (haematuria),
4. Nausea and vomiting after high I.V. dose,
5. Gonadal effects if given at or after puberty,
6. Epilation.

Uses 1. ALL 2. Lymphomas 3. Solid tumours: neuroblastoma, retinoblastoma, rhabdomyosarcoma, other soft tissue sarcomas, Ewing's tumour 4. Histiocytosis-X 5. Autoimmune disorders.

Cytosine Arabinoside

(1-β-D-arabinofuranosyl cytosine)

Abbreviations: CSA; ara-C (in U.S.A.). Trade name: Cytosar (Cytarabine).

Preparation Vials 100 mg and 500 mg of freeze-dried powder to be dissolved in 2 ml and 10 ml (respectively) of sterile water or normal saline. Solution must be used within 3 days.

Routes of administration

1. Intravenous
2. Subcutaneous
3. Intrathecal

Usual dose Intravenous intermittent: 30–40 mg/m^2 8-hourly for 4 days each month,

OR 125–200 mg/m^2 by infusion over 24 hours, daily for 3–5 days each month.

Intravenous daily: 100–120 mg/m^2 by push injection to limit of tolerance (usually 7–10 days), then reduce dosage.

Subcutaneous intermittent: 50 mg/m^2 12 hourly for 4 days each month.

Intrathecal: 25–30 mg/m^2 twice weekly (diluent must not contain benzyl alcohol).

Mechanism of action A synthetic nucleoside which rapidly inhibits DNA synthesis by blocking conversion of cytosine to deoxycytidine: an antimetabolite (antipyrimidine) action.

Toxic effects

1. Bone marrow depression, leukopenia, thrombocytopenia,
2. Megaloblastosis ± anaemia,
3. Alimentary tract: stomatitis, nausea, vomiting, diarrhoea,
4. Fever, commonly with intermittent 8-hourly injections.

Antidote Deoxycytidine

Uses 1. AML 2. ALL 3. CNS leukaemia (IT administration) 4. Lymphomas.

Dactinomycin

(actinomycin D)

Abbreviation: DTM. Trade name: Cosmegen.

Preparation Vial 500 micrograms (mcg) of lyophilized powder to be dissolved in 1·1 ml of sterile water. Solution must be freshly prepared.

Route of administration Intravenous.

Usual dose 400–600 mcg/m^2 every 3 days for 4 doses
OR 350–400 mcg/m^2 daily for 4–5 doses
(usual maximum single dose 500 mcg/m^2) } Scalp tourniquet used

Mechanism of action Inhibits messenger RNA formation.

Toxic effects

1. Nausea, vomiting; metallic taste (within hours of injection),

2. Stomatitis, abdominal pain, diarrhoea,
3. BM depression, neutropenia, thrombocytopenia,
4. Epilation,
5. Rash, accentuated radiation erythema; delayed wound healing.

} After first week of treatment

Uses 1. Wilms' tumour 2. Other solid tumours: rhabdomyosarcoma, neuroblastoma, hepatoblastoma, etc. 3. Lymphomas, especially reticulosarcoma 4. CNS leukaemia (given IV).

Daunorubicin

(daunomycin; rubidomycin)

Abbreviation: DRB. Trade name: Cerubidin.

Preparation Vial 20 mg of lyophilized powder to be dissolved in 2 ml of sterile water or normal saline. Best used freshly prepared.

Route of administration Intravenous.

Usual dose 45–65 mg/m^2 every 7–14 days
OR 15–25 mg/m^2/day for 4–5 days.

Mechanism of action Inhibits synthesis of both DNA and RNA.

Toxic effects

1. Bone marrow depression, neutropenia, thrombocytopenia,
2. Cardiotoxicity (if total dose $>$ 600 mg/m^2),
3. Nausea; mouth ulcers (rare),
4. Epilation (occasional and slight).

N.B. Urine becomes reddish in colour for 24 hours.

Uses 1. ALL 2. AML 3. Reticulosarcoma
4. Solid tumours: neuroblastoma, rhabdomyosarcoma.

Desacetmethylcolchicine

(demecolcin)

Abbreviation: DMC. Trade name: Colcemide.

Preparation Powder which is made into elixir or capsule in the appropriate dose for each child. Capsules 0·5 mg.

Usual dose 2·5–5·0 mg/m^2/day.

Mechanism of action Closely related to colchicine, it is a powerful anti-mitotic drug, arresting cell division at metaphase.

Toxic effects

1. BM depression, leukopenia, thrombocytopenia,
2. Stomatitis (rare),
3. Alopecia (slight),
4. Cholestatic jaundice and pruritus (rare).

Uses 1. CML (adult and juvenile).

Dimethyl Triazeno Imidazole Carboxamide

(imidazole-carboxamide-dimethyl-triazeno)

Abbreviations: DTIC; DIC or ICDT in U.S.A.

Preparation Ampoules 100 mg and 200 mg of white powder; must be stored at 4° or less, protected from the light. Reconstituted with 5% dextrose/water or normal saline. Solution must be used within 8 hours.

Route of administration Intravenous, as rapid injection (painful) or infusion in 75–100 ml of diluent over 30 minutes.

Usual dose 200 mg/m²/day for 5 days, repeated every 3–4 weeks.

Mechanism of action Uncertain, ?partly as alkylating agent. Major effect may be in G2 phase of the cell cycle (Fig. 6.1, p. 101).

Toxic effects

1. Nausea and vomiting for 1–3 days,
2. Bone marrow depression, leukopenia, thrombocytopenia after 2–4 weeks,
3. 'Flu-like' syndrome—fever, headache and myalgia (uncommon).

Uses 1. Malignant melanoma 2. Soft tissue sarcomas 3. Neuroblastoma.

Fluorouracil

(5-fluorouracil)

Abbreviation: 5FU. Trade name: Fluoro-uracil.

Preparation Ampoule of 5 ml each containing 250 mg 5FU (i.e. 50 mg/ml). Store in cool place, not refrigerator. Deteriorates on prolonged exposure to $T > 35°$ or $< 10°$, and to sunlight.

Route of administration Intravenous.

Usual dose Intravenous daily: 400 mg/m²/day for 5 days; may be repeated after interval.

Intravenous intermittent: 500–600 mg/m² once every 2 weeks.

Mechanism of action Inhibits DNA synthesis and to a lesser extent the formation of RNA.

Toxic effects

1. Bone marrow depression, leukopenia, thrombocytopenia,
2. Stomatitis, nausea, vomiting, gastro-intestinal ulceration and haemorrhage, diarrhoea,
3. Epilation,
4. Dermatitis.

Uses Certain solid tumours: hepatoblastoma, osteosarcoma, intestinal and ?adrenal carcinoma.

Mercaptopurine

(6-mercaptopurine)

Abbreviation: 6MP. Trade name: Purinethol.

Preparation Tablet 50 mg.
Usual dose 65 mg/m^2/day orally.
Mechanism of action Interferes with the incorporation of purines into nucleic acids. Mechanism differs from that of antifolics which interfere with the synthesis of purine and pyrimidine de novo.
Toxic effects

1. Bone marrow depression, mainly neutropenia, sometimes thrombocytopenia,
2. Nausea and vomiting (mild),
3. ?Hepatic damage (rare).

Uses 1. ALL 2. AML 3. Subacute AML and CML
4. Auto-immune disease.

Methotrexate

Abbreviation: MTX. Trade name: Methotrexate.
Preparation

Tablet 2·5 mg.
Vial 5 mg to be dissolved in 2 ml of sterile water.
Vial 50 mg to be dissolved in 20 ml of sterile water (or in 4 ml if high concentration required). Solution may be stored at room temperature for 2 weeks, but should be discarded if a precipitate forms.

Routes of administration

1. Oral
2. Intravenous
3. Intramuscular
4. Intrathecal.

Usual dose

1. Oral daily: 3·2 mg/m^2/day, Oral intermittent: 15–20 mg/m^2 twice weekly or 20–30 mg/m^2 once weekly.
2. Intravenous intermittent: 90–120 mg/m^2 every 3–4 weeks. Much higher doses are under trial in osteosarcoma.
3. Intramuscular: similar to intravenous dosage.
4. Intrathecal: 10–12·5 mg/m^2 per dose, diluted with a further 10–20 ml of normal saline, repeated as indicated.

Mechanism of action Blocks folic acid reductase, an enzyme concerned with conversion of folic acid to citrovorum factor which contributes single carbon fragments to the purine ring and to thymine.
Toxic effects

1. Oral ulceration $\pm$ diarrhoea $\pm$ GI haemorrhage,
2. BM depression, neutropenia, thrombocytopenia,
3. Megaloblastic changes $\pm$ anaemia,
4. Anorexia, nausea, vomiting,
5. Hepatitis with fibrosis,

6. Epilation (slight).

Antidote Folinic acid (citrovorum factor or Calcium Leucovorin) 3 mg amp.; give 1–3 amps. up to a maximum of 1 mg per mg of MTX given, preferably within 2 hours of the MTX dose.

Uses 1. ALL 2. Lymphomas 3. Solid tumours – sarcomas, teratoma, neuroblastoma
4. CNS leukaemia and medulloblastoma (I.T. administration)
5. Histiocytosis-X.

Mitomycin C

Abbreviation: MMC. Trade name: Mitomycin.

Preparation Ampoule 2 mg to be dissolved in sterile water or normal saline; prolonged shaking may be needed. MMC can be stored at room temperature, away from sunlight. Solution preferably used as soon as possible.

Route of administration Intravenous.

Usual dose 5–6 mg/m^2 alternate days, to a maximum of ?30 mg/m^2.

Mechanism of action Suppresses the division of cancer cells apparently by inhibiting DNA synthesis.

Toxic effects

1. Bone marrow depression, neutropenia, thrombocytopenia,
2. Nausea and vomiting,
3. Hepatic and renal disturbances (rare).

Uses 1. Hepatoblastoma 2. Lymphomas 3. Sarcomas
4. ?Carcinoma

Procarbazine

(methyl hydrazine)

Abbreviation: PCZ. Trade name: Natulan.

Preparation Capsule 50 mg.

Usual dose For remission induction, start with 25–50 mg/m^2/day, increasing gradually to 100 mg/m^2/day.

Mode of action Uncertain. There is a decrease in mitoses; cell division is inhibited as a consequence of prolonging interphase. Breaks down DNA, ?by alkylation.

Toxic effects

1. Anorexia, nausea and vomiting,
2. Bone marrow depression, leukopenia, thrombocytopenia,
3. Allergic skin reactions (rare) and alopecia (very rare).

Uses 1. Hodgkin's disease 2. Other lymphomas
3. ?Solid tumours.

Thioguanine

(6-thioguanine or 2-amino-6-mercaptopurine)

Abbreviation: 6TG. Trade name: Thioguanine.

Preparation Tablet 40 mg.

Usual dose Initially 50 mg/m^2/day orally.

Mechanism of action A purine derivative closely related to 6MP, it is an antimetabolite which blocks purine metabolism. Cross resistance exists between 6TG and 6MP.

Toxic effects

1. Nausea, vomiting, anorexia, stomatitis,
2. Bone marrow depression, neutropenia and occasionally thrombocytopenia, anaemia,
3. ?Toxic hepatitis.

Uses 1. AML 2. CML 3. ALL

Vinblastine

(vincoleukoblastine)

Abbreviation: VBL. Trade name: Velbe (vinblastine sulfate).

Preparation

Vial 10 mg to be dissolved in 5 ml of normal saline.
Solution may be stored in a refrigerator for 30 days.

Route of administration Intravenous.

Usual dose

I.V.: 3·5–6·0 mg/m^2 once weekly.

Mechanism of action Metaphase arrest of dividing cells.

Toxic effects

1. Nausea and vomiting,
2. BM depression, neutropenia, thrombocytopenia,
3. Epilation,
4. Neurotoxicity (in high dosage) with parasthesiae, abdominal cramps, constipation, etc.

Uses 1. Hodgkin's disease 2. Neuroblastoma
3. Other lymphomas 4. Histiocytosis-X
5. Monocytic and erythro-leukaemia.

Vincristine

(leurocristine)

Abbreviation: VCR. Trade name: Oncovin.

Preparation Vials 1 mg and 5 mg to be dissolved in sterile water or normal saline to give 1 mg per ml. Solution may be stored in refrigerator for 14 days.

Route of administration Intravenous.

Usual dose 1·6–2·25 (commonly 2·0) mg/m^2 once weekly (scalp tourniquet used).

Mechanism of action Metaphase arrest of dividing cells (spindle poison). May have other effects on cells.

Toxic effects

1. High-level constipation and abdominal cramps, within 2–4 days,
2. Neuritic pains, parasthesia, jaw-ache,
3. Motor weakness, wasting especially in hands,
4. Cranial nerve palsies – CN. III, IV, VII, laryngeal,
5. Mood changes, encephalopathy, convulsions,
6. Epilation (severe without, mild to moderate with, a scalp tourniquet),
7. Neutropenia,
8. Anaemia.

Uses 1. ALL 2. AML 3. Lymphomas
4. Solid tumours: Wilms', neuroblastoma, Ewing's, rhabdomyosarcoma, hepatoblastoma, etc. 5. Brain tumours.

Appendix IV. Biopsy Techniques

The role of biopsies in the diagnosis and management of children with malignant disease is outlined in Chapter 5, (p. 81). In many instances the operation is a simple matter, but some general points may be mentioned to ensure that it is performed with minimum disturbance to the child, optimum cosmetic result, and maximum information from the tissue obtained.

ANAESTHESIA

With few exceptions, e.g. aspiration of marrow, and possibly a drill biopsy of a pelvic tumour in an older child, biopsy in childhood should be performed under general anaesthesia. Local anaesthesia requires additional (and often prolonged) sedation which is less desirable than a short-acting general anaesthetic.

CHEMOTHERAPY 'COVER'

The advisability of administering cytotoxic agents before biopsy, when the diagnosis is still unknown, has been questioned, and although there may be theoretical advantages, there are no data such as better survival rates which would justify their use. One potential disadvantage is their action on the cells of a tumour, leading to a misleadingly high mitotic index which could affect the histological diagnosis (p. 25).

OPERATIVE TECHNIQUE

To obtain the best healing and the least noticeable scar, the skin incision, or the long axis of an ellipse of skin, should run parallel to the natural lines of cleavage (e.g. 'Langer's' lines now superseded, see Cox, 1941*; Kraissl, 1951†).

Dexon® or a similar suture material is the most suitable for closure; interrupted subcutaneous sutures (2/0 or 3/0) and a continuous subcuticular stitch (4/0 or 5/0) produce a scar as good as or better than any other method, with the added advantage, for a child, that there are no sutures to be removed.

The following methods of biopsy may be employed:

Excision biopsy
Incision biopsy

* Cox, H. T. (1941). The cleavage lines of the skin. *Brit. J. Surg.*, **29** : 234.

† Kraissl, C. J. (1951). The selection of appropriate lines for elective surgical incisions. *Plastic & Reconstr. Surg.*, **8** : 1.

Needle or drill biopsy
Operative ('open') biopsy
Biopsy 'in-situ' (testis)
Frozen sections (intra-operative biopsy)
Lymph node biopsy
Marrow biopsy.

Selection of the best method may be straightforward, but in some cases judgement and a knowledge of the behaviour and appearances of the tumours of childhood are a great advantage. When in doubt, the surgeon should seek the advice of an experienced histopathologist, so that the patient may be spared a fruitless or unnecessary operation, which may have to be repeated, or a more appropriate technique employed.

EXCISION BIOPSY

A superficial lesion less than 2–3 cm in maximum dimension can be completely excised, together with an ellipse of skin (not less in length than twice the width) including an adequate margin of macroscopically uninvolved tissue surrounding the lesion. When the lesion is reported to be benign, definitive treatment has been completed, and no further surgery is required.

However, the site and size of the lesion determine which method of biopsy should be used. Even a small lesion 1 cm in diameter can present difficulties when located on or near the vermillion of the lip, the cheek, nose or the pinna. In these areas an excision biopsy would require a reconstructive procedure which might prove to have been unnecessary, e.g. when the lesion is inflammatory and capable of resolving completely without any residual blemish. In such cases a needle, 'drill' or trephine biopsy, removing of one or more 'cores' of tissue, 2–3 mm in diameter and up to 1 cm long, may be preferable. Two cores, e.g. one taken vertically through the margin and a second more centrally, or horizontally beneath the lesion, will provide sufficient material for a histological diagnosis without the need for sutures. A corneal trephine and a blunt stylet to push out the core obtained, or a dermal biopsy punch (see below) is particularly suitable for skin lesions.

A subcutaneous lesion can be excised *in toto* through a skin incision, or together with an ellipse of skin if desired. Depending on the depth of the lesion, the block of subcutaneous tissue removed can be extended to the level of the deep fascia.

INCISION BIOPSY

When a tumour is too extensive to be removed completely before establishing the diagnosis, part of the lesion can be removed for examination. This has the obvious disadvantages that cells may be disseminated when the tumour is cut into, and when total excision is shown to be the appropriate method of treatment, a further operation will be required. Nevertheless, incision-biopsy has its place, and in a large superficial lesion an ellipse of skin can be fashioned so that it includes the margin of the lesion and adjacent normal tissue.

A deeper lesion, e.g. an inter- or intra-muscular swelling (p. 789), should be approached through an incision chosen to give adequate access, opening and later closing fascial and muscular planes as necessary, in short a formal exploratory operation with 'open biopsy' (see below).

NEEDLE OR DRILL BIOPSY

When incision-biopsy or a formal exploration would be an undesirable major operation, a needle or drill biopsy is preferable in some situations. Biopsy of a lesion in the scalp or on the calvarium (p. 302) can be obtained in this way, and an 'aspiration' drill biopsy of a low intrapelvic mass, e.g. in the prostate or the presacral region, can be performed with the guidance of a finger in the rectum palpating the tumour.

A Francine or other type of needle (see below) can be used to obtain a core of tissue from a tumour at a considerable depth, e.g. in the liver or kidney, although there are potential disadvantages, e.g. dissemination of tumour cells, rupture of a thin but hitherto effective capsule or 'pseudo-capsule', and subsequent bleeding if the lesion is very vascular or coagulation is impaired.

It is generally agreed that there is no place for needle biopsy of a renal tumour in childhood.

The advisability of needle biopsy of the liver largely depends on the provisional diagnosis; it is probably the method of choice in confirming or excluding hepatic metastases, e.g. in neuroblastoma (p. 547), non-neoplastic enlargement of the liver (p. 525), and disseminated histiocytosis (p. 216). On the other hand, needle biopsy is at least debatable, and condemned by some, when the most likely diagnosis is a hepatoblastoma, the risk of intraperitoneal dissemination of tumour cells outweighing the advantages of establishing the diagnosis before making preparations for hepatic lobectomy under hypothermia (p. 614). Needle biopsy is also contraindicated when hydatid disease or a hepatic haemangioma (p. 607) is a possibility, and when there is a disorder of coagulation.

OPERATIVE (OPEN) BIOPSY

A formal surgical exploration is sometimes required to obtain material for biopsy, e.g. from a hepatoblastoma (see above), a thoracotomy for a lymphosarcoma confined to the mediastinum (p. 453), to plot the extent of the disease as a guide to treatment, e.g. a staging laparotomy (p. 191) in Hodgkin's disease, or 'open' biopsy of a bone tumour.

Bone biopsy is performed in order to (a) exclude a benign conditiou (p. 727); (b) confirm a clinical and radiological diagnosis of a primary tumour, e.g. osteosarcoma (p. 751); (c) distinguish atypical osteomyelitis from a Ewing's tumour (p. 725); (d) discover the cause of an area of rarefaction, pain or pathological fracture, e.g. metastatic neuroblastoma (p. 552) or eosinophilic granuloma (p. 209); and (e) to determine whether there is local recurrence of a tumour not treated by amputation, e.g. Ewing's tumour.

The important points in the approach and operative technique of open biopsy of a suspected bone tumour are mentioned on p. 743. A hand-operated 'drill' (e.g. a Turkel trephine, see below) or a 'plug-cutter' (Stryker, see below) can be used to obtain a cylindrical biopsy from 3 to 10 mm in diameter and 0·5 to 3 cm in length. The larger diameter is ideal in a region where the affected bone will not be unduly weakened by removal of a core of this size, e.g. the pelvis.

'BIOPSY IN-SITU'

Because the majority of swellings in the testis in adults are malignant, orchiectomy (usually transecting the cord at the internal inguinal ring) has come to be considered the minimum biopsy for a testicular swelling. In prepubertal boys, most testicular swellings are benign, and cautious exploration (p. 880) to determine the nature of the swelling is, in the circumstances, preferable. In a few cases frozen sections may be required to determine whether orchiectomy is required.

'FROZEN SECTIONS'

In paediatric tumours, the need for an intra-operative diagnosis based on frozen sections is much less than in adult practice. The sites and types of tumours of childhood are quite different, for example the virtual absence of carcinoma of the breast eliminates one large group. Further, rapid paraffin processing can yield conventional sections in as little as $2\frac{1}{2}$ hours.

Paediatric tumours in which frozen sections may be required are as follows.

1. *Brain tumours* (p. 86). Because of their misleading macroscopic appearances, the diagnosis, the scope of the excision to be attempted, and the prognosis, are best determined by the microscopic findings, and a biopsy is generally obtained only at the time of craniotomy.
2. *Hepatic tumours*. Histological evidence is always required to distinguish a hepatoblastoma from a mesenchymal hamartoma of the liver or, less

commonly, a hepatocarcinoma (p. 614). The advisability of preoperative needle biopsy in this situation is the subject of debate, and the alternatives are (a) a preliminary laparotomy and 'open' biopsy or (b) reliance on cryostat sections and diagnosis as the first step towards a hepatic lobectomy. Frozen sections may also be required to determine whether involvement of the contralateral lobe rules out a standard or even an extended hepatic lobectomy (p. 618).

3. *Lymphosarcoma of the ileum.* To the naked eye, infiltration of the mesentery or mesenteric lymph nodes with lymphoblastic lymphosarcoma can be difficult or impossible to distinguish from secondary chylous or lymphatic congestion. The resectability of the primary tumour and the scope of the resection required (or its impracticality) can in some cases only be determined by evidence of frozen sections from questionable areas (p. 637).

4. *Soft tissue sarcomas.* Although amputation for primary soft tissue sarcoma arising in a limb is now less commonly performed (p. 793), it may still be necessary to determine at operation the extent of the tumour, e.g. to delineate the area to be irradiated subsequently. When the operative findings suggest that a major neurovascular bundle is infiltrated, this can be clarified by frozen sections, and the excision restricted or extended accordingly.

5. *Bone tumours.* The diagnosis and the need for amputation are usually established from paraffin sections of the tumour taken at an 'open' biopsy, but frozen sections of material from the medullary cavity are required to show that the tumour has not extended to the point where the bone is to be transected (p. 755). If positive, a more proximal point is chosen, and further frozen sections are obtained.

6. *Thyroid carcinoma.* In exploring what appears to be a single nodule in the thyroid gland (p. 375), biopsies from more than one area may be taken, and time for study of paraffin sections is usually necessary. During definitive resection for a carcinoma, frozen sections may be helpful in determining the extent of infiltration of the contralateral lobe, or the presence of metastases in cervical lymph nodes. This information will indicate whether subtotal or total removal of the contralateral lobe is required, and whether a unilateral or bilateral modified block dissection of the nodes (p. 377) should be performed.

7. *Rare tumours*, e.g. of the bile ducts (p. 621), pancreas (p. 622), retroperitoneal tissues (p. 584) or the mesenteries (p. 675) cannot be identified at operation by their macroscopic appearances alone, and in general the rarer the tumour the less reliable is the interpretation of frozen sections. Complete removal of the tumour at the initial laparotomy should be the objective, but if this is not feasible because of fixity or the extent of the resection required (e.g. pancreaticoduodenectomy), the alternative is a biopsy for detailed study, including electron microscopy if necessary.

Multiple biopsies, e.g. of lymph nodes or adjacent infiltrated viscera, are useful in determining whether an attempt should be made to remove the tumour at a second operation.

Frozen sections are definitely contraindicated (a) on lymph nodes in suspected lymphomas (except in abdominal lymphosarcoma mentioned above), including mesenteric nodes obtained during staging laparotomy for Hodgkin's disease (p. 191); (b) when the only biopsy obtainable is small in volume; in such cases the material should be processed so as to produce sections of the highest quality, and this cannot be said of even very good cryostat sections; (c) when interpretation of frozen sections will not immediately influence the surgical operation in progress.

LYMPH NODE BIOPSY

Removal of an enlarged lymph node may be undertaken; (a) to establish the diagnosis, e.g. in neuroblastoma (p. 552) or reticulum cell sarcoma (p. 182); (b) to determine the extent of dissemination as an aid in planning treatment, e.g. in abdominal Hodgkin's disease (p. 191), or the extent of metastases in retroperitoneal nodes in rhabdomyosarcoma of the testis or spermatic cord (p. 895). In all situations it is recommended that the largest or most central node of the group should be removed, for it is more likely to yield the information required than a smaller, more easily removed but less informative, 'peripheral' node.

MARROW BIOPSY

A suitable sample of marrow can be obtained from the sternum or the ilium, as a rule under local anaesthesia, but whenever possible while the child is anaesthetized for another investigation, e.g. angiography.

There are two methods and each has a specific purpose.

(a) *A sternal marrow puncture* with a Salah needle, to obtain semi-fluid material which is used to make sinears so that individual cells can be examined, and counted if necessary.

(b) *A marrow biopsy*, usually from the ilium, is obtained with a Jamshidi needle (see below), removing a solid core which can be processed, sectioned and stained by the same range of techniques as for other tissue biopsies. This method is the most appropriate when investigating the marrow for metastases in Hodgkin's disease.

As well as in leukaemia (p. 143) and the lymphomas (p. 174), a marrow aspirate should be obtained in children with a neuroblastoma (p. 558), a rhabdomyosarcoma (p. 788), particularly the alveolar type (p. 786), and in children with a disseminated tumour, as part of their assessment before deciding on a plan of treatment.

INSTRUMENTS

The following needles and drills, have been found to be satisfactory in obtaining material from tumours in a variety of sites. Most of them can be used effectively in sites other than those for which they were designed.

The dimensions are either the internal or external diameter, and as the thickness of the cutting edge is not great, these indicate the approximate diameter of the core of tissue obtained.

Francine liver biopsy needle. Gauges 14, 16, 18, 19, 20. Locally manufactured by A. J. Taylor. Supplied by 'Mayven Surgical', Melbourne.

Menghini biopsy needle. Gauges 14, 16. Mueller Corp. Code No. SU–21040. Down Bros. Code No. A 13–01 to A 13–09.

Franklin-Silverman needle. Gauge 14. (Metzoff modification, manufacturer unknown).

Vim-Silverman biopsy needle (Franklin modification). Mueller Corp. Code No. SU–21060.

Trucut® Renal Biopsy Needle, Gauge 14, Disposable. Travenol Laboratories, Code No. ZN 2704.

A long needle which can be used for biopsy of a variety of sites other than the kidney, e.g. liver, muscle, pelvic tumours, etc.

Keyes' Dermal biopsy punch.

Medicon®. Sizes 2, 4, 6 mm diameter.

Grieshaber Corneal Trephine.

1·5 mm Mueller Code No. OP5876.

2 mm Mueller Code No. OP5877.

'Salah' marrow aspiration needle. Gauges 15, 17, 19 (1″ length). Manufactured locally, H. A. Taylor, South Yarra, Melbourne.

Jamshidi 'Needle' (Kormed Inc.); a marrow trephine.

Infant size 2″ (length) Gauge 13.

Paediatric size $3\frac{1}{2}$″ (length) Gauge 13.

Regular (adult) 4″ (length) Gauge 11, the most frequently used.

Turkel Bone Biopsy Trephine. Gauges 10, 14, 17. For long bones etc. in the extremities (p. 743). Several sizes are available.

Down Bros. A-10 for biopsy of a vertebral body.

Mueller Corp. SU–21070. Gauges 14, 17.

Bone 'Plug-Cutter' (Stryker Corp.). A 'dowel' cutter, used to obtain a large biopsy, e.g. from the pelvis.

6 mm Code No. 1108–6.

8 mm Code No. 1108–8

10 mm Code No. 1108–10

Hand operated, this produces an excellent cylindrical biopsy, but so large that it is unsuitable for a long bone in an extremity, for which one of the larger Turkel trephines is preferred.

Appendix V. TNM classifications

TNM CLASSIFICATIONS, AS SPECIFIED IN 'CLINICAL ONCOLOGY'

(U.I.C.C., published by Springer-Verlag, Berlin, Heidelberg, New York, 1973).

Although primarily orientated to adult tumours, the following may be adaptable to paediatric equivalents. No TNM classification for tumours of the small bowel or neuroblastoma have as yet been formally adopted for international use.

TONSIL

- T0 No evidence of primary tumour
- T1 Tumour limited to one site
- T2 Tumour extending to two sites
- T3 Tumour extending beyond oropharynx
- N0 No palpable nodes
- N1 Movable homolateral nodes
  - N1a Nodes not considered to contain growth
  - N1b Nodes considered to contain growth
- N2 Movable contralateral or bilateral nodes
  - N2a Nodes not considered to contain growth
  - N2b Nodes considered to contain growth
- N3 Fixed nodes
- M0 No evidence of distant metastases
- M1 Distant metastases present

NASOPHARYNX

The nasopharynx is divided into three regions:

- (a) Posterior superior wall: extends from the level of the soft palate to the base of the skull
- (b) Lateral wall (fossa of Rosenmuller)
- (c) Anterior wall: consists of the choanae and the upper surface of the soft palate

T1S Pre-invasive carcinoma, so-called carcinoma *in situ*
T0 No evidence of primary tumour
T1 Tumour limited to one region
T2 Tumour extending to two regions
T3 Tumour extending beyond nasopharynx without bone involvement
T4 Tumour extending beyond nasopharynx with bone involvement, including the cartilaginous portion of the Eustachian tube
N0 No palpable nodes
N1 Movable homolateral nodes
 N1a Nodes not considered to contain growth
 N1b Nodes considered to contain growth
N2 Movable contralateral or bilateral nodes
 N2a Nodes not considered to contain growth
 N2b Nodes considered to contain growth
N3 Fixed nodes
M0 No evidence of distant metastases
M1 Distant metastases present

THYROID

T0 No palpable tumour
T1 Single tumour confined to the gland. No limitation of mobility or deformity of gland or scanning defect, in a gland normal to palpation
T2 Multiple tumours or single tumour producing deformity of gland. No limitation of mobility
T3 Tumour extending beyond the gland as indicated by fixation or infiltration of surrounding structures
N0 No palpable nodes
N1 Movable homolateral nodes
 N1a Nodes not considered to contain growth
 N1b Nodes considered to contain growth
N2 Movable contralateral or bilateral nodes
 N2a Nodes not considered to contain growth
 N2b Nodes considered to contain growth
N3 Fixed nodes
M0 No evidence of distant metastases
M1 Distant metastases present

OVARY

T1S Pre-invasive carcinoma, so-called carcinoma *in situ*
T1 Tumour limited to one ovary
T2 Tumour limited to both ovaries
T3 Tumour extending into the uterus and/or Fallopian tubes

T4 Tumour extending directly to other surrounding anatomical structures

TX Tumour cannot be assessed (laparotomy not done)

NB—No regard is paid to the presence of ascites

NX When it is not possible to assess the regional lymph nodes, the symbol NX will be used permitting eventual addition of histological information, thus: NX− or NX+

N0 No abnormal regional lymph nodes demonstrated

N1 Abnormal regional lymph nodes demonstrated

M0 No evidence of distant metastases

M1 Implantation or other metastases present

- M1a In the true pelvis only
- M1b Within the abdomen
- M1c Beyond the abdomen and pelvis

The TNM Classification must be supplemented by histological grading.

VAGINA (? applicable to sarcoma in childhood)

T1S Pre-invasive carcinoma, so-called carcinoma *in situ*

T0 No evidence of primary tumour

T1 Tumour limited to the vaginal wall

- T1a The tumour is 2 cm or less in its greatest dimension
- T1b The tumour is more than 2 cm in its greatest dimension

T2 Tumour infiltrating the paravaginal tissues, but not extending to the pelvic wall

T3 Tumour extending to the pelvic wall

T4 Tumour extending beyond the true pelvis, or infiltrating the mucosa of the rectum or bladder

NB—The presence of bullous oedema is not sufficient evidence to classify the tumour as T4.

(a) Regional lymph nodes of upper two thirds of vagina

NX It is not possible to assess the regional nodes.

Additional histological information may be added, thus: NX− or NX+

N0 No deformity of regional nodes on lymphography

N1 Regional nodes deformed on lymphography

(b) Regional lymph nodes of lower third of vagina

N0 No palpable nodes

TESTIS

T1 Tumour occupying less than one half of the testis

T2 Tumour occupying one half or more of the testis

T3 Tumour confined to the testis and producing enlargement

T4 Tumour extending to the epididymis or beyond the testis
NX When it is impossible to assess the regional nodes the symbol NX will be used, permitting eventual addition of histological information, thus: NX− or NX+
N0 No deformity of regional nodes on lymphangiography
N1 Regional nodes deformed on lymphangiography
N2 Fixed palpable abdominal nodes
M0 No evidence of distant metastases
M1 Distant metastases present

WILMS' TUMOUR

T0 No evidence of primary tumour
T1 No enlargement of kidney. Urography shows minimal calyceal abnormality
T2 Kidney enlarged with no limitation of mobility, or urography shows gross deformity affecting one or more calyces, or displacement of the ureter
T3 Kidney enlarged and mobility limited without complete fixation, or urography shows deformity of the pelvis of the kidney, or there is evidence of vascular compression (e.g. varicocele)
T4 Kidney enlarged and with complete fixation
NX When it is impossible to assess the regional lymph nodes the symbol NX will be used, thus: NX− or NX+
N0 No deformity of regional lymph nodes on lymphangiography
N1 Regional lymph nodes deformed on lymphangiography
M0 No evidence of distant metastases
M1 Distant metastases present

BLADDER (? applicable to sarcoma in childhood)

T1S Pre-invasive carcinoma, so-called carcinoma *in situ*, either papillary or sessile
T1 Tumour with infiltration of subepithelial connective tissue
T2 Tumour with infiltration of superficial muscle
T3 Tumour with infiltration of deep muscle
T4 Tumour fixed or invading adjoining organs
NX When it is impossible to assess the regional lymph nodes the symbol NX will be used
N0 No deformity of regional nodes on lymphangiography
N1 Regional nodes deformed on lymphangiography
M0 No evidence of distant metastases
M1 Distant metastases present

PROSTATE (? applicable to sarcoma in childhood)

- T1 Tumour occupying less than one half of the prostate and surrounded by palpably normal gland
- T2 Tumour occupying one half or more of the prostate
- T3 Tumour confined to the prostate but producing enlargement or deformity of the gland
- T4 Tumour extending beyond the prostate
- NX When it is impossible to assess the regional lymph nodes, the symbol NX will be used, thus: NX− or NX+
- N0 No deformity of the regional nodes on lymphangiography
- N1 Regional nodes deformed on lymphangiography
- N2 Fixed palpable abdominal nodes
- M0 No evidence of distant metastases
- M1 Distant metastases present

P—HISTOPATHOLOGICAL CATEGORIES
(determined after operation)

The following supplementary P categories are suggested for more precise grouping when histological findings are available. Whenever possible both T and P categories should be used in the reporting of results.

Tumours of the parenchyma (hypernephroma, so-called Grawitz tumour), the mostly papillary carcinomas of the pelvis of the kidney and nephroblastoma (Wilms' Tumour) should be recorded separately.

NEPHROBLASTOMA

- P1 Tumour infiltrating only the parenchyma of the kidney
- P2 Tumour extending beyond the kidney but not infiltrating intrarenal or extrarenal veins and/or lymph vessels
- P3 Tumour infiltrating intrarenal or extrarenal veins and/or lymph vessels

PAPILLARY TUMOURS

- P1 Tumour with infiltration of subepithelial connective tissue
- P2 Tumour with infiltration of muscle, or the parenchyma of the kidney, but not infiltrating intrarenal or extrarenal veins and/or lymph vessels
- P3 Tumour infiltrating surrounding tissues, or intrarenal or extrarenal veins and/or lymph vessels

Note: Multiple tumours may be indicated by the addition of the suffix (m) to the appropriate category, e.g. P2(m).

Index

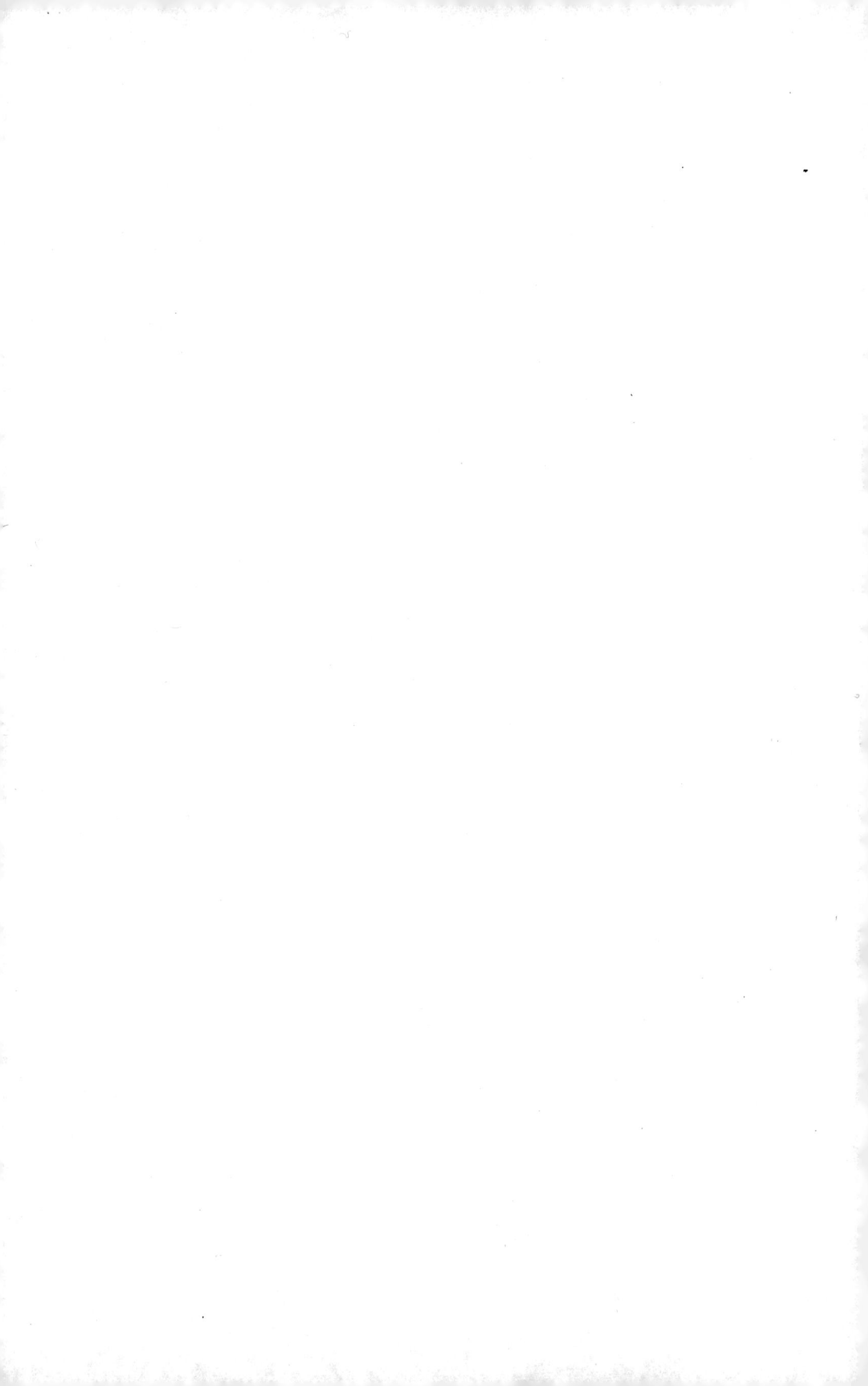